HANDBOOK OF
CULTURAL PSYCHIATRY

HANDBOOK OF CULTURAL PSYCHIATRY

Wen-Shing Tseng

University of Hawaii
Honolulu, Hawaii

ACADEMIC PRESS

San Diego   London   Boston   New York
Sydney   Tokyo   Toronto

Academic Press
A Harcourt Science and Technology Company
525 B Street, Suite 1900, San Diego, California 92101-4495, USA
http://www.academicpress.com

Academic Press
Harcourt Place, 32 Jamestown Road, London NW1 7BY, UK
http://www.academicpress.com

Library of Congress Catalog Card Number: 00-111402

International Standard Book Number: 0-12-701632-5

PRINTED IN THE UNITED STATES OF AMERICA
01   02   03   04   05   06   MM   9   8   7   6   5   4   3   2   1

Contents

Preface

Cultural psychiatry is a dynamic and newly developing subfield of psychiatry that focuses on the fascinating cultural aspects of psychiatric practice and mental health. On a clinical level, cultural psychiatry strives to provide health care for patients of diverse ethnic or cultural backgrounds in a manner that is culturally relevant. This includes a culturally sensitive assessment, an understanding of the psychological problems of the patient, and their treatment. From an academic point of view, cultural psychiatry illuminates how ethnic and cultural factors influence human behavior, determine stress and coping strategies, configurate psychopathology, and modify help-seeking behavior. Ethnicity and culture also work, consciously or subconsciously, to shape our clinical practices into what we call the art of healing.

During the past three decades, concurrent with a rising global interest in and need for serving patients of various ethnic and cultural backgrounds, it is estimated that more than 10,000 journal articles and several hundred books have been published on the subject of cultural psychiatry and mental health. Despite this surge in research and experience, most of the books are edited works with multiple authors focusing on various special subjects or collections of essays. There is no *handbook* or *textbook* on cultural psychiatry in which the material is presented in a comprehensive, systematically organized, and integrated manner. My intention is for this handbook to fill the urgent need for such a work.

Although no single publication can ever be truly comprehensive, I have carefully planned the content and theme of this book to examine cultural psychiatry from a universal perspective. The cultural focus is beyond any particular ethnic group and includes many majority and minority communities from around the world so that "cultural" issues are addressed in the broadest sense. Nearly 2000 selected works relating to cultural psychiatry and mental health are reviewed and quoted. More than 30 experts in the field of cultural psychiatry and mental health, from the East and West, were consulted on particular topics. Therefore, this book will be invaluable not only for readers in the United States, but for international scholars and clinicians as well.

The overall goal of this book is to update what is known about cultural psychiatry and to organize those theories and facts into a world perspective. The handbook begins with the cultural aspects of human behavior within the framework of the human life cycle. It moves to the cultural influences on stress and illness behavior, which provide the basic sociocultural knowledge needed by clinicians. The focus then turns toward the impact of culture on various psychopathologies, clinical assessment and practice, and psychological therapy. Culturally relevant therapies for various subpopulations and special social phenomena relevant to clinical work are then presented. The book ends with the issues of research and theoretical elaboration. Because information about existing books on cultural psychiatry is not easily accessible by computer search, an appendix of books organized by subject is provided for the convenience of the reader.

Several years, if not decades, were spent gathering the books and literature used to prepare this work. I give my deepest thanks to 30 national and internationally well-known consultants who made a substantial effort to add their vast expertise and insights to this book. I am also grateful to the many colleagues and friends who were kind enough to contribute their valuable photographs for illustrations, which add a very special quality to this book.

Special thanks are due to the publisher, Academic Press for its vision and commitment in undertaking the timely, needed publication of this handbook, particularly to the chief editor, George Zimmar, Ph.D., for his friendly guidance and assistance in preparing the work.

Throughout this academic and personal undertaking, I have been ever grateful and am forever indebted for the endless encouragement and support given by my wife, Jing Hsu, M.D. (my colleague and coauthor on previous books in psychiatry), as well as our three children: Chau-Wen Tseng, Ph.D., Chien-Wen Tseng, M.D., and Stephanie Tseng, M.D. It took me more than three years to work on the manuscript and I give my extreme appreciation to Kathy Luter Reimers for her dedication in editing the manuscript through these years. I also thank Christine Yoshida, who provided help with the references and index, and Gary Belcher for preparing the tables and figures.

I also express my sincere gratitude to the many teachers and mentors that I have been fortunate to have in my professional life. In sequence of time, I first express my great appreciation to Professor Tsung-Yi Lin, then chairman of the Neuropsychiatric Department of the School of Medicine, National Taiwan University, who inspired me to choose a career in psychiatry and guided me, as a World Health Organization fellow, to pursue advanced study abroad. I am very grateful to the late Professor Jack R. Ewalt, then superintendent of the Massachusetts Mental Health Center, Harvard Medical School, with whom I studied dynamic psychiatry and whose direct supervision stimulated me to sharpen and broaden my view and understanding of the human mind. I am also in debt to the late Professor William P. Lebra, then director of the Culture and Mental Health Program for Asia and the Pacific, East–West Center, who offered me the chance to study culture and mental health, promoting my knowledge and interest in this particular field of science. Finally, I am grateful to the late Professor Henry B.M. Murphy, then chairman of the Transcultural Psychiatry Section of the World Psychiatric Association, who inspired me to expand my vision and experience of cultural psychiatry from a world perspective.

There have also been many colleagues, experts, and friends who have kindly served as formal and informal consultants throughout countless years. They have provided expertise, shared experiences, and inspired me to broaden my knowledge in cultural psychiatry. I am very grateful for their very valuable direct and indirect contributions to this book, which I hope will serve as a landmark and a stepping stone to the further development of cultural psychiatry.

Wen-Shing Tseng, M.D.
Honolulu, Hawaii
June 5, 2000

About the Author
Wen-Shing Tseng, M.D.

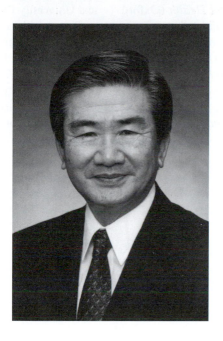

Wen-Shing Tseng, M.D., is a professor of psychiatry at the University of Hawaii School of Medicine. Born in Taiwan in 1935, he was trained in psychiatry at the National Taiwan University in Taipei and later at the Massachusetts Mental Health Center of Harvard Medical School in Boston. He was a research fellow in culture and mental health at the East-West Center from 1970 to 1971, before being recruited as a faculty member of the University of Hawaii School of Medicine, where he became a professor in 1976, and served as training director for the psychiatric residency training program between 1975 and 1982.

As a consultant to the World Health Organization and for teaching and research projects, he has traveled extensively to many countries in Asia and the Pacific, including China, Japan, Singapore, Malaysia, Fiji, and Micronesia. He served as chairman of the Transcultural Psychiatry Section of the World Psychiatric Association for two terms, from 1983 to 1993. In that capacity, he developed a wide network of colleagues around the world in the field of cultural psychiatry. Relating to the subject of culture and mental health, he has coordinated numerous international conferences in Honolulu, Beijing, Tokyo, and Budapest. He has held the position of guest professor of the Institute of Mental Health, Beijing University, since 1987.

He has conducted numerous research projects, mainly relating to the cultural aspects of assessment of psychopathology, child development, family relations, epidemic mental disorders, culture-related specific psychiatric syndromes, folk healing, and psychotherapy. The studies resulted in the publication of more than 80 articles in scientific journals and book chapters.

He has edited/coedited the books: *People and Cultures of Hawaii: A Psychocultural Profile* (University Press of Hawaii, 1980), *Chinese Culture and Mental Health* (Academic Press, 1985), *Suicidal Behaviour in the Asia-Pacific Region* (Singapore University Press, 1992), *Chinese Societies and Mental Health* (Oxford University Press, 1995), *Migration and Adjustment* (in Japanese) (Nihon Hyoronsha, 1996), *Chinese Mind and Psychotherapy* (in Chinese) (Beijing Medical University Press, 1997), *Culture and Psychopathology* (Brunner/Mazel, 1997) and *Culture and Psychotherapy* (American Psychiatric Press, 2001). He has authored the books: *Culture, Mind and Therapy: Introduction to Cultural Psychiatry* (Brunner/Mazel, 1981), *Culture and Family: Problems and Therapy* (Haworth Press, 1991), *Textbook of Psychiatry* (in Chinese) (Buffalo Book Co., 1994), and *Psychotherapy: Theory and Analysis* (in Chinese) (Beijing Medical University Press, 1994).

Presently, he is a member of the Board of Directors of the Society for the Study of Psychiatry and Culture and honorable advisor of the Transcultural Psychiatry Section of the World Psychiatric Association. Because of his research, publications, and experience, he has gained a reputation as an expert in cultural psychiatry, at both the national and international levels.

List of Consultants
(and Subjects Consulted)

(By Alphabet Order)

Renato D. Alarcón, M.D., M.P.H. *(Cultural psychiatry training)*
Professor and Vice-Chairman, Department of Psychiatry and Behavioral Sciences, Emory University School of Medicine; and Chair, Cultural Psychiatry Committee, Group for the Advancement of Psychiatry (USA).

Goffredo Bartocci, M.D. *(Religion and mental health)*
Presidente, Istituto Italiano di Igiene Mentale Transculturale (Italy); Chair, Transcultural Psychiatric Section, World Psychiatric Association.

Richard W. Brislin, Ph.D. *(Cross-cultural research methods)*
Professor and Director of Ph.D. Program in International Management, College of Business Administration, University of Hawaii; Former Research Associate, Institute of Culture Learning, East–West Center (USA).

José Cañive, M.D. *(Culture and mental health of Hispanic group)*
Associate Professor and Director of Clinical Psychiatry, Department of Veterans Affairs, Albuquerque, NM; Member of the Board of Directors, The Society for the Study of Psychiatry and Culture (USA).

Ajita Chakraborty, M.D. *(Culture and mental health in India)*
Professor and Former Head, Department of Neurology & Psychiatry, Institute of Post Graduate Medical Education & Research, Calcutta

(India); Ex-Committee Member, Transcultural Psychiatric Section, World Psychiatric Association.

Edmond Chiu, A.M., F.R.A.N.Z.C.P. *(Culture and geriatric psychiatry)*
Associated Professor and Director, Aged Psychiatry, Education & Research, University of Melbourne (Australia); President, International Psychogeriatric Association; Chair, Section of Old Age Psychiatry, World Psychiatry Association.

Juris G. Draguns, Ph.D. *(Culture and psychopathology/List of books in culture and mental health)*
Professor Emeritus of Psychology, Pennsylvania State University (USA).

Keisuke Ebata, M.D. *(Migration and adjustment)*
Superintendent, Tokyo Metropolitan Central Area Comprehensive Mental Health Center (Japan). Vice-President, Japanese Association of Transcultural Psychiatry.

F.M. El-Islam, M.D. *(Mental health in Arabic societies)*
Emeritus Professor of Psychiatry, Cairo University (Egypt); Former Secretary, Transcultural Psychiatric Section, World Psychiatric Association.

Armando R. Favazza, M.D., M.P.H. *(Scope of cultural psychiatry)*
Professor of Psychiatry, University of Missouri-Columbia; Member of the Board of Director, The Society for the Study of Psychiatry and Culture

(USA); Committee Member, Transcultural Psychiatric Section, World Psychiatric Association.

Edward F. Foulks, M.D., Ph.D. *(Culture and personality disorders)*
Professor of Psychiatry and Associate Dean, Tulane University School of Medicine; Member of the Board of Directors, The Society for the Study of Psychiatry and Culture (USA).

Ezra Griffith, M.D. *(Minority and mental health)*
Deputy Chairman for Clinical Affairs, Professor of Psychiatry and of African-American Studies, Yale University School of Medicine (USA).

Jing Hsu, M.D. *(Culture and family therapy)*
Clinical Professor of Psychiatry, University of Hawaii School of Medicine; Practicing Psychiatrist (USA).

Wolfgang Jilek, M.D., MSc, MA, FRCP(C) *(Traditional healing practice)*
Professor Emeritus of Psychiatry, University of British Columbia (Canada); Guest Professor, University of Vienna; Former Chair, Transcultural Psychiatric Section, World Psychiatric Association.

Kwang-Iel Kim, M.D., Ph.D. *(Culture and mental health in Asia)*
Superintendent, Hanyang University Kuri Hospital; Professor of Psychiatry, Hanyang University (Korea); Ex-Committee Member, Transcultural Psychiatric Section, World Psychiatric Association.

J. David Kinzie, M.D. *(Refugees and psychological trauma)*
Professor of Psychiatry, Oregon Health Science University (USA); Committee Member, Transcultural Psychiatric Section, World Psychiatric Association.

Laurence J. Kirmayer, M.D. *(Anxiety disorder and somatoform disorders)*
Professor of Psychiatry, McGill University (Canada); Editor-in-Chief; *Transcultural Psychiatry.*

Joan D. Koss-Chioino, Ph.D. *(Medical and psychological anthropology)*
Professor of Anthropology, Arizona State University; and Member of the Board of Directors, The Society for the Study of Psychiatry and Culture (USA).

Takie Sugiyama Lebra, Ph.D. *(Culture and society)*
Professor Emeritus of Anthropology, University of Hawaii (USA).

Keh-Ming Lin, M.D., M.P.H. *(Ethnicity and psychopharmacology)*
Professor of Psychiatry, UCLA; Director, Research Center on the Psychobiology of Ethnicity, Harbor-UCLA Research and Education Institute (USA).

Tsung-Yi Lin, M.D. FRCP(C) *(Culture and psychiatry in world perspectives)*
Professor Emeritus of Psychiatry, University of British Columbia (Canada); Former Senior Medical Officer Responsible for Social and Cultural Psychiatry, WHO; Former President, World Federation of Mental Health.

Roland Littlewood, M.B., D.Phil., F.R.C.Psych *(Culture and psychiatric theories)*
Professor of Anthropology and Psychiatry, and Director, University College Centre for Medical Anthropology, University College London (UK); Former President, Royal Anthropological Institute; Ex-Committee Member, Transcultural Psychiatric Section, World Psychiatric Association.

Francis G. Lu, M.D. *(Training relating to culture competence)*
Clinical Professor of Psychiatry, University of California, San Francisco; and Member of the Board of Directors, The Society for the Study of Psychiatry and Culture (USA).

Juan E. Mezzich, M.D., Ph.D. *(Classification of disorders)*
Professor of Psychiatry and Director, Division of Psychiatric Epidemiology and International Center for Mental Health, Mount Sinai Medical Center, (USA); Chair, Epidemiology Section,

World Psychiatric Association; Secretary-General, World Psychiatric Association.

Masahisa Nishizono, M.D. *(Eastern psychotherapy)*
Professor and Former Chair, Department of Psychiatry, Fukuoka University (Japan); President, Japanese Association of Transcultural Psychiatry.

Raymond Prince, M.D. *(Culture and psychotherapy)*
Professor, Division of Social and Transcultural Psychiatry, McGill University (Canada); Editor, Transcultural Psychiatric Research Review; Honorable Advisor, Transcultural Psychiatric Section, World Psychiatric Association.

Norman Sartorius, M.D., Ph.D. *(WHO-coordinated epidemiological studies of mental disorders)*
Professor of Psychiatry, Universite de Genève (Switzerland); Former Director, Division of Mental Health, World Health Organization; Former President, World Psychiatric Association; President of the Association of European Psychiatrists.

Shen Yu-Cun, M.D. *(Mental health in China)*
Honorable Director, Institute of Mental Health, Beijing University (China); Academician, The Chinese Academy of Engineering; Member of the WHO Expert Advisory Panel on Mental Health.

Ronald C. Simons, M.D., M.A. *(Culture-related specific syndrome)*
Professor Emeritus, Departments of Psychiatry and Anthropology, Michigan State University; Clinical Professor, Department of Psychiatry and Behavior Sciences, University of Washington (USA).

Jon Streltzer, M.D. *(Culture and consultation–liaison psychiatry)*
Professor of Psychiatry, University of Hawaii School of Medicine (USA).

Eng-Seong Tan, M.D. *(Culture and mental health in south Asia and Australia)*
Associate Professor of Psychiatry, University of Melbourne (Australia); Formerly Chair, Department of Psychological Medicine, University of Malaya, Malaysia.

Vijoy K. Varma, M.D. *(Indian mind and mental health)*
Visiting Professor of Psychiatry, Columbia University College of Physicians and Surgeons (USA); (Retired) Professor of Psychiatry, Postgraduate of Medical Education and Research, Chandigarh (India); Secretary, Transcultural Psychiatric Section, World Psychiatric Association.

Joseph Westermeyer, M.D., Ph.D. *(Alcoholism and other substance abuse)*
Professor of Psychiatry, Department of Veterans Affairs Medical Center, Minneapolis; Member of the Board of Directors, The Society for the Study of Psychiatry and Culture (USA).

Ronald M. Wintrop, M.D. *(Ethnic identity issues/Cultural psychiatry training)*
Clinical Professor of Psychiatry and Human Behavior, Brown University; Past-Present of the Steering Committee and Member of the Board of Directors, The Society for the Study of Psychiatry and Culture (USA).

List of Tables and Figures

ing a sacred vow to abstain in front of a model of the palace of the opium goddess. [Courtesy of Wolfgang Jilek, M.D.].

FIGURE 32-12   Treatment of drug addicts at a Buddhist temple in Thailand. (a) Performance of "purification" by herb-induced vomiting. (b) After abstinence is accomplished, a monk instructs patients on how to start new lives. [Courtesy of Wolfgang Jilek, M.D.].

FIGURE 32-13   Diviner's dream house in the southern highlands of Papua New Guinea (for diagnostic dream divination). [Courtesy of Wolfgang Jilek, M.D.].

FIGURE 32-14   Chinese divination (*Chien* drawing). (a) After a sincere pray, picking up a bamboo stick *(chien)* for divine instruction. [Courtesy of Jing Hsu, M.D.] (b) Based on the number on the stick, the corresponding divine paper is obtained, on which the divination is classified, associated with symbolism (described in a poem), and an explanation given along with a set of itemized answers. From *Kuan Yin Bodhisattva: Book of Divination,* English translation by Jinquan Zheng. Honolulu: Typeset Express, Inc., 1991. (c) An elderly person in the temple interpretating the fortune and acting as a folk counselor. [Courtesy of Jing Hsu, M.D.].

FIGURE 33-1   Morita therapy originated in Japan. (a) A Japanese psychiatrist, Shoma Morita, founded the experiential therapy, which was later named after him. (b) A young male suffering from *taijinkyofusho* resting in bed during the first stage of therapy. (c) A group of male patients doing yard work in the second stage of therapy. (d) A patient's diary with comments by his therapist in red pen as a part of the therapeutic activities. [Courtesy of Kenji Kitanish, M.D.].

TABLE 34-1   Comparison of Therapeutic Orientations, Operations, Mechanisms, and Goals among Different Indigenous and Modern Therapeutic Modes [From W.S. Tseng, *Transcultural Psychiatry, 36* (2), 131–179, 1999].

FIGURE 35-1   Pschotherapy in different cultures. (a) A group study of Mao's teachings in China during the Great Forward Movement era, utilizing political ideology for the improvement of life (source unknown). (b) Chinese child psychiatrists counseling parents at the roadside to promote child mental health in Nanjing. Privacy and confidentiality are not concerns in this public situation. [Courtesy of Tao Kuo-Tai, M.D.] (c) Medical officers in Truk, Micronesia, providing counseling to a patient with his family members around — a natural setting for family-involved therapy. (d) A psychiatrist visiting a home in the island society of Samoa to study the mental health of the family members. [Courtesy of Gail Ingram, M.D.].

FIGURE 39-1   Different therapist–couple combinations associated with cultural background.

FIGURE 49-1   Psychosociogram of man in different societies. (a) Ego boundaries are distinctly defined in individual-oriented societies. (b) Ego boundaries are relatively blurred and extend to include the surroundings in situation-oriented societies. Revised from F.H.L. Hsu, Ph.D., presented at APA annual meeting, Honolulu, 1973.

FIGURE 49-2   Cultural modifications of personality development theory. Variations on stages and themes of development.

Section A
Introduction

In order to comprehensively cover the field of cultural psychiatry, a total of nine sections are included in this book, including this introductory section. This section consists of only one chapter, which defines various terms used in this field, reviews the historical development of this newly established subfield of psychiatry, and finally describes the scope of cultural psychiatry. It provides a base for all the chapters that follow.

Section A

Introduction

1

History and Scope

I. IN THE BEGINNING: DEFINING TERMS AND CONCEPTS

A. THE DEFINITION OF CULTURAL PSYCHIATRY

Cultural psychiatry, a special field of psychiatry, is primarily concerned with the cultural aspects of human behavior, mental health, psychopathology, and treatment. At the *clinical* level, cultural psychiatry aims to promote culturally relevant mental health care for patients of diverse ethnic or cultural backgrounds. This includes culturally relevant assessment and understanding of psychopathologies and psychological problems, and culturally appropriate care and treatment. In terms of *research,* cultural psychiatry is interested in how ethnic or cultural factors may influence human behavior and psychopathology, as well as the art of healing. On a *theoretical* level, cultural psychiatry aims to expand our knowledge of human behavior and mental problems transculturally, in order to facilitate the development of more universally applicable and cross-culturally valid theories.

Culture is conceptualized as the behavior patterns and lifestyle shared by a group of people, which is

unique and different from that of other groups; it is the totality of knowledge, customs, habits, beliefs, and values that shape behaviors, emotions, and life patterns. It is learned and transmitted by the members of a society over generations. Since a cultural unit is not easily identified and labeled, for the sake of convenience, a cultural unit is often identified instead by the name of an ethnic group or a country, e.g., American, Chinese, Jewish, or Italian culture. Yet, strictly speaking, ethnicity differs from culture and they are not to be equated with each other. **Ethnicity** refers to a particular group of people that is distinctly different from other groups of people. The members of an ethnic group share a common historical path, are affiliated with each other, and may share a common language, religion, culture, racial background, or other characteristics that make them identifiable within their own group. In other words, ethnicity refers to an identified group of people, whereas culture refers to the lifestyle shared by a group of people. When considerable differences exist within groups of people in a society or even among the same ethnic groups, they are referred to as **subcultures** [cross-reference to Chapter 2: Culture and Society (Section I, A)].

Many terms with different implications have been used in the past to refer to the subfield of cultural psy-

3

chiatry. **Primitive psychiatry** was used by American anthropologist George Devereux in 1940, referring to the study of mental disorders and their methods of cure in preliterate tribes. The focus was on the study of mental illness in "primitive" societies. Similarly, **prescientific psychiatry** was used by Ari Kiev (1972). As both terms carry negative implications and concern only so-called "primitive" or "prescientific" groups, they are no longer used by most scholars. An alternative term, **ethnopsychiatry,** emerged later. Because anthropologists used the term "ethnography" to indicate a comprehensive anthropological study of a particular ethnic group, the term "ethnopsychiatry" was used to refer to the systematic study of the psychiatric theories and practices of a particular ethnic group, mainly a primitive tribe. Ethnopsychiatry concerns folk concepts of emotional disturbances, interpretations of mental illness, and traditional ways of healing those problems. Terms with similar meanings, **folk psychiatry** and **anthropological psychiatry,** were used by other scholars.

One of the pioneers of cultural psychiatry, E. D. Wittkower (1964), from McGill University in Montreal, regarded **cultural psychiatry,** as it was recognized then, as a discipline concerned with the frequency, etiology, and nature of mental illness, and the care and aftercare of the mentally ill within the confines of a given "culture unit." He coined the term **transcultural psychiatry,** which, he claimed, expanded cultural psychiatry by extending its concerns beyond the scope of one cultural unit on to others. The word "**trans**cultural" was created to emphasize its application through cultural barriers, whereas the term "**cross**-cultural" is applied to comparative and contrasting aspects of psychiatry in different cultures.

Epidemiologically oriented anthropologist J. M. Murphy and psychiatrist Leighton (1965), at Cornell University in New York, used the term **cross-cultural psychiatry** to stress that the main conceptual and methodological tool for inquiry is comparative analysis of mental disorders among various ethnic or cultural groups. Thus, emphasis is placed on cross-cultural comparisons in epidemiological studies.

Another pioneer of cultural psychiatry from Montreal, H. B. M. Murphy (1982), following Emil Krepelin's footsteps, used the term **comparative psychiatry,** as did P.M. Yap (1974) from Hong Kong. Murphy defined comparative psychiatry as "the study of the relations between mental disorder and the psychological characteristics which differentiated nations, peoples, or cultures. Its main goals are to identify, verify, and explain the links between mental disorder and these broad psychosocial characteristics" (p. 2). It is seen as an academic discipline for study, without concern for clinical applications.

A position statement made by the American Psychiatric Association (APA) (1969) used Wittkower's term **transcultural psychiatry** and described it as "the comparative study of mental health and mental illness among different societies, nations, and cultures and the interrelationships of mental disorders with cultural environments."

Thus, many terms have been used by psychiatrists as well as by behavioral scientists. All pay attention to the cultural aspects of psychiatry, but with slightly different focuses, orientations, and emphases. *Cross-cultural* is used more by psychologists to emphasize cross-cultural comparisons (as exemplified by the title of *Journal of Cross-Cultural Psychology*), whereas *transcultural* is used by many psychiatrists to stress applications through cultural barriers (as shown by the journal title of *Transcultural Psychiatry*). *Intercultural* is used to refer to interaction between two different cultures, such as intercultural marriage, or intercultural psychotherapy — the latter referring to a situation in which the therapist and the patient have different cultural backgrounds, and the therapeutic process involves the interaction of their two cultures.

Recently, the adjective *cultural* has been used more often. American cultural psychiatrist Armando R. Favazza and Oman (1978) proposed simply using the term **cultural psychiatry.** This idea was soon echoed by other scholars (Tseng and McDermott, 1981), as the term follows the way in which other subfields of psychiatry have been named, such as biological, social, and community psychiatry. The term cultural psychiatry is considered more inclusive and less exotic, and does not imply a single methodology. It does not necessarily imply that the discipline is interested merely in studying a single cultural unit, as was the case several decades ago. Rather, with the use of the word "culture," and the general orientation associated with this term, it is understood by most scholars that this field includes multiple cultural comparisons in order to highlight the dimensions of culture. Favazza (1987, 1996) even proposed the "grand" view of culture as the overriding force that provides meaning to and makes sense of biology, psychology, and social science. This gives it a synthetic and interpretative role in its application to human science. Now, the term cultural psychiatry is also preferred by Raymond Prince (1997), another pioneer in this subfield, who was closely associated with Wittkower and Murphy in Montreal when the term was first coined.

B. Boundaries and Relations among Various Sciences and Disciplines

1. Culture- and Medicine-Related Social/Behavioral Sciences

Cultural psychiatry recognizes the importance of biological factors to human behavior and mental disorders. Yet, by definition, cultural psychiatry is more oriented to the psychological, social, and cultural aspects of behavior and illness. Because of its focus, cultural psychiatry is more closely related to the academic disciplines of the social and behavioral sciences, particularly their common interests in the sociocultural aspects of human behavior, socialization, and illness behavior (Favazza & Oman, 1980; Foulks, Wintrob, Westermeyer, & Favazza, 1977; Westermeyer, 1976). It may be said that these disciplines are the sciences basic to the clinical science of cultural psychiatry (see Fig. 1-1).

a. Medical Anthropology

This is a subfield of anthropology, applied anthropology in medicine (Caudill, 1953). Although descrip-

tions of etiological beliefs and medical practices in simpler societies were important components of certain earlier ethnographic studies, much of the development of medical anthropology has occurred since World War II (Fabrega, 1972). Medical anthropology examines medical aspects of the adaptation and maladaptation of human groups to their sociocultural environment and ecology, the epidemiology of disorders, ethnomedicine (including folk disease classification and therapy), and medical aspects of social systems, as well as of illness and cultural change (Landy, 1977; Lieban, 1974).

b. Cross-Cultural Psychology

Cross-cultural psychology is concerned with the systematic study of behavior and experience as it occurs in different cultures (Triandis, 1980). It is defined as the scientific study of human behavior and its transmission, taking into account the ways in which behaviors are shaped by social and cultural forces (Berry, Poortinga, Segall, & Dasen, 1992; Segall, Dasen, Berry, & Poortinga, 1990). The adjective *cross-cultural* refers to comparisons of cultures (Marsella, Tharp, & Ciborowski, 1979). The term *cultunit* was coined to describe people who are domestic speakers of a common district dialect and belong either to the same state or the same contact group (Naroll, 1971). A major purpose of cross-cultural psychology is to test the generality of psychological laws, to develop valid psychological instruments for cross-cultural application, and to reveal the frequency of particular behaviors or particular incidents in different populations.

c. Medical Sociology

Medical sociology focuses on medical issues within the framework of society. These may include social responses to psychological problems and mental disorders, the use of treatment facilities, the role and function of mental hospitals, and social policy with regard to mental illness. When physical sickness is related to mental illness, the knowledge and con-

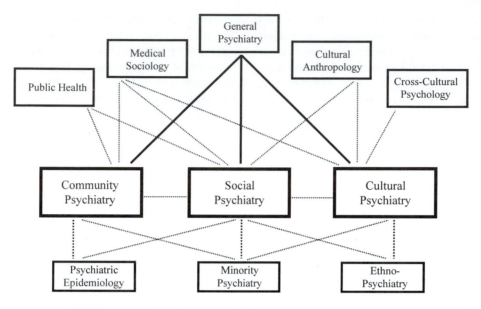

FIGURE 1-1   Scope of cultural psychiatry and its relation to other fields.

cerns of medicine and sociology begin to have common interests.

2. Other Socioenvironmentally Concerned Subfields of Psychiatry

a. Social Psychiatry

This subfield of general psychiatry, like cultural psychiatry, is primarily concerned with socioenvironmental aspects of human behavior and mental disorders (Opler, 1967). The development of social psychiatry was directly stimulated by two social factors: the disruptions of human life by World War I and the rapid social change that occurred after industrialization. Both factors had a significant impact on the mental health of people at all social levels.

According to pioneering social psychiatrists Leighton, Clausen, and Wilson (1957), social psychiatry focuses on several areas, including concepts of normality and abnormality in different societies; the relation of social environment to personality development; the effects of mental illness on social environment; modes of societal reaction to mental illness; and implications of cultural diversity for effective understanding and prevention. Ari Kiev (1969) defined social psychiatry as a discipline concerned fundamentally with the interrelationships between the sociocultural environment and the individual and the way in which the environment affects the forms, distribution, frequency, treatment, management, and prevention of psychiatric disorders. Ransom Arthur (1973) described social psychiatry as the study of the impingement of social phenomena on the genesis and manifestations of mental illness and the utilization of social forces in the treatment of mental and emotional disturbances. Jurgen Ruesch (1965) clarified social psychiatry as a point of view rather than a mode of operation. It focuses on people's social functioning; deals with individuals in groups; attempts to influence social organization; advocates a broad approach for treatment; and influences everyday life attitudes.

As indicated by its name, social psychiatry is primarily concerned with the *social* aspects of psychiatry. Its main focus is on the relation between society and mental health — how the social structure, organization, policies, and functions of a society, including its social classes, economic factors, intergroup relationships, and so on, may impact the mental health of its people and how to manipulate social factors to promote mental health.

Both *social psychiatry* and *cultural psychiatry* are concerned with the sociocultural environment, rather than the individual psychological or biological dimensions, of people. Due to differences in their basic orientations and approaches, which focus on either *society* or *culture,* they are distinguished from an academic point of view. However, in reality, they are closely related as disciplines of psychiatry.

b. Minority Psychiatry

This term is used to describe the clinical work and knowledge that focus primarily on ethnic minorities (Jones & Korchin, 1982; Littlewood & Lipsedge, 1989; Powell, Yamamoto, Romero, & Morales, 1983). Minority psychiatry takes the view that a *minority,* by definition an underprivileged subgroup of a society, tends to have special (and negative) psychological experiences, such as discrimination by the privileged majority group, cultural deprivation or uprooting, and ethnic identification problems. Minorities also tend to be underserved in the area of mental health care. Thus, there is a need to develop special clinical knowledge, experiences, and orientations for dealing with the mental health issues of minorities. Minority psychiatry can be included as a part of cultural psychiatry.

c. Community Psychiatry

As a part of social psychiatry, community psychiatry is concerned with mental health care and prevention within a defined community. It focuses on the community as a whole rather than on a single patient, family, or group. Thus, developing various mental health programs to meet primary, secondary, or tertiary mental health care needs of the community is the basic thrust of this subfield. The social resources and cultural environment of the community, including people's knowledge of and attitudes toward mental health and disease, are of major concern. Although community psychiatry has not flourished as a movement as it was originally intended in the United States in the 1960s and 1970s, the concept is still important from an academic point of view. Public psychiatry is a new term used by some clinicians to replace the term community psychiatry, indicating an emphasis on mental health at the public level.

d. Psychiatric Epidemiology

Closely related to public health and community psychiatry, psychiatric epidemiology is concerned with the frequency of mental disorders observed in communities or societies. Comparing the prevalence of mental illnesses in different societies or countries provides information about how sociocultural settings contribute to the formation and manifestation of various kinds of psychopathology. If the communities compared differ culturally, then it becomes a cross-cultural epidemiological study. However, unless cultural data, as opposed to merely demographic social background information, are specifically examined, there is no way to investigate the relation between cultural factors and the observed frequency of mental disorders. In other words, the investigation of the epidemiology of mental disorders often does not involve the study of "cultural" dimensions and does not, therefore, directly relate to cultural psychiatry in a narrow sense. However, the information obtained from cross-cultural epidemiology often becomes the basis for the investigation of cultural matters.

In summary, the core of cultural psychiatry is the analysis of cultural and its relation to psychiatry. It is based on the foundation of cultural anthropology, cross-cultural psychology, and medical sociology and exists as a subfield of general psychiatry. As a clinical science, cultural psychiatry is interested in scientific research and theoretical investigation, but its final goal is clinical application, providing culturally relevant care for patients of various ethnic/cultural backgrounds.

II. HISTORICAL DEVELOPMENT OF CULTURAL PSYCHIATRY

A. Beginning of Ethnopsychiatry (from the End of the 19th to the Early 20th Century)

Several forces promoted the development of ethnopsychiatry — the prelude to cultural psychiatry. They were as follows.

1. Differences in Psychiatric Conditions among Early Immigrants to America

The existence of ethnic or racial differences in mental illness was noticed by clinicians as early as the middle of the 18th century. According to Wittkower and Prince (1974), between 1839 and 1844, some 400,000 European immigrants flocked into the United States. Many superintendents of mental hospitals seemed to regard the immigrants of this period — mainly Irish and German peasants — as "inferior" Americans, in contrast to the immigrants of an earlier period — mainly British — and speculated that they were more susceptible to mental disorders and more resistant to treatment.

2. European Psychiatrists Discovered Unusual Syndromes in Colonized Societies

Toward the end of the 19th century, the colonizing European powers began to build and staff "lunatic" asylums in Africa, the Caribbean, and southeast Asia. Early colonial physicians, lacking anthropological and epidemiological sophistication, and often with condescending attitudes toward the natives, described unusual symptom patterns among them (Wittkower & Prince, 1974). For example, there was Arctic hysteria (Brill, 1913) among the polar Eskimo people, *amok* (Ellis, 1893) *or latah* (Fletcher, 1908) among Malay people, or (according to Edwards, 1985) *koro* (Blonk, 1895; Palthe, 1934) among Indonesians and southern Chinese. These "peculiar" or "exotic" syndromes (from

a Euro-American's point of view) were later clustered together as culture-bound syndromes (Simons & Hughes, 1985). Their discovery certainly stimulated Western-psychiatrists' interest in the cultural aspects of mental disorders [cross-reference to Chapter 13: Culture-Related Specific Syndromes (Section II, A–E)].

3. Pioneer Interest in Comparative (Descriptive) Psychiatry

For various reasons, mainly concerned with the cross-ethnic applicability of his established psychiatric classification system, Emil Kraepelin, the father of modern psychiatry, traveled to southeast Asia and other areas of the world in the 1890s. He described the differences in symptomatology that he found in different societies and established the concept of comparative psychiatry (1904) (Jilek, 1995; Kennedy, 1973). Kraepelin was planning to carry out major cross-cultural research involving seven non-European countries, but the project was prevented by World War I (Jilek, 1995). He did conduct comparative studies with American Indian, Afro-American, and Latin American patients at psychiatric institutions in the United States, Mexico, and Cuba in 1925, 1 year prior to his unexpected death.

4. Concerns about the Applicability of Psychoanalytic Concepts in Primitive Societies

As pointed out by Kennedy (1973), anthropologists, armed with evidence from nonliterate peoples, mounted a serious attack on ethnocentrism in social science in the late 19th and early 20th centuries. They documented the tremendous variability of patterns of social life around the globe and stressed the importance of cultural factors in shaping the life and behavior of an individual. During the same period, dynamic psychiatry was evolving the view that mental disorders were produced by noxious environmental factors, particularly in early childhood.

It was within this academic atmosphere in the early 20th century that Freud's psychoanalytic theory, which emphasized parent–child relationships in shaping personality and causing emotional disorders, suggested that cultures with grossly different patterns of child rearing might generate different psychiatric phenomena. In order to test Freud's theory, many cultural anthropologists were inspired to carry out field work in tribal societies. For instance, anthropologist Bronislaw Malinoski (1927) reported that the manifestation of the Oedipus complex is different in matrilineal societies. Based on his study in the Trobriand Islands, he reported that, instead of the biological father, it is the mother's brother who represents the principles of discipline, authority, and executive power in the family. He described that in a such matrilineal society, the boy's unconscious wish was to marry his sister and to kill his maternal uncle — a different version of the complex. A psychoanalyst and anthropologist, and also a student of Freud, Geza Roheim (1933), based on his field study in Australia, claimed that the classical neuroses were rare among tribal people there and conjectured that this was a result of the lesser intensity of repression in primitive races than in European societies.

B. Varied Interests in Investigating Culture and Mental Health (1930s to 1950s)

1. Enthusiasm in Studying Culture and Personality

Although the notion that culture and individual personality are interrelated is an old one, it was around the 1930s that anthropologists first made significant contributions to this subject. Anthropologist Ruth Benedict (1934), based on her field work in New Mexico, Vancouver, and Melanesia, developed the concept of "cultural configurations." Abram Kardiner (1945), a New York psychoanalyst, held the view that certain culturally established techniques of child rearing shape basic attitudes toward life that persist throughout the life of the individual. Based on this, he proposed the concept of "basic personality structure."

Later, Cora du Bois, based largely on a statistical point of view, proposed the concept of "modal personality structure." These academic views promoted an understanding of the cultural aspects of personality [cross-reference to Chapter 5: Personality and Depth Psychology (Section I,C)].

Closely associated with the interest in culture and personality was the movement to investigate cross-cultural child-rearing practices with relation to personality development. J.W.M. Whiting and Child (1953) carried out investigations to correlate ethnographic data from diverse societies. Later, utilizing standardized field work techniques, Whiting and colleagues conducted field work in six cultures to illustrate how socialization patterns differed among them (B.B. Whiting & Whiting, 1975).

2. Psychiatrists' Interest in Indigenous Healing Practices

Studies of folk healing had already been conducted in the field by medical anthropologists, and numerous volumes of literature were published on indigenous healing practices to deal with psychological problems in many preliterate societies when American psychiatrist Jerome Frank (1961) first compared folk healing with modern psychotherapy. Frank pointed out the fundamental (nonspecific) therapeutic mechanisms utilized by both folk and modern therapies, such as the cultivation of hope and the mobilization of resources. Through his study, a connection was made between witch doctors and modern psychiatry (Torrey, 1986), and the close relationship that exists between them was recognized.

3. Development of Comparative Psychiatric Epidemiology

Starting around the 1930s, many massive epidemiological studies were carried out to investigate the prevalence of mental disorders in various societies. The Thuringia study (Brugger, 1931) in Germany, the Baltimore study (Lemkau, Tietze, &

Cooper, 1941) in the United States, and the Formosa study (Lin, 1953) in Taiwan are some examples.

These epidemiological investigations, although not focused primarily on the correlation between culture and mental disorders, provided information indicating that the prevalence of mental disorders differs among societies. This provoked speculation and further interest in exploring the possible influence of culture on mental disorders.

4. Emphasis on Minor Psychiatric Disorders

Results obtained from comparative epidemiological studies, namely, that variations of prevalence were generally greater cross-culturally for minor rather than major psychiatric disorders, stimulated scholars to shift their attention more on the former from a cultural point of view. Clinical experiences also support this view. Instead of focusing on major psychiatric disorders, namely, psychoses, whose etiology is more predominantly biological, German cultural psychiatrist Wolfgang Pfeiffer (1971) emphasized the importance of studying cultural influences on minor psychiatric disorders such as neuroses or psychological problems. This view was echoed by Tseng and McDermott (1981).

C. Formal Organization of Cultural Psychiatry and Study Programs (since the 1960s)

Led by Eric D. Wittkower, a group of interdisciplinary scholars formed the Transcultural Psychiatry Division at Magill University in Montreal in 1955 (R.H. Prince, Okpaku, & Merkel, 1998). Quarterly since 1963, the division has distributed the *Transcultural Psychiatric Research Review,* one of the major journals in the world for disseminating knowledge about cultural psychiatry and promoting awareness and interest among cultural psychiatrists.

Through H.B.M. Murphy's efforts, the Transcultural Psychiatry Section was established within the World Psychiatric Association in 1971 when the World Congress of Psychiatry was held in Mexico City. The sec-

tion, chaired by Murphy for its first and second terms, was instrumental in promoting the development of cultural psychiatry around the world, particularly in developing areas. In addition to presenting Section Symposia at each World Congress of Psychiatry, the section has held international meetings periodically in different geographic regions, such as Beijing and Nanjing, China (1985), Budapest, Hungary (1991), New Deli, India, Ankara, Turkey (1994), and Rome, Italy (1997), at which colleagues from various areas, particularly developing societies, could exchange knowledge about cultural psychiatry on a global level.

Many cultural psychiatric organizations have been established at national levels during the past two decades. For instance, the Society for the Study of Psychiatry and Culture (SSPC) was founded in the United States in 1979. Many leading cultural psychiatrists, such as Ronald M. Wintrob, Joseph Westermeyers, Edward Foulk, and Armando R. Favazza, were among the original steering committee members who established the organization. The Transcultural Psychiatry Society (TPS) was formed in the United Kingdom, and Arbeitsgemeinschaft Ethnomedizin (AGEM) in Germany. Recently, the Istituto Italiano di Igiene Mental Transculturale (IMT) was founded in Italy (1984), the Chinese Society for Cultural Psychiatry (CSCP) in China, and the Japanese Society of Multiple-Cultural Psychiatry (JSMCP) in Japan, as well. All of these national associations maintain close relationships with the Transcultural Psychiatry Section of the World Psychiatric Association.

In addition to the previously mentioned *Transcultural Psychiatry Research Review* from Canada (which was changed to *Transcultural Psychiatry* in 1997), *Culture, Medicine and Psychiatry* has been published in the United States since 1977. A new journal, *Cultural Diversity and Mental Health,* was started in 1994 and renamed *Cultural Diversity and Ethnic Minority Psychology* in 1999. In the United Kingdom, the *International Journal of Social Psychiatry* has been published since 1954, featuring both social and cultural psychiatry. In Germany, there is the *Zeitschrift fur Ethnomedizin und Transcultural Psychiatrie (Journal for Ethnomedicine and Transcultural Psychiatry,* also called *Curare*) published since 1977. Besides these journals, many books have been published (mainly in English) relating to the subject of cultural psychiatry (see Appendix: Books Relating to Culture, Psychiatry, and Mental Health).

There have been numerous ongoing academic programs in different parts of the world to systematically promote the study of culture-related mental health and psychiatric issues. For instance, in the field of culture and personality, stimulated by the work of individual pioneers such as Margaret Mead, Ruth Benedice, Ralph Linton, Edward Sapir, Abram Kardiner, and others [cross-reference to Chapter 5: Personality and Depth Psychology (Section I,C)] a plan was proposed for a cross-cultural and systematic investigation involving multiple cultural units to explore the relationship between different patterns of child rearing and subsequent differences in personality. In 1953, the Committee on Social Behavior of the Social Science Research Council at Yale University sponsored a seminar and conference to discuss cross-cultural work on socialization. As a result, a field manual for the cross-cultural study of child rearing was prepared. In 1954, social scientists from Harvard, Yale, and Cornell universities participated in field research in six cultures (B.B. Whiting, 1963; B.B. Whiting & Whiting, 1975).

In Honolulu, with NIMH funding, a Culture and Mental Health for the Pacific and Asia program was conducted between 1965 and 1971 at the East-West Center. A group of anthropologists, psychologists, sociologists, and psychiatrists from around the Pacific, including North America and Asian countries, were invited to participate in the residential program and periodically held conferences whose participants included additional invited scholars. The first program was in 1965–1966, following a conference held in 1964 that resulted in a first publication (Caudill & Lin, 1969). The program continued under the leadership of cultural anthropologist William Lebra, who produced three additional volumes, published as a series, on mental health research in Asia and the Pacific (W.P. Lebra, 1972, 1974, 1976).

The national and international organizations just described, various culture and mental health programs, and the regular publication of journals and books have all been instrumental in disseminating and expanding our knowledge in the area of culture and mental health during the past several decades and in stimulating the recognition of cultural psychiatry as a formally established subfield of applied academic science.

D. Emphasis on Minority Mental Health (from the 1960s)

1. Promotion of the Minority Movement in North America

Associated with the concern for human rights and the rising of the minority movement, mainly in the United States, since the 1960s, there has been a rapid increase in concern over how to provide ethnic and culturally relevant mental health care for minority groups, such as Native Americans, African-Americans, Asian-Americans, and Latino-Americans. There has been increased recognition that minority groups encounter special psychological experiences and that there is therefore a need for ethnic-adjusted assessment and care. From a clinical point of view, there is an increased demand to pay attention to the matching of the therapist and the patient from ethnic and cultural perspectives so that the care provided will be more appropriate.

Associated with this movement, the terms culture sensitive, culture relevant, culture adjusted, and culture competent have become common professional jargon and have greatly promoted attention to the ethnic and cultural aspects of psychiatric practices. Beginning in the 1970s, numerous publications have appeared as resource books on mental health relating to various ethnic/cultural groups, as well as minority groups (Al-Issa & Tousignant, 1997; Aponte, Rivers, & Wohl, 1995; Gaw, 1993; Johnson-Powell, Yamamoto, Wyatt, & Arroyo, 1997; McGoldrick, Giordano, & Pearce, 1996; McGoldrick, Pearce, & Giordano, 1982; Powell et al., 1983; Tseng, McDermott, & Maretzki, 1974).

2. Increased Concern Regarding Minority Emigrants to Western Europe

Paralleling the situation in the United States, there was a remarkable increase in minority emigration into western Europe, particularly Germany, the United Kingdom, and France, mostly from east Europe or south Asia, due to economic reasons. The sudden increase in minorities in those developed societies brought about the need for mental health care that was appropriate and effective for the culturally diverse ethnic minorities. This stimulated a concern for, and knowledge and experience of, cultural psychiatry among general European psychiatrists (Littlewood & Lipsedge, 1989).

3. Clinical Application beyond Academic Research

Stimulated by the increased concern with providing culturally sensitive and relevant clinical care for minority groups, there was a strong interest in addressing the clinical application of cultural psychiatry, rather than simply concentrating on academic research. Many publications appeared that stressed the importance of clinical application (Comas-Diaz & Griffith, 1988; Okpaku, 1998; Tseng & McDermott, 1981), including such matters as how to comprehend and assess psychopathology (Tseng & Streltzer, 1997) and how to perform culturally relevant therapy (Abel & Metraux, 1974; Pedersen, Draguns, Lonner, & Trimble, 1989, 1996; Pedersen, Lonner, & Draguns, 1976; Tseng & Streltzer, 2001).

E. EMERGENCE OF BROAD-MINDED "CULTURAL PSYCHIATRY" (FROM THE 1970s)

1. From Isolated, Simple Societies to Developed, Complex Societies

In order to examine the relationships between culture and mental illness, scholars in the past tended to search for isolated, primitive societies where such relationships might be easier to investigate. However, as pointed out by Schwab and Schwab (1978), today we are living on a shrinking planet on which many developed and complex societies are arising. The new challenge for cultural psychiatrists is to shift their focus onto complex societies — in both the West and the East — which encompass a broad collection of subcultures. There is a practical need to examine the cultural aspects of the mental health situation in modern societies at both theoretical and clinical levels.

2. Western-Trained, Non-Western Psychiatrists' Contributions in Their Home Societies

Many non-Western psychiatrists began to have opportunities to go to western Europe or North America for further professional training, especially after World War II. After completing their training abroad, they returned to their home countries and faced the challenge of applying their Western psychiatric knowledge and experiences to non-Western settings. Such Western-trained, non-Western psychiatrists made many contributions, directly and indirectly, to cultural psychiatry at the clinical, research, and theoretical levels. For instance, the Japanese psychiatrist Takeo Doi (1973), based on his clinical work with Japanese patients, stresses that interdependent need is a part of human nature that is valued in many cultures, such as Japan, rather than being a negative behavior, as it is perceived in some Western societies, such as America. The pioneer African psychiatrist T.A. Lambo (1966) experimented with a family members-involved treatment program for inpatient care, known as the Village of Aro, not only to accommodate his native social situation, but also to illustrate, from a sociocultural perspective, a radically different approach to patient care. Similarly, the Nigerian psychiatrist T. Asuni (1967) experimented with a revised from of group therapy that fit the people of his cultural background.

Many publications address the cultural aspects of mental health and psychiatric practices among various non-Western cultures, such as the Chinese (Kleinman & Lin, 1981; Lin, Tseng, & Yeh, 1995; Tseng & Wu, 1985) and Japanese (T.S. Lebra & Lebra, 1974, 1986). Developing culturally relevant psychiatric care in different countries or geographic regions and providing culturally appropriate service for the majority of the populations of the world have become new issues (Al-Issa, 1995; Cox, 1986; Kato Price, Shea, & Mookherjee, 1995; Kleinman, 1988). These trends and insights stimulate the expansion of the view and scope of cultural psychiatry broadly from international perspectives (Desjarlais, Eisenberg, Good, & Kleinman, 1995; Lieh Mak & Nadelson, 1996).

3. Recognition of Cultural Psychiatry in (Western) Home Countries

As pointed out correctly by H.B.M. Murphy (1977), in all other branches of psychiatry, advances in theory or practice have mostly derived from, and been mainly concerned with, the major societies of western Europe and North America. In contrast, the great bulk of literature on transcultural psychiatry, at least in the past, has been concerned with other societies, principally African, Asian, and Amerindian.

This peculiar academic trend has been influenced by historical background and reflects cultural biases. Many European–American clinicians tend to believe that formal studies of a cultural nature were unnecessary in developed western European and North American societies, as their (Western) cultures are well known to the European or American psychiatrists practicing there. It is when these psychiatrists must deal with people from foreign cultures that there is a need for cultural knowledge and understanding. This bias is coupled with another fact. As pointed out by Favazza and Oman (1978), although all psychiatric disorders are to some degree culture bound, or culture related, because we (as Westerners) are intimately involved in our own (Western) cultures, we hardly realize the existence of cultural influence and find it difficult to look at culture objectively, even when we recognize its potential impact.

The biases just described and other factors challenge us to change the nature of cultural psychiatry — from merely focusing on the psychiatric matter of "other" or "non-Western" ethnic groups to including our own. Cultural psychiatry is not only for "foreign" or "alien" societies, but for our "own," including majority groups in Western societies. This new trend stimulates Western psychiatrists to pay attention to cultural factors, even when dealing with their own Western populations. For instance, attention is expanded to culture-related syndromes observed among majority groups in modern Western society (Littlewood & Lipsedge, 1986).

Another example is modifying clinical assessment and diagnosis. Following the new trend, a revision of the *Diagnostic and Statistical Manual of Mental Disorders: Fourth Edition* (DSM-IV), the formal product of the American Psychiatric Association, finally takes into consideration the cultural dimensions of the classification system, making it more applicable to Americans of multiethnic backgrounds and more useful in international situations (Mezzich, Kleinman, Fabrega, & Parron, 1996).

4. Theoretical Challenge for Worldwide Applications

Anthropologists are always concerned with how to understand human behavior from world perspectives and how to apply locally derived information and hypotheses to pan-cultural situations or on a universal level. This is one of the major tasks for cultural psychiatry as well (Mead, 1959). Many theories of psychiatry, proposed for understanding the nature of human psychology and behavior, were derived mainly from experiences with Western populations by Western scholars. There is a need for revision, modification, and expansion of these theories for worldwide application. For instance, the analytical concept of self and ego boundary needs to be revised, as the concept of "self" and its relations with others varies greatly among different cultures. The concept of personality development, which stresses sequential development by stages, from both psychosexual and psychosocial points of view, is rather culture common. However, the major theme emphasized in each stage and the pace of development from stage to stage vary among different cultures, requiring cultural modification. The concept of defense mechanisms as a whole is universal, yet the kinds of defense mechanisms that are utilized more commonly and the kinds of culture-specific defense mechanisms that exist, particularly so-called neurotic or mature mechanisms, are still awaiting future exploration [cross-reference to Chapter 49: Culture and Psychiatric Theories (Section IV, A–C)].

F. Formation of Cultural Psychiatry as a Special Field of Psychiatry (from the 1980s)

We have come a long way since psychiatrists began to show an interest in the cultural aspects of psychiatric practice. It cannot be denied that cultural psychiatry started as a discipline interested in the impact of culture on the manifestation of psychopathology. As an academic exercise, it is more concerned with research into the relationship between culture and human behavior, including abnormal behavior. Yet, associated with progress, the focus of cultural psychiatry has been expanded into clinical practice, emphasizing how to provide culturally relevant care and treatment for patients according to their cultural backgrounds (Griffith, 1988; Pfeiffer, 1994; Tseng & McDermott, 1981). Thus, cultural psychiatry is becoming a distinctly unique subfield of general psychiatry. It should be included as a part of the required curriculum in teaching and training, in the form of organized seminars and clinical consultation and supervision. The need for cultural competence to be recognized as primary to *all* psychiatric care is now being emphasized (ACGME, 2000; Psychiatric News, 1999).

Cultural psychiatry, as a subfield of psychiatry, does not focus on any special population of patients, as does child/adolescent psychiatry, geriatric psychiatry, or addiction psychiatry. While it may be more immediately useful in the care of ethnic minorities,

immigrants, and refugees from other cultures, the knowledge and skill it provides should be applied to all patients, including those from majority groups and from all other ethnic/cultural backgrounds. Similarly to social or biological psychiatry, cultural psychiatry exists as a unique branch of psychiatry, with its main orientation and focus on the cultural dimensions of psychiatric knowledge and practice.

III. THE SCOPE OF CULTURAL PSYCHIATRY

A. Past Attempts to Define the Scope of Cultural Psychiatry

1. Earlier Visions of Pioneers and Recent Views of Clinicians

From the very beginning, when cultural psychiatry emerged as a new field of academic science, its primary efforts have been focused on "research," that is, revealing how cultural factors may impact the manifestation and frequency of psychopathology. Even though the influence of culture on treatment has been recognized, attention has seldom been paid to clinical application. For instance, Wittkower and Termansen (1971) listed the themes of cultural psychiatry as examining cultural factors, such as stress, studying the frequency of mental disorders and patterns of symptomatology, and treating mental disorders. Now, their concern is with overcoming methodological problems and carrying out academic investigations of human behavior and the phenomenological aspects of psychopathology in order to increase our knowledge of cultural psychiatry. This trend is strongly reflected in numerous earlier publications by Opler (1959), de Reuck and Porter (1965), and Kiev (1972).

Greatly influenced by their clinical work in the multiethnic society of Hawaii, Tseng and McDermott (1981) stressed the importance of expanding the scope of cultural psychiatry into daily clinical application, with particular attention on assessment, diagnosis, and therapy. Their view is supported by other scholars and, particularly, by clinicians. For example, the entire scope of the discipline, according to Comas-Diaz and Griffith (1988), stresses the clinical application of cultural psychiatry, including assessment, treatment, and care delivery.

2. Defined by the American Psychiatric Association

The scope of cultural psychiatry, as defined by the Transcultural Psychiatry Committee of APA (1969), includes (1) similarities and differences in the form, course, or *manifestation* of mental illness in different societies and cultures; (2) the occurrence, *incidence,* and distribution of mental illness or behavioral characteristics in relation to sociocultural factors; (3) sociocultural factors *predisposing* to mental health, to optimal function, or to increasing vulnerability to or perpetuating or inhibiting recovery from mental illness or impaired function; (4) the forms of *treatment* or of otherwise dealing with people defined as deviant or physically or mentally ill that are practiced or preferred in various sociocultural settings; (5) the influence of sociocultural factors on the *assessment* of clinical psychiatric issues and the adaptation of established psychiatric principles to varying sociocultural contexts; (6) the relationship between culture and *personality* as it may be approached through studies of the character traits shared by members of the same society derived from exposure to similar patterns of child rearing and to positive and negative social sanctions; (7) the understanding of conflict in persons experiencing rapid social and cultural change; (8) attitudes and beliefs regarding behavioral deviance and the mentally ill, including the *labeling* of behavior; (9) the psychological and social adaptation of migrants, voluntary or involuntary, within or across national boundaries, especially as far as their cultural traits or those of the receiving society are significantly involved; (10) psychiatric or behavioral aspects of communication between individuals and groups from differing cultural or national regions; (11) response to varying culturally based *stressful* situations; and (12) cultural determinants of transnational interaction and of public policy decisions within nations.

B. REINTEGRATION OF THE SCOPE OF CULTURAL PSYCHIATRY (AS VIEWED BY THE AUTHOR)

By reviewing the different theories proposed by various scholars, the scope of cultural psychiatry can be reorganized in an integrative and comprehensive way as follows.

1. Studying Cultural Perspectives of Human Behavior

As the basis for investigation for mental health and illness-related behavior, as well as for clinical application, the first concern of cultural psychiatry is to study cultural impact on human behavior — at both universal and culture-specific levels. More precisely, cultural psychiatry may include the study of the interrelation between culture and child development, personality formation, behavior patterns, marriage and family, socialization patterns, and life cycle. It aims to increase knowledge of how culture influences the mind and behavior. In order to comprehend the social aspects of human life, the scope of study may expand to involve the examination of culture-related social phenomena, such as the mental health perspectives of cultural change, migration, minorities, interracial relations, or even religion. Based on such exploration, clinicians will have a better insight into and understanding the nature of the sociocultural environment and its impact on human life.

2. Investigating Mental Stress and Illness Behavior

Clinicians are always concerned with how an individual, a family, or a collective group encounters stress and deals with problems or conflicts. As an area of cultural psychiatry, there is a need to investigate culture-related stresses and/or culture-induced problems that exist in a society and learn the coping mechanisms provided or sanctioned by the cultural system. It is also necessary to focus on the cultural dimensions of illness behavior: namely, how patients (or their families) perceive, conceptualize, and present their problems; how they seek help; and what kinds of healing systems are available and utilized within each cultural setting.

3. Examining Psychopathology

It is important clinically to investigate from a descriptive and phenomenological point of view how cultural factors relate to the formation and manifestation of psychopathology, the clinical picture, and the frequency of certain mental illnesses, particularly minor psychiatric disorders and closely related psychological problems, which are influenced predominantly by social and cultural factors. This may also include the study of culture-related specific psychiatric conditions that are heavily influenced by culture. Although descriptive and epidemiological approaches to examining psychopathology are useful, yielding basic information for further investigation, it is important to realize that such approaches are not sufficient from a cultural point of view. A dynamic approach to examining how various factors work integratively for the formation of psychopathology is more meaningful.

4. Addressing Clinical Practice

Beyond theoretical investigation, it is currently the trend to emphasize the clinical application of cultural psychiatry — regarding evaluation, diagnosis, management, and treatment. The focus on culture is not only needed when a clinician is dealing with patients of minority or other ethnic backgrounds, or from foreign countries, but also patients who are part of the majority population of their own society. This view is based on the assumption that every person's mental life is subject to the influence of culture and that cultural attention is needed even when treating patients from the therapist's own society with the same ethnic–cultural background. Attention is not only needed on the ethnic–cultural background of

the patient, but equally on the therapist or caregiver. Cultural impact is manifested as bilateral interaction between the therapist and the patient, rather than unilateral influence. Thus, the cultural dimensions of communication, relation, and interaction between therapist and patient deserve full attention with every patient a clinician encounters. Every clinician is now expected to provide culturally sensitive, relevant, and effective clinical care and treatment for all of his patients.

5. Promoting Cultural Research

Cultural psychiatry emerged originally for scientific investigation. Without sufficient information and knowledge, scholars cannot develop meaningful theories and clinicians cannot apply that knowledge into practice. There is a continuous need to carry out research work in cultural psychiatry, with many subjects waiting for immediate study. There is a constant need to advance our knowledge and experience of cross-cultural investigations so that more meaningful and valid information can be obtained.

6. Investing in Training

How to provide urgently needed training programs for clinicians was seldom focused on or even discussed in the past. There is a need to develop formal training programs in cultural psychiatry for psychiatric residents, including a basic curriculum, core knowledge, a suitable teaching format, and desirable learning experiences. There is a further need to design advanced training for clinicians or scholars who are planning to become qualified specialists in this field.

7. Examining Theoretical Applications

Now is the time for cultural psychiatry to move from scientific research and clinical application to theoretical exploration. Many psychiatric theories are based on clinical studies and experiences with Euro-American populations. There is a need to validate or revise such Western-based theories from non-Western perspectives. Also, based on new information and clinical experiences from non-Western societies, there is reason to add to or expand psychiatric theories. It is a challenge to evaluate the universal applicability and cultural specificity of the theories and principles of psychiatry.

IV. CLOSING REMARKS

Cultural psychiatry emerged initially as the result of investigating "other" cultures, which were mainly prescientific, foreign, or exotic. The current trend is to expand the scope of cultural psychiatry into clinical application and to focus on our own society. Attention should be given to worldwide and everyday application.

From an epitomological point of view, there is always a need to stimulate cross-cultural comparisons in order to examine cultural dimensions. In general, the more homogeneous the population of a society, the less interest there will be in cultural differences. Thus, advantage should be taken of work in multiethnic societies and those with numerous minority groups, and of intercultural or international encounters and comparisons.

It is important for us to realize that the behavior of every person or group of people, no matter what his or her ethnicity or cultural background, is always influenced by cultural, as well as biological and psychological, perspectives. Cultural orientation and attention are needed, not only in dealing with ethnic minorities or people from foreign countries, but also majority people and people from our own societies.

The cultural aspects of psychiatric practice need more attention. This is because, from a worldwide perspective, there is a continuous increase in international communication, travel, and migration, and many societies are becoming multiethnic. Cultural psychiatry is becoming an essential part of general psychiatry, providing culture-relevant services for people of diverse cultural backgrounds.

REFERENCES

Accreditation Council for Graduate Medical Education (ACGME). (2000). Program requirements for residency training in pyschiatry. Chicago: ACGME.

Abel, T.M., & Metraux, R. (1974). *Culture and psychotherapy* (p.127). New Haven, CT: College & University Press.

Al-Issa, I. (Ed.). (1995). *Handbook of culture and mental illness: An international perspective.* Madison; WI: International Universities Press.

Al-Issa, I., & Tousignant, M. (Eds.). (1997). *Ethnicity, immigration, and psychopathology.* New York: Plenum Press.

American Psychiatric Association (APA). (1969). Position statement on the delineation of transcultural psychiatry as a specialized field of study. *American Journal of Psychiatry, 126*(3), 453–455.

Aponte, J.F., Rivers, R.Y., & Wohl, J. (Eds.). (1995). *Psychological interventions and cultural diversity.* Boston: Allyn & Bacon.

Arthur, R. (1973). Social psychiatry: An overview. *American Journal of Psychiatry, 130*(8), 841–849.

Asuni, T. (1967). Nigerian experiment in group psychotherapy. *American Journal of Psychotherapy, 12,* 95–104.

Benedict, R. (1934). *Patterns of culture.* Boston: Houghton Mifflin.

Berry, J.W., Poortinga, Y.H., Segall, M.H., & Dasen, P.R. (1992). *Cross-cultural psychology: Research and applications.* Cambridge, UK: Cambridge University Press.

Brill, A. (1913). Pibloktoq or hysteria among Peary's Eskimos. *Journal of Nervous and Mental Disease, 40,* 514–520.

Brugger, C. (1931). Versuch einer Geisteskrankenzahlung in Turingen. *Zeitschrift fner Neurologie und Psychiatrie, 133,* 352–390.

Caudill, W. (1953). Applied anthropology in medicine. In A. L. Kroeber (Ed.), *Anthropology today.* Chicago: University of Chicago Press.

Caudill, W., & Lin, T.Y. (Eds.). (1969). *Mental health research in Asia and the Pacific.* Honolulu: East-West Center Press.

Comas-Diaz, L., & Griffith, E.E.H. (Eds.). (1988). *Clinical guidelines in cross-cultural mental health.* New York: Wiley.

Cox, J.L. (Ed.). (1986). *Transcultural psychiatry.* London: Croom Helm.

de Reuck, A.V.S., & Porter, R. (Eds.). (1965). *Transcultural psychiatry—Ciba Foundation Symposium.* Boston: Little, Brown.

Desjarlais, R., Eisenberg, L., Good, B., & Kleinman, A. (1995). *World mental health: Problems in low-income countries.* New York: Oxford University Press.

Devereux, G. (1940). Primitive psychiatry. *Bulletin of the History of Medicine, 8,* 1194–1213.

Doi, T. (1973). *The anatomy of dependence.* Tokyo: Kodansha International.

Edwards, J.W. (1985). Indigenous *koro,* a genital retraction syndrome of Insular Southeast Asia: A critical review. In R.C.

Simons & C.C. Hughes (Eds.). *The culture-bound syndromes: Folk illness of psychiatric and anthropological interest* (pp. 169–191). Dordrecht, The Netherlands: Reidel.

Ellis, W.G. (1893). The *amok* of the Malays. *Journal of Mental Science, 39,* 325–338.

Fabrega, H., Jr. (1972). Medical anthropology. In B.J. Spiegel (Ed.), *Biennial review of anthropology.* Stanford, CA: Stanford University Press.

Favazza, A.R. (1987). *Bodies under siege: Self-mutilation and body modification in culture and psychiatry.* Baltimore: Johns Hopkins University Press.

Favazza, A.R. (1996). *Bodies under siege: Self-mutilation and body modification in culture and psychiatry* (2nd ed.). Baltimore: Johns Hopkins University Press.

Favazza, A.R., & Oman, M. (1978). Overview: Foundations of cultural psychiatry. *American Journal of Psychiatry, 135,* 293–303.

Favazza, A.R., & Oman, M. (1980). Anthropology and psychiatry. In H.I. Kaplan, A.M. Freedman, & B.J. Sadock (Eds.), *Comprehensive textbook of psychiatry, III* (Vol. 1, chapt. 5). Baltimore: Williams & Wilkins.

Fletcher, W. (1908). Latah and crime. *Lancet, 2,* 254–255.

Foulks, E.F., Wintrob, R.M., Westermeyer, J., & Favazza, A.R. (Eds.). (1977). *Current perspectives in cultural psychiatry.* New York: Spectrum.

Frank, J.D. (1961). *Persuasion and healing: A comparative study of psychotherapy.* New York: Schocken Books.

Gaw, A.C. (Ed.). (1993). *Culture, ethnicity, and mental illness.* Washington, DC: American Psychiatric Press.

Griffith, E.E.H. (1988). Psychiatry and culture. In J.A. Talbott, R.E. Hales, & S.C. Yudofsky (Eds.), *Textbook of psychiatry.* Washington, DC: American Psychiatric Press.

Jilek, W.G. (1995). Emil Kraepellin and comparative sociocultural psychiatry. *European Archives of Psychiatry and Clinical Neuroscience, 245,* 231–238.

Johnson-Powell, G., Yamamoto, J., Wyatt, G.E., & Arroyo, W. (1997). *Transcultural child development: Psychological assessment and treatment.* New York: Wiley.

Jones, E.E., & Korchin, S.J. (Eds.). (1982). *Minority mental health.* New York: Praeger.

Kardiner, A. (1945). The concept of basic personality structure as an operational tool in social sciences. In R. Linton (Ed.), *The science of man in the world crisis.* New York: Columbia University Press.

Kato Price, R., Shea, B.M., & Mookherjee, H.N. (Eds.). (1995). *Social psychiatry across cultures: Studies from North American, Asia, Europe, and Africa.* New York: Plenum Press.

Kennedy, J.G. (1973). Cultural psychiatry. In J.J. Honigmann (Ed.), *Handbook of social and cultural anthropology.* Chicago: Rand McNally.

Kiev, A. (Ed.). (1969). *Social psychiatry* (Vol. 1). New York: Science House.

Kiev, A. (1972). *Transcultural psychiatry.* New York: Free Press.

Kleinman, A. (1988). *Rethinking psychiatry: From cultural category to personal experience.* New York: Fress Press.

Kleinman, A., & Lin, T.Y. (Eds.). (1981). *Normal and abnormal behavior in Chinese culture.* Dordrecht, The Netherlands: Reidel.

Lambo T.A. (1966). The Village of Aro. In M. King (Ed.), *Medical care in developing countries. A Symposium from Makerere.* London: Oxford University Press.

Landy, D. (Ed.). (1977). *Culture, disease, and healing: Studies in medical anthropology.* New York: Macmillan.

Lebra, T.S., & Lebra, W.P. (Eds.). (1974). *Japanese culture and behavior: Selected readings.* Honolulu: University Press of Hawaii.

Lebra, T.S., & Lebra, W.P. (Eds.). (1986). *Japanese culture and behavior: Selected readings* (Rev. Ed.). Honolulu: University Press of Hawaii.

Lebra, W.P. (Ed.). (1972). *Transcultural research in mental health: Vol. 2. Mental health research in Asia and the Pacific.* Honolulu: University Press of Hawaii.

Lebra, W.P. (Ed.). (1974). *Youth, socialization and mental health: Vol. 3. Mental health research in Asia and the Pacific.* Honolulu: University Press of Hawaii.

Lebra, W.P. (Ed.). (1976). *Culture-bound syndromes, ethnopsychiatry, and alternate therapies: Vol. 4. Mental health research in Asia and the Pacific.* Honolulu: University Press of Hawaii.

Leighton, A.H., Clausen, J.A., & Wilson, R.N. (Eds.). (1957). *Exploration in social psychiatry.* New York: Basic Books.

Lemkau, P., Tietze, C., & Cooper, M. (1941). Mental hygiene problems in an urban district. *Mental Hygiene, 25,* 624–646.

Lieban, R.W. (1974). Medical anthropology. In J.J. Honigmann (Ed.), *Handbook of social and cultural anthropology.* Chicago: Rand McNailly College Publishing Company.

Lieh Mak, F., & Nadelson, C.C. (Eds.). (1996). *International review of psychiatry,* (Vol. 2.). Washington, DC: American Psychiatric Press.

Lin, T.Y. (1953). An epidemiological study of the incidence of mental disorder in Chinese and other cultures. *Psychiatry, 16,* 313–336.

Lin, T.Y., Tseng, W.S., & Yeh, E.K. (Eds.). (1995). *Chinese societies and mental health.* Hong Kong: Oxford University Press.

Littlewood, R., & Lipsedge, M. (1986). The "culture-bound syndromes" of the dominant culture: Culture, psychopathology and biomedicine. In J.L. Cox (Ed.), *Transcultural psychiatry* (pp. 253–273). London: Croom Helm.

Littlewood, R., & Lipsedge, M. (1989). *Aliens and alienists: Ethnic minorities and psychiatry.* London: Unwin Hyman.

Malinoski, B. (1927). *Sex and repression in savage society.* New York: International Library.

Marsella, A.J., Tharp, R.G., & Ciborowski, T.J. (Eds.). (1979). *Perspectives on cross-cultural psychology.* New York: Academic Press.

McGoldrick, M., Pearce, J.K., & Giordano, J. (Eds.). (1982). *Ethnicity and family therapy.* New York: Guilford Press.

McGoldrick, M., Giordano, J., & Pearce, J.K. (Eds.). (1996). *Ethnicity and family therapy,* (2nd ed.). New York: Guilford Press.

Mead, M. (1959). Mental health in world perspective. In M.K. Opler (Ed.); *Culture and mental health.* New York: Macmillan.

Mezzich, J.E., Kleinman, A., Fabrega, H., Jr., & Parron, D.L. (Eds.). (1996). *Culture and psychiatric diagnosis: A DSM-IV perspective.* Washington, DC: American Psychiatric Press.

Murphy, H.B.M. (1977). Transcultural psychiatry should begin at home. *Psychological Medicine, 7,* 369–371.

Murphy, H.B.M. (1982). *Comparative psychiatry: The international and intercultural distribution of mental illness.* Berlin: Springer-Verlag.

Murphy, J.M., & Leighton, A.H. (Eds.). (1965). *Approaches to cross-cultural psychiatry.* Ithaca, NY: Cornell University Press.

Naroll, R. (1971). The double language boundry in cross cultural surveys. *Behavior Science Notes, 6,* 95–102.

Okpaku, S.O. (Ed.). (1998). *Clinical methods in transcultural psychiatry.* Washington, DC: American Psychiatric Press.

Opler M.K. (Ed.). (1959). *Culture and mental health.* New York: Macmillan.

Opler, M.K. (1967). *Culture and social psychiatry.* New York: Atherton Press.

Pedersen, P.B., Draguns, J.G., Lonner, W.J., & Trimble, J.E. (Eds.). (1989). *Counseling across cultures* (3rd ed.). Honolulu: University of Hawaii Press.

Pedersen, P.B., Draguns, J.G., Lonner, W.J., & Trimble, J.E. (Eds.). (1996). *Counseling across cultures* (4th ed.). Thousand Oaks, CA: Sage.

Pedersen, P.B., Lonner, W.J., & Draguns, J.G. (1976). *Counseling across cultures.* Honolulu: University Press of Hawaii.

Pfeiffer, W.M. (1971). *Transkulturelle psychiatrie: Ergebnisse und probleme* (in German). Stuttgart: Thieme. (Reviewed in *Transcultural Psychiatry Research Review, 7,* 113–118 [1970].)

Pfeiffer, W.M. (1994). *Transkulturelle psychiatrie: Ergebnisse und probleme* (in German). V. Stuttgart: Thieme. (Reviewed in *Transcultural Psychiatry Research Review, 32,* 59–64 [1995]).

Powell, G.J., Yamamoto, J., Romero, A., & Morales, A. (Eds.). (1983). *The psychosocial development of minority group children.* New York: Brunner/Mazel.

Prince, R.H. (1997). What's in a name? *Transcultural Psychiatry, 34 (1),* 151–154.

Prince, R.H., Okpaku, S.O., & Merkel, L. (1998). Transcultural psychiatry: A note on origins and definitions. In S.O. Okpaku (Ed.), *Clinical methods in transcultural psychiatry* (pp. 3–17). Washington, DC: American Psychiatric Press.

Psychiatric News. Professional News; (1999). Cultural competence primary to all psychiatric care, says experts. *Psychiatric News, 34*(24), 10 and 25.

Roheim, G. (1933). Psychoanalysis and anthropology. In S. Lorand (Ed.), *Psychoanalysis today: Its scope and function.* New York: Covici-Friede.

Ruesch, J. (1965). Social psychiatry: An overview. *Archives of General Psychiatry, 12,* 501–509.

Schwab, J.J., & Schwab, M.E. (1978). Cultural psychiatry. In J.J. Schwab & M.E. Schwab, *Sociocultural roots of mental illness: An epidemiological survey,* (Chapter 16). New York: Plenum Medical Book Company.

Segall, M.H., Dasen, P.R., Berry, J.W., & Poortinga, Y.H. (1990). *Human behavior in global perspective: An introduction to cross-cultural psychology.* New York: Pergamon Press.

Simons, R.C., & Hughes, C.C. (Eds.). (1985). *The culture-bound syndromes: Folk illness of psychiatric and anthropological interest.* Dordrecht, The Netherlands: Reidel.

Torrey, E.F. (1986). *Witchdoctors and psychiatrists: The common roots of psychotherapy and its future* (pp. 73–74). New York: Harper & Row.

Triandis, H.C. (1980) Introduction to handbook of cross-cultural psychology. In H.C. Triandis & W.W. Lambert (Eds.), *Handbook of cross-cultural psychology: Vol. 1. Perspectives* (pp. 1–14). Boston: Allyn & Bacon.

Tseng, W.S., & McDermott, J.F., Jr. (1981). *Culture, mind and therapy: An introduction to cultural psychiatry.* New York: Brunner/Mazel.

Tseng, W.S., McDermott, J.F., Jr., & Maretzki, T.W. (Eds.). (1974). *People and cultures in Hawaii: An introduction for mental health workers.* Honolulu: University of Hawaii School of Medicine, Department of Psychiatry, Transcultural Psychiatry Committee.

Tseng, W.S., & Streltzer, J. (Eds.). (1997). *Culture and psychopathology: A guide to clinical assessment.* New York: Brunner/Mazel.

Tseng, W.S., & Streltzer, J. (Eds.). (2001). *Culture and psychotherapy: A guide for clinical practice.* Washington, DC: American Psychiatric Press.

Tseng, W.S., & Wu, D.Y.H. (1985). *Chinese culture and mental health.* Orlando; FL: Academic Press.

Westermeyer, J. (Ed.). (1976). *Anthroplogy and mental health: Setting a new course.* Paris: Mouton.

Whiting, B.B. (Ed.). (1963). *Six cultures: Study of child rearing.* New York: Wiley.

Whiting, B.B., & Whiting, J.W.M. (1975). *Children of six cultures: A psycho-cultural analysis.* Cambridge, MA: Harvard University Press.

Whiting, J.W.M., & Child, I.L. (1953). *Child training and personality.* New Haven; CT: Yale University Press.

Wittkower, E.D. (1964). Perspectives of transcultural psychiatry. *The Israel Annals of Psychiatry and Related Disciplines, 2*(1), 19–26.

Wittkower, E.D., & Prince, R. (1974). A review of transcultural psychiatry. In S. Arieti (Ed.-in-chief) and G. Caplan (Vol. 1) *American handbook of psychiatry* (2nd ed., Vol. 2) (pp. 535–550). New York: Basic Books.

Wittkower, E.D., & Termansen, P.E. (1971). Transcultural psychiatry. In J. Howells (Ed.), *Modern perspectives in world psychiatry* New York: Brunner/Mazel.

Yap, P.M. (1974). In M.P. Lau & A.B. Stokes (Eds.), *Comparative psychiatry: A theoretical framework.* Toronto: University of Toronto Press.

Section B
Culture and Human Behavior

After describing the scope of cultural psychiatry in Chapter 1, this section will explore the cultural aspects of human behavior in preparation for the discussion on culture and mental health in the following section.

First, the concepts of culture, society, and culture-related terms are elaborated in Chapter 2. Various marriage systems and family functions are reviewed from a cultural perspective in Chapter 3. The cultural aspects of human behavior are examined in conjunction with the human life cycle in the remaining chapters. Child development, including the process of enculturation, is analyzed in Chapter 4; the major issues relating to adulthood, i.e., personality formation and depth psychology, are discussed in Chapter 5; and basic psychology, culture-related behavior, and ethnic identity formation are analyzed in Chapter 6.

The section ends with Chapter 7, in which matters relating to the latter part of life, including aging and death, are elaborated in detail.

Thus, in a way, this section serves as a foundation for understanding human behavior from cultural perspectives, before exploring issues related to the clinical subject. It is not intended to provide an intensive review of social and cultural systems or a broad discussion of their impact on human nature. The focus is merely on presenting an introduction for clinicians in preparation for the following sections. However, this section is intended to cover the basic knowledge of the cultural aspects of human behavior and, based on this information, to move us toward an examination of clinical application.

2

Culture and Society

I. UNDERSTANDING CULTURE AND SOCIETY

A. DEFINITIONS OF CULTURE, RACE, ETHNICITY, SOCIETY, AND MINORITY

In order to explore the field of cultural psychiatry, the concept of culture should first be clarified. Several terms are often used synonymously by both laymen and professionals, but have different meanings, such as culture, race, ethnicity, and society. These terms loosely describe matters related to sociocultural issues. However, they require precise definitions and conceptual clarification in order to be applied accurately in practical situations, such as clinical work.

1. Culture

The term "culture" (*kultur* in German) was coined by a German scholar in the late 18th century to indicate the achievements of civilization. Then, in 1871 (according to Kroeber and Kluckhohn, 1952, p. 9), the British scholar E.B. Tylor, in his pioneer work, *Primitive Culture,* used the English word "culture,"

defining it as "that complex whole which includes knowledge, belief, art, law, morals, custom, and any other capabilities and habits acquired by man as a member of society."

Since then, scholars of behavioral science have defined culture in various ways. American anthropologists Kroeber and Kluckhohn (1952), after analyzing several hundred definitions and statements about culture made by anthropologists and others, summarized a reformulated concept often used by contemporary behavioral scientists. They defined the term as follows "Culture consists of patterns, explicit and implicit, of and for behavior acquired and transmitted by symbols, constituting the distinctive achievement of human groups, including their embodiments in artifacts; the essential core of culture consists of traditional ideas and especially their attached values; culture systems may, on the one hand, be considered as products of action, on the other as conditioning elements of further action."

In simpler words, in his book, *Culture and Personality* (1963, p. 5), another American anthropologist, V. Barnouw, gave the following definition: "A culture is the way of life of a group of people, the configuration of all of the more or less stereotyped patterns of

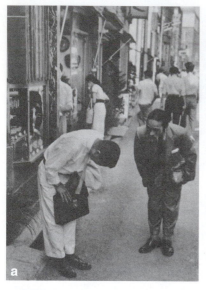 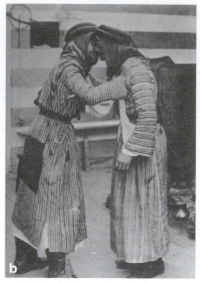 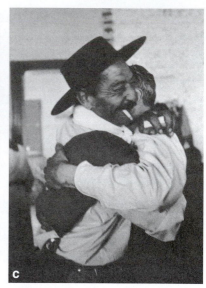

FIGURE 2-1   Culturally patterned different social greeting behavior. (a) A Japanese student keeps his physical distance and bows deeply to his professor. (b) Two Arab men rub noses. (c) The Latin American *abrazzo* emphasizes emotional expressiveness. [From *Anthropology: The study of man,* by E.A. Hoebel. McGraw-Hill, 1972, used with permission. Courtesy of (a) Marc Riboud/Magnum Photos, Inc.; (b) the American Museum of Natural History Library; and (c) Reni Burri/Magnum Photos, Inc.].

learned behavior which are handed down from one generation to the next through the means of language and imitation." (See Fig. 2-1.)

Another anthropologist, R.M. Keesing (1976, p. 138), in his textbook, *Cultural Anthropology,* emphasized that culture exists at two levels. The first is the realm of observable phenomena — the patterns of life within a community — and the second is the realm of ideas — the organized system of knowledge and beliefs that allows a group to structure its experiences and choose among alternatives. Most contemporary anthropologists view the concept of culture as ideological; culture not only guides and motivates behavior, but it provides specific meanings through which behavior and events can be constructed, de-constructed, or reconstructed. Rather than a static set of ideas, beliefs, values and perspectives on the world, culture can be negotiated or contested.

In his book, *Culture Dynamics* (1964, p. 4), Herskovits pointed out some paradoxes in the nature of culture, namely: Culture is universal in men's experiences, yet each local or regional manifestation of it is unique. Culture is stable, yet it is also dynamic and manifests continuous and constant change. Culture fills and largely determines the course of our lives, yet rarely intrudes into conscious thought.

Recently, in his textbook of *Cultural Anthropology,* Kottak (1994, 1999) delineated specific characteristics of culture: it is learned through a process of enculturation from childhood; it is transmitted through symbols, both verbal and nonverbal; and it is shared by members of groups. He pointed out that culture is not a haphazard collection of customs and beliefs; it consists of integrated, patterned systems. People use culture creatively and actively; and culture can be adaptive or maladaptive. People share experiences, memories, values, and beliefs as a result of common enculturation (see Fig. 2-2).

The current concept of culture includes the effects of "enculturation" on the mind–brain (Castillo, 1995). As a result of enculturation, every individual learns a language, a religion, or other meaning system specify-

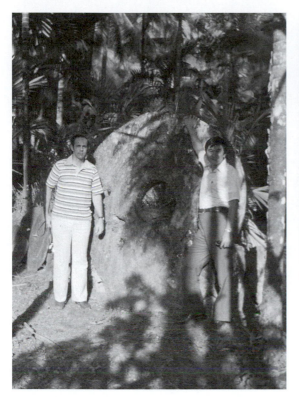

a

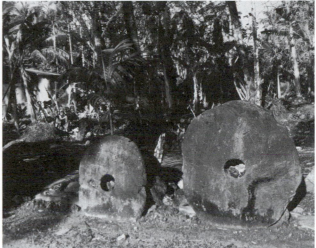

b

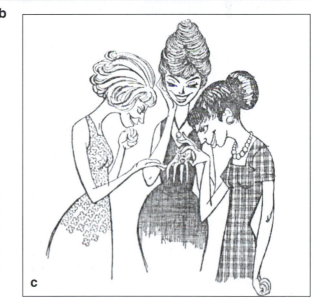

c

FIGURE 2-2 **Values emphasized in different cultures.** (a) A person-sized stone money in Yap, Micronesia, the most treasured "thing" in that culture. (b) People risked their lives sailing several hundred miles away by canoe to another island, worked hard for several years carving the stone by shell, brought it back to their island, and placed it on the roadside in the village once its credibility was established. [Courtesy of Paule Dale, M.D.] (c) A diamond is admired as a forever "thing" in some cultures; but not necessarily in others. [From *Invitation to Anthropology,* by D.L. Oliver, (1964), used by permission of Doubleday, a division of Random House.]

ing the operation of forces of nature in the world, as well as norms of behavior and patterns of experiencing the environment. All of these are structured in neural networks in the mind–brain. It has been found that the strengths of synaptic connections between individual neurons are determined by use patterns (Thompson, Doneg, & Lavond, 1986). By the habitual act of thinking in a particular language, or believing in the forms of a particular religion, those thoughts assume a type of physical reality in the organization of neural networks in the brain. In a very real sense, the social–cultural environment becomes physically structured in the brain of the individual. This process has frequently been referred to as "downward causation" (Sperry, 1987). That is, thinking as an activity pattern is "causal" in that it alters the brain at the level of dendritic branching and the strengths of neurotransmitter properties in the individual synapse. This means that the organization of culture has its psychobiological correlates in the organization of the mind–brain — in the microanatomy of the individual neuron and in the organizational formation of neural networks (Castillo, 1995).

As Castillo (1995) says: "For example, in order to speak Chinese, one must have the neural networks for speaking Chinese structured in the brain — no Chinese neural networks, no speaking Chinese. The presence of Chinese neural networks, of course, results from enculturation. Someone who is genetically Chinese, but born and raised in the United States and fully assimilated into American culture, will have American neural networks — an American mind-brain." It is these culture-specific neural organizations that in turn influence most aspects of cognitive processing by individuals, in the form of cognitive schema (Sperry, 1987). These cognitive schema structure a person's experience of the world and thus influence the development of psychopathology.

As pointed out by German ethnologist C. Brumann (1999), in the past decade, there has been major concern among scholars, including anthropologists, about the use of the term "culture" — it has even been suggested that the term be discarded — because the concept suggests boundedness, homogeneity, coherence, stability, and structure, whereas social reality is characterized by variability, inconsistencies, conflict, change, and individual agency. However, Brumann supports the view that the concept of culture should be retained as a convenient term for designating the clusters of common concepts, emotions, and practices that arise when people interact regularly.

From the point of view of application, the nature of culture can be summarized as follows:

a. Culture refers to the unique behavior patterns and lifestyle shared by a group of people, which distinguish it from other groups.
b. Culture is characterized by a set of views, beliefs, values, and attitudes toward things in life. It serves to make behavior meaningful. It is manifested in various means of regulating daily life, such as rituals, customs, etiquette, taboos, or laws, and reflected in cultural representations, such as common sayings, legends, drama, plays, art, philosophical thought, and religions.
c. Culture is learned by the process of "enculturation" and is transmitted from generation to generation through family units and social environments. Enculturation is enforced by personal child-rearing patterns, institutionalized education, and the surrounding social system.
d. Although continuity is a basic characteristic of culture, it may be subject to transient and subtle, or even acute and revolutionary, changes that may occur within the culture itself or as the result of the influence of other cultures.
e. The process of "acculturation" occurs when a group comes in contact with a new, different cultural system and, is influenced by and acquires part of it. Sometimes, a person acquires the new or dominant culture to such an extent that he or she becomes similar to its members. This phenomenon of "assimilation" may occur voluntarily or involuntarily.
f. Culture provides meanings that pattern people's behavior, but, at the same time, culture is molded by the ideas and behavior of the members of the culture. Thus, culture and people influence each other bilaterally and interactionally.
g. Culture exists as a recognizable social or institutional pattern at the macroscopic level, but is also represented in the behavior and reactions of an individual at the microscopic level, of which the individual may be consciously aware, or which may be operating at an unconscious level.

2. Race

In the past, scholars and laymen have used the term "race" to refer to a group of people characterized by certain physical features, such as color of skin, eyes, and hair, facial or body features, or physical size, that distinguish it from other groups. Anthropologists have used the term "geographic race" to indicate a human population that has inhabited a continental land mass or an island chain sufficiently long to have developed its own distinctive genetic composition, compared with that of other geographic populations (Hoebel, 1972). Based on these old concepts, laymen recognize, African (black), American (Native American), Asian (yellow), Australian, European (white), Indian, and Polynesian as some of the major geographic races of the world. Professional anthropologists have used certain terms to classify racial groups. For instance, according to anthropologist E.E. Nida (1954, pp. 57–58), the Caucasian race includes Hindu (northern India), Nordic (northern Europe), Alpine (central Europe), and Mediterranean (Mediterranean region); the Mongoloid race includes Mongolians (including Chinese, Japanese, Korean, Vietnamese, Thai, and Tibetan), Malaysian (Malay and most of Indonesia), and American Indian (often called Amerindian); the Negroid race includes Negroes (Africa), Melanesians (New Guinea, Solomon Islands, and parts of the nearby South Pacific), Negritos (including Pygmies in Africa, and similar small-statured, woolly haired people from Andaman Island, the Malay peninsula, and the Philippines), Bushman, and Hottento; and the doubtful classification group (such as Australoids in Australia, Polynesians, Ainu in Japan, and so on).

Based on these traditional views, both scholars and the general public have been conditioned to viewing human races as natural and separate divisions within the human species, based on visible physical differences. Yet, as indicated in the official statement by the American Anthropological Association (1999), with improvements in genetic study, analysis of DNA among members of different races has shown that there are greater variations *within* racial groups than *among* them. Most physical variation (about 94%) lies within so-called racial groups, whereas conventionally identified geographic "racial" groupings differ from one another only in small percentages (about 6%) of their genes. In neighboring populations there is much overlapping of genes and phenotypic (physical)

expression. Furthermore, physical traits (such as skin color, hair, shape of nose, and so on) are inherited independently of one another rather than as a related complex. For instance, skin color varies largely from light in the temperate areas in the north to dark in the tropical areas in the south — its intensity is not related to nose shape or hair texture.

As pointed out by Smedley (1999), historical records show that neither the idea of nor ideologies associated with race existed before the 17th century. The modern concept of race developed during the 18th-century colonial era. "Race" emerged as a form of social identification and stratification that was seemingly grounded in the physical differences of populations, but whose real meaning rested in social and political realities. It provided justification for colonial treatment and slavery of other groups of people. In the latter part of the 19th century, race was employed by Europeans to rank colonial people and to justify social, economic, and political inequalities (and, in its extreme, even the extermination of "inferior races").

Thus, races are socially and culturally constructed categories that may have little to do with actual biologically differences. The validity of race as a biological term has been discredited. There is a final objection to racial classification based on phenotype (Kottak, 1994, pp. 76–85). Also, given what we know about the capacity of normal humans to achieve and function within any culture, it has been concluded that present-day inequalities between so-called racial groups are not consequences of biological inheritance, but products of historical and contemporary social, economic, educational, and political circumstances (American Anthropological Association, 1999, p. 713).

3. Ethnicity

This term refers to social groups that distinguish themselves from other groups by a common historical path, behavior norms, and their own group identities. The members of an ethnic group are affiliated and may share a common language, religion, culture, racial background, or other characteristics that make them identifiable within their own group. American anthropologist George De Vos (1975, p. 9) defined an ethnic group as "a self-perceived group of people who hold in common a set of traditions not shared by the others with whom they are in contact. Such traditions typically include 'folk' religious beliefs and practices, language, a sense of historical continuity, and common ancestry or place of origin." For instance, Jewish people, based on their common faith and past history, identify themselves (and are identified by others) as the Jewish ethnic group, even though they may be scattered geographically and live in different political institutions. The same can be said of Italians, Irish, Chinese, or Japanese ethnic groups living in various parts of the world, as well as African-Americans and Hispanic-Americans from various societies in North or South America. Thus, culture refers to perspectives and meanings applied to human experience, while ethnicity refers to a group of people that shares common cultural features or a root culture. Additionally, it must be observed that ethnic groups arise not from the fact of shared cultural heritage, but from specific social and political processes that can be documented historically (Koss-Chioino & Vargas, 1999). Dominant societal groups establish boundary-setting and-maintaining mechanisms, and the ethnic groups complement their efforts by identifying themselves in a designated way. Both the boundaries and the ethnic identifications change over time as a reult of other social processes; Blacks become African-Americans, for example, with the recognition of their cultural heritage as symbolic of their difference from other groups, rather than difference being based on skin color.

Perhaps for the sake of convenience, or lack of an accurate concept, the term "ethnicity" is used by some lay people and professionals to mean "minority group." For instance, people refer to the ethnic elderly (meaning the elderly of ethnic minority groups) or ethnic restaurants (meaning restaurants that offer food of ethnic minority groups rather than of the majority group). This use of "ethnicity" seems to imply that the majority in a society does *not* have an ethnic background. Clearly it is a mistake to use the terms "eth-

nic" or "ethnicity" in this way — as if they mean only "minority." (For definition and detailed discussion of "minority," cross reference to Chapter 45: Minority by Ethnicity, Gender or Others.)

4. Society

Although the term "society" is used in close association with the term "culture," it means something different. A **society** is a social institution characterized by a particular, visible, organizational structure. It is composed of a collective group of members, organized by an administrative structure and is regulated by certain rules or systems. It performs an institutional function, including production, economic, and social functions, and self-protection of the group. Within each society, people may live a certain style of life. However, the boundaries of society and culture are not the same. Several cultures or subcultures usually exist within a single society, whereas a cultural system may be shared by people from different societies. The sizes of societies may vary. They may be small, at a community level — with several hundred inhabitants, or large, at a national level, with a population of several billion.

Thus, society refers to the community within which people live, whereas culture to the way of life lived by groups of people in the society. Therefore, these two terms refer to different perspectives of the same living environment. Culture and society are so interwoven as actual phenomena that they are often quite difficult to disentangle. It is impossible to give an adequate picture of any culture without including an account of its social structure, which almost inevitably has ramifications in economics, government, law, religion, art — in fact, touches almost every aspect of the culture (Kroeber, 1963, p. 76).

Within a society, depending on the situation, people may share one common culture, different subcultures, or even distinctively different cultures, forming a multicultural society. Culturally homogeneous societies exist only at a conceptual level or are found only in small, tribal populations. In reality, most societies contain subcultural groups. Even Japanese society and

Polish societies, believed to be rather culturally homogeneous groups, on closer examination are found to contain numerous subgroups. For instance, in Japan, there are Korean-Japanese, *burakumin,* or the Ainu who due to ethnicities, historical paths, and psychological discrimination, differ considerably from the "ordinary" Japanese and are treated by the majority as minority groups.

5. Social Class

Social class refers to the social stratification in a society. Sociologists tend to use socioeconomic status (SES) to carry out epidemiological research by dividing the population of a community into different subgroups. Commonly the variables of educational level, occupation, financial income, and ecological area of residence are used. However, some scholars (Wohlfarth & van den Brink, 1998) take the view that "social class" is different from "socioeconomic status," which has different associations with physical or mental health problems. Generally, social class is considered primarily the product of the perceptions and beliefs of about the existence of different subgroups in a society, such as upper class, middle-working class, or lower class, which are associated with certain lifestyles and values. These classes constitute a long-existing stratification that seldom changes radically. An extreme of social stratification is the caste system observed in some societies, such as India. A person's caste is inherited and never changes. It is associated with discrimination without negotiation. For example, intermarriage between different castes, while it does occur, is forbidden.

In contrast, socioeconomic status is primarily based on practical factors, such as level of education, nature of occupation, and financial income. Thus, it is changeable, i.e., a person can move up or down the social ladder depending on his or her social achievement. As pointed out by Vanneman and Cannon (1987), in United States, people tend to deny the existence of social class because America is considered a land of opportunity. Instead, racial and ethnic divisions are more prominent. In contrast, European societies, influenced by their feudal pasts, are less concerned with racial or ethnic heterogeneity, and are more preoccupied with differences and tensions among social classes.

From a health standpoint, it has been demonstrated by epidemiological studies that social class and/or socioeconomic status are among the variables associated with physical as well as mental health [cross-reference to Chapter 12: Culture and Psychiatric Epidemiology (Section III,C)]. They are also important variables that contribute to the pattern of care for patients (Molica & Milic, 1986), including the provision of psychotherapy (Acosta, Yamamoto, & Evans, 1982) and the outcome of psychiatric care (Gift, Strauss, Ritzler, Kokes, & Harder, 1986).

6. Subcultures

Subcultures refer specifically to parts of the population within a society that hold rather different cultural systems than those of the majority population. While the smaller subcultures usually have the same racial background as the majority group, they have, often, but not always, by choice, distinctly different sets of beliefs, value systems, and ways of life. They are generally voluntary in nature and, as such, are different from ethnic minorities. However, popular discourse tend to use the terms minority and subculture indistinguishably.

The best example of a subculture is the old order Amish in the United States. As described by anthropologist Serena Nanda (1980, p. 42), the Amish number about 60,000 and live mainly as farmers in the states of Pennsylvania, Ohio, and Indiana. Their religious beliefs require a simple life in a church community away from other influences. Their culture emphasizes learning through doing for the welfare of the community rather than individual competition. The Amish reject television, telephones, automobiles, radios, and other modern conveniences. Their distinctive dress and speech and their habit of manual work are symbolic of their cultural separateness and also contribute to the integration of the community. From a racial perspective, the Amish belong to the same Caucasian group as the majority of the Anglo-American population, yet they choose to maintain their unique subculture, distinct from the majority culture of the United States as a whole.

People living in a society may be a subculture simply due to social class distinctions, such as the caste hierarchy recognized in India, which as just mentioned, does not even permit intermarriage between different castes. Subcultures may be formed on the basis of occupational or financial factors. While people in the United States, people tend to deny the existence of social class, in reality, different groups of people live rather distinct styles of life mainly due to their occupation or finances. For instance, rich people, mainly successful businessmen, lawyers, or physicians, live in high end residential areas, play golf, drive expensive automobiles, fly their own airplanes, socialize at exclusive clubs, and send their children to private schools. In contrast, poor people depend on social welfare, live in poor neighborhoods, or are even homeless, use public transportation systems, and send their children to public schools. Thus, even though the rich and the poor may all watch TV and speak the same language, their life experiences, attitudes toward life, and views of the world can be quite different and place them in different subcultures within the same society.

7. Enculturation, Acculturation, Assimilation, and Uprooting

Several terms have been used to describe a person's relation to a cultural system.

a. Enculturation

This is a professional term used by cultural anthropologists to refer to the process through which an individual acquires his culture. Learning occurs through introjection and absorption of value systems from his or her parents, other family members, neighbors, friends, classmates and teachers in school, and the media. The culture incorporated is the cultural system belonging to the person's own society, or the "native" culture. Thus, it is a part of development to become a member of a society — a Russian child is enculturated to become Russian, an Italian child to become Italian [cross-reference to Chapter 4: Child Development and Enculturation (Section IV)].

b. Acculturation

In contrast to enculturation, acculturation refers to the process by which a person acquires a new set of cultural systems, either by contact with a "foreign" culture(s) or through the influence of an "outside" culture. This implies a process that occurs in adulthood, after a person has established his own "native" culture. It is the term usually used to describe how members of a minority group acquire the culture of the majority or how migrants absorb the culture of the host society. However, depending on the size of the minority group or the migrants, sometimes the members of the majority or the host society learn and acquire some cultural features of the minority or migrants. This is because bilateral interaction usually occurs when two cultures encounter each other. In Hawaii, the majority group of white people adopted the customs of hula dancing and giving lei in greeting from the minority group of Hawaiian people, even though the latter had acculturated in many ways to the dominant white culture.

c. Assimilation

This term refers to the process by which a person or a group of people, either voluntarily or by force, incorporates or assumes proportionately significant features of another cultural system — often of a majority group or a host society — so that he, or the group, assumes a role as a member of the other culture and, from a cultural point of view, belongs to the nonnative cultural system. The term is often used to describe a minority person assimilated into a majority group, colonized people assimilated into the dominant group, or an immigrant assimilated into a host society and thus, the term has political and social implications.

Different societies have various degrees of expectation with regard to the assimilation of immigrants into the host society. For instance, in the United States, immigrants becoming American citizens are only tested (by an immigration officer) on a little bit of American history and the names of some presidents. At the naturalization ceremony, they are asked to swear to be loyal to the country (as American citizens) and to pay their taxes. In Japan, immigrants are expected to change their names into Japanese names, speak Japanese, and to behave like Japanese in terms of social etiquette, public regulations, and work morale, as well as, with many more cultural requirements (Ebata et al., 1995).

d. Deculturation

Deculturation, or **(cultural) uprooting,** describes when a person or a group of people, either by accident or by force, gives up the major features of his or the group's own native cultural system and becomes like a tree that has lost its roots. Therefore, it is called uprooting. The condition does not necessarily go with acculturation or assimilation. Thus, the original culture is lost or destroyed without proper replacement by the substituted culture, causing a loss of meaning and direction in life.

Deculturation is illustrated in the following instances. Historically, when Hispanic people came to South American or Central American countries, such as Mexico, they tore down the native people's temples and built churches on the same sites, using the materials from the temples they tore down. This was done to destroy the native culture by first abolishing its native faith. Americans who originally came to Hawaii as missionaries and whalers destroyed the Hawaiian monarchy by military force. Under the influence of the Westerners, native Hawaiians lost their taboos and social etiquette, such as men and women not sitting together for meals — changing the status of men and women. The loss of native culture was accelerated by the remarkable loss of population when they encountered diseases (such as measles and syphilis) brought by the Westerners for which they had no immunological defenses. It was the combined effects of biological, political, and cultural factors that the native Hawaiians encountered that resulted in the loss of their original culture. When the Japanese took over

Taiwan from China, with the slogan of "Japanization for all the emperor's people," all the Chinese were asked to change their names to Japanese names. Furthermore, Chinese were not allowed to retain any Chinese characters from their original names in their Japanese names, even though the Chinese and Japanese use the same Chinese characters for names. It was Japan's political intention to deculturalize the native people for the "new" society.

8. Cultural Change and Cultural Diffusion

The phenomena of enculturation, acculturation, assimilation, or deculturation are viewed by people from the standpoint of their cultural systems. In contrast, cultural change or cultural diffusion, indicates how a culture as a whole is conserving its systems, making changes and reacting to other cultures it encounters. This view of culture "acting" has been replaced in anthropology by the idea that only people act through the meanings they have learned or have had communicated to them in particular situations.

Clearly, cultural change is stimulated through direct contact with other cultural systems. Cultural elements may diffuse to other cultural units through geographical routes. This spreading of cultural elements is called cultural diffusion. In the past, contact with other cultural systems through traveling, trading, migration, and war has provoked opportunities for cultural influence and diffusion. In the contemporary world, with technological advances in communication, such as movies, TV, and other mass media, culture may be transmitted to people far away, without direct contact. The borrowing of culture from others does not necessarily occur in one direction, it can be bilateral. Thus, diffusion of culture can occur on both sides (cross-reference to Chapter 43: Cultural Change and Coping).

B. Distribution and Identification of Cultural Groups

Based on anthropologists' field work, a total of 565 cultural groups have been identified around the globe and recorded in the *Ethnographic Atlas* — an anthropological filing system for world ethnographic samples established at Yale University by George Peter Murdock (1957). Cultural groups that have appeared in literature were selected and classified according to certain standard ethnographic categories. The specifications included the most populous society in the geographic area, the best described culture, examples of each basic type of economy, examples from each language stock or major linguistic subfamily found in the area, or relatively distinctive cultural systems.

Six approximately equivalent ethnographic regions were recognized around the world. Within these six regions, the distributions of cultural groups were indicated as follows:

Africa (sub-Saharan)	116
Circum-Mediterranean	78
East Eurasia	85
Insular Pacific	99
North America	110
South and Central America	77

This information indicates that a cultural unit is not an absolute category, but an artificial concept and distinguishing element. Also, even though cultural units can be identified as cultural areas on the geographic map, they do not overlap or coexist exactly with politically recognized societies or the size of populations or geography. Some cultures can be shared by a huge population, for instance, the Chinese, who number more than a billion; or merely by tribal groups with populations of several thousand, such as those in Africa or the Pacific islands. Thus, more cultural groups are recognized in geographic areas where cultural diffusion and unification among various subgroups are relatively lacking and language, geographic, or other factors exist that are barriers to cultural transmission and fusion.

As culture is an abstract term, relatively difficult to identify and distinguish, reference is customarily made by laymen to ethnicity or country. For example, Japanese culture refers to the cultural system that is shared by the people of Japan; Jewish culture to the cultural system shared by the Jewish ethnic group.

However, caution is necessary in such use, as the unit of culture is not necessarily congruent with the unit of ethnicity or country. For instance, there have been a substantial number of Koreans living in Japan for nearly a century, but even after three of four generations, due to differences in the historical backgrounds of Japan and Korea, they still identify themselves as "Korean" and are not accepted by other Japanese nationals as "Japanese." Thus, Japanese culture is not necessarily shared by "all" of the people of Japan; and Korean culture is shared not only by people living in Korea proper, but also by a group of people that are, in reality, Korean-Japanese.

Another example is found in Israel, which was inhabited by "Jewish" people after the country was established and by people who claimed to be Jewish (by faith) after mass migrations from Russia and Ethiopia. However, Ethiopian Jews comprised a distinctly different group ethnically (as indicated by their different past history) and physically (as reflected by their dark skin color and physical features) than other, light-skinned Jewish people in Israel. Thus, even though they shared the same religion, they were treated as a minority group by the majority European Jews.

C. Framework for Grouping and Comparing Cultures

Anthropologists and sociologists have tried many ways of describing and grouping cultures or societies for the sake of comparison. For instance, a society may be categorized by its primary method of production, as a hunting, agricultural, or industrialized society; by the level of development of its civilization, as a "primitive" or "civilized" society; or by its level of economic development, as an underdeveloped, a developing, or a developed society. Anthropologist E.R. Service, in his book *Profiles in Ethnology* (1978), explained that there are three primary determinants that, in combination, account for distinctive cultural diversity. They are cultural and social complexity, characteristics of the geographic environment people inhabit, and the historical continuum of tradition that they share. Based on the level of cultural and social complexity, Service categorized cultural profiles into five groups: band, tribe, chiefdom, state, and national state.

These methods of grouping are more or less based on social, rather that cultural, parameters. They only serve to divide societies into several categorical groups. They do not bring out and illustrate the characteristic natures of individual societies from a cultural perspective, particularly from the standpoint of the major emphasis on and value of behavior patterns.

1. Benedict's Grouping of Cultures

Identifying cultural characteristics and grouping different cultural system are difficult tasks. An American pioneer anthropologist, Ruth Benedict (1934), based on her own field work, compared two American Indian cultures, the Plains bison hunters and the southwestern Zuni and other Pueblo farmers. She identified and labeled the former as a Dionysian culture, after the Greek god of wine; and the latter as an Apollonian culture, after the Greek god of music and poetry. She described the people of Dionysian cultures as possessing outgoing temperaments, addicted to rushes of strong feeling, and expressing themselves in activity; the self is asserted. In contrast, the people of Apollonian cultures are characterized by calm, restrained personalities; disliking surges of emotion, vehement action, and insistence on the ego.

Later, Benedict went further and passed verdicts on cultures outside her own personal experiences: the Melanesians of Dobu Island, described by Fortune, and the Kwakiutl Indians of Vancouver Island, reported by Boas. Benedict found the Dobuan culture to be paranoid in its inclinations; the Kwakutle, megalomaniacal. Apparently, these cultures were analyzed and categorized psychologically according to the basic personalities of their members rather than according to the cultural systems as a whole. These four cultures differ in the ways described, and other cultures differ from one another in analogous ways.

It should be pointed out that another of Benedict's (1946) well-known studies was of Japanese culture.

During World War II, in order for Americans to know more about their enemy, Benedict was asked to study the Japanese. Due to the limitations of war, she was, of course, unable to visit Japan and directly study the people there. She utilized Japanese-Americans, as well as available literature, as resources for her investigation. She analyzed and examined the characteristics of Japanese culture as reflected in its behavior patterns. Through the title of her book *The Chrysanthemum and the Sword,* she skillfully identified the unique, compound features of Japanese culture through two objects that are special in Japan: the Japanese national (as well as the emperor's) flower and the samurai's sword.

However, there are limitations to categorizing culture by its characteristic trends, based on the investigator's subjective analysis and impressions. As pointed out by Kroeber (1963, pp. 130–131), Benedict herself seems to think that only some cultures can be described in this way; the majority are not sufficiently "integrated" around a single psychological trend, nor oriented exclusively in one direction. The same problem is encountered in identifying and categorizing people of different societies by their "national character."

2. Kluckhohn's Framework for Comparison

Kluckhohn (1951) proposed a conceptual framework for studying and comparing cultures comprehensively. Because its value system is the core of a culture, Kluckhohn made a proposal for the comparison of value orientations that exist in societies. Value orientations are examined from five modalities: activity, man's relation to man, time, man's relation to nature, and views about human nature. In each modality, a distinction is made according to its "preferences." Thus, variations in value systems can be described according to this framework:

Modalities	Preferences
Activity	Being, being-in-becoming, doing
Relational	Lineal, collateral, individualistic
Time	Past, present, future
Man and Nature	Subjugation to Nature, harmony with Nature, mastery over Nature
Human nature	Evil, neutral (mixture of good and evil), good

This framework offers one method of examining and comparing cultures. However, it has some limitations in practical application. Culture is such a complicated system that generalization according to a simple framework is difficult in many situations. For instance, in terms of time orientation, the Chinese may be categorized as "present" oriented. However, in their emphasis on traditional thought and past history, the Chinese are very past oriented. In their emphasis on education for their children's future, they show a great concern for the next generation and stress the importance of family continuity for the long-term future. From this perspective, they are future oriented. Thus, depending on the issues involved, the time orientation of Chinese culture varies and there is no single, simple way to describe and categorize it.

3. Different Natures of Cultures Compared

When a comparison is made between different cultural systems, it is necessary to understand the kind of systems that are being compared or else the comparison may be inappropriate and misleading.

a. "Homogeneous" vs "Heterogeneous"

The degree of variation within a cultural system may be minimal, and the culture homogeneous, or the differences may be so great that the culture is heterogeneous. If a culture is relatively homogeneous, any portion of the group will represent the total of the society, and any cultural feature may be congruently shared by the members of the culture. Thus, generalizations may be inferred. In a heterogeneous culture, however, no one fragment of the society may be taken as a reflection of the totality. A generalization of any cultural feature, as if it represents the total society, should be avoided. When a comparison is made between cultures, the degree of variation that exists within them is an important consideration.

b. "Traditional" vs "Contemporary"

Also deserving attention are the cultural patterns that have existed in the past vs those that are observed in the present. Although, by definition, it is the nature of a culture to maintain certain characteristics, culture may also evolves over time. What has been described as traditional may or may not be practiced anymore or may continue to exist in a modified form. A time reference may be needed when referring to particular value systems or unique behavior patterns in a society to avoid confusing the present with the past.

c. "Similar" vs "Dissimilar"

It is important to examine the relative similarities and differences that may exist between the cultures that are being compared (the extent of cultural difference). For instance, a comparison between a Caucasian-American and a black African-American may not reveal obvious differences that can be attributed to culture. Because they are living in the same host society, the United States, any differences that exist may be minimized. However, a comparison of a Caucasian-American and a black African living in a traditional part of Africa may show great differences between them. The wider the cultural gap, the easier it is to demonstrate the impact of cultural factors.

II. CLINICAL APPLICATION OF CULTURE

Although the terms and concepts relating to culture have been examined already, it is necessary to elaborate further on how culture is addressed, expressed, and understood by people in general and by patients and therapists in particular. It is especially important in clinical settings to know how culture is approached.

A. DIFFERENT LEVELS OF CULTURE ADDRESSED

In everyday life, culture may be perceived at different levels or in different dimensions. From the standpoint of behavior analysis, it is important to be aware of the different ways of grasping culture. From a clinical point of view, it is important to know to which levels the patient, the patient's family, and the interpreter are referring. Culture can be referred to at the following different levels for description and discussion.

1. "Ideal" Cultural Behavior

This refers to a desirable pattern of life prescribed by a certain group of people. This ideal does not necessarily match the actual behavior observed in the society. Ideal norms are generally selected and described by the members of a society in terms of group well-being and they are often violated when individual self-interest induces another course of action (Hoebel, 1972).

2. "Actual" Cultural Behavior

This is a norm of behavior actually observed in life. The real culture is what the members of a society do and think in all their activities, in fact (Hoebel, 1972). The gap between the ideal culture and the real culture may be great or small, depending on the society in question.

3. "Stereotyped" Cultural Behavior

This refers to a certain behavior pattern that is described by an outsider to the group, as if it represents the total behavior pattern of the group. The described behavior pattern is usually fragmented, exaggerated, or distorted. It may be merely a product of the outsider's own projection and not reflect the actual culture at all.

4. "Deviated" Cultural Behavior

The behavior pattern observed within a group is not necessarily homogeneous. Some of the members may manifest behavior patterns that are idiosyncratic and deviate from the pattern of the majority. Such deviated behavior may or may not be pathological.

B. DIFFERENT PERSPECTIVES OF STUDYING CULTURE: ETIC AND EMIC

The terms *etic* and *emic* are derived originally from the linguistic terms *phonetic* (sound of universal language) and *phonemic* (sound of specific language). *Etic* is used to address things that are considered universal, whereas *emic* is culture specific. In the field of cultural research, the *etic* strategy holds the view that investigation can take place anywhere in the world, as the characteristics to be studied are universal, whereas the *emic* approach takes the position that the characteristics are indigenous and distinctive and only applicable to certain cultural groups (Draguns, 1989). At another level, the *etic* approach implies that research is conducted by an outsider; the *emic* approach, by an insider. Each approach has its own inherent advantages and shortcomings. Observation by an outsider, an *etic* approach, may be more objective, able to pick up things that are taken for granted by the culture's own people, but may lose culturally relevant meaning in its interpretation. A study done by an insider, an *emic* approach, tends to be more subjective, and able to explain things from a cultural perspective, but may lose objectivity and be unaware of things that only an outsider would notice.

Applied to the clinical task of assessing psychopathology, defining abnormality, and interpreting dynamics, whether a perspective is *etic* or *emic* becomes important, as each can bring about different results. A clinician with an outside cultural background may be advantageous because he has a fresh and objective view, but disadvantageous because he misinterpretes the phenomena he observes. In contrast, a clinician with an inside cultural background will have the benefit of knowing how to give culturally meaningful explanations for what has been observed, but may be handicapped by an objective bias. Thus, the clinician should keep in mind which approach he or she is undertaking and what possible advantages or handicaps he or she is facing.

C. Various Patterns of Understanding and Interpreting Cultures

A clinician also needs to recognize that a patient has a different level of understanding of his own culture and a different pattern of using culture to explain his behavior. For instance, a patient may have no insight about his own culture or ignore the dimension of cultural influence and deny the existence of cultural impact on his thought or behavior. This is likely to occur because culture as defined, in contrast to ethnicity, race, or nationality, is a rather abstract concept, difficult for laymen to recognize. No one knows how to describe and identify his own cultural system. Thus, if you were to ask a person, What is your culture? Few people would know how to answer. Even a physician may focus on ethnic background, or religion affiliation, such as Italian-American, Catholic; or Thai people, being Buddhist.

However, some people, or patients, may be fully aware of the influence of ethnicity and/or cultural background and may use them as excuses for problems they have encountered. Many people of minority backgrounds may explain their failures as due to discrimination by the majority group or claim they are not fairly cared for by their physicians simply because of the color of their skin or their racial heritage. Clinically, it is necessary to assess to what extent these claims represent the actual situation.

Neither the complete denial of cultural influence nor the use of culture as an excuse is a healthy way to deal with problems in life. Appropriately understanding the existence and impact of culture and integrating them as a major factor in understanding thought and behavior are important even in clinical situations. The focus is not only on the patient, but also on how the therapist views his own value system and beliefs in relation to the service that he gives to his patients.

REFERENCES

Acosta, F.X., Yamamoto, J., & Evans, L.A. (1982). *Effective psychotherapy for low income and minority patients.* New York: Plenum Press.

American Anthropological Association. (1999). AAA statement on race. *American Anthropologist, 100*(3), 712–713.

Barnouw, V. (1963). *Culture and personality.* Homewood, IL: Dorsey Press.

Benedict, R. (1934). *Patterns of culture.* Boston: Houghton Mifflin.

Benedict, R. (1946). *The chrysanthemum and the sword.* Boston: Houghton Mifflin.

Brumann, C. (1999). Writing for culture: Why a successful concept should not be discarded. *Current Anthropology, 40*(Suppl.), S1–S27.

Castillo, R.J. (1995). Culture, trance, and the mind-brain. *Anthropology of Consciousness, 6,* 17–34.

De Vos, G.A. (1975). Ethnic pluralism: Conflict and accommodation. In G.A. De Vos & L. Romanucci-Ross (Eds.), *Ethnicity: Cultural continuities and change* (p. 9). Palo Alto, CA: Mayfield.

Draguns, J.G. (1989). Dilemmas and choice in cross-cultural counseling: The universal versus the culturally distinctive. In P.B. Pedersen, J.G. Draguns, W.J. Lonner, & J.E. Trimble (Eds.), *Counseling across cultures* (pp. 3–21). Honolulu: University Press of Hawaii.

Ebata, K., Miguchi, M. Tseng, W.S., Hara, H., Kosaka, M., & Cui, Y.H. (1995). Migration and transethnic family adjustment: Experiences of Japanese war orphans and their Chinese spouses in Japan. In T.Y. Lin, W.S. Tseng, & E.K. Yeh (Eds.), *Chinese societies and mental health* (pp. 123–137). Hong Kong: Oxford University Press.

Gift, T.E., Strauss, J.S. Ritzler, B.A., Kokes, R.F., & Harder, D.W. (1986). Social class and psychiatric outcome. *American Journal of Psychiatry, 143*(2), 222–225.

Hoebel, E.A. (1972). *Anthropology: The study of man.* New York: McGraw-Hill.

Keesing, R.M. (1976). *Cultural anthropology: A contemporary perspective.* New York: Holt, Rinehart & Winston.

Kluckhohn, C. (1951). Values and value orientation. In T. Parsons (Ed.), *Toward a general theory of action.* Cambridge, MA: Harvard University Press.

Koss-Chioino, J., & Vargas, L.A. (1999). Working with Latino youth: Culture, development, and context. San Francisco: Jossey-Bass

Kottak, C.P. (1994). *Cultural anthropology* (6th ed.). New York: McGraw-Hill.

Kottak, C.P. (1999). *Mirror for humanity: A concise introduction to cultural psychiatry* (2nd ed.). Boston: McGraw-Hill College.

Kroeber, A.L. (1963). *Anthropology: Culture patterns and process.* New York: Harbinger.

Kroeber, A.L., & Kluckhohn, C. (1952). Culture: A critical review of concepts and definition. *Papers of the Peabody Museum of Archaeology and Ethnology, 47*(1).

Mollica, R.F., & Milic, M. (1986). Social class and psychiatric practice: A revision of the Hollingshead and Redlich Model. *American Journal of Psychiatry, 143*(1), 12–17.

Murdock, G.P. (1957). World ethnographic sample. *American
Anthropologist 59,* 664–687.

Nanda, S. (1980). *Cultural anthropology.* New York: Van Nostrand.

Nida, E.E. (1954). *Customs and cultures.* New York: Harper.

Service, E.R. (1978). *Profiles in ethnology* (3rd ed.). New York:
Harper & Row.

Smedley, A. (1999). "Race" and the construction of human identity.
American Anthropologist, 100(3), 690–702.

Sperry, R.W. (1987). Structure and significance of the consciousness revolution. *Journal of Mind and Behavior, 8,* 37–65.

Thompson, R.F., Donega, N.H., & Lavond, D.G. (1986). The psychobiology of learning and memory. In R.C. Atkinson, R.J.
Hernstein, G. Lindzey, & R.D. Luce (Eds.), *Steven's handbook
of experimental psychology,* (2nd ed.). New York: Wiley.

Tylor, E.B. (1871). *Primitive culture.*

Vanneman, R., & Cannon, L.W. (1987). *The American perception of
class.* Philadelphia: Temple University Press.

Wohlfarth, T., & van den Brink, W. (1998). Social class and substance use disorders: The value of social class as distinct from
socioeconomic status. *Social Science and Medicine, 47*(1),
51–58.

3

Marriage and the Family

I. INTRODUCTION

The family is the basic sociocultural unit. It is a nest for the growth of an individual, a resource for social support, and the institution through which culture is transmitted. Therefore, from a cultural psychiatric point of view, the family is an appropriate arena for examining the cultural aspects of human behavior (Tseng & Hsu, 1991).

From a cross-cultural point of view, it is important to note that the term "family" has different concepts and meanings. Conventionally, a family refers to a group of people who are brought together and live together through marriage or as the product of mating. For some ethnic groups, however, the boundaries of the family are much more extended. The Micronesians have a custom of adopting each other's children (mainly those of relatives and close friends) even though they may have plenty of their own. This custom ensures the interrelation among families and increases mutual dependence and support for the sake of survival in the small island society. Within such a cultural system, there is a complicated family-compound network beyond the nuclear or extended family with which we are familiar. In Micronesia, any person living under the same roof (blood relatives or adopted children) is considered a family member (Tseng, 1986). Accordingly, the number of family members keeps changing, depending on who is living in the house at any given time. Further, among Polynesians, all young people of the same age group are addressed socially as "brother" or "sister," whether or not they are related by blood. Thus, the Polynesian definition of family is much broader than ours.

From a semantic point of view, the exact meaning of family as it is used in English may be limited or confusing when translated into another language. For example, the Japanese have one basic character that means family, but by pronouncing it differently or adding other characters, it has many variations, *ie* (house), *uchi* (the inside of a house, as opposed to the outside world), *kazoku* (members of a family, which may include only the nuclear family or a whole family clan), and *katei* (the structure and life of the family).

Marriage refers to the customs, rules, and obligations that establish a special relationship between a sexually cohabiting adult male and female, between them and any children they produce, and between the kin groups of the husband and wife (Nanda, 1980, p. 196). This traditional concept of marriage is currently being challenged by homosexual people. From a sociological point of view, marriage is considered a socially approved, formal sexual union that is intended to be permanent. It is the bond on the basis of which a family develops.

The family is a complex institution that can be investigated and understood according to various dimensions, including: the individual members of the family, the subsystem of the family, the interaction patterns of the family as a group, the life cycle of the family, and the family as a system.

Although marriage and the formation of families rest on the biological complementarity of male and female and on the biological process of reproduction, both marriage and family are cultural patterns. As such, they differ in form and function in different societies. In order to provide culturally relevant assessment and treatment for families of different cultural backgrounds, it is essential to understand the cultural aspects of marriage and family systems and functions.

II. CULTURAL VARIATIONS OF MARRIAGE

A. MARRIAGE FORMS

Anthropologists have recognized and described nearly 1000 societies around the world. Their descriptions have been recorded and collected in the *Ethnographic Atlas* for systematic scientific comparison (Murdock, 1967). Cultural anthropologists have also described the distinctions among various marriage systems by referring to parameters such as marriage forms or postmarital residence.

Marriage forms concern the number of spouses in a marriage. **Monogamy** permits a person to have only one spouse at any given time, whereas **polygamy** permits more than one spouse in the marriage. If a man has several wives, it is called *polygyny,* and if a woman is married to more than one man, it is known as *polyandry.*

According to anthropologists (Hoebel, 1972, pp. 429–430), among 854 societies described in the

Ethnographic Atlas, only 16 percent consider monogamy as an exclusively expected marriage form, 39 percent prefer both monogamy and polygamy, and 44 percent hold the polygamous family to be the norm. Polyandry (a woman married to more than one man) is found in only 4 of the 854 cultures listed. Thus, more than 80 percent of the world's societies prefer plural marriages. However, this preference does not mean that most people in these societies actually have more than one spouse. Even where polygamy is preferred, the ratio of males to females may be such that few men would be able to acquire more than one wife. Furthermore, where men must exchange wealth for wives, many cannot afford more than one wife and therefore are limited to monogamy. It should also be pointed out that the figures presented here deal with percentages of "cultural units" as identified by anthropologists and do not reflect population percentages. Some cultural units may have small populations of at most a few hundred or a thousand people, whereas others may be very large. If social units are considered in terms of number of members, it would be fair to say that the majority of the world population considers monogamy to be the expected marriage form. Monogamy is the rule in most contemporary, developed societies.

In societies where monogamy is preferred and marriage is considered closely and exclusively tied to sex and emotion, it is hard for people to understand how polygamous marriage can exist without conflict and jealousy among wives. In fact, much evidence indicates that when a man has many wives, problems usually occur among them. However, as explained by anthropologist Nanda (1980), sexual jealousy among wives might not be a great problem in societies that do not idealize romantic love and exclusive sexual rights in marriage.

Polyandry is basically different in nature from polygamy. Among the Tibetans, the Todas, and other tribes in India, where the practice of polyandry is common, several brothers usually marry the same woman (Hoebel, 1972). In societies where land and property are scarce, the division of assets among siblings can be avoided if brothers form a family by marrying a common wife. Thus, polyandry is practiced frequently as a way of coping with an economic situation (Levine & Sangree, 1980). It is not brought about by a superwoman who wants many husbands, as might be speculated.

B. Choice of Mates

Every society has certain rules pertaining to the choice of a candidate for marriage. **Exogamy** is when marriage partners must be chosen from outside one's own kin group or community. In contrast, **endogamy** is when a person is obligated to marry within his or her own culturally defined group. An example of caste-related endogamy is the social rule in India that a person must marry within his or her caste to avoid becoming "polluted" through marriage to someone outside of it.

Associated with the rule of marital choice is the process by which the marital partner is chosen. **Arranged marriage** refers to marriages in which the partners are selected primarily by someone other than the partners themselves, usually by their parents or other kin. In contrast, a marriage partner may be chosen by **self-selection** or through free love, the method preferred by young members of most contemporary societies. The main concerns in arranging a marriage are the compatibility of the family backgrounds and of the prospective partners, as well as the partners' physical condition, health, moral character, working patterns, and ability to produce the next generation (see Fig. 3-1). In free love, affection and love are the major concerns, even though other factors, such as the character and personal background of the partner, may be taken into consideration.

Different modes of acquiring a wife exist around the world. In many societies, the prevalent method of obtaining a wife is through the formal exchange of goods considered equal in value to the offspring the woman is expected to produce — the progeny price. Progeny price may partly represent compensation for the loss of the girl by her kinship group, but it is much more an act of compensation to that group for its loss

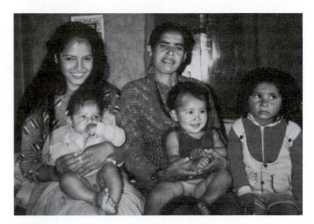

FIGURE 3-1 Arranged marriage between children in a Nepalese family. A girl in childhood is arranged to marry a boy–husband, living with and serving her mother-in-law.

of a legal claim to the children that she will bear. Well over half of all societies in the *Ethnographic Atlas* expect a progeny price to be paid to the family of the bride by the kin of the groom. Another way to obtain a wife and the rights to her future children is to work for the bride's family — suitor service.

Opposite to progeny price and suitor service is the custom that requires the bride to bring a dowry to the groom's family. The custom is based on the conception that the woman is going to be taken care of all her life by the man's family and relates to the patrilineal system, in which lineage is traced only through the male's kinship system.

C. Postmarital Residence

Another recognized parameter is the choice of residence after marriage. When the married couple lives with or near the husband's parents, it is called **patrilocal** residence. This pattern comprises 67 percent of the total world ethnographic sample (Hoebel, 1972, pp. 426–428). When the married couple lives with or near the wife's parents, it is called **matrilocal** residence. Nearly 15 percent of the sample societies follow this pattern. If the married couple lives with or near the parents of only one side, either the wife's parents or the husband's, it is called **bilocal** residence. Only 7 percent belong to this pattern. If the newly married couple lives apart from the relatives of both spouses, choosing a new place of their own, it is described as **neolocal** residence. While only 5 percent of the world sample belong to this pattern, this is the most common practice of our present industrialized and urbanized society.

The significance of postmarital choice of residence is obvious, as it affects the pattern of kinship relations as well as the power distribution and respective roles of the spouses. Why do societies practice different patterns of residence? The prime determinants of residence are ecological circumstances (Haviland, 1978). If the man's role in subsistence is predominant, patrilocal residence is the likely result. Matrilocal residence is a likely result if ecological circumstances make the role of the woman predominant in subsistence, as is found most often in horticultural societies, where political complexity is relatively undeveloped and cooperation among women is important. Bilocal residence is particularly well suited to situations in which resources are limited and the cooperation of more people is needed. Because one can join either the bride's or the groom's family, family membership is flexible, and one can go where the resources look best. Neolocal residence occurs where the independence of the nuclear family is emphasized. Because most economic activity occurs outside the family in modern, industrialized societies, and it is important for people to be able to move to where jobs can be found, neolocal residence is the pattern best suited to this type of society.

III. CULTURAL VARIATIONS OF FAMILY SYSTEMS

A. KINSHIP SYSTEM AND DESCENT GROUP

A kinship system is a system of terms used to classify different kin. It refers to the totality of relationships based on blood and marriage that links individuals through a web of rights and obligations, and the kinds of groups formed in a society on the basis of kinship. Societies differ in the categories of relatives they recognize and the principles by which kin are classified. Generation, relative age, gender, and lineality versus collaterality are some of the categories that are usually distinguished. Anthropologists have identified six basic systems of kinship terminology: Hawaiian, Eskimo, Iroquois, Omaha, Crow, and Sudanese. These systems reflect the kinds of kin groups that are considered most important.

In most societies, there is a rule of descent that defines how individuals are affiliated with sets of kin. **Patrilineal** descent affiliates an individual with kinsmen of both sexes through the males. In each generation, children belong to the kin group of the father, carry the father's family name, and lineage is traced through the grandfather, father, son, and grandson. **Matrilineal** descent affiliates an individual with kinsmen only through the females; thus, children belong to the mother's kin group and lineage is traced through the grandmother, mother, daughter, and granddaughter. **Ambilineal** descent affiliates an individual with kinsmen through either males or females so that some children belong to the kin group of the father and others to the kin group of the mother. Consequently, the descent groups show both female and male genealogical links. According to anthropologists (Hoebel, 1972), patrilineal organization is the most frequent type of descent system, constituting about 45 percent of all societies in the world. Matrilineal organization comprises only about 14 percent.

Although societies with matrilineal descent seem in many respects like mirror images of their patrilineal counterparts, they differ in one important way: who exercises authority. In patrineal systems, where the line of descent passes through the males, it is also the males who exercise authority in the kin groups. Consequently, the lines of descent and of authority converge. In a matrilineal system, however, the line of descent passes through females, but females rarely exercise authority in their kin groups. A female usually allows her husband and her brothers to exercise the power. Thus, unlike the patrilineal system, the

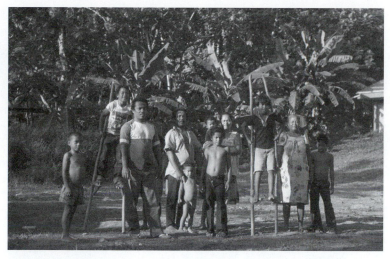

FIGURE 3-2 Micronesian family following the matrilineal system. Title is transmitted from mother to daughter, and then to granddaughter, but the power is exercised by a woman's husband and her brothers.

lines of authority and descent do not converge (see Fig. 3-2).

B. HOUSEHOLD AND FAMILY STRUCTURE

Household refers to all the persons who live in one house. Usually it is implied that they are related either by marriage or blood and share the work, financial responsibilities, and food. Several terms address various forms of households. The **nuclear family** is composed of the basic family members: parents and their (unmarried) children. This is the most frequently observed form of household in most industrialized societies. If a household is composed of a nuclear family plus the parent (or parents) of either the husband or wife, it is called a **stem family.** If, in addition to the stem family, a spouse's unmarried siblings are living with them, it is referred to as a **joint family.** If the married siblings (and their children, if any) are living in the same household (usually with the presence of their parent or parents), it is recognized as an **extended family** (see Figs. 3-3 and 3-4).

One-parent families, particularly female-headed households, are found to be widespread in various cultures. Reviewing this type of family household cross-culturally, Bilge and Kaufman (1983) regarded the one-parent family as neither pathological nor inferior. They concluded that whether or not the single-parent household becomes a personal or social disaster depends on the availability of sufficient material resources and supportive social networks, as well as culturally structured attitudes toward such a household. However, in most developed societies, such as the United States, there are not adequate institutionalized support systems for children of single-parent families, and the social conditions of such families are generally not as good as those of two-parent families. This situation is also reported in European societies, such as Denmark (Koch-Nielsen, 1980) and France (Lefaucheur, 1980).

Along with an increase in divorce and remarriage, the number of **stepfamilies** is rising remarkably in Western societies. As Visher and Visher (1982) observed, stepfamilies differ structurally from biological families in several ways: all stepfamily members have experienced important losses, all members

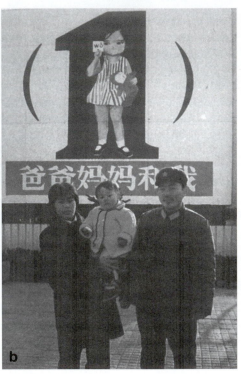

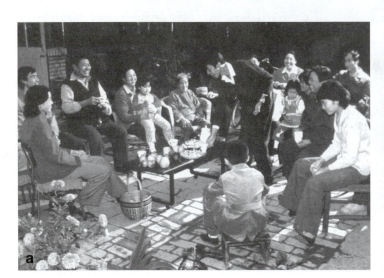

FIGURE 3-3 Traditional and contemporary Chinese families. (a) An idealized extended family with members of three generations celebrating a mid-fall festival in the family courtyard, with the children considered their parents' treasures. (b) A model family taking a picture in front of a painting on the street that advocates the one-child-per-couple family policy to avoid a potential population explosion.

come with past family histories, parent–child bonds predate the new couple relationship, there is a biological parent elsewhere (either living or deceased), children often are members of two households, and no legal relationship exists between stepparent and stepchild. Thus, from a developmental point of view, stepfamilies need to work on the reintegration of the family.

C. PRIMARY AXIS

From the perspective of loyalty and affection bonds, a particular dyad may be molded culturally as the prominent and recognizable axis in some family systems. The axis may be built on husband–wife,

father–son, mother–son, or brother–sister dyads. The presence of any particular primary axis can be recognized only when conflict and competition occur between different dyads in a family.

Based on the concept of a primary axis, psychological anthropologist F.L.K. Hsu (1972) has hypothesized that the different emphases of the primary dyad result in different family systems, which have specific, varied influences on the individuals reared in them. Consequently, many characteristic thought and behavior patterns shown by family members can be attributed to the existence of different primary bonds within a family system.

For instance, Hsu speculated that within the patrilineal, patrilocal, and patriarchal family systems that exemplify the majority of Asian peoples, including the

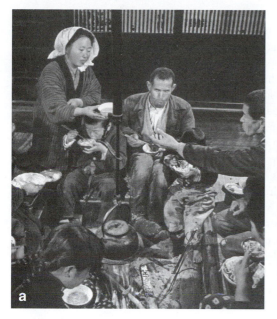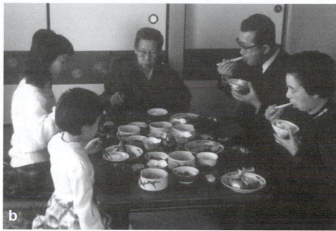

FIGURE 3-4   Japanese families in a village and in the city. (a) A wife serving food for three generations in a traditional village family. (b) A contemporary nuclear family in the city enjoying dinner together.

Chinese, Japanese, Korean, Thai, and others, the most elevated dyad is the *father–son dyad.* Characteristics associated with the father–son dyad are inclusiveness of other individuals and continuity over generations, as well as mutual dependence and mutual obligation between generations.

Although the Hindu societies of India (and possibly the Muslim groups of this subcontinent as well) also exemplify patrilineal, patrilocal, and partiarchal family systems, their most important structural relationship is the *mother–son dyad.* Associated with this dyad are the attributes of exclusiveness and discontinuity between generations. As a continuation of the mother–son relationship, unilateral dependence is encouraged and dependence upon an all-answering figure becomes the pattern.

Among the majority of Africans south of the Sahara, kinship structure is dominated by the *brother–brother dyad* across lines of descent, inheritence, and succession. The characteristics associated with such systems are horizontal orientation and ver-

tical dissociation over the generations. Because of competition among siblings, men are perceived as being unreliable.

In contrast to the just-described dyads, the kinship structure of the majority of Western people (i.e., of European origin) is usually patrilineal, patrilocal, or neolocal and, in many instances, nominally patriarchal with an egalitarian family. The most elevated dyad is the *husband–wife dyad.* The characteristics attributed to this dyad are exclusiveness of other individuals and discontinuity over generations. Individualism and self-reliance are emphasized and the independence of the children is valued.

Although Hsu's way of categorizing and analyzing various family systems is subject to criticism, his attempt to explore the potential relationship between the family systems and the patterns of life associated with each type of primary dyad deserves further investigation and validation. Awareness of the family's primary axis will at least help us understand the dynamics of the behavior observed in the family.

D. ALTERNATIVE WAYS OF FORMING A FAMILY

1. Group Marriage

Group marriage is a special marital form in which a relatively small number of adults live together, share labor, goods, and services, raise children in common, and engage in promiscuous sexual relations. According to Ember and Ember (1973), the Marquesans of the South Pacific and the Toda seem to have developed group marriages out of polyandrous marriages.

Several decades ago, small-scale group marriages were observed in various parts of the United States. Although some people were quite devoted to this family arrangement, it did not remain viable for any considerable length of time. As Ellis (1974) pointed out, a group of four or more adults of both sexes finds it difficult to live together harmoniously. Problems involving sexual or other relationships are almost certain to arise among the group members. In our present society, fewer females than males appear to be interested in group marriage.

2. Collective Communes

The collective commune as a basic living organization has been observed in different parts of the world. Communes may emerge as a result of political ideology, as in communist societies, or as a reaction to sociocultural change. In the 1960s, associated with the Hippie movement, the so-called commune movement arose in the United States as well as in Denmark. The movement attracted thousands of predominantly young followers. Most communes, however, failed after a short time. Poor planning, a general lack of organization, overidealism, excessive individualism, diversity of the members, and internal conflict were among the major factors that led to the dissolution of the communes in both countries.

The kibbutz community in Israel, a collective agricultural commune, has special historical significance and is the type most frequently studied and reported in scientific literature. The first kibbutz appeared as a unit of Jewish land settlement in the Jordan Valley. It was settled by a group of young unmarried Jews who emigrated from eastern Europe. The plan for the kibbutz called for a relationship of complete equality between husband and wife and for the economic independence of women. It was also felt that children should be reared and educated outside of the family. It was believed that such an environment would engender values of group loyalty in the children rather than the egotisms produced in the family setting. As a result, children in a kibbutz do not live with their parents, but live instead in a "children's house," where they are organized according to their age group. Full responsibility for their care is undertaken by the children's nurse, who acts as a housemother. This kind of collective commune illustrates an alternative way of organizing a family and has an interesting impact on the life of an individual.

IV. CULTURE AND FAMILY DEVELOPMENT

The stages of the life cycles of intact nuclear families in contemporary societies have been clearly defined by Western scholars. The marriage-establishment phase, the childbearing phase, the child-growing phase, the child-leaving phase, the empty nest phase, and the widowing phase are the most common subdivisions of family development. Clearly, marriage and the bearing, raising, and launching of children are important landmarks in the different stages of family development.

In different time periods, ethnic groups, or geographic locations, the stages of family development are much less clearly defined, and the changes in the phases of family life are more subtle (Berkner, 1972; Falicov & Karrer, 1980). Also, as pointed out by Rossi (1972), increased longevity and improved birth control have led to remarkable changes in family development. Women now devote a smaller proportion of their adult lives to the rearing of children, and maternity has become a very small part of the average adult woman's life.

From a cross-cultural point of view, the stages of family development may be subject to many factors, making them remarkably different from one cultural group to another (Tseng & Hsu, 1991). The ordinary age for marriage varies from culture to culture. For instance, in Nepal, a girl was traditionally married when she was about 4 or 5 years old, and her boy–husband was about 6 or 7 years old. There was actually a premarital arrangement. The girl related to her parents-in-law as if they were foster parents, and her husband was a "brother–husband" until both the girl and the boy reached young adulthood and began to relate as mates. For them, the "family" was established when they were still children. In contrast, in contemporary China, for the sake of birth control, young people are officially encouraged to marry late. The ages of the man and the woman must total more than 50 years (such as 27 and 23), otherwise the couple is not able to obtain a marriage certificate. As a result, most young people do not get married before 25, starting their families much later than in the past, when marriages were arranged for many young couples before they were even 20.

Regarding childbearing, some societies still consider it desirable to have many children. Therefore, the childbearing period is long, extending until the mother reaches the age of menopause. In contrast, in most developed societies, the number of children in a family has decreased substantially, averaging one or two. In China, one child per couple is the official policy. Thus, the childbearing period is very short, only a few years.

The autonomy of children and their departure from the family home is dealt with in various ways in different societies. In some, there are no expectations for adolescents to quickly become independent from their parents and families, either psychologically or physically. For example, the traditional Hindu family in an agricultural setting does not permit its offspring to leave the extended family household even after marriage or reaching middle age, as long as the father is still alive. In many Asian societies, it is normal for unmarried children in their 30s to continue to live with their parents. In contrast, college-age children in the United States encounter peer pressure to move out on their own, even if they attend classes in the same town where their parents live. Almost all parents of high school graduates feel that their children should move out of the family home after the age of 18 — the time for launching. Thus, there is a clear and early child-leaving phase in the Western family.

Divorce and remarriage are viewed and practiced differently in different cultures and bring about different courses of family development. In the Marshall Islands of Micronesia, separation and remarriage are viewed without prejudice, and in fact are so common that almost every couple goes through several such experiences. In other societies, these deviations from marriage occur only in exceptional circumstances and are regarded very negatively.

Social and biological changes during the 20th century have influenced the development of the distinctive stage in the family life cycle referred to as the "empty-nest" or "postparental" period. With life expectancy increasing from about 45 years at the turn of the century to about 70 years in the 1970s, the average couple can now expect to live alone without their children for more than 15 years after the last child leaves home permanently. This prolonged postparental stage of the family life cycle is a characteristic of contemporary people.

In summary, it may said that, due to differences in premarital experience, time of marriage, patterns of childbearing and childrearing, the life span of the parents, and the structure of the household, the rhythm of family development may vary in different societies. The transition between phases may be clear-cut or blurred, and the stages that are identified as "ordinary" phases of development may be short, long, or even absent. Further, due to variations in the cultural implications of critical developmental milestones, such as the formal marital union, dissolution of marital relations, the launching of children from the home, and widowhood, these milestones have different meanings and affect the lives of family members differently in different cultures. Therefore, it is necessary to examine the meaning of family development in the context of cultural background.

V. CULTURE AND FAMILY SUBSYSTEMS

There are three potential subsystems within a nuclear family: husband–wife, parent–child, and sibling–sibling. In stem or extended families, there are additional grandparents–grandchildren and in-law subsystems. The cultural aspects of the family can be examined by analyzing the cultural variations of interpersonal relations that exist in each subsystem.

A. HUSBAND–WIFE SUBSYSTEMS

From an anthropological point of view, the husband–wife subsystem is influenced greatly by the marriage and family systems. Whether the marriage of the husband and wife was arranged by their parents even before they reached puberty (as in Nepal in the past) or by their own choice after they reached young adulthood (as in most contemporary Western societies) will make a remarkable difference in the beginning of the husband–wife relationship. From the standpoint of a family system, whether a patrilineal or matrilineal system is observed will modify the husband–wife relationship significantly. For instance, in Truk, Micronesia, where the family system is matrilineal, the husband executes the authority given to him by his wife. Therefore, the performance of power is time-limited. The marriage form — whether monogamy or polygamy — will definitely shape the relationship between husband and wife. Imagine how a husband having several wives, or several brothers sharing a common wife, would affect the husband–wife subsystem.

Even in the "ordinary" marriage form of monogamy, the husband–wife relationship is modified by many factors that can be examined through various parameters, including role division, communication, affection, and so on.

1. Role Division

The role division between husband and wife is determined by the major patterns of production in a society, whether food-gathering, hunting, agricultural, or industrial. For instance, in a hunting society, it is mainly the role of the husband to go out and engage in hunting for food while the wife stays at home and does domestic work. In an industrial society, both the husband and the wife can go outside of the household to earn a living. The husband–wife relationship is thus very much shaped by the economic system.

Culture factors also have certain effects. Even though the economic systems are the same in Korea, Japan, and China, the role divisions between husband and wife have remarkable differences. In Korea, women have traditionally been discouraged from working outside of the house. Even now, when a woman is married, she is expected to stop working and become a full-time housewife. This is true even if she is well-educated, with a professional background. Less than 15 percent of Korean women continue to work outside of the house after marriage in present-day Korea. Within the household, there are clear role divisions between husband and wife. The husband never goes into the kitchen to do the cooking. The kitchen is the woman's territory. Although Japanese husbands and wives share similar relationship patterns with Korean couples, they are slightly less traditional. In Japan, about 30 percent of women continue to work after marriage, either full-time or part-time. In contrast, in mainland China, almost every wife works outside of the household, as does her husband. Both husband and wife share the domestic chores, including cooking. This is an example of how role division can vary even among different ethnic groups with similar economic systems and the common base of being Asian cultures.

2. Communication

Based on clinical experience with American families of European background, Western family therapists tend to take the view that the capacity to communicate is closely correlated with marital adjustment (Lewis, Beavers, Gossett, & Phillips, 1976). Family therapists place emphasis on teaching each marital partner to communicate effectively: speaking for themselves and articulating their own feelings rather than blaming others, engaging in calm negotiation with each other, and listening to each other with empathetic understanding. After surveying ordinary American couples, Navran (1967) pointed out that the happily married differ from the unhappily married in several aspects in terms of communication style. The happily married couples more frequently talk over pleasant things, discuss matters of shared interest, talk to each other about personal problems, and feel more frequently understood by their spouses.

In a cross-cultural investigation of differences in marital communication, Winkler and Doherty (1983) studied Israeli couples living in New York City, along with socially similar American Jewish couples, in order to compare the conflict-related communication styles of these two ethnic subgroups. They found that Israeli couples were more apt to be verbally aggressive and less apt to behave calmly during marital conflicts. These communication styles did not relate to marital satisfaction as strongly for the Israelis as for the Americans, who tend to view calm, rational approaches to communications important for a happy marriage.

3. Expressions of Affection

How feelings are shared between husband and wife, in terms of degree of expressiveness and preferred ways of sharing affection, varies among different cultures. For instance, showing intimacy in social settings is frowned upon in many conservative societies. Behaving affectionately in front of one's parents or one's own children is viewed as "disgraceful" in many Asian societies. In contrast, in the West, when a husband and wife do not show affection (such as kissing or hugging), particularly in front of friends, it is considered an indication that something is wrong with the marriage. It is considered desirable for a husband and wife to affirm their affection for each other through language (such as saying "I love you") as often as possible in private situations; in the East, for spouses to say such things, even in private, is considered awkward and even nauseating.

Concerning emotional expressiveness and marital adjustment, Ingoldsby (1980) compared couples from the United States with couples from Colombia. He found that Colombian wives were not more emotionally expressive than their husbands, as was the case with American couples. Furthermore, a positive relationship between emotional expressiveness and marital adjustment was found in the American couples, but not the Columbian ones. For the Colombian couples, it was important that the husband and wife be compatible in their levels of expressiveness.

B. PARENT–CHILD SUBSYSTEM

1. Relationships in General

Several parameters can be used conceptually for examining parent–child relationships, starting with the issue of who is the primary care provider for the children. In many cultures, it is viewed as the sole responsibility of the mother to raise the small child. The father is seldom involved in domestic work, including child rearing. This view is exemplified by traditional Japanese or Korean families. In some Chinese families, child care is shared by the father and mother to some extent. Intimacy and indulgence shown by the parents toward small children also vary among cultures. In some, close physical contact is observed with intimate relations, mainly the mother (as illustrated in many Asian families), whereas in others (such as Anglo-Saxon families), physical distance and early separation are practiced. When children become older, the extent to which parental authority and hierarchies between generations are emphasized varies among different cultures. Some stress absolute obedience and respect toward the parents, whereas others allow a more egalitarian relationship (J. Hsu, Tseng, Ashton McDermott, & Char, 1985). The relationship between parent and child is subject to many factors, including family structure, the roles of husband and wife, practical demands of the environment, cultural expectations, and the developmental stages the children go through (Tseng & Hsu, 1972). Many

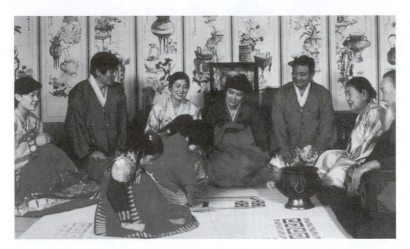

FIGURE 3-5 A Korean family showing respect for parental authority. Dressed in traditional dress, grandchildren bow to their grandparents on new year's day.

variations of parent–child relationships can be observed cross-culturally (see Fig. 3-5) [cross-reference to Chapter 4: Child Development and Enculturation (Section II, A–D)].

2. Patterns of Discipline

From a clinical point of view, one issue that deserves special attention is the way children are disciplined: in particular, to what extent corporal punishment is applied in discipline, what kind of physical discipline is permitted within cultural limits, and when it needs to be considered pathological or even physical abuse of children by parents. In other words, a culture-appropriate distinction between culturally practiced corporal punishment versus clinically considered physical abuse is necessary [cross-reference to Chapter 25: Childhood-Related Disorders (Section III, A)].

3. Triangular Relationships

Another issue that has caught the theoretical interest of scholars is how the parents–child triangular relationship (or Oedipus complex) is observed and managed in different cultures (Tseng & Hsu, 1991). From a cultural anthropological view, it has been pos-

tulated that such triangular tensions are less likely to occur in certain family systems. For instance, within the extended family, the presence of multiple adults (such as uncles, aunts, or grandparents) in addition to the father and mother make it less likely that a father–mother–child conflict of competition, favoritism, or attachment will intensify.

In matrilineal family systems, maternal uncles (the mother's brothers) have more say in major decisions regarding a boy child than the father, diluting potential conflict between father and son. In African society, when the family practices polygynous marriage, such as in Nigeria (Ebigbo & Ihezue, 1982), the father is not physically available for the children all the time. The mother usually develops intense ties with her children, particularly her sons, who serve as husband substitutes from an emotional standpoint. Naturally, the father's absence could enhance father–son tensions.

As pointed out by Hoffman (1981), there are cultural variants on triangular conflict, not only in terms of how tension is created and intensified, but also how culturally appropriate solutions are provided. In Western fairy tales, such as Snow White, Cinderella, and Jack and the Bean Stalk, the stories always end with the triumph of the children over the adult figures (the stepmother, witch, or giant). In contrast, in societies that emphasize parental authority, the stories end differently. For example, in Chinese children's stories (Tseng & Hsu, 1972) and operas (J. Hsu & Tseng, 1974), the triangular conflict theme always ends with the child, rather than the parent, being either punished or killed, appropriately complying to the traditional Chinese cultural view of parent–child relationships [cross-reference to Chapter 4: Child Development and Enculturation (Section II, D)].

C. Sibling–Sibling Subsytems

Compared to other subsystems that exist in families, the sibling–sibling subsystem has been less studied by behavior scientists and clinicians. The relationships between or among siblings can be examined according to various parameters, such as gender difference emphasized, hierarchical relation stressed, role performed, bond formed, and intimacy expressed.

Concerning gender difference, in many societies, particularly those with patrilinial and patrilocal family systems, brothers have more privileges than sisters; in matrilineal and matrilocal societies, sisters have more unspoken power than brothers. In addition, different degrees of segregation are observed between brothers and sisters. In many societies, the segregation of brothers and sisters is not heavily emphasized in young childhood, when they play and even sleep together. However, after reaching a certain age, even before puberty, segregation is practiced. The strict segregation of brothers and sisters is exemplified in Micronesia. Parallel with the importance of brother–sister relationships within the matrilineal family system is a strict segregation rule observed between male and female siblings in the form of a brother–sister taboo. For instance, if a brother and a sister find that, by chance, they are the only two people in the house, one of them has to leave right away — physical closeness between brother and sister is forbidden by the taboo.

Another parameter concerning sibling relationships is the hierarchical relation that exists within sibling-ship. In cultures that generally emphasize the importance of hierarchy within interpersonal relationship systems, hierarchical differentiation is observed in sibling relationships as well. An older sibling has more say than a younger one. Further, if the eldest son is designated as the heir to the family business or property, he has more power over his siblings. The hierarchial recognition of male siblings is well illustrated in the Japanese family system. Male siblings are often given numerical numbers as names, such as taro (first boy), jiro (second boy), saburo (third boy), siburo (fourth boy), goburo (fifth boy), and so on. The hierarchical order among siblings is identified by their first names.

With regard to age difference, the roles played by siblings may be different in various cultures. For instance, older children are expected to take care of younger children as parental substitutes. In agricultural societies, it is often the task for the older children (often the elder sister) to carry and feed her baby sibling while her mother is busy working in the field. In some Asian societies, when a family is poor and cannot afford to send all the children to school, it is often the older siblings who work at home or outside while their younger siblings go to school. Eventually, the younger siblings will have better job opportunities. In other words, due to financial limitations, the older siblings have to sacrifice their lives for their younger siblings' future occupational success.

The affection and bond between or among siblings varies from one household to another and from one culture to another. Generally speaking, in cultures where the nuclear family is the mode and personal individualization is emphasized, there is not much emphasis on close ties between siblings, as they are expected to be separated later in their individual lives. However, in cultures where the extended family is the mode and collectiveness is stressed, harmony and bonds among siblings are stressed. In reality, however, hidden competition or even openly conflicting relations may be observed despite the cultural emphasis on harmony (Nuckolls, 1993).

D. In-Law Subsystems

It is commonly recognized that the relationship between mother-in-law and daughter-in-law is one of the most difficult within the family system. It is the subsystem especially susceptible to problems in a larger family.

In a culture in which a close mother–son relationship is permitted and is a primary dyad of the family, as exemplified by traditional Hindu society, intense strain exists between the son's wife and his mother. This relationship is highly charged with potential conflict. After the marriage, by tradition, the young wife in a Hindu family is expected to subject herself to the absolute power of her mother-in-law. If she is persuasive enough to elicit her husband's support in her new family, her position becomes even more difficult. If her husband agrees with her, the delicate balance of family relationships is upset and she may suffer repercussions from the tensions created. The daughter-in-law can expect redress for her grievances only by living long enough to become a despot in turn to her own son's wife.

With the increasing preference for nuclear families over stem families and the rising emphasis on husband–wife as the primary dyad, the power of in-laws is gradually declining in many contemporary societies. In Japan, many young women prefer to marry a husband without the requirement of living with the mother-in-law after marriage. In traditional Japanese society, if there was any conflict between mother-in-law and daughter-in-law, the mother-in-law was favored. However, that is changing now. In the past, it was the daughter-in-law who, as the victim of an unresolvable conflict, attempted suicide as a last choice in coping. Now, the situation is starting to reverse. It is the mother-in-law who attempts suicide if she finds herself in an unfavorable situation with her daughter-in-law.

E. Grandparents–Grandchildren Subsystems

The relationship between grandparents and grandchildren is an important subsystem of an extended family in many cultures. Grandparents can function within a family as either the ultimate authority figures or as benign adults who tend to indulge their grandchildren. Grandparents can also interfere in the children's upbringing, especially if their relationships with their daughters- or sons-in-law are difficult ones.

VI. CULTURE AND FAMILY–GROUP BEHAVIOR

The marital dyad is the backbone of a family, and many family issues can be addressed from this perspective. However, once a couple begins to have children, the components and structure of the family are changed. It becomes relevant and necessary to deal with the family as more than just a marital dyad plus children. The family needs to be addressed, examined, and understood as a "family group." This is particularly true of families in which the children have reached an age where they have significant input and impact on the function of the whole family. In a joint or extended family, newlyweds find themselves part of a family group even before they have children of their own, as their marriage takes place within the context of a preexisting family that includes parents/parents-in-law and siblings/siblings-in-law.

The family has a number of characteristics common to all true small groups. First, the action of any member affects all group members. To function properly, the group requires unified objectives and leadership toward these objectives. Further, the maintenance of group morale requires that each member give the needs of the group some precedence over his/her own desires. Also, the group must have a structure with clarity of roles and leadership in order to carry out the group function.

The family, however, is a special kind of group because it is determined by biological background and sociocultural expectations and consists of members of different genders and generations who have intense relations for a prolonged period of time, resulting in a unique kind of commitment, bonding, and identification. The family as a group is also the basic social unit within which a society's culture is maintained and transmitted. Thus, viewing the family as a small group is another way to examine the function of the family from a cultural perspective.

The behavior and function of the family as a group can be studied using various parameters. For instance, Fleck (1980) focused on leadership, dominance, family boundaries, affectivity, communication, and task/goal performance. Lewis and his group (1976) used the parameters of the structure of the family (including overt power, parental coalitions, and closeness), mythology, goal-directed negotiation, autonomy, and family affect to assess the psychological health of the family. The family–group interaction pattern has been studied primarily by family researchers with backgrounds in psychology or psychiatry, and seldom by anthropologists. There have been a few investigations carried out from the perspective of cross-cultural comparison (J. Hsu, Tseng, Ashton, McDermott & Char, 1985; Lewis et al., 1976; Lewis & Looney, 1983), but the knowledge available is still very scarce.

A. COHESION

The degree to which family members are connected to each other is called cohesion. Family psychologists Olson and associates (1983) suggested that the spectrum of cohesion can range from "disengaged" (or separated) to "connected" (or enmeshed). According to family therapist Minuchin (1974), the "enmeshed family" is characterized by several phenomena: overinvolvement with one another, overresponsiveness to one another, diffuse interpersonal boundaries, confusion of roles, discouragement of individualization and autonomy, and low stress tolerance.

Some people have loosely used the term "enmeshed" to describe families of certain cultural groups, such as Italian or Hawaiian families, which emphasize closeness among family members.

However, in fact, neither confusion of roles nor low stress tolerance exists within close families of these cultural groups. Instead, there is always clear role

division and hierarchy in them as well as high stress tolerance. Therefore, the term "enmeshed" families should not be confused with "close" families in cross-cultural applications.

B. BOUNDARIES

Boundaries in a family refer to the borders maintained between individual family members or between subgroups that exist within the family. In a family that culturally values individualization and autonomy, there is frequent emphasis on each family member having his/her own boundaries, speaking up for his/herself, and protecting his/her own territory, both psychologically and physically. However, in a family that culturally values group togetherness, the boundaries between family members are not essential. One family member may speak up for another, particularly a senior member for a junior, and anyone overly concerned with his/her individual rights or territory is seen as acting disgracefully.

Boundaries between two families or between a family and all those outside the family also show variation cross-culturally. For example, for Pacific cultural groups that value mutual help and coexistence within the limited resources of island society, the boundaries between families as well as between the family and the community are relatively blurred. Food is usually shared among families and many belongings are loaned easily from one family to another family. Building high walls between family residences to ensure territorial rights and privacy would be a foreign custom to them.

C. ALIGNMENT

A prominent line or lines of alliance formed among particular members of a family is referred to as an alignment. When a particularly strong union is formed between parents, it is called a parental coalition. If the alignment involves a parent and a child, it is called a parent–child or cross-generation coalition.

Although the husband–wife alignment is the primary axis in most families in Western society, it is not necessarily the most prominent in other cultures. For example, the brother–sister alignment is the most important one in matrilineal Micronesian families, which trace inheritance through the mother–daughter line, while actual power is executed through the brother–sister connection.

D. POWER

Power has been defined by sociologists and family scholars as the ability of an individual to carry out his or her will within a social relationship, even in the face of the resistance from others. It is considered a dynamic process rather than a static phenomenon, and a system of property rather than an individual attribute.

From a cultural point of view, recent efforts have been made to clarify the power structure within families of different ethnic groups in the United States. For instance, Willie and Greenblatt (1978), after reviewing several studies of power relations in African-American families, pointed out that black matriarchy is a myth and that egalitarian decision-making patterns predominate in African-American families. In Mexican-American families, Hawkes and Taylor (1975) found that egalitarianism was by far the most common mode in both decision-making and action-taking among migrant farm labor families in California, indicating that the commonly held view of the dominance of the husband in Chicano families is unsubstantiated.

E. ROLE DIVISION

Many personal factors, such as age, gender, birth order, and generation, determine role division within a family. Sociocultural factors also mold the patterns determining how role division should take place within a family. In general, a considerable degree of parental role differentiation is expected between the father and the mother. For instance, an investigation by Tashakkori and Mehryar (1982) found that, in Iran, mothers tended to be dominant in the supportive-emotional areas, fathers in the authoritative-punitive matters. Among the children, girls on the whole attributed a larger share of parental decision-making to their mothers than did boys.

Lopata (1971) found that in the United States, better-educated mothers showed greater awareness of the importance of their roles in the development of their children's personalities and abilities than did less-educated mothers. Additionally, Jewish mothers tended to define role competency in terms of how the mother's personality related to and affected the other family members, whereas Catholic mothers specified the qualities of an ideal mother in terms of how well she carried out household tasks and duties. Thus, the role of the mother is perceived differently in different ethnic groups.

F. COMMUNICATION

According to family scholars, the expression and exchange of ideas among family members can be examined from various perspectives: clarity, amount, style, and congruence of communication (affect vs verbal, or statement vs context), and responsiveness (how messages are received, whether empathetically or not).

The extent to which open communication among family members is encouraged varied greatly among families of different cultural groups. In Hawaii, for example, traditional Hawaiian family custom maintains that children are to be "seen but not heard" when in the presence of their parents at family occasions, such as meals. The children are expected to listen to and learn from the adults' conversation, speaking only when they are actually invited to express their opinions. In marked contrast, American families of European ancestry commonly value conversation carried out among all family members, encouraging even the youngest children to speak up so that their opinions can be heard.

Cultural traditions greatly affect the extent to which families feel comfortable about revealing their private lives to outsiders. A comparison of families of different ethnic groups in Hawaii showed that, generally speaking, Caucasian families discussed family problems with outsiders with relative ease, whereas Hawaiian families did so less easily and Asian families with the most strain. This indicates that there would be different degrees to which families would feel ready to disclose their internal lives and private feelings to evaluators or therapists.

G. Affections

Families of different ethnic groups tend to manifest specific patterns of expression of affection. For example, whereas Italian and Latin families tend to show full emotion, Japanese and British families tend to be more reserved and constrained. Therefore, there is a need for different baselines in evaluating the emotional responsiveness of families. As pointed out by Japanese psychiatrist Doi (1973), the Japanese tend to distinguish between *omote* (public) and *ura* (private) situations in which they accordingly behave and react differently. While they tend to be very polite and restrained in public, observed situations, they tend to be relaxed, natural, and unrestrained in private settings. This twofold behavior also applies to family groups, and the discrepancy in family reaction patterns should be recognized and interpreted perceptively.

In closing, it should be pointed out that the family is a unique organization and a complex group entity. From a cultural perspective, the family needs to be examined according to family systems, family structures, family development, family subsystems, and family groups. Through these multiple dimensions, the nature of the family can be grasped comprehensively and understood cross-culturally. Based on knowledge about the cultural aspects of the family, the cultural aspects of family problems can be apprehended and relevant therapy can be offered for families of diverse cultural backgrounds (cross-reference to Chapter 40: Working with Families).

REFERENCES

Berkner, L.K. (1972). The stem family and the development cycle of the peasant household: An eighteenth-century Austrian example. *American Historical Review, 77,* 398–418.

Bilge, B., & Kaufman, G. (1983). Children of divorce and one-parent families: Cross-cultural perspectives. *Family Relations, 32,* 59–71.

Doi, T. (1973). *Omote* and *ura:* Concepts derived from the Japanese two-fold structure of consciousness. *Journal of Nervous and Mental Disease, 157,* 258–261.

Ebigbo, P.O., & Ihezue, U.H. (1982). Neurotic ties in families of Nigerians with psycho-physiologic disturbances. *International Journal of Family Psychiatry, 3,* 345–356.

Ellis, A. (1974). Group marriage: A possible alternative? In J.R. Smith & L.B. Smith (Eds.), *Beyond monogamy.* Baltimore: Johns Hopkins University Press.

Ember, C.R., & Ember, M. (1973). *Anthropology.* New York: Appleton-Century-Crofts.

Falicov, C., & Karrer, B.M. (1980). Cultural variations in the family life cycle: The Mexican-American family. In E.A. Carter & M. McGoldrick (Eds.), *The family life cycle: A framework for family therapy.* New York: Gardner Press.

Fleck, S. (1980). Family functioning and family pathology. *Psychiatric Annals, 10,* 17–35.

Haviland, W.A. (1978). *Cultural anthropology* (2nd ed.). New York: Holt, Rinehart, & Winston.

Hawkes, G.R., & Taylor, M. (1975). Power structure in Mexican and Mexican-American farm labor families. *Journal of Marriage and the Family, 37,* 807–811.

Hoebel, E.A. (1972). *Anthropology: The study of man.* New York: McGraw-Hill.

Hoffman, L. (1981). The perverse triangle in different cultures. In L. Hoffman, *Foundations of family therapy: A conceptual framework for systems change.* New York: Basic Books.

Hsu, F.L.K. (1972). Kinship and ways of life: An exploration. In F.L.K. Hsu (Ed.), *Psychological anthropology.* New Edition (pp. 509–567). Cambridge, MA: Schenkman.

Hsu, J., & Tseng, W.S. (1974). Family relations in classic Chinese opera. *International Journal of Social Psychiatry, 20,* 159–172.

Hsu, J., Tseng, W.S., Ashton, G., McDermott, J.F., Jr. & Char, W. (1985). Family interaction patterns among Japanese-Americans and Caucasian-Americans in Hawaii. *American Journal of Psychiatry, 142,* 577–581.

Ingoldsby, B.B. (1980). Emotional expressiveness and marital adjustment: A cross-cultural analysis. *Journal of Comparative Family Studies, 11,* 501–515.

Koch-Nielsen, I. (1980). One-parent families in Denmark [Special issue]. *Journal of Comparative Family Studies, 11,* 17–29.

Lefaucheur, N. (1980). Single-parenthood and illegitimacy in France. [Special issue]. *Journal of Comparative Family Studies, 11,* 31–48.

Levine, N., & Sangree, W.H. (1980). Conclusion: Asian and African systems of Polyandry [Special issue]. *Journal of Comparative Family Studies, 11*(3), 385–410.

Lewis, J.M., Beavers, W.R., Gossett, J.T., & Phillips, V.A. (1976). *No single thread: Psychological health in family systems.* New York: Brunner/Mazel.

Lewis, J.M., & Looney, J.G. (1983). *The long struggle: Well-functioning working-class Black families.* New York: Brunner/Mazel.

Lopata, H.Z. (1971). *Occupation: Housewife.* New York: Oxford University Press.

Minuchin, S. (1974). *Families and family therapy.* Cambridge, MA: Harvard University Press.

Murdock G.P. (1967). Ethnographic atlas: A summary. *Ethnology, 6,* 109–236.

Nanda, S. (1980). *Cultural anthropology.* New York: Van Nostrand.

Navran, L. (1967). Communication and adjustment in marriage. *Family Process, 1,* 173–184.

Nuckolls, C.W. (1993). *Siblings in South Asia: Brothers and sisters in cultural context.* New York: Guilford Press.

Olson, D.H., McCubbin, H.I., Barnes, H., Larsen, A., Muxen, M., & Wilson, M. (1983). *Families: What makes them work.* Beverly Hills, CA: Sage.

Rossi, A.S. (1972). Family development in a changing world. *American Journal of Psychiatry, 128,* 1057–1066.

Tashakkori, A., & Mehryar, A.H. (1982). Different roles of parents in the family: As reported by a group of Iranian adolescents. *Journal of Marriage and the Family, 44,* 803–809.

Tseng, W.S. (Ed.). (1986). *Culture and mental health in Micronesia.* Honolulu: University of Hawaii School of Medicine, Department of Psychiatry.

Tseng, W.S., & Hsu, J. (1972). The Chinese attitude toward parental authority as expressed in Chinese children's stories. *Archives of General Psychiatry, 26,* 28–34.

Tseng, W.S., & Hsu, J. (1991). *Culture and family: Problems and therapy.* New York: Haworth Press.

Visher, J.S., & Visher, E.B. (1982). Stepfamilies and stepparenting. In F. Walsh (Ed.), *Normal family process.* New York: Guilford Press.

Willie, C.V., & Greenblatt, S.L. (1978). Four "classic" studies of power relationships in Black families: A review and look to the future. *Journal of Marriage and the Family, 40,* 691–694.

Winkler, I., & Doherty, W.J. (1983). Communication styles and marital satisfaction in Israeli and American couples. *Family Process, 22,* 221–228.

4

Child Development and Enculturation

I. INTRODUCTION

Historically, laymen as well as scholars have paid little attention to psychological development in childhood. It has generally been considered that children are children, and their psychological development does not deserve attention until they become adults. According to B. B. Whiting and Whiting (1975), available reports by anthropologists, missionaries, and colonial administrators about other cultures were scant when it came to children, but there was enough material to indicate wide variations in the nature of the social and physical environment that individuals of different cultures experienced from birth to adulthood. The Freudian assumptions that experiences during infancy and childhood, associated with patterns of child rearing by primary caregivers, have a significant effect on adult personality have stimulated the study of child-rearing practices and childhood development in various cultures. Although the role of early childhood experience as the determinant for adult personality has not been considered an exclusive factor by contemporary students of personality, the importance of knowing a person's developmental background is still stressed by clinicians as one way of understanding the nature of behavior. This chapter does not intend to comprehensively review the subject of child development from a cultural perspective. The aim is rather to offer some cultural examples to illustrate how the cultural environment produces different early life experiences, which, in turn, contribute to later thought and behavior.

II. CROSS-CULTURAL STUDY OF CHILD DEVELOPMENT

First, let us realize that numerous approaches have been taken by anthropologists and behavioral scientists concerning child development and the examination of child development from a cross-cultural perspective. As indicated by pioneer anthropologists Margaret Mead and Martha Wolfenstein in *Childhood in Contemporary Culture* (1955), these approaches can be divided into field observational studies, child-rearing literature review, examination of fantasies for and about children (in fairy tales and other children's stories), analysis of children's imaginative productions, interviews with parents and children, and clinical studies. In this chapter, the cross-cultural study of child development will be examined from the following perspectives.

A. Review of Literature on Child-Rearing Practices

Different child-rearing practices can be examined and compared through existing reports by anthropologists, based on their field work around the globe. As mentioned previously [Chapter 2: Culture and Society (Section I,B)], an anthropological filing system for world ethnographic samples, the *Ethnographic Atlas,* has been established at Yale University by George Peter Murdock (1957). The atlas is based on reports from anthropologists' field work. A total of 565 cultural groups have been identified around the globe and recorded. Among the many kinds of information recorded, there is information about child-rearing practices observed in different cultures, which serves as a resource for review and investigation.

The advantage of this approach is that field samples from vast and diversified cultural units can be compared to decrease the risk of overgeneralization. However, the material from such a resource suffers from the information being gathered by different observers and reporters, who initially used their own criteria and categorizations in collecting and describing the information obtained. The reports are retrospective and do not follow standardized procedures. They rely basically on the field workers' observations and reports, which may be subject to the observers' skills, sensitivities, biases, and opportunities.

B. Observational Study of Child Development

In contrast to the method just described, observational study emphasizes the importance of direct observation by the researcher (J.W.M. Whiting & Child, 1953). The information is gathered according to predetermined methods and criteria, so it is not subjective and allows for objective comparison. There

have been several studies carried out in this way that deserve mention here.

1. Whiting and Whiting's Six-Culture Study

In order to answer the academic question, "Are children brought up in societies with different customs, beliefs, and values radically different from each other?" a well-planned field observation was conducted by a team of investigators under the leadership of Beatrice B. Whiting and John W.M. Whiting (1975). It studied children of six cultures from selected sites at Taira (Okinawa), Tarong (the Philippines), Khalapur (India), Nyansongo (Kenya), Juxtlahuuaca (Oaxaca), and Orchard Town in New England (USA). The total sample consisted of 67 girls and 67 boys between the ages of 3 and 11. Having established the daily routine, the observers began collecting samples of the behavior of the children. Each child's behavior was described in a 5-min behavior sample. No more than one observation was made per child per day, and each child was observed a minimum of 14 times over a period of several months to a year. Transcultural categories describing social interaction were used for description and coding of observed behavior. The category of social acts included acts sociably, insults, offers help, reprimands, offers support, seeks dominance, seeks help, seeks attention, suggests, acts responsibly, assaults sociably, touches, and assaults.

The analysis of obtained data yielded two dimensions for scoring: behavior Dimension A (nurturant-responsible vs dependent-dominant) and behavior Dimension B (sociable-intimate vs authoritarian-aggressive). Based on these two behavior dimensions, the social behavior of the children in the six cultures could be arranged into four groups. As illustrated by Table 4-1, children in Nyansongo (Kenya) had low scores in both Dimensions A and B; children in Khalapur (India) and Taira (Okinawa) had high scores in Dimension A, but low scores in Dimension B; children in Tarong and Juxtlahuaca had low scores in Dimension A, but high scores in Dimension B; whereas children in Orchard Town had high scores in both Dimensions A and B. This supports the view that culture has a considerable effect on the social interac-

TABLE 4-1 **Dimensions of Children's Behavior in Six Cultures**—Household structure, the socioeconomic system, and two dimensions of social behavior [From B.B. Whiting & W.M. Whiting, *Children of Six Cultures: A Psycho-cultural Analysis.* Harvard University Press, 1975, used with permission].

Household Structure

	Non-nuclear	Nuclear	
Simpler	Nyansongo (Kenya)	Tarong (Philippines) Juxtlahuaca (Mexico)	Nurturant-responsible
Complex	Khalapur (India) Taira (Okinawa)	Orchard Town (United States)	Dependent-dominant
	Authoritarian-aggressive	Sociable-intimate	

Socioeconomic System (left axis) · **Behavior Dimension A** (right axis)

Behavior Dimension B

tion patterns manifested by children of school age. The findings further illustrate that the complexity of the socioeconomic system is a cultural feature that determines the cultures falling either high or low in social behavior in Dimension A. Also, variations in household structure — either nuclear or nonnuclear — distinguish the two types of cultures whose children differed in social behavior in Dimension B.

Concerning the comparison of children of different cultures, as pointed out by B. B. Whiting and Whiting (1975, p. 174), two extreme views have been held by scholars in the past. One emphasized that because all children are human, the same developmental process and sequences apply to children of all cultures. Thus, differences in the rate of development or the development finally attained, if they occur at all, are of minor importance. The opposing view was that culture has such a profound effect that developmental sequences from one culture to another cannot be compared. Whiting and Whiting indicated that both these posi-

tions, taken in the extreme, are false, but that there is some truth in each. Their six-culture study indicated that children brought up in one type of culture behave in similar ways, but that children from contrasting types of cultures have score distributions that differ significantly. They also commented that the social behavior of the children of each cultural type usually was compatible with adult role requirements. They speculated that values are apparently transmitted to the child before the age of 6, as the younger children in their sample were already behaving in accordance with the expectations of their cultures.

2. Caudill's Study of Mother–Infant Interactional Behavior in Japan and America

In order to investigate how early in the lives of infants, and in what ways, cultural differences become manifest in behavior, an American cultural anthropologist, William Caudill, undertook a cross-cultural investigation of maternal care and infant behavior in Japan and America. Caudill and Weinstein (1969) selected a matched sample of 30 Japanese and 30 American 3- to-4-month-old infants — equally divided by sex, all first-born, and all from intact middle-class families living in urban settings — and carried out an observational study in the homes of these infants from 1961 to 1964.

Methodologically, the investigator visited the houses with the intention of observing the mother–infant interaction in their ordinary daily lives. The mother was instructed to go about her normal routine in the home, including caring for her baby. The investigator worked with each family for 2 days, 4 hr each day — in the morning on the first day and in the afternoon on the second day. A time-sampling procedure was adopted, i.e., one observation of approximately 1 sec in duration was made every 15th sec in a set of 40 predetermined variables concerning the behavior of the infant and the caretaker.

The results revealed that there are no significant differences in the amount of time awake, sucking on the breast or a bottle, or intake of food. Thus, there are areas of similarity in both cultures in terms of the biological needs of all of the infants, and the necessity for all of the mothers to care for those needs. Beyond this, however, the differences lay in the styles in which the infants and mothers behaved in the two cultures. The American mothers seemed to take more lively and stimulating approaches to their babies, positioning the infant's body and looking at and chatting with the infant more. The Japanese mothers, in contrast, were present more with the baby, in general, and seemed to have more soothing and quieting approaches, as indicated by greater lulling and more carrying in the arms and rocking.

According to their observations, the Japanese babies seemed passive and usually lay quietly, with occasional unhappy vocalizations, while the mothers tried to sooth and quiet them, and to communicate with them physically rather than verbally. However, the American infants were more active, happily vocal, and explored their environments more, while their mothers did more looking at and chatting with their babies. They seemed to stimulate their babies to activity and vocal response. Caudill explained that such patterns of mother–infant interaction correlated with cultural patterns. That is, Japanese are more group oriented and interdependent in their relations with others, whereas Americans are more individual oriented and independent.

Caudill's method of investigation—directive observation of behavior at the microscopic level—was not only a landmark for cross-cultural studies of child development, it also offered support for the theory that child-rearing patterns had a close relationship to the formation of basic personality in adulthood.

C. QUESTIONNAIRE SURVEY OF CHILD DEVELOPMENT

Direct observation of child behavior is time-consuming and applicable only to a relatively small number of subjects. In contrast, a questionnaire survey permits the study of a large sample within a relatively short time span and with a limited amount of energy. It also favors the possibility of longitudinal study by follow-up surveys to collect information about the process of development — an important perspective with regard tochildren.

1. Ten-Year Follow-Up Survey of Single and Nonsingle Children in China

In order to prevent a potential population explosion, China started a "one-couple–one-child" family planning policy in 1980. It drastically changed people's concepts and attitudes toward child-bearing — from the traditional value of "having as many children as possible to have more helpers in the household" to having "only one child for the sake of society." As a result, there has been a considerable change in family constellations and parent–child relationships, with the tendency for parents to indulge their "only" child. As these single children grow up without siblings, a challenging question for study becomes the extent to which this change in their early socialization will affect their personality development.

It was under these circumstances that a longitudinal follow-up study was undertaken in Nanjing, China (Tao et al., 1995; Tseng et al., 1988, 2000). Children of preschool age were surveyed and the study was followed up in four waves for 10 years, until the children reached the age of 15. The Chinese version of Achenbach's Child Behavior Checklist (CBCL) was used for the surveys, and information was obtained from the parents' assessments of their children's behavior. From a cross-cultural point of view, it was found that the factor structure and norm for data were considerably different from Achenbach's original study, which was based on a survey of American children. A Chinese version of the factor structure had to be applied.

The results indicated that if the nature of behavior problems was analyzed on the spectrum of introverted and extroverted, single children tended to manifest introverted behavior problems, in contrast to children with siblings, who manifested extroverted behavior problems. This was rather persistent through the different developmental stages of preschool, early school, late school, and puberty. This tendency was found to be more prominent for boys. However, when the total scores of behavior problems were examined, it revealed that, for boys, the scores tended not only to decline but the differences between single and nonsingle boys diminished when they reach adolescence. This was not so for girls; single girls maintained relatively higher scores for behavior problems than nonsingle girls even when they reached adolescence (Tseng et al., 2000). The findings supported the general observation that, in China, a son was valued as the future successor of the family. As a single child, he tended to be overprotected and indulged by his parents and grandparents while he was young, and tended to develop behavior problems of an introverted rather than an extroverted nature. However, associated with socialization after school age, the impact on a single son diminished gradually with growth. However, this was not the situation for single girls. Cultural attitudes toward the gender and number of children, plus the family constellation, affected the personality develop-

ment of children. Unfortunately, no similar study has been carried out in other cultures to determine to what extent this situation might occur in other cultural settings.

2. Cross-Comparison of Indigenous and Majority Children

Some questionnaire studies have been carried out cross-ethnically to compare not the developmental process itself, but the behavior problems between indigenous children versus majority children in the same society. In the arctic part of Scandinavia, there are indigenous people called the Samis (formerly Lapps). In Norway, they live either in the coastal or in the highland areas. The Sami in coastal regions have become a minority in the community, and many of them have lost their ethnic identity as well as their language as the result of assimilation. The Sami in the highlands have maintained their majority status because the process of assimilation was not strong. Kvernmo and Heyerdahl (1998) administered the Youth Self-Report (YSR) and Achenbach's CBCL to junior high school students of Norwegian adolescents (as the majority group) and Sami adolescents (as the indigenous group). The results indicated that Sami adolescents, particularly those living in assimilated ethnic communities in coastal areas, reported more behavior problems than Norwegian adolescents. They concluded that ethnic factors have a significant impact on behavior problems in indigenous minority adolescents living in a multiethnic context.

In Canada, a similar investigation was carried out by Dion, Gotowiec, and Beiser (1998) regarding North American native and nonnative (mostly Caucasian) children. Achenbach's CBCL and the Diagnostic Interview Schedule for Children (DISC) were used to investigate children in grades 2 and 4 in primary schools. The results showed that, according to parent ratings and child self-reports, there were no native versus nonnative differences noted in levels of conduct disorder symptoms. However, according to teachers, nonnative teachers rated higher levels of conduct disorder symptoms among native students compared with nonnative students. The investigators raised the issue that cultural distance may introduce a negative bias in teachers' cross-ethnic evaluation of native children's behavior problems.

D. Comparison of Children's Stories

Methodologically, comparing children's stories is an entirely different approach. Popular children's stories in various cultures are examined to assess the major themes emphasized. This approach takes the view that children's stories, told by adults to children, reflect the issues that concern the parents regarding their children. They also reveal the common themes that are enjoyed by children to fulfill their emotional needs. Certainly, this is an indirect way to examine the psychology of children. It is one of the most convenient ways to examine the psychological world of children cross-culturally (and by distance), as long as children's stories are available for analysis. Fairy tales, or other forms of children's stories, such as legends or myths, as "primary thinking products" usually reveal the deep-rooted emotions and drive, without the disguises of "secondary thinking products" used by adults. Folk drama or plays that are enjoyed by children can be included in the study as well. Thus, an analysis of child-related cultural products offers a convenient way to explore the in-depth psychology centering around the children. However, it should be pointed out that, methodologically, the downside of this approach is the matter of how to select representative stories and how to interpret the meanings that are expressed in them without cultural bias.

There are many children's stories and plays found in various cultures that deal with variations of the parent–child triangular theme. For instance, the story of Jack and the beanstalk, a well-known fairy tale in Europe and America, deals with a boy who conquers a giant (father figure) and takes his treasure from him, with assistance from his mother (in cutting the beanstalk and killing the giant). The peach-boy story, popular in Japan, describes a boy who, with his fol-

lowers, a dog, a bird, and a monkey, goes out to an island to conquer a devil and take his treasure also. The boy was born from a peach found floating in a river by a childless couple, but, in the story, there is no direct involvement of the mother in killing the devil. It was the boy's followers (subordinate peers) who assisted him in successfully attacking the giant devil. In an similar Chinese story of a "monkey," an omnipotent monkey (phallic symbol of a boy, born from a still stone) defies authority (the Jade Emperor and Buddha in heaven) and is punished by being put under a huge mountain. The only way for him to make up for his wrongdoing is to escort a monk on a dangerous journey to the West to bring the Buddhist bible back to China. He does this and, after completing his task, he is transformed into a human, symbolizing his growth and maturity. But there is no mother figure present in this story, from the beginning to the end. Only the issue of "omnipotence" is addressed, involving the paternal (authority)–son relation without the third figure of a mother. Thus, in these three stories, there is the common underlying thread of the triangular struggle of a boy, yet the mother figure in the stories varies from explicit presence to nonpresence.

Actually, many Western fairy tales, rooted in northern Europe, describe triangular situations involving girls. Snow White and Sleeping Beauty are two well-known stories. The triangular theme is explicit, even though the mother figure is often split into good and bad (as represented by the wicked stepmother or witch).

The *Garuda* story, a popular folk drama often performed with shadow puppets in south Asia, including Indonesia, Malaysia, and Thailand, and in India, is a triangular story as well. It describes a prince who is exiled to a jungle for 14 years by his aged father, the king, under pressure from his stepmother, the queen. The queen wants her own son to succeed as ruler of the kingdom. The young prince and his wife, joined by his sympathetic younger brother, are forced to live in the jungle for many years. One day, the wife, because of her beauty, is abducted by an evil king with magic powers from another kingdom. The prince, with assistance from the friendly king of a neighboring kingdom, who has trained monkey soldiers, is able to kill the evil king and his giant soldiers and rescue his wife. He is able to return to his home kingdom and take the crown back from his friendly half-brother, who is loyally awaiting his return. Double triangular themes appear in this popular folk drama, namely, the father–(step)mother–son triangle and the husband–wife–(evil) father. It is the father figure who is split (or projected) into the aged, good-hearted king–father and forced to exile his own son, and the evil king with magical powers who abducts the prince's pretty young wife. Despite the parent–child conflict, interestingly enough, the brother–brother relationship is portrayed as a friendly and loyal one in the story. The triangular themes are enjoyed by adults as well as children in this often-told folk story.

A psychiatrist, Julius E. Heuscher (1963), analyzed fairy tales. As a clinician, he pointed out that a dream is a psychic expression of *one individual,* whereas a fairy tale is an expression of the experiences of *a whole cultural group* (p. 31). He also stresses that all the elements of the tales, even the tiniest details, can be presumed to have been preserved because of their meaningfulness to the collective cultural group. He grouped and analyzed Western fairy tales (mostly of German origin) according to human development. For example, *Hansel and Gretel* (about two small children who are driven away from home due to a food short-age and lost in the forest) is described as a "pre-Oedipal stage" story; *Little Red Riding Hood* (about a girl who goes from home to visit her grandmother, delib-erately deviating from the path in the forest, and is almost killed by a stranger-wolf, but fortunately is res-cued by a male hunter) as an "Oedipal stage" story; and *Snow White and the Seven Dwarfs* (Snow White is taken from her castle home because her jealous step-mother–queen wants her killed, is lost in the forest, encounters a peer group of nonsexualized male dwarfs, and is finally rescued by a prince from the per-secution of her evil stepmother) as a "post-Oedipal or latent-period" story. He pointed out the similar sce-narios of leaving home and being lost in the forest (symbolic of the dangerous, but real, outer world), which may relate to the geographic setting of central

Europe, and the different themes of child develop-ment.

Inspired by Heuscher's work, Tseng and Hsu (1972) analyzed some representative Chinese chil-dren's stories relating to intergenerational relation-ships during the stages of human development. Dependency, protection, and permission were por-trayed in 24 classic stories of filial piety (except in a reversed way, with the children being filial to their parents); the transition from omnipotent fantasy to a reality orientation in the monkey *(Suen Wuh-kong)* story; the triangular conflict between a child and his parents in the *Shiue Jen-guey* opera story; and the interference by authority with the alliance of a young couple in the White Serpent *(Bai-she Zhuan)* story. The stories illustrate that, with parental authority emphasized in Chinese culture, the parental figure is so strong that children, even on the fantasy level, in children's stories, have difficulty expressing defiance of authority openly and successfully.

E. STUDY OF CHILDREN'S TEMPERAMENTS

Recently, a new subject has gained considerable attention and provoked investigation among scholars in the field of child development: child temperament. It has been discovered that, even in infancy, a baby demonstrates a certain temperament. As early as 1969, Freedman and Freedman compared the behavior of Chinese-American and Caucasian-American new-borns in New York. They reported that although new-born infants of both racial backgrounds had similar levels of central nervous system development at the time of their observation, the Chinese-American infants, in contrast to the Caucasian-American infants, were found to be calm, stable, without too much vari-ation in their responses. In 1978, in Boston, Kagan, Kearsley, and Zelazo, observed 1-year-old Asian and Caucasian babies. They reported that the Asian babies tended to make less dramatic responses to visual or auditory stimulation, were less vocal, and smiled less compared to the Caucasian babies. These studies stimulated other cross-ethnic investigations of children's temperaments.

An objective method has been developed by Kagan and Snidman (1991) to investigate infants at the age of 4 months: a standardized stimulation of language, movement objects, smell, sound, and sudden noise is given according to a specific protocol, and the responses made by the infants are recorded for study. Based on this method, studies have been conducted of infants in Boston (USA), Doublin (Ireland), and Beijing (China). According to Wang, Shen, and Chang (1997), the Chinese baby, in contrast to the American baby or the Irish baby, made fewer movement responses (11.2% vs 48.6%, and 36.7%, respectively), smiled with less vocalization (8.1% vs 31.4%, and 31/1%, respectively), and cried less (1.1% vs 7.0%, and 2.9%, respectively) in response to external stimulation during the investigation. This supports the previous reports of Freedman and Freedman (1969) and Kagan and colleagues (1978) on their observations.

In order to study small children (around the ages of 3 to 7), child psychiatrists Thomas and Chess (1968) developed the Parent Temperament Questionnaire for the study of children's temperaments in their New York longitudinal study. Based on the patterns of temperament, Thomas and Chess distinguished three basic groups of children: "easy temperament" babies, "difficult temperament" babies, and "slow-to-warm-up" babies. According to the mediate scores, the "intermediate easy" and "intermediate difficult" groups can be identified in a total of five groups. These different patterns of temperament attributed to the babies influence the way the baby is cared for by caregivers, and possibly continuously affect the formation of adult behavior. In other words, they are genetically influenced and biological in nature. However, there is still room for concern from a cross-cultural perspective. It is worthwhile to explore any difference in distribution of these identified temperament groups among different ethnic-racial groups and how the parents deal with different temperament babies in different cultural settings.

When small children's temperaments were investigated through parents' ratings using Thomas and Chess's questionnaire, data reported from American and European resources (McDevitt & Carey, 1978; Person & McNeil, 1988; Thomas & Chess, 1968) indicated that the distribution of the three major types among Caucasian children is about 9 to 16% for difficult temperament children, 33 to 43% for easy temperament children, and 4 to 17% for slow-to-warm-up children. However, among Chinese children in Beijing, Wang and colleagues (1997) reported that the distribution of easy temperament children and slow-to-warm-up children is similar to that of the Caucasian children, whereas the percentage of difficult temperament is 7%, a lower range than among Caucasian children. Thus, when babies reached the age of small children, the distribution of different temperament patterns remained the same as those found in the 4-month infant group—namely Chinese children overall tend to manifest more calm, quiet behavior than Caucasians. This supports the view that there is a biological foundation for having a different temperament based on which behavior responses are shaped by culture.

III. CROSS-CULTURAL ASPECTS OF DEVELOPMENTAL THEORIES

In order to understand individual psychological growth, different developmental theories have been proposed by scholars for the interpretation of psychological development. These include Freud's psychosexual theory, Erikson's psychosocial theory, and Piaget's cognitive theory. Among them, it is considered that the former two theories are more subject to culture influences than the latter one. Many cultural anthropologists, based on their field work around the world, have pointed out that existing developmental theories based on people in central Europe and America are biased and therefore limited from a cultural perspective and need revision and expansion (Jacobs, 1964, pp. 133–158; Shrier, Hsu, & Yang, 1996a).

These developmental theories will be elaborated here from a cross-cultural perspective.

A. Psychosexual Development Theory by Sigmund Freud

The psychosexual development theory proposed by Sigmund Freud is focused on the biological-drive aspect of individual development and is regarded by Freud and his followers as universally applicable due to the underlying biological nature of human beings. However, even Freud himself speculated that, due to the individual's unique developmental course, the drive that emerges in each developmental stage may be subject to variations.

1. Oral Stage

As described earlier, developmental study has revealed that different patterns of temperament have been observed among infants even in the earliest stage of their lives. Categorically, babies can be identified and grouped as "easy babies" and "difficult babies" according to the basic temperament they manifest. The differences of temperament not only shape the infants' behavior patterns, but, at the same time, influence the way the babies interact with and are cared for by their primary caretakers. Furthermore, cross-ethnic or -racial comparative studies have pointed out that the distribution of different temperamental groups varies among different ethnic groups. Therefore, it can be speculated that temperament will affect the child-rearing pattern during the oral stage. For instance, as Japanese babies tend to be more quiet than American babies (Caudill & Weinstein, 1969), and the Chinese have a relatively lower percentage of "difficult children" (Wang et al., 1997), it is reasonable to speculate that Asian mothers have a relatively easier job raising their babies in the early stages.

It is observed that how a baby is raised by its primary caretaker differs in different societies. In some cultures, the baby is more or less left alone in a crib or on a bed, whereas in others, the baby is carried by the mother on her back or on her side most of the time, even when the mother is working in the house or out in the field, so there is close and long-term physical contact. In many cultures, the baby is cared for by an older sister or brother, or by a grandmother, rather than by the mother, resulting in the baby being raised in a different way. As pointed out by Jacobs (1964, p. 137), grandparents, aunts or uncles, or older children are assigned responsibility for the care of babies in many societies, supplementing or even substituting for the parents. This has raised the question of the psychological consequences for babies who are cared for in the early stages of their lives by a plurality of people other than, or, at least, in addition to nuclear family members.

Even the mother–infant interaction within a nuclear family may differ in different cultures. As revealed by Caudill's observational investigation of mother–infant interaction in Japan and America (described previously), the infant's psychological development is shaped differently in different cultural settings. In Japan, a baby is raised in a way that suggests the mother wants to have a quiet and contented baby. In contrast, the American mother raises her baby as if she wants to have a vocal and active baby. Although the biological needs of the babies are similar (or universal), coupled with the potential variations of temperament, the way the babies are cared for, nourished, and gratified by their primary caretakers is subject to considerable variation.

How babies are fed, nourished, and weaned also varies in different cultural environments. For instance, in most industrialized societies, as the mother has to return to work at an outside work place, the baby is shifted early to bottle feeding, rather than being breast-fed. The baby may even be fed by bottle from the very beginning. For the sake of convenience, weaning is enforced early, whereas, in many agricultural societies, the baby is breast-fed and there is no rush to wean. Actually, the baby is allowed to suck the breast, or play with the breast, even after the baby has started to take solid food. It is not surprising to see a child of age 4 or 5 still permitted to play with the mother's breast. Although, according to Freud's theory, the different patterns of feeding may affect psychological development, by influencing different ways of gratifying oral needs, sophisticated investigation has not yet been conducted to validate such speculation.

In his work regarding child development, anthropologist J.M. Ingham (1996, pp. 70–73) has reviewed the subject of transitional objects from cross-cultural perspectives. He has pointed out that relations with inanimate objects may reflect the child's relation with his caregivers and his sense of security. The phenomena of transitional objects vary among different ethnic-cultural groups, depending on the child's experiences in his environment. Gadini (1970) carried out a study comparing 682 rural Italian children with 450 urban Italian children (living in Rome) and 52 non-Italian children (mostly Anglo-Saxon) living in Rome as family members of foreigners there. He found that only 4.9% of the rural Italian children were attached to inanimate objects, as opposed to 31.1% of the urban Italian children and 61.5% of the foreign urban children. He explained that, in Italy, more of the rural children, in comparison with foreign children, were breast-fed and they were breast-fed for more months than the foreign children who were breast-fed. More rural children slept in their parents' bed or room and more were rocked to sleep. As for the difference between rural and urban Italian children, he noted that fewer urban Italian babies were breast-fed and the ones who were breast-fed were nursed for fewer months than the children in the rural group. About the same percentage of urban as rural Italian children slept with their parents, but fewer were rocked to sleep. Based on the assumption that maternal closeness and availability correlated negatively with the occurrence of substitutive phenomena, Gaddini demonstrated clearly that, based on rural–urban and national–foreign group differences, there were substantial differences in the manifestation of transitional objects that were explained by different child-rearing patterns.

2. Anal Stage

From cross-cultural field observation, it has been demonstrated that toilet training of small children

varies in different societies. Among people living in urban settings, or close residential areas, babies tend to be toilet trained early and strictly. In rural areas, there is less concern for early toilet training. Small children are allowed to excrete at ease outside the house.

It is clear that toilet training is merely one of the aspects associated with the anal stage. As stressed by Jacobs (1964, p. 138), toilet training and weaning may comprise only a small fraction of the emotional experiences and lessons during the anal stage. From a cross-cultural perspective, numerous issues may be related to the task of motor-sphincter control during the anal stage. Walking, climbing, canoeing, swimming, or riding (in some pastoral societies) are some of the basic motor development activities required in many societies, even at this early stage, rather than toilet training.

3. Phallic Stage

As mentioned previously, after the psychosexual theory was proposed by Freud, attracting the attention of social and behavioral scientists, the question was soon raised as to what extent the concept of Oedipal phenomena can be applied to various cultures. It has been speculated that, depending on the sexual attitudes that exist in the environment, there will be different courses of psychological development in regard to the phallic stage. It is also considered that it will be subject to variations based on the family system and structures that shape the parent–child relationship.

Scholars' behavior theories may be influenced by their historical and cultural backgrounds. Jacobs (1964, p. 141) suspected that Freud's Oedipal complex theory is perhaps the cultural product of Victorian societies. The child responds to his Victorian mother's seductivenss and protectiveness and to his Victorian father's authoritarianism, jealousy, and resentment of a diminutive young rival for his wife's affection. He speculated that in Victorian Europe, Oedipal behavior was generated and magnified by culturally shaped behavior.

The cultural anthropologist B. Malinowski (1927), based on his field study of the Trobriand Islands in

Melanesia near Australia, reported that in a matrilineal society, where the family lineage is traced from mother to daughter (rather than from father to son, as in a patrilineal system), the relationship between the son and the mother's brother (maternal uncle) is more intense than between the son and his own biological father. Associated with this matrilineal family system, the bond between brother and sister is an important one. An incest taboo between brother and sister is observed to protect against this bond. The son's relationship with his own biological father is rather distant. A boy, after age 6 or 7, will visit his uncle's village and receive training in farming from the uncle. Although people there claim that they seldom have dreams, Malinowski was able to collect some dreams from children. He found that boy children tend to have dreams wishing for the death of their brothers—potential rival subjects. If they have sexual dreams, the object is usually their own sister, with whom they are forbidden to be too intimate. Thus, based on the family system, the person involved in a triangular theme will vary and the person in conflict may be replaced.

Obeyesekere (1990) reviewed myths observed in Hindu and Buddhist cultures in south Asia regarding the father–son relationship theme. By comparison, he revealed that, in Hindu mythic traditions, fathers may kill sons, whereas in Buddhist myths, sons are more apt to express hostility toward their fathers. He interpreted that this difference in father–son relations projected in cultural products may reflect the greater subordination of the son to the family in Hindu culture than in Buddhist.

Chinese-American anthropologist F.L.K. Hsu (1972), based on cross-cultural knowledge, proposed different primary bonds or dyads existing within different families such as the husband–wife dyad in European-American families, the father–son dyad in Asian families, the mother–son dyad in Hindu families, or the brother–sister dyad in matrilineal societies (such as those in Micronesia). Based on the different dyads that exist in families, Hsu suggested that different personality patterns may be observed. As an extension of this, it may be speculated that the nature of triangular conflict will probably be subject to variation.

Echoing this, cultural psychiatrists Abel and Metraux (1974) pointed out that social structure will also influence the nature of the Oedipus complex.

The impact of culture on the Oedipus complex has been discussed in terms of the solution patterns that may be proposed for the conflict. For instance, the Chinese solution of the triangular conflict, as reflected in operas and fairy tales, sometimes involves the son being defeated, punished, or killed by the father (rather than the father being killed by the son, as reflected in the Western Oedipus story—an appropriate solution to potential parent–child triangular conflict in a society that emphasizes parental respect and authority) (Tseng & J. Hsu, 1972).

4. Latent and Puberty Stages

In many cultures, particularly husbandry or agricultural societies, children are given ample opportunity to work with their parents to learn and participate in actual work, and the latent stage is relatively short for this reason. Children are expected to take adult roles as soon as they can. In contrast, in industrial societies, during the latent period, children are socialized with adults outside of their families (such as schoolteachers, boy scout leaders) and there is less opportunity for direct contact between parents and children.

In many societies, heterosexual interrelations occur very early, as soon as the youngster reaches puberty. In others, inhibition of sexual desire and activity is demanded by the culture for a rather long period, even after puberty. Regarding masturbation, many societies are unlike Europe in their lack of concern over it. As pointed out by Jacobs (1964, p. 140), there are reports that some non-Western people masturbate babies in order to soothe or quiet them. Europeans, in the past, have perceived masturbation as something evil and threatening. This view is not necessarily shared by other cultures.

Based on different family systems and practices, the age for marriage varies greatly among different societies, with that landmark for entering the adult heterosexual stage occurring in a great range of ages [cross-reference to Chapter 3: Marriage and Family (Section II, A–C)].

It needs to be pointed out that the psychosexual development theory presented by psychoanalysts is very male-child centered. The potential differences between female children and male children is not fully elaborated, only slightly in the phallic stage. However, from a cultural perspective, a great difference exists between the life of a male child and that of a female child in terms of psychological development. A thorough study of how cultural attitudes, beliefs, and behavior toward female children may affect their psychological development has not even been started and is awaiting future investigation and elaboration (Shrier et al., 1996b).

B. PSYCHOSOCIAL DEVELOPMENT THEORY BY ERIK ERIKSON

The culture-concerned child psychiatrist E. Erikson (1963), who proposed a theory of psychosocial development, has indicated that the psychosocial view of personality development needs cultural adjustment in terms of the pace of the stages that an individual may go through, and the major tasks that need to be mastered in each stage. Despite his notion, culture modification for psychosocial development has not been examined systematically. Actually, Erikson's theory has been derived merely from his field studies of two American Indian culture groups—a Sioux Indian (a hunting tribe in South Dakota) and Yuro (a fishing and acorn-gathering tribe on the Pacific coast)—in addition to his clinical work with Caucasian children. Thus, from a cross-cultural point of view, the theory is based on knowledge obtained from limited cultural units and is awaiting further expansion and validation from a cultural perspective.

Cross-cultural variations of psychosocial development have been noticed in different cultures. For instance, regarding the muscular-anal stage, it has been pointed out that a sense of shame and collaterality is emphasized with many Asian children, in addi-

tion to autonomy and mastery. Anal discipline through toilet training is less strictly performed, whereas behavior control by means of shame and collaterality is stressed (Tseng & Hsu, 1969/1970).

Margaret Mead's study of adolescent turmoil outside of Euro-American societies was a landmark investigation, revising the psychosocial developmental view. Mead, based on anthropological field work early in her career, indicated that the psychosocial lives of adolescents in Samoa are not as tumultuous as those observed in many Western societies, such as contemporary America. She described youngsters in Samoa as usually going through a relatively calm transition from childhood to adulthood, without drastic changes in the adolescent period.

Relative to the matter of gender identity at the stage of puberty and adolescence, Glimore (1990) conducted a survey of ideas about manhood in various cultures. He found that many societies emphasize masculinity for men, and a good many take this emphasis to extremes. He speculated that exaggerated masculinity tends to occur in a society where an early symbiotic union with the mother is noticed, and the exaggeration of masculinity may represent a defense against the traces of close mother–son ties. However, he also pointed out that psychological reasons alone cannot account for these tendencies. Material conditions are also important. The harsher the environment and the scarcer the resources, the more manhood is stressed as an inspiration and goal.

Concerning the Chinese adolescent, it has been pointed out that for youngsters in the latency period, diligence is stressed, with the inculcation of the desire to achieve (Bond, 1991). This creates a drastic shift in developmental requirements from earlier stages of indulgence. However, drastic psychological turmoil was not often noticed. This might be because the stage of puberty and adolescence is relatively prolonged and the entry to young adulthood delayed. Intense relations and bonds with homosexual peers are permitted and maintained whereas heterosexual relations are suppressed as long as possible (Tseng, 1995).

C. Cognitive Development Theory by Piaget

In contrast to psychosexual or psychosocial theories, Piaget's theory focuses on cognitive development that occurs through a sequence of stages. The development goes through the first (sensory-motor) stage, the second (concrete operational) stage, and the third (formal operations) stage. In each stage, various substages can be identified. Piaget contends that the pattern of cognitive development is universal in terms of the basic structure and sequence of development; physical and social environments, including cultural factors, affect only the chronological age at which the stages are attained.

There is no sufficient cross-cultural investigation yet to validate or challenge the basic assumptions made by Piaget. Yet, as summarized by Dasen and Heron (1981), from a cross-cultural point of view, there is a commonly shared view among scholars that there is little doubt about the universality of the first stage of sensory-motor development, whereas it is much less certain for the last stage of formal operation. There are still a lot of questions awaiting future investigation.

D. Integration

The cross-cultural elaborations made earlier regarding various developmental theories point out that the psychological development of an individual will be subject to basic biological needs, inherited temperament, given social conditions, and also to the cultural system. The cultural system will shape the different emphases in various stages of child development in terms of how a child is raised, what kind of psychological experiences he has to encounter, what kinds of values will be given to him to incorporate, and the kinds of models with which he has to identify in growing into adulthood and becoming a member of society.

In summary, a cross-cultural difference is noticed in terms of the pace of the stages of development, the different emphases that are placed on different stages, and the different significance that may be given to different stages of development. Thus, although it is a universal phenomenon for an individual to develop psychologically and biologically through a basic predetermined sequence, there is considerable variation in the psychological development at each stage. This view of variations in developmental theory is needed for Freud's psychosexual theory, Erikson's psychosocial theory, and perhaps also Piaget's cognitive theory. Among them, the former two theories are more subject to cultural influences and deserve more theoretical clarification, validation, modification, and expansion for cross-cultural application [cross-reference to Chapter 49: Culture and Psychiatric Theories (Section IV, B)].

IV. ENCULTURATION

"Enculturation" is a professional term used by anthropologists to refer to the process through which an individual, starting from early childhood, acquires a cultural system through his environment, particularly from his parents, family, neighbors, school, and society at large. The process occurs as an unconscious introjection or as a conscious learning of ways of thinking, attitudes toward things values, and belief systems. Thus, it is a part of psychological development and growth; however, such a process of enculturation varies from culture to culture in terms of the total cultural system incorporated and integrated.

Although enculturation is an important aspect of psychological development, this subject has not been examined systematically and intensively by behavior or social scientists as an independent variable of psychological growth. There are only fragmented views about such phenomena and processes.

The process of enculturation is considered to take place as soon as an infant starts to incorporate stimulation from outside. However, the process of encultur-

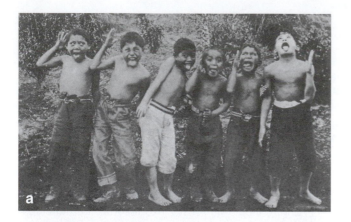

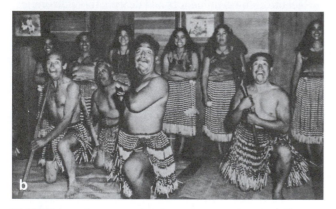

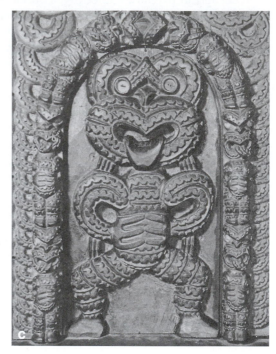

FIGURE 4-1 Encultured behavior patterns. (a) Maori boys in New Zealand practice sticking out their tongues and making sounds with popeyed looks in the belief that such gestures will threaten their enemies and chase away evil. (b) Maori adult males demonstrate the tongue-protruding gesture in the performance of a war dance. (c) These behaviors are portrayed in the image of a protective god, illustrating that culturally patterned behavior is not only practiced during childhood and performed in adulthood, but projected into a cultural product. [From *Anthropology: The study of man,* by E.A. Hoebel. McGraw-Hill, 1972. Courtesy of the American Museum of Natural History Library].

ation becomes active when a child reaches the age of 4 or 5 and has developed sufficient cognitive ability to think and perceive things differently. This coincides with the stage of socialization associated with the experience of schooling when a child is expected to learn more social matters, including etiquette, rules, and views about the community or society at large. It is also the stage when the parents and schoolteachers actively impart their views and attitudes on the youngster. However, the process of enculturation takes a passive form. It is around the adolescent stage, when

the youngster is equipped with the cognitive ability to make subjective criticisms and have preferences about things happening around him, that he or she begins the process of enculturation more or less selectively and actively (see Fig. 4-1).

Clinically, problems of enculturation are observed when a child is faced with incorporating drastically different, or even contradictory, sets of value systems and confusion results. Such confusion occurs when the family provides contradictory value systems, or the surrounding society changes rapidly, so that the value system fluctuates and changes dramatically, making it difficult for the child to follow and integrate it.

V. INITIATION CEREMONY: ENTERING ADULTHOOD

After a person goes through childhood development and reaches puberty, he is more or less ready to enter adulthood. The age for entering adulthood varies considerably in different societies. In general, in primitive or simple societies, a person is recognized as an adult as soon as he (or she) demonstrates the signs of puberty. In contrast, in more developed, modern, or industrialized societies, there is a tendency to delay the landmarks for entering adulthood.

In many primitive societies, certain rituals, such as puberty initiations, are performed to recognize a youngster's entrance into adulthood. In industrialized societies, there are no clear-cut rituals performed. However, there are some occurrences that indirectly imply the step toward adulthood. The stages set up in the educational system — from junior high to senior high, then to college and postcollege — are concrete stages through which the youngsters may progress.

Cultural anthropologists Schlegel and Barry (1979) defined an adolescent initiation ceremony as "some social recognition, in ceremonial form, of the transition from childhood into the next stage." In their review of a cross-cultural sample of over 180 societies, they found that a considerable number of societies lacked any initiations at all. Among those societies surveyed, 30 held initiations only for girls, 17 only for boys, and 46 for both sexes. Thus, initiation ceremonies are more common for females. As pointed out by Ottenberg (1994, p. 353), there is a worldwide trend toward the decreasing importance of traditional initiation rituals.

According to Ottenberg (1994, pp. 353–354), there are several psychological reasons for having initiation ceremonies. In many undeveloped societies, the death rate for children is so high that initiation has a celebratory quality. Many rites mark the change from children's aggressive and largely nonsexual competition to sexual, political, and economic competition, as well as competition over mates and fertility. Needless to say, initiations inevitably emphasize gender distinctions. J.W.M. Whiting, Kluckhohn, and Anthony (1958, p. 361) studied a sample of 55 societies to test some psychoanalytic ideas, assuming that "boys tend to be initiated at puberty in those societies in which they are personally hostile toward their fathers and dependent on their mothers." They proposed that the initiation rites prevent open revolt against the father, break the strong mother attachment, and create a shared identity with adult males. Kitahara (1974) further found out that, if the father sleeps away or in the same house as the mother, but in a different bed, there is likely to be an initiation rite, indicating the importance of sleeping arrangements and the need for a formal rite to signify that stage of development. Initiation rites for puberty have different degrees of severity. It is speculated that when a child is more attached to his parents, there is usually an initiation rite of a severe nature to indicate a clear landmark for moving into adulthood, whereas the reverse is true.

In contrast to rites for males, an important feature of female initiation is the menarche, a specifically timed indicator of potential fertility — an important function for a female. According to anthropologist Judith Brown (1963), approximately one-half of the ethnographic samples from Murdock's world ethnographic sample observed mandatory puberty rites for girls. Cross-culturally it was found that if a society performed virilocal postmarital residence (the wife normally goes to live with her husband's people), there is less chance of having female puberty rites. Removal of a girl from her parental home to her husband's sufficiently signals the status change from unmarried to married. However, if a society practices uxorilocal postmarital residence (the wife brings her husband to live with her in her parents' home) there is more chance that the culture will include female puberty rites. Such rites will help the personal identity transfer from the girl's mother (and her family) to the husband (and his) (Hoebel, 1972, p. 385).

Based on field observations of initiations performed in Papua, New Guinea, Jilek and Jilek-Aall (1978) pointed out that initiation ceremonies help the young to achieve a sense of sexual and sociocultural identity from which feelings of emotional security and social belonging are derived.

VI. MINORITY STATUS AND CHILD DEVELOPMENT

"Minority," as defined in Chapter 2, refers to a relatively smaller group identified against the majority group existing in the society. A minority group tends to be discriminated against by the majority and to suffer from underprivileged and disadvantageous conditions from social, political, economic, and cultural perspectives. The minority group could develop when the native people are invaded and taken over by (militarily superior) outsiders as the consequence of migration into a dominant foreign society or merely as the result of psychological discrimination due to historical paths [cross-reference to Chapter 45: Minority by Ethnicity, Gender, and Others (Section II, A–J)].

The minority group not only suffers from underprivileged social conditions, but also from unfavorable psychological conditions that will directly or indirectly influence the psychology of the minority people, their families, and their children, including the psychological development of the children (Greenfield & Cocking, 1994; Powell, 1983). These disadvantages are derived not only from the phenomenon of discrimination, but also from the cultural gap existing between minority and majority groups. For instance, as pointed out by J.R. Joe (1994, p. 112), many tribes of Native Americans have questioned and/or resisted the dominant (American) society's emphasis on temporal rather than spiritual values, the individual rather than the community, change rather than stability, and what seems like chaos instead of harmony. Concerning Mexican-Americans, Uribe, Levine, and Levine (1994, p. 52) indicated that, traditionally, the Mexicans, in contrast to Euro-Americans, show more hierarchy by age and gender, more emphasis on respect

and obedience, less emphasis on independence and separation during childhood, less social distance between the generation of adults in the family, and greater maintenance of kinship ties throughout the life course. There clearly is a discongruence of cultural values with the dominant group. Such differences make it difficult for the minority people to adjust to the society at large. This in turn not only affects the psychological adjustment of the adults, but also the process of development of their children.

For instance, Greenfield (1994, p. 30) pointed out that, based on the contemporary culture of industrialized society, we have assumed that encouragement of individual independence and school-based cognitive development are the universal goals of development. We fail to realize that, from a cross-cultural perspective, the opposite poles of interdependence and subsistence skills are stressed in other cultures.

It is not only the cultural gap that affects child development, but the (inferior) group identity, which either originated within the group or was given to it by the dominant group, and psychological discrimination by the majority that have a significant negative impact on the development of minority children. This is best illustrated by the situation of *burakumin's* children in Japan. As mentioned in Chapter 2, *burakumin* is a minority group that is discriminated against psychologically by the majority Japanese — simply by historical path and occupational background — even though it shares the same ethnic or racial background as the "Japanese." The children of *burakumin* are not permitted to intermarry with majority Japanese and are also not to engage in occupations other than their own traditional work as animal butchers or shoemakers, even though they may receive higher education and are qualified to work in white-collar jobs. Their parents often discourage their children from pursuing college educations because it serves no practical purpose (De Vos & Wagatsuma, 1969). The power of discrimination certainly affects the psychological development of minority children who are not permitted to seek occupational opportunities beyond their old "dirty" jobs.

VII. IMPACT OF RACE ON CHILD DEVELOPMENT

As explained previously [cross-reference to Chapter 2: Culture and Society (Section I,A,2)], scholars have now taken the view that races are socially and culturally constructed categories that may have little to do with actual biological differences. However, laymen still hold the conviction that race is characterized by certain physical features, such as color of skin, eyes, and hair, facial or body features, or physical size, that distinguishes it from other groups. It is believed that the racial background of an individual is obvious even from the time of birth. Therefore, any physical difference thought to relate to race will strongly impact the psychological development of a child. The influence of "race" on child development is illustrated in two situations: the mixed-race child and the cross-race adopted child. These situations are elaborated further.

A. THE MIXED-RACE CHILD

Clearly, a child becomes "mixed race" as the product of an interracial marriage. The best example is the black–white race-mixed child born to parents with African and Caucasian backgrounds or the Eurasian, a product of a European and an Asian parent. Associated with the increase in travel, international migration, and greater acceptance of interracial unions or marriages, there is an increase in mixed-race children.

The impact of racial mixture on child development is severalfold. How the parents and surrounding people perceive and react to racially hybrid children is one thing, how the interracially married parents are going to raise the child from a bicultural perspective is another. The interracially married couple is potentially interculturally married, i.e., they hold different cultural views, including how to raise their children. Raising and disciplining a child is a challenge for parents who have distinctively different value systems. How a child is going to see and identify himself (or herself) from a racial point of view is another matter.

As the child grows, he may have more than the usual problems achieving identification, or knowing who he is. This is particularly true in an interracial marriage where physical appearances are markedly different, for example, when an Asian-Caucasian child has long, black hair and a high nose.

In the United States in the 1960s, Stevenson and Stewart (1958) studied children's ethnic identification patterns. They found that both white and black preferred the physical characteristics of white children and had more negative attitudes toward black ones. There has been a shift in more recent years to a more positive self-esteem among African-American children in their drawings (Fish & Larr, 1972), but questions still remain. The children's identification with their parents centered on certain overvalued and ill-understood body parts, capacities, and physical characteristics. Thus, in racially mixed marriages, does the girl identify with her mother and the boy with his father, or does white identify with the white and the black with the black? Or does the black identify or seek identification with the white? How much does physical similarity influence identification, in addition to the factors of gender and interpersonal relations? These are questions awaiting further study.

B. CROSS-RACIAL ADOPTION

Cross-racial or heteroracial adoption refers to the situation in which a parent(s) adopts a child or children who has a different racial heritage from that of his adoptive parents. This in contrast to homoracial adoption, which usually occurs. Due to the racial factor, there is a distinctly noticeable difference in the physical appearances between the adoptive parent(s) and the adopted child(ren) that are recognizable from the very beginning, so that the racial issue affects the process of child rearing in certain ways. Because the color of the skin or hair or other physical features is so different, the racial identity issue is a practical one that needs special attention and management. The most common example is when a white parent(s) adopts black children or Asian children. In the process of growing up, the children themselves will react to the differences in physical appearance, as will the adoptive parents and the people surrounding them. Of particular importance will be the adoptive parent(s)' own views and attitudes toward the race of child they adopted.

Hill and Peltzer (1982) suggested that if parents are concerned about raising their heteroracially adopted children, they should examine their own self-esteem and self-concepts, identify their personal racism, and understand the individual and institutional racism in their society and how they will affect their lives.

African-American psychiatrist Ezra Griffith (1995a, 1995b), who has a special concern for this phenomenon, has extensively reviewed the subject from the literature available (Griffith & Silverman, 1995). Some empirical studies have been conducted, which indicated that, despite the concern of some experts, black children adopted by white parents are in general adjusting well. There are no problems in the area of self-esteem. Ethnic and racial identity issues often depend on how the white parents view the black children they adopted. If they openly recognize and feel comfortable about their race, their adopted black children seem to have a sound identity development regarding their racial background.

VIII. CLOSING REMARKS

In this chapter, an effort has been made to elaborate on how children from various cultures, as children of humankind, thrive and grow according to basic biological factors that seek to fulfill their universal needs for development. They also go through certain stages of psychological development in accordance with their biological and physiological conditions. Beyond that, children in different cultures also have different growth experiences associated with different child-rearing practices, parent–child relations, and the external impact of the children's surroundings, including their material, social, and cultural backgrounds. Thus, through these compound influences, children go through development with cultural variations that lead to the formation of a certain group character and the modeling of culturally patterned behavior responses. This subject will be examined further in the following chapter regarding culture and personality.

REFERENCES

Abel, T.M., & Metraux, R. (1974). *Culture and psychotherapy* (pp. 127–128). New Haven, CT: College & University Press.

Bond, M.H. (1991). *Beyond the Chinese face: Insights from psychology.* Hong Kong: Oxford University Press.

Brown, J. (1963). A cross-cultural study of femal initiation rites. *American Anthropologist, 65,* 837–853.

Caudill, W., & Weinstein, H. (1969). Maternal care and infant behavior in Japan and America. *Psychiatry, 32,* 12–43.

Dasen, P.R., & Heron, A. (1981). Cross-cultural tests of Piaget's theory. In H.C. Triandis & A. Heron (Eds.), *Handbook of cross-cultural psychology: Vol. 4. Developmental psychology* (pp. 295–341). Boston: Allyn & Bacon.

De Vos, G.A., & Wagatsuma, H. (1969). Minority status and deviance in Japan. In W. Caudill & T.S. Lin (Eds.), *Mental health research in Asia and the Pacific* (pp. 342–357). Honolulu: East-West Center Press.

Dion, R., Gotowiec, A., & Beiser, M. (1998). Depression and conduct disorder in Native and non-Native children. *Journal of the American Academy of Child and Adolescent Psychiatry, 37*(7), 736–742.

Erikson, E.H. (1963). *Childhood and society* (2nd ed.). New York: Norton.

Fish, J.E., & Larr, C.J. (1972). A decade of change in drawings by black children. *American Journal of Psychiatry, 129*(4), 421–426.

Freedman, D.G., & Freedman, M. (1969). Behavioral differences between Chinese-American and American newborns. *Nature (London), 224,* 1227.

Gadini, R. (1970). Transitional objects and the process of individuation: A study in three different social groups. *Journal of the American Academy of Child Psychiatry, 9,* 347–365.

Glimore, D.D. (1990). *Manhood in the making: Cultural concepts of masculinity.* New Haven, CT: Yale University Press.

Greefield, P.M. (1994). Independence and interdependence as developmental scripts: Implications for theory, research, and practice. In P.M. Greenfield & R.R. Cocking (Eds.), *Cross-cultural roots of minority child development.* Hillsdale, NJ: Erlbaum.

Greenfield, P.M., & Cocking, R.R. (Eds.). (1994). *Cross-cultural roots of minority child development.* Hillsdale, NJ: Erlbaum.

Griffith, E.E.H. (1995a). Culture and the debate on adoption of Black children by White families. In J.M. Oldham & M.B. Riba (Eds.), *American psychiatric press review of psychiatry,* (Vol. 14) (pp. 543–564). Washington, DC: American Psychiatric Press.

Griffith, E.E.H. (1995b). Forensic and policy implications of the transracial adoption debate. *Bulletin of the American Academic Psychiatry and Law, 23*(4), 501–512.

Griffith, E.E.H., & Silverman, I.L. (1995). Transracial adoptions and the continuing debate on the racial identity of families. In H.W. Harris, H.C. Blue, & E.E.H. Grifith (Eds.), *Racial and ethnic identity: Psychological development and creative expression.* New York: Routledge.

Heuscher, J.E. (1963). *A psychiatric study of fairy tales: Their origin, meaning and usefulness.* Springfield, IL: Charles C. Thomas.

Hill, M., & Peltzer, J. (1982). A report of thirteen groups for White parents of Black children. *Family Relations: Journal of Applied Family and Child Studies, 31*(4), 557–565.

Hoebel, E.A. (1972). *Anthropology: The study of man.* New York: McGraw-Hill.

Hsu, F.L.K. (1972). Kinship and ways of life: An exploration. In F.L.K. Hsu (Ed.), *Psychological anthropology.* New Edition (pp. 509–567). Cambridge, MA: Schenkman.

Ingham, J.M. (1996). *Psychological anthropology reconsidered.* Cambridge; UK: Cambridge University Press.

Jacobs, M. (1964). *Pattern in cultural anthropology.* Homewood, IL: Dorsey Press.

Jilek, W.G., & Jilek-Aall, L. (1978). Initiation in Papua New Guinea: Psychohygiene and ethnopsychiatric aspects. *Papua New Guinea Medical Journal, 21*(3), 252–264.

Joe, J.R. (1994). Revaluing native-American concepts of development and education. In P.M. Greenfield & R.R. Cocking (Eds.), *Cross-cultural roots of minority child development.* Hillsdale, NJ: Erlbaum.

Kagan, J., Kearsley, R.B., & Zelazo, P.R. (1978). *Infancy: Its place in human development.* Cambridge, MA: Harvard University Press.

Kagan, J., & Snidman, N. (1991). Temperamental factors in human development. *American Psychologist, 46,* 856–862.

Kitahara, M. (1974). Living quarter arrangements in polygyny and circumcision and segregation of males at puberty. *Ethnology, 13,* 401–413.

Kvernmo, S., & Heyerdahl, S. (1998). Influence of ethnic factors on behavior problems in indigenous Sami and majority Norwegian adolescents. *Journal of the American Academy of Child and Adolescent Psychiatry, 37*(7), 743–751.

Malinowski, B. (1927). *Sex and repression in savage society.* New York: International Library.

McDevitt, S.C., & Carey, W.B. (1978) The measurement of temperament in 3–7 year old children. *Journal of Child Psychology and Psychiatry, 19,* 245–253.

Mead, M., & Wolfenstein, M. (Eds.). (1955). *Childhood in contemporary cultures.* Chicago: University of Chicago Press.

Murdock, G.P. (1957). World ethnographic sample. *American Anthropologist, 59,* 664–687.

Obeyesekere, G. (1990). *The work of culture: Symbolic transformation in psychoanalysis and anthropology.* Chicago: University of Chicago Press.

Ottenberg, S. (1994). Initiations. In P.K. Bock (Ed.), *Handbook of psychological anthropology.* Westport, CT: Greenwood Press.

Person, B.L., & McNeil, L.F. (1988). Frequency and stability of temperament types in childhood. *Journal of Child Psychology and Psychiatry, 27*(5), 619–622.

Powell, G.J (Ed.). (1983). *The psychosocial development of minority group children.* New York: Brunner/Mazel.

Schlegel, A., & Barry, H., III. (1979). Adolescent initiation ceremonies: A cross-cultural code. *Ethnology, 18,* 199–210.

Shrier, D.K., Hsu, C.C., & Yang, X.L. (1996a). Cross-cultural perspective on normal child and adolescent development: Chinese and American. Part I. Introduction, historical overview, normal child and adolescent development, and future directions. In F. Lih Mak & C.C. Nadelson (Eds.), *International Review of Psychiatry* (Vol. 2) (pp. 301–334). Washington, DC: American Psychiatric Press.

Shrier, D.K., Hsu, C.C., & Yang, X.L. (1996b). Cross-cultural perspective on normal child and adolescent development: Chinese and American. Part II: special topics. In F. Lih Mak & C.C. Nadelson (Eds.), *International Review of Psychiatry* (Vol. 2) (pp.335–366). Washington, DC: American Psychiatric Press.

Stevenson, H., & Stewart, E. (1958). A developmental study of racial awareness in young children. *Child Development, 29,* 399–409.

Tao, K.T., Qiu, J.H., Li, B.L., Tseng, W.S., Hsu, J., & McLaughlin, D. (1995). One-child-per-couple family planning and child behavior development: Six-year follow-up study in Nanjing. In T.-Y. Lin, W.S. Tseng, & E.K. Yeh (Eds.), *Chinese society and mental health.* Hong Kong: Oxford University Press.

Thomas, A., & Chess, S. (1968). *Temperament and behavior disorders in children.* New York: New York University Press.

Tseng, W.S. (1995). Psychotherapy for the Chinese: Cultural adjustments. In L.Y.C. Cheng, H. Baxter, & F.M.C. Cheung (Eds.), *Psychotherapy for the Chinese. II* (pp. 1–22). Hong Kong: Chinese University of Hong Kong, Department of Psychiatry.

Tseng, W.S., & Hsu, J. (1969/1970). Chinese culture, personality formation and mental illness. *International Journal of Social Psychiatry, 16*(1), 5–14.

Tseng, W.S., & Hsu, J. (1972). The Chinese attitude toward parental authority as expressed in Chinese children's stories. *Archives of General Psychiatry, 26,* 28–34.

Tseng, W.S., Tao, K.T., Hsu, J., Chiu, J., Yu, L., & Kameoka, V. (1988). Family planning and child mental health in China: The Nanjing survey. *American Journal of Psychiatry, 145*(11), 1396–1403.

Tseng, W.S., Tao, K.T., Hsu, J., Qiu, J.H., Li, B.L., & Goebert, D. (2000). Longitudinal analysis of development among single and non-single children in Nanjing, China: Ten-year follow-up study. *Journal of Nervous and Mental Disease.*

Uribe, F. M. T., Levine, R.A., & Levine, S.E. (1994). Maternal behavior in a Mexican community: The changing environments of children. In P.M. Greenfield & R.R. Cocking (Eds.), *Cross-cultural roots of minority child development.* Hillsdale, NJ: Erlbaum.

Wang, Y.F., Shen, Y.C., & Chang, J.S. (1997). Characteristics of Chinese children's temperament: A series of studies. In W.S. Tseng (Ed.), *Chinese mind and therapy* (pp. 87–109). Beijing: Beijing University and Xieho University United Press (in Chinese).

Whiting, B.B., & Whiting, J.W.M. (1975). *Children of six cultures: A psycho-cultural analysis.* Cambridge, MA: Harvard University Press.

Whiting, J.W.M., & Child, I.L. (1953). *Child training and personality.* New Haven, CT: Yale University Press.

Whiting, J.W.M., Kluckhohn, R., & Anthony, A. (1958). The function of male initiation cermonies at puberty. In E.E. Maccoby, T. Newcomb, & E. Hartly (Eds.), *Readings in social psychology* (3rd ed.). New York: Holt.

5

Personality and Depth Psychology

I. CULTURE AND PERSONALITY

A. CONCEPT OF "PERSONALITY" IN DIFFERENT DISCIPLINES

Prior to a discussion of the cultural aspects of personality, it is important to recognize that the term "personality" is defined considerably differently by different scientific disciplines, particularly psychiatry, psychology, and anthropology.

Psychiatrists consider personality to be the total manifestation of an individual's behavior and mental functions. Very much influenced by psychoanalytic theory, personality is often analyzed from the standpoint of intrapsychic perspectives. It is considered that personality can be examined from different levels of consciousness, including the subconscious and unconscious, and different compartments of functions, namely: the id, ego, and superego. Underlying this view is the assumption that the id is biologically based and universally similar, driven by basic biological instincts and needs. The development of the ego, however, is closely related to reality and based on the patterns of child development experienced by

each individual in his or her personal life. Thus, family and the immediate environment contribute to ego development. In contrast, the formation of the superego is closely related to the ideal value system held by the parents and other members of the social environment. Thus, the concept of personality is primarily based on an individual perspective. Its function is to distinguish the maturity versus the immaturity, or the normality versus the abnormality, of the personality. It recognizes the biological, universal base of personality, yet appreciates more individual variations. Personality in the collective sense is less focused. Due to clinical applications, more attention is paid to deviated or disordered personalities, and a certain typology is used to describe different personality disorders.

Psychologists, however, view personality as an observable behavior pattern of a person that can potentially be measured objectively. Personality is usually subdivided into various parameters of behavior and psychology, such as cognition, motivation, emotion, memory, and will, and assessed as such. Thus, the personality is basically described by profile rather than by typology. The focus is on the individual as well as a group of people.

For anthropologists, personality is very oriented toward collective or group behavior patterns that are unique and distinguishable from those of other groups. Anthropologists' major interest is in finding the common behavior patterns that are shared by the people of a tribe or people living in a relatively small society. The size of the group concerned is relatively manageable and observable by direct contact. The emphasis is not so much on an individual, but on a group of people. Undoubtedly, the existence of universal or pan-cultural aspects of human behavior is recognized, closely related to birth and survival, social interdependence, and gratification and deprivation experiences (Kluckhohn & Murray, 1948). The primary interest of anthropologists is to reveal any unique or characteristic behavior that is manifested by an ethnic group. A wide variety of cultural products, such as folk tales, myths, dramas, literary fiction, customs, taboos, etiquette, and child-rearing patterns, can be used to assess personality in the cultural group from which it was collected. The collective personality may be labeled by typology if the traits are prominent enough. This usually applies to a smaller society. However, when people belong to a larger society, a description of multiple traits is given.

Given their different perspectives on personality, there will be differences in the way psychiatrists, psychologists, and anthropologists will examine the personality of an individual or a collective group. All disciplines recognize a common, universal human behavior pattern, which is rooted primarily in biological factors and subject to genetic inheritance; however, all of them concede that there are considerable differences in personalities among different groups of people that are predominantly influenced by social and cultural factors.

B. POSSIBLE RELATIONSHIP BETWEEN "CULTURE" AND "PERSONALITY"

Singer (1961) reviewed culture and personality studies through the 1950s and revealed dominant themes clustered in several areas regarding the relationship of personality and culture. Among them are the relation of culture to human nature, to typical personality, and to individual personality. Singer himself added two more areas that he thinks deserve attention: the relation of cultural change to personality change and of culture to abnormal personality.

1. Relation of Culture to Human Nature

This theme is concerned with how culture contributes to the formation of human nature as a whole at the universal level. Among anthropologists, there has been a gradual change from the view that "it is not human nature, but only culture" to the more flexible view of the "psychic unit of man." This is based on the position that there are biological similarities in growth, parent–child relations, and the need for affection among human beings. Developed human nature was not explicable entirely on the basis of modal inborn potentialities, but evolved as humans confronted similar realities and environments from birth to death (Tapp, 1981, p. 361).

2. Relation of Culture to Typical Personality

This theme is concerned with how culture contributes to the development of a typical personality among a group of people in a society. The core concept of this approach is that personality is a product of "learning, rather than genetics." This orientation was dominant in the 1940s and 1950s among behavior scientists and led to the development of many theories of configurational personality (Benedict, 1934), basic personality (kardiner, 1945), modal personality (DuBois, 1944), and national character.

3. Relation of Culture to Individual Personality

According to this approach, the study of culture and personality requires an alternating and almost simultaneous use of two different perspectives: that of culture and that of the individual person.

4. Relation of Cultural Change to Personality Change

Facing a rapidly changing society, this approach is concerned with how a change in the culture will contribute to a change in the personality. It takes the view that personality is a continuous process of growth, even after childhood, and is subject to growth and change in changing circumstances. Particularly if there is a great deal of change in the value systems within a society, its members will incorporate such changes into their individual personalities, stimulating new additions to and integrations into their personality configurations.

5. Relation of Culture to Abnormal Personality

This approach is derived from a clinical perspective and explores how culture contributes to the formation of normal and abnormal personalities. The abnormal personality is considered not so much genetically determined or organically induced as a social-norm-deviated personality. The approach is concerned with how the living environment may influence the development of a personality that deviates from the majority of the members of a society.

C. HISTORICAL TRENDS IN THE STUDY OF CULTURE AND PERSONALITY

1. 1920–1935 — Formative Period

Although anthropologists have long been interested in behavior patterns manifested in various cultural settings, the subject of "culture and personality" has been actively discussed among behavior scientists and psychiatrists since the 1920s. Greatly influenced by psychoanalytic theory, particularly the notion that early childhood experience, through patterns of child-rearing by primary caretakers, will shape the mode of behavior in adulthood, many cultural anthropologists engaged in field research. Collaboration between anthropologists and psychiatrists began, and a great deal of literature was produced.

For instance, Bronislaw Malinowski, originally from Poland, took a trip to Melanesia and lived in the Trobriand Islands for 2 years. Based on his observation of aboriginal people there, he published the book, *Sex and Repression in Savage Society* (1927). He reported on the Islands' matrilineal society, in which the family lineage is traced from mother to daughter and the son's relationship with his mother's brother (maternal uncle) is more intense than that with his own biological father. In a matrilineal family system, the bond between brother and sister is an important one. Malinowski reported that in such a society, a boy child tends to dream of the death of his uncle and of having sexual relations with his own sister. Thus, based on the family system, the people involved in a triangular situation will vary and may be replaced.

One of the favorite students of Franz Boas, a young woman anthropologist named Margaret Mead, was dispatched to a remote island in the South Pacific, Samoa, to find out whether the adolescent turmoil observed in a Western society, such as America, exists in a non-Western society. Based on her field observations while living on the island for a couple of years, she reported in her book, *Coming of Age in Samoa* (1928), that adolescents go through the transition to adulthood without the severe emotional turmoil observed in Western society. This supports the notion that child development is subject to cultural influence, particularly in the stage of adolescence.

During this period, a pioneer American woman anthropologist, Ruth Benedict, a doctoral student of Franz Boas, published her well-known book, *Patterns of Culture* (1934). Benedict came to see cultures as integrated amalgams of parts, based on the model of the individual personality. From this assumption, she portrayed the configuration of a culture in terms of integrating psychological themata, just as a clinical psychologist might describe the personality structure of a person. A landmark publication, the book (as Margaret Mead commented in the preface to the 1959 printing) widened the horizons of the comparative study of different cultures and attempted to explore the relationship between each human being with a specific hereditary endowment and life history and the culture in which he or she lived.

There were many other pioneers during this period. For instance, Edward Sapir stressed the view that different individuals make disparate psychological uses of the shared culture. Geza Roheim, a psychoanalytically trained ethnologist, did some psychoanalytic field studies in central Australia and Somaliland. Also, C.G. Seligman, the British anthropologist, carried out a study of dreams collected from Arabs. It is clear that it was the encounter of anthropology with psychoanalysis during this formative period that gave rise to the study of culture and personality.

2. 1935–1950 — Theoretical Proposal Period

Instead of studies by individual scholars, groups of scholars were formed to investigate their common interests. For example, Abram Kardiner, a psychiatrist at the New York Psychoanalytic Institute, organized a series of seminars in which anthropologists, including Cora DuBois, Ruth Benedict, and Ralph Linton, participated. A large-scale collaboration was established for research. The Indian Education Research Project was funded to study personality development among various groups of Native Americans, including Hopi, Navajo, Papago, Sioux, and Zuni.

During this period, scholars' theories and research concentrated on the relationship of culture to the typical personality. Following Benedict's proposal of the configuration of the personality in 1934, Kardiner raised the concept of the basic personality in 1945, and DuBois suggested the view of the model personality in 1944.

As pointed out by Tapp (1981, p. 345), from the late 1920s to the mid-1950s, the area was dominated by psychoanalytically oriented anthropologists of the "old" culture and personality school. The more statistically or quantitatively oriented behavioral scientists prevailed from the late 1950s into the 1960s. In the late 1960s and the 1970s, the efforts of cross-cultural researchers, primarily psychologists, in the "new" personality and culture school were more evident.

3. After 1950

Two trends were noticed during this period. The first was that instead of investigating small, primitive societies, scholars began to study culture and personality in large, modern nations, directed by Benedict (at Columbia University) and later by Mead (American Museum of Natural History).

Because of the difficulty of proving many of the ideas derived from early studies of culture and personality, there was a greater attempt to use statistics to prove the connections between child-rearing practices, personality, and other cultural patterns (Nanda, 1980, p. 33). This was the second trend that occurred during this period.

For instance, Whiting and Child (1953) used a large cross-cultural sample in an attempt to demonstrate some of these interrelationships. They tested the hypothesis that systems of curing illness would reflect techniques that had been sources of gratification in early child rearing. Thus, a culture in which children were indulged in sources of oral gratification would tend to use oral medicines for curing illnesses.

From those studies, scholars began to obtain new insights. Cultures differ in child-rearing practices, including weaning, cleanliness training, or handling of childhood sexuality, but they also differ in many other variables that contribute to personality formation. For instance, the nature of child–mother contact during the earliest period of infancy (which may be the base for socialization patterns later), the respective role of peers in the process of socialization, the structure of the family — whether nuclear or extended, for instance — will all affect the process of personality development. (Draguns, 1979).

It may be fair to say that the study of national character was stimulated by World War II, with the practical need to know our country's enemies and allies. Benedict's study of Japanese personality, resulting in the publication of *The Chrysanthemum and the Sword* (1946), is a representative example. The classic study of culture and personality reached its peak in the 1950s and then gradually faded.

D. Ethnic Character: Some Theoretical Proposals

Ethnic character refers to a common personality configuration that is manifested by the majority of members of an ethnic group and distinguishes them from other ethnic group members. It is based on the notion that every culture has a typical personality that is distinctive and characteristic of that culture, and is produced or conditioned by some aspect of the culture. Historically, three theoretical concepts have been proposed regarding ethnic character.

1. Ideal Personality or Configurational Personality

According to Ruth Benedict (1934), each society has a more or less clear idea of what constitutes the "good man" and "good woman" — the kind of person an individual ought to be. Through rewards and punishment, a society is directed toward molding all members in the image of the ideal. Thus, the ideological contours of a culture are impressed upon individuals in terms of an ideal personality type. Consequently, the personalities of the majority in any society are largely reflections of the configurational personality presented by that society's culture.

Benedict, based on her study of three primitive cultures — the Zuni, the Dobu, and the Kwakiutl — elaborates her concept of culture and personality in detail in *Patterns of Culture* (1934).

1. In every culture, there is a wide range of individual temperament types that recurs universally.
2. Every culture, however, permits only a limited number of types to flourish, and they are those that fit its dominant configuration.
3. The vast majority of individuals in any society will conform to the dominant types of that society, forming "normal" personality types.
4. A minority of individuals in every society will not "fit" the dominant types: "deviants" and "abnormals."

5. The classification and distribution of "normal" and "abnormal" personality types are relative to the configurations of particular cultures that define the criteria of "normal" and "abnormal."

A major criticism of Benedict's configuration theory of personality is that the composition of personality manifested by a collective member is always characterized by a complexity that makes it difficult to describe cultural patterns and ideal personalities, even in simple, primitive cultures; it becomes almost impossible in large, complicated societies.

2. Basic Personality Structure

Abram Kardiner, a psychoanalyst by training, proposed in 1945 that certain culturally established techniques of child rearing (primary institutional) shape basic attitudes toward life that exist throughout the life of the individual. This nuclear constellation of attitudes and behavior formed by culturally standardized patterns of child rearing in any society is the basic personality structure that is characteristic of that society. The nuclear constellations derived from primary institutions are subsequently reflected in the development of secondary institutions, such as art, folklore, mythology, religion, and social organization. Therefore, an interrelation exists between culture and personality.

According to Honigmann (1967, pp. 107–108), Kardiner's concept of "basic personality" is well illustrated by his study of Alore — Pauan pagans living in Atime-lang, a malarial village in the mountains of a small, obscure, Indonesian jungle island. According to Kardiner, during the wet season, the women's economic role allows them only about 10 to 14 days to devote themselves fully to a newborn child. The postpartum mothers resume their work in their vegetable gardens, leaving an older sibling or grandmother to care for the baby. The infant is fed by the substitute caretakers with premasticated roasted bananas and vegetables, which the infant frequently spits back, even though he remains hungry much of the time, until the mother returns in the late afternoon to offer her breast. Thus, in this way, all during infancy, maternal care remains inconsistent and undependable, leaving the infant struggling with hunger, desertion, and miscellaneous tensions. Predictably, as a result of this child rearing, characterized by poor maternal care, the children grow up to be adults who find it impossible to sustain great effort. In the face of danger and difficulty, they quickly collapse or surrender. A general mistrust governs human relations. This supports how primary institutions contribute to the formation of particular patterns of basic personality.

3. Model Personality Structure

Anthropologist Cora DuBois (1944) proposed the concept of the model personality. A wide range of variations of personalities exists within any given society. However, if the range is measured on a common baseline, data will show central tendencies that constitute the model personality for any particular culture. Thus, model personality is based on statistical constructs. Data are most easily gathered by giving psychological tests.

As pointed out by Wallace (1970, p. 153), in terms of basic personality, there was difficulty dealing with questions of frequency, whereas with model personality, there was difficulty dealing with questions of structure and patterns. Clearly, there is no single view of ethnic character that can satisfy both theoretical perspectives and practical applications, as well. Yet, each theory contributes to the understanding of culture and personality in its own way.

E. Variations of Personality

Although several attempts have been made to describe the ethnic character of national personality as a whole, it is necessary for clinicians to focus on an individual and comprehend the possible variations that are often encountered in practice in order for cultural aspects of individual and group personalities to be understood from a realistic point of view.

1. Intragroup Variability

It is necessary to understand that, within an identified cultural group, there are always meaningful variations of personality characteristics among its members. For instance, in Japan, Vogel (1963) revealed that a contrast exists in the socialization of the offspring of businessmen and those of salaried employees, clearly preparing them for different places in life and different values. Aronoff (1967) reported that the needs and personality constellations of the fishermen and cane cutters on St. Kitts in the West Indies differ sharply.

In other words, ethnic or national character is not a homogeneous phenomenon. It is heterogeneous, differing only in the degree of heterogeneity. The modes of personality described for a particular cultural group cannot give a comprehensive profile of the distribution of personality patterns existing in the subject group under consideration.

2. Intraindividual Variability

Even within an individual, there does not exist a monolithic state of "personality." As pointed out by cultural psychologist Draguns (1979), the individual personality will fluctuate according to situations (from the social-learning point of view) and across levels of consciousness (from the psychodynamic perspective).

The situation is more complicated if an individual is raised in different cultural settings. This diversified cultural impact will certainly contribute to the formation and growth of multiple levels of (cultural) personality that interact in a complex way.

F. Change of Personality

Despite the basic assumption that personality is formed when a person reaches adulthood, and the pattern of character is more less fixed through adulthood, in reality, it is better to consider personality formation as a process of change and growth that is not stagnated or fixed. This view is particularly important from a cultural perspective.

1. Individual Change of Personality

Through the stages of the life cycle, the process of maturity or life experience, an individual's personality may change to some extent. Starting when he is a small child and continuing through the process of "enculturation," an individual establishes his basic cultural system, which is the basis of how he thinks, feels, reacts, and behaves. However, the process of enculturation does not end when he grows up. It continues all his life, accumulating, revising, and adding new value systems and integrating them with those established previously. Thus, while enculturation is conceptualized as a process that takes place in early childhood, it is actually an ongoing one.

In his life experiences, an individual may encounter different cultural systems that challenge the occurrence of "acculturation" — acquiring new value systems or lifestyles that are quite different from those that are native to him, that is, those which he enculturated originally. Thus, enculturation is a process that continues wave after wave during an individual's lifetime.

However, social anthropologist LeVine (1973, p. 16), whose background is in psychoanalytic training, pointed out that another culture, very different from one's own, cannot be completely "acquired" in adulthood, if we define culture not only as the most institutionalized form of public behavior (such as customs), but also as the more private patterns of thought and emotion that accompany those behavior forms in their indigenous context and give them voluntary support, that is, the "cultural patterning of personality."

2. Intergenerational Change

It is well recognized that a generational gap exists between parents and children. The gap refers to different attitudes toward and views of things — a culture gap. The gap is attributed to age and to different life experiences encountered by the different generations. However, it also reflects the cultural environment to which people are exposed. Thus, if there is a relatively rapid and drastic change in a culture,

within one or two decades, the gap between generations could be quite wide. This is also true for a family that has migrated to a different cultural setting — grandparents, parents, and children will have considerable differences in their cultural experiences and backgrounds, contributing to a wide gap between generations.

3. Change of Group Personality

Although students of culture and personality take the view that the same group personality, either as ethnic character or as national personality, is transmitted from generation to generation, they also recognize that group character could change over time in association with cultural change. Generally, it is considered that basic personality is apt to lag behind cultural change. However, through the mechanism of intergenerational change, the group character as a whole may change. Sometimes, even within one generation, considerable change may occur. The collective change of personality among members of a society is always influenced by impinging events such as war, revolution, or cultural invasion from the outside.

G. Parallel between Culture and Personal Complexity

Cultural psychologist H.C. Triandis (1977) has proposed that there are certain parallels between culture and personal complexity, particularly in the area of cognitive structure. These are as follows.

1. Simple societies, as reflected by their simple social, political, and economic systems, produce individuals low in cognitive complexity, whereas cognitive complexity thrives in social settings characterized by specialized economic activities, elaborate systems of governance, and an intricate system of social gradation and differentiation (Triandis, 1977).

2. Societies can be viewed as having tight or loose cultures. At one end of the continuum, in a loose society, there is a great deal of ambiguity and even anomie

(i.e., loss of collective views, values, and identity) concerning divisions of labor, status, and norms of behavior. Such societies foster overt behavior, including outbursts of impulses. In contrast to this, a tight society, characterized by a system of tight prescriptions, regulates an individual and social behavior and predisposes its members toward "projective," vicarious, fantasy expression.

II. SOME NATIONAL CHARACTERS STUDIED

Instead of studying culture and personality in small, undeveloped societies, as earlier investigators did, after the 1950s, scholars were interested in culture and personality in large, modernized nations. Their efforts were called national character studies. Although it is difficult to generalize about personality in large societies composed of numerous ethnic groups, social classes, or subcultures, these attempts to study character patterns in certain nations deserve to be mentioned.

A. AMERICAN PERSONALITY

1. An Anthropologist's Look at America (Mead, 1942)

In the early 1940s, when America was about to become involved in World War II in Europe, Margaret Mead examined American culture (Caucasian-Americans) in contrast to European culture, from which American originally came. In her book, *And Keep Your Powder Dry* (1942, pp. 193–194), she summarized her view that American people have a certain character, which originated in Europe, but developed in the New World and took a shape all its own. It is a character geared toward success and movement; in which aggressiveness is uncertain and undefined; which measures its successes and failures only against near contemporaries and engages in various quantita-

tive devices for reducing every contemporary to its own structure; which sees success as the reward of virtue and failure as the stigma for not being good enough; which is uninterested in the past, except when ancestry can be used to make points against other people in the game of success; and which is oriented toward an unknown future and is ambivalent toward other cultures, which are regarded with a sense of inferiority as more coherent than our own and with a sense of superiority because newcomers in America display the strongest mark of other cultural membership in the form of foreignness.

2. Continuity and Change in National Character: Summary Review (Inkeles, 1997)

Recently, after reviewing past observations and surveys regarding the American national character, Alex Inkeles, in his book, *National Character* (1997), summarized the continuity and change of the American national character as reflected in the beliefs, attitudes, and behavior of Americans. According to Inkeles (1997, pp. 167–179), continuity is noticed in relation to several issues.

1. Self-reliance, autonomy, and independence — Numerous surveys have repeatedly shown that the belief that fate or luck significantly determines what happens to us is not a salient idea among the American people. Instead of God or luck, the great majority of Americans still believe that it is a person's own efforts that account for success or failure in life.

2. Communal action, voluntarism, and cooperation with neighbors — From the beginning of their history, Americans' propensity to form themselves into organizations and thus participate in local affairs has been outstanding. Even at present, in contrast to Europeans, such as the British, Germans, and Italians, Americans assert the obligation of the ordinary man to be active in local affairs.

3. Trust in interpersonal relations — Confidence that people can be trusted, the feeling that they care and will fulfill their obligations to you, readiness to extend the benefit of the doubt to other people even

when they are your nominal opponents, and respect for the mutual rights of others all seem to have been transmitted to the majority of Americans over the generations to the present time.

4. Innovations and openness to new experiences — The readiness to try the new and to experiment, especially in the realm of the technical and mechanical, goes back a long way in the American experience. It now extends to many other realms as well, including new forms of organization and new sensate experiences.

5. Antiauthoritarianism — Americans are still outstanding in their antiauthoritarianism, with no deep psychic need to submit themselves to a higher political authority, and a continuing propensity to assert their rights to personal autonomy as opposed to public control.

6. Equality — The sense of one's intrinsic worth and the feeling that one is equal to all others in rights before the law is one of the notable qualities always attributed to Americans.

Inkeles (1997, pp. 180–185) also described the recent change in American beliefs and attitudes in several areas, namely: an increasing tolerance of diversity; a decreasing of the ethic of hard work, temperance, and frugality; and an erosion of political confidence.

B. Japanese Personality

1. Study of Culture at a Distance (Benedict, 1946)

As mentioned earlier, during and after World War II, in order to understand America's Japanese enemy, cultural anthropologist Benedict was ordered to lead a team to study the Japanese and Japanese culture. As it was not possible to carry out field work in Japan, Benedict's study relied on literature, history, travelers' tales, movies, art, and expatriate interviews. Through this "study at a distance" and the model personality concept, Benedict completed her study of Japanese behavior. As reflected in the title of her book, *The*

Chrysanthemum and the Sword (1946), Benedict described contradictory features of Japanese psychology and behavior patterns (1946, p. 2). That is, the Japanese are, to the highest degree, both aggressive and unaggressive, militaristic and aesthetic, insolent and polite, rigid and adaptable, submissive and resentful of being pushed around, loyal and treacherous, brave and timid, and conservative and hospitable to new ways.

2. Clinical Analysis of Dependence (Doi, 1962)

Takeo Doi is an analytical psychiatrist in Japan who described the Japanese term *amae* as one of the key concepts in understanding Japanese personality structure (1962). In his Japanese language book, *Amae no kozo* (1971), later translated into English as *Anatomy of Dependence* (1973), Doi reported that, in his clinical experience of treating a bilingual Japanese–English woman, the patient used the Japanese word *amaeru* while she was in the middle of complaining in English about her son not intimately relating to her as a child. From such a trivial observation of language discrepancy between Japanese and English, Doi learned that *amaeru* is a unique Japanese word reflecting a special interpersonal relationship for the Japanese. *Amae* (adjective) and *amaeru* (verb) literally mean "sweet," but also imply "indulgence" or "dependence." A child can be indulged and dependent on *(amaeru)* his parent, or indulgent parents may treat their child sweetly *(amaeru)*. Such benevolent dependence continues into adult relationships with others, with an expectation of consideration and thoughtfulness between people and lifelong interdependency. If the need of *amae* is not satisfied, then a person, like an unhappy child, can become *hinekureru* (bitter in expressing resentfulness). Doi's work illustrated that cultural behavior or psychology can be reflected in language, and vise versa. Also, most importantly, it indicates the view that interdependency is not necessarily negative, as it is seen in Western society, but is benevolent and positive in many non-Western societies.

C. RUSSIAN PERSONALITY

1. Swaddling Hypothesis (Gorer and Rickman, 1949)

A sketch of a Russian peasant's life by American physician John Rickman, who, under special contract, worked for a couple of years as a country doctor in Russia around 1910, and, as part of the Columbia University project on Research in Contemporary Cultures, Geoffrey Gorer's study of Russians, led to a jointly published book, *The People of Great Russia: A Psychological Study* (Gorer & Rickman, 1949). They pointed out that there are marked differences in character between the Russian elite and the masses. In the book, after reviewing child-rearing patterns among rural farmers, Gorer proposed the swaddling hypothesis. He reported that rural farmers, in order to allow the mothers to work in the field at a distance, swaddled their young babies in long strips of material, holding their legs straight and their arms down by their sides. The practice was based on the idea that the baby was potentially so strong that if it were not swaddled, it would risk destroying itself or doing itself irreparable harm. Gorer postulated that such restriction on muscular movement in early childhood may contribute to the Russian peasants' character, which is able to endure physical suffering with great stoicism and is indifferent to the physical suffering of others. The peasants also tend to oscillate between unconscious fears of isolation and loneliness and an absence of feelings of individuality, so that the self is, as it were, merged with its peers in a "soul collective." The mass of the population is oppressed (by administrative authority), with diffuse feelings of guilt and hostility, but shows very little anxiety. It tends to oscillate suddenly and unpredictably from one attitude to its contrary, especially from violence to gentleness, from excessive activity to passivity, and from orgiastic indulgence to ascetic abstemiousness (Gorer & Rickman, 1949, p. 189).

2. The National Character of Great Russians (C. Kluckhohn, 1955)

A multidisciplinary group from Columbia University and the American Museum of Natural History Studies — organized originally by Ruth Benedict, but directed during most of its course by Margaret Mead — utilized literary, historical, and other published materials, personal documents, folklore, films and photographs, and some interviews with individuals who had been away from the USSR to study the national character of Great Russians. Clyde Kluckhohn (1955) summarized what seemed the most interesting generalizations in several matters. Her findings appeared in her book, *Culture and Behavior* (1962, pp. 214–215), as follows.

1. There is a sizable gap between the modal personality type advocated by the Soviet leadership and most characteristics of Great Russians in general.
2. The people are warmly human, tremendously dependent on secure social affiliations, labile, nonrational, strong but undisciplined, and needing to submit to authority.
3. The counteractive Bolshevik ideal demanded stern, ascetic, vigilant, incorruptible, and obedient personalities who would not be deflected from the aims of the Party and the state by family or personal ties and affections.
4. The attitude of the people remains, on the whole, that strong authority is both hateful and essential.

3. Brief Sketch of Modal Personality (Inkeles, Hanfmann, & Beier, 1958)

In the 1960s, Inkeles and colleagues undertook an intensive program of clinical psychological research as a part of the Harvard Project on the Soviet Social System for the study of the Russian modal personality and adjustment to the Soviet sociopolitical system. A highly selected group, almost 3000 in number, from the population of the Soviet Union at the time, namely, former citizens of Great Russian nationality who "defected" during or after World War II, was used as the subject for the psychological investigation, which included test measurements and clinical interviews. An evaluative, summary statement was derived, based on both test scores and supplementary qualitative material. The following Russian modal personality characteristics were identified by Inkeles, Hanfmann, and Beier (1958) and Inkeles (1997, pp. 139–147).

1. Central needs — The strongest and most pervasive quality of the Russian personality was a need for affiliation, intensive interaction with other people in immediate, direct, face-to-face relationships, coupled with a great capacity for having this need fulfilled through the establishment of warm and personal contact with others.

2. Modes of impulse control — On the whole, the Russians had a relatively high awareness of their impulses or basic dispositions and freely accepted them as normal or "natural" rather than as bad or offensive.

3. Typical polarities and dilemmas — The Russians showed a conscious preoccupation with the problems of trust versus mistrust in relation to others. They worried about the intentions of others, expressing apprehension that people may not really be as they seemed on the surface. Another typical polarity of Russian behavior was that of optimism versus pessimism.

4. Achieving and maintaining self-esteem — They showed rather high and secure self-esteem and were little given to self-examination and doubt of their inner selves.

5. Relation to authority — The Russians appeared to have more fear of, and much less optimistic expectations about, authority figures.

6. Modes of affective functioning — One of the most salient characteristics of the Russian personality was its high degree of expressiveness and emotional aliveness. Russians felt their emotions keenly and did not tend to disguise or deny them to themselves or to suppress their outward expression.

7. Modes of cognitive functioning — The Russians showed a keen awareness of the "other" as a distinct entity, as well as a rich and diversified recognition of his special characteristics.

It should be pointed out that this investigation was carried out with a special population of people who had defected from their country. Thus, their psychological status may be colored by their backgrounds, particularly relating to authority figures and trust of others.

D. CHINESE PERSONALITY

1. Interdisciplinary Study of Chinese Character (Li & Yang, 1974)

Led by cultural anthropologist Yih-Yuan Li and psychologist Kuo-Shu Yang, a group of interdisciplinary scholars in Taipei engaged in an academic study of the Chinese personality and published a book, *The Character of the Chinese* (1974). Based on their work, various topics have been approached by behavioral and social scientists and psychiatrists from their respective perspectives. For instance, from the perspective of value orientation, anthropologist Chung-I Wen (1974, pp. 47–78) listed respect for authority, conservatism, dependency, obedience, and being yielding, cautious, industrious, frugal, patient, and content as the basic values emphasized by the Chinese.

2. MMPI Study of the Chinese Character (Song, 1985)

In order to study the character traits of the Chinese, a research psychologist from the Chinese Academy of Science in China, Song Weizhen, led a national team in administering the MMPI (Minnesota Multiphasic Personality Inventory) to a large group of Han nationals from six major areas of China. The subjects included 1791 persons — 909 men and 882 women — whose ages ranged from 16 to 55. The results, according to Song (1985), indicated that, in contrast to data reported for American subjects, the mean profiles of normal Chinese subjects had a higher normal range for scales of D (depression) and Sc (schizophrenia). This was true for both male and female subjects. Based on these test results, Song interpreted that Chinese, in contrast to Americans, are emotionally more reserved, introverted, fond of tranquility, overly considerate, socially overcautious, and habitually self-restrained.

3. Threads of Chinese Culture That Impact Mental Health (Tseng Lin, & Yeh, 1995)

Based on their clinical experience and intuition, Tseng, Lin, and Yeh (1995, pp. 10–12) listed some characteristic Chinese cultural traits that have a direct impact on their behavior and mental health. They are harmonious attitude toward nature, balance and conservation for optimal health, the family as the basic source of support, a humanistic and interpersonal orientation, and practical and dynamic adjustment in life situations.

III. CULTURE AND DEPTH PSYCHOLOGY

In addition to personality, several parameters, such as perception, cognition, memory, emotion, and motivation, are recognized by psychologists as basic to the processes of individual psychology. Attitudes, values, communication, and group behavior are considered parameters of social psychology. Some of the parameters of individual as well as social psychology will be addressed in the following chapter. Here, from the perspective of depth psychology, the subjects of dreams and defense mechanisms will be examined from a cultural perspective. Depth psychology refers to the area of psychology that usually operates at the subconscious or unconscious levels. It is considered a fundamental part of personality and the activity of primary psychology in depth, which may rise to the surface in conscious awareness under special circumstances. Since a clinician, particularly a psychoanalytically oriented clinician, has considerable interest in depth psychology, it will addressed here after reviewing the subject of personality.

A. DREAMS

Analytically oriented psychiatrists greatly appreciate dream analysis, as dreams — as products of the primary thinking process — offer a valuable resource for understanding a person's deep-seated instincts, drives, thoughts, affects, concerns, and conflicts. Anthropologists have traditionally paid attention to the dreams and dream-related behavior of preliterate peoples. Professionally, anthropologists are interested in the study of dreams for several reasons. Dreams serve as channels for exploring secret or mythical materials that are otherwise often considered forbidden subjects that are revealed to outside investigators. It is also considered that dreams can be used to secure or support interpretations of social personality.

From an anthropological point of view, the study of dreams can be focused on several areas, namely, exploring any cultural patterns in the dream content; any patterns of the methods of interpreting dreams; and any common patterns of reacting to dream experiences, including the degree of reality that is attributed to dream experiences (Bourguignon, 1954).

Dreaming is a universal human experience, yet its themes, styles, and outcomes are individually determined. In addition, culture contributes to the content and themes of dreams, the symbolic interpretation of dreams, and the reactions toward such mental products.

Methodologically, the cross-cultural study of dreams is limited to the investigation of the "manifested" dream material. The interpretation of dreams is relatively difficult to study cross-culturally, as it is subjective and also requires a certain quality of investigator, who has a professional background in both psychoanalysis and anthropology.

1. Culture and Dream Experience

The impact of culture on dreams is illustrated not only by how the content and theme of dreams are shaped by the actual reality and cultural environment, but mostly by how the symbols of dreams are interpreted by the dreamer as well as by the members of his culture. From her field work, Eggan (1952) has demonstrated this point. For instance, one of her Hopi informants reported a frequent anxiety-laden dream of a dark canyonlike passage. According to analytic thought, one may easily associate such a theme as sexual symbolism. However, the informant was living in a desiccated canyon country. Her personal history revealed that, during her childhood, while she was traveling with her adored mother, her mother often stopped at the dark entrance to a plaza to dry her eyes. Her mother cried when she was forced to travel to other villages to visit relatives, which she resented. From such an early experience, she developed a fear of the dark. Eggan pointed out that, without reference to the geographic and cultural background of the dreamer, as well as her own associations, we may have misinterpreted the symbol of "canyonlike passage." Similarly, Honigmann (1961) reported one of his Native-American informant's dreams of a big white bear. The bear, as big as a house, appeared in the dream and the dreamer was not able to kill the beast. The informant associated a past fearful experience that he had had on a winter moose hunt when he had lost his matches and had nothing to eat for 2 days. From his life history, it became clear that the fearsome, huge, white bear had a special meaning, namely the dreamer's anxiety about his family's food supply and his perception of himself as an ineffectual hunter.

Concerning people's attitudes toward dreams, American anthropologist Bourguignon (1954) examined how the people in Haiti attribute dream experiences to reality. He reported that for Haitians, dream experiences, together with possessions, tend to validate their belief in the gods and to establish a two-way communication with supernatural beings. In other words, the reality of the dream world is placed on the same plane as that of waking experience.

2. Some Cross-Cultural Studies of Dreams

a. Comparison of Dream Content Distribution between Jewish and Arab Subjects

Clinical psychologists from Israel, Giora, Esformes, and Barak (1972) carried out a comparison of common dream situations reported by Jewish and Arab high-school students in Israel. Students from a

kibbutz were utilized for the Jewish subjects. Questionnaires used by Griffith, Miyagi, and Tago (1958), which contained 52 typical dream situations, were administered to the subjects from the two ethnic groups. The results indicated that, for the Jewish students, falling, being attacked, sexual experiences, water, helping others, and school were the six most frequent dreams. In contrast, water, school, solving a problem, running to play, finding money, and a dead person were the most frequent dream images for the Arab students. From these findings, Giora et al. interpreted that the dominant conflicts of kibbutz high-school students appeared to be the longing for maternal support and the fear of losing it. The Arab high-school students, however, in general lacked internalized conflicts. They expressed their affects without intrapsychic conflicts.

b. Cross-Cultural Study of Hunger and Thirst Motivation Manifested in Dreams

Based on the assumption that manifested dream content reveals the nature of motivational states in dreams, the American psychologist C. W. O'Nell (1965) conducted a survey of dreams among male students of four ethnic-culture groups: Ethiopians Orthodox Christian, fasting Nigerian Muslims, nonfasting Nigerians, and Americans. These four groups were selected because they represented wide variations in food and drink patterns. The former two groups maintained stringent attitudes and customs with regard to fasting and its public manifestation. Results revealed that the percentage of respondents showing manifest hunger were 63.8% for Ethiopians, 43.8% for fasting Nigerians, 33.7% for non-fasting Nigerians, and 14.5% for Americans. This cross-cultural datum illustrates that the rankings of food and drink deprivation are positively associated with the levels at which hunger and thirst motivations are manifested in group dreamers.

c. Exploration of the Oedipus Dream Theme in the East and West

In order to operationalize psychoanalytic theory in terms of manifested dream content, Calvin S. Hall and associates conducted a variety of studies. C.S. Hall (1963) found a greater frequency of hostile interactions with male strangers in the dreams of American males, and interpreted this as consistent with the Oedipal theory, which predicts father–son conflict. Subsequently, C.S. Hall and Van De Castle (1965) found more frequent acquisition of penislike objects in the reports of girls, as confirmation of the analytic concept of penis envy in the female, C.S. Hall and Domhoff (1963) extended the study into cross-cultural material, including the Australian aboriginal Yir Yiront and the American southwest Hopis. They claimed that, in all three cultures, men dreamed primarily about male characters, ranging from 64 to 77% in the various samples. However, they reported that, in the dreams of the females, both sexes appeared in approximately equal proportions.

Later, Grey and Kalsched (1971) carried out a content analysis regarding the frequency of opposite-sex figures among university students in India and the United States. They indicated that, in Indian society, the interpersonal friendship patterns of Indian men and women can be characterized as more "isophilic" than in most Western societies, especially the United States. Isophilic means nonsexual friendship preferences for one's own sex (or nonsexual homosexual partnership). The results supported their hypothesis. That is, there was a consistent tendency for the men to favor their own sex in dreams, whereas the women dreamed almost equally of both sexes. This indicates that the nature of intersexual relationships will shape the frequency of opposite-sex figures that appear in dreams.

In summary, a cross-cultural investigation of dreams illustrates that dreams are universal experiences. There is some common, and perhaps universal, content or situations in dreams, such as falling or being chased or attacked, indicating some basic human anxiety. However, based on the real world, including geographic, interpersonal, and culture contexts, the frequency of certain content or themes tends to vary to some extent. Furthermore, culture contributes to the matter of symbolism and how the dreams may be interpreted and experienced. This is analogous to the experience of psychiatric symptoms, namely culture has psychoplastic as well as psychoreactive effects [cross-reference to Chapter 11: Culture and Psychopathology: Overview (Section II,C and F)].

B. DEFENSE MECHANISMS

"Defense mechanism" is a psychoanalytic term referring to the psychic apparatus utilized by the ego to cope with anxiety. It is regarded as a mental process that operates at an unconscious level. However, some defense mechanisms may occur at the conscious level. Based on the degree of maturity, defense mechanisms are subdivided hierarchically into psychotic (or narcissistic), immature, neurotic, and mature. As parameters of depth psychology, defense mechanisms are assumed by psychoanalysts to be universally observed mental functions.

Recently, there has been an increasing awareness that the operation of defense mechanisms is subject to cultural influence. Although fewer cross-cultural variations are observed at the level of psychotic or immature defense mechanisms (the mechanisms mainly operate when a person is suffering a mental breakdown, with major psychiatric disorders), it is speculated that there are some cultural variations at the level of neurotic and mature defense mechanisms (the mechanisms primarily utilized by normal people or people with minor psychiatric disorders) in terms of which neurotic or mature defense mechanisms are used more commonly than others. In other words, cultural factors contribute to the frequent choice of mechanisms utilized. For instance, among neurotic defense mechanisms, it is reported that Russian people, under the Soviet political system, tended to use political denial and indifference or apathy in dealing with the world of reality. It is well known that the Indian hero Gandhi utilized a "passive-aggressive" mechanism to successfully defeat British control over India, illustrating that this kind of mechanism can be used by people in certain societies such as India, but can also be rather adaptive defense mechanisms.

"Humor" is considered one of the mature mechanisms for dealing with anxiety or tension. It is often used skillfully by Americans in private as well as public situations. Humor is used even by scholars to start their lectures and by politicians in their official speeches. However, in conservative societies, humor may be considered undersirable and disgraceful on serious occasions. Thus, it is clear that there are different attitudes toward the operation of various "mature" mechanisms.

It is not only the frequent choice of certain defense mechanisms that is influenced by cultural factors, but also the categorization and definition of defense mechanisms into subgroups according to the poles of pathology. For instance, in Western societies, "somatization" as a defense mechanism is categorized as an "immature" mechanism; however, in many non-Western societies, it is a mechanism commonly utilized by ordinary people and is hardly considered "immature." It may be regarded as slightly "neurotic," at worst. Another example is "dissociation," which is definitely considered a neurotic defense mechanism in the West, believed to be used only by neurotic (dissociated) patients. However, in some non-Western societies, such as Bali, dissociation is commonly used in daily life and is considered a nonneurotic mental phenomenon.

Furthermore, it has been pointed out that cultural factors contribute to the use of culture-specific defense mechanisms that are not listed among presently recognized defense mechanisms derived from analytic work with mainly Euro-American populations.

For instance, an "A-Q style" defense mechanism is a culture-specific defense mechanism that is often used by the Chinese. A-Q is a fictional person's name from a short essay written by a famous Chinese writer, Lu Xun, at the beginning of this century. In the essay, in a cynical way, Lu Xun described A-Q as his "passive-rationalization" used to cope with the frustration and insults that he received from others.

In summary, defense mechanisms are universal mental phenomena. It is generally agreed that there is a range of mechanisms, from the psychotic (narcissistic) to the mature. From a cross-cultural point of view, however, it is recognized that there is some variation in the usage of certain mechanisms. Also, the degrees of immature, neurotic, or mature depend on the values of the people in the different cultures, and the categories for subgrouping may vary. Furthermore, some culture-specific mechanisms observed in non-Western societies should be added to the presently recognized list of Western defense mechanisms [cross-reference to Chapter 49: Culture and Psychiatric Theories (Section IV, C)].

IV. CLOSING REMARKS

In this chapter, the personality and depth psychology of an individual have been elaborated from cultural perspectives. From the standpoint of "culture and personality," it has been shown that attempts to identify a model personality for any given society or ethnic group have faded since the peak observed in the 1950s. This has resulted from the realization that a group of people in a society or an identified ethnic or cultural group is often so heterogeneous that, from a practical point of view, it is difficult to describe a typical or model personality for it unless it is a relatively small group whose members manifest rather unique and homogeneous behavior patterns. From a clinical point of view, it is important to deal with each person individually. It is also necessary to clarify whether the described group personality is an ideal one, a stereotype, or a reflection of an actual one. Otherwise, we may be biased by such a personality description. In general, however, it is useful to know the common characteristics of a particular ethnic or cultural group. A general description and background knowledge will help the clinician to understand an individual's personality, specifically in the context of culture.

Here, the dream, as part of the depth psychology of an individual and the product of the primary thinking process, has been examined from a clinical point of view. The individual's unconsciously operated defense mechanisms have been reviewed from a cultural perspective. Clearly, there are still many questions awaiting answers, and there is room for expansion and further exploration in the future regarding the cross-cultural aspects of depth psychology.

REFERENCES

Aronoff, J. (1967). *Psychological needs and cultural systems: A case study.* Princeton, NJ: Van Nostand-Reinhold.

Benedict, R. (1934). *Patterns of culture.* Boston: Houghton Mifflin.

Benedict, R. (1946). *The chrysanthemum and the sword.* Boston: Houghton Mifflin.

Bourguignon, E.E. (1954). Dreams and dream interpretation in Haiti. *American Anthropologist, 56,* 262–268.

Doi, T. (1962). Amae—A key concept for understanding Japanese personality structure. In R.J. Smith & R.K. Beardsley (Eds.), *Japanese culture: Its development and characteristics.* Chicago: Aldine.

Doi, T. (1971). *Amae no kozo.*Tokyo: Kobundo.

Doi, T. (1973). *The anatomy of dependence.* Tokyo: Kodansha International.

Draguns, J.G. (1979). Culture and personality. In A.J. Marsella, R. Tharp, & T.J. Ciborowski (Eds.), *Perspectives on cross-cultural psychology* (pp. 179–207). New York: Academic Press.

DuBois, C. (1944). *The people of Alor.* Minneapolis: University of Minnesota Press.

Eggan, D. (1952). The manifest content of dreams: A challenge to social science. *American Anthropologist,54*(4), 469–485.

Giora, Z., Esformes, Y., & Barak, A. (1972). Dreams in cross-cultural research. *Comprehensive Psychiatry, 13*(2), 105–114.

Gorer, G., & Rickman, J. (1949). *The people of Great Russia: A psychological study.* London: Cresset Press.

Grey, A., & Kalsched, D. (1971). Oedipus East and West: An exploration via manifested dream content. *Journal of Cross-Cultural Psychology, 2*(4), 337–352.

Griffith, R.M., Miyagi, O., & Tago, A. (1958). The universality of typical dreams: Japanese vs. Americans. *American Anthropology, 60,* 1173–1179.

Hall, C.S. (1963). Strangers in dreams: An empirical confirmation of the Oedipus complex. *Journal of Personality, 31,* 336–345.

Hall, C.S., & Domhoff, B. (1963). A ubiquitous sex difference in dreams. *Journal of Abnormal and Social Psychology, 66,* 278–280.

Hall, C.S., & Van De Castle, R.L. (1965). An empirical investigation of the castration complex in dreams. *Journal of Personality, 33,* 20–29.

Honigmann, J.J. (1961). The interpretation of dreams in anthropological field work: A case study. In B. Kaplan (Ed.), *Studying personality cross-culturally.* New York: Harper & Row.

Honigmann, J.J. (1967). *Personality in culture.* New York: Harper & Row.

Inkeles, A. (1997). *National character: A psycho-social perspective.* New Brunswick, NJ: Transaction Books.

Inkeles, A., Hanfmann, E., & Beier, H. (1958). Modal personality and adjustment to the Soviet sociopolitical system. *Human Relations, 11*(1), 3–22.

Kardiner, A. (1945). The concept of basic personality structure as an operational tool in social sciences. In R. Linton (Ed.), *The science of man in the world crisis.* New York: Columbia University Press.

Kluckhohn, C. (1995). *Recent studies of the "national character" of Great Russians.* (Human Development Bulletin). Papers presented at the sixth annual symposium, Chicago. Kluckhohn, (1962). In R. Kluckhohn (Ed.), *Culture and behavior.* New York: Free Press.

Kluckhohn, C., & Murray, H.A. (1948). Personality formation: The determinants. In C. Kluckhohn, H.A. Murray, & D.M. Schneider (Eds.), *Personality in nature, society, and culture* (2nd ed.), New York: Alfred A. Knopf.

LeVine, R.A. (1973). *Culture, behavior, and personality.* Chicago: Aldine.

Li, Y.Y., & Yang, K.S. (Eds.). (1974). *The character of the Chinese.* Taipei, Taiwan, China: Institute of Ethnology, Academia Sinica.

Malinowski, B. (1927). *Sex and repression in savage society.* New York: International Library.

Mead, M. (1928). *Coming of age in Samoa.* New York: Morrow.

Mead, M. (1942). *And keep your powder dry: An anthropologist looks at America.* New York: W. Morrow.

Nanda, S. (1980). *Cultural anthropology.* New York: Van Nostand.

O'Nell, C.W. (1965). A cross-cultural study of hunger and thirst motivation manifested in dreams. *Human Development, 8,* 181–193.

Singer, M. (1961). A survey of culture and personality theory and research. In B. Kaplan (Ed.), *Studying personality cross-culturally.* Evanston, IL: Row, Peterson.

Song, W.Z. (1985). A preliminary study of the character traits of the Chinese. In W.S. Tseng & D.Y.H. Wu (Eds.), *Chinese culture and mental health* (pp. 47–55). Orlando, FL: Academic Press.

Tapp, J.L. (1981). Studying personality development. In H.C. Triandis & A. Heron (Eds.), *Handbook of cross-cultural psychology: Developmental psychology* (Vol. 4) (pp. 343–423). Boston: Allyn & Bacon.

Triandis, H.C. (1977). Cross-cultural social and personality psychology. *Personality and Social Psychology Bulletin, 3,* 143–158.

Tseng, W.S., Lin, T.-Y., & Yeh, E.K. (1995). Chinese societies and mental health. In T.-Y. Lin, W.S. Tseng, & E.K. Yeh (Eds.), *Chinese societies and mental health* (pp. 3–18). Hong Kong: Oxford University Press.

Vogel, E. (1963). *Japan's middle class.* Berkeley: University of California Press.

Wallace, A.F.C. (1970). *Culture and personality,* (2nd ed.). New York: Random House.

Wen, C.I. (1974). Chinese national character as revealed in value orientation. In Y.Y. Li & K.S. Yang (Eds.), *The character of the Chinese.* Taipei, Taiwan, China: Institute of Ethnology, Academia Sinica.

Whiting, J.W.M., & Child, I.L. (1953). *Child training and personality.* New Haven, CT: Yale University Press.

6

Psychology, Customary Behavior, and Ethnic Identity

I. INTRODUCTION

After discussing cultural aspects of personality and depth psychology in Chapter 4, this chapter explores some parameters of individual and social psychology, such as emotion, communication, attitude, value, group behavior, and culture-rooted customary behavior (rituals, etiquette, taboos, and other cultural regulations). Finally, the subject of ethnic identity will be examined from the perspective of its formation and its relation with mental health functioning.

Psychologists distinguish the basic processes of individual psychology and social psychology. "Social psychology" refers to the study of behavior and experience with respect to social stimuli, especially associated with people's interaction with other people. Traditionally, attitudes and values are considered core topic areas of social psychology, as people acquire attitudes and values through interaction with others (Brislin, 1980). However, some psychological parameters, considered basic to the process of individual psychology, such as emotion and communication, usually occur in a social context, are closely related to social situations, and are

seldom observed as simply as an individual's intrapsychic process. Thus, the distinction between individual and social psychology can be arbitrary. In this chapter, the two are not separated, and only some of the parameters that are more relevant to clinical situations, such as emotion, communication, values, and group behavior, will be discussed from a cultural perspective.

II. INDIVIDUAL AND SOCIAL PSYCHOLOGY

A. EMOTION

Psychiatrists, as clinicians, are interested in the psychological parameters of emotion, as they deal professionally with patients who suffer from emotional problems, such as anxiety, depression, or anger. The relationship between culture and emotion is becoming an important and popular topic of study from a cultural perspective, although there are still many factors, including the translation of emotion into language, that limit meaningful investigations cross-culturally (Leff, 1977).

1. Universality and Cultural Variations

According to Izard (1980), cross-cultural studies have developed strong evidence for the universality of certain (fundamental) emotional expressions, as all human beings recognize these expressions and attribute to them the same experiential significance. It tends to be believed that the expressions and inner experiences that characterize the fundamental emotions are innate and universal.

In order to investigate emotions systematically, Woodworth (1938) pioneered the categorization of facial expression, proposing a six-step linear scale that included love, surprise, fear, anger, disgust, and contempt. Following this, Schlosberg (1941) proposed that the facial expression of emotion could be presented in a circular fashion with two axes of dimensions: pleasantness–unpleasantness and attention–rejection. Later, he added a third dimension, sleep–tension. These were two attempts made to systematically identify and classify fundamental emotions. However, some scholars, such as Leff (1973), hold the view that the differentiation of emotional states may vary among different cultures and that some factors, including culture, complexity of society, and language development, might contribute to differences in the range and differentiation of emotion, as well as its expression.

By combining the impact of innate factors and cultural influence, Ekman and Friesen (1972) proposed the "neuro-cultural" theory, stating that facial expression is one of the biological substrates of emotion in the individual, but that one learns stimuli for triggering specific emotions and how to modify the resulting behavior. Izard (1980) indicated that cultures have different rules for displaying various emotions under different conditions. Boucher (1974) gave a case example to illustrate that, in Malay culture, a son-in-law cannot display anger toward his father-in-law, even if the former is scolded by the latter for being a fool. It has also been pointed out that emotionally aroused Japanese inhibit much of their facial behavior when in the presence of others ("outsiders" or superior persons), but when alone (or in private settings with "insiders" or peers) they display expressions very freely. This supports Doi's (1973) notion that Japanese tend to behave in two ways: one in

soto (front or *public* settings) and the other in *ura* (rear or *private* settings).

As pointed out by Izard (1980), different cultures vary significantly in their attitudes toward various emotions. For instance, kissing a sexual partner in public is customary behavior for Westerners, who consider it desirable to show signs of affection between a man and a woman; however, for many non-Westerners, it is considered disgusting to show such private feelings in front of strangers, such behavior should be reserved only for private situations. In some cultures, when a significant person dies, people close to the deceased, particularly women, such as wives or daughters-in-law, are expected to cry loudly and *display* their grief in public. Otherwise, they may criticized by other members of the society as not having feelings for the deceased. In contrast, in other cultures, it is considered undesirable to not *restrict* the expression of sad emotions on such occasions. These different attitudes toward various emotions, in turn, affect socialization practices and subsequent adult personality traits.

2. Language and Differentiation of Emotion

British psychiatrist Leff (1973), who was interested in the subject of culture and expression of emotion, utilized language describing emotion to investigate the differentiation of emotion. He pointed out that there is variety in the range of words used to describe such things as color or snow in the languages of different cultures. For instance, English has only one word for snow, whereas the native language of Eskimo people, who live in an environment of snow year-round, has words to describe many different kinds of snow. This reflects different degrees of differentiation at the levels of perception, experience, and concerns in the matter of "snow." Based on this concept of differentiation in language, Leff attempted to explore the differentiation of emotion as reflected in language used to describe emotion.

By utilizing the research material derived from the WHO's International Pilot Study of Schizophrenia conducted in nine centers around the globe, Leff (1973) examined how patients responded to language relating to the emotions of anxiety, depression, and irritability (anger), which were included in the questionnaire of the Present State Examination (PSE). He attempted to illustrate that there is a strong link between the availability of appropriate words for various emotions and the ease with which people distinguish among their experiences. As a result of the study, he reported that people in "developed" countries (Denmark, England, the USSR, Czechoslovakia, and the United States) showed a greater differentiation of emotional states than people in "developing" countries (India, Colombia, Nigeria, and China). However, it should be pointed out that he linked language with the degree of socioeconomic development (indicated by the terms "developed" and "developing") of the societies, rather than their cultural backgrounds, including the histories of their written languages and civilizations. He also failed to recognize factors relating to the language of the questionnaire, which was originally designed in English. The words referring to anxiety, depression, and irritability (anger) in the questionnaire were translated more easily and appropriately into the languages of the so-called "developed" societies that had their roots in Indo-European language; whereas in some of the societies categorized as "developing" societies, which used entirely different language systems, it was difficult to appropriately translate the language of emotions used in the English questionnaire. Therefore, the questionnaire was biased by an "emic" use of (English) language for "etic" application. Finally, he ignored the cultural factor. Culture differs not only in the matter of description, but in the matter of comfortableness in admitting certain kinds of emotion, or emotion as a whole, to strangers (investigators) in a formal examination setting.

3. Cultural Variations of the Meaning of Emotional Expression

Some cross-cultural examples of emotional expression of an extreme nature are listed here to support the notion that, beyond its physiological and innate nature, emotional expression is subject to cultural impact, particularly in terms of its meaning and function.

For instance, laughter is not necessarily always an expression of joy, but can be used to communicate an entirely different sublinguistic meaning. According to La Barre (1947), G.Gorer in 1935 reported in his book about Africa that, in some parts of the country, laughter is used by the local people to express surprise, wonder, embarrassment, and discomfort. Thus, even though the physiological behavior of certain emotions may be the same, their cultural and emotional functions may differ. Perhaps, in this case, there is a need to know how to distinguish the different kinds of laughter expressed within a culture — whether they are expressions of joy, surprise, or embarrassment.

As pointed out by La Barre (1947), the European behavior of sticking out the tongue (often at the same time as "making a face") is an insulting, almost obscene act of provocative challenge and mocking contempt toward an adversary, so undignified as to be used only by children. Yet, in Bengali, statues of the dread black mother goddess Kali show her tongue protruding to signify great, raging anger and shock. Chinese children stick out their tongues playfully in mock terror or to make fun of others. Among Chinese women, it is an expression of embarrassment. For Maori, Polynesian people living in New Zealand, sticking out the tongue and making a sound is a way of scaring and chasing away evil and enemies. It signifies fierceness and challenge. Therefore, children learn to stick out their tongues and make noises while they are playing, and adults continue such behavior in their performance as warriors.

In Japan, hissing is a polite deference to social superiors — the Basuto applaud by hissing — but in England, hissing is considered rude and is used to show public disapprobation of an actor or a speaker. Thus, the same emotion-related expression means exactly the opposite, or incommensurate things, in the two different cultures (La Barre, 1947).

4. Some Empirical Studies of Emotions across Cultures

Several quantitative studies have been carried out in the past to examine the cross-cultural aspects of the perception (or recognition) of expressed emotions. For instance, Dickey and Knower (1941) used photographs of posed emotional expressions to examine the ability of schoolchildren in Mexico and Minneapolis, in the United States, to recognize emotions. The photographs were of American men and women, and the students had to choose a label from a list of names of emotions. The results indicated that, despite the photos of American people, the average accuracy (as defined by the investigators) on individual photographs was 65% for Mexican children and higher than 50% for American children. Furthermore, they found out that both groups showed nearly total accuracy in judging photographs labeled laughter–glee–merriment, and both were least accurate on photographs of pity–sympathy–kind helpfulness.

Vinacke (1949) conducted a study in Hawaii involving groups of Japanese, Chinese, and Caucasian ethnic origin. He selected photos from magazines of spontaneous expressions shown by Americans and presented them to subjects on slides as whole pictures (with background situations) and as faces alone, without environmental cues. The results indicated that there was a greater scattering in judgment of the faces alone compared to the whole pictures, which included situations as well as body gestures. Female subjects showed consistently greater agreement than males, which was more pronounced regarding the faces alone than the whole pictures. According to ethnicity, the males and females differed only in terms of how much they agreed that a given expression represented a particular emotion.

Following this, Vinacke and Fong (1955) carried out another, similar investigation in Hawaii, but used photographs of spontaneous expressions shown by Asians. The results revealed that, in every analysis, the Japanese and Chinese subjects showed more agreement on the nature of the expressions than did the Caucasians, indicating that familiarity made a difference in the comparison. They also found from their investigation that educated Asian-Americans were as good at judging emotions shown by Caucasians as were educated Caucasians. However, educated Caucasians were inferior to educated Asian-Americans in

their judgment of emotional expressions on Asian faces. It may be suspected that this was related to familiarity rather than level of education. In general, educated Asian-Americans have more exposure to Caucasian people than vice versa.

5. Debate over Specific Emotions: Shame and Guilt

There has been some debate among scholars and clinicians over the matter of shame and guilt from the standpoint of culture. This might have been stimulated by the early observation of the pioneer psychiatrist, Kraepelin, that the manifestation of guilt was rarely observed among depressed patients in Indonesia, in contrast to those in Germany. It was speculated that those without a well-internalized superego tended to control their behavior through shame rather than guilt. Shame and guilt were seen as emotional states closely associated with behavior control. Coupled with analytic concepts, guilt was conceived as a psychological condition arising within the self, without relation to others. It was considered the result of self-blaming, whereas shame was interpreted as an emotional condition that occurred in relation to others produced by the fear of being accused by others. Thus, guilt occurred without outside control, whereas shame was a response to outside criticism. Based on this theory, anthropologists in the past even tried to distinguish between guilt societies and shame societies. Such a dichotomized view of shame and guilt is not accepted today. Problems started with the assumption that shame was a psychological state functioning only as a response to external criticism, that it was not an "internalized" response to self-criticism. Close examination of people belonging to what were categorized as shame-oriented societies showed that they had internalized self-control. However, people in societies categorized as guilt oriented did not necessarily demonstrate an internalized power of self-control. Thus, the distinction between shame and guilt was not as simple and clear-cut as it had originally seemed. After examining the psychocultural aspects of self among the Japanese, T. S. Lebra (1983) pointed out that, even though Japan had been categorized as a shame-oriented society by anthropologists in the past, shame and guilt were actually equally pervasive there. Furthermore, he noted that Japanese tended to stress guilt feelings in expressing their emotions. What they experienced as shame they were therefore likely to talk and think about as guilt.

6. Argument over Psychologized and Somatogized Expressions of Emotion

Scholars have also argued about the expression of emotions through psychologically or somatically oriented language. Disagreement originated with the view that emotion expressed by psychological terms was much more "sophisticated" and "psychologically minded" than expression through body language. This view was based on the evolutionary concept that spoken language was more developed than body language. It also derived from the assumption that they occurred as separate entities in a dichotomized way.

Based on their clinical observations, psychiatrists remarked that Western patients tended to communicate their emotional problems with psychological terms, such as depression and anxiety, whereas many non-Westerners tended to express their emotions through body discomforts, such as headaches, insomnia, back pain, and other somatic complaints. This was true to some extent; however, psychiatrists failed to understand that somatic presentation by a patient may involve numerous factors (Tseng, 1975), including culturally shaped problem-presenting patterns. For instance, in many non-Western cultures, when a person indicates he is "depressed," he is subjected to the criticism that he is "weak" or regarded as merely encountering ordinary daily life problems and ignored by others. Somatic presentation may also be related to a patient's medical orientation in association with help-seeking behavior. Treating a depressed person is generally not considered to be a physician's job; depression is related to daily life problems rather than medical problems. It is considered more appropriate to present somatic symptoms to physicians, including psychiatrists, who can offer treatment for the patient's health as defined by the body rather than the mind.

From a different perspective, some people believe that it is more "sophisticated" to refer to the condition of the body than to bluntly reveal personal and private emotions. They thus communicate their emotional states indirectly in many elaborate ways. As revealed by Liang (1939), Chinese use elaborate organ-language to indicate their emotions. For instance, *hang-xin* (cold heart) indicates disappointment, *rh-xin* (ill-feeling in the heart), disgust, *xu-xin* (empty heart), feeling down, *te-chang* (iron intestines), callousness, *da-dan* (big gall bladder), courage, *dan-po* (ruptured gall bladder), intense fear, *fa-pi-qi* (lost spleen spirit), losing one's temper, and *gan-fuo-da* (elevated liver fire), bad temper or irritation. These terms are derived from ancient concepts, according to which certain organs correspond to certain emotions.

Furthermore, clinical observation (Tseng, 1975) has indicated that when Chinese patients present somatic complaints, they are always associated with psychological complaints. It would take a skillful clinician to inquire into the concomitant presence of psychological symptoms and complaints. Otherwise, it would appear that the Chinese patient was presenting only somatic symptoms or complaints. This view has been supported by an epidemiological study of minor psychiatric disorders of the Chinese. Based on a systematic inquiry of existing symptoms of anxious or depressed patients, the study revealed that, in addition to somatic symptoms, patients acknowledged the presence of psychological symptoms (Cheng, 1988). Thus, a clinician would have to work on the culture-patterned problem presentation [cross-reference to Chapter 10: Illness Behavior: Reaction and Help-Seeking (Section I) and Chapter 16: Somatoform Disorders, including Neurasthenia (Section I,B and C)].

B. COMMUNICATION

Communication is another psychological parameter that often concerns clinicians, as clinical practice always deals with communication between people and, in particular, between the therapist and the patient. Communication involves interpersonal interaction and transmission of a message through a wide range of means, including language, sublingual or nonverbal communication, and emotional communication.

1. Culture and Verbal Communication

According to linguists, more than 4000 languages exist around the world. According to Katzner (1977/1995, pp. viii–ix), American Indian languages number more than a thousand, the languages of African close to a thousand, and those of the single island of New Guinea some 700 more. India has over 150 languages, Russia about 100, and China several dozen. At the same time, as Katzner pointed out, it needs to be understood that fewer than 100 languages are spoken by over 95% of the Earth's population. The remaining 5% speak thousands of different languages — many languages spoken by very small numbers of people. Linguists recognize and subdivide language into different families, such as Indo-European (Germanic, Italic, Slavic, Indo-Iranian, etc.), Sino-Tibetan (Chinese, Tibetan, Tah, etc.), Malayo-Polinesian, Niger-Congo, Afro-Asiatic, and so on. Of course, within each language there are always subgroups or local dialects related to geographic and historical conditions. As with the distribution of race or culture, a language system can be indicated by a map of language distribution, although the boundaries are often not absolute and clear. Also, written language is manifested in various ways, by phonetic systems, such as those of the English or Koreans, the morphological-phonetic systems of the Chinese or Egyptians, or others.

While numerous issues are involved in verbal communication, only a few that are related most closely to clinical situations will be briefly touched on here from a cross-cultural point of view.

a. Style of Interpersonal Communication

When two persons are involved in verbal communication, different styles are observed, such as symmetrical or asymmetrical communication. The former refers to partners speaking to each other interactionally, revealing and exchanging information in a symmetrical fashion. This pattern generally occurs between friends, siblings, or spouses. The latter refers to communication in which one of the speakers dominates the other in talking or revealing information or offering opinions. This may observed when a person in a superior position is talking to a person in an inferior position. From a cultural point of view, social habits and cultural rules will determine which style of communication people use in which circumstances. Otherwise, the communication deviates from the norm and may be dysfunctional from a clinical point of view. For instance, American husbands and wives are supposed to communicate symmetrically, as otherwise their relationship is considered to be without intimacy and unhealthy. Even parents and small children are encouraged to communicate symmetrically. In non-Western societies in which hierarchy is stressed and gender difference is emphasized, husbands and wives are not expected to express opinions symmetrically. Husbands have more say, at least in public. Between parents and children, it is culturally expected that parents will give advice and instructions to children and seldom communicate with them symmetrically. Otherwise, the parents are viewed as losing the authority required to serve in their parental roles.

b. Gender and Status Differentiation

From a linguistic point of view, in many cultures language is used differently according to the gender and status of the speaker. For instance, in Japanese, the term for "self" is normally *boku* for a man, whereas for a woman it is *watashi*. A person in a superior position, when talking to a person in an inferior position, addresses himself as *watakushi*. The Japanese emperor, in official documents, addresses himself as *"chin."* This illustrates that language reflects the thoughts, attitudes, and rules of a culture.

Among Japanese-Americans who migrated to Hawaii almost a century ago, all of whom speak primarily English now, Johnson, Marsella and Johnson (1974) observed that their behavior still retains many aspects of Meiji-era Japanese culture. In their verbal behavior, themes relating to a strong sense of gender difference, a concern for hierarchy and status, an emphasis on self-effacement, and a focus on nonverbal communication are still strong. Johnson and colleagues pointed out that, in social communication, there is a relatively high awareness of distinctions in status between conversational partners. There is a very conscious attempt to identify the status of one's partner and to accord him or her the degree of respect and consideration that ordinarily would accompany such a position. Because general American norms emphasize egalitarianism, directness, and, at times, a populist kind of arrogance toward those of superior status, the high concern for status and respect shown by Japanese-Americans can be misunderstood by Caucasian-Americans from Western backgrounds.

c. Range or Differentiation of Words

As described previously, associated with the needs and customs in a culture, certain words are much more elaborated and differentiated than others. The Eskimos have many words relating to snow so that they can communicate about the different kinds of snow in their environment, which has snow year-round. In the same way, there are several terms for "clouds" among the island people of Micronesia, who rely heavily on the prediction of weather through clouds. Concerning terms for kin, in English, all blood-related male siblings of the father and mother are referred to as "uncle." In contrast, the Chinese clearly distinguish paternal uncles from maternal uncles, and whether they are older or younger than one's parents. The Chinese use the terms *bobo* and *shu-shu* for uncles on the father's side and *jiu-jiu* for those on the mother's side. The same applies to the terms for cousin, brother, and sister. They are differentiated to reflect the Chinese concern with the kinship system, gender, and seniority. As mentioned in the section on emotion, the words for emotion are differentiated in accordance with the differentiations of emotion, as are the words for kin.

d. Equivalence of Words in Translation

Due to the varying degrees of differentiation and meaning attached to words, it is difficult to translate them from one language to another. Clinically, how the emotion of "depression" is expressed in language is often debated, as well as how to translate it accurately and appropriately for the purposes of cross-cultural research. When the same word, "depression," is used, does it reflect the same internal experience of emotion or not? In order to answer this delicate question, Tanaka-Matsumi and Marsella (1976) used a word association method to investigate the subjective experience of depression among college students of different ethnic groups. They reported that among Japanese students in Japan, 40% associated the word "depression" with the words "rain" and "cloud," 22% with "dark" and "gray," and nearly 19% with words relating to somatic function and illness: "disease," "tiredness," "headache," and "fatigue." Most of the Japanese-American students in Hawaii gave responses that reflected internal moods (56.3% "sadness" and 25.3% "loneliness"). The Japanese-American associations were very similar to those given by Caucasian-American students on the United States mainland. The authors concluded that the same word for an emotion is associated differently by Japanese and Americans. This indicates that the problem of the equivalence of words among different language systems is not only related to finding equivalent semantic words, but is also concerned with the feelings and emotions associated with the words.

This is why the translation of poems and jokes transculturally is often difficult: the feelings and emotions attached to words cannot be transmitted through simple semantic translation. A Japanese poet, Basho, in his famous *haiku,* expressed the poetic mood with the simple words, "*Puton* [sound of water]! A frog jumped into a pond!" A famous Chinese poet, Wang Yang-Ming, wrote: "Raise your head, see the blue mountain, lower your head, see the fence with yellow flowers." He used words of body movement and concrete subjects in nature to create the poetic atmosphere and to transmit the deep feeling, which disappear easily when the poem is translated into another language as the concrete subjects of head, mountain, fence, and flowers.

2. Cultural Variations of Sublinguistic Communication: Gestures and Distance

In addition to verbal communication, human beings, like primates and other animals, utilize gestures, posture (including spacial distance), and other body language to express meaning in communication. Such nonverbal or sublinguislistic communication is considered very important from cross-cultural and clinical perspectives, as it expresses underlying emotions and attitudes explicitly, without the barriers of language.

Based on his review of anthropological literature, La Barre (1947) gave numerous examples to stress that gestures in communication are very much shaped by culture. Despite our assumption that the nodding of the head to indicate affirmation and shaking the head for negation are universal gestures, cultural examples demonstrate that this is not so. According to La Barre, A. H. Landor in 1893 described that Ainu people living in northern Japan use unique hand signs to indicate yes and no. For negation, the right hand is used, passing from right to left and back in front of the chest; for affirmation, both hands are used, gracefully brought up to the chest and waved downward with palms upward. Further, La Barre notes, W.W. Skeat and C. O. Blagden in 1906 reported that the Semang, pygmy Negros of interior Malaya, thrust their heads sharply forward to indicate "yes" and cast their eyes down for "no." People in Micronesia raise their eyebrows to indicate affirmation.

Even though it is a universal custom for men to express friendliness when they meet each other in social settings, the expression of friendly greetings varies greatly among different cultures. In Japan, when people encounter each other on the street, they bow to each other. A certain distance is maintained without physical contact. The number of bows is determined by their roles and the hierarchy between

them. It is an unspoken rule that the subordinate person will bow continuously until the superior person stops. In contrast, Englishmen shake hands with each other to indicate their friendship. Spanish-American men greet one another with a stereotypical embrace, putting their heads over each other's right shoulders, giving each other three pats on the back, putting their heads over each other's left shoulders, and giving three more pats.

Maintaining a certain distance from others and the implications of territorial space are matters of concern among experts specializing in communication, as well as among clinicians. Scholars have distinguished four kinds of interpersonal distance — intimate distance, personal distance, social distance, and public distance — for the purpose of examining distance between people. Based on these categories, various kinds of interpersonal distance may be observed and analyzed from social and cultural perspectives, according to who is involved, on what occasion, between the poles of close and far, and for what purpose.

For instance, ordinary Japanese husbands and wives must maintain some physical distance in the presence of other family members, even at home. It is always proper etiquette for subordinates and superiors to keep a certain distance, even in personal situations. However, it is all right for peers or friends of the same sex to maintain a close distance, even to have physical contact, not only in social settings, but also in public situations. The etiquette for Amercians is different. If a husband and wife do not maintain a physical closeness to each other, even in social settings, other people may suspect that they are not intimate. If peers or friends have physical contact, such as holding hands in public, other people may wonder about the nature of their relationship. In clinical settings, how far the physician should sit from the patient and whether he should hold the patient's hand while they are talking are issues with many implications that need to be evaluated case by case, depending on the age, gender, and past relationship of the parties involved. These matters should also be considered from a cultural point of view, i.e., their implications from a cultural perspective.

C. Attitude, Beliefs, and Values

For the sake of professional elaboration, psychologists conventionally distinguish attitudes, beliefs, behavior, and values as separate parameters of psychology. However, in fact, those parameters are often closely interrelated. As explained by Davidson and Thomson (1980, p. 25), a person acquires *beliefs* about an object on the basis of life experiences. The affective value of these beliefs influences the person's *attitude* in a positive or negative direction. The attitude, in turn, is related to the favorableness of the individual's set of *behaviors* concerning the object. *Values,* as defined by Zavalloni (1980), refer to orientations toward what is considered desirable or preferable socially. As such, they express some relationship between environmental pressures and human desires.

Let us look at some examples of how attitudes, beliefs, and values may differ in different cultural systems. For instance, in the Christian bible, sex is considered to originate with the primary sin; in Buddhist thought, sexual desire, the same as other desires, is regarded as nothing but "empty"; in Confucian thought, sex, as an appetite, is viewed as natural.

In Bali, Indonesia, local people pay high regard to the volcanic mountain, believing that it is where god resides. The part of their houses that faces toward the north, toward the volcano, is kept as a sacred place, with an altar for worshiping the god. Some people even build their villages inside the volcano's crater, although the volcano erupts once in a while. While they are devoted to the mountain, they are not fond of the sea. They regard the deep sea as a dark, dangerous place where evil resides and build their houses far away from the beach. In contrast, the people of Micronesia are fond of the sea. They consider it a source for food and build their villages near the beach so that they have access to it. However, they are not fond of the high mountains and avoid going to them, fearing they are dangerous. Thus, the Balinese and Micronesians, based on their past life experiences, have developed almost opposite attitudes and beliefs about their natural environments. These attitudes and beliefs, in turn, shape their behavior and living patterns.

Attempts have been made by scholars to develop methods for the systematic comparative study of value systems as a whole as they exist in any society. As mentioned previously [Chapter 2: Culture and Society (Section I, C, 2)], Kluckhohn (1951) proposed a framework for studying and describing alternatives in value orientations in five areas.

1. The *man–nature* orientation—subjugation to nature, harmony with nature, mastery over nature
2. The orientation toward *time*—represented by past, present, and future
3. The *activity* orientation—emphasizing being, being-in-becoming, and doing
4. The interpersonal *relational* orientation—emphasizing lineal, collateral, or individualistic goals
5. The *nature of man* orientation—assumed to be good, bad, or neither

Conceptually, this is a useful framework for categorizing various values systematically. However, in reality, it is difficult to categorize value systems in such a simple way, even with regard to an individual, because, depending on the subject and circumstance, a person's attitudes, beliefs, and values may alternate. Such categorization becomes more complicated with regard to society at large. From a sociological point of view, society is seen as a field that creates conflicting values, is dominated by opposing cultural agents, and thus reproduces and creates incompatible choices.

D. Group Behavior

An individual seldom behaves alone in his life. His behavior is always related to others and involves interaction within the context of a group, whether a family, a work group, or a social group. The form and function of a group take on an entirely different perspective in the examination of human behavior. Because group relations and behavior are social matters, they are also closely related to cultural issues.

As described by Mann (1980, pp. 155–157), in all societies, people belong to small primary groups that enforce conformity to norms and require cooperation to achieve group goals. Most work on cross-cultural aspects of small-group behavior, therefore, has sought to test differences among cultures in the scope and intensity of conformity and cooperative behavior. Cultures also vary in other aspects of group functioning, namely: the nature of the pressures imposed by groups on deviate members to elicit adherence to group norms; the power of the group to produce attitude and value change by means of group discussion and decision; and the effects of variations in leadership and communication structure on group productivity and morale.

It is interesting to note that, according to Mann (1980, p. 158), studies of work groups have shown that in some cultures democratic forms of leadership and participatory types of communication structures are the most preferred and effective, whereas in others, such as India (Meade, 1967) and Japan (Misumi, 1972), autocratic and centralized styles of leadership and communication are preferred. Mann also pointed out (1980, p. 158) that while groups are naturally occurring, universal human phenomena, their continued significance for the individual may vary considerably across cultures. In small traditional societies, the individual may belong to one major group that controls virtually all that affects him; whereas in larger, modern societies, he may be a member of many groups, some small and intimate, others large and amorphous, with the freedom to join groups or leave them or to form others. Any attempt to compare small-group behavior cross-culturally must take this fundamental difference into account.

III. CUSTOMARY BEHAVIOR

Conceptually, any behavior is subject to cultural impact and is, therefore, more or less culture related. However, there are special sets of behavior that are deeply rooted in culture and consciously prescribed for members to follow in their daily lives, regulating their behavior within the society. Such customarily observed, culture-rooted behavior is referred to here as **customary behavior.** Customary behavior may include rituals, customs, etiquette (superstitions), belief-related behavior, taboos, or other culture-regulated behaviors. As a member of a society, a person's behavior — in addition to biological factors, individual psychology, and personality (as discussed earlier) — is always subject to customary regulating factors derived from sociocultural dimensions. These regulating factors are exercised and enforced through rituals, etiquette, customs, taboos, or laws. They can vary tremendously from culture to culture and may therefore not be applicable cross-culturally. Let us examine some customary behavior that impacts people's minds and shapes their behavior in daily life.

A. RITUALS, ETIQUETTE, AND CUSTOMS

1. Rituals

In every society, people traditionally observe and practice certain sets of rites, or prescribed ceremonies, in public situations. This is a formal way of enforcing rules or prescribed customs. In association with the life cycle, there are usually rituals related to birth, ceremonies recognizing puberty (such as initiation rites), formal wedding procedures, and funerals for deaths.

Initiation rites are stressed in some cultures to recognize the growth and maturity of the young people. As mentioned previously [cross-reference to Chapter 4: Child Development and Enculturation (Section V)], the intensity of initiation rites for boys is often related to the degree of closeness between mother and son during childhood. Psychologically, initiation rites serve to break these close ties and enable the boy to move into the stage of adulthood.

For Americans, birthday celebrations are emphasized for all age groups, with considerable stress on the birthday of children. Adults' birthday celebrations are often considered successful if they are in the format of a "surprise" party. In contrast, the Chinese traditionally celebrate the birthdays mainly of parents and the elderly rather than the children. Birthday celebrations, particularly for the elderly, are planned formally and publicly, without any secrecy. They are intended to show respect as a part of filial behavior. Children's birthdays were not celebrated annually in the past. In some rural areas, birthdays were not observed until the children reached preschool age. It was feared that announcing the existence of small children by holding birthday celebrations might catch the attention of the god-in-hell, who would come and take away the children's lives. Such precautions were considered necessary in the past, when the mortality rate for children was high.

2. Etiquette

This refers to the forms and manners established by convention as acceptable or required social relations in public settings. Many different etiquettes are observed in various cultures.

For instance, Westerners once considered it a virtue for gentlemen to open doors for ladies and to escort ladies in public settings. Now, in societies that emphasize women's liberation, to open a door for a woman or to yield a seat for a lady may be regarded as an unwelcome act of male chauvinism. In societies where the superiority of men is traditionally stressed, women are not expected to be treated by men in a polite way. It is considered correct etiquette for the wife to walk in the street, several steps behind, not to precede her husband or to walk side by side with him.

In Micronesia, with its matrilineal family system, the brother–sister bond is considered very important. However, in order to protect this culturally prescribed bond, a certain etiquette needs to be observed. If a brother and sister happen to be together in a room, without the presence of other people, one of them has to leave right away. This is true even when they are grown up and married. This etiquette of avoidance serves as a protection against intimacy between them.

At the dinner table, Hawaiian children are told to follow the etiquette of "listening but not talking," i.e., listening to the adults' conversation and learning from it, not speaking up and disturbing it. In contrast, contemporary Westerners, at least in America, consider it a virtue for family members to carry on conversations that include small children. For them, dinner is considered a precious time of intimate socialization and communication among close family members.

3. Customs

Customs are habitual ways of behaving carried out by tradition and enforced by social sanctions. There are endless examples of customs observed in various cultures. Only some examples are mentioned here for the sake of discussion.

Among different cultural groups, different customs are observed with regard to the exposure of body parts. For instance, Muslim women cover their faces with veils in the belief that it is not a virtue to expose their facial features to anyone other than their husbands. Westerners do not mind exposing their upper chests, including part of the breasts, but take care not to expose their legs on formal occasions. In contrast, Easterners, such as Chinese, consider it alright to expose women's lower legs when they wear traditinal *qipau* clothes, even on public occasions. However, they consider it disgraceful for women to expose their upper chests, particularly in low-necked dresses. Interestingly enough, Japanese women, when they wear traditional *kimono,* while coverring almost all part of body, may expose the back of neck for sexual attraction (see Fig. 6-1).

Based on their religious thought, Muslim people do not eat pork; Buddhists avoid eating any meat; whereas Asian farmers customarily do not eat buffalo meat — based on their belief that the buffalo have worked hard for the farmer and it is not kind to eat their meat after they die. Mormons do not drink alcohol or coffee, believing that such substances will affect their brains, and that it is not right to do so. Even regarding food, there are diversified customs among different cultural groups.

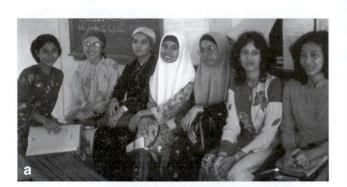

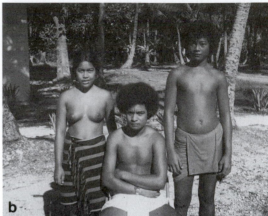

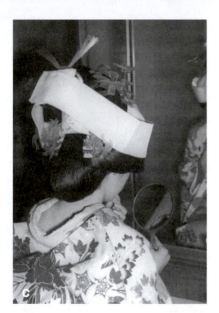

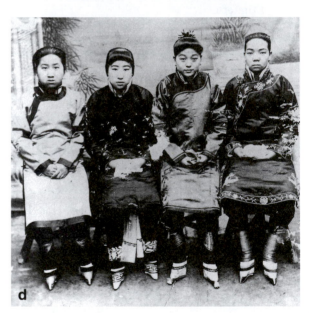

FIGURE 6-1 Customary behavior in different cultures. (a) Malay ladies, following Islam custom, cover their hair to conceal their sexual attractiveness from the opposite sex. (b) Micronesian ladies in the past were not concerned with exposing the tops of their bodies, but carefully covered the area between the umblica and the knees. (c) Japanese woman in a traditional *kimono,* exposing the back of her neck as a sign of sexual beauty. (d) Chinese young ladies from affluent families had their feet bound from childhood to show their well-bred backgrounds as well as a sign of beauty for their future husbands.

B. Taboos and Superstitions

1. Taboo

This is a social prohibition or restriction that is derived from convention or tradition. Breaking a taboo is considered socially undesirable, with the belief that certain ill effects might result.

Many different taboos are observed in various cultures. Following are some examples. In Micronesia, people traditionally follow a pregnancy taboo, i.e., if a wife becomes pregnant, she returns to her home of origin and avoids any labor. Her husband is allowed to visit her, is expected to bring nutritious food for her, but is not permitted to have intimate relations with her. It is believed that sexual relations with the pregnant wife will have ill effects on her as well as on the fetus. Not only during pregnancy, but even after the baby is born, until it is 1 year old, and knows how to dip its head into the water and hold its breath (basic survival skills for island people) — the taboo continues and the wife stays in her own home. This may be considered a culturally prescribed method of protecting pregnant women and new babies or a measure of population control for the islanders (see Fig. 6-2).

According to Australian cultural psychiatrist John Cawte (1976), the aborigines who inhabited the Wellesley Islands of the Gulf of Carpentaria, Australia, observed a sea–land territorial taboo. The people believed there was a mutual antipathy between the land and the sea. A person who entered the sea without washing his hands after handling land food ran the risk of succumbing to *malgri* — a special kind of sickness. According to this taboo, if the precautions were neglected, the totemic spirit that guarded that particular territory was believed to invade the belly "like a bullet." In many cultures, particularly in Africa, a severe form of punishment was believed to occur in the form of voodoo death if a person broke certain taboos prescribed by their culture [cross-reference to Chapter 13: Culture-Related Specific Syndromes (Section II,A,4)].

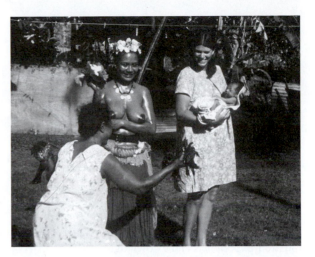

FIGURE 6-2 Pregnancy taboo in Micronesia. Traditionally a wife who becomes pregnant has to return to her family of origin not only for the period of gestation, but also for the first year of child rearing. This is a custom to ensure the health of the mother and child. The photograph illustrates public showing of the healthy mother and the birth of a lively new child—the most important issues for the island people.

2. Superstitious Beliefs and Avoidance

The term "superstitions" refers to a set of beliefs collectively held by a group of people that are considered by people outside of the group to have no basis in reality or cannot logically be explained by scientific knowledge. Therefore, they are labeled "superstitions" by outsiders. Although they might not be believed by outsiders, the people inside the culture are psychologically influenced by such beliefs, which are manifested in their emotions and behavior. "Superstitious avoidance" is a set of customarily observed avoidance behaviors based on superstitious beliefs. It is closely related to a taboo, yet differs in that there is no serious punitive action taken when the regulation is broken. It is merely considered undesirable if the avoidance is not observed.

Many Christians, based on historical events described in the bible, believe that Friday the 13th is an unlucky day. Some Christians avoid going out on that day. There is no 13th floor in some hotels and no bed

No. 13 in some hospitals in the strong (superstitious) belief that the number is unlucky. The Japanese do not care about the number 13, but they try to avoid the number 4 if they can, as the sound of "four" is similar to that of "death." The Chinese favor the number 9, as "nine" sounds the same as "long," implying longevity. In Hong Kong, many people are willing to pay a fortune for a car license plate that includes many nines.

Depending on how you interpret it, some Chinese still strongly believe in *fensui* — a geographic concept that the position of a mountain, the direction of a subject, plus the natural force of wind and water will affect practical situations in life, bringing bad or good luck. This concept may have originally reflected accumulated experience and knowledge about the effects of the physical environment. However, for some Chinese, it has become such a strong (superstitious) belief that they have to consult an "expert" to select the location of a building, the arrangement of furniture, and so on, including which direction their heads should be pointing when they are in bed.

The Chinese observe certain superstitious avoidances. It is considered bad luck to break something on New Year's day. If someone does, other people will say "*sui-sui ping-an*" in Chinese. The Chinese pronunciation of "*sui*" means "things broken (into pieces)" as well as "year." Saying the phrase "*sui-sui ping-an*" (which literally means "year-year peace!") is a customary way of undoing the unlucky event.

C. CULTURAL REGULATIONS AND LAWS

1. Cultural Regulations

These are certain regulations prescribed traditionally by culture for people to observe and follow. They are unwritten, but almost formally and publicly recognized practices demanded of people.

In India, after the death of her husband, no matter how young she is, the wife is expected to be confined socially for the rest of her life — not to interact with any men besides her father-in-law or brothers-in-law, and to avoid social activity outside of her household. This derives from the concept that a woman who has

lost her husband is "evil" in a certain sense. It is also a cultural way of enforcing the male-dominated patrilineal family system.

For traditional Chinese, following Confucian rites and mourning for parents has to be observed for at least 2 years. During this period, no wedding is permitted for filial sons. The only way to avoid this rule is to apply the exception, which allows a young adult son to marry immediately, within 1 month of his parent's death. It is considered that the happiness of the marriage will neutralize some of the sorrow. Thus, some young men arrange to find a potential wife and get married within that time period, rather than waiting for a couple of years until the mourning is completed.

Although the traffic regulation of driving on one side of the road is a modern one, which side is driven on, whether the left or the right, is very much rooted in historical path and political situation, as well as in practical matters, and there is cultural pride in maintaining the choice. Thus, the world is divided into the British custom of driving on the left side and the non-British custom of driving on the right side, with no compromise between them. This makes things rather complicated if you are traveling and driving in different countries. On Okinawa island, during the American military occupation after World War II, driving was changed to the right side of the road (the American way) rather than the left (the Japanese way). However, almost four decades later, when the island was returned to the Japanese government's administration, traffic was rearranged in a single day and converted back to driving on the left side.

It is assumed by modern man that 1 day has 24 hours. It is quite true that all the clocks produced in any country today have faces that are subdivided into 12 sections for 12 hours — for daytime or nighttime, totaling 24 hours per day. This is a universally accepted regulation. Also, the pointers, or hands, for hours and minutes are all supposed to turn "clockwise" — namely, from the viewer's standpoint, the pointers turn toward the right and down, then left and up. However, if you travel to Venice, Italy, on the old clock tower you will find that historically it was not always this way. The face of the clock on the tower has more than 12 subdivisions. Also, it was designed in such a way that the hands turned "counterclockwise," opposite to the modern clock. This illustrates that, in the past, there was a different regulation for subdividing the hours of the day at least in ancient Italy. Fortunately, the regulation of time has been universalized so there is no confusion internationally.

2. Law

This is a formal regulation set up through administrative procedure by the justice system and enforced by law-enforcement agencies. Based on historical background and social setting, different legal systems are observed in different countries — Euro-continental law and American law, for instance. Some of the differences are derived from purely professional matters, others from societal and practical matters, and still others are reflections of cultural beliefs and attitudes. For instance, whether a pregnant woman is permitted by law to terminate her pregnancy — the right to life or abortion — is a subject of hot debate in the United States at present. People are divided into opposite positions and argue emotionally on the matter, even using bombings as threats (and actual murder) to insist on "life protection!" However, in Italy, while abortion is prohibited by the Catholic Church, it is commonly practiced by most women. There is no oppositional argument in society, no bomb threats against abortion clinics as in the United States. In China, related to its national policy for population control, abortion is required if a woman, after having one child, is found to be pregnant. Thus, abortion is considered a legitimate way of carrying out the national policy of family planning. There are many other examples of how, based on their cultural views, people take different positions in regard to public law. Laws on life-related matters, such as organ transplants, the definition of legal death, or euthanasia (physician-assisted suicide), are still debated in many cultures [cross-reference to Chapter 42: Working with Medically Ill Patients (Section II, D, 5)].

This review of customary behavior helps us to understand that, in our daily lives, particularly in social relations, we are led to behave or think in certain ways without knowing how much our behavior is shaped by our culture. Unless we take the position of an "outsider," we may not be able to objectively comprehend the nature of our ordinary daily behavior. Although only some examples of culture-rooted customary behavior are described, it is hoped that a review of these examples will increase our insight into how culture influences our behavior.

IV. ETHNIC IDENTITY

A. ETHNIC IDENTITY FORMATION

Ethnic identity refers to the psychological way in which a person identifies his own ethnic background and how he feels about his own ethnicity. In contrast to an individual or personal identity, ethnic identity is one kind of group identity. American anthropologists De Vos and Romanucci-Ross (1975) clarified ethnic identity by saying that: "It is essentially subjective, a sense of social belonging and ultimate loyalty; is a form of role attribution, both internal and external" (p.3). Further, they pointed out that "ethnic identity is in essence a past-oriented form of identity, embedded in the cultural heritage of the individual or group" (p.363). From a psychological perspective, it needs to be pointed out that prejudice plays a big part in how one self-identifies ethnically, as well as in terms of race, nationality, social class, or religious group.

In general, a person has to deal with identities on various levels. These include "personal identity," which is concerned with how a person identifies himself as a "person"; "family identity," which focuses on how a person identifies and views his own "family"; or other "group identities," relating to community, school, occupation, religion, society, or nation. Ethnic identity is one kind of group identity dealing with the psychological function of identification at the "ethnic" level. Cultural identity is close to ethnic identity, except that from the time a person is a child, from a cognitive perspective, he is usually unable to perceive and conceptualize his own cultural system, as it is an abstract entity. However, ethnicity, in the same way as race, is more or less an objectified subject that can be perceived, conceptualized, and identified so that, in practice, ethnic or racial identity can become an operational concept with a recognizable existence.

As with personal, family, or other kinds of group identity, a sound and positive ethnic identity is important for an individual's psychological well-being and health. To know one's origins is to have not only a sense of provenance, but, perhaps more importantly, a sense of continuity in which one finds to some degree the personal and social meaning of human existence (De Vos & Romanucci-Ross, 1975, p. 364). Thus, developing a healthy ethnic identity is a matter of concern from a mental health point of view.

Theoretically, the process of ethnic identification and/or racial identity starts to take place at an early age — when cognitive function becomes such that a child is able to perceive, understand, and identify the differences of ethnicity or race that are expressed by the external characteristics of behavior or appearance. Aboud (1987) reported that racial differences are recognized by children at the ages of 3 and 4, whereas ethnic differences are not recognized until age 7. However, the formation and function of group identity is subject to numerous reality factors, and the process tends to fluctuate.

First of all, group identity formation and maintenance — although intrapsychic phenomena — depend greatly on external stimuli. When other distinguishable groups and stimulation for the need to distinguish the differences exist, the sense of group identity is provoked. In other words, as indicated by Devereux (1975), "ethnic identity develops only after an ethnic group recognizes the existence of others who do not belong to the group." For instance, a group of schoolmates will obtain a sense of their "school identity" when their school is in competition with other schools in sports or other activities. The process of identifying with his own school with a sense of loyalty will be stimulated. A citizen will

increase his "national identity" and demonstrate loyalty toward his own country when it is in open conflict (such as war) with other countries. If the external stimulation is rather longstanding, such as discrimination against an underprivileged minority, the stimulation for identity formation will become rather continuous. If there has been a long history of conflict and hostile relations between different groups — exemplified with the situation for the Irish Protestant and Irish Catholic in North Island — the antagonism and conflict continues for centuries.

The ethnic identity is also strongly influenced by political factors. Based on the circumstance, ethnic identity may change over time. This is well illustrated in the situation for people in Russia, identifying with former Soviet for many decades, but changed overnight to Russia.

In general, the process of identity development is a dynamic one and will fluctuate with vicissitude depending on the external situation (Devereux, 1975). This is true for the whole life cycle. However, associated with the developmental stage, adolescents tend to be more sensitive to the matter of ethnic identification and may react to related issues with psychological turmoil.

B. FUNCTIONAL OR DYSFUNCTIONAL ETHNIC IDENTITY

The nature of ethnic or racial identity can be discussed in terms of whether it is positive or negative, functional or dysfunctional. Needless to say, if an ethnic or racial group is looked down upon by other groups, or by the dominant group, its members will tend to develop an inferior image of their group, forming a negative ethnic or racial identity. Such a negative identity will greatly influence the mental health of the group's members.

Depending on the situation, ethnic or racial identity can be changed. This is well illustrated by the situation of African-Americans in the United States. Numerous studies have reported that African-American children have had a more positive image of themselves as African-Americans recently than they did several decades ago. Ward and Braun (1972) reported that, in the 1950s and early 1960s, studies of racial preference of children consistently showed black children choosing white models and rejecting dark models. However, a study of black children growing up since 1963 indicates a reversal of this position, with blacks choosing more dark models. Similarly, Fish and Larr (1972) compared human figure drawings by African-American children before 1960 and after 1970, indicating that more black racial indicators are included in current drawings than in the past. All the findings are interpreted to mean that African-American children are more positively aware and accepting of their racial and ethnic background now than they were before 1960 (Harris, Blue, & Griffith, 1995).

Ethnic identity usually has both positive and negative components, to some extent. As in the case of personal, family, or other group identity, a positive ethnic identity will contribute greatly to the psychological well-being of a person. Generally speaking, the ethnic identity should be suitable, objective, and balanced. Otherwise it can be dysfunctional at both individual and social levels.

Dysfunctional ethnic identity is usually illustrated by extreme ethnocentrism, i.e., taking an extremely ethnic, self-centered view associated with a very negative attitude toward ethnic groups other than one's own. Good examples of such dysfunctional ethnic identity are the Germans in Hitler's era, who believed that German was the most superior ethnic group and discriminated against and even tried to exterminate Jewish people; the Japanese in World War II, who believed that they were blessed ethnically by the existence of the Japanese emperor and used this idea to "rescue" colonized people and start the war in Asia; and the KKK groups in the United States, who believe that minority groups, particularly blacks, should be discriminated against and excluded from the society.

As explained by De Vos and Rommanucci-Ross (1975), how a person maintains a healthy ethnic identity if he or she is living as a member of a minority group within a pluralistic society becomes a mental health concern. The offspring of interethnic or interra-cial marriage will face issues of mixed ethnic identity. As pointed out by De Vos and Romanucci-Ross, a dual or combined identity is not denied but encouraged. For instance, the Mestizos in Mexico are a recognized ethnic group whose members are graded according to the degree of their racial mixture and their Spanish or Indian cultural behavior. In the multiethnic society of Hawaii, as a result of mixed marriages among different ethnic groups, the offspring identify themselves merely as a "mixed" group without psychological problems associated with that identification.

How we identify with self, family, a small group, or a large collective group, including a society, ethnicity, race, or culture, has a direct impact on our psychology and mental health. However, in the past, little effort has been made to understand the process of ethnic identity formation and its relation to mental health (Sue & Sue, 1990). What constitutes normal and healthy ethnic identity versus abnormal or dysfunctional ethnic identity is a subject awaiting further exploration.

REFERENCES

Aboud, F.E. (1987). The development of ethnic self-identification and attitudes. In J.S. Phinney & M.J. Rotherman (Eds.), *Children's ethnic socialization: Pluralism and development* (pp. 29–51). Newbury Park, CA: Sage.

Boucher, J.D. (1974). Culture and the expression of emotion. *International and Intercultural Communication Annual, 1*, 82–86.

Brislin, R.W. (1980). Introduction to social psychology. In H.C. Triandis & R.W. Brislin (Eds.), *Handbook of cross-cultural psychology: Vol. 5. Social psychology* (pp. 1–23). Boston: Allyn & Bacon.

Cawte, J.E. (1976). *Malgri:* A culture-bound syndrome. In W.P. Lebra (Ed.), *Culture-bound syndromes, ethnopsychiatry, and alternate therapies* (pp. 22–31). Honolulu: University Press of Hawaii.

Cheng, T.A. (1988). A community study of minor psychiatric morbidity in Taiwan. *Psychological Medicine, 18,* 953–968.

Davidson, A.R., & Thomson, E. (1980). Cross-cultural studies of attitudes and beliefs. In H.C. Triandis & R.W. Brislin (Eds.), *Handbook of cross-cultural psychology: Vol. 5. Social psychology* (pp. 25–71). Boston: Allyn & Bacon.

Devereux, G. (1975). Ethnic identity: Its logical foundations and its dysfunctions. In G. De Vos & L. Romanucci-Ross (Eds.), *Ethnic identity: Cultural continuities and change* (pp. 42–70). Palo Alto, CA: Mayfield.

De Vos, G., & Romanucci-Ross, L. (Eds.). (1975). *Ethnic identity: cultural continuities and change.* Palo Alto, CA: Mayfield.

Dickey, E.C., & Knower, F.H. (1941). A note on some ethnological differences in recognition of simulated expressions of the emotions. *American Journal of Sociology, 47,* 190–193.

Doi, L.T. (1973). *Omote* and *ura:* Concepts derived from the Japanese two-folds structure of consiousness. *Journal of Nervous and Mental Disease, 157,* 258–261.

Ekman, P., & Friesen, W.V. (1972). The repertoire of nonverbal behavior—Categories, origins, usage and coding. *Semiotica, 1,* 49–98.

Fish, J.E., & Larr, C.J. (1972). A decade of change in drawings by black children. *American Journal of Psychiatry, 129*(4), 421–426.

Harris, H.W., Blue, H.C., & Griffith, E.E.H. (Eds.). (1995). *Racial and ethnic identity: Psychological development and creative expression.* New York: Routledge.

Izard, C.E. (1980). Cross-cultural perspectives on emotion and emotion communication. In H.C. Triandis & W. Lonner (Eds.), *Handbook of cross-cultural psychology: Vol. 3. Basic process* (pp. 185–221). Boston: Allyn & Bacon.

Johnson, F.A., Marsella, A.J., & Johnson, C.L. (1974). Social and psychological aspects of verbal behavior in Japanese American. *American Journal of Psychiatry, 131*(5), 580–583.

Katzner, K. (1995). *The languages of the world* (New ed.). London: Routledge. (Original work published 1977)

Kluckhohn, C. (1951). Values and value orientation. In T. Parsons (Ed.), *Toward a general theory of action.* Cambridge; MA: Harvard University Press.

La Barre, W. (1947). The cultural basis of emotions and gestures. In J.M. Starr (Ed.), *Social structure and social personality.* Boston: Little, Brown.

Lebra, T.S. (1983). Shame and guilt: A psychocultural view of the Japanese self. *Ethos, 119*(3), 192–209.

Leff, J.P. (1973). Culture and the differentiation of emotional states. *British Journal of Psychiatry, 123,* 299–306.

Leff, J.P. (1977). The cross-cultural study of emotions. *Culture, Medicine and Psychiatry, 1*(4), 317–350.

Liang, P. (1939). A preliminary note on verbal expressions of emotion in Chinese. In R.S. Lyman, V. Maeker, & P. Liang (Eds.), *Social and psychological studies in neuropsychiatry in China.* Peking: Peking Union Medical College.

Mann, L. (1980). Cross-cultural studies of small groups. In H.C. Triandis & R.W. Brislin (Eds.), *Handbook of cross-cultural psychology: Vol. 5. Social psychology* (pp. 155–209). Boston: Allyn & Bacon.

Meade, R.D. (1967). An experimental study of leadership in India. *Journal of Social Psychology, 72,* 35–43.

Misumi, J. (1972). *Group dynamic in Japan.* Fukuoka, Japan: Kyushu University, The Japanese Group Dynamics Association, Faculty of Education.

Schlosberg, H. (1941). A scale for the judgement of facial expressions. *Journal of Experimental Psychology, 29,* 497–510.

Sue, D.W., & Sue, D. (1990). Racial/cultural identity development. In D.W. Sue & D. Sue *Counseling the culturally different: Theory and practice.* New York: J Wiley.

Tanaka-Matsumi, J., & Marsella, A.J. (1976). Cross-cultural variations in the phenomenological experience of depression. I. Word association studies. *Journal of Cross-Cultural Psychology, 7,* 379–396.

Tseng, W.S. (1975). The nature of somatic complaints among psychiatric patients: The Chinese case. *Comprehensive Psychiatry, 16,* 237–245.

Vinacke, W.E. (1949). The judgment of facial expression by three national-racial groups in Hawaii. I. Caucasian faces. *Journal of Personality, 17,* 407–429.

Vinacke, W.E., & Fong, R.W. (1955). The judgment of facial expressions by three national-racial groups in Hawaii. II. Oriental faces. *Journal of Social Psychology, 41,* 185–195.

Ward, S.H., & Braun, J. (1972). Self-esteem and racial preference in black children. *American Journal of Orthopsychiatry, 42*(4), 644–647.

Woodworth, R.S. (1938). *Experimental psychology.* New York: Holt.

Zavalloni, M. (1980). Values. In H.C. Triandis & R.W. Brislin (Eds.), *Handbook of cross-cultural psychology. Vol. 5. Social psychology* (pp. 73–120). Boston: Allyn & Bacon.

7

Late Adult Life: Aging and Death

I. ADULT LIFE CYCLE

The life cycle after a person has reached adulthood has seldom been explored seriously by scholars in the past, with the general assumption that life is the same once one has grown up and become an adult. An exception was made by the ancient Chinese scholar Confucius. Based on his own personal adult development, he said: "At 15 I set my heart upon learning. At 30, I had planted my feet firmly upon the ground. At 40, I no longer suffered from perplexities. At 50, I knew what were the biddings of Heaven. At 60, I heard them with a docile ear. At 70, I could follow the dictates of my own heart; for what I desired no longer overstepped the boundary of right." He described beautifully how he grew up psychologically and became more mature as a scholar through his own personal life. Then, what about an ordinary person's life cycle? Is there a universal pattern for a person in growing up as an adult? Associated with the longer lives of contemporary people, is there any change in the latter part of life? Any cultural differences? These are issues that need to be addressed.

Modern psychologists are increasingly interested in the life cycle as a unit of study and in such questions as whether adult development, like child development, is to be perceived as a succession of stages. As behavior scientist specializing in human development, Neugarten (1979) has pointed out that a stage theory of adult development seems oversimplified for several reasons. The timing of life events is becoming less regular for modern man, and age is losing its customary social meaning. Psychological themes and preoccupations reported by adults in different age groups do not follow a single, fixed order. Further, intrapsychic changes occur slowly with age and not in stepwise fashion. Despite this, it cannot be denied that the life of an adult changes in association with increased age, whether explicitly or not, and there are certain common issues that need to be faced.

According to Birren and Renner (1977), it is useful to differentiate three aspects of human age and aging: biological, psychological, and social age. The biological age of an individual can be defined as an estimate of the individual's present position with respect to his potential life span; psychological age refers to the adaptive capacities of the individual; and social age refers to the roles and social habits of an individual with respect to other members of a society. From a cultural point of view, we are more concerned with the latter two, particularly social age.

Through the work of pioneer cultural anthropologists, it has become clear in this century that development, including adulthood, is, indeed, a cross-cultural phenomenon (Colarusso & Nemiroff, 1981, p. 170). Nevertheless, David Gutmann (1977) has sought to find the similarities in development among various cultures represented by five different groups: men in Midwest America; men of the Navajo Indian nation; men in the lowland and men in the highland Mayan cultures of Mexico; and men of an Islamic sect, the Druze of Israel. Based on his investigations, he identified three stages of adult development, each with characteristic attitudes toward the relationship between the world and the self. The first stage, labeled "active mastery," encompasses roughly the years from 35 to 54 and is characterized by a productive orientation focused on actively dealing with and changing externals. The second stage, called "passive mastery," covers the decade from 54 to 64. During this stage, the man now views the world as a place where there are many things that he cannot change, and where his sources of pleasure and ways to meet his needs are most often not in his control, but in the hands of forces or powers larger than himself. The final stage, referred to as "magical mastery," beginning around age 65, is colored by the tendency to move toward regression, receptivity, and magical solutions to problems. Gutmann views culture as the modifier of these underlying universal developmental phases. Further, as Colarusso and Nemiroff pointed out (1981, p. 171), societal effects on development lead to later adulthood with culture specificity.

In the introductory chapter of the book *Anthropology and Aging,* edited by Rubinstein, Keith, Shenk, and Wieland (1990, p. 1), it is pointed out that an awareness of national and international "graying," and its accompanying problems and potentials, is widespread. Anthropologists are playing an increasingly vital role in the study of later life, not only because the graying of the planet is widespread and cross-cultural, but also because of the increasing recognition of the significance of culture and cultural differences in human life, even in its later stages (Cohen, 1992).

II. APPROACHING THE STAGE OF THE AGED

A. Views and Attitudes about Aging

The views and attitudes toward aged people are rather negative in contemporary American society, and the term "ageism" is even used (K.S. Berger, 1994, p. 586). Ageism is similar in many respects to racism and sexism, in the sense that it is based on subjective, stereotyped, falsified, negative views of a particular group without a base in reality and is harmful to the group against which the prejudiced is directed. The main reason for the strength of ageism in the contemporary United States is the culture's emphasis on youth, strength, and success. The aged person is viewed as a negative or an obstacle in striving toward such a cultural ideal. Thus, as Butler and Lewis (1982) have pointed out, any sign of a person's "beginning to fail" is feared and exaggerated in its seriousness.

As mentioned earlier, "age," and particularly "aging," can be viewed from three perspectives: biological, psychological, and social. Behavior and social scientists tend to take the view that aging represents one of many aspects of reality that are socially defined and that old age is a social category whose properties and problems are constructed within the context of shared expectations particular to specific groups. This is well illustrated by the study by Bengtson, Kasschau and Ragan (1977). They conducted subjective assessments of age among populations living in southern California. The results revealed that self-categorization of aging varied considerably by ethnic group membership. For example, over 30% of the Mexican-Americans identified themselves as "old" at age 57. The same percentage of African-American respondents was not reached until age 63, and of Caucasian-Americans until nearly age 70. In discussing contrasts between African-American and Caucasian-American elderly, Jackson (1970). suggested that, in the United States, minority group members perceive themselves as "old" at a considerably earlier chronological age than the majority group because of the repeated hardships they have faced through a lifetime of economic and social disadvantage.

B. Coping with Some Aging Landmarks

1. Menopause

It has been noticed that, associated with the improvement of living conditions in modern societies, the onset of puberty among youngsters is occurring several years earlier than in the past, whereas the age of menopause is coming later, increasing the span of reproductive years from a biological standpoint as reflected in chronological age. Strictly speaking, menopause is a physiological change that occurs in women at the end of the reproductive stage. It occurs as the result of hormonal changes associated with a cluster of somatic symptoms, such as flushing, heavy sweating, and so on.

Concerning possible influences of race of the onset of menopause, a study has been carried out by Goodman, Grove, and Gilbert (1978) in Hawaii, comparing age at menopause in relation to reproductive history in Japanese-Americans, Caucasian-Americans, Chinese-Americans, and Hawaiian women living in Hawaii. Their results indicated that there were no noticeable differences among them in terms of age of menarche, or age of menopause. There were no interactions of ethnic group with age at menarche, parity, or months spent breast-feeding. Because they were living in more or less similar social settings, the age for menarche and menopause seemed similar among the different ethnic or racial groups.

However, medical investigation has revealed that the severity of menopausal symptoms and complaints varies cross-ethnically. It has been found that this is related mainly to food-intake patterns rather than to psychological factors. For instance, Japanese women were found to have less severe menopausal symptoms, related to their high intake of tofu, which is rich in "vegetable estrogen" — a substance that could reduce the symptoms associated with menopause.

Despite the biological basis for menopause, there still exist cultural factors that influence reactions to the occurrence of menopause, with different meanings for the arrival of menopause depending on how people interpret it. It may be seen as the termination of the reproductive stage, with reproduction an important function for women in some cultures, or a signal for relief of the burdens associated with reproduction, including the cyclic occurrence of menstruation. Menstruation is viewed in some cultures as a "dirty" discharge, with many ways developed to avoid its contamination.

2. Middle-Age Adjustment

The concept of a middle-age crisis is rather popular in Western society, where youth is valued and the signs of aging in middle age produce relatively serious psychological reactions. This may not be true in societies where middle age is considered a time for people to enjoy social status and power in their lives.

Authors of the book *Adult Development,* Colarusso and Nemiroff (1981, pp. 122–124) identified several factors involved in the midlife transition. They are bodily changes, changes in time perceptions, changes in marital relationships and relationships with children, and social and financial change. Considering marital change, it can be pointed out that, associated with the family system, family structure, and the practices of separation, divorce, and remarriage, different courses of marital relationships will be observed during middle age. For instance, in a society where the production of children is encouraged and divorce is not permitted, adults at middle age will be surrounded by many children and living with a spouse — whether or not the person feels happy. In contrast, in a society where the bearing of children is not valued and divorce is easy, there is a higher chance for a middle-age person to be living alone, without a spouse and with few children. Again, whether or not the person feels gratified with his life, it is certainly a different way to go through the midlife stage and to encounter different natures and degrees of crisis.

From social and financial perspectives, it is easy to understand that in the individual-oriented capitalist society, a person needs to depend on his own financial achievement in middle age. His source of security is his own individual effort and success. In contrast, in a society where financial achievement is the product of collective effort, and there is a solid public system of support even after people become old, they will have different social and financial experiences in middle age.

3. Retirement

The system of retirement is a product of industrialized society. For most of human history, no one stopped working until their health failed. This was true in hunting or agricultural societies where no artificial line was drawn to indicate when a person stopped his productive work. Today, however, the vast majority of people in developed societies work for three decades or more and then stop when late adulthood begins — going through the developmental landmark of "retirement" and adjusting to postretirement life. According to Quinn and Burkhouser (1990), in the United States, the majority of retirees leave the work force because they want to and their employers encourage it. Most retirees not only adjust well to their change in lifestyle, but even improve in health and happiness. The exceptions are primarily among those who retire prematurely and involuntarily, and are abruptly severed from their major source of status and social support.

III. THE AGED AND THE FAMILY

A. Aging and the Family: Developmental Change

Paralleling personal and family development, there is a considerable shift in and evolution of an individual's relation to the family. Most people in Western society have passed the stage of launching grown-up children when they reach middle age and encounter the stage of the empty nest. Later, most people will relate with their adult children as aged parent(s) and,

sooner or later, encounter the stage of widowhood. In terms of intrafamily interpersonal relationships, a person loses his relations with his own parents when they pass away and relates to his own adult children when he reaches old age.

In terms of personal and family development, two characteristic relationships need to be adjusted in accordance with aging: the husband–wife relationship and the parent–children axis. A spouse has to relate to changes that include widowhood, and an aged parent has to adjust to how he or she relates with his or her adult children.

B. Spousal Relations between Aged Husband and Wife

Although a shift of power from husband to wife in association with increased age is noticed to some degree among families of various ethnic groups, it is more noticeable among some Asian couples. By tradition, the husband has more authority and power within his family, particularly over his submissive wife. However, this is only true when they are relatively young. After they reach a certain age, particularly after their children have grown up and the wife becomes a mother-in-law, her status increases considerably. As a woman, she not only reverses her previous submissive role toward her own mother-in-law, becoming a dominant mother-in-law herself, but the tendency to express a dominant role is manifested in the marital relationship as well. As he ages, the husband tends to become less dogmatic and authoritative, allowing his wife to have more power in expressing her opinions and contributing to decision making.

C. Intergenerational Relations between Aged Parents and Adult Children

Although the occurrence of a gap between generations has been noticed after children reach adolescence, this intergenerational gap continues to exist when the children are adults and their parents become aged, except that the nature of the problems change. When the younger generation is still young, the parents are more experienced and have more power to influence the parent–child relationship. However, when the children grow up and become adults and the parents age, the situation is reversed. The adult children have accumulated sufficient experience in their lives and have also begun to have considerable power in their opinions, whereas the aged parents' views tend to be seen as "out of date," losing their creditability.

The reversed parent–child relationship becomes more prominent if they encounter considerable cultural change, a change that may occur within a society, or associated with transcultural migration. In the latter situation, the aged parents usually suffer from language problems and are less experienced and familiar with the host society, putting them at a disadvantage. There are usually increased communication problems between aged parents and their adult children, with a wider gap in their value systems and reversed parent–child roles. This phenomena has been noticed among various Asian immigrants to the United States, including Japanese-American elderly (Osako & Liu, 1986), Chinese-American elderly (Yu & Wu, 1985), and Korean-American elderly (Kiefer et al., 1985). Most of the studies tend to indicate that filial piety toward parents is an ideal concept among Asian people, but, in reality, coupled with many other factors, including socioeconomic and working conditions, filial behavior toward aged parents is far from what is traditionally expected.

Examining family interactions with the elderly, Mitchell and Register (1984) compared African-Americans and Caucasian-Americans, pointing out that Caucasian-American elderly see their children and grandchildren more frequently than African-American elderly; however, African-American elderly are more likely to receive help from their children and grandchildren and take children into their homes to live. They commented that giving help to children and grandchildren is influenced more by socioeconomic status than race factors among the subjects studied.

IV. ADJUSTMENT OF THE AGED

A. SOCIOCULTURAL ASPECTS OF RISK FACTORS FOR THE AGED

Numerous risk factors can be encountered by the elderly, including physical, psychological, and social ones. Here, only some of the risk factors that are closely related to social and cultural factors will be discussed.

Bengtson and associates (1977) conducted a study of the major problems encountered in old age among residents of southeastern California. Among three ethnic groups living there — Caucasian-Americans, African-Americans, and Mexican-Americans — they found that there were cross-ethnic similarities as well as differences. All three ethnic groups reported finances as the number one problem and health as the second. After these two factors, ethnic differences became evident. Over one-quarter of the African-Americans identified crime in the community as a problem; about the same percentage of the Mexican-Americans volunteered the cost of food as a specific difficulty. More Caucasian-Americans indicated problems of morale: loneliness, isolation, or feeling "blue."

Regarding residential relocation, Brand and Smith (1974) studied a group of subjects aged 65 and over who experienced involuntary relocation because of urban renewal projects. The subjects were low-rent tenants forced to move for new housing projects. The subjects were composed of two racial groups, Caucasians and African-Americans. The survey, carried out over a 2 to 3 year period after the relocation, revealed that the elderly showed greater life dissatisfaction, as measured by the Life Satisfaction Index, than the control group. Between the two racial groups surveyed, the African-American elderly seemed to adjust better after relocation than the Caucasian group. The investigators pointed out that the amount of social interaction of the elderly with their environment was affected by the relocation. Compared to the nonrelocated group, the relocated elderly were generally less active and had fewer social contacts. This study suggests that an involuntary change of residence at an aged stage may disrupt social networks and lead to deleterious consequences in the life adjustment of the elderly.

Linn, Hunter, and Perry (1979) conducted a study of a group of elderly living in Miami, Florida, from 1976 to 1978. The group was composed of three ethnic subgroups: Caucasian, African-American, and Cuban. The results revealed strong differences among these subgroups. The African-American elderly, who were mostly local-born residents, showed the best adjustment when social class and level of disability were held constant. The Cuban group, which had migrated from Cuba, suffered from cultural displacement and showed the most negative adjustment, whereas the Caucasian group, which had moved from other areas of the country to Miami after retirement, was in between. The investigators interpreted the differences in the psychosocial adjustment of the elderly as possibly the indirect result of relocation.

B. Availability and Utilization of Support Systems

The social care system for the elderly involves publicly funded formal services and informal services provided by family, friends, and neighbors. In order to understand the patterns of informal social support utilization by the elderly, Fleishman and Shmueli (1984) conducted a survey in Baka, in Jerusalem, Israel. Data obtained were compared with that reported from studies carried out in Europe and America. They commented that the characteristics observed in the Jewish community, such as long-term commitment, a multigenerational permanent membership group, and close physical proximity exhibited by the principal helper, permit the performance of a wide range of informal assistance activities by kin, and the elderly need not seek help from nonkin. In contrast, in other countries, especially in the United States, residential distance from offspring more often forces the elderly to develop informal social support systems in which neighbors play an important role.

Chatters, Taylor, and Jackson (1986) conducted a study of elderly African-Americans concerning

choice for an informal help network by impaired elderly adults. Nine categories of helpers were examined: spouses, sons, daughters, fathers, mothers, brothers, sisters, friends, and neighbors. They reported that the results indicated that marital status is important in selecting the categories of sister, friend, and neighbor. The presence of children decreased the likelihood that siblings and friends would be chosen. Also, perceived family closeness facilitated the selection of siblings, but inhibited the choice of friends. This supports the view that membership in sociodemographic subgroups influences the use of specific informal helpers.

Utilizing publicly available facilities for living, i.e., nursing homes, is a financial, psychological, and cultural issue. People in general hold negative views about nursing homes, considering them terrible places to live when you get old. It is quite true that the condition of some nursing homes is not desirable, but many are improving. Still, in general, people prefer to stay at home if they can when they get old. This is particularly true in a society where it is still strongly believed that a family home is the primary place to live and that the family should take care of family members in need of care (Beland, 1984). However, due to social structures and employment conditions, it is getting difficult for many adults to cope with taking care of their aged and disabled parents in their homes (Pace & Anstett, 1984; Poulshock & Deimling, 1984). Sending them to live in nursing homes is becoming a necessary choice for many, particularly in industrialized, urban societies. Making such a choice is becoming a new cultural challenge (Strong, 1984).

C. Sexual Activity, Interest, and Attitude

Knowledge about sexual behavior in old age is still very scant. There is almost no cross-cultural data, and only fragments of information that allow us to make some speculations.

In the United States, Pfeiffer, Ver woerdt, and Wang (1968) conducted a sexual behavior survey of men and women in their 70s. A structured interview was carried out with community volunteers residing in North Carolina. The subjects ranged in age from 60 and 94 (average age 71) with a mixed racial composition of Caucasians and African-Americans. On the basis of cross-sectional data, they found a gradual decline in both sexual activity and interest with advancing age. The age when sexual intercourse stopped ranged from 50 to 85 for men, with a median age of 68, and 45 to 75 for women, with a median age of 60. This indicated that the women ceased having sexual intercourse nearly a decade earlier than the men. Among reasons for stopping sexual intercourse, for men, 42% were due to their spouses (death, illness, or loss of interest) and 58% were due to self (loss of potency or illness). For women, 86% were due to their spouses, and only 14% due to self. Interestingly enough, longitudinal data revealed that, contrary to the general pattern obtained from cross-sectional data, a significant percentage of aged individuals showed rising patterns of sexual activity and interest.

Portonova, Young, and Newman (1984) did a survey in the 1990s of a group of Caucasian elderly women who were residing in a small town in northeastern Pennsylvania. The subjects were aged 60 or older, with a median age of 69. The survey showed that, in general, elderly women had positive attitudes toward sexual activity among older men and women. In particular, their attitudes were more positive if the persons engaged in sexual activity were married. Many women in their later years expressed a desire for male companionship.

However, this view may not be shared cross-culturally. In general, among conservative societies, there is a cultural prejudice against the expression of sexual desires and activities in old age. As a result, as pointed out by Berezin (1978), elderly people themselves view their own sexual desires, fantasies, and feelings negatively.

D. Integration: Older People in Social and Cultural Contexts

Despite the universal phenomena observed around the world about the lives of old people, there are numerous variations noted cross-culturally (Bergener,

Hasegawa, Finkel, & Nishimura, 1992). Maddox (1978) described such variations within social and cultural contexts. In general, the status of the aged is high in societies in which there is a high reverence for or worship of ancestors. It also tends to be high in agricultural societies and lower in urbanized societies. It is high in societies in which the extended form of the family is prevalent and lower in societies that favor the nuclear form of the family and neolocal marriage. The stability of residence favors high status of the aged; mobility tends to undermine it. The status of the aged is inversely proportional to the rate of social change; the adjustment of the elderly is significantly affected if there is rapid cultural change. Retirement is a modern invention, found chiefly in modern, high-productive societies. The roles of widows tend to be clearly ascribed in primitive societies, but such role ascriptions decline with modernization; the widow's role in modern societies tends to be flexible and ambiguous. The individualist value system (of Western society) tends to reduce the security and status of older people.

V. DEATH AND MOURNING

A. Views and Attitudes toward Death

Even though death, from a narrow perspective, is primarily a biological phenomenon, i.e., the end of the life of an organism, it is associated greatly with psychological matters. Death can have many meanings: it can be seen merely as a biological event, a rite of passage, an inevitable natural occurrence, or many other things. Needless to day, culture contributes to the perspectives on death and dying (A. Berger et al., 1989; Ross, 1981).

In most African traditions, as pointed out by Opaku (1989), elders take on an important new status through death, joining the ancestors who watch over their own descendants, as well as the entire village. Therefore, everyone in the village participates in a funeral to prepare the deceased's journey to the ancestral realm. The death of the individual becomes an occasion for the affirmation of the entire community, as members jointly celebrate their connection with each other and with their collective past.

In contrast, in many Muslim societies, death affirms their faith in their god, Allah. People are taught that the achievements, problems, and pleasures of this life are transitory and ephemeral and that everyone should be mindful of, and ready for, death at any time. In Buddhist societies, such as Thailand, based on their religious thoughts of incarnation, the present life is considered part of the whole circulating cycle. Death is simply an entrance to another part of the cycle. In Hindu societies, such as India, helping the dying to relinquish their ties to this world and prepare for the next is a particularly important obligation for the immediate family (Firth, 1989).

From the examples just mentioned, it is clear that attitudes toward death and reactions to the loss of a close person are shaped by religious thought or philosophy of life. However, as Eisenbruch pointed out (1984), when we look at how the individual actually feels and deals with his predicament, the suffering individual is not content with theological thought or philosophical explanation. Further, Eisenbruch stated that, even within any "one" religious denomination, there can be many different explanations of the meaning of death that will be mirrored by that group's characteristic ways of grieving. This is illustrated by the variety that exists within Christian groups.

In the past, throughout most of Western society, death was an accepted, familiar event that usually occurred at home. In 20th-century North America and western Europe, death came to be withdrawn from everyday life. More and more people died alone in hospitals rather than at home among family members (K.S. Berger, 1994, p. 680).

B. Grief, Mourning, and Widowhood

1. Grief and Mourning Customs Practiced in Different Cultures

Although the loss of a significant person in life is always an emotional event, there are numerous diversified customs prescribed by different cultures for people to guide their reactions when they encounter a close person's death (Rosenblatt, Walsh, & Jackson, 1976).

According to the customs of Orthodox Jews, relatives must remain with a dying family member so that the soul does not leave while the person is alone. Jews do not leave a dead body unattended, as that would be a sign of disrespect (Rabinowicz, 1979). In the Jewish tradition, those who are making condolence visits are advised to enter the house and sit silently unless the mourners show a desire to speak of their loss (Chafetz, 1980).

Who mourns for whom is a basic question that sometimes needs to be addressed because of different family systems. For example, according to Fulton (1977), among the Ifaluk people living in Micronesia, a wife was not expected to grieve for her husband. Within that matrilineal society, a woman's emotional ties remained with male members of her maternal family and she was culturally expected to grieve for her father, her brothers, but not for her husband.

In China in the past, following a custom established in Confucius' time, a different period of time for mourning was expected for different people, e.g., 3 years for parents, 1 year for a husband, and 1 month for children. Also, it was generally expected that women would show their feelings of sorrow openly in the public. It was almost a ritual for a female to cry loudly at the time of the funeral. When a parent(s) died, in addition to the daughter(s), it was considered a daughter-in-law's primary job to cry loudly to show how the family missed the deceased parent-in-law.

2. Widowhood in Cross-Cultural Perspectives

Widowhood, losing a lifelong marital partner, is a major event affecting development in many adults. The developmental tasks for people in widowhood are to mourn emotionally; to form new life patterns in regard to daily activity and work, if still working; to become reinvolved with others in new ways; and possibly to remarry or to reform intimate relations with a new life partner.

According to Colarusso and Nemiroff (1981, p. 178), Goin and Burgoyne in 1980 reported that in many healthy individuals the emotional attachment to a dead spouse may remain for years. This leads us to hypothesize that the mourning process in later life may be qualitatively different than that in earlier stages of development, being more prolonged and more difficult to complete.

Different experiences of widowhood have been described cross-culturally by Mathison (1970) as follows. India has a strong patrilineal social organization in which women are devalued. The Hindu religion has decreed that a widow shall not remarry, although a widower is urged to remarry as soon as possible. The situation is worsened by another Hindu custom: girls are frequently betrothed while still very young to much older boys or even to men. With the age differential and the death rate in India, it is not uncommon for a girl to become a widow before the marriage is even consummated. Throughout history, the life of a widow in India has been dismal. She can stay with her husband's family, but is then regarded as the most menial of all the other persons in the household. She cannot attend ceremonies of rejoicing, as her presence is considered a bad omen. As pointed out by Mathison (1970), at least part of the rationale behind the dehumanizing treatment of widows lies in the Hindu belief that the husband's death has in some way resulted from the sins the wife has committed in a past life.

In contrast, the fate of widows among the Trobriand Islanders in New Guinea is consistent with matrilineal social organization, in which women occupy a more prestigious position than in other societies. The widow is provided with highly structured rituals to observe during her bereavement. During the several days of funeral rites, the widow is required to mourn ostentatiously and dramatically, shaving her head and howling loudly with grief. After this, she enters a small cage built into her home and remains in the dark for a period of 6 months to 2 years. This is said to keep the husband's ghost from finding her. Kinsmen are with her at all times. Once the period of mourning is terminated, she is ceremonially washed and dressed in a gaily decorated grass skirt. She is then considered to be available for remarriage.

Because women in this culture control material goods through the matrilineal descent system, and are thus an economic asset to men, remarriage is highly likely (Mathison, 1970).

Examining individual grief and mourning processes across cultures through a review of ethnographic literature, Rosenblatt and associates (1976) found that societies which performed final ceremonies sometime after a person's death lacked prolonged expressions of grief, whereas grief is prolonged (and often disturbed) in societies that lack final postburial ceremonies.

Comparing bereavement in Samoan and American communities, Ablon (1971) brought up the issue that Samoans view death as natural, even in the experiencing of life. In contrast, death in the United States is a subject that is generally hidden, or at least ignored as much as possible.

C. EUTHANASIA, OR PHYSICIAN-ASSISTED SUICIDE

Associated with the extension of life spans and the increase of deteriorated physical or mental conditions for some aged persons, the possibility of actively ending someone's life has become a consideration, and physician-assisted suicide, or euthanasia, has become a controversial topic in many societies (Coomaraswamy, 1996). There is a need to distinguish between "active" and "passive" euthanasia. In the former, the physician takes an active role in ending a person's life, using medical means to end the life of a person wishing to die. In the latter, the physician withdraws any medical methods of sustaining a person's life so that the person will eventually die.

After reviewing the situations in Germany, Holland, and the United States, Battin (1991) pointed out that, although they are alike in having aging populations that die primarily of deteriorative diseases, the end-of-life dilemmas are handled differently in these three countries. In the United States, up to now, withholding and withdrawing of treatment were the only legally recognized means of aiding dying. In Holland, voluntary active euthanasia is practiced by physicians.

In Germany, assisted suicide is a legal option, but is usually practiced outside of a medical setting.

Clearly, the way we deal with a person wishing to end his life is a complicated issue that needs to be carefully thought about and decided upon. It involves philosophical, practical, medical, legal, and culture matters that are awaiting examination and answers in the near future.

REFERENCES

Ablon, J. (1971). Bereavement in a Samoan community. *British Journal of Medical Psychology, 44,* 329–337.

Battin, M.P. (1991). Euthanasia: The way we do it, the way they do it [Special issues]. *Journal of Pain and Symptom Management, 6*(5), 298–305.

Beland, F. (1984). The decision of elderly persons to leave their homes. *The Gerontologist, 24*(2), 179–185.

Bengtson, V.L., Kasschau, P.O., & Ragan, P.K. (1977). The impact of social structure on the aging individual. In J. Birren & K.W. Schaie (Eds.), *Handbook of the psychology of aging.* New York: Van Nostrand-Reinhold.

Berezin, M.A. (1978). The elderly person. In A.M. Nicholi, Jr. (Ed.), *The Harvard guide to modern psychiatry* (pp. 541–549). Cambridge, MA: Harvard University Press.

Bergener, M., Hasegawa, K., Finkel, S.I., & Nishimura, T. (Eds.). (1992). *Aging and mental health disorders: International perspectives.* New York: Springer.

Berger, A., Badham, P., Kutscher, A.H., Berger, J., Perry, V.M., & Beloff, J. (Eds.). (1989). *Perspectives on death and dying: Cross-cultural and multi-disciplinary views.* Philadelphia: Charles Press.

Berger, K.S. (1994). *The developing person through the life span* (3rd ed.). New York: Worth.

Birren J.E., & Renner, V.J. (1977). Research on the psychology of aging: Principles and experimentation. In J.E. Birren & K.W. Schaie (Eds.), *Handbook of the psychology of aging.* New York: Van Nostrand-Reinhold.

Brand, F.N., & Smith, R.T. (1974). Life adjustment and relocation of the elderly. *Journal of Gerontology, 29*(3), 336–340.

Butler, R.N., & Lewis, M.I. (1982). *Aging and mental health: Positive psychosocial and biomedical approaches* (3rd ed.), St. Louis, MO: Mosby.

Chafetz, P. (1980). Jewish practices in death and mourning. *Death Education, 3*(4), 367–369.

Chatters, L.M., Taylor, R.J., & Jackson, J.S. (1986). Aged blacks' choice for an informal helper network. *Journal of Gerontology, 41*(1), 94–100.

Cohen, L. (1992). No aging in India: The uses of geontology. *Culture, Medicine and Psychiatry, 16*(2), 123–162.

Colarusso, C.A., & Nemiroff, R.A. (1981). *Adult development: A new dimension in psychodynamic theory and practice.* New York: Plenum Press.

Coomaraswamy, R.P. (1996). Death, dying, and assisted suicide. In G.J. Kennedy (Ed.), *Suicide and depression in late life: Critical issues in treatment, research, and public policy.* New York: Wiley.

Eisenbruch, M. (1984). Cross-cultural aspects of bereavement. I: A conceptual framework for comparative analysis. *Culture, Medicine and Psychiatry, 8*(3), 283–309.

Firth, S. (1989). The good death: Approaches to death, dying, and bereavement among British Hindus. In A. Berger et al (Eds.), *Perspectives on death and dying: Cross-cultural and multi-disciplinary views.* Philadelphia: Charles Press.

Fleishman, R., & Shmueli, A. (1984). Patterns of informal social support of the elderly: An international comparison. *The Gerontologist, 24*(3), 303–312.

Fulton, R. (1977). The sociology of death. *Death Education, 1*(1), 15–25.

Goodman, M., Grove, J.S., & Gilbert, F., Jr. (1978). Age at menopause in relation to reproductive history in Japanese, Caucasian, Chinese and Hawaiian women living in Hawaii. *Journal of Gerontology, 33*(5), 688–694.

Gutmann, D.L. (1997). The cross-cultural perspectives: Notes toward a comparative psychology of aging. In J.E. Birren & K.W. Schaie (Eds.), *Handbook of the psychology of aging.* New York: Van Nostrand-Reinhold.

Kiefer, C.W., Kim, S., Choi, K., Kim, L., Kim, B.L., Shon, S., & Kim, T. (1985). Adjustment problems of Korean American. *The Gerontological Society of America, 25*(5), 477–482.

Jackson, J.J. (1970). Aged negroes: Their cultural departures from statistical stereotypes and rural-urban differences. *The Gerontologist, 10,* 140–145.

Linn, M.W., Hunter, K.I., & Perry, P.R. (1979). Differences by sex and ethnicity in the psychosocial adjustment of the elderly. *Journal of Health and Social Behavior, 20,* 273–281.

Maddox, G.L. (1978). The social and cultural context of aging. In G. Usdin & C.K. Hofling (Eds.), *Aging: The process and the people.* New York: Brunner/Mazel.

Mathison, J. (1970). A cross-cultural view of widowhood. *Omega, 1,* 201–218.

Mitchell, J., & Register, J.C. (1984). An exploration of family interaction with the elderly by race, socioeconomic status, and residence. *The Gerontologist, 24*(1), 48–54.

Neugarten, B.L. (1979). Time, age, and the life cycle. *American Journal of Psychiatry, 136*(7), 887–894.

Opaku, K.A. (1989). African perspectives on death and dying. In A. Berger et al. (Eds.), *Perspectives on death and dying: Cross-cultural and multi-disciplinary views.* Philadelphia: Charles Press.

Osako, M.M., & Liu, W.T. (1986). Intergenerational relations and the aged among Japanese Americans. *Research on Aging, 8*(1), 128–155.

Pace, W.D., & Anstett, R.E. (1984). Placement decisions for the elderly: A family crisis. *The Journal of Family Practice, 18*(1), 31–46.

Pfeiffer, E., Verwoerdt, A., & Wang, H.S. (1968). Sexual behavior in aged men and women: I. Observations on 254 community volunteers. *Archives of General Psychiatry, 19,* 753–758.

Portonova, M., Young, E., & Newman, M. (1984). Elderly women's attitudes toward sexual activity among their peers. *Health Care for Women International, 5,* 289–298.

Poulshock, S.W., & Deimling, G.T. (1984). Families caring for elders in residence: Issues in the measurement of burden. *Journal of Gerontology, 39*(2), 230–239.

Quinn, J.F., & Burkhouser, R.V. (1990). Work and retirement. In R.H. Binstock & L.K. George (Eds.), *Handbook of aging and the social sciences* (3rd ed.). San Diego, CA: Academic Press.

Rabinowicz, H. (1979). The Jewish view of death. *Nursing Times, 75*(18), 757.

Rosenblatt, P.C., Walsh, R.P., & Jackson, D.A. (1976). Grief and mourning. In P.C. Rosenblatt, R.P. Walsh, & D.A. Jackson *Cross-cultural perspective.* New Haven, CT: HRAF Press.

Ross, H.M. (1981). Societal/cultural views regarding deathand dying. *Topics in Clincal Nursing, 3,* 1–16.

Rubinstein, R.L., Keith, J., Shenk, D., & Wieland, D. (Eds.). (1990). *Anthropology and aging: Comprehensive reviews.* Dordrecht, The Netherlands: Kluwer Academic Publishers.

Strong, C. (1984). Stress and caring for elderly relatives: Interpretations and coping strategies in an American Indian and White sample. *The Gerontologist, 24*(3), 251–256.

Yu, L.C., & Wu, S.C. (1985). Unemployment and family dynamics in meeting the needs of Chinese elderly in the United States. *The Gerontological Society of America, 25*(5), 472–476.

Section C
Culture and Mental Health

Following a review of the cultural aspects of human behavior in general (in Section B), and prior to examining the impact of culture on psychopathology (in Section D), this section aims to elaborate on several issues that have direct relevance to the matter of mental health and clinical care from cultural perspectives.

There are three chapters altogether. Chapter 8 will address how culture impacts stress and modes of coping with stress. Then, Chapter 9 reviews how mental illness is perceived, explained, and grouped by laymen with folk knowledge. This is followed by an elaboration in Chapter 10 on illness behavior, including how people react to mental illness and how they seek help for their problems.

8

Stress and Coping Patterns

I. THEORETICAL CONSIDERATIONS AND APPLICATIONS

A. DYNAMIC NATURE OF STRESS

From a biological point of view, Selye (1982) defined stress simply as the nonspecific result of any demand upon the body, whether mental or somatic. From an epidemiological perspective, Kasl (1996, pp. 14–15) indicated that stress can be formulated in various ways: as environmental stress, susceptible to objective definition and measurement; as a subjective perception or appraisal of an objective environmental condition; as a particular response or reaction; or as a particular relational term linking environmental characteristics and personal characteristics, particularly environmental demands in excess of the individual's capacity to meet them. Here "stress" is used as a generic term for psychological stress, referring to a condition that creates outstanding psychological problems, burdens, pressures, traumas, frustrations, or conflicts to which the subject must react with excessive effort, inducing a considerable disturbance of his or her emotional state. Thus, it is psychological in nature and subject to cultural influence. However, before discussing cultural input on stress, let us first clarify the basic concepts of the dynamic nature of stress.

According to McCubbin and Patterson (1982), concerning family adaptation to crises, Hill proposed his ABCX formula in 1949 to illustrate that the relationship between stressful events and resulting crisis is of a dynamic nature. It is an interactive result of variables, including the stressful event itself(A), supporting resources available to the subject for coping with stress (B), and the perception of stress by the subject (C). These factors interact to produce the outcome of the crisis (X). Additional factors may be added, including the strength of the subject who encounters the stress and his method of coping with it.

Culture is involved in each of these variables. That is, culture influences the occurrence of stress, modifies the perception or appraisal of the stress, is involved in the selection of a coping style, and has an impact on the supporting resources available to the subject. In other words, culture has a broad impact on stress in multiple dimensions.

B. Measurement of Stress

It is recognized by most scholars that stress, due to its dynamic and complicated nature, is difficult to delineate as a discreet condition for scientific measurement. However, numerous methods have been developed to attempt to measure stress. The Social Readjustment Rating Questionnaire (SRRQ) developed by Holmes and Rahe (1967) is one way to assess stress quantitatively. The questionnaire was constructed by culling events "observed to cluster at the time of disease onset" from the life charts of more than 5000 medical patients. It was composed of 43 items of identified life events. The respondents were asked to use their experience to rate certain life events according to the relative degree of readjustment they required.

The method of investigation by life events has been criticized by many scholars for several inherent problems. Schwab and Schwab (1978, p. 257) pointed out that most studies of life events have been retrospective and, thus, their findings may lack reliability. Some of the events identified as "stress" may be the results of stress, or symptomatic of mental illness, and may not be preceding factors. For instance, for SSRQ, "divorce" may be the consequence of mental illness, and "loss of job" may be due to personality or emotional problems. Such variables will confuse the study of the relationship between stress and mental illness. From a cultural point of view, various cultural groups may assign different values to the same event identified as "stress." Therefore, cross-cultural applicability for very diverse cultural groups is questionable.

The Psychiatric Epidemiology Research Interview (PERI) Life Events Scale was constructed by eliciting nominations of actually experienced stressful life events from subjects living in New York City (B.S. Dohrenwend, Krasnoff, Askenasy, & Dohrenwend, 1978). It is composed of 102 life events. It was reported that an analysis of these ratings suggests that there are group differences, with more differences due to ethnic background than to sex or social class.

Goldberg and Comstock (1980), with backgrounds in public health and epidemiology, have commented

that, because different subgroups of the population experience different frequencies of total life events and particular individual events, life-event scores can vary considerably from group to group, depending on demographic composition and the appropriateness of the list of life events for each subgroup. If not adjusted for, such relationships could lead to coincidental associations between life events and health-related outcomes. Their comments can be extended into situations involving groups of diverse cultural backgrounds.

Instead of major life events, Kanner, Coyne, Schaefer, and Lazarus (1981) used the Hassles and Uplifts Scale in their study. The Hassles and Uplifts Scale includes items that define the irritating, frustrating, distressing demands that to some degree characterize everyday transactions with the environment. It includes annoying practical problems, such as losing things or traffic jams, and fortuitous occurrences, such as inclement weather, as well as arguments, disappointments, and financial and family concerns. Kanner and colleagues applied the measurement to a community sample of middle-age white adults in the United States, claiming that the Hassels Scale was a better predictor of concurrent and subsequent psychological symptoms than the life-event scores.

Burnam, Timbers, and Hough (1984) carried out a community survey in El Paso, Texas, and Ciudad Juarez, Mexico, to investigate ethnic and social predictors of psychiatric disorders. Psychological distress was assessed with the Langner Scale (Langner, 1962) and the Psychiatric Epidemiologic Research Interview (PERI) Demoralization Scale (B.P. Dohrenwend, Shrout, Egri, & Mendelsohn, 1980). The Demoralization Scale was constructed with such items as dread, anxiety, sadness, helplessness, hopelessness, psychophysiological symptoms, perceived physical health, poor self-esteem, and confused thinking. In their study, four ethnic/residential groups were compared: Anglo-Americans, Mexican-Americans raised in the United States, Mexican-Americans raised in Mexico, and Mexicans. They reported that the two scales yielded different results. Anglo-Americans reported lower levels of psychological distress with the Langer Scale than the three groups of Mexicans, but no differences were found with the Demoralization Scale. Ethnic differences in Langer Scale scores were greatest among older adults and were attenuated when controlled for socioeconomic status. They explained that the discrepancy between the two scales may be attributed to response bias and different perceptions of symptoms, as well as scoring differences. It was their interpretation that social demographic and methodological factors may mediate ethnic–origin differences. It should be pointed out that these two scales utilize the occurrence of psychiatric symptoms as an index for measuring psychological stress — a method that does not truly reflect the nature of the stress encountered in life and does not distinguish possible ethnic differences.

C. STRESS AND PSYCHIATRIC DISORDERS

As pointed out by B.S. Dohrenwend and Dohrenwend (1984), we have learned from clinical case studies that life stressors can play a part in causing serious illness and even death. Further, specification of the kinds of life events that affect health have been made in relation to certain disorders. For instance, Paykel (1974) identified a class of events in which a person leaves the social field of the subject (i.e., death of a close family member, marital separation, divorce, family members leaving home, child getting married, and son drafted). He found that the presence of one or more events in this category was strongly related to the onset of depression. Theorell (1974), in a retrospective study, found that work events were closely related to cardiac patients. Later (1976), in a prospective study, he revealed that "increased responsibility at work during the last year" was associated with subsequent myocardial infarctions.

This view has been echoed by Cooke and Hole (1983). They suggested that the effects of specific types of life events on specific psychiatric disorders are of great importance. They reviewed various studies conducted by others to investigate possible rela-

tions between stressful events and psychiatric disorders. They pointed out that, in many investigations in which "general" life events were used to relate to "overall" psychiatric morbidity, the extent of variance ranged mostly at the level of 5 to 10%. However, in Finlay-Jones and Brown's study (1981), the investigators empirically distinguished psychiatric disorders arising from anxiety and depression cases. In addition, they divided stressful life events into "loss events" and "danger events." The "loss events" were related to depression and the "danger events" to anxiety with a variance of 23 and 25% respectively. Cook and Hole used these results as an example to stress their view that particular types of events appear to have etiological significance for particular types of psychiatric disorders.

The impact of life changes on psychiatric disorders has been studied by various investigators (Rahe, 1979). For instance, Jacobs, Prunsoft, and Paykel (1974) compared patients' life-change events prior to the onset of schizophrenia to life-change events prior to depression. The investigators found that although both depressives and schizophrenics, upon their first hospital admissions for their diseases, showed increased recent life-change experiences compared to controls, depressives reported more "exits" from the social field as well as a greater variety of undesirable events than schizophrenics. In the interpretation of Jacobs and colleagues, recent life events have a "precipitating" capacity in the lives of schizophrenics, and life-change events play a "formative" role in the symptom pictures of depressives.

Regarding minor psychiatric disorders, Tennant and Andrews (1978) found, in a community sample of adults in Sidney, Australia, a significant relationship between patients' recent life-change experience and the onset of neurotic impairment. The investigators found that neither the number of recent life-change events nor life-change scaling results correlated independently with impairment; a subjective distress score, however, did correlate independently with levels of neurotic symptoms in the group studied. Their view supports the notion that it is not the life event itself but the appraisal of the event by the subject that has a more direct psychological impact, which in turn has a greater relation to the formation of psychiatric disturbance of a functional nature.

D. VARIOUS WAYS CULTURE INFLUENCES STRESS

Regarding its dynamic nature, as mentioned earlier, stress needs to be understood as a complicated issue that is influenced by multiple and compound factors, including the occurrence of stress itself and its appraisal by the subject experiencing it, as well as supporting resources for coping and the strength to cope available to the subject that enable him to face the stress. Here, let us elaborate the various ways in which culture impacts stress.

1. Culture Itself Produces Stress or Problems

Psychological stress or problems can be directly produced by the cultural system itself. Through commonly shared beliefs and group attitudes, a society may induce stress in its members. This will be elaborated in detail in Section II.

2. Culture Influences the Perception of Stress or Appraisal of Problems

How cultural factors influence the perception of stress or problems is well illustrated by Masuda and Holmes' cross-cultural study of Japanese and Americans (1967). They used the Social Readjustment Rating Questionnaire (SRRQ) to rank items that were perceived as stressful and required considerable readjustment in subjects' lives. Data obtained were arranged in order of the severity of the items.

The results indicated a high concordance between the Japanese and the American samples in the manner in which they establish a relative order of magnitude of life events. For instance, "death of spouse" was ranked first by both Japanese and Americans. "Divorce" was second for Americans and third for Japanese. However, it was also evident that from the

common bases manifested by these two industrialized societies, cultural variants were derived that distinguished one from the other. In the study, 17 of the 42 life-event items were found to be scored significantly differently by Japanese and Americans. For instance, "detention in jail" was ranked second by Japanese and sixth by Americans. "Minor violation of the law" was ranked 28th by Japanese and 43rd by Americans. This is in keeping with one of the prime facets of Japanese culture, the obligation of the individual to his family, his name, and his position. "Mortgage or loan over $10,000" (a considerably large debt at the time of the investigation in the 1960s) was ranked higher (17th) by Japanese, in contrast to 28th by Americans. This reflected that, in Japan, going to a bank to borrow money was uncommon. People usually tried to borrow money from relatives or close friends first. To borrow money from a bank was considered a last resort and an unfavorable way to manage financial debts.

In contrast to these findings, several items, such as "marital separation," "marital reconciliation," and "change in number of arguments with spouse," all relating to conflictive transactions with a spouse, were ranked higher (3rd, 10th, and 15th, respectively) by the Americans, who emphasize the husband and wife axis as the primary family relationship, than they were by the Japanese (7th 15th, and 33rd, respectively).

Following Masuda and Holm's investigation, Rahe (1969) added a survey of additional cultural groups, namely African-American, Mexican-American, Hawaiian, Danish, and Swedish in his comparative study (for the latter two groups, the samples were Danish and Swedish university students studying in the United States). Again, even though the investigator claimed that general patterns were similar for all the subject groups studied, there were considerable differences among the groups. For instance, "divorce" appeared to be less of a life change for the African-American (13th ranking order) and Mexican-American (10th ranking order) groups than for the other samples: Caucasian-American (second ranking order), Japanese (third), and

Danish and Swedish (both fourth). "Marriage" was considered to be below many other life changes only in the Swedish sample (15th ranking order); in other groups, the ranking order ranged between first and sixth. "Jail term" appeared to represent less of a life change for the Mexican-American (19th ranking order) and Hawaiian (10th ranking order) groups; in contrast to second ranking order for the Japanese, Danish, and Swedish, and sixth ranking order for Caucasian-Americans. Being "fired from work" seemed relatively less of a life change for the African-Americans (16th ranking order), whereas it was 7th to 10th for the other groups. Thus, it is clear that, associated with their different life situations, the life events that could have caused life changes had considerably different ranking orders in the various cultural groups investigated.

It is important to point out that, although there are some methodological issues in those cross-cultural studies (Fairbank & Hough, 1981), including the original investigators' intention to conclude a "concordance" of rating patterns, considerable differences do exist among different cultural groups in terms of how stressful they perceive life events to be. Another level of caution is needed in considering to what extent an event really is stressful if the life event does occur. However, it does prove that stress is "perceived" differently by different cultural groups depending on their life circumstances, as well as how they view problems.

3. Culture Shapes Reactions to and Coping Patterns for Stress or Problems

How culture may mold the pattern of reaction to and coping with stress is best illustrated by ethnic differences in reacting to pain. Even though pain is considered a universally recognized somato psychological stress, which is usually reacted to differently due to individual factors, including a patient's personality, sensitivity to and threshold of pain, and psychological needs in coping with suffering, culture shapes the reaction patterns among different ethnic groups. For instance, it has been pointed out by

Zborowski (1952) that Old Americans (of Anglo-Saxon background) have a matter-of-fact orientation toward pain. In contrast, Jews express a concern for the implications of pain and distrust palliatives. Italians, however, express a desire for the relief of pain, whereas the Irish inhibit expressions of suffering and concerns for the implications of pain. Closely related to ethnic character and cultural attitudes toward physical suffering, diverse pain reactions can be noticed among different ethnic groups [cross-reference to Chapter 16: Somatoform Disorders, including Neurasthenia (Section II, E).

Concerning the kinds of coping strategies used by widows regarding widowhood-related problems, Ide, Tobias, Kay, Monk, and de Zapien (1990) examined Mexican-Americans and Anglo-Americans. They reported that the Mexican-American widows used nonconfrontational "intrapsychic strategies" most frequently (60%), confrontational modes of "direct action" and "information seeking" next (37 and 35%, respectively), and "inhibition of action" strategies least frequently (14%). In contrast, Anglo-Americans favored all these mentioned strategies almost equally (24, 22, 24, and 28% respectively). It was interpreted that as Mexican-American tend to have family members living with them or nearby after widowhood, "direct action" coping modes (seeking assistance from others) work well for them. In contrast, Anglo-Americans, who tend to live alone and have a more diffuse social network, more often chose "inhibition of action" as best for coping.

4. Culture Effects Supporting Resources Available for Managing Stress

Finally, culture affects stress through the supporting resources it offers for coping with problems. The nature of supporting resources varies greatly; it may be of a private or public nature, it may come from neighbors, the family, community, or government or it may be material or emotional. No matter what it is, cultures may differ in terms of the availability of supporting resources for those facing stress, which in turn influences the outcome of coping with problems.

II. CULTURAL CONTRIBUTION TO STRESS AND PROBLEMS

Behavior scientists have recognized and investigated various kinds of exogenous stressors. They are related to the physical environment, such as natural disasters or overcrowding; psychological conditions, such as sensory deprivation, long-term imprisonment, nontraumatic but wearing events, population pressure, examination, loss of an important person, bereavement, or uncertainty; or cultural factors, such as taboo transgression, culture change, or role conflicts.

The specific cultural factors of stress have received considerable attention among scholars in the past (Leighton & Hughes, 1961; Wittkower & Dubreuil, 1973). Let us list in detail the different ways culture contributes to the occurrence of stress, problems, or vulnerability.

Here, "stress" refers to the occurrence of severe psychological strain at a particular time. Thus, it is more time limited. In contrast, a "problem" implies that the ill-condition exists continuously, without a limited time period. The distinction is an arbitrary one without clear-cut boundaries. "Vulnerability" means that an individual person, a group of people, or a society as a whole has certain weaknesses to face in dealing with the stress or problems they encounter.

A. CULTURE-PRODUCED STRESS

1. Stress Created by Culturally Formed Anxiety

Culture may contribute to the occurrence of stress directly through the beliefs that are held by the members of a society. There are numerous examples that illustrate this. The folk belief that excessive or inappropriate sexual outlets will cause shrinkage of penis into the abdomen, threatening death, is an example of a culture-induced anxiety resulting in *koro,* a panic attack among some Chinese and Thai people, and people in Bangladesh, sometimes in epidemic form. Similarly, the belief that leaking of semen through urina-tion as a result of excessive masturbation will result in serious illness is another example of culture-derived anxiety (referred to as *Daht* syndrome) among some young people in India. Cross-territorial anxiety relating to sea and land, causing multiple somatic pains *(malgri),* observed among aborigines in Australia, or voodoo death as the result of taboo breaking, are also examples of how culture can cause severe anxiety and even panic-related death [cross-reference to Chapter 13: Culture-Related Specific Syndromes (Section II, A)]. Fear of vampires, the end of the world, UFO invasion, heart attack, contamination from nuclear radiation, the hazards of smoking, or the ill-effects of being overweight are other examples of anxiety that may originate from supernatural beliefs, scientific knowledge, or reality. Such group-shared anxieties can escalate or decline according to the attitudes and degrees of concern shared by people in a given time and place.

2. Stress Induced by Culturally Prescribed Special Roles and Duties

In a society, some members are prescribed certain roles and duties from a cultural perspective. If the role prescribed is an inferior one and the duties are hard to perform, the person concerned may suffer a stressful life experience. Such situations are exemplified by the following examples.

In China in the past, it was the custom that if a family was poor and had too many children, the parents would give up their youngest daughter for adoption to another family for monetary payment. This "adopted daughter," even though she was still young, was expected to work hard as a domestic maid for the adoptive parents. In other words, she was sold to work as a maid. Until she was grownup and ready for marriage, she had to wake up early and stay up late doing all the chores in the household. She had to obey her adoptive mother and was subjected to harsh discipline if she did not perform well. There are stories describing such miserable "adopted daughters" living their youths with tears in their eyes all the time. This is similar to the situation of African-Americans brought to work as slaves in the United States in the past, who suffered from their underprivileged roles and harsh duties.

In Muslim culture, a husband was allowed to have more than one wife, while it is considered a woman's main function to bear children. If a woman failed to bear children after marriage, she faced the breakup of her marriage. This caused stress-induced anxiety and has been described as one kind of culture-bound neurosis (El-Islam, 1975).

In India, as previously described (Chapter 3), when a woman became a widow, she was considered subconsciously by others as an "evil" woman who had caused her husband's death. Thus, she was treated as an unfavorable person in the household. This was reinforced by the cultural attitude that, under the patrilineal family system, a woman is nothing but an accessory of a man. The widow was confined to her domestic environment and not permitted to socialize outside of the house. She was given a lifelong sentence of confinement, even if she was still young. Remarriage was out of question.

In a less dramatic example, it has been pointed out that, even in our present society, adult children are more or less culturally expected to take care of their elderly parents if they become disabled. This often causes a daily-life burden and emotional stress for adult children.

3. Stress Produced by Culturally Demanding Performance

Although a certain amount of pressure regarding performance is necessary for individuals and society at large, sometimes the demand is so excessive that it may cause culture-produced stress in the individuals as well as in the society as a whole.

The American behavioral scientist Vogel (1962), who studied emotional disturbances in Japanese society, has described the psychological pressure that youngsters encounter there, particularly relating to school entrance examinations (see Fig. 8-1). The problem of gaining admission to good academic institutions is not peculiar to Japan; the tension surrounding admission is probably found in every society. However, what is peculiar to Japan, according to Vogel, is the severity and intensity of the problem. He reported that most middle-class Japanese, even if they are short of funds, will struggle to provide their children with desks and other facilities conducive to long hours of study. A tutor is hired for perhaps a year or

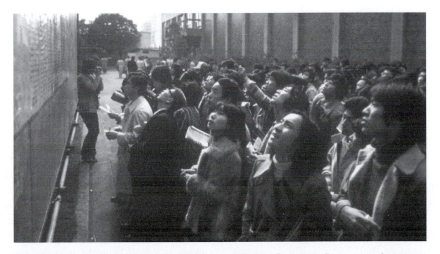

FIGURE 8-1 Stress created by culturally demanded performance. Japanese students nervously search for their names on the college bulletin board for the results of the entrance examination—the most anxious time in their lives.

two to work regularly with the child in preparation for the examination. A high school student may stop various other kinds of activities and settle down to a life of serious study, studying many hours a day after school.

There is a cultural reason for this emphasis on entrance examinations in Japan. Historically, the best way to obtain competent people for government offices was to select them from certain institutions of higher learning. Indeed, as Vogel explained, which educational institution a person attended was used as the main universal criterion for employment in government. Furthermore, Japanese firms generally make a life commitment to an employee at the time of hiring. An employee of one company almost never leaves to work at another company. Each firm seeks to obtain men of considerable competence because they will be committed to these men for life. Because the best students will almost invariably try to get into the best universities, the most reliable single factor for judging competence is the university attended. Very much determined by the historical and social structural characteristics of Japanese society, Japanese mothers will put considerable pressure on the child for school performance, even starting from kindergarten. It is viewed by the society that a good kindergarten leads to a good grade school, a good grade school leads to a good high school, and then to a good university, which, in turn, leads to a good company for life.

Coupled with the pressure for (college) entrance examinations, there is the associated phenomenon of graduation phobia observed in Japan. According to Kasahara (1974), a large number of college seniors have postponed their graduations. This has been particularly true of students in the literature department. For instance, according to a 1970 survey at Kyoto University, one of the ivy-league schools in Japan, over a quarter of the senior class had postponed graduation for more than 1 year. Mental health counselors in colleges are concerned about so-called *ryunen* students, who continuously stay in college and postpone their graduation for more than 3 years. Thus, they are called *ryunen* (literally meaning stagnation year after year), staying in the senior class as a "precipitated"

group with no intention to graduate. This group of students tends to show a lack of interest in their major field of study and indifference to social activity, and complains of feelings of emptiness and intellectual impotence. As explained earlier, once a student graduate and enters a company, he is expected to work with that company for life, with little chance of trying other companies. Thus, students ready to graduate intentionally postponed their graduation with the hope of getting better jobs if they failed to find desirable ones before graduation. Kasahara gave the additional interpretation that those students, usually male, were not sure of their masculinity in their protected school life and were not ready to face the tough adult life awaiting them in the real world.

4. Stress Imposed by Cultural Limitations on Behavior Expression

In contrast to the situations just described, in which culture demands certain behavior performance and achievement, are circumstances in which culture limits behavior expression and discourages social performance, contributing to the occurrence of stress among those who encounter the limitations. Such situations can occur in subtle or explicit ways. An illustration of the former is the circumstance in which women are not permitted to pursue higher education and are expected not to perform outside of their domestic environments. The latter is well exemplified by the situation of American women living in Saudi Arabia. As described by Becker (1991), there is tendency of prohibition against women in Muslim societies, such as Saudi Arabia, enforcing the dependency of women on men. This restrictive aspect of Saudi society often creates stress among American women, who are raised in their home cultures to behavior independently from men and to express themselves in social settings. Facing such cultural limitations, many American women feel confined and helpless in this foreign setting. Depression or anger may develop. The anger is often brought into the marital relationship, which is further stressed because of the lack of outside outlets to diffuse tension and conflicts.

B. CULTURE-RELATED PROBLEMS

1. Problems Due to Cultural Restrictions on the Range of Behavior

This refers to cultural systems that create tight restrictions on the lives of all members of the society. This is a matter of relative comparison with other ethnic or culture units. The cultural restrictions on the range of behavior may be associated with a religious background, military situation, or political condition. Probably the best example is that of the people of the Hutterite religious sect living in certain areas of Canada and the United States. Their dress is prescribed and their duties as farmers, sheepherder, cooks, tailors, or shoemakers are assigned. Their children are not allowed even to ice skate. Their choice of husbands or wives must be approved by the brethren; the request for permission to marry is ritualized. The preparation and eating of food follow traditional sex-segregation etiquette. Contacts with nearby towns are limited to necessity. The Hutterites do not necessarily suffer from their restricted life patterns. If there is little opportunity for them to compare their lifestyle with that of others, they may not complain and may accept it. Or, perhaps because the Hutterites as a group formed their own restrictions, the limited range of behavior expresses the group's own wishes and personality. However, outsiders who come to live with them may have psychological difficulty following their cultural restrictions.

2. Problems Due to Cultural Regulations of Choice

Instead of restrictions on life behavior as a whole, problems may be limited to certain choices in special matters that have a significant impact on life. The choice of a mate, of a professional career, or of staying in one's own country or migrating to another place are some examples. If the choices are determined by the culture, through taboo, custom, or cultural regulation, and are outside of an individual's own will, they are going to affect an individual's mental life significantly.

Even now, many societies still practice marriage by arrangement. It is usually the parents who find a suitable marriage partner. The idea is that the parents will screen the person for negative factors and consider the favorable conditions for selection of a lifelong marital partner. The parents may or may not consider whether the partners concerned are fond of each other. They may base their choice entirely on other perspectives, such as the families on both sides, financial or health factors, and so on. Affection between the man and the woman may not be part of the picture. Arranged marriage does not necessarily bring an unhappy end. On the contrary, it works well for many couples. However, being forced to marry someone you dislike or having to marry someone simply for the sake of family, financial, or political reasons tends to be associated with emotional unhappiness.

The incest taboo is observed in most societies, but the scope of incest relations is defined differently by different cultures. In Chinese and Korean culture, it is considered taboo to marry someone who has the same family name. By definition, a person who has the same family name belongs to the same "family" (clan). They may be your cousin or niece if you trace the family clan back for a hundred or a thousand generations. Thus, they are "relatives" by definition. This concept is "arbitrarily" observed only in paternal family systems, as, when a woman married, according to the culture, she belongs to her husband's family and is excluded from her family of origin. At any rate, a taboo against marrying a person with the same family name does not cause problems if there are many family names in a society, as there are in Japan and in Western societies. There is little possibility of a Mr. Yamamoto falling in love with a Ms. Yamamoto or of a Mr. Smith dating a Ms. Smith. There is a wide range of choices of people to date. However, among Chinese, there are only several dozen common family names, such as Chang, Chen, Lin, Wang, and so on. In Korea there are also only a few family names, such as Kim, Pak, Lee, and Kang. Despite this, there is a strict cultural rule that defines as incestuous relations between a man and a woman who have the same family name. Thus, if two people who are in love have the same family name, they are not permitted to marry. Such cases often end in tragedy, with the lovers committing suicide together. In such cultures, it is important to clarify a person's name before you start dating to avoid serious trouble.

3. Problems That Arise from Sociocultural Discrimination

Societies have a dismaying habit of dividing themselves into the accepted and the not accepted, the chosen and the outcast, the favored and the merely tolerated. The majority group looks down on the minority, the superior caste discriminates against the lower castes. Groups such as the Vietnamese "boat people" and Cuban refugees, first given sympathy and help by others, soon began to be seen as financial burdens and threats to job-seekers; discrimination against these victims of tragedy grew rapidly.

African-Americans have been liberated politically, but many of them still suffer from less education and employment, poor housing, and long-existing racial discrimination. Jews are still subject to social slights. In Hawaii, where many ethnic groups live without outward discord, disdain still finds expression. Some Japanese still look down on Okinawans. There are still mutual feelings of inferiority among a few members of different Chinese subethnic groups, such as between Bendi (local) people and Hakka (guest) people, or mainland Chinese and Taiwan-Chinese. Discrimination may be between ethnic or subethnic groups or within a group. Such intergroup discrimination often causes tension, affects interpersonal relations and social involvement in a subtle way, or induces conflicts or riots in an explicit way. It may affect the self-image of a group or individual, influencing mental health.

A unique race-related stress is elaborated by Loo, Singh, Scurfield, and Kilauano (1998) in connection with the experiences of Asian-American soldiers during the Vietnam War. In combat situations in Vietnam, American soldiers were required to respond to ambiguous visual stimuli with split-second decisions for survival — judging whether the Asian-looking people they encountered were threatening or friendly.

Negative racial stereotypes of Asians were socially conditioned by the association of fear of the enemy with fear of Asians in general. As a result, due simply to their physical similarity to the "enemy" (Viet Cong), Asia-American soldiers were exposed to various kinds of stress. As a result of combat indoctrination, dehumanization, and racial hatred, they were subjected to hostility and estrangement as the "enemy"; exposed to a greater potential of and actual life threats; and, afraid of being suspected of disloyalty to their fellow American soldiers, they might have dehumanized Vietnamese civilians in ways that led to later feelings of regrets or remorse.

Rather than ethnicity or race, intergroup discrimination may be based on gender or other factors, such as physical handicaps or occupational status. The best example is the *burakumin* in Japan. *burakumin* is a group of Japanese who are discriminated against by the majority of Japanese simply because of their occupational backgrounds as butchers, tanners, saddle makers, caretakers of the dead, or grave diggers. According to Shinto belief, these are "dirty" jobs. Therefore, the people doing them are discriminated against by the majority of the Japanese people, even though they belong to the same (Japanese) ethnic group. They are not permitted to seek white-collar jobs even if they receive college educations. They are not welcome to marry the majority Japanese, and even try to conceal their "dirty" backgrounds [cross-reference to Chapter 45: Minority by Ethnicity, Gender, and Others (Section II,D)].

4. Problems Induced by Rapid Cultural Change

It is commonly recognized that when a society goes through rapid cultural change within a short period of time, resulting in radical changes in value systems, lifestyles, and behavior norms, psychological problems tend to occur among the people due to difficulties in adjustment. These problems may be illustrated by a wide generational gap, misbehavior of youth, and confusion of the adults and will be elaborated in detail later [cross-reference to Chapter 43: Cultural Change and Coping (Section IV,A–C)].

If a person moves to live, either temporarily (as a visitor) or permanently (as an immigrant), in a society that has a radically different cultural background, he or she will experience "culture shock." According to Mumford (2000), the term "culture shock" was originally coined by anthropologist Kalervo Oberg in 1960 and referred to an occupational disease of people who have been suddenly transplanted abroad. Taft (1977) expanded and elaborated on the transcultural situation in which a person experiences considerable strain due to the effort required to make necessary psychological adaptations to the new culture; a sense of loss and feelings of deprivation regarding to friends, status, profession, and possessions that a person had in the original culture; rejection by and/or rejecting members of the new culture; confusion of role, role expectations, values, feelings, and self-identity; and feelings of impotence due to the inability to cope with the new environment.

Regarding transcultural adaptation, a British psychiatrist, David Bardwell Mumford (2000), carried out an interesting study. He examined British high-school graduates who had been accepted by the GAP Activity Project for placement in 27 different countries worldwide. GAP is an educational charity that offers overseas voluntary work opportunities to high-school graduates in these different countries during the "gap" year between high school and higher education or training — more or less similar to the American Peace Corps Project. In addition to the Culture Shock Questionnaire, the Culture Distance Index was administered to the students. A strong correlation was found between the volunteers' scores on the Culture Shock Questionnaire and the "cultural distance" they had traveled from Britain. For the British subjects assigned to the 27 countries, Germany, Australia, and Canada were cultures closest to their own, whereas India, Nepal, and Pakistan were most distant and associated with greater culture shock scores.

5. Problems Related to Cultural Uprooting or Destruction

If the occurrence of cultural change is so great that it almost results in the loss of a society's cultural roots, or the cultural system is almost completely destroyed by others, people will suffer from cultural uprooting. They will encounter emotional pain and psychological suffering, loss of meaning and direction in their lives, and confusion about the way to live. These results of cultural destruction produce what is called a state of "anomie" by scholars. According to Spencer (2000, p.8), the sociologist Durkheim claimed that social life is "nomic," i.e., governed by a set of rules, mostly unwritten, shared by the collective consciousness of a group. "Nomie" exists when individual interests are subordinated to the common interests, resulting in social stability and mental well-being. However, if there is gross and rapid change in society resulting in cultural uprooting, called "anomie," people will suffer from the loss of long-established life patterns with feelings of demoralization and dispossession. These phenomena are often observed among indigenous people everywhere who encounter the invasion of a more powerful dominant culture, creating personal conflict and social distress. Unsatisfactory relief is sought through a variety of strategies such as substance use and antisocial behavior. For instance, Spencer (2000) pointed out that the aboriginal people in Australia remained disadvantaged socially, professionally, and educationally after the arrival of Western people there for several centuries. Imprisonment rates for aboriginal people exceed by severalfold those of the rest of the population. Infant mortality rates are four to five times greater, whereas life expectance is 15 to 20 years shorter. Maternal deaths, alcoholism, obesity, diabetes, smoking, and substance abuse are just some of the many disorders on this very depressing list of high prevalence rates.

C. CULTURALLY INHERENT VULNERABILITY

1. Vulnerabilities within the Cultural System Itself

Due to characteristic traits or beliefs inherent in a cultural system, a society may be exposed to certain kinds of vulnerability in dealing with problems it encounters, particularly when it is invaded by outsiders. The best example is the situation of the Hawaiian people. For generations, Hawaiians cherished two great beliefs. One was the fundamental belief in the spiritual force called *mana*. All men had some of this force, but the gods had infinitely greater *mana*. The other belief was that their god, Lono, who had left his people in the dim past, would someday return. Legend said that Lono was fair of face and would return on a "floating island." It was based on this legend and the cultural trait of "aloha" (love) that when (British) Captain Cook came to Hawaiian shores on his floating island of a ship, the Hawaiian people thought that Lono had indeed returned. Because Lono had high and sacred *mana*, so too must every member of his crew. Instead of reacting suspiciously toward the strange visitors, the Hawaiian people showed warm hospitality to the white-skinned "god." Young women swam out to the ship; fathers sent their daughters to spend the night with the sailors because they thought they would have high *mana* babies. Instead they acquired syphilis and gonorrhea (Pukui, Haertig, & Lee, 1979). After the door was opened to these outsiders, there followed missionaries, whale hunters, and businessmen. The Hawaiians offered them the use of their land, women had sexual relations with them, and, very soon, a major portion of the population was wiped out due to its lack of immunity to the foreigners' diseases (such as measles and syphilis). Later, the people even lost their monarchy to the outsiders' military power.

This is in contrast to the situation of the Japanese when they were forced by the black ships led by the American naval admiral Perry to open their harbors for trading. Although the Japanese were scared of Perry's advanced military power, they continued to treat the Westerners as *gaijin* (foreigners), despising intermarriage with them. They were only interested in learning and adopting Western industrial and military strengths, even undertaking government-led revolutionary change in the Meiji era, but they retained the core of their traditional culture and ethnocentrism, even to the present. These two examples illustrate how different cultural heritages — either vulnerability or

strength — determined the course of the societies' histories, including the physical and mental health of the people.

2. Culturally Inherent Personal Vulnerability

Culturally influenced vulnerability can exist not only at a societal level, as described earlier, but also at an individual level. An individual may inherit a certain psychological vulnerability as a result of certain patterns of personality development molded by culture. Anthropologists found a good example of this among the Alore people living on the jungle island of Indonesia. According to Honigmann (1967, pp. 107–108), postpartum mothers have to resume work in their vegetable gardens soon during wet season, often leaving older siblings to care for their infants. The infants consequently suffer from hunger, desertion, and tension. Thus, due to poor maternal care in early childhood, adult personalities are characterized by a low ability to sustain great effort. They are vulnerable to stress and, in the face of difficulty, they collapse or surrender quickly due to a low threshold for frustration. This illustrates how a culture, through its primary institutions, can contribute to the formation of vulnerable basic personality among a group of people.

III. CULTURE AND COPING PATTERNS

A. BROAD CATEGORIES OF COPING PATTERNS

Although the concept of "coping" is clearly understood and the term "coping pattern" is now used frequently even by laymen, its distinction from defense mechanism is not necessarily clear. In general, a defense mechanism refers to the intrapsychic mechanism used by an individual to cope with internal anxiety or external stress; it operates generally at the unconscious or subconscious level. In contrast, a coping pattern implies a cognitive, attitudinal, and behavioral reaction of an individual or a collective group for dealing with external stress or problems, which can be undertaken as a conscious or rational choice. From a cultural point of view, the word "pattern" is used to imply that a certain coping method is utilized more frequently by the members of a culture. The term "coping strategy" is used to refer to a plan or maneuver used to solve the problems or difficulties encountered by an individual or by an organized group of people. The term will be used interchangeably with coping pattern here.

While there are numerous ways of coping with problems, there is not yet any systematic description and detailed classification of coping patterns or strategies offered by behavior scientists and psychiatrists. Lazarus and Folkman (1984, pp. 150–152) mentioned that several emotion-focused forms of coping strategies are recognized, such as avoidance, minimization, distancing, selective attention, positive comparison, and wresting positive value from negative events. Problem-focused forms of coping can be described as those directed at the environment and those directed at the self. The former strategies include altering environment pressures, barriers, resources, procedures, and the like. The latter are directed at motivational or cognitive changes, such as shifting the level of aspiration, reducing ego involvement, finding alternative channels of gratification, developing new standards of behavior, or learning new skills and procedures. From a cross-cultural point of view, a comprehensive study of coping patterns is still lacking.

B. Culture-Related Specific Coping Patterns Observed in Some Societies

Despite the difficulty of categorizing various coping patterns utilized by individuals in different cultures, there are many examples available to illustrate some specific coping patterns or strategies that have been utilized by certain societies in particular eras from a historical point of view. In the previous section, examples from Hawaii and Japan were used to illustrate how people react and deal with the intrusion of foreigners in quite different ways, with different coping reactions resulting in different outcomes. Such culture-related specific coping patterns or strategies exercised by a society will be described here to illustrate how coping patterns, deeply embedded in cultural ideology and social circumstances, will vary in different social settings.

1. Passive-Resistance Coping Method in India

It is well known that Indians, led by Gandhi, successfully eliminated British colonial control through nonviolent passive resistance. Instead of an aggressive, bloody revolution, the Indian people, following their political and philosophical leader, made good use of their cultural heritage of endurance and patience to fight the British administration successfully without a drop of blood.

2. Kamikaze (Self-Destructive) Coping Choice Advocated by the Japanese Military

Toward the end of the Pacific War, when Americans mobilized their forces to take over the island of Okinawa — one step before landing on the Japanese islands proper — the Japanese coped with the critical situation in a desperate way, adopting the strategy of *kamikaze* attacks. Many young pilots were asked to go on self-destructive missions to attack the enemy. This military strategy could take place only in a society whose culture expected complete obedience toward superiors and loyalty to authority (the emperor). It was also based on the belief that it was a duty and an honor for a soldier to sacrifice his individual life to save the country as a whole. Actually, even before the Pacific War had started, the Japanese navy had planned and executed minisubmarine suicide attacks on Pearl Harbor — when it was not yet at a point of desperation.

Near the end of the war, the collective suicides of Japanese civilians were performed here and there in Manchuria and on Okinawa and Saipan. With the cultural belief that "it is better to be a broken jade rather than to survive as a complete piece of brick," people

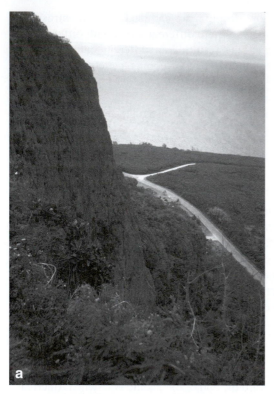
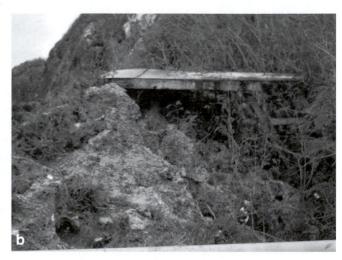

FIGURE 8-2 Culture-advocated coping: Collective suicide in Saipan. (a) At the end of the Pacific War, by order of the army, many Japanese civilians ended their lives by jumping from a cliff in Saipan, Micronesia, shouting "banzai." The cliff is now called Banzai cliff by local people. (b) Three decades after the war ended, the wooden jumping board is still left in the memorial site of the suicide cliff.

were indoctrinated to die rather than surrender to the enemy. In order to carry out the suicides, cyanide was offered in Manchuria, hand grenades were distributed in Okinawa, and in Saipan, several hundreds or thousands of civilians were ordered by military personnel to jump from a suicide cliff shouting "banzai" (10,000 years' life) for the emperor (see Fig. 8-2).

3. "Mr. Sai's Horse's" (Reality-Accepting) Coping Attitude Utilized in China

There is a common Chinese saying, *"Sai-weng-zhi-ma,"* which literally means, "An old man, Mr. Sai's horse." The saying is derived from a story about an old man, Mr. Sai, whose fate alternately changed

for the better and for the worse after he lost his horse. One day, according to the proverb, an old man lost his domesticated horse. Many friends came to comfort him, but the old man said that there was nothing to be sad about. Several days later, the lost horse not only returned home but was accompanied by a wild horse. When his friends congratulated him for this unexpected gain, the old man said that there was nothing to be happy about. Several days later, when his son tried to ride the wild hose, he fell and injured his leg and became crippled. When the old man's friends came to comfort him for his misfortune, the old man said there was no need to feel frustrated. Several months later a war started and most of the young men in the village went to fight and lost their lives, but the old man was spared the tragedy of losing his son, who, with his crippled leg, did not have to fight (Tseng, Lu, & Yin, 1995, p. 289).

This saying is used frequently by Chinese to remind themselves that life is unpredictable, fluctuating between good and bad luck, and that they need to take a philosophical view in dealing with things that happen. The saying offers a reality-accepting coping attitude that is based on the Chinese philosophical view.

4. Iron-Curtain (Self-Isolation) Coping Pattern Applied in the USSR

In Russia, during Stalin's era, the country was shut off from the outside for several decades. The "iron curtain" was built so that people inside were not accessible to news from the outside, including how affluent life was in the capitalistic societies in the West. It helped the government control the people and maintain a certain social stability, even though people were suffering from communism and dictatorship. A similar kind of self-isolation was enforced in China, with the so-called "bamboo curtain." This was a politically derived coping method utilized to control people's minds and lives. It took a certain cultural mentality for people to accept and comply with such self-isolation.

5. Externalizing-the-Enemy Coping Maneuver Used by the Nazis

A historically well-known politically derived coping maneuver has been identifying an outside enemy in order to maintain a strong cohesion internally and create social or national unity despite the preexistence of fragmentation or instability within the society or nation. By identifying an outside enemy, the people's anger, fear, or resentment was projected outward and gave them an excuse to express their aggression externally. This coping method was best exemplified in the Nazi era in Germany. Greatly stirred up by Hitler and his party, the German people were motivated to wage war against their neighboring countries, fulfill their

ambition to unite Europe, and carry out the massive execution of the unwelcome Jewish ethnic group. Beyond the fanatical political leader, it also involved a certain national character — who were willing to obey authority without question. A similar strategy was utilized by the Japanese army in starting the Pacific War as part of World War II. In order to fulfill their military ambition, the political rational was used of chasing Western imperialism out of Asia for the sake of "coexistence and peace for Asians" — a slogan that was never appreciated by any Asian people during or after the war but was firmly believed by the Japanese people themselves.

For the sake of convenience, all the examples just given were, or are, operating more or less at the societal level. However, they indirectly illustrate that the choice of coping patterns can be shaped by culture at the individual level as well. It is important for clinicians to recognize and understand the cultural impact on a patient's reaction patterns for coping with stress.

REFERENCES

Becker, S. (1991). Treating the American expatriate in Saudi Arabia. *International Journal of Mental Health, 20*(2), 86–93.

Burnam, M.A., Timbers, D.M., & Hough, R.L. (1984). Two measures of psychological distress among Mexican Americans, Mexicans and Anglos. *Journal of Health and Social Behavior, 25,* 24–33.

Cooke, D.J., & Hole, D.J. (1983). The aetiological importance of stressful life events. *British Journal of Psychiatry, 143,* 397–400.

Dohrenwend, B.P., Shrout, P.E., Egri, G., & Mendlesohn, F.S. (1980). Nonspecific psychological stress and other dimensions of psychopathology. *Archives of General Psychiatry, 37,* 1229–1236.

Dohrenwend, B.S., & Dohrenwend, B.P. (1984). Life stress and illness: Formulation of the issues. In B.S. Dohrenwend & B.P. Dohrenwend (Eds.), *Stressful life events and their contexts.* New Brunswick, NJ: Rutgers University Press.

Dohrenwend, B.S., Krasnoff, L., Askenasy, A.R., & Dohrenwend, B.P. (1978). Exemplification of a method for scaling life events: The PERI Life Events Scale. *Journal of Health and Social Behavior, 19,* 205–229.

El-Islam, M.F. (1975). Culture bound neurosis in Qatari women. *Social Psychiatry, 10,* 25–29.

Fairbank, D.T., & Hough, R.L. (1981). Cross-cultural differences in perception of life events. In B.S. Dohrenwend & B.P. Dohrenwend (Eds.), *Stressful life events and their contexts.* New York: Prodist.

Finlay-Jones, R., & Brown, G.W. (1981). Types of stressful life events and the onset of anxiety and depressive disorders. *Psychological Medicine, 11,* 803–815.

Goldberg, E.L., & Comstock, G.W. (1980). Epidemiology of life events: Frequency in general populations. *American Journal of Epidemiology, 111*(6), 736–752.

Hill, R. (1949). *Families under stress.* Connecticut: Greenwood Press.

Holmes, T.H., & Rahe, R.H. (1967). The social readjustment rating scale. *Journal of Psychosomatic Research, 11,* 213–218.

Honigmann, J.J. (1967). *Personality in culture.* New York: Harper & Row.

Ide, B.A., Tobias, C., Kay, M., Monk, J., & de Zapien, J.G. (1990). A comparison of coping strategies used effectively by older Anglo and Mexican-American widows: A longitudinal study. *Health Care for Women International, 11*(3), 237–249.

Jacobs, S.C., Prusoff, B.A., & Paykel, E.S. (1974). Recent life events in schizophrenia and depression. *Psychological Medicine, 4,* 444–453.

Kanner, A.D., Coyne, J.C., Schaefer, C., & Lazarus, R.S. (1981). Comparison of two modes of stress measurement: Daily hassles and uplifts versus major life events. *Journal of Behavioral Medicine, 4*(1), 1–39.

Kasahara, Y. (1974). "Graduation phobia" in the Japanese university. In W.P.Lebra (Ed.), *Youth, socialization, and mental health: Vol. 3. Mental health research in Asia and the Pacific.* Honolulu: University Press of Hawaii.

Kasl, S.V. (1996). Theory of stress and health. In C.L. Cooper (Ed.), *Handbook of stress, medicine, and health.* Roca Raton, FL: CRC Press.

Langner, T.S. (1962). A twenty-two item screening score of psychiatric symptoms indicating impairment. *Journal of Health and Human Behavior, 3,* 269–276.

Lazarus, R.S., & Folkman, S. (1984). *Stress, appraisal, and coping.* New York: Springer.

Leighton, A., & Hughes, J.H. (1961). Cultures as causative of mental disorder. In A. Leighton & J.H. Hughes *Causes of mental disorders: A review of epidemiological knowledge.* New York: Milbank Memorial Fund.

Loo, C.M., Singh, K., Scurfield, R., & Kilauano, B. (1998). Race-related stress among Asian American Veterans: A model to enhance diagnosis. *Cultural Diversity and Mental Health, 4*(2), 75–90.

Masuda, M., & Holmes, T.H. (1967). The Social Readjustment Rating Scale: A cross-cultural study of Japanese and Americans. *Journal of Psychosomatic Research, 11,* 227–237.

McCubbin, H.I., & Patterson, J.M. (1982). Family adaptation to crisis. In H.I. McCubbin, A.E. Cauble, & J.M. Patterson (Eds.), *Family stress, coping, and social support* (pp. 26–47). Springfiled, IL: Charles C. Thomas.

Mumford, D.B. (2000). Culture shock among young British volunteers working abroad: Predictors, risk factors and outcome. *Transcultural Psychiatry, 37*(1), 73–87.

Paykel, E.S. (1974). Life stress and psychiatric disorder: Applications of the clinical approach. In B.S. Dohrenwend & B.P. Dohrenwend (Eds.), *Stressful life events: Their nature and effects.* New York: Wiley.

Pukui, M.K., Haertig, E.W., & Lee, C.A. (1979). *Nana I Ke Kumu (Look to the source),* (Vol. 2). Honolulu: Hui Hanai (Queen Lili'uokalani Children's Center).

Rahe, R.H. (1969). Multi-cultural correlations of life change scaling: America, Japan, Denmark and Sweden. *Journal of Psychosomatic Research, 13,* 191–195.

Rahe, R.H. (1979). Life change events and mental illness: An overview. *Journal of Human Stress, 5*(3), 2–10.

Schwab, J.J., & Schwab, M.E. (1978). Stress and life events. In J.J. Schwab & M.E. Schwab *Sociocultural roots of mental illness: An epidemiological survey* (chap. 14). New York: Plenum Medical Book Company.

Selye, H. (1982). History and present status of the stress concept. In L. Goldberger & S. Breznitz (Eds.), *Handbook of stress: Theoretical and clinical aspects.* New York: Free Press.

Spencer, D.J. (2000). Anomie and demoralization in transitional cultures: The Australian aboriginal model. *Transcultural Psychiatry, 37*(1), 5–10.

Taft, R. (1977). Coping with unfamiliar cultures. In N. Warren (Ed.), *Studies in cross-cultural psychology,* (Vol. 1). London: Academic Press.

Tennant, C., & Andrews, G. (1978). The pathogenic quality of life event in neurotic impairment. *Archives of General Psychiatry, 35,* 859–863.

Theorell, T. (1974). Life events before and after the onset of a premature myocardial infarction. In B.S. Dohrenwend & B.P. Dohrenwend (Eds.), *Stressful life events: Their nature and effects.* New York: Wiley.

Theorell, T. (1976). Selected illness and somatic factors in relation to two psychosocial stress indices—a prospective study in middle-aged construction building workers. *Journal of Psychosomatic Research, 20,* 7–20.

Tseng, W.S., Lu, Q.Y., & Yin, P.Y. (1995). Psychotherapy for the Chinese: Cultural considerations. In T.-Y. Lin, W.S. Tseng, & Y.K. Yeh (Eds.), *Chinese societies and mental health.* (pp. 281–294). Hong Kong: Oxford University Press.

Vogel, E.F. (1962). Entrance examination and emotional disturbances in Japan's "new middle-class." In R.J. Smith & R.K. Beardsley (Eds.), *Japanese culture: Its development and characteristics.* Chicago: Aldine.

Wittkower, E.D., & Dubreuil, G. (1973). Psychocultural stress in relation to mental illness. *Social Science and Medicine, 7,* 691–704.

Zborowski, M. (1952). Cultural components in response to pain. *Journal of Social Issues, 8,* 16–30.

9

Mental Illness: Folk Categories and Explanation

I. CATEGORIES AND GROUPING OF MENTAL ILLNESSES

There is good reason to speculate that mental illness has existed from the beginning of the history of human beings. However, in terms of the history of medicine, the formal concept of mental disorders and the terminology and categorization of specific disorders (such as epilepsy, delirium, melancholia, and hysteria) did not appear until around 5th or 6th century B.C. in Western medicine, which originated in Greece, and around 6th or 7th century B.C. in Chinese traditional medicine (Tseng, 1973). Unlike other medical disorders (such as measles, typhoid fever, or malaria), mental sickness is less likely to manifest typified clusters of symptoms or follow patterned courses of illness. Therefore, it is relatively difficult even for professionals to identify and categorize, much less laymen. In addition, the manifestation of psychic disturbance is often mysterious and beyond ordinary knowledge, and its actual cause unclear, giving rise to speculation and subjective interpretation. Thus, there is also good reason to consider that the perception, recognition, grouping, and interpretation of mental illnesses are influenced greatly by societal and cultural factors, in addition to medical knowledge.

It has been pointed out by American anthropologists Good and Good (1982) that folk concepts of illness are not based on simple grounds. They can be formed according to etiological categories, such as illness caused by fright, loss of soul, intrusion of wind, possession by evil; by descriptive categories, such as falling sickness, excited insanity, idiocy; or a mixture of both, such as the Samoan term *ma'i aitu* (describing a person who speaks rudely to an authority figure or physically assaults other family members as a result of being possessed by an evil spirit). Further, it should be noted that folk terms of disordered mental conditions may refer to specific conditions or may be used generically, without distinguishing clearly among various kinds of disorders. There is often no attempt to establish clear boundaries among different sicknesses, as there is in professional practice, and there may be much overlapping. Also, a similar condition may be labeled informally and differently at different times or in different regions within the same society. Good examples are the terms "hurrying-pig sickness," "sickness of the hasty organ," or "deceiving sickness," all of which refer tohysterical attacks, but were labeled differently by traditional Chinese physicians during different dynastic periods. This practice may be complicated further by the labeling of similar morbid conditions according to folk names that are quite different in different societies, making it difficult to trace and identify the possible relationship among the terms. For instance, concerning illness occurring as a result of fright, the term *saladera* is used in the Peruvian Amazon, *lanti* in the Philippines, and *susto* among people of Hispanic background in Central and South America. Without a clear definition of these folk terms, a clinical description of the condition, and semantic knowledge, confusion is invited. These are issues that need to be kept in mind in studying and elaborating on folk concepts of mental illness.

This chapter will first review the criteria used by laymen to identify mental illness (mainly for psychotic conditions), examine the kinds of mental illness that have been recognized and labeled, and analyze the folk interpretations of mental illnesses in various cultures.

A. FOLK CRITERIA FOR CONSIDERING MENTAL ILLNESS

The ways in which people in different societies recognize and label mental illness is an interesting subject in cultural psychiatry. Several studies have been carried out in the past in diversified cultural settings that give us a glimpse into this matter.

1. Four East African Societies (Edgerton, 1966)

Concerning African's own conceptualization of mental disorders primarily of psychoses, Edgerton (1966) conducted an investigation in several tribal groups in east African societies. These included the Sebei of southeast Uganda, the Pokot of northwest Kenya, the Kamba of south central Kenya, and the Hehe of southwest Tanganyika. The economies of the four tribes are varied, ranging from predominantly pastoral to almost exclusively agricultural. Using probability sample techniques, about 130 subjects were interviewed from each tribe. Except for the Kamba, virtually all of whom said they have seen psychotics, approximately half of the respondents had not actually seen anyone who was psychotic.

When the respondents were asked to describe their concepts of psychoses, aside from a few tribal differences, the general pattern was remarkably similar for all four tribes. One notable emphasis was upon nudity: among all respondents, 20% of the Kamba, 14% of the Sebi, 12% of the Hehe, and 6% of the Pokot indicated that it was a sign of being psychotic. Apparently, exposing the genitalia is shameful and shocking, and to "walk naked without shame," particularly for women, is a social index of a mental breakdown. The act of murder or attempted murder, as well as serious assault, is another sign of insanity. Obviously, overtly violent behavior, which disrupts the social order, is indicative of a mental disorder. It is noteworthy that hallucinations (either auditory or visual) are seldom mentioned. Perhaps such intrapsychic pathology is not sufficiently visible for inclusion in a list of psychotic behaviors.

Some differences were noted among the tribes. For instance, "sleeps and hides in the bush" was mentioned by many (40%) of the Hehe respondents, but very few (from 2 to 5%) of the respondents from the other three tribes. "Talking nonsense" was mentioned more often by the Pokot and Sebi respondents (16 and 12%, respectively), and less by the Kamba and Hehe (6 and 5%, respectively). The reasons for these tribal differences are unknown and are awaiting future investigation — perhaps by increasing the number of subjects investigated to minimize errors of probability.

The investigation pointed out valuable information. On the one hand, it indicated that the African folk concept of psychoses is quite similar to that of western European psychoses, particularly regarding the constellation of mental disorders known as schizophrenia, characterized by gross, strange behavior and loss of contact with social reality. On the other hand, it also pointed out that the emphasis in folk criteria is relatively different from a professional emphasis, which pays more attention to certain overt behavior disorders that become dystonic with the sociocultural norm.

2. Survey of Rural Laos (Westermeyer & Wintrob, 1979a)

To study the "folk" criteria of local people to identify mentally ill persons in the community, American cultural psychiatrists Westermeyer and Wintrob (1979a) carried out a field survey of villagers in rural Laos. Family members, neighbors, village elders, and Buddhist monks were asked on what basis they assigned the social label of *baa* (insane) to an individual. As a result, they found that the categories of criteria for considering a person insane (psychotic), in order of importance, are danger to others and property, danger to self, nonviolent socially disruptive behavior (such as unable to work, wandering, or running away), problems in speech and communication, socially dysfunctional behavior (strange, unexpected, or embarrassing behavior), impaired psychological functioning ("wrong ideas" or "false beliefs"), affective disturbance, and somatic signs and symptoms (such as insomnia, weight loss, or weakness).

Westermeyer and Wintrob commented that, in Laos, a folk diagnosis of mental disorder is made on the strength of not one criterion, but several. In contrast to medical–professional criteria, it is noted that the criterion of hallucinations is absent. They emphasized that folk criteria for mental illness (psychosis) are determined primarily by the persistence of socially dysfunctional behavior rather than by disturbances in thought and affect.

3. Perception of Mental Illness by Mexican-Americans (Edgerton & Karno, 1971)

In order to comprehend why Mexican-Americans, in contrast to Anglo-Americans, are strikingly underrepresented in mental health service systems, Mexican-American psychiatrists Karno and Edgerton (1969) carried out a study to examine their perception of mental illness. A series of psychiatric case vignettes (illustrating disorders of depression, schizophrenia, juvenile delinquency) were given to Mexican-American and Anglo-American subjects in household interviews. Surprisingly, it was found that there were no significant differences between the two ethnic groups. However, when data were reanalyzed by subdividing the Mexican-Americans into two groups — Spanish-speaking (born in Mexico, less educated) and English-speaking (born in the United States, with more education) — the results showed many significant differences (Edgerton & Karno, 1971) The English-speaking group far more often saw the source of depression as "loneliness," whereas the Spanish-speaking group saw it as a "nervous" condition. The English-speaking group tended to refer to schizoprenia as a "mental" illness, whereas the Spanish-speaking group attributed it to "nerves." Regarding the nature of mental illness, the Spanish-speaking subjects, in contrast to their counterparts, believed more in the inheritance of mental illness and that it could be cured by prayer. Thus, although the subjects were of the same ethnic group, there were considerable differences in their perception and understanding of mental illness, according to their subcultural backgrounds.

B. Recognized Categories of Mental Illnesses

1. Mental Illnesses Recognized in Rhodesia, Africa (Brelsford, 1950)

By examining local language, Brelsford (1950) identified the names of types of mental illness recognized by the Bemba tribal people in the Northern Province of northern Rhodesia (now Zambia) in Africa. They are:

Problems with the brain (idiocy): *Icipuba* (no ability to eat or clothe oneself), *kapupushi* (no sense to do a job properly)

Madness: *Ukupena* or *ukufunta* (madness with violent conduct), *lya mukoli* (dangerous madness, needing confinement by ropes)

Fits: *Icipumputu* (violent fits, frothing at the mouth, falling down on the fire)

Hearing voices: *Waluba* (hearing voices that tell one to do things, even to kill or to burn huts)

Melancholic: *Alwalo mutima* (sick in the heart or spirit)

Eccentric: *Napuntuka* (queern without being mad)

Apathetic: *Uluntanshe* (a wanderer who has no aim in life)

This list illustrates that, in this case, even in laymens' minds, a rather wide range of mental illnesses exists, including major categories of mental disorders that are recognized by modern professional psychiatry.

2. Mental Disorders as They Appeared in Samoan Semantics (Clement, 1982)

Using ethnosemantic techniques, American anthropologist Clement (1982) carried out a field survey in American Samoa, in the South Pacific. She reported that the Samoans used the term *na'i valea* to lump together all mental conditions that are severe and apparently incurable. Beyond this general term, Samoan representations of mental disorders can be largely broken into three subsets.

1. **Conditions due to brain abnormalities:** *Ma'i o le mafaufau* (abnormality present from birth, result of a blow to the head, the result of illness in another part of the body).
2. **Conditions due to spirit possession:** *Ma'i aitu* (a person speaks rudely to an authority figure or physically assaults other family members as the result of being possessed by an evil spirit).
3. **Conditions caused by experiencing an excess of emotion:** This is subdivided further into worry sickness (*Ma'i popole;* depression, anxiety, and lack of confidence due to anticipation of losing something of value, encountering unavoidable dreads); depressed sickness, (*Ma'i manatu;* strong feeling of depression and sadness caused by separation from a loved one); and anger sickness (*Ma'i ita;* outburst of anger associated with sadness or the influence of alcohol).

3. Psychiatric Disorders Recognized in Traditional Chinese Medicine (Tseng, 1973)

A review of traditional Chinese medical books reveals that certain terminology appeared historically to describe mental disorders (Tseng, 1973) (cross-reference to section III,A). There was a separation of medicine from divination in the beginning of the Chou dynasty, around 10th century B.C., and a medical document, *The Classic of Internal Medicine,* appeared around 7th century B.C. — one or two centuries before the time of Hippocrates in Greece. In this ancient document, medical theory was built on the yin-yang theory, the idea of the five elements, and the microcosm–macrocosm concept (see Section III, A). Among various medical disorders (such as typhoid fever, measles, tuberculosis, and apoplexy), several medical terms appeared that described the mental disorders of delirium (caused by fever or other organic conditions), excited insanity (probably related to manic conditions or psychotic confusion, which were interpreted as the result of excessive yang element), and falling sickness (referring to epilepsy, which was interpreted as the result of losing the yang element, resulting in excessive yin). This is in contrast to Western medicine, which started in Greece at the time of Hippocrates (about 5th to 6th century B.C.), when the morbid conditions of delirium, melancholia, and epilepsy were also recognized. Later, in Soranus's time, around first century A.D., the term mania was added to the list of mental disorders.

It is interesting to note that, during Hippocrates' time, the sudden onset of emotional turmoil was labeled "hysteria." It was considered that the illness occurred as the result of a wandering uterus. In China, toward the end of the Han dynasty, around 1st century A.D., the medical documents *Treatise on Fevers* and *Golden Box Summary* appeared. In these documents, descriptions of "hurrying-pig sickness" or "sickness of the hasty organ (uterus or heart)" appeared, all referring to hysterical outbursts of emotional disorders. This indicates that the sudden onset of emotional turmoil manifested by females had caught the attention of physicians even in the early stages of medical development.

Interestingly enough, when the medical document *Treatise on Symptoms of Various Illnesses* was written in the 6th century, during the Sui dynasty, equivalent to the period of "Theological Medicine" in the West, the medical terms "ghost-evil insanity" and "ghost-bewitched insanity" appeared, attributing insanity to supernatural causes, even though the separation of divination and medicine had taken place as early as 10th century B.C. This terminology later disappeared.

When the medical document *Chin-Yue's Medical Book* was printed in the early Ming dynasty, around the 14th century, in addition to the term "deceiving sickness" (referring to hysterical conversion), the medical term "depression" appeared, even though the term of "stagnation" of vitality was mentioned in *The Classic of Internal Medicine,* about one or two centuries before Hippocrates' time, when melancholia was described. Even though the medical term "depression" came later in traditional Chinese medicine, there were detailed descriptions of depressive states. The author, Jing-Yue, recognized three kinds of depression: anger depression, apprehension depression, and melancholic depression. Anger depression was depression that occurred after an outburst of excessive anger; apprehension depression was due to excessive brooding; and melancholic depression was brought about by excessive worry.

From a historical point of view, it was noted that various kinds of mental disorders were recognized in a certain order in both the East and the West. Mental confusion associated with a feverish condition (delirium), illness characterized by a sudden fall (epilepsy), overexcitement (either mania or excited insanity), and an outburst of emotional turmoil (hysterical attack) were recognized earlier historically. Those disorders were characterized by the occurrence of gross mental confusion and sudden onset, easily caught people's attention and were easy to distinguish, or they were associated with relatively clear causative factors (such as feverish sickness) and thus were easily comprehended as disorders. Minor psychiatric disorders, or neuroses, such as neurasthenia,

hypochondriasis, or even depression (in the East) were not conceived as mental disorders until rather recent history.

4. Survey of Mental Symptom Clusters in Senegal, West Africa (Beiser, Ravel, Collomb, & Egelhoff, 1972)

The American psychiatrists Beiser, Ravel, Collomb, and Egelhoff (1972) investigated stress-related mental symptoms described by the people of Senegal, west Africa. Instead of using existing symptom questionnaires designed by Western psychiatrists for Western populations, the investigators constructed an indigenous questionnaire based on local ways of expressing disturbance. This helped them avoid the danger of forcing data into categories or scales that existed in their own minds. Collected data were factor-analyzed, and four clear-cut factors emerged: physiological anxiety, topical depression, health preoccupation, and episodic anxiety. These four groups represented the spectrum of mental disturbance described by the local people, which was different from the mental spectrum presented by other cultural groups, particularly of Western backgrounds. This *emic* approach (culture-specific) for identifying mental symptoms not only overcame the shortcomings of an *etic* approach (universal method), but also allowed the investigators to gather information focusing on severe psychopathologies (such as insanity), which usually occur in the study of preliterate societies, and to cover minor psychopathologies as well (anxiety disorders and other minor emotional problems), making the scope of the study more comprehensive.

As a part of this investigation, Beiser, Burr, Ravel, and Collomb (1973) identified three major types of "illness of spirit" recognized and interpreted as such by the local people. *O'Bodah* means someone with no idea in his head, one who thinks like a child, talks to himself, and is easily influenced; *O'Dof* refers to someone who shows agitation, destructive behavior, habit deterioration, and visual and auditory hallucination; and *M'Befedin* describes a person subject to periodic attacks characterized by falling, thrashing movements of the limbs, tongue biting, incontinence, and especially foaming at the mouth — an illness felt to be contagious through the saliva of affected people.

5. Naming and Grouping Illnesses in Feira, Brazil (Ngokwey, 1995)

In order to understand the sociocultural construction of illness, Ngokwey (1995) carried out an investigation of the popular medicine of Feira de Santana, a city in northeastern Brazil. Data indicated that illnesses are named after their dominant symptoms, such as *fraqueza* (weakness) and *febre* (fever); their anatomical location, such as *dor de* (pain of) *cabeca* (head) or *doenca de* (illness of) *figado* (liver); or the interpreted cause of their occurrence. Many mental problems are attributed to supernatural causes. Examples are *encosto,* a condition caused by a spirit leaning upon the victim; *obsesso,* a spirit "obsessing" its victim; or *olhado,* a condition caused by an evil eye. Ngokwey commented that although folk illness categorizations appear to be incoherent and inconsistent, it is important to recognize that folk terms are used by people according to their needs and purposes. Indeed, a particular illness episode is negotiated in the process of social interaction; hence, there is flexibility in illness categorization.

II. EXPLANATIONS FOR MENTAL ILLNESSES

A. VARIOUS EXPLANATIONS FOR MENTAL PROBLEMS

1. Supernatural Explanations

This group of explanations is based on supernatural beliefs. It attributes the causes of sickness to supernatural powers, which are beyond human understanding and control. Supernatural explanations of illnesses take many forms.

a. Object Intrusion

In a concrete way, sickness is interpreted as the result of the intrusion of certain undesirable objects, which can be simply tiny bones, bits of leather, coagulated blood, insects, or hairs. All are considered evil in nature and prove to be the causes of illnesses in a concrete and convincing way for the people who believe in this theory. It is based on magical thought, which is different from the nature-orientated pathogenic object theory. According to Clements (1932), this is perhaps one of the most primitive ways of interpreting the causes of sickness.

b. Soul Loss

"Soul" here refers to the supernatural being of "self," which usually resides in our bodies. This is a view held by many people in preliterate societies. It is believed that for some reason, such as being frightened, hit on the head (where the soul resides), sneezing, or experiencing troubled sleep, the soul will leave the body and be unable to return. It is considered that when a person has lost his individual "soul" he will behave and feel differently and, in extreme conditions, become sick. The *susto* concept held by Latin people is one example. Prayer or a ceremony is required to bring back the lost or wandering soul.

c. Spirit Intrusion and Possession

This explanation takes the view that sickness is due to the presence in the body of evil spirits. Although the presence of spirits or other supernatural beings does not necessarily cause sickness all the time, the intrusion of malicious spirits does. When a person speaks and talks as if he has been taken over by a supernatural being, he is described as "possessed." This is a special form of spirit intrusion. The disorder of fox possession *(kitsune-tsuki)* described in Japan (Eguchi, 1991) is one special example that is commonly recognized and labeled by laypersons. Certain ceremonies can be performed to satisfy the intruding or possessing spirit's demands, asking it to leave the body, or exorcisms can be conducted to chase it away.

d. Breach of Taboo

This explanation sees sickness as a punishment by the gods for the breach of religious prohibitions or social taboos that have divine sanction. The breach may be unintentional or even unknown to the sufferer, but is still interpreted as the cause of the illness. Voodoo death is often attributed to breach of taboo. According to this interpretation, there are certain ways to undo the punishment, including confession.

e. Sorcery

This interpretation considers sickness to be the result of the manipulations of persons skilled in magic or having supernatural powers. It is suspected that illness is induced with malicious intent by the acts of others, through the use of supernatural powers. The mechanism of projection is used to affect others, and interpersonal conflict often exists. However, an underlying belief in supernatural powers is necessary for this to occur. Repairing troubled interpersonal relations is one way to remove the effects of the sorcery; performing counteracting sorcery is another.

2. Natural Explanations

These explanations stem from the basic assumption that there are underlying principles of the universe that govern all of nature, including man's life, behavior, and health. When physical or mental illness, misfortune, or great unhappiness occur, the causes are thought to be related to natural matters in several ways, as follows.

a. Disharmony of Natural Elements

It is assumed that certain homeostatic conditions exist in the world of nature by means of the harmonic balancing of various elements. If there is disharmony among these natural elements, illness as an undesirable condition will occur. The humoral view of Greek medicine and the five-element theory of Chinese medicine are both rooted in this basic concept. The theory of the five elements in Chinese medicine proposes that everything in the human body and in nature belongs to one of five categories, which are represented by the five elements of wood, fire, earth, metal, and water. The five viscera (liver, heart, spleen, lungs, and kidney), five emotions (anger, joy, worry, sorrow, and fear), and five climatic factors (wind, heat, humidity, dryness, and cold) all correspond respectively to the five elements. The idea of the correspondence between microcosm and macrocosm holds that human beings are governed by the principles that rule nature. The excessive existence of a certain element, such as the fire element, will stimulate the liver organ and cause the individual to lose his temper easily. Extraordinary external conditions of wind, cold, heat, humidity, and dryness, as well as extraordinary internal conditions of joy, anger, worry, sorrow, and fear, were seen as contributing to the causes of illness. This is similar to the humors theory of Greek medicine, according to which the human body contains four basic humors: blood, black and yellow juices, and sputum. Imbalance of these four humors causes certain disorders. For instance, excessive black juice from the gall bladder will cause depression.

b. Incompatibility with Natural Principles

Closely related to the concept of the correspondence between microcosm and macrocosm, some people believe that misfortune or illness is brought about by incompatibility with natural principles. Astrologers may interpret misfortune as the result of unusual movement of your designated star in the sky. Geometrists (or *feng-shui* masters) may explain that you suffer from a chronic illness because your ancestor was buried in a place that does not fit geometric, or *feng-shui* principles. A fortune teller may interpret frequent marital problems as the result of the mismatching of the animal natures of the husband and wife. For instance, a man with a horse nature does not fit with a woman with a tiger nature, as a tiger will not be subordinate to but will only threaten a horse all the time. It offers explanations symbolically regarding the concept of harmony versus antagonism — the basic principle elaborated by the yin and yang theory.

c. Philosophical Explanations and Acceptance

The occurrence of illnesses, particularly malicious or untreatable ones, may be attributed to fate, with the philosophical attitude of accepting and tolerating it. For instance, if a person attempts suicide repeatedly, it may be explained that he or she has a predetermined fate to end his or her life early.

d. Noxious Factors in the Environment

In this view, when any natural element, such as wind or water, is excessive or unnatural, it becomes noxious and is thought to be the cause of mental illness. Cold air is considered to be the cause of "catching cold," even by modern man at present. Apoplexy was thought to occur as the result of the intrusion of "wind" in Chinese medicine. Thus, the condition was labeled *zhong-fun,* which literally means "attack by wind."

3. Somato-Medical Explanations

This group of explanations views sickness as the result of undesirable conditions existing within our own bodies. It considers certain conditions necessary for the organism to function. Any factors that are not favorable to these conditions will result in sickness.

a. Physical-Physiognomy Problems

In this view, a person faces illness as the result of some physical problem, such as physical appearance or structure. The person is often born with the problem, and it may cause him difficulty in life. For example, a person with a flat nose is considered to lack a strong will and have difficulty carrying out tasks. A person with long ears is considered to have a successful future, with good fortune in both in wealth and achievement.

b. Distress or Dysfunction of Certain Visceral Organs

This explanation is based on the belief that certain visceral organs are closely related to certain emotional or mental functions. Due to distress or other reasons, dysfunction of particular organs may occur, which in turn lead to the occurrence of certain somatoemotional disturbances. The heart distress conceived by Iranian people (Good, 1977), the kidney-deficiency syndrome of the Chinese, based on traditional concepts (Wen, 1995), and neurasthenia, or exhaustion of the nervous system observed by Western psychiatrists at the turn of the 19th century, are some examples.

c. Physiological Imbalance or Exhaustion

A badly balanced diet, exhaustion, or inappropriate activity, especially in sexual life, is considered to cause physiological disturbances that result in mental disorders. Loss of energy through excessive sexual activity has been held responsible for psychiatric conditions in both the Eastern and the Western world. An elevated fire element in the body, causing an irritated temper and anger (labeled *hwa-byung* by Koreans) is an example.

Based on the Greek humoral concept of pathology — according to which the four bodily fluids or "humors" were characterized by a combination of hot or cold with wetness or dryness — people in Latin America today classify most foods, beverages, herbs, and medicines as "hot" or "cold." By extension, illness is often attributed to an imbalance between heat and cold in the body (Currier, 1966).

d. Insufficient Vitality

It is believed that a person, as an organism, needs a certain force, vitality, or energy to function. Many terms have been used to describe the concept of such a force or vitality in different societies, such as *mana* for Hawaiians, *Jing* and *qi* for Chinese, *dhat* for Indians, for Japanese, and so on. No matter what term is used, the basic underlying concept is that it is important to acquire, maintain, and reserve this biological–mental force in order for a person to function effectively. If there is insufficiency or excessive loss of the force, it will often result in sickness, and a resupply of the force will be needed.

e. Inborn or Acquired Pathologies

This explanation takes the view that mental illness occurs as the result of a physical handicap or vulnerability that was inborn or acquired through infection, trauma, intoxication, or other organic causes. This is an organic view held even by medical professionals.

4. Psychological Explanations

This group of explanations is entirely different from those described previously in that it takes the view that the mental sickness is an ill-function of the mental condition that can be induced by an undesirable mental affect. Thus, it is based on the psychogenic theory of mental illness.

a. Fright

If a person is subject to excessive and undesirable emotional excitement, such as fright, it may cause disturbance in his mental balance and result in mental sickness. The conditions causing fright vary. A person may be frightened by lightning, encountering a ghost, or witnessing a horrifying situation, such as murder.

b. Overburdening

Very much related to the homeostatic view of organisms, it is held that if a person uses his brain in an excessive way, he will exhaust it and cause an overburdened condition. Naturally, mental rest as well as nutritional supplements are considered ways to help the brain recuperate from such an exhausted condition.

c. Excessive Discharge of Emotion

Based on daily life observation, it is believed that excessive emotional discharge, in the form of anger, sorrow, or even excitement, particularly for long periods of time, will bring ill effects on the body. Therefore, it is recommended that a person maintain a certain regulation of emotional expression, and not be excessively angry, happy, or sad. This is a psychosomatic view of sickness.

5. Societal Explanation

This explanation attributes the causes of mental problems to society as a whole. Tension, confusion, disorder, or pressure within a society are blamed for the occurrence of certain kinds of mental problems, such as substance abuse, drinking problems, violent or criminal behavior, and so on. This view is held by some professional people, such as Thomas S. Szasz (1961), who claimed that the concept of mental illness is a myth and should be regarded as the expression of man's struggle with the problem of how he should live.

Although the societal explanation applies to certain kinds of mental problems, such as substance abuse, drinking problems, and criminal behaviors that are attributed predominantly to sociocultural factors, it does not explain many other mental disorders, such as psychoses, which are mainly attributed to biological factors. Thus, contemporary psychiatrists do not entertain the extreme view of social etiology or cultural causes for all mental problems or disorders. From an anthropologcal point of view, the societal explanation is seldom given by laymen.

B. Geographic Distribution of Folk Explanations among "Primitive" Societies

In order to understand how mental illness is perceived and explained by the people of preliterate cultures, Clements (1932) carried out an extensive study. He identified the explanations of sickness given by "primitive" people into the categories of sorcery, breach of taboo, disease-object intrusion, spirit intrusion, and soul loss. Then, by utilizing available ethnographic records, he examined how such explanations of the causes of mental sickness are distributed geographically among various "primitive" cultures. He reported that the belief in disease-causing sorcery is distributed literally to the ends of the earth, even though the forms of sorcery vary considerably. The interpretation of breach of taboo is scattered rather widely around the world, but it is noted that people in Polynesia attach real importance to this concept and link it with confession as a way of treating mental sickness. The concept of disease-object intrusion (supported by the actual presence in the body of a tangible, supposedly pathogenic substance) is almost universal in the New World, but its distribution in the Old World is not so continuous. The distribution of spirit intrusion is continuous in Europe, Africa, all of southern Asia, and most of Oceania, but more sporadic in the New World. In contrast to this, the interpretation of possession as the cause of sickness exists widely in the Old World, plays a great part in Oceanic religion, exists over most of Africa, India, and China, yet is not reported in North America and only a single case has been noted in South America. Clements' interpretation is that possession may be a more recent development than spirit intrusion from a historical perspective. Finally, while the distribution of the interpretation of soul loss is enormous, its occurrence is not universal. It is noted that it occurs very widely in Siberia, being by far the most important theory of disease.

C. DISTRIBUTION OF VARIOUS EXPLANATIONS WITHIN A SOCIETY

It is rather difficult to examine systematically the ways various explanations of mental illness are distributed among different societies. Because there are different kinds of healing practices involved, explanations of illnesses will vary according to the nature of the practices. However, some fragmented reports are available that offer us a glimpse into this matter.

1. Explanation by Shaman in Korea (Kim, 1973)

Interested in the explanations of illness given by shamans, a Korean cultural psychiatrist, Kwang-Iel Kim, conducted a survey in Korea (1973). He reported that by utilizing the categories proposed by Clements, the most frequent explanation given by shamans for the causes of illness was spirit intrusion (59.4%),

breach of taboo (21.3%), and soul loss (9.7%). He pointed out that explanations of sorcery (0.8%) as well as object intrusion (0.8%) were both rare.

2. Explanations by Patients and Families in Rural Laos (Westermeyer & Wintrob, 1979b)

When Westermeyer and Wintrob (1979a) interviewed mental patients and their relatives and neighbors in rural Laos to investigate the folk criteria used by people concerning insanity (psychoses), they also studied the explanations given by others for such disorders (1979b). They obtained a total of 54 explanations. They categorized them into subgroups according to the nature of the explanations. Of the total explanations, 15 focused on supernatural causes (such as offending ghosts or spirits or being harmed by witchcraft or sorcery), 15 on physical causes (such as problems in the brain, fever, trauma, or excessive bleeding), 14 on social problems (dissension between or separation of lovers, family problems, job dismissal), and 10 on psychological states (mental strain, death of a husband, panic from a bomb blast, etc.) They commented that the range of folk explanations was quite correlated to psychiatric concepts of mental disorders.

3. Puerto Ricans in Connecticut (Gaviria & Wintrob, 1976)

In order to explore Puerto Rican folk interpretations of mental illness, Gaviria and Wintrob (1976) conducted interviews with 20 patients and 40 nonpatients among Puerto Ricans living in an urban community in central Connecticut. They used two approaches, direct and indirect, to explore the informants' beliefs about the causes of mental illness. Using the direct approach, they found that the majority of the respondents (65% of the patient group and 39% of the nonpatient group) gave psychological factors, such as family turmoil, marital problems, and excessive worry, as the causes of mental illness. Following this, 20% of the patient group and 34% of the nonpatient group listed biological factors, such as heredity, head injury, weakness of the brain, substance abuse, and others. Some of them (10% of the patient group and 18% of the nonpatient group) considered sociological causes to be responsible: financial problems and stressful working conditions. There were a few (5% of the patient group and 9% of the nonpatient group) who believed that supernatural factors (such as *susto, dano,* and witchcraft) were the causes of mental illness. (*Susto* means loss of one's soul, whereas *dano* means the malicious effects of others who are jealous of you.)

These data were obtained by a direct interview approach. When the information was solicited by an indirect approach — the informants were presented with a list of factors possibly related to mental disorders and were asked to estimate the extent to which people in their community would agree that such a relationship was valid evidence for the existence of mental illness — a combination of "natural" and "supernatural" factors were cited as causative explanations. The percentage of supernatural explanations increased remarkably. The majority of patients as well as the nonpatient group supported the reasons of spiritualism (90 and 80%, respectively), witchcraft (50 and 60%, respectively), bad luck or fate (50 and 55%, respectively), and *dano* (30 and 40%, respectively). In Gavira and Wintrob's interpretation, it was when the indirect approach allowed respondents to project their own views on the community that the beliefs in supernatural reasons emerged clearly as important causative factors.

4. Attributions of Heart Distress in Iran (Good, 1977)

Specifically concerning "heart distress" — a folk illness in Iran — American behavior scientist Byron J. Good conducted a field survey to explore the factors to which people attributed the illness, commonly observed mostly among women. He revealed that most of the causes were considered to be sadness, worry, and anxiety occurring in life (40%), which can be subdivided into worry about poverty (7%), inter-

personal problems (7%), fright or anger associated with the evil eye (7%), and sadness associated with mourning (5%). Other causes given were weakness, with too little blood (11%), side effects from taking contraceptive pills (10%), pregnancy, too many childbirths, sexual activity (9%), nerve problems (8%), physical disease (7%), or old age (6%). According to Good, those factors can be reduced into two most important fields of symbols and experience: the problems of female sexuality and the oppression of daily life. In other words, the illnesses with which people were frequently concerned were directly linked to the typical stresses of life in their society.

III. TRADITIONAL MEDICINE: KNOWLEDGE AND CONCEPTS

Any medical systems that are outside of formally recognized, modern medicine are labeled "traditional" medicine. They were established in the past with formal, systematic theories, knowledge, and accumulated experiences of practice that deserve attention. Let us examine some of the most well-established traditional medical systems.

A. CHINESE TRADITIONAL MEDICINE

1. Historical Development

Chinese traditional medicine is considered one of the most well-established traditional medical systems in the world. It has a history of several thousand years and is still officially recognized and clinically practiced in contemporary China (Tseng, 1999).

The earliest Chinese medical text, *The Classic of Internal Medicine (Huang-Di Nei Jing),* supposedly authored by the legendary Yellow Emperor in the Shang Dynasty, about 2000 to 3000 years B.C., was considered by historians to actually have been written in the Warring States Period, during the Zhou Dynasty, two to three centuries before Christ. With the passing of time and improvements in medical knowledge, several important medical books appeared, yet all were based on the theories and concepts described in *The Classic of Internal Medicine.*

2. Fundamental Concepts

The basic theoretical system of traditional Chinese medicine is characterized by several conceptual thoughts.

a. The Concept of Yin and Yang

This theory takes the view that the human body, like the cosmos, can be divided fundamentally into a positive force (yang) and a negative force (yin), which are complementary to each other. In the cosmos, the sun symbolizes the positive force, whereas the moon is the negative. Among living beings, the male symbolizes yang and the female, yin. Even food is subdivided into two categories. Spicy foods, tonics, and meat are considered "hot," or yang foods; whereas most green vegetables and fruits are "cold," or yin foods.

The concept of positive and negative forces applies not only to physiology, but also to psychopathology and treatments for it. If the two forces are balanced and in harmony, good health is maintained; if not, illness will result. For example, excited insanity is the result of excessive positive force, whereas falling sickness (i.e., epilepsy) or *koro* is caused by excessive negative force. In treatment, reduction of the positive force is considered necessary for excited insanity, whereas supplementing the positive force is needed for falling sickness or *koro* attacks. Yin and yang are thus interpreted as the dual forces operating in the nature, as well as in human beings, and emphasize the principle of balance.

b. The Theory of Five Elements

This proposes that everything in nature, including human bodies, belongs to one of five categorical elements, represented by *water, wood, fire, earth,* and *metal.* In nature, the five climatic factors of *wind, heat, humidity, dryness,* and *cold* are considered to be related to these five elements. In humans, the five primary visceral organs, *liver, heart, spleen, lungs,* and *kidneys,* correspond to the five elements, which in turn are related to the five basic emotions of *anger, joy, worry, sorrow,* and *fear* (see Fig. 9-1).

According to this theory, certain orderly relationships exist among the five elements: *water* creates wood, *wood* creates fire, *fire* creates earth, *earth* creates metal, and *metal* creates water. Therefore, circular relationships exist among them. At the same time, there is antagonism between *water* and fire, *fire* and metal, *metal* and wood, *wood* and earth, and *earth* and water (see Fig. 9-2).

Because each element as a concept represents many aspects of things, including the structure and functions of the body, the relationships among these aspects are revealed by the relationships among the five elements. The basic idea emphasized by the theory of five elements is the interactional relationship among things, with circular input and paired antagonism. It attempts to explain the complicated relationships that exist in the world, as well as in the body and mind.

c. Basic View of the Visceral Organs

Without the knowledge and techniques for examining the body physiologically, as is done in modern times, everything occurring in the body and mind was

The Theory of Five Elements

Element	Water	Wood	Fire	Earth	Metal
Climatic factors	Humidity	Wind	Heat	Dryness	Cold
Visceral organs	Kidney	Heart	Liver	Spleen	Lung
Emotions	Fear	Joy	Anger	Worry	Sorrow

FIGURE 9-1 **The theory of the five elements in Chinese traditional medicine.**

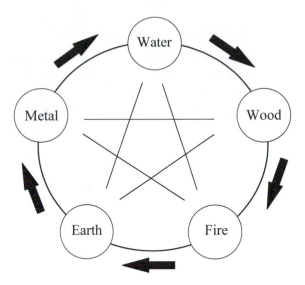

FIGURE 9-2 Circular relations and paired antagonisms among the five elements.

d. The Idea of Correspondence between Microcosm and Macrocosm

This idea takes the view that human beings are governed by the principles that rule nature. Therefore, phenomena occurring inside of a person can be understood in terms of phenomena manifested in nature. As the four seasons and five climatic elements — wind, heat, humidity, dryness, and cold — manifest changes in nature, so also in the body are changes in the five viscera and the five spirits expressed in emotions such as joy, anger, worry, sorrow, and fear. In other words, a person's emotions are viewed as equivalent to the weather in nature (see Fig. 9-3).

This view sees extraordinary conditions of wind, cold, heat, humidity, and dryness as *external causes,* and extraordinary conditions of joy, anger, worry, sorrow, and fear as *internal causes* of illness. This pathological view stresses the critical influences of natural phenomena externally and affection internally. As a whole, this view emphasizes the significance of harmony and stability.

e. Three Categories of Etiology for Illness

The causes of disorders were subdivided simply into three categories: external, internal, and others,

interpreted as an expression of the visceral organs — the parts of the human body existing in the trunk, which could be observed easily. The *heart* was thought to house the superior mind, the *liver* to control the spiritual soul, the *lungs* the animal soul, the *spleen* ideas and intelligence, and the *kidney* vitality and will. When vital air was concentrated on the *heart,* joy was created; on the *lungs,* sorrow; on the *liver,* anger; on the *spleen,* worry; and on the *kidney,* fear. Thus, it was considered that various emotions were stirred through the visceral organs. In accordance with this medical knowledge, in daily life, many organ-related sayings were used by the common people, such as "elevated liver fire," "losing spleen spirit," "hasty heart," or "exhausted kidney," to denote becoming angry and irritated, losing one's temper, being anxious, or generally fatigued, respectively.

This also reflects a holistic view of body and mind and the common acceptance of somatic presentation of emotion. It deserves mention that this parallels modern psychosomatic approaches and sharply contrasts the dual concepts of psychic and somatic in contemporary Western psychiatry.

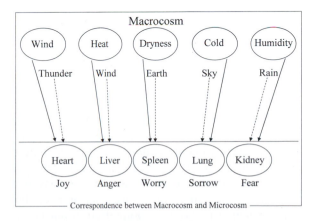

FIGURE 9-3 The idea of correspondence between microcosm and macrocosm.

which included those that could not be categorized as either external or internal. Based on the medical knowledge of the time, there was no concept of organism-caused infection as one etiology of disorders. External causes referred to any illness factors arising from nature in the form of weather conditions, such as extraordinary wind or humidity or excessive heat or cold, as well as injury. Internal causes referred to factors arising from inside a person, i.e., improper emotional experiences. It was believed that physical disorders would affect the emotions, but at the same time, unnatural emotional experiences would result in illness. In other words, a psychogenic view of somatic illness was not only recognized, but was very much emphasized from the beginning of Chinese traditional medicine.

f. The Concept of Vital Energy and Vital Air

Vital energy, called *Jing,* refers to the essence of the life force that exists in the body and regulates the vitality of the organism. When a person is full of vital energy, he or she functions efficiently both mentally and in bodily productivity. Without sufficient vital energy, illness may occur and even death. Conservation of *Jing* becomes an important practice for the preservation of health. Paralleling *Jing* is vital air, *Qi,* which is considered an abstract energy that gives strength to the body and mind. Proper conservation and an adequate supply of these vital forces or energies are cardinal to maintaining health.

3. Impact on Psychiatric Practice

Because traditional medicine has been practiced for so long in China, its concepts and knowledge not only influence clinicians, but also patients and other laymen. In other words, traditional medicine does not merely function as one kind of medical system influencing the pattern of professional practice, but is also deeply a part of the culture itself. From a sociocultural perspective, it has a strong impact on the illness-behavior of patients, including their help-

seeking behavior. Several general trends that might be observed from a psychiatric perspective are:

1. Patients are very likely to have a holistic orientation and are not used to making a dichotomatized distinction between body and mind.

2. Patients, even though clearly aware of their psychological state or emotional problems, may use somatic and organ-oriented concepts and terms to describe their emotional states.

3. Patients, following traditional medical practices, may expect their doctors to inquire about their somatic symptoms, to perform a physical examination, and to even take their pulse, but will feel unfamiliar and uncomfortable if they inquire about their social history or personal and family lives. This is particularly true for those who have had no experience in visiting psychiatrists.

4. Patients usually expect the physicians to prescribe medicines as remedies for their illnesses. Western medicine is generally considered effective, but too strong, with side effects, and even harmful to the body; herb medicine, however, is welcomed because it is perceived as more gentle, with the primary aim of balancing vitality and restoring strength.

5. Based on the yin and yang theory, patients may inquire as to what kind of food, either hot or cold, should be consumed, and whether it is necessary to take a tonic to regain their strength. These issues are influenced by traditional medical concepts of illness and treatment.

6. In the area of psychotherapy, based on the concept of the preservation of life, the need to regulate the emotions and manage behavior for the sake of health is easily understood by patients and their families, whereas the dynamic concepts of "adjustment" and "coping" are often foreign to them. Also, the concept of complying with nature and accepting things as they are, including suffering and illness, is understandable to patients and useful in the application of psychotherapy. This is quite a contrast to the Western approach, which emphasizes the resolution of problems, conquering the difficult, and removing obstacles. Emphasizing an individual's responsibility to cope with his situation can sometimes become a bur-

den for the patient and his family. An alternative approach needs to be considered for certain patients and their families.

B. AYURVEDIC MEDICINE

Ayurveda, the traditional Indian system of medicine, has its root in *Atharva Veda,* an older, prehistorical, oral medical tradition, which is still active and vibrant today as folk medicine. *Vedas* are the ancient sacred books of knowledge of the Hindus, containing cosmogony, philosophy, religious scriptures, codes of conduct, and such. Historically, ancient Indian medical knowledge and practices were on a par with those of China and Egypt in their original state. In India, these were codified, systematized, and written down between 8th and 6th centuries B.C., when the great schools arose (Kutumbiah, 1962). Practices of this period drew parallels with Greek and Persian medicine.

As pointed out by Kutumbiah, *ayurveda* is an extremely rational, logical, and coherent system of medicine based on the "logicist or rationalist school of Indian philosophy." Based on the humoral theories, it has a fundamental similarity with other traditional medical systems. Its emphasis on the listing of names, metonymy, synonymy, and poetic elaboration, linking it to the social and cultural constructions of symbols and relations, is unique.

Conceptually, the basis of the diagnoses, pathology, and therapeutics of *ayurveda* is the doctrine of *tridosa.* It envisages the body as composed of the elemental ingredients, called *bhutas,* of space, air, fire, water, and earth. These interact and are modified to support the body with *dhatus* formed from ingested food. The waste products of food, *vayu, pitta,* and *kaph* (roughly equivalent to wind, bile, and phlegm, respectively), support the *dhatus* when they are in proper measure and balance. However, they become *dosas* (disease) when they vitiate *dhatus* through imbalance.

It is interesting to note that the great teacher Charaka classifies diseases into three groups: physical, accidental, and mental. Physical disease arises from abnormal conditions of the body. Accidental diseases are from the action of spirits, poisons, wind, fire, and violence done to the body. Mental diseases *(manasa)* are those that arise from nonattainment of objects desired or coveted. Excessive anger, grief, fear, joy, and malice are all part of mental distemper. This exposition is very simplified. However, it is worth noting that the psychological attributes of sickness were well recognized in ancient times.

Ayurveda covers every aspect of medicine, from gynecology to dentistry. Surgery developed as a parallel system. Psychiatry, however, should be given the pride of the place in *ayurveda.* The world's first tranquilizer, the rawlfia serpentina, has been used by it for mental disease since antiquity. *Ayurveda* gives elaborates classifications to mental disorders. It recognizes endogenous causes (imbalances of the humors in the body interacting with the elements or *dhatus*) as well as exogenous causes (bad spirit, magic, and sorcery). Though the latter are discounted in modern times as "superstition," social causation is implicit in them, as treatment of disorders in this group involves the community. Folk medicine, however, is more dominant in this sphere. Apart from treatment with herbs and chemicals, *ayurveda* contains elaborate psychotherapeutic prescriptions for mental diseases. *Ayurveda's* strongest point is that, being holistic, it equates stability, balance, and equilibrium with health. It considers mental health as an integral part of life. Medicine only helps to maintain a long and healthy life.

According to a cultural psychiatrist from Calcutta, India, Ajita Chakraborty (personal communication 2000), *ayurveda,* together with all other traditional knowledge and practices, went into decline during the British colonial period (1757 to 1947). The reasons were not only competition from modern sciences but also their systematic downgrading and devaluation by the colonial authorities. The national government's efforts to revive it have ensured its survival, but the process was tardy. However, *ayurveda* remains very much alive and active as an alternative medicine. The effects of its systems of thought are seen in the way patients present their symptoms. Somatization is, after all, the patient's language based on cultural understanding. There are other features, such as the belief that "heat" (symbolizing temper, irritation, or anger) in the body or the head denotes mental problems. Patients' attitudes toward drug dosages are also reflections of prevalent beliefs — *ayurveda* follows a very stringent regimen and drugs need to be finely calibrated for individual patients. Above all, people strongly believe that affection, love, and care from close people are more effective in treating mental disease than doctors and medicine.

C. GALENIC–ISLAMIC MEDICINE

The backbone of traditional Galenic–Islamic medicine is the humoral theory, according to which illness arises from an excess or deficiency of the humors, or the basic qualities of life. The heart is perceived as an organ of emotional functioning or the seat of the vital soul, providing "innate heat" and "vital breath" to the body. Consequently, malfunctioning of the heart provides the cultural framework for focusing attention on the heartbeat, establishing causal links between irregularities in heartbeat and specific personal and social conditions. According to Good (1977, p. 32), heart distress clinically ranges along a continuum from mild excitation to chronic sensations of irregularities to fainting and heart attack. Thus, a cluster of emotional disorders is linked to the distress of the "heart" organ. Further, when the possible causes of heart distress were surveyed, Good found a long list of answers offered by laymen. This included feelings of sadness and anxiety; situational difficulties relating to death, debts, poverty, quarrels, and family illness; problems associated with old age, pregnancy, delivery and miscarriage, or usage of contraceptives; or somatic reasons of lack of blood, low blood pressure, too few vitamins, nerve problems, and so on. Through statistical analysis, the two most important fields of symbols and experiences that emerged were "the problematic of female sexuality" and "the oppression of daily life" — two of the most common psychological problems encountered by females in that culture.

IV. INTEGRATION AND THEORETICAL SPECULATIONS

A. FOLK AND PROFESSIONAL MENTAL DISORDERS RECOGNIZED AND CATEGORIZED

From the review of mental disorders recognized by folk people, including preliterate people, it becomes obvious that there is a certain degree of difference in the ways laymen and professional therapists conceive the sickness from which a patient is suffering. The scope of mental sickness covered by ordinary people and medical professionals is different. Ordinary people tend to be concerned with sicknesses that are more explicitly recognizable and may bring more gross disturbance to the community; whereas professional therapists tend to focus on sicknesses that are more or less treatable. Ordinary people follow the rules of reality, whereas therapists follow the dictates of biomedical professional knowledge. Also, as indicated by Eisenbruch (1990), explanations given by common folk tend to be personal; those given by professionals tend to be imperson.

Numerous factors contribute to identifying mental sickness. In general, it is attributed to medical knowledge and experience, the sensitivity and perception of people toward certain disorders, or the tolerance they have toward certain deviant or abnormal mental conditions. The latter reasons fall under the influence of cultural factors.

B. POPULAR AND PROFESSIONAL EXPLANATIONS

Comparing various explanations given by laymen and professionals, it is found that there are certain differences in the explanations offered by lay people, traditional or folk healers, and contemporary professionals. The different and overlapping range of explanations offered by folk people and professionals are illustrated by Fig. 9-4.

		Folk Concept	Professional Concept
Supernatural Explanations	Object intrusion	++	−
	Soul loss	+++	−
	Spirit possession	+++	−
	Breach of taboo	++	−
	Sorcery	++	−
Natural Explanations	Disharmony of nature	+++	±
	Incompatibility with natural principles	++	+
	Fate in life	++	−
	Noxious features in the environment	+	+
Somato-Medical Explanations	Insufficient vitality	++	±
	Physical-physiognomy problems	++	+++
	Dysfunction of visceral organs	+++	++
	Physiological imbalance or exhaustion	+++	+++
	Inborn or acquired pathologies (heredity)	+	+++
Psychological Explanations	Fright	++	±
	Excessive discharge of emotion	+	±
	Overburdening or exhaustion	+	++
	Psychological trauma	±	+++
Societal Explanations	Social disorder or pressure	−	++
	Cultural confusion	−	++

FIGURE 9-4   Range of explanations offered by folk people and professionals.

C. SOME THEORETICAL SPECULATIONS

1. Evolution of Illness Explanations

When Clements (1932) attempted to review the geographic distribution of illness explanations around the world, referring only to "primitive" societies, he was quite aware of the scarcity of approaches of this kind; however, a lack of reports in ethnographic records does not necessarily mean that such phenomena do not exist. However, examining the geographic distribution of explanations for causes of sickness, coupled with the knowledge of the relative historical antiquity of primitive societies, he speculated that, for human beings, the disease theory might have evolved through a sequence of disease-object intrusion, soul loss, spirit intrusion, and breach of taboos, in that order. It started with a concrete object cause shifting toward a more abstract cause, paralleling the cognitive development noted for an individual and possibly followed by humankind as a group.

2. Cultural Variations in the Selective Elaboration of Illness

The review given earlier reveals that mental sickness is categorized differently in different societies. There are numerous reasons for this. Disease may be influenced by medical knowledge and professional tradition. Certain systems of classification have been utilized through medical training and clinical practice. Illness is attributed to historical path, cultural factors, and experiences in life. It is closely related to concepts and semantics regarding illness. Cultural factors influence people to decide where the focus will be and how the illness will be elaborated. They also reflect the problems that people encounter in real life.

This point is well illustrated by Good (1977) in his study and analysis of "heart distress" — a folk illness in Iran. Rooted in the traditional Iranian folk concept of "heart" — the organ that provides "innate heat" and "vital breath" to the body and is the seat of the emotions, particularly fear and anger (rather than an organ of circulation, as it is viewed in scientific physiological and anatomical terms) — heart-distress disorder occurs when the organ is in distress and symptoms and complaints are elaborated and expressed through it. Heart-distress disorder has become a prominent and prevalent illness recognized and categorized by Iranians. As noted earlier, it covers a wide spectrum of illnesses, including mild excitement of the heart, chronic heart irregularities, fainting, and heart attack.

In contrast, as Wen indicates (1995), the Chinese place great emphasis on the kidneys. Based on traditional medical concepts, they are the organs that store vitality. The sexual and excretory organs were combined in traditional medical thought. As a result, it was believed that an excess or inappropriate discharge of semen (a source of vitality) through sex-related activity would exhaust a person's energy and make him vulnerable to sickness. There is a cluster of illnesses considered to be related to the folk illness of "kidney insufficiency syndrome" (*shen-kui* is the traditional medical term), including *nao-shenjing shuairuo* (brain neurasthenia), *shenkui* (chronic fatigue or general neurasthenia), *pa leng* (frigophobia, excessive fear of catching cold, which results in losing the yang element), and *suoyang* (*koro,* a morbid fear derived from the belief that shrinkage of the sexual organ will result in death). Thus, for various reasons, in each society, based on its cultural concerns and beliefs, people tend to elaborate and categorize different clusters of illnesses.

3. Possible Association between Culture and Modes of Illness Explanation

In a manner similar to Clements in 1932, Denko (1966) reviewed the material available in human relations area files regarding how preliterate societies around the world explain mental illness. Based on his study, he made the theoretical speculation that explanations for mysterious phenomena (such as disturbed behavior) might parallel with other attitudes in a culture. For instance, he suspected that societies with high standards of personal responsibility and conduct might reasonably attribute misfortunes to punishment for failing to live up to societal standards, whereas cultures that emphasize a deterministic philosophy would be more likely to place the blame on inscrutable spirits. Furthermore, highly integrated societies with complicated interactions and interdependencies might attribute disordered behavior to a breakdown of these interpersonal relationships, whereas societies of rugged individualists might resort less to explanations involving other persons (sorcery) and more to spiritual forces (ghosts, deities) or to the results of unacceptable behavior. These suppositions sound possible but, as Denko himself pointed out, they are awaiting future study for confirmation.

As indicated by Fabrega (1989), social sciences have been influential in developing the concept of "cultural relativism," referring to the differences in beliefs, feelings, behaviors, traditions, social practices, and technological arrangements that are found among diverse peoples of the world. Thus, culture influences not only basic human characteristics, but presumably the "illnesses" to which humans are susceptible. From an academic point of view, there are two positions dealing with culture and psychiatric illness depending on whether an *etic* or *emic* approach is taken [cross-reference to Chapter 2: Culture and Society (Section II, B)]. An *etic* approach takes the view that all psychiatric illnesses in societies can be conceptualized, reliably measured, and studied across societies as a function of cultural differences. An *emic* approach takes the position that the medical phenomena of a particular group of people needs to be studied according to their cultural background because it is subject to the power of cultural differences. Fabrega is correct in pointing out that each approach has its own merits and limitations.

V. CLINICAL IMPLICATIONS

A. DISTINCTION BETWEEN "ILLNESS" AND "DISEASE"

From the review just given, it is evident that the way laymen perceive and conceptualize their physical disorders or mental problems is not necessarily congruent with the way they are defined and conceived by contemporary physicians. Through their field experience, this difference was pointed out by some scholars and clinicians quite some time ago (Clements, 1932; Lipowski, 1969; Mechanic, 1962). However, the need to make a conceptual distinction between "illness" and "disease" was advocated only recently, beginning with American social psychiatrist Leon Eisenberg (1977). It is suggested that the two terms, "illness" and "disease," be distinguished and used differently. Artificially, "illness" is assigned to the sickness that is experienced and conceived by the patient or his family. It is subjective, experiential,

and stems from the folk point of view. It is based on personal knowledge, folk concepts, and the cultural interpretation of how a laymen describes suffering, attributes the cause of his problems, and reacts and copes with the ill condition.

In contrast, "disease" refers to the morbid condition or pathological entity that is defined and conceptualized by modern physicians (and psychiatrists). A certain etiological cause is considered (or speculated, even if it is still unknown). It is assumed that the disease will manifest certain patterns, creating an identifiable clinical picture, and will take a predictable clinical course with a certain prognosis. Also, based on the diagnosis, a specific treatment can be prescribed, if such a remedy is available. Thus, there are two systems operating on the same patient or on the same sickness: "illness" from the patient's perspective and "disease" from the physician's point of view. They may overlap or be incongruent with each other (Fig. 9-5).

For example, a person who suffers from headaches and back pain, cannot concentrate at work, loses his temper easily, cannot sleep well at night, and feels tired most of the day may consider himself to be suffering from nervous exhaustion. He may try a herb medicine or rest and recuperation, hoping that his weakened nervous system will recover and regain strength. If the same person consulted a psychiatrist, he might be diagnosed as suffering from depression and an antidepressant might be prescribed for him. A parent whose child is suffering from irritability, frequent nightmares, poor appetite, and loose stools and is not responding to ordinary available remedies may perceive the problems to be the result of his child losing his soul due to fright. A folk healer may be consulted to call back the lost soul. If the child were brought to see a pediatrician, it might be suggested that he go through a series of laboratory tests to see if he is suffering from some kind of medical disease.

Thus, the physician looks for certain objective evidence to meet the diagnostic criteria that has been established, based on professional knowledge and accumulated experience, and then makes plans for

	Disease	**Illness**
Definition	Pathological entity conceptualized by professionals	Morbid condition experienced and conceived by patient and family
Orientation	Objective observation of disorder	Subjective experience of suffering
Foundation	Biomedical foundation	Personal-sociocultural orientation
Phenomena	Manifest certain pattern with identifiable clinical picture and predictable course	Dysfunctional phenomena with disturbance to self, family, community
Help-Seeking	Visit modern health facilities	Consult folk healers
Assessment	Diagnosis by objective evidence	Comprehend by intuition
Explanation	Scientific explanation	Folk, supernatural interpretation
Remedy	Specific treatment to be prescribed	Magic and symbolic maneuver
Therapy	Direct treatment for etiology	Indirect, subtle intervention
Goal	Cure of disorder Regaining health	Help the person from suffering or solve the problems

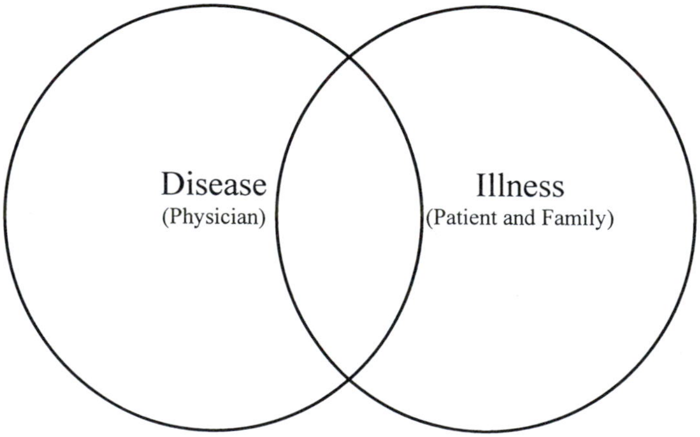

FIGURE 9-5   Conceptual distinction between "disease" and "illness."

treatment accordingly. The diagnostic criteria may change according to a change in medical knowledge and professional views (as illustrated by the periodical revising of official classification systems); however, physicians hold the view that "disease," as an "entity," exists, and, based on their accumulated professional knowledge, they know how to identify it accurately and treat it effectively. The physician's knowledge is objective, oriented toward scientific logic, and is characterized by a biomedical foundation. This is quite different from the perspective of the patient, who is subjective, even speculative, but, to him, the illness is "actual," subject to individual as well as traditional views and cultural interpretation.

Thus, it is important for the clinician to recognize the potential differences that exist between the way the patient and the therapist perceive and interpret the sickness and conceptualize the problems. It is a clinical art to be able to integrate the realities of illness and disease that are conceived by the patient and the therapist.

B. Definition of "Normality" and "Pathology"

Closely related to the folk view of illness is the issue of how to distinguish between "normal" and "abnormal" or "health" and "pathology." From a psychiatric point of view, it has been pointed out (Offer & Sabshin, 1974) that there are four ways to distinguish pathology from normality. They are by professional definition, by deviation from the mean, by assessment of function, and by social definition. These will be discussed in detail later (cross-reference to Chapter 27: Clinical Assessment and Diagnosis). However, it is appropriate to elaborate briefly here on how social and cultural factors contribute to the distinction between pathology and abnormality, health and normality.

The Samoan term *Ma'i aitu* (a person who speaks rudely to an authority figure or physically assaults other family members as the result of being possessed by an evil spirit) is a good example of how abnormal behavior is defined by a societal code of behavior. In a society such as Samoa, where respect toward authority figures in a family, a village, or a community as a whole is considered important, if a person breaks this cultural code, his behavior is clearly defined as "abnormal" and is interpreted as the result of possession by an evil spirit — otherwise, it would be unthinkable for a person to lose his mind and act in such a culturally unacceptable way. A similar situation was noted in the Soviet Union. If someone dared to protest against the government, it was interpreted as "insane" behavior and the person was hospitalized under a politically created clinical diagnosis of "vague schizophrenia." It is not only politically incorrect but also politically "insane" for a person

to voice an opinion against a political administrator in an extremely autocratic society that does not allow any member to have a different opinion from that of the government. In other words, within each society there is some culturally sensitive area. If someone breaks the code of social expectation, cultural taboo, or political views, it is relatively easy to be labeled abnormal and to be treated as such.

It may be said, in general, that if a person acts outwardly strangely or destructively in such a way that he disturbs the harmony or integration of the family, village, community, or society at large, his behavior will tend to be perceived as "pathological" and he will be treated to control it. However, if a person manifests his problems inwardly in such a way that he does not disturb his surroundings too much, even if his behavior is not favorable to himself, his family and the community will tend to accept or tolerate it and not hurry to deal with it. Thus, the rule of reality operates in defining normality from pathology.

C. The Effects of "Naming" and "Labeling"

A competent and skillful clinician, particularly a psychiatrist, needs to understand the meaning and effect of labeling sicknesses. Clearly, there is an association between the effects of "naming" and giving a diagnosis. Identifying the nature of a problem and giving a name to it serves several functions for the patient and his family (as well as for the physician and care deliverers). The patient and his family will be released from the anxiety of the unknown. They will know what the problem is and how to act accordingly. Whether or not the diagnosis is "accurate," it directs the patient to take action, which in turn eliminates anxiety and provides hope for a cure. In other words, it is important psychologically for the illness to have some kind of label that will direct the patient's energy and efforts to cope with it. This explains why folk labels of illnesses still exist and affect patients' lives. Magical factors are involved in giving a diagnosis if it is offered in a culturally correct way.

On a cultural level, it is important that the name of the sickness be familiar and meaningful to the patient so that he will accept it and work within the framework of the proposed solution. That is why a modern therapist should not only identify the medical disease on a professional level, but should also pay attention to the folk term and concepts used by the patient in understanding it, minimizing the potential gap that might exist between the patient and the therapist.

D. COMPLEMENTS BETWEEN FOLK AND PROFESSIONAL SYSTEMS OF ILLNESS CONCEPTS

Obviously a certain gap exists between folk and medical systems in conceiving mental disorders and offering explanations for their causes. Folk systems involve magic, extend into the supernatural realm, are based on intuition, and are meaningful to the people who believe in them. In contrast, professional systems are characterized by logical thinking, operate according to scientific approaches, are based on clinical experience, tend to be inhuman and mechanical, and are not necessarily meaningful to laymen. However, beyond their different natures, many features of folk and professional systems are parallel or correlated.

The question of the possible relationship that exists between the two systems, or their influence on each other, was raised by Westermeyer and Wintrob (1979b). They speculated that, historically, there must have been some kind of dynamic and continuing exchange between folk and scientific realms of explanation. They further pointed out that differences between folk and psychiatric perspectives do not imply an innate conflict between the two. Rather than being mutually exclusive, the two systems can provide complementary explanations of mental and behavioral phenomena that we encounter. This is a point that deserves to be taken into consideration by clinicians when they are dealing with patients and their families, particularly those of divergent cultural backgrounds.

As White (1982) pointed out, while it was largely cross-cultural investigations that stimulated the aware-

ness of cultural impact on the recognition and understanding of mental illness, this impact by no means occurs only in exotic societies or to minority ethnic groups. Cultural beliefs concerning mental illness and psychological problems are an important ingredient in ordinary, everyday explanations of disorders, as well as in clinical practice.

REFERENCES

Beiser, M., Burr, W.A., Ravel, J.L., & Collomb, H. (1973). Illnesses of the spirit among the Serer of Senegal. *American Journal of Psychiatry, 130*(8), 881–886.

Beiser, M., Ravel, J.L., Collomb, H., & Egelhoff, C. (1972). Assessing psychiatric disorders among the Serer of Senegal. *Journal of Nervous and Mental Disease 154,* 141–151.

Brelsford, W.V. (1950). Insanity among the Bemba of Northern Rhodesia. *Africa, 20,* 46–54.

Clement, D.C. (1982). Samoan folk knowledge of mental disorders. In A.J. Marsella & G.M. White (Eds.), *Cultural conceptions of mental health and therapy* (pp. 193–213). Dordrecht, The Netherlands: Reidel.

Clements, F.E. (1932). Primitive concepts of disease. *University of California Publications in American Archaeology and Ethnology, 32,* 185–252.

Currier, R.L. (1966). The hot-cold syndrome and symbol balance in Mexican and Spanish-American folk medicine. *Ethnology, 5*(3), 251–263.

Denko, J.D. (1966). How preliterate peoples explain disturbed behavior. *Archives of General Psychiatry, 15,* 398–409.

Edgerton, R.B. (1966). Conceptions of psychosis in four East African societies. *American Anthropologist, 68,* 408–425.

Edgerton, R.B., & Karno, M. (1971). Mexican-American bilingualism and the perception of mental illness. *Archives of General Psychiatry, 24,* 286–290.

Eguchi, S. (1991). Between folk concepts of illness and psychiatric diagnosis: Kitsune-tuski (fox possession) in a mountain village of Western Japan. *Culture, Medicine and Psychiatry, 15,* 421–451.

Eisenberg, L. (1977). Disease and illness: Distinctions between professional and popular ideas of sickness. *Culture, Medicine and Psychiatry, 1*(1), 9–23.

Eisenbruch, M. (1990). Classification of natural and supernatural causes of mental distress: Development of a mental distress explanatory model questionnaire. *Journal of Nervous and Mental Disease, 178*(11), 712–719.

Fabrega, H., Jr. (1989). Cultural relativism and psychiatric illness. *Journal of Nervous and Mental Disease, 177*(7), 415–430.

Gaviria, M., & Wintrob, R. (1976). Supernatural influence in psychopathology: Puerto Rican folk beliefs about mental illness. *Canadian Psychiatric Association Journal, 21,* 361–369.

Good, B.J. (1977). The heart of what's the matter: The semantics of illness in Iran. *Culture, Medicine and Psychiatry, 1*(1), 25–58.

Good, B.J., & Good, M.D. (1982). Toward a meaning-centered analysis of popular illness categories: Fright-illness" and "heart distress" in Iran. In A.J. Marsella & G.M. White (Eds.), *Cultural conceptions of mental health and therapy* (pp. 141–166). Dordrecht, The Netherlands: Reidel.

Karno, M., & Edgerton, R.B. (1969). Perception of mental illness in a Mexican-American community. *Archives of General Psychiatry, 20,* 233–238.

Kim, K.I. (1973). Traditional concept of disease in Korea. *Korea Journal, 13*(1), 12–18.

Kutumbiah, P. (1962). *Ancient Indian medicine.* Calcutta, India: Orient Longmans.

Lipowski, Z.J. (1969). Psychological aspect of disease. *Annals of Internal Medicine, 71*(6), 1197–1206.

Mechanic, D. (1962). Some factors in identifying and defining mental illness. *Mental Hygiene, 46,* 66–74.

Ngokwey, N. (1995). Naming and grouping illnesses in Feira (Brazil). *Culture, Medicine and Psychiatry, 19,* 385–408.

Offer, D., & Sabshin, M. (1974). *Normality: Theoretical and clinical concepts of mental health* (2nd ed). New York: Basic Books.

Szasz, T.S. (1961). *The myth of mental illness: Foundations of a theory of personal conduct.* New York: Hoeber-Harper.

Tseng, W.S. (1973). The development of psychiatric concepts in traditional Chinese medicine. *Archives of General Psychiatry, 29,* 569–575.

Tseng, W.S. (1999, August 6–11). *Chinese traditional medicine: Relevance to psychiatry.* Plenary presentation at the 11th World Congress of Psychiatry, Hamburg, Germany.

Wen, J.K. (1995). Sexual beliefs and problems in contemporary Taiwan. In T.-Y. Lin, W.S. Tseng, & E.K. Yeh (Eds.), *Chinese society and mental health* (pp. 219–230). Hong Kong: Oxford University Press.

Westermeyer, J., & Wintrob, R. (1979a). "Folk" critieria for the diagnosis of mental illness in rural Laos: On being insane in sane places. *American Journal of Psychiatry, 136,* 755–761.

Westermeyer, J., & Wintrob, R. (1979b). "Folk" explanations of mental illness in rural Laos. *American Journal of Psychiatry, 136,* 901–905.

White, G.M. (1982). The ethnographic study of cultural knowledge of "mental disorder." In A.J. Marsella & G.M. White (Eds.), *Cultural conceptions of mental health and therapy* (pp. 69–95). Dordrecht, The Netherlands: Reidel.

10

Illness Behavior: Reaction and Help-Seeking

I. WHAT IS ILLNESS BEHAVIOR?

The term "illness behavior" is used to describe how a person behaves when he becomes ill. In a broad sense, it covers a set of sequential behaviors, including how the person recognizes, perceives, and interprets the discomfort or suffering and reacts against it; how he seeks help, attention, or treatment from others; how he communicates and presents his problems or illness to his family, healers, and others; how his role changes when he is sick, including how he is cared for by family members, friends, or others; how he reacts to therapy prescribed or treatment offered by healers, including compliance and adherence to it; and how he accepts or reacts to the results of treatment and the prognosis of his disorders. Thus, illness behavior includes several identifiable elements that are involved in the process of illness (Chrisman, 1977).

From a clinical point of view, it is necessary to pay attention to a patient's illness behavior, as it will significantly influence the process of treating him as well as the course and outcome of the disorder. From a cultural perspective, it is important to know how cultural factors contribute to a patient's behavior and to his behavior in seeking help, including how he utilizes the healing systems that are available. It is believed that illness behavior is shaped by culture to a great extent, and that such behavior varies considerably among societies with different cultural backgrounds.

When we are discussing illness behavior, a conceptual distinction between "illness" and "disease," as discussed previously [Chapter 9:Mental Illness (Section V, A)], is very useful. It is also important to comprehend that the "illness behavior" manifested by the patient is going to interact with the "treatment behavior" undertaken by the therapist, resulting in the clinical phenomena observed. The modern physician is trained to inquire into the patient's symptoms, to detect the manifested signs of his illness, to obtain the needed laboratory data, and, based on this information, to make a clinical diagnosis. Then he is expected to prescribe a treatment plan and predict the course and outcome of the patient's disorder. This "treatment behavior" is often undertaken by clinicians, particularly those who are biologically medically oriented. Clearly, there is a wide gap between the illness behavior of the patient and the treatment behavior of the therapist. How these two sets of behavior interact with each other and result in the total outcome should be a major concern of the competent clinician. The purpose of this discussion is to explore ways to compromise between or integrate these two sets of behavior to make treatment more relevant, meaningful, and effective.

II. PERCEPTION AND INTERPRETATION OF ILLNESS

A. SENSITIVITY TOWARD ILLNESS AND TOLERANCE OF MENTAL SICKNESS

Every person has his own sensitivity to and tolerance of the illness from which he suffers. It is commonly observed that men are more likely than women to deny their problems and often have to submit involuntarily to the imposition of help from others (Horwitz, 1977). Generally speaking, hypochondriacal patients tend to perceive any physical sign as serious and react with exaggeration, whereas adolescent patients tend to deny and conceal their psychological problems. Thus, various factors, including individual personality, gender, age, and medical knowledge, shape the process of illness behavior. Beyond these factors, cultural views of illness certainly mold how one perceives and reacts to suffering.

It is speculated that people of different ethnic groups will perceive, tolerate, and react differently to the same somatic symptom, such as pain. Zborowski (1952), a pioneer in the study of culture and pain, investigated veterans with chronic pain in New York. For the sake of cross-ethnic comparison, he divided the subjects into "Old Americans" (Anglo-Saxon Protestants whose families had lived in the United States for several generations), Jewish people, and Italians. He pointed out that Old Americans tended to be stoic in responding to pain, whereas Jewish and Italian people did not hesitate to complain about it. They responded to painful experiences expressively and emotionally. However, the Jews and Italians differed from each other in other respects. The Italians were eager for pain relief, whereas the Jews were fearful of pain medication. They perceived pain as an indication of how their illness was doing.

How patients complained about or tolerated pain and how such illness behavior was perceived by the medical staff were investigated from a cross-ethnic point of view in Hawaii by Streltzer and Wade (1981). In order to standardize the severity and nature of pain, they focused on patients who experienced acute pain after undergoing an elective gall bladder removal operation. Instead of a subjective description of the severity of pain, which was difficult to measure, this investigation examined the amount of postoperative pain medication used by the patients. It was found that Caucasian-American patients received the most pain medication, whereas Filipino-, Japanese-, and Chinese-Americans received the least. Hawaiians were intermediate. In addition to the factors of age, sex, surgical complications, and other medical variables, ethnicity was found to be one of the contributing variables, i.e., there was a difference in pain medication according to ethnic groups. Further analysis revealed that the differences were not related to the surgeon who prescribed the pain medication "to be taken as needed," but that it was the nurse who decided whether to give the medication in response to the patient's complaints of pain. In other words, the actual use of pain medication was at the nurse's discretion. In response to the ethnicity-shaped, pain-complaining behavior, the nurses, as the actual bedside care deliverers, perceived the need for pain medication differently for patients of different ethnic groups.

Related to their cultural backgrounds, people of different ethnic groups demonstrate different patterns in presenting the symptoms from which they suffer. In a comparison of Irish and Italian outpatients in the United States, medical sociologist I.K. Zola (1966) disclosed that the Italians reported symptoms in greater detail and included disruptions of interpersonal relationships as part of their complaints. The Irish gave truncated responses and denied any impact of symptoms on interpersonal relations.

People react to certain stresses and problems with different intensity based on their orientation and viewpoint. As discussed previously [Chapter 8: Stress and Coping Patterns (Section I, D, 2)] Masuda and Holmes (1967) carried out a comparative study of life stresses between Japanese and Americans. The study showed that, in contrast to Americans, the Japanese, who lived in a law-and-order-sanctioned society, considered "detention in jail" a relatively serious problem, whereas "argument with spouse" was less serious because husband–wife relations were not regarded as priorities in their emotional lives.

Depending on their backgrounds, people perceive and tolerate certain mental symptoms or psychopathologies in different ways. For instance, depression is considered a potentially serious matter for those who emphasize emotional life and regard happiness as their goal in life. In contrast, for those who view life as full of misery and depression as nothing but an expected part of life, the occurrence of depression is not regarded as critical.

In a society where drinking is a normal part of life and drunken behavior is common, the problems of alcohol abuse or alcoholism are less alarming. In contrast, in a society that emphasizes sobriety and despises the intake of alcohol, excessive drinking behavior will alarm the family and community.

In general, in a society that is very concerned with interpersonal harmony, family and other members of society have less tolerance for outwardly disturbing behavior (such as destructive or violent behavior), but have a better acceptance of dysfunctional behavior that is manifested inwardly (such as withdrawal or asocial behavior).

B. Interpretation of Illness

As elaborated previously (Chapter 9: Mental Illness: Folk Categories and Explanation), there are many systems according to which the patient and his family may explain his illness. The interpretations may be supernatural, natural, somatomedical, psychological, or societal.

The choice of explanatory models is based on numerous factors and is influenced by the common beliefs of the society or culture. Loss of semen through urination, loss of the soul due to fright, the intake of imbalanced (hot and cold) food, lack of exercise, inheritance of pathological genes, and abuse by parents in early childhood are some of the culture-patterned, fashionable explanations given by society to explain illnesses.

1. Dynamic Meaning of Illness-Interpretation

Interpretation of illness can also relieve the burden blame for the illness from the patient or his family. Identifying ill fate, bad inheritance, or early trauma can alleviate the responsibility of the "self" as the cause of the problems. The explanation model will be altered depending on whether the society believes the individual should take responsibility for his own actions.

2. Interpretations Contributing to Illness-Coping Patterns

How a patient's view and interpretation of illness shape different patterns of coping with illness is well illustrated by a breast cancer study conducted by Baider and Sarell (1983) in Israel, even though it is not related to psychiatric illness. In Israel, the morbidity of breast cancer is 65 cases per 100,000 — one-fourth of all malignancies in women. Dividing all the Israeli women in their study into Western Jews (born in Europe or America) and Oriental Jews (born in the predominantly Muslim countries of North Africa and the Middle East), the investigators disclosed that the "Oriental" Jewish women tended to be aware of their cancer diagnoses but did not assume individual responsibility in their new roles as cancer patients. Rather, they responded fatalistically, feeling helpless, resigned, and submissive. Their illness was seen as uncontrollable and irreversible. However, the "Western" women were also mostly aware of their cancer diagnoses, but responded by mobilizing their own energies, trying to control their bodies and behaviors, and trusting the resources of medical science and its professionals. They did not blame themselves or others for their illnesses and were not guilt-ridden.

In India, Banerjee and Banerjee (1995) examined the help-seeking behavior of epileptics. They found that a belief in the supernatural cause of epilepsy combined with family input in making decisions tended to lead patients to seek help from indigenous healers, whereas those who believed that epilepsy had a physical cause and who participated in a social network in their decision making tended to see practitioners of modern medicine.

Wahass and Kent (1997) examined public attitudes concerning the psychiatric experience of auditory hallucinations in Britain and Saudi Arabia. Patients seeing their general practitioners were utilized for the study. It was revealed that those living in Saudi Arabia were most likely to believe that hallucinations were caused by Satan or magic and that religious assistance would be most effective. In contrast, people in the United Kingdom were more likely to cite schizophrenia or brain damage as the cause of these psychic experiences and to support medication and psychological therapies for their treatment.

Furnham and Murao (1999) compared laypersons' views of schizophrenia in Japan and the United Kingdom. They found that the Japanese, who have more taboos about mental illness in general than the British, tended to see patients suffering from schizophrenia as more dangerous, "morally insane," and difficult to deal with. They saw institutional care as the best way to help schizophrenics. In contrast, the British were more concerned with the human rights of schizophrenic patients and viewed them as less dangerous and abnormal than the Japanese. They stressed individual care and consideration as more relevant. Thus, due to cultural influence, the same psychiatric condition is viewed and reacted to differently by laypeople from different cultural backgrounds.

3. Illness-Interpretation and Treatment Compliance

It is considered that patients' compliance in therapy (particularly in psychotherapy) is a function of the degree to which they share their therapists' view of the causes of their illness. In order to test this hypothesis, Foulks, Persons, and Merkel (1986) carried out a survey. Utilizing outpatients of the psychiatric clinic at

the University of Pennsylvania hospital, they administered a cause of illness inventory questionnaire that they developed. The items included in this questionnaire were divided into two groups: "medically congruent explanations" and "medically noncongruent explanations." The former group referred to explanations of the causes of mental illness that were consistent with the biopsychosocial model widely used by contemporary psychiatrists. Examples included being upset too often, having tension in the family, and being mistreated by others. The latter group was not consistent with modern psychiatrists' views. Examples included eating too many hot foods, God's will, being hexed, and having committed too many sins. In a clinical follow-up study of the patients, it was disclosed that those who endorsed more medically congruent explanations made more visits to the clinic and ended treatment in a more compliant manner, whereas those who tended to hold more medically noncongruent explanations did not.

III. SICK ROLE AND THE REACTIONS OF OTHERS

From a sociological point of view, "role" refers to the behavioral expectations of others regarding the individual in question as determined by general cultural norms of proper behavior and the individual's particular social identity (Twaddle, 1972). In each society, a person suffering from illness is delegated a certain "sick role" to play and receives certain reactions and treatments from others. As elaborated by Parsons (1951, p. 436), a sick person is generally exempted from normal social responsibilities. Society generally recognizes that the sick person cannot get well by himself and needs certain kinds of care and help. At the same time, the state of being ill is itself regarded as undesirable and carries with it the obligation to "want to get well." If a person becomes sick, it is generally considered necessary for him to seek technically competent help.

In general, if a person suffers from an acute physical illness with somatic distress, he may be regarded as a "sick" person, receiving comfort and care from others. However, if a person suffers from a chronic disability, is unable to take care of himself, is disturbing others' lives, and is being a burden to family members or staff who offer care, he may be perceived as an undesirable patient and be subjected to neglect or even abuse. Depending on the nature and severity of their disorders, psychiatric patients may be responded to by others in different ways. For instance, charming and hysterical patients, who know how to get attention from others, may receive considerable care from their service deliverers. A hypochondriacal patient may be reacted to positively or negatively by others, depending on whether he is liked or disliked. Strangely behaving psychotic patients, particularly socially disturbing ones, will often be stigmatized or treated in a negative way. Thus, how the patient manifests his problems, and how the people around him react to him, will affect the pathways to treatment, the course of therapy, and the outcome of care.

In Western society, if a person complains that he is "depressed," he will get considerable attention from others. At his work place, he will be permitted to take a less severe work load, at least temporarily. He will receive care from and the concern of family members or his spouse, if they have a good relationship. At a clinic, he will get attention from the therapist and will prompt him to ask if he has any suicidal thoughts. It is common medical practice (as well as a medical–legal requirement) for a therapist to do so. If the answer is yes, then the therapist will consider the need for the patient to be hospitalized, to be protected from taking suicidal action, and to receive needed treatment. In contrast, in other cultures, where people are struggling for a living, worrying about food and shelter, if a person mentions that he is "depressed," he will receive a "so what?" kind of reaction. His depression will be viewed as a part of everyday life, nothing to be alarmed about, or something about which nothing can be done. In a society where people are expected to work hard and take responsibility for their own lives, others may react to a person's depression as if it were his own fault because he did not have enough will power or a strong enough character to resolve his own

problems. He will not receive any special attention or sympathy from others, but will be considered a "weak" person. Thus, different patients who are suffering from the same pathology may be reacted to differently by professionals and others and be assigned different "sick" roles.

Psychiatrists from the city of Tagane in Japan and Shanghai in China did a cross-cultural comparison of schizophrenic patients. Among many variables, their major concern was how the patients' illnesses were viewed by their families, who referred the patients for psychiatric treatment, and the way the patients were brought to the treatment center (Bunai, Asai, Asai, Zheng & Wang, 1988). The results revealed that, in Shanghai, families were still very concerned with having a member who was mentally ill, with more than one-third of them (38%) trying to keep it a secret from others. It was usually the parents (43%) who took the patient to the psychiatric service, and nearly half of the patients (48%) were not told by their parents that the visit was for psychiatric care. In contrast, in Tagane, fewer families (12%) tried to keep the illness a secret. In addition to arrangements made by his parents (28%), the patient might be referred to a psychiatric service by a family physician, colleagues, or others. Fewer patients (18%) were not informed that the visit was a psychiatric one. The investigators concluded that, in China, a stigma is still strongly attached to psychiatric illness. The patients often find it difficult to get married, particularly females, have trouble finding employment, and are stigmatized by others. The existence of such attitudes and undesirable consequences explains the ways the patients were handled.

IV. HELP-SEEKING BEHAVIOR AND PATHWAYS

"Help-seeking behavior" is a part of overall illness behavior. It particularly refers to how the patient (or his family) seeks help for the care of his illness. Help-seeking behavior is determined by multiple factors, including, for instance, how the patient perceives the nature and severity of his illness; how he is motivated to seek help from the health system; how he understands the appropriate health service for his illness and whether he knows such a service is available; how he feels about visiting a care-delivery service; what the sociocultural implications will be of receiving health care; and the economical effects of receiving service delivery. Needless to say, these factors will also be influenced by the availability of the service system that exists in the community. From the standpoint of the community health system, examining a patient's help-seeking behavior is a major issue, as it will reveal the general pattern of how the patient utilizes the health system and whether he does so relevantly, adequately, and effectively. From a cultural perspective, it is useful to know the stylized pattern that is adopted by the patient in seeking help in his cultural setting. Such knowledge will offer us an opportunity to alter it if necessary for improvement.

A. Help-Seeking Pathways

As indicated by Rogler and Cortes (1993), help-seeking pathways mean the sequence of contacts made with individuals and organizations by the distressed person and the efforts of his or her significant others in seeking help, as well as the help that is supplied in response to those efforts. As pointed out by Rogler and Cortes, help-seeking pathways are not random: they are structured by the convergence of psychosocial and cultural factors.

It is a clinical impression that, in many societies, both East and West, patients who have mental illnesses or emotional problems often seek help from folk healers or alternative health systems before they visit psychiatrists (Kleinman, Eisenberg, & Good, 1978).

1. Prevalent Utilization of Folk Healing: Example from the United States

Even though the United States is considered one of the most economically developed and scientifically advanced societies, as pointed out by Ness and Wintrob (1981), many people living there still frequently utilize folk-healing methods to deal with their mental problems. For instance, faith-healing practices are common to a number of Christian denominations (Hufford, 1977). One of the more intense, group-oriented forms of faith healing is practiced by American fundamentalist Protestant congregations. Rootwork refers to beliefs and practices used to cope with the physical and psychological effects of malign magic — an evil spell cast by others that may cause grave misfortune, illness, or death. Rootwork beliefs incorporate elements of European witchcraft, west African sorcery, and west Indian voodoo. According to Whitten (1962), such beliefs and practices are encountered mainly in the southeastern United States among both Caucasian-American and African-American. *Curanderismo* is a system of beliefs commonly found among Mexican-Americans concerning the causes and management of personal and social misfortune, including illness. These beliefs are an interweaving of Iberian Catholic and indigenous Mexican traditions. *Espiritismo* (or spiritism) is a syncretized system of Spanish, African, and Indian folk-healing practices based on the belief that the visible and invisible worlds are inhabited by spirits that are temporarily encased in a human body in the material world. This system and related healing practices are observed among Puerto Ricans living in the northeastern United States. Based on the prevalent utilization of religion–magical healing systems in advanced societies, Ness and Wintrob (1981) indicated that contemporary medical interventions are limited in their scope, i.e., they deal mainly with the proximal causes and manifestations of problems, while the patient is concerned with a complex physical–social–spiritual problem involving not only himself, but also his family, his social network, and his relations with the spirit world.

2. Tracing Help-Seeking Pathways in Japan

A comprehensive investigation was carried out by Japanese psychiatrist K.H. Asai (1984) concerning the pathways taken by psychiatric patients in Japan. The study included 121 patients who were admitted consecutively over a 3-month period in 1980 to the Asai Mental Hospital in Togane City, Chiba prefecture, near Tokyo. Based on data obtained, Asai indicated that, in Japan, family members play a decisive role in perceiving the occurrence of mental problems and motivating the patient to seek professional help. He indicated that, contrary to expectation, the role played by public agencies was relatively insignificant and infrequent. The role of family doctors in community care has long been regarded as very important in Japan; however, in cases involving psychiatric problems, the intervention of family doctors is very limited. They also have a tendency to retain psychiatric patients under their care for an unduly long time before referring them to psychiatric institutes for proper treatment.

3. Different Pathways within the Same Society: A Study in Taiwan

In Taiwan, Hwang, Wu, Wen, Hwang, and Rin (1983) carried out a study of help-seeking pathways taken by patients there. The patients were divided into those with major psychiatric disorders (psychoses), minor psychiatric disorders (neuroses), severe medical disorders (cancer or uremic disorders), and a health-examination group (admitted to the hospital for routine health exams). The study was conducted in two settings, one in Taipei in the northern part of Taiwan and the other in Kaohsiung city in the south. The study produced several findings. First, it was disclosed that, although only 17% of the health-examination patients had previously visited temples to consult fortune-tellers or health advisers, 44% of the severe medical cases had demonstrated such help-seeking behavior. Historically, people living in the southern part of Taiwan tended to have a stronger belief in supernaturally oriented folk healing than those living in the north. Data obtained were compared according to geographic differences. It was found that 84% of the psychotic patients and 34% of the neurotic patients who lived in southern Taiwan had previously visited temples for their health problems compared to only 38% of the psychotic patients and 26% of the neurotic patients in northern Taiwan. This indicates that, overall, it is a common practice for people in Taiwan to visit temples to obtain divine consultation in the care of their illnesses. This is particularly true for psychotic patients in the south, where people tend to believe more in folk healing and where adequate mental health care facilities are relatively lacking.

It was revealed that none of the health-examination group had ever consulted shamans, whereas 39% of the severe medical cases had. Among psychiatric patients, 36% of the psychotics and 25% of the neurotics in the south and 9% of the psychotics and 5% of the neurotics in the north had contacted such supernaturally oriented folk healers prior to visiting psychiatrists. This showed that when a patient suffered from a severe illness, either medical or mental, he tended to seek help from a shaman. Again, there were considerable differences between patients in the south and north, with the former tending more toward supernatural folk healing.

As for visiting traditional medical doctors, 28% of the health-examination group had previously had such previous experiences. Among severe medical cases, 58% had sought advice from traditional doctors. Among psychiatric patients, 39% of the psychotics and 52% of the neurotics in the south and 9% of the psychotics and 32% of the neurotics in the north had visited traditional medical doctors. In general, patients who suffered from minor psychiatric problems, in contrast to major disorders, tended to utilize traditional medicine prior to or coinciding with their visits to Western psychiatrists.

This investigation illustrates that it is rather common for people in Taiwan to seek alternative healing systems before they reach out to modern mental health facilities. This is quite true in many other societies as well, including developed societies such as the United States, as described earlier (Ness & Wintrob, 1981). The Taiwan study supports the view that, even in the same society, depending on their social backgrounds (as reflected in the location in this study) and the nature and severity of the illness, patients tend to take different pathways to obtain health-related help (Tseng, 1975; Wen, 1985).

In another study, a cultural psychiatrist from Taiwan, Jung-Kwang Wen (1990), reported that a temple called Lung Hwa Tang (The Hall of Dragon Metamorphoses) had been converted into an indigenous asylum for the chronically mentally ill in the southern city of Taiwan. In addition to the asylum being founded and organized by a monk trying to rehabilitate chronic psychotic patients through religious and work activities, there is the following interesting fact from the perspective of help-seeking behavior and community mental health. Because of a shortage of public mental health institutions for the custodial care of chronically mentally ill patients in Taiwan, and because many families could not afford to keep their ill family members in an expensive private facility over a long period of time, in their desperation, they kept the patients in this temple–asylum. The families were expected to make a certain monetary donation and the temple would keep the patients for the rest of their lives. Thus, in a way, families who had exhausted their energies and finances, as a last resort in dealing with the patients, left them in the care of the monks, hoping that they would take care of them. This reflected a shortage of modern mental facilities, as well as a lack of satisfaction toward professional service.

B. REASONS FOR SELECTING DIFFERENT HEALING SYSTEMS

1. Why Patients Go to See Psychiatrists: Investigation in Malay

Why patients go to see psychiatrists is a legitimate question from both clinical and administrative points of view. Cultural psychiatrist, Jin-Inn Teoh, Kinzie and Tan carried out a survey in Malaysia (1972) to explore this issue. There was a newly built university hospital in Kuala Lumpur, the capital of Malaysia. It is a multiethnic city inhabited by Malays, Chinese, and Indians. The investigators interviewed patients to find out their reasons for visiting the psychiatric clinic. The patients' stated reasons were categorized into three groups: "subjective distress" (the patient felt personally upset or had symptoms primarily limited to himself that did not involve interpersonal relationship problems), "interpersonal or social distress" (the patient was displaying disruptive or deviant behavior that his family or social group could not cope with), and "for assessment" (the patient gave no complaints of his own, but was referred by his family, relatives, or others for assessment). The results revealed that, among the three ethnic groups, a large number of the Indians (61%) visited psychiatrists for subjective distress, 23% due to social distress, and 16% for assessment. In contrast, of the Chinese, 43% visited for subjective distress, but more than half (51%) for social distress and only 6% for assessment. Of the Malays, 43% visited for subjective distress, 43% for social distress, and 13% for assessment. This showed that, within the same society, the Indian patients tended to visit a psychiatrist more because of their own suffering, whereas the Chinese visited more because of distress at disturbing others around them.

2. Why Patients Consult Folk Healers: Explanations According to Medical Anthropology

In some societies, because of the lack of modern psychiatrists, the local people still utilize folk healers as the major source of help in dealing with mental problems. However, in many societies, even though modern psychiatrists are relatively available, patients still utilize folk healers as alternative sources of help. The medical anthropologist Castillo (2000), after examining various forms of alternative therapies, pointed out that there are several reasons for this phenomenon. Cultural congruence, orientation to treating illness, and familiarity were some of the reasons listed. This does not mean that there were no disadvantages to consulting folk healers. Some negative consequences were mentioned, such as neglect or delaying "proper" treatment, suffering from financial fraud at the hands of greedy, unethical healers, or other malpractices, including improper sexual behavior toward female clients by male healers. Still, many people, particularly those who were not satisfied with modern psychiatric service, sought help from alternative therapists that they could believe in (cross-reference to Chapter 32: Culture-Embedded Indigenous Healing Practices).

V. SERVICE UTILIZATION AND COMPLIANCE

We all know that many social factors significantly affect the pattern of mental health service utilization. Financial factors, including the medical insurance system, the cost of visits, and the availability of service, are some of the social factors that have a direct impact on how the services are utilized by a patient. Beyond these factors, there are ethnic, racial, and cultural factors as well.

Many investigations conducted in the United States have pointed out that, in contrast to the majority group of Caucasian-Americans, many minority groups tend to underutilize the existing (modern) mental health system (K.M. Lin, Inui, Kleinman, & Womack, 1982; T.-Y. Lin, Tardiff, Donetz, & Goresky 1978; Sue, 1977) and also tend not to adhere to the service if they do connect with it. For example, Sue and Zane (1987) reported that among ethnic minorities, more than 50% dropped psychotherapeutic treatment after their first appointment. Wells, Aough, Golding, Burnam, and Karno (1987) reported that less acculturated Mexican-Americans tended to use outpatient mental health services less frequently (one-seventh as much) than non-Hispanic Caucasian-Americans in the Los Angeles area.

Many explanations have been offered for these phenomena. For instance, Karno and Edgerton (1969) have pointed out that due to their perception and definition of mental illness, Mexican-Americans tend to seek treatment for obviously psychiatric disorders from family physicians. The patients' orientation to and understanding and expectation of psychiatric therapy affect their patterns of utilization. Cultural incongruities between the patient and treatment are considered to play a role in the results among Hispanic patients (Miranda, 1976). Language barriers are always cited as major problems. The utilization of interpreters in psychiatric settings, particularly in psychotherapy, tend to disrupt and delay the work, making it difficult. Finally, therapists' cultural insensitivity is another reason that needs to be considered.

Culturally relevant psychiatric care is a crucial need in clinical reality. This subject will be elaborated in further detail in Section E: Culture and Clinical Practice, Section F: Culture and Psychological Therapy, and Section G: Culture and Therapy with Special Subpopulations.

REFERENCES

Asai, K.H. (1984). Pathways of help-seeking of psychiatric patients in Japan: A research study in Togane City. *American Journal of Social Psychiatry, 4*(2), 38–44.

Baider, L., & Sarell, M. (1983). Perceptions and causal attributions of Israeli women with breast cancer concerning their illness: The effects of ethnicity and religiosity. *Psychotherapy and Psychosomatics, 39,* 136–143.

Banerjee, T., & Banerjee, G. (1995). Determinants of help-seeking behaviour in cases of epilepsy attending a teaching hospital in India: An indigenous explanatory model. *International Journal of Social Psychiatry, 41*(3), 217–230.

Bunai, S., Asai, K.H., Asai, T., Zheng, Z.P., & Wang, Z.C. (1988). A cross-cultural study of patterns of help-seeking: Schizophrenic patients in Japan and China. *Japanese Journal of Social Psychiatry, 11*(1), 71–81 (in Japanese).

Castillo, R.J. (2000). Lessons from folk healing. In W.S. Tseng & J. Streltzer (Eds.), *Culture and psychotherapy: A guide for clinical practice* (pp. 81–101). Washington, DC: American Psychiatric Press.

Chrisman, N.J. (1977). The health seeking process: An approach to the natural history of illness. *Culture, Medicine and Psychiatry, 1*(4), 351–377.

Foulks, E.F., Persons, J.B., & Merkel, R.L. (1986). The effect of patients' beliefs about their illness on compliance in psychotherapy. *American Journal of Psychiatry, 143*(3), 340–344.

Furnham, A., & Murao, M. (1999). A cross-cultural comparison of British and Japanese lay theories of schizophrenia. *International Journal of Social Psychiatry, 46*(1), 4020.

Horwitz, A.V. (1977). The pathways into psychiatric treatment: Some differences between men and women. *Journal of Health and Social Behavior, 18,* 169–178.

Hufford, D. (1977). Christian religious healings. *Journal of Operational Psychiatry, 8,* 22–27.

Hwang, W.S., Wu, W.L., Wen, J.K., Hwang, M.G., & Rin, H. (1983). The study of psychiatric patients' help-seeking behavior. *Mental Health, 26,* 25–31 (in Chinese).

Karno, M., & Edgerton, R.B. (1969). Perception of mental illness in a Mexican-American community. *Archives of General Psychiatry, 20,* 233–238.

Kleinman, A., Eisenberg, L., & Good, B. (1978). Culture, illness, and care: Clinical lessons from anthropologic and cross-cultural research. *Annals of Internal Medicine, 88,* 251–258.

Lin, K.M., Inui, T.S., Kleinman, A.M., & Womack, W.M. (1982). Sociocultural determinants of the help-seeking behavior of patients with mental illness. *Journal of Nervous and Mental Disease, 170,* 78–85.

Lin, T.-Y., Tardiff, K., Donetz, G., & Goresky, W. (1978). Ethnicity and patterns of help-seeking. *Culture, Medicine and Psychiatry, 2,* 3–14.

Masuda, M., & Holmes, T.H. (1967). The social readjustment rating scale: A cross-cultural study of Japanese and Americans. *Journal of Psychosomatic Research, 11,* 227–237.

Miranda, M.R. (1976). *Psychotherapy with the Spanish-speaking: Issues in research and service delivery,* [Monograph No. 3]. Los Angeles: Spanish-Speaking Mental Health Research Center.

Ness, R.C., & Wintrob, R. (1981). Folk healing: A description and synthesis. *American Journal of Psychiatry, 138,* 1477–1481.

Parsons, T. (1951). *The social system.* Glencoe, IL: Free Press.

Rogler, L., & Cortes, D.E. (1993). Help-seeking pathways: A unifying concept in mental health care. *American Journal of Psychiatry, 150*(4), 554–561.

Streltzer, J., & Wade, T.C. (1981). The influence of cultural group on the undertreatment of postoperative pain. *Psychosomatic Medicine, 43,* 397–403.

Sue, S. (1977). Community mental health services to minority groups: Some optimism, some pessimism. *American Psychology, 32,* 616–624.

Sue, S., & Zane, N. (1987). The role of culture and cultural techniques in psychotherapy: A critical reformulation. *American Psychology, 42,* 37–45.

Teoh, J.I., Kinzie, J.D., & Tan, E.S. (1972). Why patients attend a psychiatric clinic: Breaking the barrier. *International Journal of Social Psychiatry, 18,* 301–307.

Tseng, W.S. (1975). Traditional and modern psychiatric practices in Taiwan. In A. Kleinman, P. Kunstadter, E.R. Alexander, & J.L. Cale (Eds.), *Medicine in Chinese cultures: Comparative studies of health care in Chinese and other societies* (pp. 311–328). Washington, DC: U.S. Department of Health, Education and Welfare, Public Health Services.

Twaddle, A.C. (1972). The concept of the sick role and illness behavior. *Advancement in Psychosomatic Medicine, 8,* 162–179.

Wahass, S., & Kent, G. (1997). A comparison of public attitudes in Britain and Saudi Arabia towards auditory hallucinations. *International Journal of Social Psychiatgry, 43*(3), 175–183.

Wells, K.B., Hough, R.L., Golding, J.M., Burnam, M.A., & Karno, M. (1987). Which Mexican-Americans underutilize health services? *American Journal of Psychiatry, 144,* 918–922.

Wen, J.K. (1985). Mental disorders and help-seeking behavior: Problems and strategies. *Chinese Journal of Mental Health, 2*(1), 36–45 (in Chinese with English abstract).

Wen, J.K. (1990). The hall of dragon metamorphoses: A unique, indigenous asylum for chronic mental patients in Taiwan. *Culture, Medicine and Psychiatry, 14,* 1–19.

Whitten, N.E. (1962). Contemporary patterns of malign occultism among Negro in North Carolina. *Journal of American Folklore, 75,* 311–325.

Zborowski, M. (1952). Cultural components in response to pain. *Journal of Social Issues, 8,* 16–30.

Zola, I.K. (1966). Culture and symptoms: An analysis of patients' presenting complaints. *American Sociological Review, 31,* 615–630.

Section D
Culture and Psychopathology

As a part of their clinical practice, psychiatrists and related mental health workers are concerned about the psychopatholgy manifested by their patients. By fully understanding the mental disorders or mental health problems from which the patients are suffering, relevant clinical care may be given. In general, psychopathology is attributed to various factors, ranging from the biological to the psychological to the sociocultural. In this section, various kinds of cultural influences on psychopathology will be reviewed and examined in detail.

This section starts with Chapter 11, which provides an overview on the different ways in which culture impacts psychopathology, namely its pathogenetic, -selective, -plastic, -elaborative, -facilitate, and -reactive effects. Next, the cultural aspects of psychiatric epidemiology are reviewed in Chapter 12. This is followed by the elaboration of different categories of psychopathology, starting with culture-related specific syndromes (Chapter 13) and epidemic mental disorders (Chapter 14), the disorders that are most influenced by cultural factors, to other kind of mental disorders. There is no intention to cover all mental disorders, but to review as many as possible based on the information available. Although significant cultural contributions on certain disorders, such as sexual disorders, violent behavior, or antisocial behavior are speculated, such disorders are not reviewed due to limited cross-cultural knowledge available at present. The aim of this section is to give a paramatic view on how culture impacts various kinds of mental disorders in terms of development, manifestation, and prevalence.

11

Culture and Psychopathology: An Overview

I. INTRODUCTION: CONCEPT OF PSYCHOPATHOLOGY

In contrast to other fields of medicine, psychiatry is still far from knowing the exact etiological causes for various mental disorders. While medical knowledge has increased remarkably, most explanations of the causes of psychiatric disorders are still at the stage of speculation and hypotheses. However, the study of the relationship between sociocultural variables and psychopathology has enjoyed a remarkable growth in populatity among a broad spectrum of medical and behavioral science disciplines and professions during the past several decades (Marsella, 1993). It is generally considered by contemporary psychiatrists that multiple factors, including biological (such as hereditary and organic), psychological (relating to the individual and/or his family), and social–cultural factors, in different combinations and in an integrative, dynamic way, all contribute to the occurrence of mental sickness.

The term "psychopathology" implies simply a psychological condition that is pathological and different from the normal. It includes psychiatric disorders that are viewed as morbid entities manifesting certain pathological mental conditions. Severe mental symptoms or signs recognized by professionals (such as disorientation, hallucination, delusion, depression, anxiety) are present, leading to the distress or disability of the person concerned. It also includes abnormal behavior that may belong to the category of mental disorders, but certainly deviates from normal behavior and is considered dysfunctional (such as extreme shyness, suspicious, or explosive behavior). Such behavior not merely deviates from social norms, but is intolerable or disturbing from the point of view of the society in which it occurs. From a mental health perspective, clinicians pay attention to emotional or behavior problems in a broad way, encompassing many daily life problems (such as school maladjustment, marital problems, acculturation problems).

As pointed out by Berrios (1994), since the beginning of modern psychiatry, clinicians and scholars have debated on the matter of the "continuity" and "discontinuity" of pathology. According to the continuity model, there exists a continual spectrum from normal (nonpathological) to pathological psychic phenomena. Manifestations of mild degrees of anxiety, fear, or depression fit this model. Intellectual impairment, drinking behavior, or personality problems can exist within the continuity spectrum as well. The discontinuity model holds that there are pathological psychic symptoms that have no counterparts in normal behavior. Bizarre psychotic symptoms or pathognomonic organic mental conditions belong to this model and are explained according to the concept of mental disease, rather than viewed merely as exaggerations of normal into abnormal behavior.

Depending on their professional backgrounds and orientations, psychiatrists, as clinicians, prefer to use the term "pathology," implying that the disordered condition is related to the morbid entity of disease, whereas behavioral scientists, such as psychologists, tend to use the term "abnormality," meaning dysfunctional behavior that measurably deviates from the normal range. Here, the term and concept of "psychopathology" are used to refer broadly to any pathological mental condition or abnormal behavior.

According to Tanaka-Matsumi and Draguns (1997) and Berry, Poortinga, Segall, and Dasen (1992), clinical psychologists may be divided into three groups according to the way in which they conceptualize the interplay of abnormal behavior and culture: absolutist, universalist, and relativist. The absolutist posits invariance of psychopathological phnomena across cultures. The universalist takes the view that psychopathology exists universally, with variations due to cultural impact. The relativist believes that abnormal behavior exists only relative to how it is perceived by a society. It is becoming a common trend to recognize that culture exerts some degree of influence on psychopathological processes and manifestations. The debate tends to center around the extent of the influence, from trivial and superficial to pervasive and fundamental.

II. DIFFERENT WAYS CULTURE CONTRIBUTES TO PSYCHOPATHOLOGY

Recognizing that psychopathology is attributed to multiple factors, including biological, psychological, and sociocultural ones, here we are going to focus primarily on cultural contributions to psychopathology.

From a conceptual point of view, depending on how the impact occurs, there are six different ways that culture can contribute to psychopathology. They are in the form of pathogenic, pathoplastic, pathoselective, pathofacilitative, and pathoreactive effects. Let us examine how culture impacts psychopathology in these different ways.

A. PATHOGENIC EFFECTS

Pathogenic effects refer to situations in which culture is a direct causative factor in forming or "generating" psychopathology. As elaborated previously [Chapter 8: Stress and Coping Patterns (Section II, A), there are several ways that cultural ideas and beliefs can contribute to stress, which, in turn, produces psychopathology. Stress can be created by culturally formed anxiety, e.g., the folk belief that death will result if the penis shrinks into the abdomen, inducing the *koro* panic, or the popular anxiety over the "harmful" leaking of semen, leading to the development of the *daht* syndrome. Stress can be produced by culturally demanded performance, such as the expectation for a wife to give birth to a boy to carry on the family lineage, causing anxiety and insecurity in women who fail to do so; and family pressure on youngsters to succeed in college entrance examinations in societies where success is determined heavily by education. Stress may be induced by special culturally prescribed roles and duties, e.g., a widow, viewed as an "evil" woman who caused her husband's death, is treated unfavorably by her family and is expected to live a confined social life, which tends to induce depression for the rest of her life.

In cases such as these, culture is considered to be a causative factor, as culturally shared specific beliefs or ideas contribute *directly* to the formation of a particular stress, which, in turn, induces a certain mode of psychopathology. Without such a formal, culturally rooted idea or belief, the psychopathology would not occur. This is exemplified by the "territory taboo anxiety" (*malgri* syndrome) (Cawte, 1976) caused by the "land–sea" trespassing taboo, or the "*koro*" panic" induced by the fear of death from shrinkage of the penis into the abdomen based on the *yin-yang* concept, even in its epidemic form (Tseng et al., 1988). Sudden death brought about by breaking taboos or curses occurs only in societies in which people strongly believe in a supernatural power and the fatal consequences of taboo breaking (Eastwell, 1982).

Because the cultural beliefs that cause psychopathology are often culture specific, culture-induced psychopathology tends to be unique to the cultures that hold those beliefs. In other words, culture contributes to the development of an entirely unique psychopathology that is observed only in certain cultural environments and cannot phenomenologically be categorized into (or even closely related to) any diagnostic group that exists in current (Western) classification systems.

As such disorders are heavily related to culture, the disorders are considered to be culture-related specific psychiatric syndromes [cross-reference to Chapter 13: Culture-Related Specific Syndromes (Section II, A, 1–5)]. They comprise only a small number of psychiatric disorders that are recognized in the field of psychiatry, yet the pathogenetic effects of culture are vividly illustrated by these rare and unique clinical conditions.

B. PATHOSELECTIVE EFFECTS

At an individual level, we can analyze how a person, influenced by personal factors, such as personality and other psychological conditions, "selects" certain patterns of reaction toward stress, choosing a certain type of psychopathology. At a cultural level, it can be understood that a group of people in society, as a result of cultural influences, tends to select certain reaction patterns, resulting in the manifestation of certain psychopathologies.

This can be elaborated by utilizing a hypothetical case of running *amok,* as observed in the Muslim society of Malaysia. When a man discovers that his wife is unfaithful to him, he feels insulted socially and has a choice of reactions to this grave embarrassment: he

can become angry and hit his wife, who brought the disgrace on him; attack or kill the man who stole his wife; become a monk and withdraw to a mountain to live a hermetic life; become depressed; or end his life by committing suicide. Thus, there are "choices" of psychopathologies, including violent behavior, social withdrawal, depression, or suicide.

Influenced by individual personal factors, such as personality and psychological conditions and social factors, a person can choose different means for coping with his emotional pain. If he lives in a society in which religious beliefs do not permit suicide (such as Muslim society), such a choice would be out of the question. If the society would view him as a "coward" if he withdrew into the mountains and tried to resolve his psychological pain by relying on spiritual healing, he might not make that choice. If he were to become depressed, he might be perceived by his friends as a "weak" man. However, if there is cultural permission, and even the expectation, for him to express his sorrow, shame, and anger by killing others, even on a mass scale, and being killed himself for his violent behavior, he may make such a choice. In other words, he may choose the culturally expected way of killing himself through the random killing of others.

Another example is the so-called "family suicide" still often observed in Japanese society. A hypothetical situation is that of a husband who finds himself unable to pay his mortgage and keep his house. He tries in vain to borrow money from relatives or friends. The bank is not willing to loan him money without sufficient credit. Facing such a hopeless situation, he suggests the idea of suicide to his wife, who agrees to join him and end their lives together. Further, they make plans to die with their two young children. They tie themselves with ropes to the seats of their car, drive the car into the sea, and all drown. This is a typical case vignette of *"ikka-shinju"* (family suicide) observed in Japan (Ohara, 1963). Even though the parents' double suicide and homicide of their children is against the law, such family deaths still occur rather frequently.

What would other choices be if the husband faced this situation in another culture, such as the United

States? The answer is simple: claim bankruptcy, and no one would be responsible for the financial situation, but this would not work in Japan. It would be a life-long disgrace to claim bankruptcy. Being unable to borrow money from your own relatives and friends is already a very grave sign that you are not a welcome person in the society. There is no way to move to another place to hide from your responsibilities. Household records are so tight that there is no easy way to hide from law enforcers. Suicide seems the best way to resolve your problems, but why kill your young children when you want to end your life? It sounds cruel, but there is a cultural reason behind this action. Japanese, like many other Asians, believe that "blood is thicker than water." Based on this concept, there is a fear that orphans will not be well taken care of after the deaths of their parents. It is considered more "thoughtful" to take the children's lives together with their parents — to go to the other world together as a family rather than leaving them to suffer without their parents.

Without their knowing it, culture has a powerful influence on the choices people make in reacting to stressful situations and shapes the nature of the psychopathology that occurs as a result of those choices. Of course, this only applies to minor psychiatric disorders, particularly of culture-related specific syndromes, not to major psychiatric disorders, but it is clearly illustrated in the extreme cases described earlier that culture plays a significant role in determining the patterns of our reactions and the manifestations of our psychopathology.

C. PATHOPLASTIC EFFECTS

Psychopathoplastic effects refer to the way in which culture contributes to modeling or "plastering" of the manifestations of psychopathology. This can occur on two different levels.

1. Shaping the Content of Symptoms

Culture shapes symptom manifestation at the level of the content presented. The content of delusions, auditory hallucinations, obsessions, or phobias are subject to the environmental context in which the pathology is manifested. Cultural beliefs and attitudes toward life contribute to the content of symptoms. For instance, an individual's grandiose delusions may be characterized by the belief that he is a Russian emperor, Jesus Christ, Buddha, or the president of the United States, depending on which figure is more popular or important in his society. If a person develops a delusional disorder with persecutor ideas, based on his social background, the subject who follows him, tries to poison him, or otherwise persecutes him may be either a member of the CIA, the KGB, a communist, a political enemy, a deceased person's malicious spirit, an evil spirit, or an agent from outer space. In addition to personal knowledge and experiences, social and cultural elements contribute to the formation of symptoms. As long as there is sufficient clinical evidence to meet the nosological criteria for a delusional disorder, the diagnosis of persecutor delusion will not be affected, no matter who the patient believes is following or spying on him. In the same way, when a person becomes depressed, he may feel "guilty" for sins he has committed or "ashamed" for socially noncompliant performance or neither guilty nor ashamed.

A phobic patient may be preoccupied with the fear of many things. He may be afraid of being contaminated by germs, viruses, placental fluid, menses, bewitched subjects, or nuclear toxins, depending on what subjects are viewed as "dirty" or "dangerous" by the members of his society at a particular time. Fear of passing gas, exposing one's own body smell, or having one's face flush in front of others can be serious, obsessive social phobias if it is believed that such occurrences are very embarrassing in social situations.

Some psychiatric symptoms are emotional in nature, such as anxiety, depression, fear, or anger, whereas another group of symptoms is closely related to matters of thought, such as obsessive, phobic, or delusional ideas. The content of the thoughts is subject to the plastic effects of the external environment. Culture thus has psychopathoplastic effects on thought-related symptoms.

2. Modeling the Clinical Picture

The effect of cultural factors on psychopathology could be observed at the level of the presence (or exaggeration) or absence of certain symptoms that modify the total manifestation of the clinical picture to some extent.

It is commonly known that an emphasis on guilt or shame in the larger society shapes the nature of the depressive guilt idea (or even delusion) that may form in one of its susceptible members. There is less experience (or even absence) of guilt feelings, idea, or delusion in depressive patient in some societies in which the concept of "guilt" is not emphasized so heavily. At the end of the 19th century, Emil Krepeline, the founder of the modern psychiatric classification system, compared depressive patients in Indonesia to those in Germany. He pointed out that even with the same depressive disorder, the guilt delusion is seldom noticed among Indonesian patients, therefore, the clinical picture differs from that of the German patients (Jilek, 1995).

Fundia, Draguns, and Phillips (1971) commented that hospitalized patients in Argentina, in South America, and elsewhere exhibit more passive and socially oriented symptomatology than their counterparts in the United States.

Certain differences were even found in the clinical pictures of schizophrenic patients of different ethnic groups from the same society. An American anthropologist and sociologist, Marvin K. Opler (1959), carried out a cross-ethnic comparison of the symptomatology of schizophrenia between hospitalized Italian- and Irish-American patients in New York City. He reported that more Italian than Irish patients manifested behavior problems, rejected authority, and displayed overt homosexual tendencies during psychotic episodes. In contrast, more Irish than Italian patients were preoccupied with sin and guilt, manifested chronic alcoholism, and had fixed delusional thoughts. Opler's study showed that ethnic background (contributing to ethnic personality) shaped the total clinical picture, even though the differences described represented merely secondary symptoms or behavior

problems and had nothing to do with the core of the schizophrenic disorder.

Another example is anorexia nervosa. It has been pointed out by Chinese psychiatrists (Lee, Ho, & Hsu, 1995) that Hong Kong Chinese with anorexia nervosa are seldom concerned with being physically overweight. This is different from the anorexia nervosa recognized in Western society and is called "nonfat-concerned anorexia."

There are more examples to suggest that psychopathology is often shaped by social and cultural factors so that the clinical picture does not necessarily manifest uniformly at the universal level or similarly to the way it manifests in Western populations. *Taijinkuofusho* (fear of interpersonal relation disorder), a pathological concern over not being able to relate to others, is a special form of "social phobia" found in Japan. Japan is characterized by close social relations and emphasis on proper social behavior in public. In this cultural background, the disorder of *taijinkyofusho* is prevalent. The brain fag syndrome described by Prince (1960) among Africans is characterized by complaints of intellectual impairment, as well as somatic complaints of pain in the head or neck. It often occurs among students, who attribute phenomena such as "fatigue of the brain" to excessive mental work. It may be considered an African version of anxiety disorder, neurasthenia, or a subtype of somatoform disorder.

Depending on the intensity of the plastic effect and the degree of modification of symptomatology, culture will affect the psychopathology in such a way that the disorders could be recognized as "atypical," "subtypes," or "variations" of disorders officially recognized in the current (Western) classification system. Some of them will be included as culture-related specific syndromes, if cultural attention is considered important.

D. PATHOELABORATING EFFECTS

While certain behavior reactions (either normal or pathological) may be universal, they may become exaggerated to the extreme in some cultures through cultural reinforcement (Simons, 1996). Some mental conditions are not necessarily pathological and fulfill certain needs of the individual as well as the society; others are clearly pathological and are intensely elaborated by the culture.

The concept of pathoelaborating effects is well illustrated by the unique mental phenomenon latah, which is mainly observed in Malaysia. The phenomenon is characterized by the sudden onset of a transient dissociative attack induced by startling. Malaysia is a society in which modesty is emphasized and the interaction between men and women is conservative. However, many women develop a habit of *latah* attacks. During these dissociated, uninhibited mental states, they imitate things other people say or follow others' commands, saying words that have sexual overtones or manifesting socially forbidden sexual behavior toward men. The person is often provoked on social occasions and acts like a clown, providing social entertainment. Thus, culture supports the *latah* attack and elaborates the function of this unique mental condition. A similar situation is observed in Bali, Indonesia, where transient trances or possession states occur during religious ceremonies to fulfill a social function.

In the United States, it is observed that, at present, many people are very concerned with body weight in relation to health. Many methods of diet control and instruments for physical exercise have been developed. In addition to health-related concerns, the culture-shaped body image belief that "slim is beautiful" is certainly at the root of body weight anxiety.

Regarding previously mentioned *taijinkuofusho* — culture-related unique "social phobia" — its clinical picture is not only shaped by culture through pathoplastic effect, its existence is also very much elaborated by the culture. Clinically, descriptions of its symptoms are elaborated greatly by both patients and professionals and it is commonly spoken of by laymen in everyday language. Patients tend to manifest a particular set of symptoms in a stereotypical way that is very familiar to clinicians and easy to diagnose (Tseng, Asai, Kitanish, McLaughlin, & Kyomen, 1992). Special clinics have been set up and special

treatment approaches, such as Morita therapy, have been developed. Thus, this disorder is not only the product of a situationally oriented society that is very concerned with how others view your behavior — forming a culturally shaped, unique social phobic syndrome (Kasahara, 1974; Kimura, 1983), there is also cultural elaboration of the disorder [cross-reference to Chapter 13: Culture-Related Specific Syndromes (Section II, C, 1)].

E. PATHOFACILITATIVE EFFECTS

These imply that although cultural factors do not change the manifestation of the psychopathology too much, i.e., the clinical picture can still be recognized and categorized without difficulty in the existing classification system, cultural factors do contribute to the frequent occurrence of certain mental disorders in a society. In other words, the disorder potentially exists and is recognized globally, yet due to cultural factors, it becomes prevalent in certain cultures at particular times. Thus, it "facilitates" effects, making it easier for certain psychopathologies to develop and influencing their frequency.

It needs to be pointed out that there are many factors related to prevalence other than biology. The acceptance of a disorder by the society, the availability of support, and the existing care system all impact the prevalence of the disorder. Schizophrenia, a major psychiatric disorder, is predominantly determined by biological factors and its incidence rate tends to have a narrow range of variation among different societies (Lin, 1953). In contrast, many psychiatric disorders that are tied intimately to psychological and sociocultural variables in their development tend to have a wider range of variation of prevalence. Suicidal behavior (Kok & Tseng, 1992), alcoholism (Day, 1995), and substance abuse (Anthony & Helzer, 1995) are examples of disorders whose frequency varies among different societies and whose occurrence is influenced significantly by sociocultural context.

It is considered that general life patterns and attitudes toward certain issues may facilitate the occurrence of certain psychopathology, which may have its own biophysiological or other (still unknown) primary etiological factor, but is provoked more frequently by the secondary catalytic effect of a particular social milieu or cultural attitude. The excessive concern with body weight and the perception of slimness as beauty may facilitate the occurrence of excessive dieting and even a pathological eating disorder; a liberal attitude toward weapons control may result in more weapon-related violence or homicidal behavior (Westermeyer, 1973); and cultural permission to consume alcohol freely may increase the prevalence of drinking problems.

In extreme situations, the social and cultural environment will determine the occurrence of epidemic mental disorders. They may occur in certain cultural environments, but may be extremely rare in others. Mass hysteria, particularly involving youngsters, collective panic, or group-shared delusions are some of the epidemic mental disorders that are attributed to social and cultural factors (cross-reference to Chapter 15: Epidemic Mental Disorders).

From a social psychiatric point of view — mainly derived from the findings obtained from epidemiology — numerous hypotheses have been proposed to explain why certain disorders tend to occur in certain societies or subgroups of society. Theories of cultural disintegration, social disorganization, or social drift are some examples and will be elaborated in detail later (see Section III, B).

It should be cautioned that the high prevalence of a certain psychiatric disorder in a society does not necessarily mean that it is influenced directly by social or cultural factors. Culture may have no "direct" and "causative" contribution to the frequent occurence at all. However, culture may contribute to the increased prevalence of certain disorders in "indirect" ways. For instance, in Belau, Micronesia, an island country with a population of 20,000 or so, the high prevalence of schizophrenia, nearly 7.6 cases per 1000 adults (Dale, 1981), is considered the result of the cultural encouragement of intramarriage, in addition to the limitations of living in an isolated island society. The intramarriage (or endogamy) among the people leads to the transmitting and accumulating of the genes that lead to this mental disorder. In other words, the lifestyle enhances the transmission of the genes that cause the development of predominantly biologically determined mental disorders. However, culture is not a direct or etiological cause of the prevalent occurrence of schizophrenia.

F. Pathoreactive Effects

These effects indicate that although cultural factors do not affect the manifestation or frequency of the mental disorder directly, they influence people's beliefs and understanding of the disorder and mold their "reaction" toward it. Culture influences how people label a disorder, how they react to it emotionally, and then guides them in expressing their suffering. Consequently, the clinical picture of the mental disorder is colored by the cultural reaction — at a secondary level — to the extent that the total process of the illness varies.

Studies indicate that the prognosis of schizophrenia may vary in different societies. It tends to have a poor prognosis in highly developed, industrialized, urban societies, but better outcomes in less developed, rural, farming societies. It is considered that the social environment, particularly family and community attitudes toward the patient, determines how well the person suffering from a schizophrenic disorder will rehabilitate into social and family life, thus affecting the prognosis of the disorder.

Posttraumatic stress disorder associated with war is another example. How the society perceives the disorder and reacts to the emotional sequel — with a sympathetic attitude, many social welfare benefits, or none — will influence how many people will claim to have such a disorder and how they will describe the severity of their suffering.

It is generally observed that the frequency of certain disorders, such as conversion and dissociation disorder, is gradually decreasing. It is speculated that laypeople's understanding of and attitude toward such disorders will change their prevalence significantly.

III. CULTURAL IMPACT ON DIFFERENT GROUPS OF PSYCHOPATHOLOGY

We have clarified how culture contributes to psychopathology in different ways. Next, it is important to recognize the different nature of cultural impact, depending on the different groups of disorders or the nature of psychopathology. Generally speaking, psychopathology that is predominantly determined by biological factors is less influenced by cultural factors and any such influence is secondary or peripheral. In contrast, psychopathology that is determined predominantly by psychological factors is attributed more to cultural factors. This basic distinction is necessary in discussing different levels of cultural impact on various types of psychopathology. Let us try to elaborate on this, according to different groups of psychopathology, as follows.

A. ORGANIC MENTAL DISORDERS

By definition, organic mental disorders are caused by organic etiological factors. Thus, culture does not have a "direct" causal effect on these disorders. However, cultural factors, such as a unique lifestyle collectively shared by a group of people, may contribute "indirectly" to the occurrence, or influence the prevalence, of certain organic mental disorders.

A good example is the degenerative disease of the nervous system called *kuru* among the Fore tribespeople of New Guinea. About 1% of the population, mainly women, die annually from this fatal disease. The Fore people maintain *kuru* is caused by sorcery. However, study has shown that *kuru* is a disease caused by a virus that attacks the central nervous system after a long incubation period. The Fore people have a custom of eating human brains, which contain a virus that causes the disease. It is most interesting to note, as pointed out by Keesing (1976), that it was the custom for Fore women to ritually eat the bodies and brains of their dead relatives. Consequently the disease was transmitted through the females. This illustrates clearly that while culture does not cause this disease of the central nervous system, the culture-rooted habit of eating human brains contributes significantly, though secondarily, to the transmission of the organic mental disorder.

Another example is sexual behavior related to organic mental disorders, such as neurosyphilis, gonoencephalitis, or AIDS-related neuropsychopathy. Culture is not an etiological factor in these organic mental disorders, yet a society's attitude toward sexual behavior, particularly outside of marriage, and its tolerance of promiscuity will certainly affect the sexual behavior of its members. This, in turn, will influence the prevalence of sexually transmitted diseases and resulting mental complications.

Through psychopathoplastic effect, culture may influence the content of organic mental symptoms, such as confabulation. However, its impact is minimal and peripheral, not important enough to change the manifestation of the psychopathology of the disorders.

B. FUNCTIONAL PSYCHOSES

In the past, clinicians and scholars were interested in investigating possible differences in the prevalence of functional psychoses among people of different ethnic, racial, or cultural backgrounds. However, cross-cultural epidemiological findings tend to indicate that the range of differences is not very great, supporting the notion that functional psychoses are not affected predominantly by psychology and culture as etiological factors.

In general, it is considered that, at most, culture may contribute psychopathoplastic effects to the psychopathology of functional psychoses, shaping the content of psychotic symptoms, particularly delusional thoughts or disorganized thought content. In the early stages of exploration, Marvin K. Opler (1959) compared the symptomatology of Italian and Irish male schizophrenic patients hospitalized in New York City. As mentioned earlier, there were several significant variables between Irish and Italian patients. For example, more Italian psychotic patients manifested overt homosexual tendencies, whereas more Irish patients manifested chronic alcoholism and were preoccupied with sin and guilt ideation. However, it should be pointed out that these differences were reflections of ethnic personality differences rather than the schizophrenic disorder itself. That is, they were not at the core of the schizophrenia, but represented secondary symptoms or behavior problems associated with the psychotic condition.

Later, the International Pilot Study of Schizophrenia was carried out by the World Health Organization (WHO) (1973) in nine study centers around the world, with the primary concern of identifying the common symptomatology of the disorder. The average percentage scores were very similar in all the centers. All had high scores on lack of insight, predelusional signs, flatness of affect, auditory hallucinations (except the Washington center), and experiences of control. Although there was no intention to examine cultural aspects of the disorder, coupled with prevalence rates from many other epidemiological studies, the results indirectly inferred that schizophrenia, as a functional psychosis, is less influenced by social or cultural factors in its occurrence and manifestation.

However, the follow-up study carried out by the WHO (Sartorius, Jablensky, & Shapiro, 1978) revealed that the level of social development has a certain relation to the short-term prognosis of schizophrenia; cases in more developed societies have less favorable outcomes. It has been speculated that the family, social, and cultural factors may have psychopathoreactive effects on certain functional psychoses, such as schizophrenia, resulting in different prognoses.

C. SUBSTANCE ABUSE AND DEPENDENCY

Mental disorders associated with substance abuse and/or dependency are basically biophysiological in nature, yet there is room for psychological input in such disorders. Culture has psychopathoselective and psychopathofacilitative effects on the prevalence of abuse. For instance, it is well illustrated that if a society takes a firm attitude toward drinking, such as most societies with Muslim backgrounds, alcohol consumption is very low and problems with alcohol are relatively rare. In contrast, if a society takes a relatively liberal attitude

toward drinking, such as most of Euro-American societies, as well as Korea and Japan in Asia, alcohol consumption is very high and the prevalence of alcohol-related problems tends to be higher. Indulgence in alcohol (as well as other substance) intoxication as a way of dealing with stress becomes a culturally available or favored choice (cross-reference to Chapter 21: Alcohol-Related Problems).

It is generally observed that when there is rapid sociocultural change, particularly associated with cultural uprooting, substance abuse tends to increase sharply, particularly among the youngsters. Numerous examples illustrate that among many culturally deprived minority groups, the problems of substance abuse and dependency among young people are often very prevalent and serious.

It has been shown in the past that through socio–political–cultural measurement, the problem of abuse and dependence can be controlled rather effectively. This is evidenced by the situation in China several decades ago. When mainland China was taken over by the communists, a political campaign was undertaken to eradicate the problem of opium that had troubled China for nearly a century. Backed by political forces, a very firm antiaddiction program was launched to stop the abuse and rehabilitate the addicted. In less than half a decade, China successfully solved the long-standing problem of opium addiction (Shen, 1980; Tseng, 1986). However, recently, when, after reopening its doors to the outside world, the problems of addiction began to recur in the border regions (cross-reference to Chapter 20: Alcohol-Related Problems and Chapter 21: Substance-Related Problems Other than Alcohol).

D. MINOR PSYCHIATRIC DISORDERS AND EPIDEMIC MENTAL DISORDERS

In contrast to major psychiatric disorders, culture has a broader and more direct effect on minor psychiatric disorders at all the levels of genetic, selective, plastic, elaborating, facilitating, and reactive effects.

Among all minor psychiatric disorders, conversion and dissociation disorders are good examples of the rich effects of culture. The prevalence of conversion or dissociation varies greatly among different societies (due to facilitating effects). It is also clear that in some societies, in contrast to other forms of psychopathology, it is preferable to deal with stress (selective effects) by repressing or dissociating the painful emotion. Although some theories have been proposed to explain why certain cultural traits or certain child-rearing patterns favor the occurrence of conversion or dissociation (genetic effects), there is not yet any solid data to support such speculation. However, it is obvious that different societies have different reactions to the phenomena of conversion or dissociation (reactive effects), which, in turn, may facilitate the occurrence of such psychopathology. These points will be elaborated further when each disorder is examined in the following chapters, respectively (cross-reference to Chapters 15, 16, and 17).

It needs to be pointed out that when minor psychiatric disorders occur in an epidemic or collective manner, such as mass hysteria, it becomes clearer that social and cultural factors play a significant role in the occurrence of these rather unique mental pathologies. Psychopathogenic, selective, plastic, and facilitating effects are all significantly involved (cross-reference to Chapter 14: Epidemic Mental Disorders).

E. Culture-Related Specific Syndromes

By definition, the development of culture-related specific syndromes is influenced heavily by cultural factors. In most cases, the psychopathogenic, selective, plastic, elaborating, facilitating, and reactive effects of culture all work together to some extent to contribute to the occurrence of such specific syndromes. Among them, psychopathogenic effects are characteristically at work in some disorders. That is, cultural beliefs or attitudes have direct and etiological effects on the development of psychopathology. This is particularly true in the case of *koro, malgri, daht* syndromes and many others. Cultural input is so significant that culture-related specific syndromes are

often unevenly distributed, concentrated in certain cultural regions that offer the cultural conditions for forming them. This illustrates psychopathoselective and facilitating effects in their extreme.

In the past, it has been believed by some scholars that culture-related specific syndromes are "bound" to particular ethnic groups or cultural units. Thus, they were called "culture-bound syndromes." Recently, this view has changed. Based on cross-cultural literature and findings, scholars have come to realize that such syndromes may be closely related to certain cultural features, but not necessarily "bound" to any particular ethnic group or "cultural entity." The syndromes may occur across the boundaries of ethnicity, society, or cultural units, as long as they have common cultural "traits," "elements," or "themes" that contribute directly to the formation of such pathologies (cross-reference to Chapter 13: Culture-Related Specific Syndromes).

In summary, there are different kinds and levels of cultural impact on various groups of psychopathology, ranging from organic mental disorders, functional psychoses, substance abuse and dependency, and minor psychiatric disorders to culture-related specific syndromes. It is fair to say that, overall, culture has a moderate, but not unlimited, impact on psychopathology (Draguns, 1980), depending on the cultural group involved and the nature of the culture influence.

IV. FURTHER ELABORATION OF SOME CONCEPTUAL ISSUES

The following issues still await further elaboration and final integration.

A. Relationship between Culture and the Nature of Psychopathology

The possible relationship between culture and the nature of psychopathology has been studied by behavior scientists. Draguns (1980) has listed various speculations that have been made in the past. Following are some examples.

1. Possible Relation between Normal and Abnormal Behavior

From a sociocultural standpoint, there are basically three possible relationships between normal and abnormal behavior observed in a culture: (a) abnormal behavior represents an exaggeration of the typical adaptive behavior of its given milieu; (b) abnormal behavior stands in contrast to the culture and is manifested as social negativism; and (c) abnormal behavior varies across cultures, but in a manner independent of variations in normal behavior.

2. Possible Cultural Implications and Functions of Abnormal Behavior

What, if any, are the implications for becoming insane or certain functions for behaving abnormally? From a cultural perspective, several possibilities are hypothesized (Draguns, 1980): (a) abnormal behavior may express the themes, concerns, wishes, and illusions of the time and place; (b) the symptomatology of psychiatric patients may express the implicit philosophy of the culture at a specific time; and (c) abnormal behavior may act out the myths of the culture.

3. Abnormal Behavior as an Indicator of Unresolved Social Problems

In this view, various measures of psychological disturbance may serve as social indicators of the culture in which they occur. Suicide rates, prevalence of substance abuse, frequency of violent or criminal behavior, or child abuse rates are examples of measures that are used to reflect the level of mental health in a society.

From a clinician's point of view, there are some inherent problems in the just-mentioned speculations regarding "abnormal behavior." First, all mental disorders are included in the broad term "abnormal behavior," without distinguishing among various kinds of psychopathology. They are treated as if they are a single unit with the same nature. Further, in this view, all psychopathologies are "functional" in nature. Biologically and psychologically based "disease entities" are not recognized and the position is taken that all psychopathologies are merely "quantitative" deviations from normal behavior, without a "quality" difference from a normal mental condition.

Once presented and clarified, the just-described speculations can be considered for discussion, as long as they are specified for "certain" psychopathologies — mostly those that are functional in nature or predominantly psychologically determined minor psychiatric disorders, including mild abnormal behavior disturbances.

B. SOCIAL CONTRIBUTIONS TO THE OCCURRENCE OF PSYCHOPATHOLOGY

Mainly from a social psychiatric perspective several hypotheses have been proposed in the past to explain some epidemiological findings, i.e., why psychopathology is more prevalent in some societies than in others. Following are some theories offered by pioneers in the field.

1. The Social Disorganization Hypothesis

Faris and Dunham (1939) observed that the majority of psychiatric patients admitted to a mental hospital near Chicago came mainly from inner city areas. Based on this observation, they speculated that extreme social disorganization, characterized by poverty, communication breakdown, high mobility and transiency, racial conflict, social isolation, or other unfavorable social conditions, may contribute to high rates of psychopathology, particularly schizophrenia.

Alexander Leighton (1959) developed a psychosocial theory trying to link psychopathology to "social disintegration." He proposed that human beings are striving toward an essential condition to meet the basic needs of physical security, sexual satisfaction, affection, and so forth. However, if the society disintegrates or if there is a breakdown in its capacity to function as an adaptive resource for the essential conditions for living, psychopathology will increase.

Many social reasons can contribute to the occurrence of disintegration. Rapid social–cultural change occurring within a society, social disasters associated with revolution or wars, invasion by outsiders, transcultural migration of refugees, sociopolitically deprived minorities, or socioculturally uprooted aboriginals are some examples. Poverty, secularization, cultural confusion, fractured social relationships, inadequacies in leadership, increase of substance abuse, and failure to control crime and delinquency are among the criteria used to indicate social disorganization or disintegration.

Generally speaking, among all psychiatric disorders and abnormal behavior, minor psychiatric disorders, such as anxiety or depressive disorder, as well as drinking problems and other substance abuse, criminal behavior problems are more prone to social disintegration. More biologically attributed severe mental disorders, such as schizophrenia, are less influenced by sociocultural change (Lin, Rin, Yeh, Hsu, & Chu 1969).

2. The Social Drift Hypothesis

The social disorganization hypothesis was questioned by many scholars, who pointed out that it was *not* undesirable social conditions that contributed to major mental disorders, but that severe mental patients, who have difficulty surviving in ordinary communities, tended to *drift* and live in poor and disorganized community settings (Clausen & Kohn, 1959; Meyerson, 1941).

In order to test this idea, British researchers Goldberg and Morrison (1963) carried out a generational study to compare the social class backgrounds of schizophrenic patients and their fathers. A documentary survey of a national sample of males aged 25–34, on their first admission to mental hospitals in England and Wales for schizophrenia, showed a usual excess of patients in social class V (with class I as the most desirable, class V as least desirable, from the standpoint of economics, educational, occupation, or other social indexes). However, the social class distribution of their fathers at the time of the patients' births was

very similar to that of the community population as a whole. A clinical study confirmed these findings. It pointed out that there was an apparent decline in occupational status both from father to son and in the patient's own history. The discrepancies in social performance between father and son were mainly attributed to the disease process. That is, due to disability associated with disease, the patients drifted into less desirable social settings. This theory only applies to severe disabling psychotic conditions, such as schizophrenia, as affective disorders were found to be relatively more prevalent in upper social classes.

3. Social Attraction Hypothesis

Instead of viewing mental patients as drifting into undesirable social settings, Robert Hare (1956) speculated that certain kinds of patients, associated with the nature of the psychopathology from which they are suffering, were attracted to so-called "undesirable" social environments. His theory was based on an epidemiological study he carried out in Bristol, United Kingdom. Hare pointed out that the inner city of Bristol contained both rich and poor people. However, despite this, Hare found that there were areas where schizophrenic patients congregated. This phenomenon led him to hypothesize that the social disorganization of some inner city areas can attract (schizophrenic) individuals who find social contact aversive.

4. Social Cohesion as Protection Theory

As opposed to social disintegration, social cohesion was considered a significant protective factor for patients suffering from mental disturbances. Chance (1964) conducted a cross-cultural survey to assess the degree of social cohesion observed in various societies, with correlations to the frequency of depression. He reported that there was a significant correlation between social cohesion and depression, namely severe feelings of worthlessness and guilt tended to occur among members of highly cohesive groups.

One issue that needs to be commented on and clarified is that even though certain social conditions may contribute to a higher prevalence of mental disorders, this does not mean that certain social conditions "etiologically" cause mental disorders, they only facilitate or make certain groups of people more vulnerable to psychopathology. In other words, they may increase a person's susceptibility or vulnerability, but not as etiology. An analogy is found in medical disease. That is, poor social hygiene will make people susceptible to pulmonary tuberculosis or hepatitis, but these diseases are not "caused" etiologically by social conditions, they are caused by tuberculosis bacteria or hepatitis virus. This is a conceptual matter that needs to be clarified. Otherwise, it may lead some people to take a "sociogenic" view of mental disorders and "socialize" psychiatric diseases, claiming that emotional disturbances are nothing but the products of society.

Many people who live in so-called "undesirable" social conditions — perceived and defined by outsiders as poverty, low living standards, or social disintegration — will not necessarily develop psychopathologies. Furthermore, "undesirability" is a relative and subjective matter. It is not necessarily "pernicious" to the inhabitants. For some, it is a challenge and an acceptable living situation. An analogy is the saying that "Richness does not guarantee happiness; poverty does not necessarily make you feel miserable."

Another point is that there are numerous kinds of mental disorders that need to be distinguished in discussing contributions to their occurrence. There is a great difference between major psychiatric disorders and minor psychiatric disorders. From the perspective of psychopathology, suicidal behavior is considerably different from substance abuse or personality disorders. There are even different kinds of depression, those that are predominantly endogenous and others that are reactive. Some suicidal behavior is associated with complications of severe endogenous depression, whereas some behavior is a hysterical reactive attempt at self-killing without a clinical depressive picture. Therefore, there is a need to differentiate when discussing social contributions to psychopathology.

C. The Spectrum of Psychopathology and Different Natures of Cultural Impact

From the discussion just given, it is obviously a mistake to consider all psychopathologies together simply as "mental disorders" without distinguishing among various groups. From a cultural perspective, it is useful to consider the existence of a spectrum of psychopathology. At one end is severe pathology (customarily referred to as a major psychiatric disorder), determined predominantly by biological causal factors, only indirectly related to culture, and characterized by disability. At the other end, the pathology is less severe, without gross reality distortion (thus, it is labeled a minor psychiatric disorder). It is determined predominantly by psychological causal factors, is characterized by suffering from distress, and tends to be closely related to culture. This is a hypothetical conceptual spectrum, placing different groups of psychopathology between two extreme poles. From a cultural point of view, it helps to clarify the different roles culture plays in different groups of psychopathology.

This view is illustrated in Fig. 11-1. Figure 11-1 shows the various ways culture impacts psychopathology, namely in a genetic, selective, plastic, elaborating, facilitating, or reactive way, and identifies different degrees of involvement in various groups of psychopathology within this conceptual spectrum — from predominantly biologically determined to predominantly psychologically determined to predominantly socioculturally determined mental disorders.

It can be said that there is a range of universally uniform psychopathologies versus culture-elaborated specific psychopathologies. The degree of cultural input varies between the extremes of distantly culture-related to closely culture-related psychopathology. These integrated conceptual views will assist in elaborating the subject of "culture and psychopathology" without confusion or ambiguity.

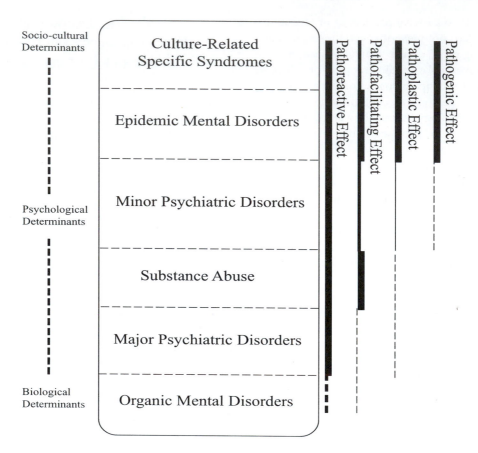

FIGURE 11-1   **Spectrum of psychopathology: Different natures of determinants and their cultural impact.**

D. CLUSTERS OF PSYCHOPATHOLOGY RELATING TO UNDERLYING COMMON CULTURAL THEMES

Another issue that has seldom been discussed by scholars or clinicians is the existence of a group of psychopathologies that can be tied together as a cluster through the common underlying cultural theme that contributes to its formation. A careful examination of various psychopathologies that exist in a single society, particularly folk-labeled disorders, will reveal that they are actually related as a cluster of sicknesses,

manifesting basically similar culture-related problems. Although they may manifest different levels of severity and different forms of psychopathology, they belong to the same cluster of disorders. Following are some examples.

In China, closely associated with the traditional medical concepts of yin and yang and the balance and conservation of energy, there is a group of disorders known by the folk terms: *nao-shenjing shuairuo, shenkui, pa leng,* and *suoyang* (Wen, 1995). The so-called *nao-shenjing shuairuo* literally means "brain-nerve weakness (or exhaustion)" and refers to a condition of poor concentration, poor memory, dizziness, blurring of vision, inability to study, and insomnia — a frequent complaint of students, office clerks, or intellectuals who are involved in intense mental work. It is often attributed by laymen to overwork or overstudy, resulting in exhaustion of the brain. According to herb doctors, it is associated with excessive masturbation, which exhausts yang energy in the brain.

Closely associated with this is *shenkui,* which literally means "weak kidney," referring to "kidney vitality insufficiency syndrome." According to traditional medical concepts, the kidney, as one of the five viscera and an "excretory and sexual" organ, stores and excretes semen (essence of vitality), which represents the *yang* element. An excessive excretion of semen exhausts the kidney and causes excessive loss of the *yang* force. Many people, particularly young people, are led to believe this concept and complain of clouded urine, back pain, and weak legs, in addition to dizziness, poor memory, and poor concentration. Sexual abstinence and a supply of tonic are often prescribed as remedies for this morbid loss of semen.

Another folk-conceptualized disorder, *pa leng,* literally means "fear of cold" and is labeled "frigophobia" by modern psychiatrists. The patient becomes excessively sensitive toward coldness or a fear of catching cold. "Cold" is tied to the cold–hot concept of the yin-yang theory. Catching cold is interpreted as an overintake of the yin element, which is not good for a vital organism. As a result, the patient wears excessive clothing, even in a hot climate. Many measures are taken to prevent the intrusion of cold, such as wearing a belt around the abdomen, closing windows, wearing a heavy coat, or covering the body with a quilt, even though it is summertime. Clinically, this is a rather rare condition, but it is still found occasionally (Chang, Rin, & Chen, 1975).

Suoyang (shrinkage of the yang organ), the Chinese term for *koro,* was mentioned earlier. It is derived from the folk belief that shrinkage of the penis into the abdomen, a sign of excessive shortage of the *yang* element, or overflooding of the yin, can be fatal. Thus, severe anxiety or panic develops if the patient believes that his penis or another protruding organ (such as the nose or ear) is shrinking excessively. This is considered an extreme state of yin-yang imbalance due to excessive loss of semen.

Thus, clusters of psychopathologies involving the kidneys, sexual organs, and the brain are categorized and labeled according to underlying traditional medical concepts and beliefs. Even though they have different degrees of severity and different clinical manifestations, they form a cluster of pathologies centered around the themes of losing vitality and the imbalance of *yin-yang* forces. From another perspective, it may be said that according to basic health–sick concepts, many different forms of illness are elaborated and differentiated through the pathoelaborating effects of culture, as discussed previously.

Another example derives from Iran. Medical anthropologist Good (1977) described a folk illness called *narahatye qalb* (heart distress). It is a common illness among women, particularly those from the lower social classes. According to classic humoral theory, the backbone of traditional Galenic–Islamic medicine, the illness arises from an excess or deficiency of the humors, or the basic qualities. The heart is perceived as an organ of emotional functioning or the seat of the vital soul, providing "innate heat" and "vital breath" to the body. Consequently, malfunctioning of the heart provides the cultural framework for focusing the attention of individuals on the heartbeat, establishing causal links between irregularities in heartbeat and specified personal and social conditions. According to Good (1977, p. 32), the heart distress ranges along a clinical continuum from mild excitation to chronic sensations of heart irregularities to fainting and heart attack. Thus, a cluster of emotional disorders is linked by the distress of the "heart" organ. Furthermore, when the possible causes of the heart distress were surveyed, Good found that there was a long list of answers offered by the layperson, which included feelings of sadness and anxiety; situational difficulties relating to death, debts, poverty, quarrels, and family illness; problems associated with old age, pregnancy, delivery, and miscarriage or use of contraceptives; or somatic reasons of lack of blood, low blood pressure, too few vitamins, nerve problems, and so on. Through statistical analysis, the two most important fields of symbols and experiences that emerge are "the problematic of female sexuality" and "the oppression of daily life" — two of the most common psychological problems encountered by females in that culture.

The existence of a culture-related cluster of psychopathologies is not necessarily observed in every society. It can be discovered only in a society where there are prominent medically related cultural themes that profoundly affect the thoughts of the people, even in the area of psychopathology. Without such traditional medical beliefs, the phenomenon of clustered psychopathologies would not be found and elaborated.

E. The Evolution and Vicissitudes of Certain Psychopathologies

From the perspective of medical history and cross-cultural study, it is noted that certain mental disorders that were prevalent in the past are becoming less frequent among European–American societies. Perhaps one of the best examples is women's fainting behavior, commonly observed among Western women in the last century. It was even shown in the famous movie *Gone with the Wind* several decades ago. This culturally patterned and expected emotional reaction of women toward stress has disappeared almost completely from contemporary Western society.

Beyond such minor abnormal behavior observed in daily life, several clinical conditions are observed as well. Among major psychiatric disorders, the catatonic or hebephrenic (or disorganized) subtype of schizophrenia is becoming less frequent than it was only a half-century ago. Modern Western psychiatrists almost never witness cataleptic signs. Among various minor psychiatric disorders, conversion and dissociation are now observed only rarely in Western clinical settings. However, they are still observed in some underdeveloped non-Western societies. It is speculated that, associated with modernization, socioeconomical development, and knowledge of mental health, certain groups of psychopathologies will grad-

ually change. Instead of self-induced dissociation, substance-induced dissociation has become popular in many developed societies. Instead of conversion, repressing pain and conflict, as interpreted analytically, depression has become prevalent, a condition that results from feeling helpless in dealing with pain and frustration.

The vicissitudes of certain psychopathologies call for an explanation. Do they indicate that psychopathology is changing in association with the evolution of the human mind or can they be interpreted merely from social and cultural perspectives? These are scientific questions waiting for answers. It is tempting to offer explanations from a cultural perspective. However, caution is necessary not to "socialize" or "culturalize" mental disorders. There are still many unknown factors that contribute to and regulate the vicissitudes of psychopathology.

REFERENCES

Anthony, J.C., & Helzer, J.E. (1995). Epidemiology of drug dependence. In M.T. Tsuang, M. Tohen, & G.E.P. Zahner (Eds.), *Textbook in psychiatric epidemiology* (pp. 361–406). New York: Wiley-Liss.

Berrios, G.E. (1994). The history of descriptive psychopathology. In J.E. Mezzich, M.R. Jorge, & I.M. Salloum (Eds.), *Psychiatric epidemiology: Assessment concepts and method.* Baltimore: Johns Hopkins University Press.

Berry, J.W., Poortinga, Y.H., Segall, M.H., & Dasen, P.R. (1992). *Cross-cultural psychology: Research and applications.* Cambridge, UK: Cambridge University Press.

Cawte, J.E. (1976). *Malgri:* A culture-bound syndrome. In W.P. Lebra (Ed.), *Culture-bound syndromes, ethnopsychiatry, and alternate therapies* (pp. 22–31). Honolulu: University Press of Hawaii.

Chance, N. (1964). A cross-cultural study of social cohesion and depression. *Transcultural Psychiatric Research Review, 1,* 19–24.

Chang, Y.H., Rin, H., & Chen, C.C. (1975). Frigophobia: A report of five cases. *Bulletin of the Chinese Society of Neurology and Psychiatry, 1*(2), 9–13 (in Chinese).

Clausen, J.A., & Kohn, M.L. (1959). Relations of schizophrenia to the social structure of a small city. In B. Pasamanick (Ed.), *Epidemiology of mental disorders.* Washington, DC: American Association for the Advancement of Science.

Dale, P. (1981). Prevalence of schizophrenia in the Pacific island population of Micronesia. *Psychiatric Research, 16,* 103–111.

Day, N.L. (1995). Epidemiology of alcohol use, abuse, and dependence. In M.T. Tsuang, M. Tohen, & G.E.P. Zahner (Eds.), *Textbook in psychiatric epidemiology* (pp. 345–360). New York: Wiley-Liss.

Draguns, J.G. (1980). Psychological disorders of clinical severity. In H.C. Triandis & J.G. Draguns (Eds.), *Handbook of cross-cultural psychology: Psychopathology* (pp. 99–174). (Vol. 6). Boston: Allyn & Bacon.

Eastwell, D. (1982). Voodoo death and the mechanism for dispatch of the dying in East Arnhem, Australia. *American Anthropologist, 84,* 5–18. (Reviewed by E.A. Gomez in *Transcultural Psychiatry Research Review, 21*(1), 66–67 [1984])

Faris, R., & Dunham, H. (1939). *Mental disease in the Chicago area.* Chicago: University of Chicago Press.

Fundia, T., Draguns, J., & Phillips, L. (1971). Culture and psychiatric symptomatology: A comparison of Argentine and United States patients. *Social Psychiatry, 6,* 11–20.

Goldberg, E.M., & Morrison, S.L. (1963). Schizophrenia and social class. *British Journal of Psychiatry, 109,* 785–802.

Good, B.J. (1977). The heart of what's the matter: The semantics of illness in Iran. *Culture, Medicine and Psychiatry, 1*(1), 25–58.

Hare, R. (1956). Mental illness and social condition in Bristol. *Journal of Mental Science, 102,* 349–357.

Jilek, W.G. (1995). Emil Kraepellin and comparative sociocultural psychiatry. *European Archives of Psychiatry and Clinical Neuroscience, 245,* 231–238.

Kasahara, Y. (1974). Fear of eye-to-eye confrontation among neurotic patients in Japan. In T.S. Lebra & P.L. Lebra (Eds.), *Japanese culture and bahavior* (pp. 396–406). Honolulu: University Press of Hawaii.

Keesing, R.M. (1976). *Cultural anthropology: A contemporary perspective* (p. 219). New York: Holt, Rinehar & Winston.

Kimura, S. (1983). *Nihonjin no taijinkyofushio [Japapanese anthrophobia].* Tokyo: Keso Shobo.

Kok, L.P., & Tseng, W.S. (Eds.). (1992). *Suicidal behavior in the Asia-Pacific region.* Singapore: Singapore University.

Lee, S., Ho, T.P., and Hsu, L.K.G. (1995). Fat phobic and non-fat phobic anorexia nervosa — A comparative study of 70 Chinese patients in Hong Kong. *Psychological Medicine, 23,* 999–1017.

Leighton, A.H. (1959). *My name is Legion. Vol. I of the Stirling County Study.* New York: Basic Books.

Lin, T.-Y. (1953). An epidemiological study of the incidence of mental disorder in Chinese and other cultures. *Psychiatry, 16,* 313–336.

Lin, T.-Y., Rin, H., Yeh, E.K., Hsu, C.C., & Chu, H.M. (1969). Mental disorders in Taiwan, fifteen years later: A preliminary report. In W. Caudil & T.-Y. Lin (Eds.), *Mental health research in Asia and the Pacific.* (pp. 66–91). Honolulu: East-West Center Press.

Marsella, A.J. (1993). Sociocultural foundations of psychopathology: An historical overview of concepts, events and pioneers prior to 1970. *Transcultural Psychiatric Research Review, 30*(2), 97–142.

Meyerson, A. (1941). Review of mental disorders in urban areas. *American Journal of Psychiatry, 96,* 995–997.

Ohara, K. (1963). Characteristics of suicides in Japan, especially of parent-child double suicide. *American Journal of Psychiatry, 120*(4), 382–385.

Opler, M.K. (1959). Cultural differences in mental disorders: An Italian and Irish contrast in schizophrenia—U.S.A. In M.K. Opler (Ed.), *Culture and mental health: Cross-cultural studies* (pp. 425–442). New York: Macmillan.

Prince, R. (1960). The "brain fag" syndrome in Nigerian students. *Journal of Mental Science, 104,* 559–570.

Sartorius, N., Jablensky, A., & Shapiro, R. (1978). Cross-cultural differences in the short-term prognosis of schizophrenic psychoses. *Schizophrenia Bulletin, 4,* 102–113.

Shen, Y.C. (1980). The development of modern psychiatry in our country. In Beijing Medical School (Ed.), *Psychiatry* (pp. 9–12). Beijing: People's Medical Publishing Company (in Chinese).

Simons, R.C. (1996). *Boo!—Culture, experience, and the startle reflex.* New York: Oxford University Press.

Tanaka-Matsumi, J., & Draguns, J.G. (1997). Culture and psychopathology. In J.W. Berry, M.H. Segall, & C. Kagitçibasi (Eds.), *Handbook of cross-cultural psychology* (2nd ed., Vol. 3). Boston: Allyn & Bacon.

Tseng, W.S. (1986). Chinese psychiatry: Development and characteristics. In J.L. Cox (Ed.), *Transcultural psychiatry* (pp. 274–290). London: Croom Helm.

Tseng, W.S., Asai, M.H., Kitanish, K.J., McLaughlin, D., & Kyomen, H. (1992). Diagnostic pattern of social phobia: Comparison in Tokyo and Hawaii. *Journal of Nervous and Mental Disease 180,* 380–385.

Tseng, W.S., Mo, K.M., Hsu, J., Li, L.S., Ou, L.W., Chen, G.Q., & Jiang, D.W. (1988). A sociocultural study of koro epidemics in Guandong, China. *American Journal of Psychiatry, 145*(12), 1538–1543.

Wen, J.K. (1995). Sexual beliefs and problems in contemporary Taiwan. In T.-Y. Lin, W.S. Tseng, & E.K. Yeh (Eds.), *Chinese societies and mental health* (pp. 219–230). Hong Kong: Oxford University Press.

Westermeyer, J. (1973). On the epidemicy of *amok* violence. *Archives of General Psychiatry, 28,* 873–876.

World Health Organization (WHO). (1973). *The international study of schizophrenia.* Geneva: WHO.

12

Culture and Psychiatric Epidemiology

I. INTRODUCTION

A. THE NATURE OF PSYCHIATRIC EPIDEMIOLOGY

Psychiatric epidemiology, as indicated by its name, is a subfield of psychiatry with a special focus on the frequency of mental disorders. Examining the frequency of mental disorders in certain communities or societies and the social demographic variables of the subjects examined, such as age, gender, educational level, occupation, marital status, socioeconomic status, social class, and ethnic or racial background, will reveal the variables that contribute to the frequency of mental disorders. This will be useful clinical knowledge and community information on which public health policies and measurements can be based. Thus, psychiatric epidemiology is closely related to social psychiatry, community psychiatry, and public health psychiatry. Certain detailed aspects of psychiatric epidemiology, including methodologies and the major findings of investigations, have been elaborated in numerous publications (Lin & Standley, 1962; Mezzich, Jorge & Salloum, 1994; Pasamanick, 1959; Schwab & Schwab, 1978; Tsuang, Tohen, & Zahner

1995). In this chapter, the discussion will focus more on issues relating to the cultural perspectives of psychiatric epidemiology.

In a strict sense, psychiatric epidemiology does not relate closely to cultural psychiatry, even when cross-ethnic, -racial, -societal, or -national comparative epidemiological studies are carried out, unless the epidemiological investigations are conducted in conjunction with an examination of core cultural variables, namely the beliefs, values, and attitudes of the subjects, their families, or others in the community surveyed. Such studies have seldom been done in the past. Nevertheless, if a comparative epidemiological study is carried out among subjects of different ethnic or racial groups, or in different cultural settings, the findings obtained will often be useful. Because they are based on such epidemiological data, certain cultural speculations and further examinations can be made.

B. HISTORY AND EVOLUTION OF METHODS OF INVESTIGATION

The investigation of psychiatric epidemiology started around the beginning of the 20th century. According to Schwab and Schwab (1978), in 1916,

A.J. Rosanoff conducted a community survey of a small district of Nassau County in New York in the United States. Between 1929 and 1933, C. Brugger carried out a survey in a large rural area of Thurningia, Germany; and in 1931, O. Graemiger conducted a study in St. Gallen, Switzerland. In terms of the increased sophistication of survey methods, scholars distinguish three generations of psychiatric epidemiology studies, from the turn of the century to the present (Dohrenwend, 1995).

1. First-Generation Studies

These cover the era between the turn of the 20th century and World War II. Methodologically, they are characterized by the reliance of investigators on key informants in the community and agency records to supply the information needed to identify psychiatric cases. Needless to say, this is a relatively easy and inexpensive way to carry out an investigation. However, from the standpoint of validity, this method tends to ignore untreated cases of disorders as well as minor disorders that are often less recognized by others. Data obtained tend to underreport the actual cases that exist in the community. The pioneer studies carried out in Thuringia, Germany, by Brugger (1931), on Hachijo Island, Japan, by Uchimura and his associates (1940), and in Baltimore, Maryland, by Lemkau, Tietze, and Cooper (1941) are examples of this generation of studies.

2. Second-Generation Studies

This group was mostly conducted from after World War II until the 1980s. Methodologically, targeted subjects in the community were surveyed through direct interviews, even though data from key informants and official records may have been utilized as supplementary information in identifying cases. For case findings, a single psychiatrist or a small team headed by a psychiatrist conducted personal interviews of subjects. In general, clinical judgment was utilized for decisions and the interview procedures were not standardized. The Stirling

County study and the Midtown study carried out by a research team from Cornell University in the 1950s are representative of this generation of studies. Stimulated by cross-cultural interest, there were several epidemiological studies carried out, not in the investigators' own countries but in other societies, particularly underdeveloped or developing ones. The studies of the Serer in Senegal (Beiser, Ravel, Collomb, & Egelhoff, 1972) and the Yoruba in Africa (Leighton et al., 1963) are two examples. Such epidemiological studies in foreign societies by outside investigators have brought about many methodological challenges.

3. Third-Generation Studies

This group of studies occurred after the 1980s. Semistructured diagnostic interviews and rating examinations were developed for field surveys of targeted subjects. Thus, the method of collecting information and the criteria for identifying cases were standardized. This is a rather expensive and time-consuming method of study. There have not been too many investigations of this kind, even though it is a more sophisticated way of gathering valid epidemiological data. The Collaborative Study on the Determinants of Outcome of Severe Mental Disorders (DOS) conducted by the World Health Organization (WHO) and the Epidemiologic Catchment Area (ECA) study conducted by the National Institute of Mental Health in the United States in the 1980s are typical examples of third-generation studies.

C. PROBLEMS INHERENT IN CROSS-CULTURAL COMPARATIVE EPIDEMIOLOGY

When epidemiological data are available from different culture settings, there is always a certain limitation in cross-cultural comparisons. The information obtained needs to be carefully interpreted, as there are often inherent methodological problems, such as the following.

1. Different Methodology of Investigations

One of the most critical problems existing in epidemiological data for cross-cultural comparison is that investigations carried out in different social or cultural settings are often conducted by different investigators using different methods of investigation (or methods of different levels of sophistication) for gathering data, and different ways are used to analyze the collected information. This makes it difficult to make direct cross-comparisons for meaningful interpretations. Unless the collection of data across cultural sites is standardized, the investigators from different centers trained for reliability, and the same transculturally applicable instrument used, such as in WHO collaborative studies, the comparison of obtained data is limited in its validity.

2. Findings Might be Attributed to Many Other Variables

Any findings that illustrate there is a substantial difference in certain kinds of psychopathologies between, or among, subjects of different ethnic, racial, or cultural backgrounds should not be immediately attributed to "ethnic" or "cultural" factors. Many other factors, including biological or social, should first be considered. For instance, on the Micronesian island of Yap, in the middle of the Pacific Ocean between Hawaii and the Philippines, there is an extraordinarily high prevalence of schizophrenia. The rate for persons over age 15 reaches 9.7 per 1000 adult population — the highest ever reported in the world (Dale, 1981). Instead of attributing this to any unique lifestyle or family system of the Yapese people, it is better to consider biological or environmental factors, such as special infectious factors, the contamination of particular foods (fish or rice) that are consumed, or hereditary factors resulting from centuries of endogamy that might have accumulated in the gene pool and contributed to the development of schizophrenia. The latter is one of the most probable explanations that is currently under investigation.

Another example is from the WHO's International Pilot Study of Schizophrenia (IPSS). It was unexpectedly discovered the prognosis of schizophrenia was better in developing societies than in developed societies (World Health Organization [WHO], 1973). Thus, among many social variables, close family and other relationships in the community were speculated to contribute to favorable outcomes for schizophrenic patients in developing societies, particularly in rural settings. This seemed like a reasonable speculation. However, in a subsequent study on DOS carried out by WHO, the investigation of numerous factors, including social and family relations, failed to reveal any that might contribute to a better prognosis for schizophrenic patients in developing societies (Jablensky et al., 1991).

3. Cultural Variables Often Neglected in Investigations

From a cultural perspective, another common problem observed in psychiatric epidemiological studies in the past is that most did not include the study of cultural information. Even when data were compared with data from different cultural settings, in an attempt at "cross-cultural" comparison, most of the investigations focused on social or demographic data, which are not the same as cultural variables. Ethnic or racial background, social class, economic level, and religious background may indirectly reflect the attitudes, beliefs, or values of the subjects, but they are not a direct reflection of the culture. They only allow us to make some inferential interpretations. Unless the subjects' (or their family members') views about mental illness, their interpretations of and attitudes toward mental problems, their patterns for coping, and so on are directly investigated in association with the study of the frequency of the illness, it is impossible to evaluate the possible impact of culture on the illness.

4. The Need for Culturally Sensitive Epidemiological Research

Finally, no matter how sophisticated the methodology, there are still many issues that need to be considered from a cultural perspective in order to perform culturally sensitive and relevant epidemiological studies.

This is true when you are going to conduct a survey with subjects of different ethnic–cultural backgrounds within multiethnic or -racial societies or in foreign settings where people use different languages, live different lifestyles, and are not used to community surveys. As pointed out by Rogler (1994) and Parry (1996), there are several areas that need special consideration and careful management in order to conduct culturally sensitive epidemiological studies. These are areas of language, examination setting (with or without the presence of family members), style of interviewing, the cultural pattern of the subject's reaction toward the interview and questionnaire survey, confidentiality, the choice and revision of the questionnaires to be used, and the analysis and interpretation of data obtained. These issues will be elaborated further in Chapter 48 [Cross-Cultural Research (Sections I, B and II, A)].

II. SOME EPIDEMIOLOGICAL INVESTIGATIONS

A number of psychiatric epidemiological surveys have been conducted in various parts of the world at different times using different generations of methodology. While many were conducted in selected communities within societies, data obtained may be compared indirectly with comparable data from investigations in other societies. Some research was carried out by the same investigators using the same methodology in communities with different social, ethnic, or racial backgrounds to allow direct cross-comparisons. Only rarely did investigations involve longitudinal follow-ups of the same communities after social change had occurred in order to examine the possible effects of social and cultural change. Some of the studies will be reviewed briefly here from the standpoint of historical interest and cross-cultural perspectives.

A. EPIDEMIOLOGICAL STUDIES IN THE EARLY 1950S IN NORTH AMERICA

The two epidemiological investigations outlined in this section were undertaken in the 1950s in north-

eastern America, studying a Western population. They were related projects with similar methodologies, but focused on different social settings and tested slightly different social hypotheses.

1. The Stirling County Study

According to J.M. Murphy and Leighton (1965, pp. vi–viii), the project was directed by Alexander H. Leighton and conducted by the Department of Sociology and Anthropology of Cornell University in 1955. Its primary focus was a rural community population. The site selected was Stirling County in one of the Atlantic provinces of Canada — a fishing, lumbering, and subsistence-farming region inhabited by two main ethnic groups, English and French Acadian. Although interested in the full range of psychiatric disorders, including psychoses, psychoneuroses, behavior disturbances, and mental deficiency, more focus was given to psychoneuroses and psychophysiological disorders among the nonhospitalized population. Questionnaire interviews were employed as one means of case finding. A probability sample of 1010 adults was surveyed to elicit sociocultural information and data on both physical and psychiatric health.

The analysis of sociocultural environment focused on contrasts in cultural background and differences in degree of social "integration and disintegration." It was hypothesized that "social disintegration" affects mental health and mental illness. Social disintegration was considered the result of combined factors of poverty, secularization, cultural confusion, fractured social relationships, and rapid sociocultural change, as well as inadequacies in leadership, recreation, associations, communication, and control of crime and delinquency.

2. The Midtown Study

According to J.M. Murphy and Leighton (1965, pp. vii–viii), this project was originally instituted by Thomas A.C. Rennied. After his death, it was completed under Leighton's directorship. The project was based at the Cornell University Medical College in New York City. Methodologically it was similar to the

Stirling County project, except that it was concerned with an urban setting. A section of Manhatten (Midtown) in New York City was chosen for investigation, and it was, therefore, called the Midtown Study. The area is a complex and heterogeneous society, with several ethnic groups, including Irish, Italian, German-Austrian, Hungarian, Czechoslovakian, Polish, British, Old American, and others. A probability sample of 1660 adults was surveyed. The concept of "socioeconomic status" was employed as a way of quartering the environment in order to uncover sociocultural patterns.

J.M. Murphy and Leighton (1965, p. viii) reported some conclusions that were obtained from the Stirling County and Midtown studies, i.e., the differences in environment encompassed by the terms "urban" and "rural" and the division of Western society into ethnic groups (such as French, English, Irish, and Italian) did not parallel major differences in the prevalence of psychiatric disorders in the two sample populations studied.

B. Studies in the 1950s and 1960s in Asia

Several epidemiological studies were carried out in Japan (Akimoto, 1942; Uchimura et al., 1940) in the early 40s. Stimulated by this, two epidemiological studies were implemented in Taiwan that offered very valuable information concerning the Chinese population.

1. Fifteen-Year Follow-Up Study in Taiwan

Led by Tsung-Yi Lin (1953) from the School of Medicine of the National Taiwan University, the Taiwan project was carried out from 1946 to 1948 in three communities (Baksa, Simpo, and Ampeng). One of the intentions of the study was to compare different subethnic groups and urban/rural differences in the three regions. However, it was found there were no substantial regional differences. Data from the total population were compared with data from previous studies in other countries, including Germany (Brugger, 1931), Denmark (Strömgren, 1938), Sweden (Sjoegren, 1948), and the United States (Lemkau et al., 1941; Roth & Luton, 1943) in the West and Japan (Akimoto, 1942; Uchimura et al., 1940) in the East.

The comparison revealed that, in general, the distribution of the prevalence of various psychiatric disorders among the Chinese in Taiwan was comparable to that of other countries in the West and East. In particular, it was noted that the range of prevalence rates for schizophrenia was rather narrow, from 1.7 to 4.6 per 1000 population, as reported by Roth and Luton (1943) from Tennessee and Sjoegren (1948) from Sweden, respectively. The rest of the rates were somewhere in between: 1.9 reported by Brugger (1931) for Germans, 2.1 by Lin (1953) for the Chinese, 2.1 by Akimoto (1942) for the Japanese, and 2.9 by Lemkau et al. (1941) for Americans in Baltimore. These findings suggest that schizophrenia, as a psychosis predominantly determined by biological factors, did not show a great variation of prevalence among different ethnic or cultural groups.

Fifteen years later, a follow-up study was repeated from 1961 to 1963 by the same research team led by Lin (Lin, Rin, Yeh, Hsu, & Chu, 1969) in the same three communities. Since the initial study, the residents had experienced rapid sociocultural change. When the communists took over the mainland, the national government retreated to Taiwan. There was a massive influx of Chinese mainlanders and intense military tension across the strait. On Taiwan, there was a dramatic change in the political situation and the educational system, followed by rapid industrialization and urbanization. During this period of social upheaval, people experienced subcultural changes as well.

The follow-up study revealed that there was no increase observed in psychotic disorders over the 15-year period, in striking contrast to the significant increase in nonpsychotic disorders, especially psychoneuroses. The prevalence rate of psychoneuroses rose from 1.2 to 7.8 per 1000 population. It seemed that psychotic disorders were less affected by environmental changes than nonpsychotic disorders. This supports the view that some innate genetic or biological factors play a more important role in the etiology of psychotic disorders than in that of neurotic disorders (Lin et al., 1969).

During these 15 years, associated with urbanization, there was considerable internal movement among the original (Taiwanese-Chinese) inhabitants, as well as the migration of mainland Chinese into the area. Dividing the subjects into "original Taiwanese inhabitants," "Taiwanese migrants," and "mainland migrants" for subgroup comparisons, it was found that the rate of psychoneuroses increased with the increased intensity of migration: 6.9, 12.1, and 16.1 per 1000 population for the three subgroups. It was the opposite for mental deficiency. The rates were 5.1, 3.7, and 2.9 for the three groups, indicating that mental deficiency was found more among the original inhabitants and less among the migrants. Perhaps people with low intelligence were screened out in the process of migration.

2. Cross-Comparison between Aboriginal and Han Chinese in Taiwan

The same research team, Rin and Lin (1962), undertook another epidemiological study in Taiwan from 1949 to 1953. This time the subjects were members of the aboriginal population. Prior to the migration of the Chinese (Han nationals) from mainland China, Taiwan (also known by Westerners by its Dutch name, Formosa), around the end of the Ming dynasty in the 17th century, was inhabited by people of Malayo-Polynesian stock who had drifted in from the South Pacific some 10 to 20 centuries before. These aboriginal tribespeople retreated to the rugged mountain areas after the massive influx of Chinese Han nationals. This epidemiological investigation was aimed at the aboriginal population with comparison of data obtained previously from the Chinese (Han national) group (Lin, 1953). Although they were living on the same island, the aborigines had a different racial background than the Chinese, they were a minority group, lived in mountainous areas with less favorable social conditions and hygiene, and relied on hunting and subsistence farming for their survival.

A total of 11,442 subjects were studied. The results of the survey revealed that, in contrast to the Chinese group (which lived mostly in the plains area and was of majority status, with more favorable socio-economic conditions), the aboriginal group had a higher prevalence rate of organic psychoses (1.9% vs 0.7%), epilepsy (3.9% vs 1.3%), and alcoholism (1.1% vs 0.1%), but slightly less of schizophrenia (0.9% vs 2.1%) and psychoneurotic cases (0.8% vs 1.2%). Organic psychoses were caused by malaria.

Although the method of investigation was of the second-generation type, the strength of the study was that it was carried out by the same research team using the same screening methods and diagnostic criteria for case identification. The study revealed that even among groups living on the same island, due to different racial backgrounds and living conditions, the prevalence of mental disorders differed considerably — with mental disorders of an organic nature being more prevalent among the aboriginal group who lived in the mountain areas with less favorable living conditions.

C. Two Unique Studies in the 1960s

Numerous epidemiological studies have been conducted in various parts of the world, including Europe. Two will be mentioned here that shed light on theoretical considerations from a sociocultural perspective.

1. Social Class and Mental Illness Study in New Haven, Connecticut

Concerning the effects of social class on the occurrence and treatment of mental illness, Hollingshead and Redlich (1958) undertook a study of mental patients who were receiving treatment in the greater New Haven area in Connecticut. A stratified random sample of 3559 households was examined. Subjects were defined as "mental patients" who, during a 6-month time period (between May 31 and December 1,

1950), were receiving either outpatient or inpatient psychiatric care from private practitioners, agencies, and hospitals. Social class was determined by the ecological area of residence, occupation, and education and was grouped into five categories: classes I, II, III, IV, and V (I=high, V=low). The results revealed a define inverse relation between social class and being a psychiatric patient. The prevalence rates per 100,000 population were 553, 528, 665, and 1668 for classes I–II, III, IV, and V, respectively, with a much higher prevalence for the lower class V. Further, it was found that in the upper classes I and II, about 35% of the cases were diagnosed psychotic and 65% neurotic. This was in remarkable contrast to class V, in which about 90% were diagnosed psychotic and only 10% neurotic. Almost all class I–II patients with neuroses were treated by private practitioners or in private hospitals, whereas almost all class V patients with neuroses were treated in public clinics, including military, Veterans Administration Hospitals, or state hospitals. The study illustrated clearly that the prevalence of mental disorders, the categories of disorders that led the patients to receive care, and the nature of the service provided differed according to the social class of the patients.

2. Study of the Hutterite Society in the United States

Socioculturally, the Hutterites are a unique group of people living in scattered colonies in remote parts of the Dakotas and Montana in the United States and Alberta and Manitoba in Canada. According to Schwab and Schwab (1978, pp. 188–190) the sect originated in Switzerland in the early 16th century. During the next few centuries, it moved to various locations in central Europe and southern Russia to escape persecution, and finally emigrated to the United States in the latter part of the 19th century. Its members are pacifists and its colonies each contain about 100 persons. They believe in communal ownership of all property and government by consensus. Farming is the only industry and every person is expected to work. The members have similar lifestyles

and clearly defined roles. They have shared the same beliefs and continued the same lifestyle for more than four centuries. They prize the simple life and have a reputation for good mental health.

In order to study how such a unique life pattern might affect mental illness, Eaton and Weil (1955) undertook a community survey. A total of 8542 subjects were studied. The results revealed that, per 1000 population, the rate for psychoses was 6.2; neuroses 8.1; mental deficiency 6.0; epilepsy 2.3; and personality disorders 0.7 Eaton and Weil concluded that despite the good mental health reputation of its members, the Hutterite way of life provided no immunity from severe psychiatric disorders. Furthermore, they indicated that the Hutterites's social structure and way of life was associated with particular forms of psychopathology: guilt feelings among those who feared they might not live up to group expectations and a high frequency of depression, mostly on a neurotic level.

Eaton and Weil did not conduct thorough genealogical studies. However, as pointed out by Schwab and Schwab (1978), because the Hutterite society is endogamous, the significance of genetic factors would appear to be great. Furthermore, only those with certain personality traits — high-principled, rigid, restrictive persons who internalize their emotions — can adhere to its pacifistic doctrines and restrictive way of life. Thus, as Schwab and Schwab commented, the genetic and cultural factors conjoined to produce a homogeneous cultural group in which certain personality traits were common and a significant number of persons were afflicted with (hereditary) mental disorders, even though the society was relatively stress free.

D. WHOs International Multicenter Studies since the 1970s

1. International Pilot Study of Schizophrenia

In the 1960s, the World Health Organization carried out a well-planned systematic study of schizophrenia, involving nine study centers around the world: Aarhus (Denmark), Agra (India), Cali (Colombia), Ibadan (Nigeria), London (UK), Moscow (USSR), Prague (Chechoslovakia), Taipei (Taiwan, China), and Washington (USA). It was the first formal comparative study involving multiple cultural sites using standardized methods for the collection of data. The project, led by T.Y. Lin (then Who's director of mental health) and his associate, N. Sartorius, was implemented in 1965 and completed in 1971. Its primary mission was to investigate the clinical manifestation of schizophrenia across different cultures. The results were reported in 1973 (WHO, 1973).

Methodologically, at least 125 patients were identified for the study at each site, according to the operational inclusion criteria of schizophrenia. The instrument of Present State Examination (PSE) was used to assess the mental status of the patients. The instrument was translated carefully into different languages for use in each site. The interviewers from each field study center were trained in interview procedures and the collection of clinical information to assure interrater reliability.

The results revealed that the average percentage scores were very similar across all the centers. All had high scores on lack of insight, predelusional signs, flatness of affect, auditory hallucinations (except the Washington center), and experiences of control. This landmark study not only proved that it is possible to carry out cross-cultural studies of functional psychosis in multiple societies through carefully designed methodology, it also validated schizophrenia as a functional psychosis that manifests basically similar clinical pictures (or symptoms) among patients from different societies with diverse cultural backgrounds.

2. Collaborative Study on the Determinants of Outcomes of Severe Mental Disorders

A 2 year follow-up study was conducted as the second phase of the IPSS. It was unexpectedly found that the prognosis of the schizophrenic patients differed among societies with different levels of socioeconomical development. More favorable prognoses were indicated in developing than in developed societies. A few years later, stimulated by this finding and supported by the National Institute of Mental Health in the United States, the World Health Organization launched another study, the Collaborative Study on the Determinants of Outcomes of Severe Mental Disorders.

Twelve study sites in 10 countries were involved: Asrhus (Denmark), Agra and Chandigarh (India), Cali (Columbia), Dublin (Ireland), Honolulu and Rochester (USA), Ibadan (Nigeria), Moscow (USSR), Nagasaki (Japan), Nottingham (UK), and Prague (Czechoslovakia). Six of these centers had taken part in the original IPSS. The DOS was based on the IPSS in its methodological approach. The goal of the study was to investigate not only the prognosis of severe mental disorders (the primary concern was schizophrenia), but also the incidence of the disorders. Therefore, methodologically, all individuals from a defined catchment making a first contact with a specified psychiatric, medical, or other agency due to symptoms of a possible schizophrenic illness were identified, assessed, and followed up for 2 years.

The study provided several findings (Jablensky et al., 1991). Using a broad definition of schizophrenia (according to CATEGO S), the incident rates of schizophrenia were found to be significantly different among the centers investigated. Nevertheless, the rates ranged only from 1.5 to 4.2 per 10,000 population aged 15–54. If a strict definition of schizophrenia was used (according to CATEGO class S+), the incidence rates would not differ among the centers, with a range from 0.7 to 1.4 per 10,000 population aged 15–54.

Regarding prognosis, the study confirmed the previous finding that the outcomes for schizophrenic patients were better in developing societies. In this study, much more social and family information was collected than in the IPSS, but, even so, no fundamentally different findings emerged to clarify the kinds of factors that contributed to a favorable prognosis.

3. Depressive Disorders in Different Cultures

Although depressive disorders occur in all parts of the world and depressive patients constitute a significant proportion of all people who need mental health care, a lack of a common language among investigators and clinicians who deal with depressive disorders prevents a wider sharing of information. In order to remove this obstacle, WHO launched a collaborative study on standardized assessments of depressive disorders (Sartorius et al., 1983). Five study areas were selected: Basle (Switzerland), Montreal (Canada), Nagasaki (Japan), Teheran (Iran), and Tokyo (Japan). In these centers, a total of 573 patients with depressive disorders were selected and assessed in a uniform and standardized way. The WHO Schedule for Standardized Assessment of Depressive Disorders (WHO/SADD) was used.

This collaborative study revealed that if the study patients were accepted as typical of the usual caseload of the centers involved, the patients who sought psychiatric treatment for depressive illnesses in the five study areas were strikingly similar in many respects. With regard to symptomatology, the patients in all the centers exhibited a "core" of depressive symptoms that were present in 76 to 100% in both diagnostic groups. Only a few symptoms appeared with markedly different frequency at the different centers [cross-reference to Chapter 18: Disorders of Depression (Section III,A,2)].

4. Psychological Problems in General Health Care

A multipurpose international collaboratory study was carried out by WHO to examine the "psychological problems in general health care" (Üstün & Sartorius, 1995). A total of 15 study centers in 14 countries around the world were involved. They were Ankara (Turkey), Arthens (Greek), Bangalore (India), Berlin (Germany), Groninge (Netherlands), Ibadan (Nigeria), Mainz (Germany), Manchester (UK) Nagasaki (Japan), Paris (France), Rio de Janeiro (Brazil), Santiago de Chile (Chile), Seattle (USA), Shanghai (China), and Verona (Italy). Nearly 5500 patients were assessed in detail, using the General Health Questionnaire (GHQ) as the instrument for clinical assessment and diagnosis according to ICD-10 criteria. In addition to the questionnaire diagnosis, the patients' presenting complaints, the proportion of the psychological disorders recognized by the treating physicians, and other variables were studied.

The results revealed that (Üstün & Sartorius, 1995) the complaints presented by the (medical) patients in general health care clinics (as illustrated in Table 12-1) differed remarkably if the complaints were subdivided arbitrarily into categories of psychological, fatigue/sleep problems, pain, and other somatic complaints. It was noted that among patients who visited general health care facilities, psychological problems were presented more frequently in the study centers in European countries, such as the Netherlands (12.8%), France (11.0%), and the United Kingdom (9.4%), as well as some countries in South America: Chile (13.2%) and Brazil (7.6%). In contrast, psychological problems were presented less frequently by patients from China (0.2%), Japan (1.3%), Greece (2.2%), Nigeria (2.3%), and Turkey (2.6%) (cross-reference Chapter 16: Anxiety Disorder, for a discussion of these findings).

The diagnosed prevalence of mental disorders — mostly of so-called "minor" psychiatric disorders, such as alcohol dependence, harmful use of alcohol, depression, dysthymia, agoraphobia, panic disorder, generalized anxiety disorder, somatization disorder, hypochondriasis, and neurasthenia as defined by ICD-10 — varied among the centers investigated. In addition to the expected wide variation of alcohol dependence — 7.2% for Germany vs 0.4% for Nigeria — there was also a broader range of prevalence in other disorders, such as depression — 29.5% for Chile vs 2.6% for Japan — and somatization disorder — 17.7% for Chile vs 0.1% for Italy. It is also worth noticing that neurasthenia was found in all the centers studied, even though it did not have a very high percentage (cross-reference to Chapter 15: Anxiety Disorder; Chapter 16: Somatoform Disorder; and Chapter 18: Disorders of Depression, respectively, for further discussion on these findings).

TABLE 12-1 Psychological Problems Presented in General Health Care[a]

	Study Centers														
	Ankara, Turkey	Athens, Greece	Bangalore, India	Berlin, Germany	Groninge, Netherlands	Ibadan, Nigeria	Mainz, Germany	Manchester, United Kingdom	Nagasaki, Japan	Paris, France	Rio de Janeiro, Brazil	Santiago de Chile, Chile	Seattle, United States	Shanghai, China	Verona, Italy
I. Presenting complaints															
Psychological	2.6	2.2	1.3	3.7	12.8	2.3	3.6	9.4	1.3	11.0	7.6	13.2	2.6	0.2	6.4
Fatigue/Sleep	5.6	5.1	8.0	5.2	5.7	9.0	0.6	13.4	9.5	8.4	5.1	3.6	1.6	13.3	3.7
Pain	80.5	21.9	35.1	32.3	28.2	51.4	28.0	24.8	21.3	25.3	42.1	17.4	17.0	26.2	25.9
Other Somatic	44.4	33.5	17.7	36.0	37.0	31.0	33.5	38.2	22.8	39.6	16.9	31.6	15.8	52.9	25.6
II. ICD diagnoses															
Alcohol dependence	1.0	1.0	1.4	5.3	3.4	0.4	7.2	2.2	3.7	4.3	4.1	2.5	1.5	1.1	0.5
Harmful use of alcohol	0.8	3.5	0.6	4.0	5.5	0.8	3.0	1.4	2.5	5.0	1.7	10.0	8.6	1.6	2.6
Current depression	11.6	6.4	9.1	6.1	15.9	4.2	11.2	16.9	2.6	13.7	15.8	29.5	6.3	4.0	4.7
Dysthymia	0.9	1.4	9.8	0.5	1.8	1.3	0.9	2.0	0.4	3.6	2.4	4.2	0.3	0.6	2.0
Agoraphobia	1.2	0.9	0.1	1.5	2.7	0.1	1.6	3.8	0.0	2.2	2.7	3.9	1.3	0.1	0.6
Panic disorder	0.2	0.7	1.0	0.9	1.5	0.7	1.7	3.5	0.2	1.7	0.0	0.6	1.9	0.2	1.5
Generalized anxiety disorder	0.9	14.9	8.5	9.0	6.4	2.9	7.9	7.1	5.0	11.9	22.6	18.7	2.1	1.9	3.7
Somatization disorder	1.9	1.3	1.8	1.3	2.8	0.4	3.0	0.4	0.1	1.7	8.5	17.7	1.7	1.5	0.1
Hypochondriasis	0.2	0.2	0.2	0.4	1.0	1.9	1.2	0.5	0.4	0.1	1.1	3.8	0.6	0.4	0.3
Neurasthenia	4.1	4.6	2.7	7.4	10.5	1.1	7.7	9.7	3.4	9.3	4.5	10.5	2.1	2.0	2.1
One or more mental disorders	17.6	22.1	23.9	25.2	29.0	10.4	30.6	26.2	14.8	31.2	38.0	53.5	20.4	9.7	12.4
All patients (%)	100.0	100.0	100.0	100.0	100.0	100.0	100.0	100.0	100.0	100.0	100.0	100.0	100.0	100.0	100.0
III. ICD-10 disorders[b] (Percentage)	8.2	11.6	16.2	32.5	27.0	27.9	33.0	28.1	4.8	30.3	20.4	58.5	19.7	5.4	47.3

[a] Psychological Problems Presented in General Health Care: WHO's International Study [Revision from T.B. Üstün and N. Sartorius (Eds), *Mental illness in general health care: International study*. John Wiley & Sons, 1995].

[b] Recognized by treating physicians as a psychological case

This study produced very useful epidemiological data for cross-cultural comparison, as almost no investigations had been done previously on minor psychiatric disorders using standardized methods of investigation and multiple cultural sites. Nevertheless, this study had certain inherent methodological problems. Because minor psychiatric disorders by definition are based on the patient's subjective complaints, it is difficult to know to what extent the obtained information was affected by the patient's complaining patterns rather than the disorders from which they suffered. It was also difficult to evaluate the revealed data without knowing to what extent it was influenced by the health care system, particularly the availability of (psychiatric) service as a specialty vs the nature and function of the general health care system within each of the societies investigated. The population would be influenced greatly by the health care system as well as the patient's help-seeking behavior. These are the inherent problems associated with the study of minor psychiatric disorders through clinical populations.

E. CATCHMENT-AREA STUDIES IN THE 1980S IN THE UNITED STATES

In order to disclose how many patients are suffering from mental disorders in America, who they are, the kind of disorders from which they are suffering, and the kinds of treatment that they need, the ECA study was launched by the National Institute of Mental Health (NIMH) in the United States in the 1980s. Its aim was to examine the frequency of various types of specific mental disorders present in the society so that proper mental health services could be planned (Regier et al., 1984).

As reported by Regier and Kaelber (1995), it was decided to select investigators at multiple collaborating sites. Five investigators were selected from Yale University, Johns Hopkins University, Washington University, Duke University, and the University of California at Los Angeles to survey communities and institutions in New Haven, Baltimore, St. Louis, Durham, and Los Angeles, respectively. This approach permitted utilization of community variations with access to special populations (e.g., African-American, Hispanics, the elderly, and urban and rural populations).

It was decided that a new instrument would be developed for the ECA program so that trained staff could administer the questionnaire-based survey of the large populations selected — at least 200,000 persons at each site. Based on the Renard Diagnostic Interview (Helzer, Robins, Croughan, & Welner, 1981), the NIMH Diagnostic Interview Schedule (DIS) was developed, which incorporated coverage of DSM-III diagnostic criteria for selected mental and behavioral disorders. As pointed out by Regier and Kelber (1995), while the DSM-III encompassed over 120 diagnoses for adults, the DIS included only a portion of these disorders, focusing on those that had greater frequency and for which the diagnostic criteria were explicit enough to be evaluated from a single interview.

Numerous findings were obtained from the study. Only those that have sociocultural implications will be mentioned here. Among all the mental disorders included in the study, phobias and alcohol abuse were found to be the most prevalent. While the high prevalence of alcohol abuse among Americans was not news, that of phobic disorders was. Surprisingly, over 14% of the persons surveyed reported a phobia during their lifetime and nearly 9% during the past year (Robins, Lock, & Regier, 1991). This was in contrast to data obtained from other cultures, such as Taiwan, for instance, where the incidence was only 3.5% in rural villages and 5.7% in townships (Yeh, Hwu, Lin, 1995). Concerning only social phobias, the lifetime prevalence obtained from the ECA for the United States was 2.4%. Although that for New Zealand was also high (3.9%), it was only 1.0 for Italy, 0.6% for Korea, and 0.4–0.6% for Taiwan (Horwath & Weissman, 1997). The possible reason for the high prevalence rate of phobic disorders among Americans is still a question awaiting investigation.

In the ECA program, with its catchment-area design, the ethnic minority groups of African-Americans and Hispanic-Americans were included. It was found that there were higher rates of all mental disorders studied among African-Americans in terms of both lifetime prevalence (38%) and active in the last year (26%) than among Caucasian-Americans (32 and 19%) or Hispanic-Americans (33 and 20%), respectively (Regier & Kaelber, 1995, pp. 142–143). However, when social economic status (SES) was controlled, rates for African-Americans were not higher than for Caucasian-Americans.

Regier and Kelber (1995) indicated that there were some methodological shortcomings in the ECA program, including that not all psychiatric disorders were considered by the DIS. The diagnosis relied entirely on data collected through the questionnaires (rather than on the clinical judgment of the psychiatrists who performed the interviews, as in second-generation studies), and, because the persons interviewed varied in their willingness and ability to answer questions accurately, there may have been limitations in defining cases. There were also nonrandom refusals to be interviewed and, finally, the five collaborating sites did not represent random samples of the U.S. population. Not all minority groups were included sufficiently for comparison. Despite these limitations, the ECA program produced data that was not only valuable in creating a national mental-health service plan, but was also available for international comparison.

Adopting methodology similar to that of the ECA, several epidemiological studies were undertaken in other cultures including the study of a city (Seoul) and rural areas in Korea (Lee et al., 1990a, 1990b) and different geographic areas in Taiwan, China (Compton et al., 1991; Yeh et al., 1995), which produced valuable data for cross-cultural comparison. They offered the opportunity to make East–West comparisons based on the same third-generation methodology.

III. GENERAL FINDINGS DERIVED FROM CROSS-CULTURAL STUDIES

A. PSYCHIATRIC DISORDERS FOUND IN MOST SOCIETIES

It is generally found that except for some (culture-related) specific or unique psychiatric syndromes, most psychiatric disorders or abnormal behaviors rec-

ognized by contemporary psychiatric classification systems exist in most of the societies investigated, regardless of geographical location, the nature of the society, its culture, and its level of (economic) development. This tends to support the view that there are certain degrees of "culture-common" psychopathology observed in humankind as a whole.

However, there are certain disorders that are prevalent in some societies and rare in others. This is not because the disorders are unique or culturally related and "culture specific" (such as *koro*, cargo cult, *and amok*), but because they can be attributed to certain diagnostic criteria (such as neurasthenia, posttraumatic stress disorder, or borderline disorders), because of social sensitivity to the fluctuation of certain psychopathologies (such as substance abuse and drinking problems), or because of the vicissitude of psychopathology, i.e., the fluctuation of psychiatric disorders within a society or within humankind as whole (such as catatonic subtypes of schizophrenia, hysterical conversion, or dissociation).

B. DIFFERENCES IN RANGE EXIST IN THE PREVALENCE OF DISORDERS

It is also obvious that there are different ranges of frequency among the psychopathologies investigated. Some of them demonstrate a rather narrow range of prevalence and others a relatively wide range. Severe psychoses, such as schizophrenia, belong to the former group, whereas substance abuse and suicidal behavior belong to the latter. These findings indirectly support the idea that there are biological vs psychological determinants of psychopathology.

C. SOCIAL PARAMETERS ATTRIBUTED TO CERTAIN GROUPS OF MENTAL DISORDERS

Several social parameters are recognized as contributing factors for certain groups of mental disorders, particularly those that are susceptible to sociocultural environment. The social parameters are social class (Hollingshead & Redlich, 1958), urban/rural environmental differences, social disintegration (J.M. Murphy & Leighton, 1965, p. viii), and migration (H.B.M. Murphy, 1977).

Psychiatric epidemiological studies have demonstrated that stratification by SES is often closely associated with mental problems or disorders. In addition to the pioneer study made by Hollingshead and Redlich (1958) in the United States, there have been continuous investigations carried out around the world. It has been reported from Brazil that socioeconomic differences are associated inversely with arterial blood pressure and depressive symptoms (Dressler, Balieiro, & Dos Santos, 1998). In the Netherlands, a higher prevalence of unfavorable personality profiles and more negative coping styles were found in subjects who grew up in lower social classes, supporting the view that there are associations between social class in childhood and adult mental health (Bosma, van de Mheen, & Mackenbach, 1999). In Britain, it was revealed that alcohol-related mortality rates were higher for men in manual occupations than in nonmanual occupations, but the relative magnitude depended on age — greater (10–20 times more) for men aged 25–39 and less (only 2.5–4 times) for those aged 55–64. Among women, younger women in the manual classes were more likely to die from alcohol-related causes, but among older women, those in the professional class suffer elevated mortality. Thus, social class is a risk factor for alcohol-related mortality, although it is mediated by age and gender (Harrison & Gardiner, 1999). Concerning the impact of socioeconomic factors on various groups of psychiatric disorders, Koppel and McGuffin (1999) carried out an investigation in the county of South Glamorgan in the United Kingdom. Standardized psychiatric admission ratios (SAR) for different diagnostic groups were calculated for a 5-year period. It was revealed that psychiatric morbidity reflected in SAR was related inversely to socioeconomic deprivation for both sexes. The relationship was most marked for schizophrenia, delusional disorders, and substance abuse, closely followed by personality disorders, and less

for affective and neurotic disorders. Utilizing data from two surveys, the National Comorbidity Survey (1990–1992) and Epidemiologic Catchment Area Follow-up (1993–1996) Muntaner, Eaton, Dalia, Kessler, & Sorlie, (1998) examined the association between social class and common types of psychiatric disorders in the United States. They reported that from the former survey data, there was an inverse association between financial and physical assets and mood, anxiety, alcohol, and drug disorders; and from the latter survey data, anxiety, alcohol, and drug disorders as well.

D. THEORIES OF SOCIAL CAUSATION, SELECTION, AND ATTRACTION

Based on epidemiological studies, several social theories have been proposed for the possible relation between social factors and the prevalence of mental disorders. As elaborated in a previous chapter, there are hypotheses of social causation (through sociocultural disintegration), social selection (or drift), and social attraction [cross-reference to Chapter 11: Culture and Psychopathology (Section III,B)].

E. CULTURAL CONTRIBUTIONS TO SOME GROUPS OF DISORDERS

Most epidemiological studies have not addressed cultural variables directly. Cultural dimensions have been explored indirectly through the ethnic/racial or religious backgrounds of the subjects examined or through cross-comparisons of data derived from different cultural settings. Occasionally, certain parameters, such as rapid cultural change or confusion, have been taken into consideration. There have been almost no studies that directly examined the possible relationship between certain cultural attitudes, beliefs, or values held by the subjects and the formation of certain psychopathologies. Tseng and colleagues (1992) attempted to examine sex-related folk beliefs and their relation to the prevalence of the *koro* epidemic disorder in China.

Nevertheless, it is generally considered that culture, in close conjunction with social variables, has a significant impact on the occurrence of certain psychopathologies. This is supported by many epidemiological findings relating to sociocultural variables; e.g., a persistent, unique style of life, such as that of the Hutterites (Eaton & Weil, 1955); rapid sociocultural change, illustrated by the rise of neurotic disorders found in a longitudinal study in Taiwan (Lin et al., 1969); the fluctuation in suicide rates associated with sociocultural change in Japan (Yoshimatsu, 1992); the remarkable rise in the suicide rate of youngsters in Micronesia (Rubinstein, 1992); or cultural disintegration associated with social change (J.M. Murphy & Leighton, 1965).

This chapter has presented a brief overview of psychiatric epidemiology, with particular reference to socioculture perspectives, and summarized the general findings of epidemiological studies. Epidemiological data relating to specific disorders (such as anxiety, somatoform, dissociation, depression, and suicide) will be elaborated more in Chapters 16 to 26, respectively.

REFERENCES

Akimoto, H. (1942). Demographische und psychiatrische Undersuchung der abgegrenzten Kleinstadtbevolkerung. *Psychiatria et Neurologia Japonica, 47,* 351–374.

Beiser, M., Ravel, J.L., Collomb, H., & Egelhoff, C. (1972). Assessing psychiatric disorders among the Serer of Senegal. *Journal of Nervous and Mental Disease, 154,* 141–151.

Bosma, H., van de Mheen, H.D., & Mackenbach, J.P. (1999). Social class in childhood and general health in adulthood: Questionnaire study of the contribution of psychological attributes. *British Medical Journal, 2,* 18–22.

Brugger, C. (1931). Versuch einer Geisteskrankenzahlung in Turingen. *Zeitschrift fuer Neurologia und Psychiatrie, 133,* 352–390.

Compton, W.M., III., Helzer, J.E., Hwu, H.G., Yeh, E.K., McEvoy, L., Tipp, J.E., & Spitznagel, E.L. (1991). New methods in cross-cultural psychiatry: Psychiatric illness in Taiwan and the United States. *American Journal of Psychiatry, 148,* 1697–1704.

Dale, P.W. (1981). Prevalence of schizophrenia in the Pacific island populations of Micronesia. *Journal of Psychiatric Research, 16*(2), 103–111.

Dohrenwend, B.P. (1995). "The problem of validity in field studies of psychological disorders" revisited. In M.T. Tsuang, M.

Tohen, & G.E.P. Zahner (Eds.), *Textbook in psychiatric epidemiology.* (pp. 3–20). New York: Wiley.

Dressler, W.W., Balieiro, M.C., & dos Santos, J.E. (1998). Culture, socioeconomic status, and physical and mental health in Brazil. *Medical Anthropology Quarterly, 12*(4), 424–446.

Eaton, J.W., & Weil, R.J. (1955). *Culture and mental disorders: A comparative study of the Hutterites and other populations.* New York: Free Press of Glencoe.

Harrison, L., & Gardiner, E. (1999). Do the rich really die young? Alcohol-related mortality and social class in Great Britain, 1988–1994. *Addiction, 94* (12), 1871–1880.

Helzer, J.E., Robins, L.N., Croughan, J.L., & Welner, A. (1981). Renard diagnostic interview: Its reliability and procedureal validity with physicians and lay interviewers. *Archives of General Psychiatry, 38,* 393–398.

Hollingshead, A.B., & Redlich, F.C. (1958). *Social class and mental illness: A community study.* New York: Wiley.

Horwath, E., & Weissman, M.M. (1997). Epidemiology of depression and anxiety disorders. In M.T. Tsung, M. Tohen, & G.E.P. Zahner (Eds.), *Textbook in psychiatric epidemiology* (pp. 317–344). New York: Wiley.

Jablensky, A., Sartorius, N., Ernberg, G., Anker, M., Korten, A., Cooper, J.E., Day, R., & Bertelsen, A. (1991). *Schizophrenia: Manifestations, incidence and course in different cultures: A World Health Organization Ten-Country Study* (Psychological Medicine, Monograph Supplement No. 20). Cambridge, UK: Cambridge University Press.

Koppel, S., & McGuffin, P. (1999). Socio-economic factors that predict psychiatric admissions at a local level. *Psychological Medicine, 29*(5), 1235–1241.

Lee, C.K., Kwak, Y.S., Yamamoto, J., Rhee, H., Kim, Y.S., Han, J.H., Choi, J.O., & Lee, Y.H. (1990a). Psychiatric epidemiology in Korea. Part I. Gender and age differences in Seoul. *Journal of Nervous and Mental Disease, 178*(4), 242–246.

Lee, C.K., Kwak, Y.S., Yamamoto, J., Rhee, H., Kim, Y.S., Han, J.H., Choi, J.O., & Lee, Y.H. (1990b). Psychiatric epidemiology in Korea. Part II. Urban and rural differences. *Journal of Nervous and Mental Disease, 178*(4), 247–252.

Leighton, A.H., Lambo, T., Hughes, J.M., Leighton, D., Murphy, J., & Macklin, D. (1963). *Psychiatric disorder among the Yoruba.* Ithaca, NY: Cornell-University Press.

Lemkau, P., Tietze, C., & Cooper, M. (1941). Mental hygiene problems in an urban district. *Mental Hygiene, 25,* 624–646.

Lin, T.-Y. (1953). An epidemiological study of the incidence of mental disorder in Chinese and other cultures. *Psychiatry, 16,* 313–336.

Lin, T.-Y., Rin, H., Yeh, E.K., Hsu, C.C., & Chu, H.M. (1969). Mental disorders in Taiwan, fifteen years later: A preliminary report. In W. Caudil & T.Y. Lin (Eds.), *Mental health research in Asia and the Pacific.* (pp. 66–91). Honolulu: East-West Center Press.

Lin, T.-Y., & Standley, C.C. (1962). *The scope of epidemiology in psychiatry.* (Public Health Papers No. 16). Geneva: World Health Organization.

Mezzich, J.E., Jorge, M.R., & Salloum, I.M. (Eds.). (1994). *Psychiatric epidemiology: Assessment concepts and methods*. Baltimore: Johns Hopkins University Press.

Muntaner, C., Eaton, W.W., Diala, C., Kessler, R.C., & Sorlie, P.D. (1998). Social class, assets, organizational control and the prevalence of common groups of psychiatric disorders. *Social Science and Medicine, 47*(12), 2043–2053.

Murphy, H.B.M. (1977). Migration, culture and mental health. *Psychological Medicine, 7,* 677–684.

Murphy, J.M., & Leighton, A.H. (Eds.). (1965). *Approaches to cross-cultural psychiatry*. Ithaca, NY: Cornell University Press.

Parry, C.D.H. (1996). A review of psychiatric epidemiology in Afirca: Strategies for increasing validity when using instruments transculturally. *Transcultural Psychiatric Research Review, 33*(2), 173–188.

Pasamanick, B. (Ed.). (1959). *Epidemiology of mental disorders*. Washington, DC: American Association for the Advancement of Science.

Regier, D.A., & Kaelber, C.T. (1995). The Epidemiologic Catchment Area (ECA) Program: Studying the prevalence and incidence of psychopathology. In M.T. Tsung, M. Tohen, & G.E.P. Zahner (Eds.), *Textbook in psychiatric epidemiology* (pp. 135–155). New York: Wiley.

Regier, D.A., Myers, J.K., Kramer, M., Robins, L.N., Blazer, D.G., Hough, R.L., Eaton, W.W., & Locke, B.Z. (1984). The NIMH Epidemiologic Catchment Area Program: Historical context, major objectives, and study population characteristics. *Archives of General Psyciatry, 41,* 934–941.

Rin, H., & Lin, T.-Y. (1962). Mental illness among Formosan aborigines as compared with the Chinese in Taiwan. *Journal of Mental Science, 108,* 134–146.

Robins, L.N., Lock, B.Z., & Regier, D.A. (1991). An overview of psychiatric disorders in America. In L.N. Robins & D.A. Regier (Eds.), *Psychiatric disorders in America*. New York: Free Press.

Rogler, L.H. (1994). Culturally sensitive research in mental health. In J.E. Mezzich, M.R. Jorge, & I.M. Salloum (Eds.), *Psychiatric epidemiology: Assessment concepts and method*. Baltimore: Johns Hopkins University Press.

Roth, W.F., Jr., & Luton, F.H. (1943). The mental health program in Tennessee. *American Journal of Psychiatry, 99,* 662–675.

Rubinstein, D.H. (1992). Suicidal behavior in Micronesia. In L.P. Kok & W.S. Tseng (Eds.), *Suicidal behavior in the Asia-Pacific Region*. (pp. 199–230). Singapore: Singapore University Press.

Sartorius, N., Davidain, H., Ernberg, G., Fenton, F.R., Fujii, I., Gastpar, M., Gulbinat, W., Jablensky, A., Kielholz, P., Lehmann, H.E., Naraghi, M., Shimizu, M., Shinfuku, N., & Takahashi, R. (1983). *Depressive disorders in different cultures: Report on the WHO collaborative study on standardized assessment of depressive disorders*. Geneva: World Health Organization.

Schwab, J.J., & Schwab, M.E. (1978). *Sociocultural roots of mental illness: An Epidemiologic survey*. New York: Plenum Medical Book Company.

Sjöegren, T. (1948). Genetic-statistical and psychiatric investigation of a West Swedish population. *Acta Psychiatrica et Neurologica, Supplementum, 52,* 1–103.

Strömgren, E. (1938). Beiträge zur psychischen erblenre. *Acta Psychiatrica et Neurologica, Supplementum, 19,* 1–259.

Tseng, W.S., Mo, K.M., Hsu, J., Li, L.S., Chen, G.Q., Ou, L.W., & Zheng, H.B. (1992). Koro epidemics in Guandong, China: A questionnaire survey. *Journal of Nervous and Mental Disease, 180*(2), 117–123.

Tsuang, M.T., Tohen, M., & Zahner, G.E.P. (Eds.). (1995). *Textbook in psychiatric epidemiology*. New York: Wiley.

Uchimura, Y. et al. (1940). Uber die vergleichend-psychiatirsch und erbpathologiesche Untersuchung auf einer Japanischen Insel [Comparative psychiatric and inherited-pathologic study of an Japanese island]. *Psychiatria et Neurologia Japonica, 44,* 745–782.

Üstün, T.B., & Sartorius, N. (Eds.) (1995). *Mental illness in general health care: An international study*. Chichester: Wiley (on behalf of WHO).

World Health Organization (WHO). (1973). *The international study of schizophrenia*. Geneva: WHO.

Yeh, E.K., Hwu, H.G., & Lin, T.-Y. (1995). Mental disorders in Taiwan: Epidemiological studies of community population. In T.-Y. Lin, W.S. Tseng, & E.K. Yeh (Eds.), *Chinese societies and mental health* (pp. 247–265). Hong Kong: Oxford University Press.

Yoshimatsu, K. (1992). Suicidal behavior in Japan. In L.P. Kok & W.S. Tseng (Eds.), *Suicidal behavior in the Asia-Pacific Region* (pp. 15–40). Singapore: Singapore University Press.

13

Culture-Related Specific Syndromes

I. TERMINOLOGY, DEFINITION, AND SUBGROUPING

A. DEFINITION AND HISTORICAL TRENDS

Culture-related specific syndromes, also called culture-bound syndromes, refer to mental conditions or psychiatric syndromes whose occurrence or manifestation is closely related to cultural factors and thus warrant understanding and management primarily from a cultural perspective. Because the presentation of a culture-related syndrome is usually unique, with special clinical manifestations, it is called a culture-related specific psychiatric syndrome. From a phenomenological point of view, such a condition is not easily categorized according to existing psychiatric classifications, which are based on clinical experiences of commonly observed psychiatric disorders in Western societies, without adequate orientation toward less frequently encountered psychiatric conditions and diverse cultures worldwide.

Around the turn of the 20th century, during a period of colonization by Western societies, Western ministers, physicians, and others visited faraway countries where they encountered behaviors and unique psychiatric conditions that they had never experienced at home. Most of these conditions were known to the local people by folk names, such as *latah, amok, koro, susto,* and so on, and were described by Westerners as "exotic," "rare," "uncommon," or "extraordinary" mental disorders (C.T.H. Friedmann & Faguet, 1982; Meth, 1974), mental illnesses "peculiar to certain cultures" (Yap, 1951), or "folk illnesses." This indicates how extensively psychiatric classifications were based on Anglo-Saxon patient populations in Europe and North America. Any clinical pictures manifested by patient populations outside of those "main" populations were seen as unusual or atypical. It also shows that psychiatric classifications were the result of Westerners' ethnocentric views of psychopathology; anything beyond their commonly observed phenomena was considered exotic or peculiar.

In 1967, P. M. Yap, a Chinese cultural psychiatrist from Hong Kong, suggested the term "culture-bound reactive syndrome" to describe the various psychopathologies or atypical syndromes bound to certain cultures. The following year, he omitted the word "reactive" and changed the term to "culture-bound syndrome." Since then, this term has been used by psychiatrists to refer to psychiatric syndromes that are closely related to culture and are "bound" to a particular cultural region, such as *amok* among Malaysian people and *koro* among the southern Chinese. Recently, however, cultural psychiatrists have realized that such psychiatric manifestations are not necessarily confined to particular ethnic–cultural groups. For instance, epidemic occurrences of *koro* (penis-shrinking panic) occur among Thai or Indian people, not only among the southern Chinese; and sporadic occurrences of *amok* attacks (mass, indiscriminate homicidal acts) are observed in the Philippines, Thailand, Papua New Guinea (Burton-Bradley, 1975), and in epidemic proportions in many places in south Asia, in addition to Malaysia (Westermeyer, 1973). Terrifying examples of *amok* have occurred with frequency on school campuses and in workplaces in the United States (see Fig. 13-1).

Thus, the term "culture-bound" does not seem to apply, and it has been suggested that "culture-related specific psychiatric syndrome" would be more accurate to describe a syndrome that is closely **related** to certain *cultural traits* or *cultural features* rather than **bound** specifically to any one *cultural system* or *culture unit* (Tseng & McDermott, 1981). Accordingly, the definition has been modified to "a collection of signs and symptoms that is restricted to a limited number of cultures, primarily by reason of certain of their psychosocial features" (Prince & Tcheng-Laroche, 1987). In this chapter, the shorter term, "culture-related syndromes," will be used to refer specifically to psychiatric conditions that are strongly related to certain cultural traits, even though it is recognized that every psychopathology is influenced by culture to a certain degree.

Associated with the increased interest in and awareness of cultural psychiatry, particularly culture-related specific syndromes, many clinicians around the world overuse or use the term loosely, reporting syndromes that may not meet the definition of "culture-related specific syndrome" in a strict sense. Hundreds of psychiatric conditions have been reported by scholars in the past as folk illnesses (Simons & Hughes, 1985). However, folk labels for mental disorders do not necessarily imply that the disorders are culture-related syndromes.

B. CRITERIA FOR CONSIDERATION

Clear definitions and operational criteria are necessary to make discussion meaningful. "Culture-related specific syndromes" are defined here as psychiatric syndromes that are closely related to certain cultural features in their formation or manifestation of psychopathology. The clinical manifestations tend to be unique and different from those of psychiatric disorders that fit within existing psychiatric classifications. These syndromes tend to be observed more frequently in certain cultural areas that share common cultural traits, or features than in others. Whether they are prevalent or infrequent in those areas is not as much of an issue in determining whether special clinical attention is warranted as the importance of cultural factors in their formation and the significance of local people's reactions to them.

As discussed previously [cross-reference to Chapter 11: Culture and Psychopathology (Section II,A–F)], cultural influences on psychiatric syndromes can occur in six ways: through (1) pathogenetic effect, in which cultural beliefs induce stress and anxiety, which cause the development of the disorders; (2) pathoselective effect, in which the culture chooses unique (pathological) patterns of coping with stress or anxiety; (3) pathoplastic effect, in which culture shapes the content of symptoms and manifestations of the clinical picture; (4) pathoelaborating effect, in which culture exaggerates certain mental conditions to an elaborate level, where they become unique; (5) pathofacilitating effect, in which culture influences the frequency with which the pathology occurs in a particular society; and (6) pathoreactive effect, in which culture impacts the patient's, family members', or the community's reactions to the disorder, including how it is interpreted and managed, and often influences its outcome.

Regions / Syndrome	Africa	Central America	South America	Arctic	Asia	South Asia	Australia New Zealand	Pacific
Koro					South China	Indonesia (?)		
(Koro Epidemic)					South China	Singapore Thailand India		
Daht Syndrome						India		
Frigophobia					Taiwan, China			
Voodoo Death	Africa		South America				Australia New Zealand	Pacific Islands
Malgri							Wellesly Is. Australia	
Amok						Malay, Laos, Thailand, Phillipines		Papua New Guinea
Family Suicide					Japan			
Cargo Cult								Melanesia
Taijinkyofusho					Japan Korea			
Brain Fag Syndrome	Nigeria, Uganda							
Arctic Hysteria				Greenland and other Arctic areas				
Malignant Anxiety	Nigeria and others							
Ataques de Nervios		Puerto Rico	Latin America					
Latah (Imu)					Hokkaido, Japan	Malay, Burma Indonesia Thailand Phillipines		
Hwabyung					Korea			
Susto			Latin America					

FIGURE 13-1   Regional distribution of recognized culture-related specific syndromes.

Based on this framework, the criteria of culture-related specific syndromes may be examined in detail as follows: among the six ways that culture can influence disorders, the first — pathogenic effect (cultural influence on the formation of a disorder) — is the essential and sufficient element for defining a syndrom as culture-related and specific. Closely associated is the second, or psychoselective effect (culture selecting certain coping patterns to deal with stress). If the chosen pattern is culture related and rather unique, it also meets the criteria. The psychoplastic (culture modifying the manifestation), pathoelaborating (culture elaborating mental conditions into a unique nature), and psychofacilitating (culture promoting the frequency of occurrence) effects also contribute to the development of the specific syndrome, but they are not sufficient conditions by themselves. The psychoreactive effect (culture shapes folk responses to the clinical condition) does not alone meet the criteria for culture-related specific syndromes because there is no specific or unique pathological condition involved and the cultural impact is secondary, merely interpreting and labeling the phenomenon.

These six ways in which culture influences psychopathology are not necessarily mutually exclusive; actually, culture often impacts syndromes in multiple ways. Recognizing these will help us examine the operational criteria for culture-related psychiatric syndromes. It should be clarified that cultural factors impact *every* kind of psychopathology to some extent — whether or not it is predominantly psychological or biological in nature. However, unless cultural impact is very significant and deserves special attention, there is no point in identifying and labeling a pathology as a "culture-related specific syndrome."

C. DIFFERENT SUBGROUPING SYSTEM FOR SYNDROMES

In order to organize and categorize various culture-related syndromes, several different subgrouping systems have been proposed by different scholars in the past. Following are some examples.

1. Subgrouping by Cardinal Symptoms

This method of subgrouping was suggested by Hong Kong cultural psychiatrist P.M. Yap in 1967. Identifying the cardinal symptoms and referring to the "typical" prototype of the pathology as it was already recognized in the existing classification system, he suggested subgroups of primary fear reactions (including malignant anxiety, *latah,* psychogenic or magical death), hyperidic rage reaction *(amok),* specific culture-imposed nosophobia *(koro),* and trance dissociation *(windigo* psychosis).

2. Subgrouping by "Taxon"

Similarly, in 1985, Ronald C. Simons, an American cultural psychiatrist, and his anthropological colleague, Charles C. Hughes, suggested classifying and categorizing all culture-related syndromes by "taxon." As in the field of biology, taxon refers to a category or unit that arranges a group of objects according to a common factor. Based on this approach, they suggested the startle-matching taxon (including *latah, imu*); the sleep-paralysis taxon; the genital-retraction taxon *(koro);* the sudden-mass-assault taxon *(amok);* the running taxon *(pibloktoq, grisi siknis,* arctic hysteria); the fright-illness taxon *(susto);* and the cannibal-compulsion taxon *(windigo* psychosis).

3. Subgrouping by Relationship to Culture

In 1981, Tseng and McDermott suggested an entirely different way of categorizing culture-related syndromes. They proposed subgrouping the syndromes according to how they might be affected by cultural factors. This approach is more meaningful for addressing and understanding the disorders from a cultural perspective. German cultural psychiatrist Wolfgang Pfeiffer (1982) also emphasized that when we categorize syndromes according to their clinical manifestation, we lose the basis for dealing with them as products of culture.

D. Proposed Subgrouping of Various Syndromes

For the sake of discussing the way in which cultural factors contribute to syndromes, and how the syndromes are related to culture, the following subgroupings are suggested. There is no intention to classify culture-related syndromes into certain diagnostic categories. Also, as it is impossible to review all the syndromes claimed by scholars to be culture bound or related, only some will be reviewed here, based on the availability of information on and familiarity with them.

Group A: Culture-Related Beliefs as Cause for the Occurrence

This group includes syndromes that, according to currently available knowledge, are caused primarily by psychological stress stemming from cultural beliefs. The belief explicitly exists and is consciously recognized by the folk people involved. In other words, the syndromes are the direct result of the pathogenic impacts of culture-belief-induced anxiety. Culture plays a role in the etiological formation of the disorder through **pathogenic effect.** These syndromes include:

Koro — Anxiety or panic attack resulting from the folk belief that excessive shrinking of the penis into the abdomen will cause death.

Dhat syndrome — Anxiety based on the belief that excessive semen loss will result in illness.

Frigophobia — A fixated morbid fear of catching cold based on the folk belief that excessive cold will result in serious effects on health.

Voodoo death — Intense fear that often results in sudden death based on the belief that breaking taboos or curses will cause fatal outcomes.

Malgri — Anxiety due to the belief that breaking sea-land territorial food taboos will cause sickness.

Group B: Culture-Patterned Specific Stress-Coping Reactions

This group includes psychiatric conditions that reflect culture-shaped specific coping patterns. While there are potentially numerous ways of coping, culture — through its belief, values, and customs — influences the choice of certain patterns of coping with stress. Such patterns are seen as unique by people from other cultures. In other words, culture contributes to the selection of patterns for coping with stress through **pathoselecting effects.** This group includes:

Amok — Indiscriminate, mass homicidal attacks in reaction to stress or loss.

Family suicide *(ikkashinjiu)* — The whole family commits suicide together as a way of coping with stress.

Cargo cult syndrome — A group of people collectively gives up its customary work, believing that the worship of a supernatural power will bring the benefits (cargo) it needs for survival.

Group C: Culture-Shaped Variations of Psychopathology

While the manifestation of a psychopathology of any kind is more or less shaped by sociocultural factors that result in variations of clinical symptomatology, the culture-related specific syndrome is more remarkably influenced by cultural factors in the formation of the clinical condition. The degree of pathoplastic effect is so significant, and the manifested clinical condition so different from "ordinary" psychiatric disorders, that it is manifested as an "atypical" or "unique" variation. Culture contributes to the modification of disorder manifestation through **pathoplastic effects.**

Anthrophobia *(taijinkuofusho)* — A unique type of social phobia involving excessive concern with and phobia about interpersonal relations with intermediately familiar persons (such as friends or colleagues), but often not with strangers.

Brain fag syndrome — Culturally shaped anxiety–somatoform disorder with predominately somatic symptoms of the central nervous system.

Arctic hysteria *(pibloktoq)* — A unique type of hysterical attack observed in arctic areas.

Malignant anxiety — A severe form of anxiety often associated with violent behavior toward others.

Ataques de nervios (attack of nerve) — Unique emotional reaction to stressful situations with anxiety–hysterical features.

Group D: Culturally Elaborated Unique Behavior Reactions

Although certain behaviors may be observed universally, they are exaggerated to extreme forms in some cultures through cultural reinforcement. The occurrence of such behaviors or mental conditions is not necessarily pathological and often fulfills certain needs of the individual as well as the society. Culture plays the role of elaborating such unique or pathological behaviors through **pathoelaborating effects.** Examples of this group are:

Latah — Transient dissociative attacks provoked by startling for social amusement.

Body-weight-concerned behavior — Excessive concern over body image associated with anxiety about being overweight, resulting in excessive or pathological food-intake control.

Group E: Culture-Provoked Frequent Occurrence of Pathological Conditions

In this group, there is no uniqueness (or specificity) about the psychopathologies manifested. However, due to sociocultural influence, certain disorders become prevalent in certain cultural settings at given times. Associated with sociocultural attitudes, the frequency of the occurrence of these disorders varies significantly, indicating cultural impact on them through

pathofacilitating effects. The disorders are not necessary "specific" — they may be potentially universal, but the influence of cultural factors results in their frequent occurrence. Therefore, they are heavily culture-*related* (but not as *specific* psychiatric syndromes). Common examples are:

Massive hysteria — In reaction to collectively shared stress, a group of people develops a transient hysterical attack with features of dissociation, conversion, or emotional turmoil that act contagiously.

Alcohol-related problems — Very much influenced by cultural attitudes toward drinking, alcohol-related problems have a wide range of prevalence among different societies.

Substance-abuse behavior — The occurrence of substance abuse is provoked by sociocultural conditions and its prevalence varies greatly among different cultures, or even in the same society at different times.

Group F: Cultural Interpretation and Reaction to Certain Mental Conditions

Local people react to certain clinical mental conditions in particular ways, with cultural interpretations of their causes, familiar labels, and culturally prescribed ways of dealing with them. The clinical condition concerned does not have specific manifestations of any kind, and often has a mixed or multiple nature; therefore, it does not fit the label of a specific syndrome. Cultural influences are observed as folk responses to the disorder through **pathoreactive effects.** Idiosyncratic labeling occurs as a part of the illness behavior. In a strict sense, this group is not composed of culture-related "specific syndromes" even though folk illness terms are used.

Hwabyung — Interpretation of a morbid emotional condition resulting from a "fire" sickness.

Susto — Interpretation of and reaction to the folk concept of loss of soul.

Group G: Other (Questionable) Conditions

There were several mental conditions reported in the past as "culture-bound syndromes" for which there was no clear evidence to support that they were strongly culture-related, manifested specific symptoms, or actually existed at all. Examples are:

Spirit possession — Possession disorder in which the patient behaves as if possessed by a spirit or is interpreted by others as such.

Windigo psychosis — Cannibalistic possession psychosis "claimed" to occur among people living in arctic areas. There is no clinical study to support the existence of such a condition.

Multiple-personality disorder — The increased occurrence of multiple-personality disorder in Western societies is "interpretated" to be culture related. However, its actual relation to cultural factors is not yet clearly understood.

It is obvious that the proposed groupings are not clear-cut and fixed; there is always a possibility of overlapping because the influence of cultural factors can be multiple. Also, new knowledge and information obtained in the future concerning cultural impact may lead to modifications of the groupings at any time. Most of the culture-related syndromes indicated in Fig. 13-2 are positioned according to two parameters: the degree and nature of cultural impact and whether the syndromes are specific. It should be noted that although many of the syndromes manifest special clinical features and are therefore called specific syndromes, some are, rather, mixed syndromes or have nonspecific clinical conditions from a phenomenological standpoint. However, the latter are still included as culture-related syndromes because they are heavily related to cultural impact, mainly through pathoreactive effects.

Based on the suggested groupings, various kinds of culture-related syndromes, either specific or nonspecific, will be discussed in detail in the following section. If there is clinical material available, case vignettes are added to illustrate and clarify the syndromes.

II. VARIOUS KINDS OF CULTURE-RELATED SPECIFIC SYNDROMES

A. CULTURE-RELATED BELIEFS AS CAUSES OF THE OCCURRENCE

1. Koro *(Genital-Retraction Anxiety Disorder)*

a. Definition and Historical Review

Koro refers to the clinical condition in which the patient is morbidly concerned that his penis is shrinking excessively and dangerous consequences (such as death) might occur. The manifested symptoms may vary from simple excessive concern to obsessive/hypochondriac concern, intense anxiety, or a panic condition. Clinically, this is usually a benign (nonpsychotic) condition that occurs in individual, sporadic cases, but occasionally it may grow to epidemic proportions. The majority of cases are young males who fear that their penises are shrinking, but the organ concerned may be any protruding part of the body, such as the nose or ear (particularly when patients are prepuberty children) or the nipples or labia (in females). The patient may simply be concerned that his penis is shrinking, with some vague idea that there may be ill results, but some believe specifically that excessive shrinking of the penis into the abdomen may result in death. Therefore, they panic, anxiously seeking life-saving remedies (see Fig. 13-3). Based on local folk beliefs, different treatments may be undertaken. For example, the patient might drink a hot substance, such as ginger juice or chili pepper jam, to supplement the needed yang element; physically hold or pull the shrinking organ, to avoid the fatal effect; or make noise to chase away the possessing evil — if he or she believes that the attack is the result of possession by an evil spirit.

Koro is a Malay term of uncertain origin, which means "to shrink." The related Malay words *kuro* and *kurg,* meaning tortoise, have been suggested as possible origins (Gwee, 1968; van Wulfften Palthe, 1934).

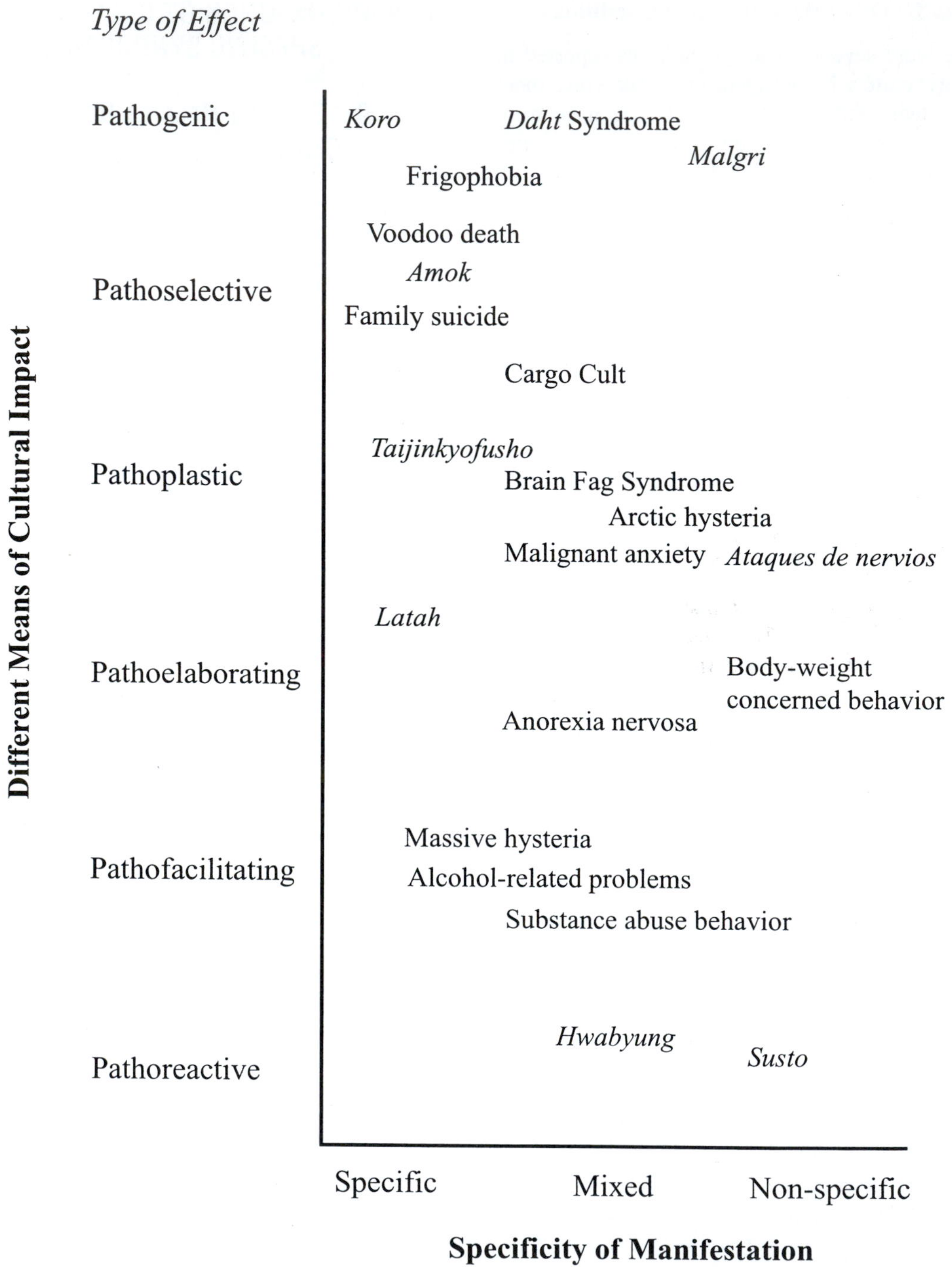

Type of Effect

Different Means of Cultural Impact				
Pathogenic	*Koro*	*Daht* Syndrome		
			Malgri	
		Frigophobia		
Pathoselective	Voodoo death			
	Amok			
	Family suicide			
		Cargo Cult		
Pathoplastic	*Taijinkyofusho*			
		Brain Fag Syndrome		
		Arctic hysteria		
		Malignant anxiety	*Ataques de nervios*	
	Latah			
Pathoelaborating			Body-weight concerned behavior	
		Anorexia nervosa		
Pathofacilitating	Massive hysteria			
	Alcohol-related problems			
		Substance abuse behavior		
Pathoreactive		*Hwabyung*	*Susto*	
	Specific	Mixed	Non-specific	

Specificity of Manifestation

FIGURE 13-2   Position of culture-related syndromes according to two parameters.

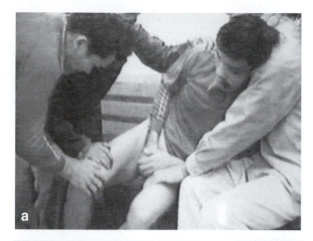

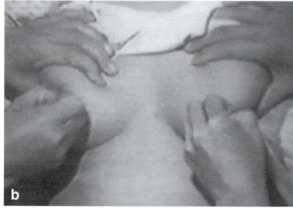

FIGURE 13-3 *Koro* in southern China. (a) During an epidemic in Leizhou Peninsula in 1985, a Chinese man, suffered from a *koro* panic attack, shouting for help in the fear that his penis would shrink into his abdomen and he might die, while his wife and friends tried to "rescue" him. (b) A Chinese female, suspected to be suffering from *koro,* was "rescued" by her female friends, who held her and pulled at her "shrinking" nipples. [Courtesy of Mo Gan-Ming, M.D.].

Both the Malays and the Chinese use the head of a tortoise to symbolize the penis. The Chinese use the term *suo-yang* (in Mandarin, literally, shrinking of the yang organ, i.e., the penis) to refer to the condition. The most ancient and traditional Chinese medical book, *Huang-Di Nei-Jing* (Yellow Emperor's Classic of Internal Medicine), believed to have been written around 200–300 B.C., states that "As *yang* (the male

genital) retracts into the abdomen, death is inevitable" (Tseng et al., 1988). Some traditional physicians later interpreted this brief statement, which was perhaps merely describing the sign of a terminal condition, as the fatal disease *suo* (or *suoyang*), caused by the shrinking of the penis or other protruding (yang) organs. In laymen's minds, it provoked the idea that the shrinking of the penis is dangerous and any means should be utilized to stop it from occurring.

According to Chinese psychiatrists from Gunazhou, G.M. Mo and associates (1987), an 1862 record was found in the local chronicle, *Ya-zhou Zhi,* of the Ya state, on Hainan Island in southern China, which stated that: "In the eleventh year of the Xinyou regime in the Qing dynasty (1862), *suo* illness had spread; men's genitalia shrank, females' breasts, ears, tongues, or other protruding parts shrank. To rub with ginger or set firecrackers off will stop it." Hainan Island is well known as a place where *suoyang* epidemics have occurred in the past. This is probably the earliest record of the *suoyang (koro)* epidemic disorder.

According to Edwards (1985), the term *koro* was first introduced by J.C. Blonk to Western science in 1895, referring to a malady indigenous to southern Sulawesi (an island of Indonesia, formerly known as Celebes). A brief spate of articles appeared in the 1930s (such as van Wulfften Palthe, 1934), but it was not until the 1960s when Gwee (1963) in Singapore and Yap (1965) in Hong Kong used the term in their articles that *koro* become popular among psychiatrists as a culture-related specific syndrome.

In addition to using the folk terms *koro* or *suoyang* to refer to this disorder, there is also a tendency to use English terms, such as "genital retraction syndrome" (Chowdhury, 1994; Edwards, 1985) or "impotence panic" (Tseng & McDermott, 1981). However, these terms do not accurately convey the nature of the disorder. For instance, "genital retraction syndrome" implies that the patient is actually suffering from the retraction of the genital organ. In fact, the patient does not have such a physiological or psychophysiological disorder. Nothing happens to the organ, rather it is an anxiety disorder in which the patient develops a psychological fear, anxiety, or panic reaction, believing that his genital organ may morbidly retract, with serious consequences. Thus, it will be referred to here as "genital-retraction anxiety disorder" to describe it accurately from a nosological point of view.

b. Case Illustration

Case A (abstracted from Rin, 1965) — Mr. A, a 32-year-old single Chinese cook, originally from Hankow in central China, migrated to Taiwan in 1945 (when mainland China was taken over by the communists) and visited a psychiatric clinic with complaints of panic attacks and somatic symptoms of palpitations, breathlessness, numbness of limbs, and dizziness. One month prior to his visit, he had seen a traditional Chinese herb doctor, who diagnosed him as suffering from *shenkui* ("kidney deficiency," indicating insufficient vitality) and prescribed the drinking of a young boy's first-morning urine and eating human placenta as a way to supply *qi* (vitality). Around this time, the patient began to notice his penis shrinking and withdrawing into his abdomen, usually a day or two after having sexual intercourse with a prostitute. He became anxious about the condition and ate excessively to relieve intolerable hunger pangs.

The patient's history revealed that he had been brought up in a small town on the Yang-zi River. The eldest of five sons, he was his mother's favorite child. He had little contact with his father, who worked on a junk and was seldom at home. His father died of an unknown disease when the patient was 7. His mother remarried, but the stepfather disliked the patient and frequently abused him physically.

Under these circumstances, the patient became an apprentice barber at age 11, and started to learn cooking when he was 16. He was soon able to support himself, but he spent most of his earnings gambling and in brothels, upsetting his mother greatly. At the age of 18, he worked as a cook on a steamboat. According to the patient, because of excessive masturbation, he became emaciated. He took more than 20 kinds of herb medicines, with no relief, until he followed the

herb doctor's suggestion and started drinking his own first urine every morning, which cured him in 4 months.

After he migrated to Taiwan at the age of 22, he worked in a bakery, and once again started gambling and going to brothels when he lost his money. For several years he had sexual intercourse every night to relieve the mounting sexual tension. The thought of saving money and marrying never occurred to him.

At age 30, he had his first attack of breathlessness and palpitations. A physical examination by a modern physician showed nothing, and he was given a vitamin B injection. He wandered from one doctor to another for vitamin injections, believing that they supplemented a vital element for him. Later, he consulted the herb doctor, and was warned that he was suffering from *shenkui* and would eventually die if he continued going to prostitutes.

Almost irresistible sexual desire seized him whenever he felt slightly better, yet he experienced strange "empty" feelings in his abdomen when he had sexual intercourse. He often found his penis shrinking into his abdomen, became very anxious, and held on to his penis in terror. Following the herb doctor's prescription, for 4 months he drank a cup of his own urine each morning, and this helped him a great deal.

Case B (a female case from an epidemic episode, Tseng et al., 1988) — Ms. B was 20 years old and living in a remote village in Leizhou Peninsula, Guanzhou, China, when the epidemic occurred there in 1985. Both her mother and father died when she was young. She lived with her aunt for a year or so but was mistreated and was later adopted by foster parents. When she reached 20, her foster parents arranged for her to marry a young man she did not know. For 2 weeks before the wedding, following the local custom, she was joined by her female friends to cry in the evening — a ritual to express sorrow at leaving her family of origin. But she cried very loudly, with genuine tears, thinking about her pitiful past experiences and her future as the wife of a poor groom.

Ms. B's nightly crying coincided with the spread of the *suoyang* epidemic in the neighboring villages. Villagers were already apprehensive about the speading of a *suoyang* attack from one village to another. Upon observing that the girl cried so seriously and endlessly, the people in the village became suspicious that she might be bewitched by a female ghost and wanted to examine her breasts for symptoms of *suoyang (koro)*.

The day of the wedding, when she was escorted to the sedan-chair to be carried to the groom's house, she became pale and fainted. The people surrounding her immediately assumed that she was possessed by the fox ghost that causes *suoyang*. They tried to pull her nipples to prevent them from shrinking. A fishnet was placed over her head and she was beaten with a green tree branch (which was believed to contain the yang element) to exorcise the evil spirit until she shouted loudly that she was not possessed by any evil ghost.

The marriage ceremony was held after her recovery 10 days later. The marriage went well, without any complications, and she gave birth to a baby a year later.

c. Common Clinical Manifestation

Most of the sporadic *koro* cases involve young male patients, who are mostly single — as illustrated by case A. At the core of the symptoms is the concern that the penis is shrinking or is going to retract into the abdomen. There may be an accompanying fear of impending death. Based on the severity of the fear, clinically the patient may manifest anxiety, hypochondriacal concern, or a panic state, with some somatic complaints. In sporadic cases, the condition may become chronic, but in epidemic cases, it is usually transient, with full recovery.

Sporadic occurrences of female *koro* cases have never been reported. However, in *koro* epidemics, a small portion of the victims may be female (Chowdhury, 1994; Tseng et al., 1988). In those cases, the female patients demonstrate slightly different clinical pictures, mainly focusing on the retraction of the nipples and some on the labia. The clinical condition is characterized by a more or less hysterical panic, associated with multiple somatic symptoms; a bewitched feeling or, as shown in case B, the misinterpretation or accusation by others of being bewitched may occur during an epidemic.

d. Geographical and Ethnic Group Distribution

Cultural psychiatrists originally considered *koro* (or *suoyang*) to be a culture-bound disorder related only to the Chinese (Gwee, 1963, 1968; Rin, 1965; Yap, 1965). The American psychiatrist Kobler, who worked in China after World War II, reported one case that he encountered in 1948 in Fushan (Fatshan), Guangtong. Chinese-Singaporean psychiatrist A. L. Gwee (1963) presented three Chinese-Singaporean cases he observed in Singapore; Yap (1965) reported that he was able to gather 19 (Chinese-Hong Kong) cases in Hong Kong during his 15-year practice there; and Rin (1965) described two cases in Taiwan — with one patient originally from Hankow (Hankou) and the other from Kiangsu (Jiangsu) province, both areas of central China. Tsai (1982), from Guangdong, reported five cases of *suoyang* that he observed over a period of 4 years. It is the general impression that *suoyang* cases are found more in southern China, particularly among the coastal provinces of Fujien, Guangdong, and Hainan, and is relatively rare in northern China. Most Chinese investigators have taken the view that the disorder is related to the Chinese cultural belief in *suoyang*. Gwee (1963), Yap (1965), and Tan (1981) speculated further that the occurrence of *koro* among people in south Asian countries, such as Malay and Indonesia, was the result of Chinese migrants. However, this cultural-diffusion view is doubted now, as *koro* epidemics have been reported in Thailand and India, as well, involving non-Chinese victims.

As a result of the dissemination of knowledge about *koro* as a culture-bound syndrome, there is increased literature reporting so-called *koro* cases from various ethnic groups around the world. For instance, Barrett (1978) reported a 33-year-old engineer, born and living in London, who, after awakening early one morning, suddenly developed an intense feeling of impending doom, associated with the physical awareness that his penis had become very small and was shrinking into his body — a typical *koro* attack. Ang and Weller (1984) described two cases they encountered in the United Kingdom: one an immigrant from the West Indies and the other from

Greece. Both were suffering from schizophrenia with *koro* symptoms, namely the conviction that their penises were shrinking into their abdomens. Ede (1976) reported an Anglo-Saxon Canadian patient who, after having surgery for a coccygel cyst, complained of the distressing symptoms of having difficulty reaching orgasm via masturbation and the feeling that his penis was shrinking.

In Israel, Hes and Nassi (1977) described two cases among Jewish immigrants, one from Yemen and the other from Georgia, Transcaucasia. Chiniwala, Alfonso, Torres, and Lefer (1996) reported that a Muslim west African man, who migrated to New York from Guinea, developed an acute psychotic condition associated with the belief that his penis was retracting into his body. His psychotic onset coincided with the holy month of Ramadan and was an expression of guilt over having had sex with prostitutes.

Berrios and Morley (1984) reviewed literature that described *koro*-like symptoms in a total of 15 non-Chinese subjects. They pointed out that among the cases reported, all suffered from many psychiatric conditions: affective disorders, nonaffective psychoses (schizophrenia), and anxiety disorders, as well as drug abuse and organic brain disorders. They referred to the cases as having "*koro*-like symptoms," which is not exactly the same as the "*koro* syndrome" presented by Chinese patients. Reviewing the *koro* symptoms presented by the Canadian patient, Ede (1976) explained that the Chinese *koro* cases from South Asia usually present "typical" conditions, including three cardinal manifestations: a feeling of the penis shrinking into the abdomen, severe anxiety, and the belief in ultimate death if the penis should disappear into the abdomen. He pointed out that non-Asian patients usually manifest *koro*-like *symptoms,* but not the "typical" koro *syndrome.*

e. Subgrouping of Clinical Phenomena

The above discussion makes it clear that we need to recognize that *"koro"* is referred to on different levels or according to different subgroups, as follows.

1. *Koro* (genital-retraction concern/anxiety) as a **symptom.** Genital shrinkage is presented merely as a concern, or as a part of other anxious, depressive, or delusional symptoms. It is *symptomatic* in nature. There is usually a primary or cardinal psychiatric disorder, either a psychosis or an affective or anxiety disorder. The symptoms themselves are probably global, reflecting the common human experience of anxiety without cultural impact (Adeniran & Jones, 1994).

2. *Koro* (genital-retraction anxiety/panic) as a **syndrome.** The fear of the penis shrinking is the cardinal picture of the syndrome. Based on this fear, the patient manifests various symptoms of anxiety, hypochondriac tendencies, or even a panic condition. Underlying his fear is the belief or conviction that if the genital organ shrinks excessively, it will result in a serious, and possibly fatal, outcome. Therefore, the patient becomes overly sensitive and anxious, with obsessive concerns about his genital condition, and even panics. The patient may seek folk remedies to avoid the fatal consequence. His beliefs may seem "delusional" and his behavior "strange," however, if viewed from the standpoint of a cultural belief system, they will "make sense" from an emic point of view. Clinically, they are considered "neurotic" in nature (as defined in the past) and not psychotic — not out of touch with "reality." The course of this syndrome may be benign and brief or it may be chronic. One thing is clear: the syndrome is psychogenic and strongly related to cultural beliefs in the etiological formation of and reaction to the illness. It may, after careful analysis, illustrate certain personality predispositions (such as a dependency pattern and insecure feelings about the self) as well as a personal background that indicates psychosexual developmental problems or sexual adjustment difficulty.

3. *Koro* (genital-retraction panic/hysteria) as an **epidemic disorder.** A *koro* endemic or epidemic is hysterical in nature. Most victims develop transient *koro* panic through a contagious process, influenced by other victims or the surrounding atmosphere (see Fig. 14-3). *Koro* as an epidemic disorder is primarily manifested as a panic reaction in a single attack, but, for some, it may be recurrent. Most of the victims are

considered "normal" in terms of premorbid conditions. After recovery from the attack, most of them regain their original conditions quickly, without any sequels. There is hardly any sign of preexisting psychosexual problems. Social stress is the primary reason for the occurrence, whether interracial conflict, fear of an outside enemy, or pending natural disaster. Cultural belief is the foundation for the occurrence and spreading of the morbid condition (Tseng et al., 1988). From a social psychological perspective, Bartholomew (1994b) suggested to view koro epidemic as a collective misperception (rather than a syndromes) — a rational attempt at problem-solving [cross-reference to Chapter 14: Epidemic Mental Disorders (Section III,A)].

f. Theoretical Considerations

According to Edwards (1985), as soon as the *koro* case was reported in literature by Blonk in 1895, it rapidly engendered psychoanalytic interpretations by other colleagues (such as Brero, 1896). Due to its focus on the male genital organ, castration anxiety was one of the natural dynamic speculations made by some clinicians (Kobler, 1948; Rin, 1965).

Among the Chinese, as Wen (1995) pointed out, *suoyang* as a genital-retraction anxiety disorder can be viewed as a part of a cluster of culture-related sexual-somato-anxiety disorders that includes *nao-shenjing shuairuo* (brain neurasthenia), *shenkui* (kidney-deficiency disorder), and *pa leng* (frigophobia). These morbid conditions, although manifested symptomatically in different ways, share the common underlying concern with the weakness or vulnerability of a person (lacking vitality or yang deficiency). They can also be considered part of a pathological spectrum, including various hidden psychosexual disorders. These concerns are based on two interrelated cultural beliefs: (1) the yin and yang theory, according to which excessive loss of the yang element (through semen discharge) will result in sickness, and (2) that an evil spirit, such as the fox spirit, wanting the yang element, may disguise itself as a pretty young female who seduces a male to obtain his yang element. A man seduced by

such an evil spirit will become sick and even die from the excessive loss of his yang element — a common theme that appears frequently in the folk ghost stories of *Liao-Zhai* (see Fig. 13-4).

Similarly, Carstairs (1956) has suggested that the *dhat* syndrome and *koro* share a common pathology: the former concerned with the excessive leaking of semen, the latter the retraction of the genital organ — both vulnerable conditions for a man.

g. Clinical Implications

i. Diagnostic Considerations   Clinicians habitually try and fit pathologies into certain diagnostic categories. However, as explained previously, when we try to categorize culture-related specific syndromes according to the existing nosologically oriented classification system, their meaning and purpose are lost. However, in order to satisfy professional curiosity and clarify the concept, some comments will be made here, from a diagnostic point of view, regarding *koro,* or genital-retraction anxiety disorder.

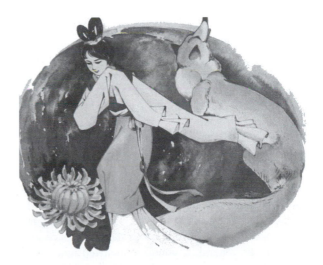

FIGURE 13-4   Picture from the Chinese folk ghost story of *Liao-Zhai* about an evil fox spirit disguised as a pretty woman who seduces young men, absorbing their yang element—the core concept associated with *suoyang (koro)* problems.

Because the patient, based on "misinterpretation" (from an etic point of view), is morbidly preoccupied with the idea that certain ill effects may occur due to the excessive retraction of his genital organ, the condition may, in a broad sense, be classified as a hypochondriac disorder as defined in DSM-IV. The condition is also similar to a body dysmorphic disorder, as the patient is preoccupied with a culturally induced, imagined defect in his physical condition. If the focus is on how the patient reacts emotionally — how he responds to the culture-genic stress, with fear, anxiety, or a panic state — anxiety disorder may be considered. Although depersonalization was originally proposed by Yap (1965), most cases do not exhibit such altered states of consciousness.

Also, as elaborated earlier (Section III,A,e), *koro* may merely refer to a symptom or may imply a syndrome. In the former case, certain psychiatric disorders can usually be identified, including psychoses or other psychiatric disorders. In the latter, *koro* appears as the cardinal feature within the anxiety, hypochondriac disorder, or panic state. Thus, various diagnoses may be given, depending on the major clinical manifestations of each case. *Koro* can manifest as an endemic or epidemic situation in which the clinical manifestation is predominated by a panic state or a hysterical attack. Categorization into existing classifications will vary accordingly. In summary, if the clinical symptomatology is focused on making a diagnosis, as it is in DSM-IV, various diagnostic categories can be considered (Chowdhury, 1996; Rubin 1982).

ii. Therapy for Sporadic Individual Cases

Assurance may be provided or medical knowledge offered in the form of educational counseling to eliminate the patient's concern about impending death. This supportive therapy may work in many cases, but for someone who firmly believes the *koro* concept, it may not. In general, a young, unmarried male, who lacks adequate psychosexual knowledge and experience, will respond favorably to therapy. If necessary, it is desirable to work on issues such as the patient's self-image, self-confidence, or his masculinity.

iii. Management and Prevention of Epidemics

Because the epidemics usually occur in a hysterical, contagious manner, the distruption of the panic atmosphere in the community is critical. Educational guides and assurance of the laymen in the society are essential in stopping the spread of epidemic [cross-reference to Chapter 14: Epidemic Mental Disorders (Section III,A)].

2. Dhat *Syndrome (Semen-Loss Anxiety)*

Very closely related to the genital-retraction anxiety disorder (*koro*) is the semen-loss or semen-leaking anxiety disorder, or spermatorrhea, also known by its Indian folk name, *dhat* syndrome. According to Indian psychiatrists Bhatia and Malik (1991), the word *dhat* derives from the Sanskrit *Dhatu,* which refers to the elixir that constitutes the body. Of the seven types of *Dhatus* described, semen is considered the most important. In the Indian system of medicine, *Ayurveda,* it is suggested that disturbances in the *Dhatus* result in an increased susceptibility to physical and mental disease.

The term "*dhat* syndrome" was first used by the Indian psychiatrist N.N. Wig in 1960 and by J.S. Neki in 1973. The syndrome refers to the clinical condition in which the patient is morbidly preoccupied with the excessive loss of semen from an "improper form of leaking," such as nocturnal emissions, masturbation, or urination. The underlying anxiety is based on the cultural belief that excessive semen loss will result in illness. Therefore, it is a pathogenically induced psychological disorder. The medical term "spermatorrhea" is a misnomer, as there is no actual problem of sperm leakage from a urological point of view.

From a clinical point of view, the patients are predominantly young males who present vague, multiple somatic symptoms such as fatigue, weakness, anxiety, loss of appetite, and feelings of guilt (about having indulged in sexual acts such as masturbation or having sex with prostitutes). Some also complain of sexual dysfunction (impotence or premature ejaculation). The chief complaint is often that the urine is opaque, which is attributed to the presence of semen (Paris,

1992). The patient attributes the passing of semen in the urine to his excessive indulgence in masturbation or other socially defined sexual improprieties (Bhatia & Malik, 1991). Clinically, the patient is characterized as anxious or hypochondriacal. As part of the illness behavior, the patient will ask the physician to examine his urine to determine whether there is leaking of semen or not. The patient also always asks for a tonic or other remedy to regain the vitality lost due to excess leakage of semen.

According to Bhatia and Malik (1991), the syndrome is also widespread in Nepal, Sri Lanka (where it is referred to as *prameha* disease), Bangladesh, and Pakistan. In Taiwan, Wen (1995) considers *shenkui* ("kidney deficiency," or insufficient vitality due to excessive loss of semen), prevalent among young Taiwanese men, as the counterpart of the *dhat* syndrome observed among the Chinese. The *shenkui* disorder in traditional medical terminology is often considered equivalent to the neurasthenia referred to by modern Chinese psychiatrists.

Whether it is called the *dhat* syndrome in India, *prameha* in Sri Lanka, or *shenkui* in China, there is a common characteristic among these syndromes: they are based on folk beliefs that excessive loss of semen will result in illness. Akhtar (1988) pointed out that according to the religious scriptures of the Hindus, "Forty meals produce one drop of blood, 40 drops of blood give rise to one drop of bone marrow, and 40 drops of marrow form one drop of semen." Variations on this saying are found in the other cultures where semen-loss anxiety disorder is observed. These cultural beliefs that conservation of vitality is important and loss of semen is harmful to the health create culture-genic stress and contribute to the formation of semen-loss anxiety.

It should be explained that the concept of conserving semen as the main resource of vitality is not specific to Asian culture (Bottéro, 1991). Nocturnal emissions were also considered symptoms of excessive venery in European society during the 19th century. However, as noted by Malhotra and Wig (1975), Asian culture condemns all types of orgasms because they involve semen loss and are therefore "dangerous." In contrast, the Judo-Christian cultures of the 18th and 19th centuries in Europe considered most types of sexual activities outside marriage to be "sinful."

3. Frigophobia

a. Description of the Condition

"Frigophobia," or "morbid fear of catching cold," is a clinical condition described by Chinese psychiatrists as a culture-related syndrome of the Chinese (Rin, 1966). In Chinese (Mandarin) it is called *pa-len* or *wei-han* (literally, fear of cold). Such a morbid condition is not very prevalent. Only sporadic cases have been reported since attention was given to the condition as a culture-bound syndrome. Chang, Rin, & Chen reported five cases in Taiwan in 1975; Chiou, Liu, Chen, and Yang cited two cases in 1994. Among the five cases reported by Chang and colleagues, four of the subjects were born in various parts of mainland China and migrated to Taiwan after the mainland was taken over by the communists. Up to now, few reports from mainland China have appeared in literature. Perhaps professional attention has not been paid to the disorder there as a culture-related specific disorder.

This unique disorder is characterized by the patient's excessive concern with and morbid fear of catching cold. According to Chinese traditional theory of yin and yang, an imbalance between yin and yang will result in disorders. Excessive yin, caused by cold air or excessive eating of cold food (such as watermelon), will result in weakness and sickness. The chilling sensation of cold sweat is interpreted as a sign of weakness due to excessive yin. Based on these folk concepts, even ordinary people will avoid cold air, cold rain, eating too much cold food, and will wear belly bands around their abdomens to protect them from catching cold, particularly in cold whether.

At the extreme of this concern, a patient who develops frigophobia will overdress in warm clothes (even in hot weather), wearing a heavy hat to protect his head, surrounding his neck with a warm neckerchief, and wearing many layers of clothing to keep his body from catching cold. In an extreme case, the patient will wrap himself up with a blanket or heavy quilt and stay in bed, afraid to go outside and be exposed to the cold air.

Clinical examination of patients often reveals psychiatric manifestations of depression, hypochondriasis, phobia, and anxiety with panic tendency, in addition to the morbid fear of catching cold. In other words, the morbid fear of cold is part of a compound clinical picture rather than the total picture. However, because of the patient's excessive concern with and fear of catching cold, many "odd" maneuvers for protecting the body from catching cold, including inappropriate heavy dress, become so obvious that frigophobia becomes a prominent part of the clinical condition and warrants such a specific diagnosis. The personal histories in such cases often reveal that, during their early lives, the subjects were overprotected by their mothers and developed anxious or dependent personalities. The fear of catching cold usually developed as a reaction to a crisis or a significant loss in the patient's life that provoked feelings of insecurity.

b. Case Illustration

Case A (abstracted from Tseng & Hsu, 1969/1970) — Mr. A was born the eldest and only son of a rich, traditional, extended family. He slept with his grandmother until the age of 11 and was babied by her. Like every Chinese mother and grandmother, she was concerned with his bodily health, especially his warmth. She kept him overdressed and wearing a belly band even in adult life. He was not permitted to leave the bed at night. Arrangements were made for him to urinate into a chamber pot until he was 11 years old as a precaution against catching cold.

When he was grown up, borrowing power from his father, he became a general when he was only in his early 30s. It was arranged for him to marry a woman older than himself, whereas it is usual for a Chinese man to marry a younger woman. His family thought that an older woman would take good care of him. Because of wealth and social status, he was later able to have several concubines. When the communists took over mainland China, he fled to Taiwan, taking with him only his money and one of his concubines.

Several years later, he learned that his father had been persecuted by the communists and his mother had died of sickness after the tragedy. This precipitated his first attack of frigophobia when he was 35. He presented himself at the hospital in the heat of the summer swathed in many layers of clothing and quilts and complaining of feeling cold (see Fig. 13-5a). He did not complain of feelings of sadness, loneliness, or depression. Similar attacks occurred twice more, each time following a loss. In one instance it was a loss of money, in the other the loss of his concubine.

Case B (abstracted from Chang et al., 1975, case #2) — Mrs. B was a 47-year-old married woman. She was born to an affluent farmer in Guandong. She was the youngest of five children. For reasons unknown to her, she was adopted by her foster mother when she was very young. She recalled that her foster mother had been very fond of her since her childhood. The foster mother suffered from asthma attacks, usually at night, and the patient, as a young girl, always tried to take care of her. After finishing normal school, Mrs. B became a schoolteacher. At the age of 21, due to the civil war in China, she evacuated to Taiwan with her husband, leaving her two young children in her hometown. After settling down in Taiwan, she had several miscarriages. Later, she finally gave birth to two daughters. However, when Mrs. B was 34, her youngest daughter, at 4 years old, died from illness. Mrs. B reacted to this loss severely, blaming herself. One year later, she caught cold after having a stillbirth. Since then, she began to be afraid of catching cold. She usually covered her head with a woolen cap, wrapped her neck with a towel, and held several thick cloths in front of her chest to keep her body warm (see Fig. 13-5b). She used her hand to cover her mouth while she was talking, for fear that cold air might intrude into it. Her excessive fear of catching cold had become severe during the past 3 years. She often stayed at home, closed the windows tightly, even in the hot summer, for fear that cold air might enter the room. She often hid under a quilt, asking doctors to make home visits to give her injections to supply her with nutrients or tonics. She was very concerned that she was losing her vitality through chills and sweating.

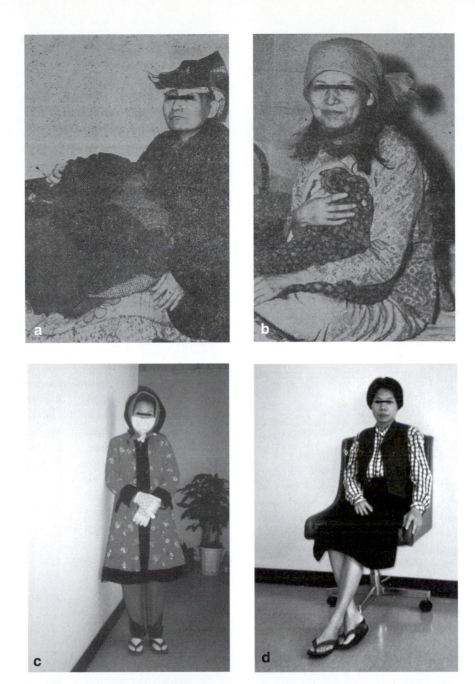

FIGURE 13-5   Frigophobia reported from Taiwan. (a) Case A: wearing a wool hat and a cotton-padded overcoat and covering his body with quilts during the hot summer for fear of catching cold. (b) Case B: covering her head with a wool scarf, wrapping her neck with a towel, and holding heavy clothes to protect her throat and abdomen from catching cold while ordinary people are wearing short-sleeved summer clothes. [From *Bulletin of the Chinese Society of Neurology and Psychiatry, 1* (2), 1975. Courtesy of Yen-Huei Chang, M.D.] (c) Case C: wearing heavy socks, gloves, a coat, and a face mask to protect herself when she was suffering from a fear of catching cold. (d) Dressed in an ordinary way after recovering from her frigophobia. [Courtesy of Nien-Mu Chiou, M.D.].

From a psychological perspective, it seemed that the patient was suffering from loss, loneliness, and insecurity. However, she believed that her body must be "weak," causing her to experience frequent miscarriages and stillbirths, needing nourishment to supply her body with vitality.

Case C (abstracted from Chiou et al., 1994, case No. 1) — Mrs. C, a 46-year-old divorced woman, called an ambulance for emergency care with chief complaints of fear of cold, palpitations, and cold sweats after she was exposed to cold evening air. Although it was summer, she wore a heavy coat, socks, gloves, and a face mask to protect herself from catching cold (see Fig. 13-5c). She was very anxious and panicky. After admission to the hospital, she requested intrevaenous injections to suppy a tonic element for her "insubstantial" condition.

Her history revealed that she was born in Taiwan, the daughter of a farmer. Her brother suffered from a schizophrenia-like disorder and her sister from an emotional disturbance with a history of suicide attempts. Her father was described as a mean person who lost his temper easily and did not care for children. As a child, Mrs. C did not get along with her family, including her mother, and left home to work as a maid as soon as she finished grade school. She married, had one child, but did not get along with her husband and mother-in-law, and deserted her family. Since then, she had lived alone, had done many kinds of odd jobs to suport herself; but, at the same time, had been frightened by terrifying events many times, such as being robbed, threatened with a knife by a villain, and daunted by a drunken customer at a dance hall where she worked. Nine years before, after her first episode of being terrified, she began to suffer from an extreme fear of catching cold, associated with somatic discomfort such as dizziness or headache. It was her interpretation that she was suffering from a deficiency of vitality and she frequently tried tonics such as *danggui* and *renshen.*

Clinically it was found that she was not depressed. Although she experienced panic-like attacks, the episodes were not frequent enough to be considered primary disorders. Frigophobia with panic feature was

the diagnosis. Loneliness and feelings of insecurity from repeated terrified trauma was considered to be her major problem. In addition to psychotherapy, antidepressants for her panic condition (imipramine and, later, clomipramine) were tried and produced considerable improvement, enabling her to dress in an ordinary way again (see Fig. 13-5d).

c. Elaboration

As pointed out by Chang and associates (1975), as well as Tseng and Hsu (1969/1970), there is a common tendency for Chinese patients to manifest their psychological problems with somatized symptoms. However, in some cases, the somatization is not manifested merely as a somatic symptom, but as an elaborate way of being concerned and complaining about a morbid somatic condition. Fear of catching cold is one such example. The disorder of frigophobia was based on the traditional concepts of hot and cold and folk beliefs about the importance of maintaining vitality, avoiding catching cold, and keeping the body warm to preserve vitality. Even though the disorder is not very prevalent, and only a handful of cases have been collected, these few cases illustrate how basic folk beliefs can model unusual clinical manifestations, such as the tip of an iceberg above the sea. It may be said that loss underlies the two cases illustrated. Instead of manifesting their problems as depression, through the effects of culture, the patients manifest their conditions as a unique and elaborate fear of cold syndrome.

4. Sorcery Fear and Voodoo Death
   (Magic-Fear-Induced Death)

a. Definition

The peculiar phenomena of "voodoo death" refers to the sudden occurrence of death associated with taboo-breaking or curse fear. It is based on the belief in witchcraft — the putative power to bring about misfortune, disability, and even death through "spiritual" mechanisms (Hughes, 1996). If someone breaks a taboo, or is cursed by others, he or she will be punished by death. A severe fear reaction may result from such beliefs, which may actually end in death. From a psychosomatic point of view, it would be psychogenically induced death. From a cultural psychiatric perspective, it is another example of culture-induced morbid fear reaction.

b. Case Report

Case A — A young African man on a journey in the Congo lodged at a friend's house for the night. The friend had prepared a wild hen for their breakfast, a food strictly banned by a local rule that was supposed to be inviolably observed by the young. The young man inquired whether it was indeed a wild hen, and when the host answered, "No," he ate heartily and proceeded on his way. A few years later, when the two met again, the old friend asked the young man if he would eat a wild hen. He answered that he had been solemnly charged by a wizard not to eat that food. Thereupon the host began to laugh and asked him why he refused now after having eaten it at his table before. On hearing this, the young man immediately began to tremble, so greatly was he possessed by fear, and in less than 24 hr he was dead. [According to Cannon (1957), this case was reported by Merolla in his voyage to the Congo in 1682 and was cited by Pinketon (1814).]

Case B — A 33-year-old black man from a rural area near Little Rock, Arkansas, was admitted to a university hospital. The patient had been having seizures recently, becoming irritable, confused, and almost delirious. He was very fearful whenever people approached him and began to hallucinate. All neurological findings, including a brain scan, proved normal. However, after 2 weeks, the patient suffered a cardiac arrest and died. An autopsy provided no reason for the death. After he died, the patient's wife told staff members that her husband had been seeing a "two-headed" — an older woman considered by the local community to be a witch who cast spells. The widow stated that her husband had angered the two-headed and that she had caused his death (Golden, 1977).

c. Clinical Discussion

Modern physicians (Engel, 1971) have recognized sudden death related to psychological stress occurring during experiences of acute grief, the threat of the loss of a close person, personal danger, or other stressful situations. Instead of considering these instances of psychogenic death, there has been speculation on the mechanism of death, for instance, the possibility of death resulting from natural causes coincidentally or the possible use of poisons in association with sorcery or witchcraft. Investigating the medical records and interviewing aboriginal medical field workers in Australia, Eastwell (1982) speculated that the victims, secondary to excessive fear reaction, died from dehydration or existing physical illness, particularly the elderly patients. No matter what the direct cause of death, the psychological fear of sorcery by the victim, his family, or other people around him certainly contributed to the intense emotional fear and fatalistic reactions. Such psychological reactions will in turn contribute to physical ill effects, such as not eating or drinking water, or provoke the aggravation of underlying physical illnesses and become fatal.

A caution is needed in understanding how the concept of sorcery is related to actual deaths. If the malicious results of breaking a taboo or sorcery are firmly believed, they may strongly affect the psychological and physiological condition (psychopathogenetic effect as illustrated by case A). Thus, the cultural belief has a primary role and is directly responsible for the ill effects or deaths. However, the concept of sorcery or malicious magic may be used merely to interpret the occurrence of misfortune. (In case B, the patient might have been suffering from an organic-induced delirious condition associated with psychotic features. His death was primarily due to physical reasons, but cultural belief was used secondarily by his surviving wife to interpret her view of the phenomenon, i.e., pathoreactive effect.)

According to Cannon (1957), voodoo death is widely observed among the natives of Africa, South America, Australia, New Zealand, and the islands of the Pacific. However, this phenomenon is not rare, even in contemporary Americans (Golden, 1977).

5. Malgri *(Territorial Anxiety Syndrome)*

Another interesting psychiatric syndrome attributed to culture-induced stress is the so-called *malgri* originally reported by Australian cultural psychiatrist John Cawte (1976). *Malgri* is a local name for aborigines who inhabit the Wellesley Islands of the Gulf of Carpentaria, Australia. The central theme in *malgri* is a mutual antipathy between land and sea. The local people believe that a person who enters the sea without washing his hands after handling land food runs the risk of succumbing to *malgri*. If the precautions are neglected, the totemic spirit that guards the particular littoral is believed to invade the belly "like a bullet." The victim grows sick, tired, and drowsy. He suffers from headaches, a distended abdomen, and groans in pain. Clinical symptoms cover a range of Western diagnoses. The local people have special remedies to treat this "sickness of intruders." A grass or hair belt is unraveled to provide a long cord, one end of which is tied to the victim's foot, while the other end is run down to the water — to point the way home for the intruding spirit.

Based on a field study of the Yolngu aborigines living on Elcho Island, in Arnhem Land, north Australia, American anthropologist Arthur Hippler also reported a similar (but unnamed) occurrence of territorial anxiety syndrome observed among the Yolngu people. Hippler and Cawte (1978) pointed out that this phenomenon did not seem to be an isolated or localized affliction. It may be necessary to understand it from the standpoint of the cultural personality of a hunter–gatherer–raider society. In the Yolngu culture, the importance of the group in determining behavior is so great that it might be said that most personal controls are externalized. The externalized social controls reflect an internal psychic reality of the Yolngu. The people believe that if you travel to a different area and feed yourself on the food belonging to the people of that area without going through the proper ceremony, you will become sick. Hippler and Cawte raised the view that the malgri territorial anxiety syndrome could be a primitive form of agoraphobia — an insecurity disorder characterized by an unaccountable fear of new places and leaving secure locations.

From a clinical point of view, the basic question of whether the victim's morbid condition occurs as a psychosomatic response to a culture-induced anxiety or is interpreted as the result of breaking a taboo and treated as such is unclear. If it is the former, then *malgri*, as a territorial taboo anxiety disorder, offers another example of a culture-related disorder through pathogenic effects. Otherwise, it may be merely a pathoreactive effect on somatic disorders. This is a question awaiting further investigation.

B. CULTURE-PATTERNED SPECIFIC COPING REACTIONS

1. Amok *(Indiscriminate Mass Homicide Attacks)*

a. The Nature of the Behavior

Amok is a Malay term that means "to engage furiously in battle" (Westermeyer, 1973). Cultural psychiatrist P. M. Yap, who brought attention to this phenomenon as one of the mental diseases "peculiar to certain cultures" (1951), defined *amok* as "an acute outburst of unrestrained violence associated with (indiscriminate) homicidal attacks, preceded by a period of brooding and ending with exhaustion and amnesia." *Amok* homicides are distinct from other murders: The killer chooses an extremely destructive weapon, a crowded location, and insanely and indiscriminately kills a large number of people (Westermeyer, 1972).

Running *amok* has been noticed in Malay in the past and has even been described in a book (see Fig. 13-6a). There has been much speculation as to why *amok* behavior tends to occur in Malay society. One explanation is its connection to the religious background of the people. Muslims are not permitted to commit suicide, which is considered a most heinous act in the Mohammedan religion (Ellis, 1893). Amercian cultural psychiatrist Joseph Westermeyer (1982) has reviewed past explanations about the nature of *amok* from multiple perspectives, including biological, psychological, social, and cultural. Aggressive-

a

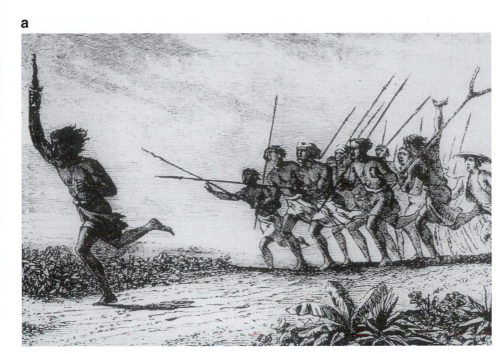
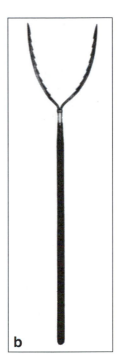

FIGURE 13-6 *Amok* **in Malay.** (a) A picture from an old book showing a Malay man with a knife in his hand running *amok* and being chased by the villagers with weapons. [Artist: George Cohen, from *Running Amok: A Historical Inquiry* by John C. Spores. Reprinted with permission from Ohio University Press, Athens, Ohio.] (b) A specially designed, fork-shaped weapon, kept in a police station in Malaysia in the past, for catching dangerous men who had run *amok*. [Courtesy of Eng-Seong Tan, M.D.].

homicidal behavior influenced by infectious diseases has been considered, along with malaria, dengue, neurosyphilis, epilepsy, and so on, as biological in some cases. From a psychological point of view, an extraordinary sensitivity to hurt and the tendency to blame others for one's own difficulties are considered possible causes for the phenomenon. Loss of social standing — by way of insult, loss of employment, or financial loss — has been posited as a precipitating event for *amok*.

From a cultural perspective, behavioral scientist J. E. Carr (1978) has done a detailed analysis to explain the relation between *amok* behavior and Malay culture. According to Carr, there is a great emphasis on being passive, unemotional, nonconfronting, and obedient in Malay culture. Hence, the people in Malay, especially those in traditional rural areas, are inexperienced and unprepared to cope with social stress in the form of interpersonal confrontation, social or economic frustration, and psychological assault. According to social expectations, a person must comply and withdraw until the conditions for exercising traditional options for retaliation (in the form of *amok*) and subsequent social sanctions (explained as "insanity") are fulfilled. As Carr points out, the culture itself, evolved to reduce tensions, may contribute significantly to the stress of its members. Still, the cultural system does provide, in its own way, the means by which threatening phenomena can be defined and explained, corrective measures applied, and favorable outcomes anticipated. In other words, *amok* behavior is purposive, motivated, and subtly sanctioned coping behavior (Carr & Tan, 1976; Tan & Carr, 1977) by means of pathoselective effects.

Because *amok* is a phenomenon commonly observed in Malay in the past, a special weapon has been designed and placed in all police stations for dealing with *amok* people (see Fig. 13-6b). It is a trident-like weapon in the shape of a two-forked prong attached to a long handle, which allows police to press an *amok* runner against a wall and capture him without having to grapple with him.

b. Psychiatric Examination of Subjects

The Chinese-Malay psychiatrist Een-Seong Tan has had the opportunity to carry out psychiatric examinations of surviving *amok* runners. According to Tan (1965), during a 3-year period (1962–1965) at Tampoi Mental Hospital in Johore Bahru, Malaya, there were 107 remanded criminal cases. Among them, 15 cases involved homicidal behavior. Of these, 5 were recognized as *amok* cases, and all were diagnosed as schizophrenia. As mental health specialists of the South Pacific commission, Schmidt, Hill, & Guthrie (1977) were able to study 24 cases of *amok* found between 1958 and 1969 in Sarawak, east Malaysia. According to them, all of the subjects warranted psychiatric diagnoses that included paranoid schizophrenia (7 cases); paranoia and endogenous depression (3 cases each); chronic schizophrenia, anxiety reaction, and neurosyphilis (2 cases each); and paranoid reaction, paranoid personality, involutional melancholia, manic-depression, and epilepsy (1 case each). As they pointed out, it is apparent that *amok* behavior does not appear in conjunction with one specific psychiatric disorder. Because many of the people who run *amok* may be killed during their violent behavior, there is no opportunity to examine them. Only those who are caught alive are available for psychiatric assessment. Therefore, there is no way to clinically assess the kind of people *amok* runners are as a whole.

c. Evolution of the Phenomenon

The Chinese-Malay cultural psychiatrist Jin-Inn Teoh (1972) raised the issue of the changing psychopathology of *amok*. He reviewed the early litera-

ture and reported that a British administrator in Malay, Swettenham, noted in 1895 that the *amok* state was the war cry of Malay pirates in the "olden days"; plunder was their object and their action was socially allowed and regarded as honorable. In 1893, the medical superintendent of the lunatic asylum in Singapore, W. G. Ellis, recorded that, because of the high frequency of *amok,* an English judge in 1864 posed the question of whether an *amok* runner should be apprehended and hanged. This resulted in legislation in 1893 in Penang that ruled all *amok* subjects should be apprehended and tried in court. From that date onward, the rate of *amok* behavior dropped markedly. Teoh pointed out that, in Malay, as a result of negative sanctions by society, the clinical picture of *amok* has evolved from a deliberate, conscious, frenzied, socially tolerated attack to an unconsciously motivated psychiatric disorder.

A Canadian cultural psychiatrist who has worked in south Asia, H. B. M. Murphy (1973), also did an extensive historical review of *amok* in Malay society. Murphy's opinion supported Teoh's view that the *amok* syndrome showed a historical evolution over a 400-year period. During the 16th and 18th centuries in southeast Asia, reports of the behavior indicated that the *amok* runner initiated his actions consciously and deliberately; that there was very often a connection between some precipitating event and the episode; that he often undertook the action as political terrorism, attacking only identified "enemy-subjects" and avoiding injuring his own relatives and friends; that no signs of mental illness were noted before or after the *amok* attack; and that society often saw such an individual as an invincible hero and gave approval to his acts. During the first half of the 19th century, the nature of the behavior seemed to change. An *amok* episode became sudden and unpremeditated; the mass killings occurred in a dissociated state, with subsequent amnesia. Since the latter half of the 19th century, the frequency of *amok* has declined, *amok* runners have much more frequently had a history of long-term psychosis, and *amok* has become a manifestation of psychoses rather than the act of a normal individual or the result of a dissociated reaction.

Because much of this behavior is unrecorded, it is difficult to estimate the frequency of *amok* observed in a society, particularly from a historical perspective. Teoh (1972) managed to review the *amok* cases that were reported in the *Straits Times Press,* the major English newspaper of Malaysia, in the period 1935 to 1970. He found that by dividing the years into 5-year cohorts, the number of cases reported were as follows: 12 (1993–1939), 2 (1940–1944), 22 (1945–1949), 26 (1950–1954), 42 (1955–1959), 40 (1960–1964), and 45 (1965–1970). Although a caution is needed — because the numbers show the cases "reported" in the newspaper and not necessarily the actual cases — it is noted that the number of reported cases increased during the past four decades. At least, this is evidence that *amok* is still prevalent in Malaysia. Also, during World War II, the number of reported cases dropped sharply, to only 2 between 1940 and 1944. This follows the general observation that the incidence of suicide and homicidal behavior within a society declines during wartime.

The most important finding revealed by Teoh (1972) is that, although in the past *amok* occurred among indigenous Malay people, recently, beginning in the 1940s, Malay people comprised only 46.2% of the subjects reported in this survey, ethnic Chinese 44.5%, and Indians and other ethnic groups 9.3%. This illustrates that the phenomenon has occurred among residents of different ethnic origins in the same Malay society. This also supports the notion that reacting to emotional frustration with violent homicidal behavior becomes a culturally selected, shaped, and available (if not sanctioned) coping mechanism utilized by residents cross-ethnically. Most investigators agree that *amok* may serve as a socially prescribed escape from an irremediable problem (Burton-Bradley, 1968; Westermeyer, 1972).

d. Amok Behavior in Other Areas

The outburst of aggressive (mass) homicidal behavior is not necessarily confined to one cultural area, but can potentially be observed elsewhere. As the only psychiatrist available in the territory of Papua and New Guinea, B. G. Burton-Bradley (1968) reported seven cases of *amok* syndrome that he observed over his 8-year service there, between 1960 and 1968. His report challenged the notion that *amok* is culturally bound to Malay society.

In 1972, the American cultural psychiatrist J. Westermeyer, after serving as a consultant to Laos for many years, studied a total of 32 homicidal cases. Among them, 20 were considered *amok* cases. By comparing *amok* and non-*amok* homicidal cases from this cohort, he pointed out that *amok* homicides can be distinguished from other homicides by objective criteria, such as the large number killed and/or wounded, the choice of weapon used (*amok* generally involves the use of the most destructive ordnance available), and the choice of a crowded location. He further indicated that despite similarities in premorbid personality and other personal factors, as well as the precipitating event, the outcomes for the two groups differ markedly. The non-*amok* homicidal person, after killing one or two people, is usually arrested and ends up in prison, whereas *amok* involves an average of 10 victims and the *amok* person generally commits suicide.

Reviewing the *amok* behavior reported in various societies, including Thailand, the Philippines, Malaysia, and Indonesia, plus his own field observations in Laos, Westermeyer (1973) challenged the previous view that *amok* occurs endemically within a particular society. He indicated that *amok* could happen in a fashion by "communicability" and through "transmission" from one population to another. He also pointed out that *amok* homicide tends to wax and wane in epidemic proportions over time. During periods of momentous political, social, and economic upheaval there could be increased rates of *amok* in a society.

During the past decade in the United States, there have been increasing episodes of massive (and aimless) killing of people in neighborhoods, workplaces, and of teachers/students in schools by deadly military weapons. The episodes are occurring so frequently, in such a "fashionable" manner, that they have caused anxious concern in many communities. These are American versions of *amok* attacks.

2. Family Suicide

a. Brief Description

When parents encounter severe difficulty (such as financial debt or a disgraceful event), they may decide to commit suicide together with their young children. This stress-coping method is based on the cultural belief that it would be disgraceful to live after a shameful thing had happened and that the shame would be relieved by ending one's life. This is coupled with the belief that the children, if left as orphans, would be mistreated by others. Therefore, it would be better for them to die with their parents. This unique way of solving problems by dying together as a family was often observed in Japan in the past and even continues at present [cross-reference to Chapter 22: Suicide Behavior (Section III,A,2)].

b. Case Reports (from Japanese Newspapers)

Case A — Mr. A borrowed some money from friends for investments, hoping that he would be able to return it soon. However, his investments failed, and there was no way to return the money. He tried to get help from his relatives, but was refused. He decided to commit suicide to pay for his mistake. When he explained the situation to his wife, she indicated her wish to die with him. As a result, they planned a family suicide, asking their 14-year-old son and 7-year-old daughter to sit with them in their car, where they would die together from exhaust fumes (see Fig. 13-7a).

Case B — In order to buy a house, Mr. and Mrs. B borrowed money from a loan shark because the mortage they obtained from the bank was not enough.

a

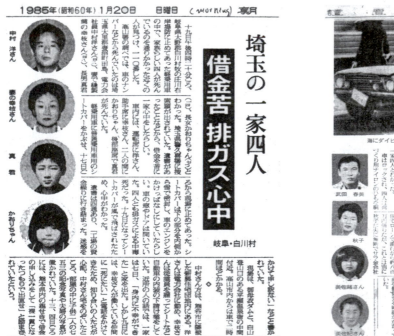

b

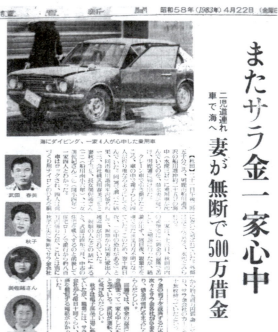

FIGURE 13-7 Family suicide in Japan. (a) Case A: a husband and wife and their son and daughter died together from their car exhaust fumes because they were unable to pay their debts. (b) Case B: parents and their two daughters commited suicide together by driving their car over a cliff into the sea. [From Japanese newspapers. Courtesy of Shingo Takahashi, M.D.].

Their financial situation became worse, and the loan shark came after them to repay the debt. They asked for help from relatives, but were politely refused. They planned a family suicide to deal with the embarrassing situation. With their two daughters (11 and 10 years old), they drove their car over a cliff into the sea. The event was reported in the newspaper, with the headline: "Another family suicidal event" (see Fig. 13-7b).

3. Cargo-Cult Syndromes (Millenniary Delusions)

a. General Description

Numerous social and behavior scientists have noted that, historically, there have been occurrences of "crisis cults" in many different countries. The Taiping (Great Peace) Rebellion in China, Kikuyu maumau in Kenya, and the Ghost Dance of the Plains Indians of North America are some examples. Central to all these cultures are marked feelings of inferiority, conflict, and anxiety among the member–participants after being exposed to other, superior cultures and an attempt to renovate their self-images. Underlying these nonlogical, magic–religious endeavors is a strong wish for resolution of their social, economic, and political problems and for a new and better way of life, such as that of the invading, superior cultures.

One kind of crisis cult is the "cargo cult" that has repeatedly arisen in Melanesia over the past century as a means of obtaining the manufactured articles possessed by European invaders (Lidz, Lidz, & Burton-Bradley, 1973). "Cargo" is a neo-Melanesian or pidgin word that designates all of the manufactured goods, including canned foods and weapons, possessed by the Europeans, which are greatly desired by the indigenous people. Without knowing how the "cargo" was manufactured in the home countries of Europe, based on their own folk beliefs, the local people thought that it was given to the white people by their powerful ancestors through the performance of proper rituals. Accordingly, the local people tried to perform the white people's rituals, such as worshiping the cross, or practiced their own indigenous rituals, such as sacrifices, in the hopes that their ancestors would send them a lot of cargo and their lives would eventually be full of wealth.

To describe this phenomenon, B. G. Burton-Bradley, a cultural psychiatrist practicing in Papua New Guinea, presented the term "cargo-cult syndrome" in 1975. Basically, the term referred to people who believed in the cargo cult and were possessed by the magical, grandiose idea that they could communicate with and eventually receive cargo from the gods. Most of the people lived in the highlands (see Fig. 13-8a) where they saw the "big bird" (airplane) deliver cargo to the airport — the only way to transport material to the area (see Fig. 13-8b). It was their misinterpretation that if they followed the white people's behavior, they would also receive things that they wanted from the gods. In order to achieve their goal, they practiced various odd rituals, usually imitating white people's behavior, such as building a cross in the backyard for worship (see Fig. 13-8c), imitating a foreign soldier's march (see Fig. 13-8d), or clearing their back yards (as if building an airstrip), hoping that the "big bird" would land with cargo for them. Some would perform the traditional ritual of sacrificing a human being to please the gods. This behavior might be individual or it might involve a group of followers that gave up their normal lives to perform religious rituals, waiting for the arrival of the cargo, not only for several months, but for many years. They would become collectively deluded and led by a cult leader.

b. Case Illustration (Abstracted from Burton-Bradley, 1975)

Case A — A young male in his mid-20s was threatened with dismissal from work for not cooperating with his European supervisor. He attacked the supervisor and bit him on the buttock. He left the workplace and returned to his village, claiming that the spirit of his dead grandfather appeared before him and told him to go home to look after the village cemetery. Then he commenced to dig a deep hole in a certain place. He said that in due course he would come upon a big snake with skin like a white man

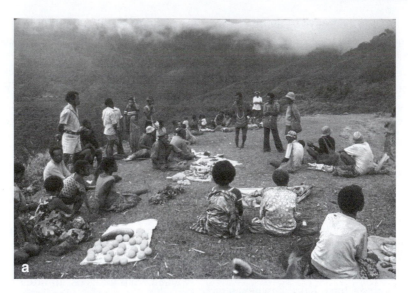

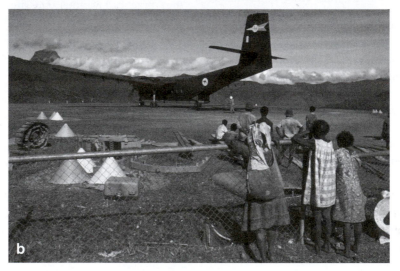

FIGURE 13-8   Cargo cult in Papua, New Guinea. (a) People living in the highland area where the airport is the main place to interact with the outside world. (b) The airport with a "big bird" arriving and delivering cargo. [Courtesy of Nicholas C. Demetry, M.D.].

and that the snake would lead him to paradise. While there he would find a thousand dollars. While he was digging, many villagers came to support him and join in. He did nothing but continue his digging for 3 years. The hole ended up about 20 feet deep, but nothing was found. With the passage of time, the taunts of villagers began to increase. One woman laughed at him many times. He became upset, threw a spear into her thorax, and killed her with an axe. After he was convicted of murder and diagnosed as

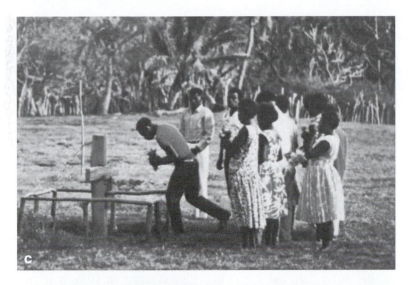

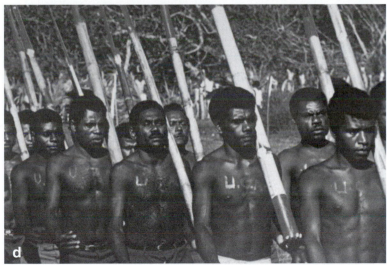

FIGURE 13-8 (Continued) (c) The local people, believing in the cargo cult, built a cross in imitation of the white people's worshiping of the almighty god. (d) Local people marching like U.S. soldiers in imitation of a white people's "ritual." [Source unknown.]

a paranoid schizophrenic, he was confined to a mental hospital. His followers assisted him when he escaped from the hospital so that he could return to his village and continue his digging. The case occurred in an area where the cargo cult was not unfamiliar to the village people. During World War II, when Japanese soldiers landed there, the local people completely stopped working, killed pigs and dogs, and spent a lot of time dancing. They believed that the whole world was turning over, with the Europeans fighting, and they celebrated the arrival of their anticipated new lives.

Case B — An elderly male was admitted to a psychiatric hospital for assessment after killing his friend in a ritual of human sacrifice. The patient and his friend (the victim of the sacrifice) had discussed for years various ways of raising their status to that of the industrialized (white) people, with all their material appurtenances. The patient, who was also a mission catechist, decided that the only way to do this was to emulate the Christian Passion, on the assumption that the advent of Christianity was responsible for the wealth and standing of Europeans. His friend readily agreed that this was so. The patient arranged the erection of an enclosure in the village with a platform in the center from which he addressed his followers. He obtained a long American bush knife, and led his friend to the center of the enclosure. His friend raised his hand to "the sun, the moon, and the stars," to inform these cosmic forces of what was about to happen. The friend offered his neck, and the patient made one quick, violent blow with the knife. Most of those present (including their followers) were surprised by what had happened and ran away. Later, in explanation, the patient stated that, some years previously, his friend had asserted that the spirit of God had appeared before him and said he must die and shed his blood as did Jesus Christ to ensure a wonderful series of changes in the lives of the people. In his trial, the patient was found guilty but insane.

c. Clinical Discussion

A report from Burton-Bradley's investigation (1975, 1982) indicated that many people involved in cargo cults, particularly the cult leaders, could be considered clinically psychotic cases — suffering from schizophrenia, delusional disorders, or mania. Some manifested their cargo-cult behavior alone, but, often, there were many followers, and the phenomenon needed to be considered a collective mental disorder (cross-reference to Chapter 14: Epidemic Mental Disorders).

From an emic standpoint, the worldview of the indigenous people, their interpretation of the arrival of the cargo, and their desire and expectation to have the cargo are understandable; from their perspective, their levels of cognition and knowledge, and their life experiences, their behavior is not as "illogical" as it is from an etic point of view, i.e., from an outsider's perspective. However, the behavior can be seen as pathological from a socially functional perspective, as its goal was never reached and the lives of the followers were disturbed. The core of the phenomenon should be comprehended as a manifestation of a people coping with social stress, although in a dysfunctional way.

As a culture-related specific syndrome, it may be understood that culture contributed to the stress that was encountered and also shaped the unique, pathological pattern of coping with it — a combination of pathogenic and pathoselective effects. Because there were no further reports of cargo cults after Burton-Bradley's initial report in 1975, it is unclear whether this phenomenon is still observed in Papua New Guinea.

C. CULTURE-SHAPED VARIATIONS OF PSYCHOPATHOLOGY

This category includes a group of disorders that manifests a clinical picture that is considerably "different" from the "ordinal" symptomatology of identified disorders described in current psychiatric classifications (of Euro-American origin). It is considered that the uniqueness of the symptomatology may be culturally attributed, i.e., to cultural pathoplastic effects. Culture affects not only the content of symptoms, but, even more, the total clinical picture by the absence, addition, or variation of symptoms, resulting in considerable change in the manifestations of variations or subtypes of universally recognized psychiatric disorders.

1. Anthrophobia (Interpersonal Relation Phobia)

a. Definition and Nature of the Disorder

"Anthrophobia" is the English translation for the Japanese term *taijin-kyofu-shio*. In Japanese, *taijin* means interpersonal, *kyofu* means phobic, and *shio* means syndrome or disorder. Therefore, *taijin-kyofu-shio* literally means the disorder with fear of interpersonal relation. (In this sense, the English term anthrophobia — fear of "human subject" — is an incorrect translation.) *Taijinkyofusho* as a psychiatric diagnostic term was invented by Japanese psychiatrists to address a special type of neurosis commonly observed among Japanese patients.

In the 1920s, when Japanese psychiatrist Shoma Morita, the founder of Morita therapy, established his classification system of *shinkei-shitsu* (nervous temperamental disorders), he classified *taijinkyofushio,* in addition to obsessive-compulsive disorder, paroxysmal neurosis (panic disorder), and general neurosis (neurasthenia), as a subcategory of *shinkeishitsu* (nervous temperament) (Kitanish & Mori, 1995). Since then, the term *taijinkyofushio* has become a subject for Japanese psychiatrists. It refers to the condition of a person who becomes excessively concerned and phobic about "interpersonal relations," with symptoms of flushing, concern about his or her body smell, or eye contact with others.

Taijinkyofushio is said to be prevalent among Japanese and is considered a culture-related psychiatric disorder. In Tokyo, among outpatients with minor psychiatric disorders (such as anxiety, obsessive, or hypochondriac disorders) who visited one of the metropolitan psychiatric hospitals, 11% were diagnosed as anthrophobic (Iwa, 1982). Yamashita (1977/1993) reported that, in Hokkaido, among the outpatients who visited the university psychiatric clinic, 7.8% were given this diagnosis. Kasahara (1974) reported that among 430 college students who received mental health services at the student health service of Kyoto University in 1968, one-half were neurotic and, among them, 18.6% could be classified as *taijinkyofushio* cases (of the rest, 24% were depression and 20% were psychosomatic disorders). At the Morita Clinic setup in Jikey University in Tokyo, specializing in residential treatment for *shinkeishitus* (neurotic patients), 34.2% of the total population was diagnosed as *taijinkyofushio* cases, 35.3% as obsessive-compulsive, and 20.2% as having anxiety disorders (Mori & Kitanishi, 1984).

b. Major Clinical Picture

There are several clinical studies reported by Japanese psychiatrists that provide overviews of the clinical picture of the disorder. Yamashita (1977/1993) has reviewed 100 consecutive cases of *taijinkyofushio* under his care at the university clinic. According to data, the onset of illness was early as 10–14 years old (18%), mostly between 15 and 19 years (44%), some later, at 20–24 years (26%), and a few after 25 years (12%). In his series of cases, there were 76 males and 24 females, showing that the disorder is more prevalent among males, with a ratio of roughly 3:1. The cardinal symptoms manifested by the patients are fear of one's bodily odors (28%), fear of flushing (22%), fear of showing odd attitudes toward others (18%), fear of eye contact with others (15%), concern about others' attitudes toward oneself (9%), and fear of body dysmorphia (5%).

Kato (1977, p. 30) reviewed the medical charts of 560 cases of *taijinkyofushio* who visited one of the mental hospitals specializing in the treatment of *taijinkyofushio* in Tokyo during the years 1953 to 1955 and 1962. According to him, the age distribution was concentrated at 15–19 years (33%) and 20–24 years (46%). The chief complaints, allowing for multiple calculations, were fear of flushing (50%), fear of crowds (45%), fear of making a public speech (36%), fear of interacting with the opposite sex (35%), fear of carrying on a conversation with others (34%), fear of eye contact with others (31%), feeling inferior (31%), fear of socialization (26%), and fear of relating with authority (24%). The sex ratio was also 3:1, but, based on Kato's clinical experience, it was his impression that female cases were increasing slightly after the war.

In summary, the majority of the patients suffering from *taijinkyofushio* were teenagers or young adults. Males were three times more likely than females to suffer from this disorder.

c. Case Illustration

Case A (from Tseng, Asai, Kitanish, McLaughlin, & Kyomen, 1992) — Mr. A was a 26-year-old, single, male college graduate and a company employee who had been taking excessive sick leave for 1 year. He presented problems of feeling uneasy about maintaining eye contact with others and experiencing difficulty in relating to his colleagues and friends. His problems started at age 16, when he moved from his freshman to sophomore high school class. He found that most of his classmates had changed and he had difficulty talking to the teachers and his new classmates, particularly the females. He was concerned about how others might feel about him. Someone had commented to him that he had a severe look in his eyes, and from then on he always looked into mirrors to check his eyes.

He was accepted into college, but through his 4 years of college life he was always in seclusion and avoided close contact with others. After graduation, he was employed by his present company. He worked for 1 year, although he was always concerned about other people's attitudes toward him. The previous year, there had been a rearrangement of the company and he was moved to a new and larger office. Here, he had more difficulty relating to his colleagues, especially the women. He was also uncomfortable with his new superior. Therefore, he went on sick leave and has not since returned to work.

Case B (from Tseng, Asai et al., 1992) — Mrs. B was a 25-year-old housewife who had been married for 3 years. When she was 14 and a second-year student in junior high school, her closest friendship was severed due to a minor misunderstanding. During the disagreement, this special friend had made a comment about the patient's "ugly face." Since then, she had become seriously concerned about her "ugly face." Although she did not actually have any facial deformity, she was uncomfortable about facing her classmates in the classroom.

She managed to graduate from high school and went to work at a factory, but she continued to feel uncomfortable when people stared at her and had difficulty maintaining eye contact with them. She coped with the situation by wearing glasses. Despite her difficulties, she met and married her husband. Her condition did not improve much even after her marriage.

d. Dynamic Interpretation and Culture Formulation

Morita theory takes the view that *shinkeishitsu* (including *taijinkyofushio*) is caused by the combined factors of temperamental predisposition, hypochnidical tendency, and "psychological interactional effects." The term "psychological interactional effects" refers to a person's excessive attention to certain (body) sensations or external stimulation. As a result, the sensations are alerted and, in turn, lead to more attention. Through this vicious interactional cycle of morbid preoccupation and obsession (called *toraware* in Japanese), a person becomes overly sensitive to and fixated on the morbid condition. The main focus of Morita therapy is to disrupt the cycle of over-attention by learning to ignore the sensations or stimulation.

Kasahara (1974) brought out an important point: the characteristic of *taijinkyofushio* is that the fear is induced in the presence of classmates, colleagues, or friends — those who are neither particularly close (such as family members) nor totally strange (such as people in the street). In other words, subjects are concerned with how to relate to people of intermediate familiarity. It is toward these people that a person must exercise delicate social etiquette.

Kasahara explained further that Japan is a situationally oriented society, very much concerned with how others see your behavior. Japanese parents often discipline their children by saying, "neighbors are watching whatever you do." Also, it is considered that the act of staring at the person to whom one is talking is quite extraordinary and considered to be rude. Thus, there are cultural characteristics that cause Japanese to be hypersensitive about "looking at" and "being looked at."

Kimura (1982) pointed out that patients who were suffering from *taijinkyofushio* were not phobic toward human subjects. On the contrary, they were eager to socialize with others. However, because they were concerned with how they were perceived by others, particularly their friends, they became embarrassed and nervous when relating to them. They were not so concerned about strangers or close family members, just semiclose friends. Within Japanese society, there is such a strong demand to be sensitive to interpersonal interactions that sensitivity is heightened.

Taijinkyofushio is a psychological disorder of the adolescent. It is closely related to the problems associated with psychological development in the area of socialization. The Japanese child is raised in an atmosphere of indulgence and trust. However, when this protected child enters the wider world of junior high school, he or she faces multiple tasks: coping with conflict between biological needs and social restrictions, personal identity problems, and an increasing need for acceptance and love by others in social settings. This intensifies a feeling of unworthiness, making him or her more concerned about other's sensibilities and reactions (Yamashita, 1977/1993).

e. Diagnostic Considerations

From a diagnostic point of view, Yamashita (1977/1993) clarified that although sufferers of both hypochondriasis and *taijinkyofushio* complained about their physical conditions, the symptoms of the former were related to the physical self and of the latter to the social self, which is the basic difference between them.

In order to test the way in which American mental health professionals diagnosed Japanese anthrophobia, Tanaka-Matsumi (1979) gave six Japanese case descriptions of *taijinkyofushio* to American clinical psychologists and psychiatric residents for their diagnostic impressions. It was found that American mental health professionals grouped the Japanese cases of *taijinkyofushio* into a number of heterogeneous categories, including schizophrenia, paranoid personality, anxiety neurosis, phobic neurosis, and others.

In order to further investigate the cross-cultural aspects of clinical diagnosis, a comparison was made between the diagnoses of social phobia by Japanese psychiatrists in Tokyo and American psychiatrists in Hawaii (Tseng, Asai et al., 1992). A brief segment of videotaped interviews and written case histories of Japanese patients from Tokyo and Japanese-American

patients from Hawaii, who were clinically confirmed as social phobic cases by their psychiatrists, was blindly presented to the clinicians for their diagnoses. It was found that Japanese psychiatrists tended to diagnose social phobia congruently in the Japanese cases but not in the Japanese-American cases (from Hawaii). The American psychiatrists tended to diagnose incongruently in various categories (including anxiety disorder and avoidance personality disorder, in addition to social phobia) for patients from both Tokyo and Hawaii. This study illustrated that the diagnostic patterns for social phobia varied considerably between the psychiatrists of these two countries. In addition to the unique nature of the psychopathology and the patients' stylized patterns of presenting problems, the clinicians' professional orientations and familiarity with the disorder had a strong impact on the results.

f. Anthrophobia in Other Areas

For many years, Japanese psychiatrists held the view that anthrophobia was a culture-bound disorder especially related to Japanese culture. This view was challenged when Korean psychiatrist S.H. Lee (1987) reported that anthrophobia is found to be prevalent in Korea as well. Later, a similar view was mentioned by psychiatrists from mainland China (Y.H. Cui, personal communication, 1996). Based on this new information, it may be said that *taijinkyofushio* is not a psychiatric condition "bound" to Japanese society (or culture). It is a psychiatric problem that can be observed in various societies in Asia in which there are certain cultural traits, i.e., where there is overconcern about interpersonal relations with intermediately surrounding persons and a child development pattern that tends to make it difficult for adolescents who were overprotected in childhood to deal with delicate social relations after entering young adulthood.

2. Brain Fag Syndrome

This syndrome was described by Canadian cultural psychiatrist Raymond Prince (1960), who worked as a medical officer in Nigeria in the 1950s. According to Prince, a very common minor psychiatric disorder occurring among the students of southern Nigeria is characterized by subjective complaints of intellectual impairment, (visual) sensory impairment, and somatic complaints, mostly of pain or a burning sensation in the head and neck. The student–patients often used the word of "brain fag" to complain that they were no longer able to read, grasp what they were reading, or recall what they had just read, basically stressing their difficulty in mentation. The term "brain fag" syndrome was suggested by Prince (1960) for this distinct clinical mental condition.

According to Prince, the patients were mostly students in secondary school or university or teachers or government clerks who were studying in their spare time to raise their educational levels. The patients generally attributed their illnesses to fatigue of the brain due to excessive mental work. Actually, most often the symptoms commenced during periods of intensive reading and study prior to or after examinations. In addition to the subjects' faulty study habits, spending long hours poring over their books with little relaxation, Prince explained that the syndrome was in some way related to the imposition of European learning techniques upon the Nigerian personality. European learning techniques emphasize isolated endeavor, individual responsibility, and orderliness, activities and traits that are foreign to the Nigerian by reason of the collectivist society from which he derives, with its heightened "oralness" and permissiveness. Prince noted that in Nigeria, education was often a family affair, in which one of the brighter children was supported financially by family members; the educated member in turn was expected to be responsible for other family members when the need arose. Because of this family aspect of education, the student was burdened by the responsibility of maintaining the family's prestige. Thus, his or her academic success or failure was associated with great stress. Prince (1990) considered it more relevant to understand this condition as "adjustment disorder."

Two decades after Prince's initial report on this syndrome in 1960, R. O. Jegede (1983), a psychiatrist from Nigeria, claimed that the disorder was not necessarily confined to students and that excessive studying for examinations may be just one of several possible precipitating factors. For instance, some of the patients with these complaints were housewives. Further, Jegede reported that patients who were sophisticated enough to explain their symptoms in more psychologically oriented terms were less likely to complain of the somatic symptoms associated with brain fag. He suggested that brain fag syndrome did not constitute a single disease entity, as the patients were, in a way, suffering from anxiety neurosis or depressive neurosis.

Twenty-five years after he first described this disorder among the Yoruba, Ibo, and other ethnic groups in southern Nigeria, Prince indicated that it was subsequently observed in Uganda, Liberia, the Ivory Coast, and Malawi (Prince, 1990). Based on this, Prince confirmed that brain fag syndrome was a widespread and prevalent stress disorder among students in Africa south of the Sahara.

It should be mentioned that, in China, many students and intellectuals who are excessively competitive academically or under great occupational demands develop a similar kind of "brain-exhausted" syndrome, labeled "brain neurasthenia" by the Chinese (Wen, 1995).

3. *Arctic Hysteria* (Pibloktoq)

a. *General Description*

Arctic (or polar) hysteria, also known by the local name *pibloktoq,* refers to a unique hysterical attack observed among the polar Eskimo people living in Arctic areas. According to Gussow (1960/1985), A. A. Brill (1913) published the first account of the disorder in psychiatric literature, introducing this native Eskimo illness found in northwestern Greenland.

The clinical condition is characterized by the sudden onset of loss or disturbance of consciousness. During the attack, as summarized by Gussow (1960/1985) and Foulks (1972), the patient may show various abnormal behaviors, such as tearing off his or her clothing, glos-

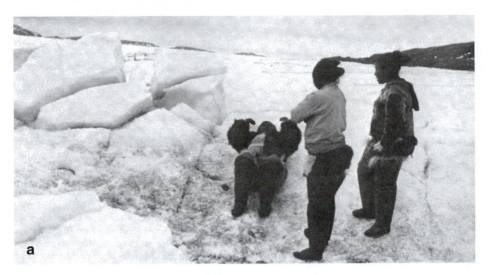

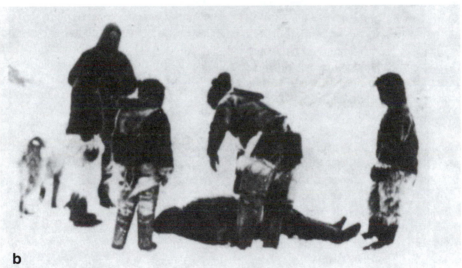

FIGURE 13-9 Arctic hysteria *(pibloktog)* in Greenland. (a) An Eskimo woman suffered from a *pibloktog* attack, falling on the ground and demonstrating a carpo-pedal spasm. (b) No one knew exactly what to do with her. [From *The Arctic hysterias,* by Edward F. Foulks, M.D., American Anthropological Association, 1972. Courtesy of the American Museum of Natural History Library].

solalia, fleeing (nude or clothed), rolling in the snow, throwing anything handy around, performing mimetic acts, convulsion, or other bizarre behavior (see Fig. 13-9). This emotional outburst occurs predominantly in women, but occasionally among men.

No specific precipitating causes are noted. It has been speculated that the reaction is a manifestation of the basic Eskimo personality. Because the reaction is prevalent in winter, it is also thought that it may be related to increased threats of starvation or higher accident rates. Generally it is suspected that the disorder is due to some basic, underlying anxiety, triggered by severe, culturally typical stresses: fear of certain impending situations, fear of loss, or fear of losing emotional support, including the sense of being on safe, solid, familiar ground.

b. Case Illustration

Case A (abstract from Foulks, 1972, case No. 7) — Mrs. A is a 30-year-old woman who has had periodic episodes of "strange experiences" in the past 3 years (since her mother's death). Three years ago, in the winter, during her first episode, she was acutely assaultive and tried to harm herself. The attack lasted about 15 min and she remembered nothing about it afterward. Two years ago, she had her second attack, which lasted about half an hour, during which time she ran from her home into the snow, tearing off her clothing. This winter, her husband returned home and found her clawing at the bed and looking "quite wild." She said she was talking to her dead mother. In a few minutes she recovered and became sensible.

Mrs. A's parents are both dead. She remembers that they were very old-fashioned people. Her father hunted, trapped, and went whaling for a living. He maintained a very strict mode of living for his children, yet all of them were attracted to Western lifestyles. Actually, all Mrs. A's brothers and sisters had moved away and were living in Western cities. When Mrs. A was young and in school, she was always very shy. Ten years ago, after her father's death, she lived with her mother. Several years later, she took a trip to the city to visit her sister. There she met a Western man and fell in love with him. People in the village did not approve of the outsider and considered the love affair scandalous. They felt girls from the village should marry local men. Mrs. A was the subject of many comments and jokes. Finally, she married the young man. Her husband wished to return to the city with Mrs. A, but she was torn. She did not want to leave her mother alone. After the marriage, many of the villagers would not speak to her or her husband. During the past 3 years, since her mother's

death, with her siblings in other places, Mrs. A has felt unsupported against the gossip and distrust of the people in her village. She has felt lonely and depressed, yet reluctant to leave her home village. She is unable to make an acceptable life for herself in either the village or the faraway city.

c. Diagnostic and Etiological Considerations

Because a *pibloktoq* attack is usually brief and followed by complete remission, with the subject claiming amnesia, it can be classified as a hysterical attack. In a certain way, it may be understood as a culturally patterned emotional reaction to stress or trauma. The geographic environment of the polar area may contribute to its occurrence.

From an entirely different angle, some scholars entertain the theory that Arctic hysteria may represent behaviors associated with hypoglycemia. Lack of adequate dietary calcium and low levels of vitamin D synthesis during the Arctic winter are among the reasons considered (Foulks, 1972).

4. Malignant Anxiety

a. Clinical Condition

A special, intensified form of anxiety disorder observed in Africa was reported by Nigerian psychiatrist T. Adeoye Lambo (1960, 1962). He described the condition as characterized by intense anxiety, extreme irritability, restlessness, and intense fear, and, therefore, named it malignant anxiety. It was referred as frenzied anxiety as well. Often, the patient claimed that there was a change in his sense of self and reality, but there was no sign of personality deterioration or disintegration and no latent or overt psychotic symptoms. However, patients often suffered from intense feelings of anger that led to homocidal behavior. The condition usually occurred in sporadic cases, but occasionally as an endemic.

Lambo (1962) explained that the occurrence of the disorder was situationally related, associated with adaptational problems to new and stressful life situations. Very often the patients were culturally "marginal" persons, who were in the process of renouncing their age-old cultures but had failed to assimilate the new.

5. Ataques de Nervios *(Attack of Nerves)*

The folk name, *ataques de nervios,* literally meaning attack of nerves, refers to a stress-induced, culturally shaped unique emotional reaction with mixed anxiety–hysterical features (Guarnaccia, Rubio-Stipec, & Canino, 1989; Oquendo, Horwath, & Martines, 1992). This is an illness category used frequently by Hispanic people. Initially observed among Puerto Rican army recruits, it was also labeled "Puerto Rican syndrome" (Fernández-Marian, 1959; Mehlman, 1961).

According to Guarnaccia and associates (1989), this condition typically occurs at funerals, in accidents, or in family conflicts, and calls forth family or other social supports. Commonly experienced symptoms include shaking, palpitations, a sense of heat rising to the head, and numbness, symptoms resembling a panic attack (Liebowitz et al., 1994). The individual may shout, swear, and strike out at others, and finally fall to the ground, manifesting convulsion-like movements.

As part of a major study of the psychological consequences of the 1985 floods and mudslides that caused considerable damage and death in Puerto Rico, a question was added to the Diagnostic Interview Schedule/Disaster Supplement concerning *ataques de nervois.* From this study, Guarnaccia, Canino, Rubio-Stipec, and Bravo (1993) reported that those subjects identified as *ataques de nervois* cases were more likely to be female, older, and less educated. Their clinical conditions were more likely to meet the criteria for anxiety and depressive disorders rather than panic disorders.

Based on their clinical samples, Salmán and colleagues (1998) reported that most of the patients (about 80%) were female. From a clinical, diagnostic point of view, according to DSM-III-R criteria, the condition belongs to many subtypes of disorders, including panic disorder (41.3%), recurrent major

depression (19.3%), generalized anxiety disorder (8.3%), nonspecific anxiety disorder (8.3%), and others. If Salmán and colleagues' description of the syndrome is correct, then, because the clinical picture is of a mixed, rather than a specific nature, it may be interpreted simply as a folk label of an emotional reaction. That is, it should be listed in the group (F), with *susto* or *hwabyung,* as a cultural interpretation of a mental condition caused by pathoreactive effects. Guarnaccia (1993) stressed the point that *ataques de nervois* refers to an acute episode of social and psychological distress related to upsetting or frightening events in the family sphere. Focusing on symptoms alone misses what is most salient and meaningful about illness categories.

D. CULTURALLY ELABORATED OR REINFORCED UNIQUE BEHAVIOR

1. Latah *(Startle-Induced Dissociative Reaction)*

a. Defining the Condition

Latah is a Malay word referring to the condition in which a person, after being startled by external stimuli, such as being tickled, suddenly experiences an altered consciousness and falls into a transient, dissociated state, exhibiting unusual behavior (such as echolalia, echopraxia, or command automatism), including explosive verbal outbursts, usually of erotic words that are not ordinarily acceptable. The phenomenon has been observed in other places around the world and has been given various folk names — in Burma (where it is called *yaun*), Indonesia, Thailand *(bah-tsche)* (Suwanlert, 1988), the Philippines *(mali-mali),* indigenous tribes in Siberia, Russia *(myriachit),* and among the Ainu in Japan (who call it *imu*). However, this phenomenon has been found more frequently among the people in Malay, and literature reporting the "mental malady of the Malay" (Ellis, 1897) appeared as early as the end of the 19th century.

The *latah* reaction is found predominantly among women, although men may occasionally be involved. Chiu, Tong, & Schmidt (1972) conducted a compara-

tive study of psychiatric disorders among the three
ethnic groups of Malay, Iban, and Chinese in Sarawak
in eastern Malaysia. As a side product, they evaluated
the cases of *latah*. They reported a total of 50 *latah*
cases, all of them women. A subtotal of 37 out of 3386
female subjects was of Malaysian background; 17 of
3627 were Iban female subjects; and none were from
the Chinese group. According to this study, the crude
prevalence indices for *latah* would be 1.5% for female
Malays and 0.5% for female Bans.

Winzeler (1995) carried out field work in the
Kelantan state of mainland Malaysia and Sarawak on
the island of Borneo. He reported that in a village of
about 800 people he surveyed, 40 were regarded as
latah by their neighbors. It was found that *latah* tends
to run in families. The overwhelming majority of
cases were female. The men who had *latah* experiences were not known to be transvestites or in any
way distinctly feminine, as had previouly been
thought.

In the past, it was primarily young women who
were involved in *latah*. Most of the subjects found
now are beyond middle age. Most cases are found in
rural areas. Some develop *latah* reactions insidiously,
without any precipitating events, whereas others occur
after enduring psychologically stressful events. The
loss of a significant person usually occurs shortly
before the first experience of *latah* reaction. Once the
reaction is experienced, it becomes habitual, and,
thereafter, any sudden stimulation may provoke it.
Hearing a sudden noise or being suddenly touched or
poked by others may cause *latah*. Throwing a rope or
other snake-like object in front of the person or simply
shouting "snake!" will sufficiently startle the person to
start a *latah* reaction. During the reaction, the subject
will imitate the words of other people *(echlalia)*,
repeat other people's actions *(echopraxia)*, follow others' commands, such as barking like a dog (autonomic
obedience), sing in a euphoric mood, say words that
have sexual overtones, or try to touch or hit a man,
which is against cultural dictates (see Fig. 13-10).

The condition may last for several minutes or several hours if the person is continuously provoked.
After the dissociative reaction is over, the subject usu-

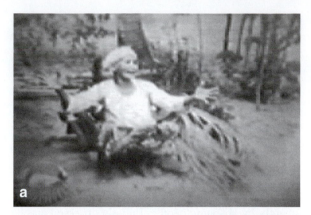

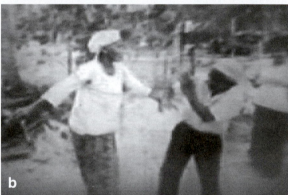

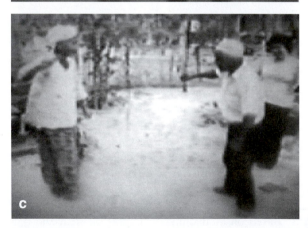

**FIGURE 13-10 A Malay woman provoked into having a *latah*
attack.** (a) A Malay woman was startled and, with both her hands
raised upward, began to fall into a *latah* attack. (b) The woman tried
to hit the man who provoked her. (c) Joyfully imitating her provoker's
gestures (echopraxia), as well as repeating whatever he said (echol-
aria). From a documentary film made by Ronald Simons, M.D.

ally claims amnesia and is puzzled about what had happened. Often, the subject is very apologetic and embarrassed for the (socially) "inappropriate" things he or she may have said (sexually colored "dirty" words) or done (such as touching men) during the attack.

Observing *latah* cases within an extended family, anthropologist Bartholomew (1994a) interpreted the *latah* reaction as a "ritual of deception." He noticed that the "teasers" are always close relatives who ensure that the "victim" does not do anything too outrageous, such as stabbing someone with a knife. Also, the *latah* condition is almost always terminated when both physical and verbal cues indicate that the person is tired.

It should be pointed out that in contrast to altered states of consciousness (such as those exhibited in meditation or shaman performances), which are induced through the mental mechanisms of monotonous stimulation (such as quiet chanting or simple, repetitive rhymes) and/or intensive concentration (meditation), the dissociated state of *latah* is induced (or conditioned) by sudden stimulation.

b. Case Illustration

Case A — Mrs. A was a 40-year-old woman who had been working at a university cafeteria for many years. She was known among her co-workers as having *latah* attacks. According to her, she married her husband when she was 20 and bore three children. As a wife and mother, she had a typical life. However, about 10 years earlier, she learned that her younger brother had been killed in a traffic accident while riding his motorcycle. She was shocked at this bad news and became sad. One day, while she was gazing into the air, thinking about her deceased brother, someone nearby startled her by touching her from behind. She suddenly became dissociated and manifested strange behavior — talking nonsense for a while, imitating others' behavior. The condition lasted for about 10 min. She felt slightly dizzy after the episode. After that, every time she was startled by others, either by being poked suddenly or hearing a noise, she fell into

this *latah* condition. People around her began to notice this and would provoke her once in a while for the sake of amusement. She begged her co-workers not to disturb or startle her, as she wanted to keep her job. She had been working at the university cafeteria for almost a decade and was successful in concealing her *latah* from her supervisor (see Figure 13-11).

Case B — Mrs. B was about 30 years old. She worked at the university cafteria with Mrs. A. She recalled that one evening several years earlier, her husband had suddenly touched her, inducing a startled reaction. Since then, her husband liked to startle her sometimes at night before they went to bed. He enjoyed having her become dissociated and acting joyfully and freely before they had intimate relations. However, at her workplace, hardly anyone knew that she had a *latah* tendency and no one bothered her (see Fig. 13-11).

c. The Nature of the Reaction

Actually, there is a debate among scholars as to whether the *latah* condition should be regarded as a culture-related "mental disorder" or merely as an "unusual behavior response" found in some cultures. According to Chinese-Malaysian psychiatrist T. H. Woon (1988), who has practiced psychiatry for more than two decades, no patient has ever sought psychiatric help for *latah;* also, among 20 *latah* subjects he investigated in a field study, he found only one subject who had ever sought help from a traditional healer *(bomoh)* for this phenomenon. No healing suggestion was offered by the healer, as she was not considered to be suffering from an illness, but just exhibiting entertaining behavior. In other words, local people as well as healers do not view this condition as a problem or an "illness." Woon pointed out that it is mainly Western physicians, unused to observing dissociative episodes in daily life, who categorize and report the condition as a "mental disease."

According to T.H. Woon (personal communication, 1980), the majority of subjects who experience the *latah* condition are considered "ordinary" people. Except during their *latah* reactions, they function

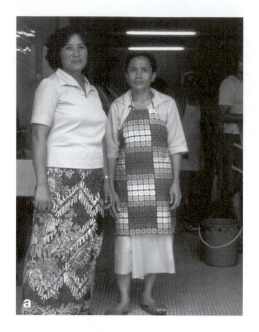

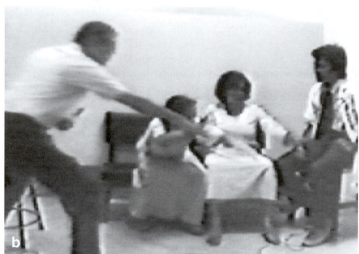

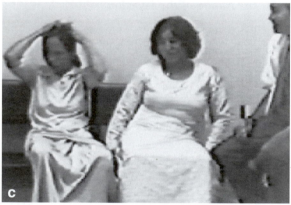

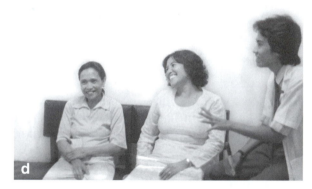

FIGURE 13-11   Two Malay women demonstrated *latah*. (a) Two ordinary Malay women (Mrs. A and Mrs. B), who worked in a university cafeteria and were found to have histories of *latah,* agreed to be provoked together in front of camera and be videotaped. (b) After being startled by a provoker, who pointed toward a nearby man's leg and said it was a "snake," the woman on the left rushed toward the man, trying to hit his legs (culturally impolite behavior). (c) In their trance states, they made "monkey-like" gestures, scratching their hair with rhythmic mannerisms and imitating monkey sounds. (d) After they recovered from their attacks and were shown the videotape of their behavior, they felt embarrassed for hitting a man. [Courtesy of Woon Tai-Hwang, M.D.].

effectively in the community. However, there have been a few cases in which it was difficult to control (or terminate) the dissociated condition of the subjects, and they injured themselves or became aggressive or homicidal toward others. These reactions were labeled "malignant," as opposed to "regular," *latah.*

T.H. Woon (personal communication, 1980) reported that there are actually three types of *latah* recognized by local people. *Latah gembira* (happy *latah*) is often seen during wedding ceremonies and on other joyful occasions. Well-known *latah* subjects are usually invited to attend and, after the serious part of the ceremony is over, they are provoked by the participants for "entertainment." *Latah marah* (angry *latah*) occurs when the subject is teased in a socially inappropriate place and time or in a disturbing way and becomes abusive, aggressive, and even violent. *Latah berbahaya* (dangerous *latah*) refers to situations when the *latah* reaction is provoked while the subject is involved in potentially dangerous activities, such as handling knives or standing next to boiling cooking oil. When provoked, the subject may grab the knife and injure others or burn herself with the fire or boiling oil. It is necessary to recognize that the *latah* reaction involves a range of behavior, from benign to socially entertaining to annoying or even dangerous.

While subjects are seldom involved in criminal acts during *latah* states, they do occasionally injure others by using nearby weapons in startled reflex actions or at the criminal suggestions of others. Whether or not the person in the *latah* state was criminally responsible in such situations had become a forensic issue as early as the beginning of the century (Fletcher, 1908).

d. Etiological Speculations

From an etiological point of view, various theories have been proposed. Because most of the examples of *latah* were reported among indigenous groups from south Asia, including aboriginal tribes in Siberia and northern Japan, it has been speculated that race is the essential factor in the etiology. According to Yap (1952), early investigators, such as Czaplicka (1914) and Galloway (1922), have stressed that this disorder might have something to do with the character of the Mongol race. However, as pointed out by Yap, the "jumpers" (or "shakers") phenomenon — the ritualistic jumping, shaking, and also the utterance of incoherent gutturals by a group of religious folk, originating from the Methodist Congress of Wales and spread to North American in early stage, with vague resemblance of *latah* — has historically been observed

among Caucasians. It has also been indicated that Chinese people living in Malaysia never showed the reaction unless they were brought up in a basically Malaysian cultural milieu. A similar phenomenon was noted among Japanese nationals, a majority of whom never succumbed to *imu* unless they were raised by Ainu parents — an aboriginal minority ethnic group living in northern Japan. These findings favor a cultural attribution to the condition.

According to Yap (1952), several scholars (such as Loon, 1927; Repond, 1940; Winiarz & Wielawski, 1936) have considered *latah* from a psychological point of view as a primitive form of fear reaction, or a primitive psychoneurosis among "uncivilized people."

Anthropologists have tried to understand the *latah* condition from a cultural point of view. Regarding the incidence of *latah* among the Javanese, Geertz (1968) has pointed out that Java culture is characterized by four themes: the value of elegant and polite speech, a concern with social status, sexual prudery, and the dread of being startled. The *latah* reaction is remarkably congruent with the cultural themes emphasized, but in a paradoxical way. Geertz's view was echoed by Kenny (1983), who indicated that the *latah* condition has a profound internal relationship with Malay-Indonesian culture. He stressed the meaning of *latah* as a peculiarly appropriate means of communicating marginality to others. R.L.M. Lee (1981) contended that *latah* subjects are engaging in a "performance," "a role," and "theater" — a culture-specific idiom expressing marginality while simultaneously reaffirming normative boundaries. Bartholomew (1994a) examined 37 cases of *latah* and reported that 33 belonged to the "habitual" category — *latah* as a culturally conditioned, cathartic stress response to sudden startling; the remaining four cases belonged to the "performance" category — *latah* as a form of ritualized social gain. He stressed that *latah* was mistakenly labeled in medical terms as "mental illness" due to the misunderstanding of this behavior by outsiders.

As pointed out by Chiu and colleagues (1972), the traditional polygamous Malay extended family structure is male dominated. Within this cultural system, *latah* is socially accepted as a female attention-seeking response, one of the few permissible overt, excitable, aggressive, and/or sexual demonstrations. In other words, *latah* is a culturally sanctioned emotional outlet for females.

American cultural psychiatrist Ronald C. Simons (1980, 1996), after carrying out intensive fieldwork in Malay, hypothesized that most or all human populations contain individuals who can be easily and strongly startled. However, in some cultures, such a hypersensitive startle response is sanctioned and utilized for social purposes. According to Simons, the *latah* reaction is a culture-specific exploitation of a neurophysiologically determined behavioral potential. The condition, similar to fainting, is frequent in populations whose cultures notice, expect, shape, and elaborate on such behavior and is rare but not absent in populations that do not pay special attention to it.

e. Similar Behavior in Other Areas

i. *Imu* (Possession Attack) among the Ainu in Japan. The Japanese psychiatrist Uchimura (1956) reported the phenomenon of *imu* among the Ainu, an aboriginal minority ethnic group inhabiting the northern Japanese island of Hokkaido. *Imu* in the Ainu language literally means "possessed." Uchimura, Akimoto and Ishibashi (1938) estimated that there were 111 cases of *imu* among the 17,500 Ainu people living in northern Japan at the time of his field investigation in the 1950s. The *imu* subject is commonly startled by hearing the word "snake" or seeing snake-like creatures (see Fig. 13-12). In viewing the silent film made by Uchimura, it was noticed that *imu* was similar to the *latah* condition observed in Malaysia — induced by startling, manifesting echolalia and ecopraxia in an altered state of consciousness — even though from an ethnic or racial point of view Ainu and Malay people are not related. Local people believe that the serpent spirit can expel evil spirits from people. According to psychiatrists working in Kokkaido, Daiguji and Shichida (1998), the phenomenon of *imu* among the Ainu has declined and is rarely observed today.

ii. Other *Latah*-like Conditions As mentioned earlier, numerous conditions reported in the literature are similar to the *latah* phenomenon. *Mali-mali* in the Philippines (Musgrave & Sison, 1910), *young-dah-het* in Burma (Still, 1940), *bah-tsche* in Thailand (Simons, 1980), *or myriachit* in Siberia are some examples.

2. Body-Weight-Concerned Behavior and Anorexia Nervosa

Excessive concern with being overweight is currently observed in many European and American societies. It is primarily based on health-related concerns, but it is also rooted in the cultural view that "keeping the body in good shape is important." In order to live up to this cultural standard, many diets have been developed to ensure eating the proper low-calorie foods and many exercise programs have been designed to maintain an ideal body weight. Many diet cookbooks have been published and the sale of exercise machines has become a good business. In other words, in addition to being healthy, people are under cultural pressure to be slim and beautiful, and develop elaborate ways to meet these expectations.

Although the causes of eating disorders are still not clear, it is speculated that they may be more likely to happen in some cultures than others. First, in some societies, food is so scarce that people are anxious to obtain it for survival. It is unlikely for people in such a society to not want to eat food. Eating disorders will only be prevalent in societies where food is reasonably abundant. The second observation is crucial: how people perceive the body, particularly the female body. In some cultures, it is considered beautiful to be "fat" — in Hawaii, Samoa, and other Pacific Islands, for instance; in some cultures, being fat is considered a sign of being fortunate or blessed, such as in many Oriental countries, where statues of Buddha depict him as a fat person with a large belly. Obviously, there is no concern about being "overweight" and thus there is no reason for suffering from anorexia nervosa.

In contrast, in contemporary European and American societies, there is a tendency to emphasize "slimness" as a sign of beauty or good health. The popular

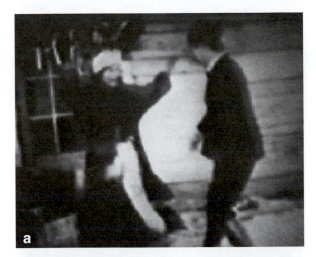

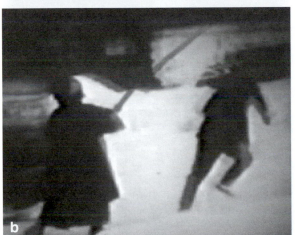

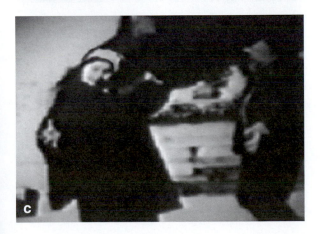

models are usually tall and slim — to the extent that, by other cultures' perceptions and standards, they look "anorexic." Based on this sociocultural factor, anorexia nervosa is considered a culture-related specific syndrome observed mainly in European or American societies (Gordon, 1990; Swartz, 1985). The psychopathological condition is nourished, elaborated, and enforced by the value systems existing in these societies (cross-reference to Chapter 23: Eating Disorders)

E. CULTURAL INFLUENCE OF PREVALENT OCCURRENCE OF DISORDERS

This category includes several conditions that are commonly known as psychiatric disorders. There is nothing particular about them in terms of clinical manifestation (thus, they are not *specific* or *unique* disorders). However, their prevalence is influenced strongly enough by cultural factors that they may be viewed as heavily culture-related syndromes rather than merely *ordinary* psychiatric disorders. Culture may also vary the issues related to these problems. From the perspective of examining the impact of culture on these psychopathologies, there is room for discussion, even though, in a strict sense, they are not considered culture-related *specific* syndromes.

1. Massive Hysteria or Group Suicide

When a group of people in the community collectively develops a hysterical outburst, in the form of dissociation, conversion, or emotional turmoil, as a reaction to group-shared stress, it is referred to as mass hysteria — most frequently observed in epi-

FIGURE 13-12 *Imu* **studied in Hokaido, northern Japan in the 1940s.** (a) A man (Dr. Uchimura) dropped his towel in front of an Ainu woman and shouted "snake." The woman startled, raised up her hands, and fell into an *imu* (possessed) state. (b) The woman picked up a stick and chased after the male provoker (ordinarily impolite behavior). (c) Later, she playfully imitated the provoker's motions (echoplaxia). [From a documentary film made by V.Y. Uchimura, M.D.].

demic mental disorders. While such occurrences are by no means rare, and are even occasionally observed in many developed societies, they tend to occur in societies where direct emotional expression, especially toward authority, is traditionally discouraged and there is no other choice but to burst into somatic conversion. Thus, the cultural environment favors and facilitates the occurrence of this unique social mental phenomenon [cross-reference to Chapter 14: Epidemic Mental Disorders (Section III,B)].

Suicidal behavior itself is commonly observed. However, if suicidal behavior occurs in a contagious way and if a group of people in a community commits suicide within a relatively short period of time, it is called mass, group, or collective suicide, which is strongly attributed to sociocultural factors, and may be viewed as a culture-related specific syndrome [cross-reference to Chapter 22: Suicide Behavior (Section III,A,3)].

2. Alcohol-Related Problems

Excess consumption and abuse of alcohol is not a unique problem and is widespread around the world. There is a broad range in the amount of consumption in different cultures, depending on their attitudes toward drinking behavior [cross-reference to Chapter 20: Alcohol-Related Problems (section II,B)]. However, alcohol-related problems may become unique when they are aggravated and manifested in certain ways, due to sociocultural factors, and then warrant the label of culture-related syndromes.

This is observed in Micronesia, where alcohol intake was strictly forbidden during the German and Japanese occupation during World War II, and regulations became quite liberal after the war. As a trust territory of the United States, a large amount of alcohol, mainly beer, was imported from the United States, and everybody was allowed to drink, even small children (as if they were drinking Coca Cola, see Fig. 13-13a). Empty beer cans were piled up in front of people's houses to show how much they could afford to drink and had consumed (see Fig. 13-13b).

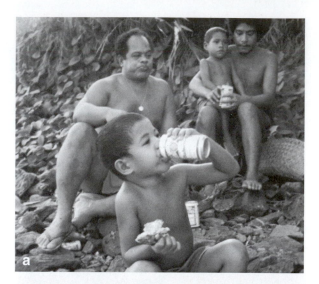

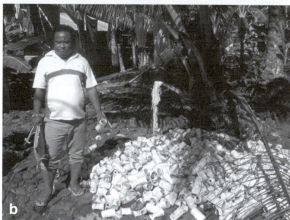

FIGURE 13-13 **Culturally patterned drinking behavior in Micronesia.** (a) When the drinking prohibitions of the past were removed after World War II, small children learned how to drink beer like their parents. (b) Beer cans were piled up in the front yard of almost every household, showing off how much beer had been consumed. [Courtesy of Boyd Slomoff, M.D.].

A pattern of drinking developed in which people would often gather socially on the weekend and, as a group, consume as much beer as they could until the supply was exhausted. In this group drinking pattern, with episodic high consumption, no alcohol dependence was noted; however, many people experienced acute intoxication associated with violent behavior. Thus, in addition to high consumption, this unique drinking pattern caused behavior problems. On weekends, after they got drunk, many young people were involved in fights, injured, and sent to hospital emergency rooms, earning them the label "weekend warriors" by the local people (see Fig. 13-14).

3. Substance Abuse

It is quite clear among psychiatrists and public health workers that the clinical manifestations and formation of dependence in substance abuse are based on biological factors. However, it is also obvious that its prevalence and epidemiology are very much dependent on sociocultural factors. Normally, no one considers substance abuse a culture-related "specific" syndrome, as it is potentially universally observed. However, it is salient that social and cultural factors stimulate and nourish substance abuse, particularly when a society encounters difficult times [cross-reference to Chapter 21: Substance-Related Problems Other Than Alcohol (Section II,A–D)].

Several examples illustrate this. It is known that the Chinese had a history of opium abuse. However, many people are not aware that Western imperialism at the end of the Chin dynasty contributed greatly to opium addiction becoming a serious social problem. For economic benefit, the British government supported the British East India Company in its importing and selling of opium in China (Fields & Tararin, 1970; Lowinger, 1973). This provoked the Chinese–British Opium War. The Chinese lost, and the British government was allowed to support the opium business for many decades, until China become a republic and opium abuse was strictly forbidden. In Japan, after its defeat in World War II, everybody worked very hard to recover from the war's destruction. During this period, many Japanese abused the stimulants that had been used by soldiers in the war (Kato, 1990). In the United States, substance abuse became prevalent and severe when the country was involved in the Vietnam War, which brought distress and confusion to the society.

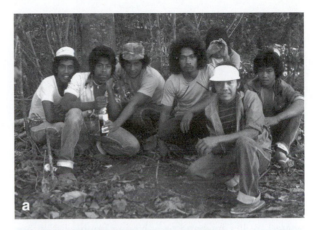

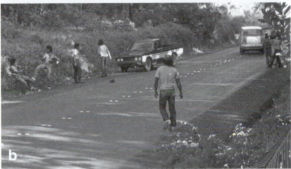

FIGURE 13-14 Alcohol-related youth problems in Micronesia. (a) Adolescent boys drinking liquor in the bush in Truk, Micronesia. (b) The same group of adolescents, after getting drunk, started fighting in the street, damaging a passing car and injuring others.

F. Cultural Interpretation of Certain Mental Conditions

1. Hwabyung (Fire Sickness)

Hwa-byung in Korean language literally means "fire *(hwa)* sickness *(byung)*." Based on a traditional Chinese medical concept that is still prevalent in Korea — that an imbalance among the five elements within the body (metal, wood, water, fire and earth) may cause physical disorders — laypeople in Korea use the folk term "fire sickness" to describe ill conditions. This is a folk idiom of distress characterized by a wide range of somatic and emotional symptoms. According to Korean psychiatrist Si-Hyung Lee (1977), three-fourths of the patients that complained of *hwabyung* were women, who linked their conditions to anger provoked by domestic problems, such as their husbands' extramarital affairs and strained in-law relationships. As pointed out by Pang (1990), the occurrence of *hwabyung* was interpreted when distressed emotions developed in association with intolerable and tragic life situations. Min and Lee (1988) explained that male chauvinism has always been dominant in Korean society, and women tend to suffer from their vulnerable status. When a housewife is mistreated by her husband or is having troubles with her in-laws, according to Korean culture, she has to suppress her emotional reactions so that there will be no disturbance in the stability of the family. As a woman, she is taught to accept defeat, bear frustration, and suppress her hatred. As a result, accumulated "resentment" (*hahn* in Korean) becomes a major issue for some women. Min and Lee interpreted this as the core dynamic for understanding *hwabyung*.

The patients who alleged that they were suffering from *huabyung* usually presented multiple somatopsychological symptoms. Min and Lee (1988) examined 100 Korean patients who claimed that they were suffering from the *hwabyung* condition. The common somatic symptoms they complained about were feeling oppressed in the chest (93%), heart pounding (86%), sighing (78%), fire sensation rising within the body (77%), sleeping problems (62%), pain in the body (54%), dry mouth (50%), an obstructive sensation of mass in the upper abdomen (38%), indigestion (36%), anorexia (34%), dizziness (33%), and others. Emotional symptoms were feeling mortified (53%), worry (44%), feeling frustrated (36%), anger or resentment (37%), feeling depressed (35%), feeling hateful (34%), anxiety (25%), and others. These data illustrate that the manifested condition is a mixture of anxiety-depressive and psychosomatic states. Min and colleagues (1986) tried to make clinical diagnoses of 56 psychiatric outpatients who believed that they were suffering from *hwabyung*. Based on the criteria of DSM-III, they claimed that these patients could be diagnosed as having combined depressive and somati-

zation disorders. In addition, general anxiety, panic attacks, and phobias are associated diagnoses. In other words, there is no specific, homogeneous clinical syndrome associated with the claimed condition of *hwabyung*.

In order to study how Korean folk-illness labels were used by Korean Americans, K.M. Lin and colleagues (1992) carried out interviews of 109 Korean American subjects in the Los Angeles area. They reported that a relatively high proportion (12%) of the subjects said they had suffered from *hwabyung*. Based on their assessment, Lin and associates reported that more *hwabyung* than non-*hwabyung* subjects fulfilled the diagnosis of major depression. They speculated that *hwabyung* may be a culturally patterned way for Koreans to express major depression and related conditions. It was also suggested that a more prominent role be given to "anger" in depression, as anger and the suppression of anger were identified as the main features of *hwabyung* by Koreans.

It seems that it is better to understand *hwabyung* as a "cultural interpretation" of suffering (through pathoreactive effects). Cultural factors may contribute indirectly to the occurrence of particular psychological problems that are encountered by Korean women, but they do not contribute to the formation of particular psychiatric syndromes (pathogenetically) with unique manifestations (through pathoplastically). Almost any emotional reaction was labeled by laymen as an indication of "fire sickness" (*hwabyung*). Therefore, this disorder was placed in group F because culture contributes to the folk interpretation of its cause.

From a clinical point of view, particularly among Korean-Americans (as an immigrant population) in the United States, it would be useful for clinicians to know about the folk interpretations of patients so that appropriate treatment could be offered in psychotherapy for underlying emotional conflicts and medication for symptomatic treatment (K.M. Lin, 1983; Pang, 1990).

2. Susto (Soul loss)

Susto is a Spanish word that literally means "fright." The term is widely used by people in Latin

America to refer to the condition of loss of soul (Rubel, 1964; Rubel, O'Nell, & Collado, 1985). It is based on the folk belief that every individual possesses a soul, but, through certain experiences, such as being frightened or startled, a person's soul may depart from the body. As a result, the soul-lost person will manifest certain morbid mental conditions and illness behavior. The remedy for such a condition, naturally, is to recapture the soul through certain rituals.

George Murdock (1980), based on the study of a world sample of 139 societies from his *Ethnographic Atlas* (Murdock, 1967), identified 13 theories of natural and supernatural causes of illness. Among them, one theory of the cause of sickness was attributed to fright, resulting in soul loss. Thus, it is not surprising that the concept of loss of soul as a cause for sickness is prevalent and that terms similar, or equivalent, to *susto* are found widely distributed across many different cultural groups, such as *el miedo* (fright) in Bolivia (Hollweg, 1997), *lanti* in the Philippines (Hart, 1985), or *mogo laya* in Papua New Guinea (Frankel, 1985).

It should be pointed out that although the cause is uniformally attributed to spiritual–psychological reasons relating mostly to a frightening experience or misfortune, from a clinical point of view, the manifested syndrome is quite heterogeneous, without a commonly shared syndrome (Gillin, 1948). The victim may manifest loss of appetite, sleep disturbance, reduced strength, absentmindedness, headache, dizziness, or many other somatic symptoms, as well as emotional symptoms of depression, anxiety, or irritability. Therefore, strictly speaking, it is not a culture-related "specific syndrome" derived from psychogenic or psychoplastic effects. It is culture related *only* in the sense that the morbid condition is "interpreted" after the fact according to folk concepts of "etiology" and certain ways of regaining the lost soul, such as rituals, are offered. Therefore, the role of culture is interpretation of and reaction to the illness.

3. Other Folk Illness

There are almost countless mental disorders labeled by folk names (Simons & Hughes, 1985). This is particularly true in societies in which modern psy-

chiatry is not prevalent and contemporary mental health service is lacking. Therefore, folk names still play an important role in identifying morbid conditions and in deciding how to manage them. They often determine the reaction of the patient, his family, and the community to such illnesses, shaping the pattern of problem presentation and management, as well as the possible outcome of the condition, and are therefore called pathoreactive effects. Whether the morbid conditions described by local folk names need to be considered "culture-related specific syndromes" depends on the extent to which culture impacts the formation of the condition and the specificity of the psychopathology manifested.

G. Questionable Conditions

For the time being, several of the clinical conditions listed in this group are considered "questionable" because, based on current information, their status as culture-related specific syndromes is unclear and awaiting further elaboration and discussion.

1. Spirit Possession

Many people in different societies around the world develop the disorder of possession. A person may talk and behave as if possessed by another being and announce that he or she is possessed or it is often family, friends, neighbors, or other onlookers who claim that the person is possessed. The being possessing a person may be a deceased family member, a local god, or even an animal spirit. Based on the local language and the possessing being, numerous terms used in various societies have been reported by clinicans and scholars. For instance, *phii pob* (spirit possession) has been reported in Thailand (Suwanlert, 1976), *kitsune-tsuski* (fox possession) in Japan (Daiguji, 1993; Eguchi, 1991; Sasaki, 1969), and *shiebing* (evil sickness) in Taiwan (T.-Y. Lin, 1953).

While spirit possession syndrome is becoming rare in developed European and American societies, it is frequently observed in many other societies, particularly where most people still strongly believe in the possibility of an individual becoming possessed by a supernatural being (Castillo, 1994; Pak, 1996). Pathoreactive effects are clearly observed in such a condition, in terms of how the dissociated/possessed behavior is interpreted, perceived, and responded to, and the possibility of pathoplastic effects should be considered. However, to what further extent the condition is attributed to specific cultural features is awaiting future study.

2. Windigo Psychosis

One kind of possession disorder is known as *windigo* psychosis. The term *windigo* (Ojibwa) or *witiko* (Cree) refers to a folk monster that eats human flesh. It has been speculated that hunters living in the pole area, when they failed at hunting and were starving, may have developed a dissociated state as a result of the desire to eat human fresh, believing they were possessed by the *windigo* monster.

Reviewing the literature carefully, Marano (1985) disclosed that an Oblate missionary, J.E. Saidon (1928), who worked among the Cree of the western James Bay area in the early part of this century, was the first and only individual to observe a *windigo* victim and report his observations in print. Saidon observed a woman who wished not to see anyone outside her immediate family because strangers looked like wild animals to her and she experienced urges to kill them in self-defense. Saidon identified the phenomenon of fearing becoming *windigo* as a "sickness." Later, another priest, J. M. Cooper, in 1933, based solely on Saidon's description and no firsthand observations of his own, published a brief communication in a journal in which he applied the term psychosis to the *windigo* phenomenon. Very soon, misunderstandings snowballed among scholars. A diagnosis and classification had been made with no observation of an actual case based on the fragmented accounts of informants or nonprofessional people. As pointed out by Marano (1982/1985), there never were any *windigo* psychotics in the sense that cannibalism and murder were committed to satisfy an obsessive craving for human flesh. American cultural psychiatrist Robert

Kraus (personal communication, 1996), who worked in the pole area for many years, commented that he never encountered or heard of any *windigo*-like clinical case in his field experiences.

3. Multiple-Personality Disorder

There are increased reports among Western societies of the phenomenon of multiple-personality disorder. Instead of the animal or spirit possession found in developing societies, possession by an "other" self or selves is described in developed societies, where animal or spirit possession is not believed. Whether it is the substitute or variation of dissociation or possession disorder is unclear. Why such a disorder becomes more prevalent, or obtains professional attention in developed societies, is a question we are challenged to answer.

III. COMMENTS AND SUGGESTIONS FOR FUTURE STUDY

A. Culture "-Bound" or "-Related" Issues

Although the term "culture-bound syndrome" was originally invented to refer to the existence of specific psychiatric syndromes "bound" to particular cultural groups (Yap, 1967), recent studies favor the view that such syndromes are not necessarily bound to particular cultural groups and can be observed among various ethnic groups across different geographic areas. Good examples are the sporadic and epidemic occurrences of mass, nondiscriminatory murderous behavior *(amok)* observed in many south Asia societies (such as Laos, the Philippines, and Thailand) beyond Malay (Westermeyer, 1973), as well as in developed societies such as the United States. *Koro* epidemics have been noted beyond south China, in India, and in Thailand (Tseng et al., 1988). The *latah* behavior found in Malay is also observed as *imu* among Ainu in northern Japan (Uchimura, 1956). *Taijinkyofushio,* considered special to the Japanese, is now claimed to also exist among the Koreans (S.-H. Lee, 1987).

Thus, a culture-bound syndrome is not always "bound" to a particular culture unit or system identified in association with ethnicity, but can be observed among several different ethnic groups in different geographic areas (Westermyer & Janca, 1997). Such syndromes need to be reformulated as heavily "related" to certain cultural traits that can be found in different geographic areas, or across ethnicity or cultural unit or systems, which share the common cultural view, attitude, or elements attributed to the formation of the specific syndrome. Based on this new understanding, the term should be changed to "culture-related specific syndromes" to reflect its nature accurately (Tseng & McDermott, 1981).

There are nearly 200 folk names for mental conditions that are recognized and listed by Simons and Hughes (1985). Among them, some are culture-related specific syndromes, whereas others are merely folk terms used by local people to refer to certain mental conditions or disorders. Unless there is sufficient information to support its culture relatedness, a condition should not be regarded as a "culture-related syndrome" simply because it has a folk label.

B. THEORETICAL APPLICATION OF THE TERM AND CONCEPT

Cultural psychiatrists are advised to use the generic term culture-related specific syndrome carefully and not to include in it too many psychiatric conditions. In particular, it is necessary to consider in what way cultural factors contribute to the syndrome — in terms of pathogenic, -selecting, -plastic, -elaborating, -facilitating, or merely -reactive effects? It is suggested that, in a restricted way, unless there is sufficient evidence to support that the syndrome is heavily related to cultural factors in psychogenic or psychoselective ways, with unique complex manifestations, the syndrome should not be labeled a "culture-related specific syndrome" (Prince, 1985). Otherwise, hundreds or thou-

sands of syndromes known by their folk names could potentially be listed as culture-related specific syndromes, while they do not meet the theoretical constructs of such syndromes. If we are too anxious to include syndromes in this category, we will lose its meaningfulness and usefulness.

C. DIAGNOSIS AND CLASSIFICATION ISSUES

Associated with the increased awareness of the impact of culture on psychiatric classifications, as reflected in the recently published American classification system DSM-IV, there is controversy regarding how to deal with culture-related specific syndromes from a diagnostic point of view (Hughes, 1996). Some clinicians feel strongly that various known culture-bound syndromes (such as *koro* or *hwabyung*) should be officially recognized and included in the present classification system.

However, it needs to be pointed out that the present DSM classification system is based on the descriptive approach: categorizing psychiatric disorders by certain sets of manifested symptomatology. If we try to fit culture-related specific syndromes into the categories of the existing classification system or try to create new categories of disorders, they will be classified as NOS (not otherwise specified) or, at best, as "variations" of presently recognized disorders. Many culture-related syndromes are ill-defined or manifested by multiple psychiatric conditions that are difficult to categorize (Chowdhury, 1996). Most importantly, by squeezing the culture-related specific syndromes into the descriptive-oriented classification system, we will lose the unique meaning of the syndromes from a cultural perspective (Guarnaccia, 1993; Pfeiffer, 1982). As pointed out by Hughes (1998), once cultural considerations are accepted as part of all diagnostic categories in the classification system (of DSM-V), it will no longer be necessary to group specific culturally determined behavior patterns into the disjunctive category of "culture-bound syndromes" in the DSM-IV.

Furthermore, it needs to be emphasized that most culture-related specific syndromes are relatively rare, even in the cultures in which they occur. This is particularly true of those syndromes that occur through pathogenetic effects, such as *koro,* frigophoabia, or *voodoo* death. Therefore, adding such rarely observed mental conditions into the presently existing classification system would not be very useful from a practical point of view. Psychiatric classification should be aimed for clinicial usage at the majority of psychiatric disorders. Culture-related syndromes deserve theoretical elaboration and clinical attention, but their significance will not be changed by trying to fit them into a classification system that is basically descriptive in nature.

From a diagnostic point of view, it is necessary to be careful in labeling "peculiar behavior" as a "disorder" simply because it is not familiar to you in your culture. A good example is a case relating to the *latah* phenomenon. Behavior scientists (mainly with anthropological backgrounds) favor the view that *latah* as a social behavior is not necessarily a "disorder" from an etic point of view, even though some psychiatrists have considered it a psychopathological condition and offered various clinical diagnoses, such as hysterical dissociation or even hysteria psychosis. If you had the opportunity to actually observe an episode of *latah* in its social setting, you would not label it a "psychotic condition" and very likely you would doubt the validity of categorizing it as a "psychiatric disorder," unless the person was subjectively suffering from the mental episode.

Also, many behavioral scientists and clinicians who do not have sufficient psychiatric knowledge or direct clinical observation of actual cases, and who simply rely on others' reports, have tried to lump together various morbid conditions into one similar entity. For instance, Arctic hysteria observed among Eskimo people in Alaska, *latah* reaction observed in Malay, and the so-called *windigo* psychosis are categorized together as hysteropsychoses. Although these three disorders may share "hysterical" elements, they involve entirely different mental conditions (C.T.D. Friedmann, 1982). Clinical specula-

tions and elaborations should not be made without direct clinical observation and examination merely on the basis of other people's reports, particularly those of writers with nonprofessional backgrounds or clinicians without cultural sensitivity. It is necessary to have culturally oriented psychiatric knowledge and experience in order to grasp the nature of culture-related disorders in an appropriate and meaningful way.

D. CULTURE-RELATED SYNDROMES IN WESTERN SOCIETIES

The last point that must be made is that, by definition, culture-related specific syndromes should be able to be discovered everywhere — as every society has its own culture. However, the trend has been to consider that most culture-related specific syndromes (such as *koro, amok,* or *dhat* syndromes) occur in non-Western societies. This is due to two reasons: they were considered "peculiar" phenomena observed in areas previously colonized by Western people or they simply did not fit the classification system developed for Euro-American populations. This trend is now changing. There is an increased interest among Western cultural psychiatrists (such as Littlewood & Lipsedge, 1986) to recognize syndromes in "our own" Western cultures that are heavily culture related. Several psychiatric disorders have been suggested by various scholars for consideration as Western culture-related syndromes. These include anorexia nervosa (Littlewood & Lipsedge, 1986; Palazzoli, 1985; Swartz, 1985), obesity (Ritenbaugh, 1982), drug-induced dissociated states, multiple personality, and even premenstrual syndrome (Johnson, 1987) — disorders that are seldom observed in non-Western societies. Because these conditions are already recognized in the existing Western nosological system, they are, in a sense, not viewed as "specific" syndromes. However, they can be viewed as "culture-related" psychiatric conditions that are influenced by the pathoelaborative, pathofacilitative, or pathoplastic effects of Western culture.

E. Suggestions for Future Research

Looking back, we see that the majority of the work of clinicians regarding culture-related syndromes has been in the area of the clinical description of certain phenomena and speculation on how culture might contribute to them. It is suggested that future efforts should be made in the following two areas.

1. Comprehensive Psychiatric Case Study for Dynamic and Cultural Understanding

There is a need to carry out more comprehensive studies of individual cases in order to understand the psychodynamics of the disorders. We should not merely collect data on the clinical manifestations of a group of victims, but carry out intensive clinical evaluations of individual cases in order to understand the personal histories, family backgrounds, psychological development, and stress and coping patterns, as well as possible cultural contributions to the formation of the disorders. Guarnaccia and Rogler (1999) have commented that instead of concentrating on diagnostic issues, such as how to subsume the syndromes into psychiatric categories, future research needs to focus on the nature of the phenomena.

2. Mass-Survey Studies

In addition to the clinical collection of demographic information about a group of subjects suffering from a particular culture-related syndrome, it is desirable to carry out well-designed questionnaire surveys of the subjects using variables to test certain hypotheses, particularly regarding the ways in which culture may contribute to the disorders. The hypotheses may be related to personality patterns, common psychological problems, shared culture beliefs or attitudes, and the sociocultural meaning of the psychopathology manifested (Tseng, Mo et al., 1992). In other words, the time is ripe for clinicians to move one step further and carry out more comprehensive clinical studies. It is hoped that, by doing so, we may accumulate more information on how culture contributes to psychopathology and how to deal with the pathology when it occurs. This is the main purpose for recognizing and studying culture-related syndromes.

3. Sociocultural Understanding of the Phenomena

As pointed out by Jilek and Jilek-Aall (1985), echoed by Bartholomew (1994b), in future evaluations of culture-related specific syndromes, we have to look beyond individual psychodynamics and culture-specific personal traits to the total geopolitical, socioeconomic, and ideological circumstances of the society in which the phenomena occur. This will give us a more meaningful understanding of the metamorphosis of culture-related syndromes: how individuals respond to culture-related stress with culture-conditioned reactions within a particular sociocultural climate.

REFERENCES

Adeniran, R.A., & Jones, J.R. (1994). Koro: Culture-bound disorder or universal symptom? *British Journal of Psychiatry, 164,* 559–561.

Akhtar, S. (1988). Four culture-bound psychiatric syndromes in India. *International Journal of Social Psychiatry, 34,* 70–74.

Ang, P.C., & Weller, M.P.I. (1984). Koro and psychosis. *British Journal of Psychiatry, 145,* 335.

Barrett, K. (1978). Koro in a Londoner. *Lancet, 8103,* 1319.

Bartholomew, R.E. (1994a). Disease, disorder, or deception? Latah as habit in a Malay extended family. *Journal of Nervous and Mental Disease, 182*(6), 331–338.

Bartholomew, R.E. (1994b). The sociology of 'epidemic' koro. *International Journal of Social Psychiatry, 40*(1), 46–60.

Berrios, G.E., & Morley, S.J. (1984). Koro-like symptom in a non-Chinese subject. *British Journal of Psychiatry, 145,* 331–334.

Bhatia, M.S. & Malik, S.C. (1991). Dhat syndrome—A useful diagnostic entity in Indian culture. *British Journal of Psychiatry, 159,* 691–695.

Bottéro, A. (1991). Consumption by semen loss in India and elsewhere. *Culture, Medicine and Psychiatry, 15,* 303–320.

Burton-Bradley, B.G. (1968). The *amok* syndrome in Papua and New Guinea. *Medical Journal of Australia, 1,* 252–256.

Burton-Bradley, B.G. (1975). Cargo cult. In B.G. Burton-Bradley (Ed.), *Stone age crisis: A psychiatric appraisal* (pp. 10–31). Nashville, TN: Vanderbilt University Press.

Burton-Bradley, B.G. (1982). Cargo cult syndromes. In C.T.H. Friedman & R.A. Faguet (Eds.), *Extraordinary disorders of human behavior.* New York: Plenum Press.

Cannon, W.B. (1957). "Voodoo" death. *Psychosomatic Medicine, 19,* 182–190.

Carr, J.E. (1978). Ethno-behaviorism and the culture-bound syndromes: The case of *amok. Culture, Medicine and Psychiatry, 2,* 269–293.

Carr, J.E., & Tan, E.K. (1976). In search of the true *amok: Amok* as viewed within the Malay culture. *American Journal of Psychiatry, 133*(11), 1295–1299.

Carstairs, G.M. (1956). *Hinjra and Jiryan:* Two derivatives of Hindu attitudes to sexuality. *British Journal of Medical Psychology, 29,* 128–138.

Castillo, R.J. (1994). Spirit possession in South Asia: Dissociation or hysteria? Part 1. Theoretical background. *Culture, Medicine and Psychiatry, 18*(1), 1–22.

Cawte, J.E. (1976). *Malgri:* A culture-bound syndrome. In W.P. Lebra (Ed.), *Culture-bound syndromes, ethnopsychiatry, and alternate therapies* (pp. 22–31). Honolulu: University Press of Hawaii.

Chang, Y.H., Rin, H., & Chen, C.C. (1975). Frigophobia: A report of five cases. *Bulletin of the Chinese Society of Neurology and Psychiatry, 1*(2), 9–13 (in Chinese).

Chiniwala, M., Alfonso, C.A., Torres, J.R., & Lefer, J. (1996). Koro in an immigrant from Guinea with brief psychotic disorder. *American Journal of Psychiatry, 153*(5), 736.

Chiou, N.M., Liu, C.Y., Chen, C.C., & Yang, Y.Y. (1994). Frigophobia: Report of two cases. *Chinese Psychiatry, 8*(4), 297–302 (in Chinese).

Chiu, T.L., Tong, J.E., & Schmidt, K.E. (1972). A clinical and survey study of latah in Sarawak, Malaysia. *Psychological Medicine, 2,* 155–165.

Chowdhury, A.N. (1994). Koro in females: An analysis of 48 cases. *Transcultural Psychiatric Research Review, 31,* 369–380.

Chowdhury, A.N. (1996). The definition and classification of koro. *Culture, Medicine and Psychiatry, 20,* 41–65.

Cooper, J.M. (1933). The Cree Witiko psychosis. *Primitive Man, 6,* 20–24.

Daiguji, M. (1993). *Psychopathology of possession: Modern clinical study* (in Japanese). Tokyo: Seiwa.

Daiguji, M., & Shichida, H. (1998, October). *Imu phenomena observed among the Ainu people in northern Japan: Past and present.* Presented at the Second Pan Asia-Pacific Mental Health Conference, Beijing.

Eastwell, D. (1982). Voodoo death and the mechanism for dispatch of the dying in East Arnhem, Australia. *American Anthropologist, 84,* 5–18 (Reviewed by E.A. Gomez in *Transcultural Psychiatry Research Review, 21*(1), 66–67 [1984].)

Ede, A. (1976). Koro in an Anglo-Saxon Canadian. *Canadian Psychiatric Association Journal, 21,* 389–392.

Edwards, J.W. (1985). Indigenous koro, a genital retraction syndrome of Insular Southeast Asia: A critical review. In R.C. Simons & C.C. Hughes (Eds.), *The culture-bound syndromes: Folk illness of psychiatric and anthropological interest* (pp. 169–191). Dordrecht, The Netherlands: Reidel.

Eguchi, S.Y. (1991). Between folk concepts of illness and psychiatric diagnosis: Kitsune-tsuki (fox possession) in a mountain village of western Japan. *Culture, Medicine and Psychiatry, 15*(4), 421–452.

Ellis, W.G. (1893). The *amok* of the Malays. *Journal of Mental Science, 39,* 325–338.

Ellis, W.G. (1897). Latah: A mental madady of the Malays. *Journal of Mental Science, 43,* 33–40.

Engel, G.L. (1971). Sudden and rapid death during psychological stress: Folklore or folk wisdom? *Annals of Internal Medicine, 74,* 771–782.

Fernández-Marian, R. (1959). The Puerto Rican syndrome: Its dynamic and cultural determinants. *Psychiatry, 24,* 79–82.

Fields, A., & Tararin, P.A. (1970). Opium in China. *British Journal of Addiction, 64,* 371–382.

Fletcher, W. (1908). Latah and crime. *Lancet, 2,* 254–255.

Foulks, E.F. (1972). The Arctic hysterias of the North Alaskan Eskimo. In D.H. Maybury-Lewis (Ed.), *Anthropological studies,* (No. 10). Washington, DC: American Anthropological Association.

Frankel, S. (1985). *Mogo laya,* a New Guinea fright illness. In R.C. Simons & C.C. Hughes (Eds.), *The culture-bound syndromes* (pp. 399–404). Dordrecht, The Netherlands: Reidel.

Friedmann, C.T.D. (1982). The so-called hystero-psychoses: Latah, windigo, and pibloktoq. In C.T.H. Friedmann & R.A. Faguet (Eds.), *Extraordinary disorders of human behavior.* New York: Plenum Press.

Friedmann, C.T.H., & Faguet, R.A. (Eds.). (1982). *Extraordinary disorders of human behavior.* New York: Plenum Press.

Geertz, H. (1968). Latah in Java: A theoretical paradox. *Indonesia, 5,* 93–104.

Gillin, J. (1948). Magical fright. *Psychiatry, 11,* 387–400.

Golden, K.M. (1977). Voodoo in Africa and the United States. *American Journal of Psychiatry, 134*(12), 1425–1427.

Gordon, R.A. (1990). *Anorexia and bulimia: Anatomy of a social epidemic.* Cambridge, UK: Basil/Blackwell.

Guarnaccia, P.J. (1993). Ataques de nervios in Puerto Rico: Culture-bound syndrome or popular illness? *Medical Anthropology, 15,* 157–170.

Guarnaccia, P.J., Canino, G., Rubio-Stipec, M., & Bravo, M. (1993). The prevalence of *ataques de nervios* in the Puerto Rico Disaster Study: The role of culture in psychiatric epidemiology. *Journal of Nervous and Mental Disease, 181*(3), 157–165.

Guarnaccia, P.J., & Rogler, L.H. (1999). Research on culture-bound syndromes: New directions. *American Journal of Psychiatry, 156*(9), 1322–1327.

Guarnaccia, P.J., Rubio-Stipec, M., & Canino, G.J. (1989). *Ataques de nervios* in the Puerto Rican Diagnostic Interview Schedule:

The impact of cultural categories on psychiatric epidemiology. *Culture, Medicine and Psychiatry, 13,* 275–295.

Gussow, Z. (1985). Pibloktoq (hysteria) among the Polar Eskimo: An ethnopsychiatric study. In R.C. Simons & C.C. Hughes (Eds.), *The culture-bound syndromes.* (pp. 271–287). Dordrecht, The Netherlands: Reidel. (Original work published 1960)

Gwee, A.L. (1963). Koro: A cultural disease. *Singapore Medical Journal, 4,* 119–122.

Gwee, A.L. (1968). Koro: Its origin and nature as a disease entity. *Singapore Medical Journal, 9,* 3–6.

Hart, D.V. (1985). Lanti, illness by fright among Bisayan Filipino. In R.C. Simons & C.C. Hughes (Eds.), *The culture-bound syndromes.* Dordrecht, The Netherlands: Reidel.

Hes, J.P., & Nassi, G. (1977). Koro in a Yemenite and a Georgian Jewish immigrant. *Confinia Psychiatrica, 20,* 180–184.

Hippler, A., & Cawte, J. (1978). The *malgri* territorial anxiety syndrome: Primitive pattern for agoraphobia. *Journal of Operational Psychiatry, 9*(2), 23–31.

Hollweg, M.G. (1997). Main culture bound syndromes in Bolivia. *Curare, 20*(1), 23–28.

Hughes, C.C. (1996). The culture-bound syndromes and psychiatric diagnosis. In J.E. Mezzich, A. Kleinman, H. Fabrega, Jr., & D.L. Parron (Eds.), *Culture and psychiatric diagnosis: A DSM-IV perspective* (pp. 289–307). Washington, DC: American Psychiatric Press.

Hughes, C.C. (1998). The glossary of 'culture-bound syndromes' in DSM-IV: A critique. *Transcultural Psychiatry, 35*(3), 413–421.

Iwa, H. (1982). *Shinkeisho (Neuroses).* Tokyo: Nihonbunka Kagakusha.

Jegede, R.O. (1983). Psychiatric illness in African students: "Brain fag" syndrome revisited. *Canadian Journal of Psychiatry, 28,* 188–192.

Jilek, W.G., & Jilek-Aall, L. (1985). The metamorphosis of "culture-bound' syndromes. *Social Science Medicine, 21*(2), 205–210.

Johnson, T.M. (1987). Premenstrual syndrome as a Western culture-specific disorder. *Culture, Medicine and Psychiatry, 11*(3), 337–356.

Kasahara, Y. (1974). Fear of eye-to-eye confrontation among neurotic patients in Japan. In T.S. Lebra & P.L. Lebra (Eds.), *Japanese culture and bahavior* (pp. 396–406). Honolulu: University Press of Hawaii.

Kato, M. (1977). Japanese characteristics of neurosis. In *Shakai to Seishinbyori [Society and psychopathology]* (pp. 23–34). Tokyo: Kobundo (in Japanese).

Kato, M. (1990). Brief history of control, prevention and treatment of drug dependence in Japan. *Drug and Alcohol Dependence, 25,* 213–214.

Kenny, M.G. (1983). Paradox lost: The latah problem revisited. *Journal of Nervous and Mental Disease, 171*(3), 159–167.

Kimura, S. (1982). *Nihonjin no taijinkyofushio [Japanese anthrophobia]* (in Japanese). Tokyo: Keso Shobo.

Kitanish, K. & Mori, A. (1995). Morita therapy: 1919 to 1995. *Psychiatry and Clinical Neurosciences, 13,* 31–37.

Kobler, F. (1948). Description of an acute castration fear, based on superstition. *Psychoanalytic Review, 35,* 285–289.

Lambo, T.A. (1960 December 10). Further neuropsychiatric observations in Nigeria: With comments on the need for epidemiological study in Africa. *British Medical Journal,* pp. 1696–1704.

Lambo, T.A. (1962). Malignant anxiety: A syndrome associated with criminal conduct in Africans. *Journal of Mental Science, 108,* 256–264.

Lee, R.L.M. (1981). Structure and anti-structure in the culture-bound syndromes: The Malay case. *Culture, Medicine and Psychiatry, 5,* 233–248.

Lee, S.-H. (1977). A study on the *"hwabyung"* (anger syndrome). *Journal of the Korean General Hospital, 1,* 63–69.

Lee, S.-H. (1987). Social phobia in Korea. In *Social phobia in Japan and Korea. Proceedings of the First Cultural Psychiatry Symposium between Japan and Korea.* Seoul: The East Asian Academy of Cultural Psychiatry.

Lidz, R.W., Lidz, T., & Burton-Bradley, B.G. (1973). Culture, personality and social structure: Cargo cultism—A psychosocial study of Melanesian millenarianism. *Journal of Nervous and Mental Disease, 157*(5), 370–388.

Liebowitz, M.R., Salmán, E., Jusino, C.M., Garfinkel, R., Street, L., Cárdenas, D.L., Silvestre, J., Fyer, A.J., Carrasco, J.L., Davies, S., Guarnaccia, P., & Klein, D.F. (1994). Ataque de nervios and panic disorder. *American Journal of Psychiatry, 151,* 871–875.

Lin, K.M. (1983). *Hwa-byung:* A Korean culture-bound syndrome? *American Journal of Psychiatry, 140*(1), 105–107.

Lin, K.M., Lau, J.K.C., Yamamoto, J., Zheng, Y.P., Kim, H.S., Cho, K.H., & Nakasaki, G. (1992). Hwa-byung: A community study of Korean Americans. *Journal of Nervous and Mental Disease, 180*(6), 386–391.

Lin, T.-Y. (1953). An epidemiological study of the incidence of mental disorder in Chinese and other cultures. *Psychiatry, 16,* 313–336.

Littlewood, R., & Lipsedge, M. (1986). The "culture-bound syndromes' of the dominant culture: Culture, psychopathology and biomedicine. In J.L. Cox (Ed.), *Transcultural psychiatry* (pp. 253–273). London: Croom Helm.

Lowinger, P. (1973). How the People's Republic of China solves the drug abuse problem. *American Journal of Chinese Medicine, 1*(2), 275–282.

Malhotra, H.K., & Wig, N.N. (1975). Dhat syndrome: A culture-bound sex neurosis of the Orient. *Archives of Sexual Behavior, 4*(5), 519–528.

Marano L. (1985). Windigo psychosis: The anatomy of an emic-etic confusion. In R.C. Simons & C.C. Hughes (Eds.), *The culture-bound syndromes* (pp. 441–448). Dordrecht, The Netherlands: Reidel. (original work published 1982).

Mehlman, R.D. (1961). The Puerto Rican syndrome. *American Journal of Psychiatry, 118,* 328–332.

Meth, J.M. (1974). Exotic psychiatric syndromes. In S. Arieti & E.B. Brody (Eds.), *American handbook of psychiatry: Vol. 3. Adult clinical psychiatry* (pp. 723–739). New York: Basic Books.

Min, S.K., & Lee, H.Y. (1988). *A clinical study on hwabyung.* Presented at the Fourth scientific meeting of the Pacific Rim College of Psychiatry, Hong Kong.

Min, S.K., Lee, M.H., Shin, J.H., Park, M.H., Kim, M.K., & Lee, H.Y. (1986). A diagnostic study on *hwabyung. Journal of Korean Medical Association, 29*(6), 653–661.

Mo, G.M., Li, L.S., & Ou, L.W. (1987). Report of koro epidemic in Leizhou Peninsula, Hainan Island. *Chinese Journal of Neuropsychiatry, 20,* 232–234 (in Chinese).

Mori, W., & Kitanishi, K. (1984). Morita-shinkeishitsu to DSM-III [Morita nervous temperament disorders and DSM-III]. *Rhinshoseishin-igaku 13,* 911–920 (in Japanese).

Murdock, G.P. (1967). *Ethnographic atlas.* Pittsburgh: University of Pittsburgh Press.

Murdock, G.P. (1980). *Theories of illness: A world survey.* Pittsburgh: University of Pittsburgh Press.

Murphy, H.B.M. (1973). History and evolution of syndromes: The striking case of *latah* and *amok.* In M. Hammer, K. Salzinger, & S. Sutton (Eds.), *Psychopathology.* New York: Wiley.

Musgrave, W.E., & Sison, A.G. (1910). Mali-mali, a mimic psychosis in the Philippine Islands: A plenary report. *Philippine Journal of Science, 5,* 335–339.

Neki, J.S. (1973). Psychiatry in South-east Asia. *British Journal of Psychiatry, 123,* 256–269.

Oquendo, M., Horwath, E., & Martines, A. (1992). Ataques de nervios: Proposed diagnostic criteria for a culture specific syndrome. *Culture, Medicine and Psychiatry, 16*(3), 367–376.

Pak, O.K. (1996). Spirit possession in East Asia. *Transcultural Psychiatric Research Review, 33*(1), 81–87.

Palazzoli, M.S. (1985). Anorexia nervosa: A syndrome of the affluent society. *Transcultural Psychiatric Research Review, 22*(3), 199–205.

Pang, K.Y.C. (1990). *Hwabyung:* The construction of a Korean popular illness among Korean elderly immigrant women in the United States. *Culture, Medicine and Psychiatry, 14,* 495–512.

Paris, J. (1992). Dhat: The semen loss anxiety syndrome. *Transcultural Psychiatric Research Review, 29*(2), 109–118.

Pfeiffer, W.M. (1982). Culture-bound syndromes. In I. Al-Issa (Ed.), *Culture and psychopathology.* Baltimore: University Park Press.

Prince, R. (1960). The "brain fag" syndrome in Nigerian students. *Journal of Mental Science, 104,* 559–570.

Prince, R. (1985). The concept of culture-bound syndromes: Anorexia nervosa and brain-fag. *Social Science and Medicine, 21*(2), 197–203.

Prince, R. (1990). The brain-fag syndrome. In K. Pelzer & P.O. Ebigbo (Eds.), *A textbook of clinical psychiatry in Africa.* Enugu, Nigeria: Chuka.

Prince, R., & Tcheng-Laroche, F. (1987). Culture-bound syndromes and international disease classifications. *Culture, Medicine and Psychiatry, 11,* 3–19.

Rin, H. (1965). A study of the aetiology of *koro* in respect to the Chinese concept of illness. *International Journal of Social Psychiatry, 11,* 7–13.

Rin, H. (1966). Two forms of vital deficiency syndrome among Chinese male mental patients. *Transcultural Psychiatric Research Review, 3,* 19–21.

Ritenbaugh, C. (1982). Obesity as a culture-bound syndrome. *Culture, Medicine and Psychiatry, 6*(4), 347–361.

Rubel, A.J. (1964). The epidemiology of a folk illness: *Susto* in Hispanic America. *Ethology, 3,* 268–283.

Rubel, A.J., O'Nell, C.W., & Collado, R. (1985). The folk illness called *susto.* In R.C. Simons & C.C. Hughes (Eds.), *The culture-bound syndromes* (pp. 333–350). Dordrecht, The Netherlands: Reidel.

Rubin, R.T. (1982). *Koro (shook yang):* A culture-bound psychogenic syndrome. In C.T.H. Friedmann & R.A. Gaguet (Eds.), *Extraordinary disorders of human behavior* (pp. 155–172). New York: Plenum Press.

Salmán, E., Liebowitz, M.R., Guarnaccia, P.J., Jusino, C.M., Garfinkel, R., Street, L., Cárdenas, D.L., Silvestre, J., Fyer, A.J., Carrasco, J.L., Davies, S.O., & Klein, D. (1998). Subtypes of ataques de nervios: The influence of coexisting psychiatric diagnosis. *Culture, Medicine and Psychiatry, 22,* 231–244.

Sasaki, Y. (1969). Psychiatric study of the shaman in Japan. In W. Caudil & T.-Y. Lin (Eds.), *Mental health research in Asia and the Pacific.* (pp. 223–241). Honolulu: East-West Center Press.

Schmidt, K., Hill, L., & Guthrie, G. (1977). Running *amok. International Journal of Psychiatry, 23*(4), 264–274.

Simons, R.C. (1980). The resolution of the latah paradox. *Journal of Nervous and Mental Disease, 168*(4), 195–206.

Simons, R.C. (1996). *Boo!—Culture, experience, and the startle reflex.* New York: Oxford University Press.

Simons, R.C., & Hughes, C.C. (1985). *The culture-bound syndromes: Folk illnesses of psychiatric and anthropological interest.* Dordrecht, The Netherlands: Reidel.

Still, R.M. (1940). Remarks on the aetiology and symptoms of young-dah-hte with a report on four cases and its medical-legal significance. *Indian Medical Gazette, 75,* 88–91.

Suwanlert, S. (1976). *Phii pob:* Spirit possession in rural Thailand. In W.P. Lebra (Ed.), *Culture-bound syndromes, ethnopsychiatry, and alternate therapies* (pp. 68–87). Honolulu: University Press of Hawaii.

Suwanlert, S. (1988). A study of *latah* in Thailand. *Journal of the Psychiatric Association of Thailand, 33*(3), 129–133.

Swartz, L. (1985). Anorexia nervosa as a culture bound syndrome. *Transcultural Psychiatric Research Review, 22*(3), 205–207.

Tan, E.S. (1965). *Amok:* A diagnostic consideration. *Proceedings of the Second Malaysian Congress of Medicine,* pp. 22–25.

Tan, E.S. (1981). Culture-bound syndromes among overseas Chinese. In A. Kleinman & T.-Y. Lin (Eds.), *Normal and abnormal behavior in Chinese culture* (pp. 371–386). Dordrecht, The Netherlands: Reidel.

Tan, E.S., & Carr, J.E. (1977). Psychiatric sequelae of *amok. Culture, Medicine and Psychiatry, 1*(1), 59–67.

Tanaka-Matsumi, J. (1979). Taijin kyofusho: Diagnostic and cultural issues in Japanese psychiatry. *Culture, Medicine and Psychiatry, 3*(3), 231–245.

Teoh, J.-I. (1972). The changing psychopathology of *amok*. *Psychiatry, 35,* 345–351.

Tsai, J.B. (1982). *Suoyang* disorder: Five cases report. *Zhunguo Senjing Jjingsenbin Zazhi 4,* 206 (in Chinese).

Tseng, W.S., Asai, M., Kitanish, K., McLaughlin, D.G., & Kyomen, H. (1992). Diagnostic patterns of social phobia: Comparison in Tokyo and Hawaii. *Journal of Nervous and Mental Disease, 180,* 380–385.

Tseng, W.S., & Hsu, J. (1969/1970). Chinese culture, personality formation and mental illness. *International Journal of Social Psychiatry, 16*(1), 5–14.

Tseng, W.S., & McDermott, J.F., Jr. (1981). *Culture, mind and therapy: An introduction to cultural psychiatry.* New York: Brunner/Mazel.

Tseng, W.S., Mo, G.M., Hsu, J., Li, L.S., Chen, G.Q., Ou, L.W., & Zheng, H.B. (1992). Koro epidemics in Guandong, China: A questionnaire survey. *Journal of Nervous and Mental Disease, 180*(2), 117–123.

Tseng, W.S., Mo, G.M., Hsu, J., Li, L.S., Ou, L.W., Chen, G.Q., & Jiang, D.W. (1988). A sociocultural study of koro epidemics in Guandong, China. *American Journal of Psychiatry, 145*(12), 1538–1543.

Uchimura, V.Y. (1956). Imu, eine psychoracktive Erscheinung der ainu-Frauen [*Imu,* a psychoactive pnenomenon of *ainu*-women]. *Nervenarzt, 12,* 535–540.

Uchimura, V.Y., Akimoto, & Ishibashi, (1938). The syndrome of *imu* in the Ainu race [Comment]. *American Journal of Psychiatry, 94,* 1467–1469.

van Wulfften Palthe, P.M. (1934). Koro: Een eigenaardig angstneurose. *Geneeskundi Tijdschrift voor Nederlandsch-Indie, 74,* 1713–1720.

Wen, J.K. (1995). Sexual beliefs and problems in contemporary Taiwan. In T.-Y. Lin, W.S. Tseng, & E.K. Yeh (Eds.), *Chinese societies and mental health* (pp. 219–230). Hong Kong: Oxford University Press.

Westermeyer, J. (1972). A comparison of *amok* and other homicide in Laos. *American Journal of Psychiatry, 129*(6), 703–709.

Westermeyer, J. (1973). On the epidemicy of *amok* violence. *Archives of General Psychiatry, 28,* 873–876.

Westermeyer, J. (1982). *Amok.* In C.T.H. Friedmann & R.T. Faguet (Eds.), *Extraordinary disorders of human behavior.* New York: Plenum Press.

Westermeyer, J., & Janca, A. (1997). Language, culture and psychopathology: Conceptual and methodological issues. *Transcultural Psychiatry, 34*(3), 291–311.

Wig, N.N. (1960). Problem of mental health in India. *Journal of Clinical and Social Psychiatry (College of Lucknow, India), 17*(2), 48–53.

Winiarz, W., & Wielawski, J. (1936). Imu: A psychoneurosis occuring among Ainus. *Psychoanalytic Review, 23,* 181–186.

Winzeler, R.L. (1995). *Latah* in *Southeast Asia: The ethnography and history of a culture-bound syndrome.* Cambridge, UK: Cambridge University Press. (Reviewed by M.G. Kenny in *Transcultural psychiatry Research Review 33,* 43–54 [1996]).

Woon, T.H. (1988). *The latah phenomena.* Presented at the annual meeting of Pacific Rim College of Psychiatry, Hong Kong.

Yamashita, I. (1993). *Taijin-kyofu or delusional social phobia.* Sapporo: Hokkaido University Press. (English translation of Japanese book originally published in 1977, Tokyo: Kanehara) (Reviewed by S.C. Chang in *Transcultural Psychiatry Research Review, 2,* 283–288 [1984]).

Yap, P.M. (1951). Mental diseases peculiar to certain cultures: A survey of comparative psychiatry. *Journal of Mental Science, 97,* 313–327.

Yap, P.M. (1952). The latah reaction: Its pathodynamics and nosological position. *Journal of Mental Science, 98,* 515–564.

Yap, P.M. (1965). Koro—A culture-bound depersonalization syndrome. *British Journal of Psychiatry, 111,* 43–50.

Yap, P.M. (1967). Classification of the culture-bound reactive syndromes. *Australia and New Zealand Journal of Psychiatry, 1,* 172–179

14

Epidemic Mental Disorders

I. INTRODUCTION

From a cultural point of view, next to specific culture-related syndromes, epidemic mental disorders are probably among the most interesting psychopathological conditions. Because their development is closely related to social and cultural factors, they have attracted keen attention from cultural psychiatrists. "Epidemic mental disorders" refer to mental disorders or pathological psychological reactions that occur among groups of people in a contagious way within a relatively short period of time in a particular social setting. The mental disorders may involve a small number of subjects or hundreds or even thousands collectively through the process of contagion in an endemic or epidemic fashion, and are therefore called "contagious" or "epidemic." Because the mental disorders are transmitted or spread from one person to another, involving tens, hundreds, or thousands of people, the nature of the transmissions is understood to be psychological, closely related to the social atmosphere and community setting at the particular time and the common beliefs or attitudes shared by the group of people involved, and a part of the mechanism of group psychology. Therefore, it is also called "mass

psychogenic illness." The psychiatric symptoms are usually manifested as hysterical conversion reactions (such as fainting, paralysis, or convulsions) or panic states (such as fear of disaster, danger, or death). However, they may also take the form of collective depressive or delusional states or a mixture of various disturbances.

II. HISTORICAL SURVEY

Epidemic mental disorders have been manifested, if not defined, since before the Middle Ages. According to historical reports, for centuries the Western world has witnessed numerous group exhibitions of "peculiar behavior." From the early 1300s through the 16th century, dancing epidemics occurred, for example, in Metz, Cologne, and Aix-la-Chapelle in 1377 and in Strasbourg in 1412 (Kagwa, 1964). Burton's *Anatomy of Melancholy* (1628/1961) gave this description: "It is strange how long they will dance, and in what manner, over stools, forms, tables; even great bellied women sometimes … will dance so long that they can stir neither hand nor foot, but seem to be quite dead."

Western Europe called the dance manias St. John's dance or St. Vitus' dance. The epidemic had spread to Italy by the late 1600s. In 1844, Hecker wrote that those with this condition first became morose, withdrawn, and apathetic, but, at the sound of music, began to dance and jump (Tan, 1963). In Italy, the mania inspired folk accounts of its cause and cure. It was said to be caused by the bite of a tarantula and relieved only by the spirited music called *Tarantella.* Thus, it was called Tarantism. Outbreaks in Spain were called *Jota* (Ivanova, 1970). In psychiatric terms, it was mass hysteria.

In the 17th century, hysterical outbreaks occurred in religious frameworks, several involving nuns. One conspicuous episode occurred at a convent in Loudun, France. The hysteria centered on beliefs of *incubi* and possession. At that time, it was believed that demonic spirits could take the form of a man, obtain semen (some said from a corpse), and actually impregnate a sleeping victim. The word "nightmare" comes from the Latin *incubo* and its literal meaning, "to lie upon." A 1651 prayer ended with the entreaty that the devil would not molest one during sleep, "especially in those members designed for procreation" (Robbins, 1959).

In the Loudun incident, the belief in possession by demon made possible what seems to have been a combination of deliberate maliciousness and genuine hysteria. It began with a plot to punish a priest, Father Grandier, for insulting the powerful Cardinal Richelieu. Several nuns were persuaded to pretend that they were possessed. Father Grandier, who they said caused their possession, was forced to exorcize them in public. Some sources say that one nun, who cherished an unrequited love for the priest, told her *incubi* possession story to the other nuns and they became convinced that they, too, were possessed (Sirois, 1974). The public exorcisms inspired their own mass hysteria. Before the episode ended, Father Grandier was tried for witchcraft, tortured, and burned alive. Two of the priests who tortured him died insane and a third was later banished from France. A doctor who acted as a "witch hunter" died in delirium. Had the nuns been only acting at the beginning, and then,

cloistered, caught up in their own dramatics, and given appreciative, hysterical audiences, become genuinely hysterical? History suggests that both the performers and the onlookers who recorded the events were hysterical. Reports said that the nuns' faces were "so frightful one could not bear to look at them," that they uttered loud cries and obscenities, that "their eyes remained open without winking," and that one young nun was "in convulsions" and, falling on the ground and "lifting her petticoats … displayed her privy parts without shame" (Robbins, 1959).

A half-century after the Loudun incident, Louis XIV ordered an end to witchcraft trials in France. But in 1692, in the village of Salem, Massachusetts, in the young American colonies, an infamous chapter in hysteria began. A few bored teenage girls fueled a cycle of suspicion, accusation, revenge, and panic, putting on exhibitions of "fits" and eccentric behavior. They then accused a Negro slave, a pipe-smoking woman beggar, and a crippled woman of "bewitching" them. At their trial, one of these scapegoats named another as the witch who had caused the trouble. The cycle began, with neighbors accusing neighbors. Some of those accused panicked and confessed to witchcraft; some named others as witches, thereby aligning themselves with the "innocent." Accused became accuser, and by the time the last witchcraft trials had ended, more than 30 men and women and two 7-year-old children had been put to death (Robbins, 1959).

Were these incidents merely historical curiosities or reflections of beliefs or ignorance in developing countries? The answer, based on the phenomena of later years in established civilizations, is a decided *no.* For example, Schuler and Parenton (1943) cited Schutte's 1906 description of a "trembling disease" that affected children in several schools in Meissen, Germany. The children's hands and arms shook spasmodically for a few minutes and, in some cases, for as long as an hour. The seizures lasted for weeks, with random, symptom-free periods in which the children felt completely well.

Just before Halloween in 1938, panic threatened much of the United States when CBS radio broadcast the Mercury Theater's version of H. G. Wells' *War of* the Worlds (Cantril, 1940). Some of us still remember that Sunday evening when we were lulled at first by a simulated "remote broadcast" of dance music. "News bulletins" interrupted, announcing that a strange object — perhaps a meteor — had fallen in New Jersey. A news announcer was sent to the scene. His voice, at first professionally calm, rose in convincing mock hysteria as he described a "strange machine" from which, he said, came "monsters from Mars," devastating the land. Later "bulletins" came, declaring that neither troops nor air attack could halt the monsters. Then, for a moment, the radios were silent. It was terrifying. CBS — the silence implied — no longer existed.

Thousands of listeners did not wait long enough to hear the reassuring station-break announcement. Panic had set in. In New Jersey, hundreds of cars clogged the highways as people fled. Some told police they had *seen* the Martians and their machines, and they were ready to cross the Hudson River and take New York City. In Georgia, frantic phone calls to the police and newspapers reported variously that "monsters" had killed anywhere from 40 to 7,000 people. A church service in Indianapolis ended abruptly so that people could go home, while in Virginia, people gathered together to pray. Pennsylvania bridge players fell on their knees to pray. Five college students in North Carolina fainted, as did two girls riding in their father's car in Michigan. In Pittsburgh, genuine tragedy was narrowly averted when a man came home just in time to stop his wife from swallowing poison.

III. RECENT EPIDEMIC EPISODES

During the past several decades numerous cases of mental epidemics have been reported in scientific literature in both the East and the West. Those that were reported during or after the 1960s and were well investigated and described in terms of the dynamics of epidemic occurrence are noted here to illustrate possible correlations between elements of a particular culture and the type of mass behavior that occurred. For the sake of comparison, the epidemics are grouped according to the cardinal symptoms manifested.

A. EPIDEMICS OF GENITAL-RETRACTION PANIC (KORO)

As described in Chapter 13, *koro* is a special kind of mental illness characterized by the belief that if the penis shrinks into the abdomen, death will result. This fear can be manifested as anxiety or a state of panic. The disorder has various local names, such as *suoyang* in Mandarin (literally, shrinking of the yang organ, or penis), *sukyang* or *sookyang* in Cantonese, and *koro* in Malay. In the Malay language, *koro* means the head of a turtle, symbolizing the male sexual organ. Among scholars, the Malay term *koro* is used to refer to this morbid condition, which usually occurs in sporadic cases, but sometimes develops collectively as an endemic or epidemic *koro*. As an epidemic, it is manifested as a panic state rather than an anxiety or obsessive state. According to scientific reports, epidemic *koro* has been observed in several areas in southern Asia and in India (see Fig. 14-1).

1. Suoyang *(Koro)* Epidemic in Singapore

According to Ngui (1969), a collective occurrence of suoyang, or *koro,* was observed in Singapore in 1967. Swine fever had broken out, and a program to inoculate pigs was publicized and carried out. Several months later, a case of *suoyang* suddenly appeared. Unfortunately, a rumor that eating inoculated pork could cause *koro* created public panic. Soon the incidence of *koro* assumed epidemic proportions. At the peak of the epidemic, as many as a hundred cases were seen at general hospitals in a single day. It was speculated that nearly a thousand people claimed that they were attacked by *suoyang* during the epidemic, which lasted a couple of months.

A total of 536 *suoyang* victims who visited one general hospital were investigated by a research team (Ngui, 1969). Of the total, 95% were Chinese males, with only 2.2% Malays and Indians. Singapore is a

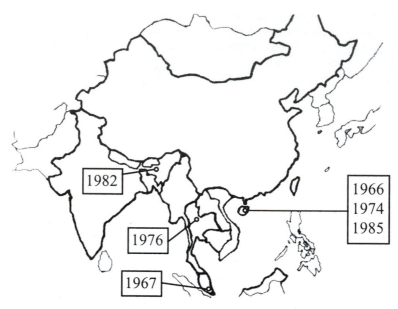

FIGURE 14-1 **Geographic locations of** *koro* **epidemics in the past:** 1952, 1962, 1966, 1974, and 1984–1985 in Hainan, China; 1967 in Singapore; 1976 in northeast Thailand; and 1982 in West Bengal and Lower Asam in India.

multiracial society. The percentage distribution of population by racial groups at the time was about 75% Chinese, 15% Malay, 8% Indian, and 3% Eurasian and others. Clearly, it was mainly the Chinese ethnic group that contracted *suoyang*. In addition to rushing to the hosptial for "emergency care," some used folk methods to prevent the shrinkage of the penis into the abodomen (see Fig. 14-2).

According to Ngui, six of the *suoyang* victims were small children, one of them only 7 months old. The children were brought to the hospital by their parents, who feared that their children's penises were shrinking and that the children might die.

The occurrence of swine fever and the accompanying rumor that it could cause *suoyang* may have precipitated the mass epidemic in Singapore. However, Ngui points out that the shared folk concept of *suoyang* among the Chinese ethnic group was an important ground for shared panic. It was speculated that some interracial tension may have existed and

been aggravated prior to the occurrence of the epidemic, mainly between the Chinese and the Malay groups. It was taboo for the Malay, who were Muslim, to eat pork, an important meat for the Chinese. The rumor that eating infected pork would cause illness might have been related to the racial tension.

2. Wartime *Koro* Epidemic in Thailand

A *koro* epidemic erupted in northeast Thailand in November 1976, shortly after the war started in Vietnam Suwanlert & Coates, 1979; Suwanlert, Sugondhabhirom, Pimpaniti, & Chaiyasit, 1978). During the war, many Cambodian refugees migrated from their country to Thailand. The Thais feared a communist invasion. There was also tension between local Thais and the refugees who disrupted their communities. In this atmosphere of political and military apprehension, a rumor spread that communists had put a certain herb into the food, mainly the rice, that would make

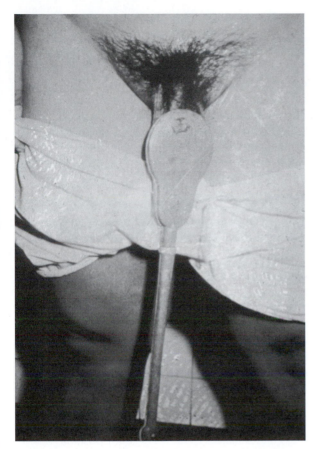

FIGURE 14-2 Koro epidemic in Singapore, 1967. A Chinese-Singaporean using a traditional Chinese weight case to clamp the penis during *a koro* attack. From Koro Study Team. [Courtesy of Gwee Ah Leng, M.D., with permission from Kua Ee Heok, M.D.].

Thai males sexually impotent, thus making it easy for the communists to seduce Thai women. Men allegedly suffering from *koro* began to ask for treatment. More than a thousand cases were reported during the epidemic. The government had to form a health team in the region to counteract the rumor and calm the panic.

According to Suwanlert (1983), a brief koro endemic reoccurred in February 1982 in two provinces in northeast and central Thailand. A local newspaper reported that several victims complained about penile shrinkage possibly caused by the intake of certain foods and smoking. The news spread and 40 victims in 1 day appeared at a hospital clinic with koro-related anxiety. They were all male, teenagers or young adults below the age of 30. The endemic subsided within a couple of days. Although most of the victims investigated were aware of the epidemic that had occurred 6 years before, the direct cause of this brief recurrence was unclear.

3. *Koro* Epidemic and Endemic in India

Although from an anthropological point of view the people of India are remarkably different from the people of south Asia, with different faiths (mainly Hindu and partly Muslim), they share common concerns about sexual matters. Both believe that it is important for men to conserve semen, and that its excessive discharge may harm their bodies. It is well known that Indian males suffer from *dhat* syndrome (or spermrrharia, fear of losing semen by leakage) — a unique psychosomatic disorder that is based on this sex-related belief. Also reflecting this concern were outbreaks of *koro* epidemics in the eastern part of India in 1982.

According to Phookon Dutta, and Das (1982) and Chakraborty (1982, 1984), a koro epidemic occurred in India in 1982 from the latter part of June to the middle of September. The epidemic seems to have started in the foothills of the Himalayas and affected West Bengal and four districts (Goalpara, Kamrup, Darrang, and Nowgong) in the neighboring state of Assam, rapidly spreading from west to east and to the south, eventually engulfing the suburbs of Calcutta. The affected areas were mostly semitribal and agricultural. The epidemic seemed to jump from one village to another, lasting for about 3 to 5 days in each place, then vanishing, only to reappear in a neighboring region. In the small town where the condition first appeared, hundreds of people were affected within a day or two.

As most of the victims did not contact medical facilities, there were no data to indicate how many were actually involved. Dutta and associates (1982) interviewed 83 cases who were seen by investigators either in medical clinics or in study tours of the affected areas. It was found that, among these 83 cases, 46 (55.4%) belonged to the 20- to 29-year age group and 29 (34.9%) to the 10- to 19-year age group, indicating that most of the victims were young adults or teens. Among them, 64 cases (77.1%) were male and 19 (22.9%) were females, showing that *koro* is preponderant in the male sex. The clinical picture was basically similar to *koro* attacks described elsewhere, in which victims became anxious or panicked, with the fear that the penis (for males) or nipples (for females) would shrink, with impending death. The local people in Assam used the folk term *jinjinia* (tingling) because the attack would start with a tingling sensation in the foot; *kattao* (cut off) was used in north Bengal. Among all the subjects studied, 60 (72.3%) had heard about, discussed, or witnessed a *koro* case on the same day or a few days prior to the onset of their illness. Most cases admitted apprehension or fear of contracting this "dreadful killer disease."

It is interesting to note that, regarding the religious background of the victims investigated, 69 cases (83.1%) were Hindus, 13 (15.7%) were Muslims, and the remaining 1 case was Christian. Among these, nearly two-thirds were Assamese and one-quarter Bengalis. There were Chinese among them. These findings contradict the previous belief that *koro* is a culture-bound disease confined to people of Chinese origin in southeast Asia.

In order to combat the epidemic, massive reassurance and health education measures were undertaken by the government through various mass media, including microphones. Following this official propaganda, the epidemic suddenly came to a halt in the middle of September, almost 3 months after it started.

Some people suspected that the initial cases of this epidemic may have been provoked by serious illnesses and deaths that had occurred recently in the areas. However, according to Chakraborty (1982, 1984), the areas hit by the epidemic had recently experienced severe interracial strife. A heavy influx of economically active and industrious Hindu refugees from what is now Bangladesh had changed landownership and created collective anxieties among the local tribal people. Around the time of the *koro* outbreak, the tribes-

men had prepared a militant action against the immigrant Bengalis that was aborted by government intervention.

Noticing a similar situation surrounding the Thai epidemic, i.e., the social threat of migrants from a neighboring country, Jilek (1986) proposed a theory that the individual with *koro* anxiety responds to the collective fear of genocidal extermination by a well-defined enemy who is perceived as threatening the survival of one's ethnic–national group by attacking its procreative capability.

4. Recurrent Suoyang *(Koro)* Epidemics in Southern China

The first Western report of a *koro* epidemic was published in a French medical journal in 1908 by J. Legendre (R. Bartholomew & Gregory, 1996; Jilek, 1986). It described an endemic episode among school students in the Sichuan province in central China diagnosed as *so-in-tchen* (*suo-yin-zheng* in Chinese, meaning "shrinking of private part sickness"). However, according to Chinese psychiatrists (Mo, Chen, Li, Tseng, 1995), recurrent instances of *suoyang* epidemics had been noted on Hainan Island and the neighboring Leizhou Peninsula of Guangdong in south China about 130 years before. *Suo-yang* in Chinese literally means shrinkage of the yang organ (penis), which is equivalent to the clinical condition of *koro* as it is known in medical literature. According to Mo and colleagues, in *Ya-zhou Zhi* (the local chronicle of the Ya state, Hainan), it was recorded that: "In the eleventh year of the Xinyou regime in the Qing dynasty (1862), *suo* illness had spread; men's genitalia shrank, females' breasts, ears, tongues or other (protruded) parts shrank. Rubbing with ginger or set firecrackers off will stop it." Two years later, an epidemic was also recorded in the *Dan-xian Zhi* (the local chronicle of Dan county, Hainan). According to that record, "In the second year of the Tong-zhi regime, *suo* disease occurred. Trembling and shrinkage occurred of patients' ears, noses, hands, feet, men's private parts, or women's breasts, and patients fell unconscious. Need many people to beat gong or drum and to hold the shrinking part (of the body), and pour on ginger juice for immediate cure." According to the *yin-yang* theory, protruding parts of the body, such as the ears, nose, feet, or penis, are considered *yang* organs, whereas concave areas, such as the mouth, nostrils, or vagina, are *yin* organs. Ginger, pepper, or any green vegetables are regarded as foods rich in the *yang* element and are good remedies for *yang*-deficient physical conditions.

No official record of a *suoyang* occurrence has been noted since then. However, Mo and associates (1995) reported that five major epidemics were noted in Hainan in 1952, 1962, 1966, 1974, and 1984. According to the recollections of old residents, the 1952 epidemic appeared during the period of land reform under the Communist regime, in which landlords' properties were confiscated and redistributed to the farmers — a time of severe social tension. The 1962 epidemic occurred after the Great Leap Forward movement, in which there was economic crisis throughout the country. The 1966 epidemic broke out at the beginning of the cultural revolution, when there was serious conflict and turmoil in the country. The 1974 epidemic started under the menace of an outbreak of encephalitis. The epidemic of 1984 occurred in an atmosphere of fear, when local fortune-tellers predicted a bad year for farmers. It seems that a specific social tension was related to the occurrence of each *suoyang* epidemic. Most of the people in the epidemic areas believed that all social disasters would ultimately result in a *suoyang* occurrence.

From a sociological point of view, it is noted that more than half the population of Hainan Island and Leizhou Peninsular are peasants and fishermen. Most of them live in remote village areas and have little formal education. People in Hainan and Leizhou are very religious. There are many temples, and people are still considerably influenced by supernatural beliefs of the past. Most of them still retain sex-related beliefs, such as the traditional medical concept of conserving semen to maintain the balance of *yin* and *yang*. They also believe that ghosts in hell are anxious to obtain human protruding body parts, particularly men's penises, which contain the rich *yang* force. The ghosts

have lost their *yang* element and are anxious to get *yang* force to enable them to return to the human world. Therefore, local people believe that a ghost disguised as a fair lady comes to collect men's penises. A ghost in the form of a fox spirit is also thought to possess a victim in order to take away his *yang* force.

In the summer of 1984, the rice did not grow well in Hainan. Local fortune-tellers predicted it would be a troublesome year, in which the people would suffer from many disasters. It was in this uneasy atmosphere that the first case of *suoyang* appeared on the north coast of the island near Tan county — a place with a historical record of *suoyang* epidemics since the Qing dynasty. An epidemic gradually spread westward, involving whole villages and towns, ending on the south coast of the island. A second wave of the epidemic started at Haikang Town in Leizhou Peninsula when the news reached there. It spread southward and northward (see Fig. 14-3). It usually involved a village for several days to a couple of weeks, with a dozen or more victims, then spread to a nearby village. In a period of 6 months, it was estimated that more than 3000 people became victims of *suoyang*. All the victims were Han nationals. There were no cases in the central mountainous part of the island, inhabited by Li and Miao nationals, who did not share the concept of *suoyang* (Tseng et al., 1988).

When a *suoyang* case broke out in a village, several to several dozen of people might be affected (see Fig. 14-4a). The people in the community usually became hysterical, particularly when numerous victims were found at the same time. The villagers would strike drums, gongs, or anything that made loud noises, or set off firecrackers to scare off the evil ghosts (see Fig. 14-4b and 14-4c). The men would carry knives, swords, spears, or other weapons, and patrol the streets. They would block the village gate to stop outsiders from entering. They were afraid that a ghost disguised as a human might infiltrate the village. As soon as a new case occurred in a neighboring village, the original village was set free because people believed that the evil ghosts had gone on to the other village.

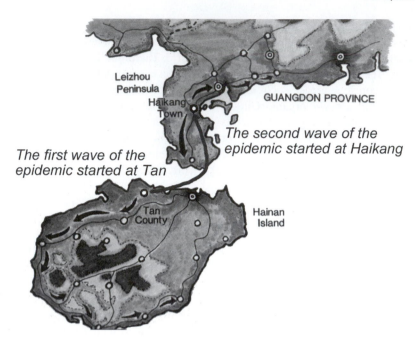

FIGURE 14-3   Epidemic spread of *koro* in Guangdong, China, in 1984–1985. An epidemic originated in a village near Tan County in Hainan Island, spreading from one village to another southward in the coastal area of the island; the news of the disaster was brought to Haikang Town on Leishou Peninsula, where a second wave started, spreading southward and northward on the peninsula. [Revised from W.S. Tseng et al., *American journal of psychiatry, 145*(12), 1988].

A field study was carried out by a research team in one selected part of the epidemic area (Haikan county). Among 232 cases investigated, it was found that 195 (84%) were men and 37 (16%) were women. Most of the victims were between the ages of 10 and 25 years. About two-thirds had elementary school educations.

Later, a total of 214 victims were randomly recruited from Hainan and Leizhou for a questionnaire survey (Tseng et al., 1992). Data from this *koro* group were compared with a total of 56 anxiety cases that had visited the psychiatric clinic (the clinic group) and 153 cases of non-*koro*, nonclinic cases (the control group) recruited from the same area. Comparison of these three groups revealed several things. As reflected by the symptom checklist, the symptom profile of the *koro* group was characterized by anxiety with phobic

tendencies, but was not similar to that of the clinic group. A study of personality profiles from Cattell's Sixteen Personality Factor test showed that *suoyang* victims were different from usual anxiety disorder cases and, as a group, had lower intellectual endowments than the control group.

Because *suoyang* epidemics tended to occur in the Guangdong area and not in other parts of China, a comparison of folk beliefs held in different regions in China was carried out in 1992. In order to determine whether there were any differences in sex-related folk beliefs and the *suoyang* concept held by people in different regions of China, the same folk belief questionnaire was administered to subjects in Jilin, northeastern China, and Taiwan, as well as in Guangdong. The results revealed that although people in Jilin, Taiwan, and Guangdong were all aware

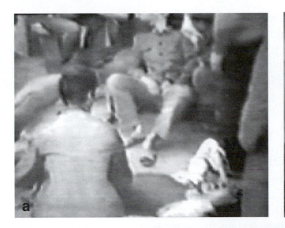
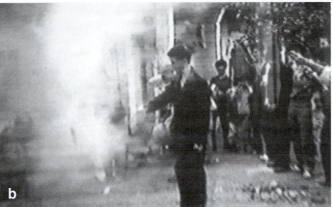
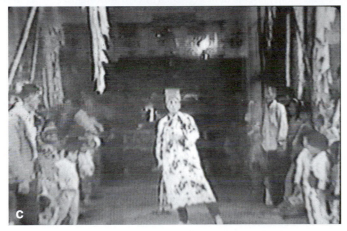

FIGURE 14-4 *Koro* **epidemic in southern China, 1984–1985.** (a) Two Chinese men simultaneously suffered from attacks through contagion during the epidemic—one sitting on the street holding his "shrinking" penis and the other lying on the ground shouting for help. (b) Scared villagers set off firecrackers to scare off the evil ghost, believing that the ghost had infiltrated the village to steal the yang element. (c) A Daoist monk performing a ritual to chase away the evil from the village. [From Guangdong Suoyang Epidemic Research Team. Courtesy of Mo Gan-Ming, M.D.].

of the rumors of *suoyang* in the community, there were major differences in how dangerous a condition the subjects considered it to be — the subjects in Guangdong considered the potential danger of contracting *suoyang* more serious. The findings illustrate that there are different degrees of belief in and attitudes toward the *suoyang* folk concept among Chinese in different geographic areas and in different subcultures. The findings support the view that the belief in *suoyang* in Hainan and Leizhou of Guangdong is one of the major reasons for the recurrence

of *suoyang* epidemics in those regions (Tseng et al., 1993).

B. Mass Hysteria (or Epidemic Conversion/Dissociation Attacks)

Mass hysteria is one of the most common collective mental disorders observed and reported in scientific literature in both the East and the West. Hysteria is used here in a restrictive sense, referring to the sudden occurrence of conversion reaction (manifested with symptoms of motor dysfunctions, sensational disturbances, fainting, and other converted somatic symptoms) and/or dissociation reaction. Following are some examples.

1. Nervous Twitching Epidemic in Baltimore, Maryland

Schuler and Parenton (1943) reported an occurrence of an epidemic in Baltimore, Maryland, in 1939, involving a group of high school girls. A few days before the onset of the epidemic, the school had converted physical education classes into social dancing classes. The outbreak started with one of the most popular girls in the senior class, who did not dance well. At the school's homecoming dance, she merely watched the others. It was then that she suddenly developed a nervous twitching and jerking in her legs. The spasmodic twitching recurred occasionally at school during the next several weeks. Three weeks later, two other girls developed similar symptoms. After several days, more girls followed suit. The episode reached its climax when agitated parents, after hearing about "strange things going on in the school," drove to the school and demanded that their children return home. Panic broke out at the school. Investigators interpreted the first case as a somatic expression of avoiding the stress of trying to dance. The other girls may have unconsciously identified with the first girl and, as a result, developed the same symptoms. Reporting this episode, investigators stressed that the "mental epidemic" is not exclusively historical, nor is it confined to ignorant and backward populations.

2. Hyperventilating Attack in Blackburn, England

According to Moss and McEvedy (1966), hyperventilating became epidemic among girls at a secondary school in Blackburn, England, in 1965. The episode began after 20 girls fainted during a ceremony that kept the entire student body standing for 3 hr. The students' discussion of the fainting and dizzy feelings promoted a massive outbreak of complaints. The next day, 85 girls were sent by ambulance to the hospital for hyperventilating attacks. Approximately a third of the 550 girls in the school were affected before the episode ended.

3. Mass Hysteria in an Arab Culture

Although there have been few published reports on the phenomenon of epidemic hysteria in the Middle East, Amin, Hamdi, and Eapen (1997) described the circumstances surrounding an outbreak of mass hysteria among first-year female university students in an Arab culture. The outbreak was precipitated by a state of panic over the possibility of a fire, which turned out to be harmless fumes from a locally used burning perfume. A total of 23 cases presented to a hospital emergency room with symptoms of respiratory distress accompanied by marked emotional reactions.

4. Endemic Hysteria in Malaysia Schools

Tan (1963) mentioned that epidemic hysteria was a rather common occurrence in the Malay area. In 1971 alone, a total of 17 episodes were noted by psychiatrists. Even a rare case of collective hysteria among family members was reported by Woon (1976).

Teoh, Soewondo, and Sidharta (1975) reported an episode of endemic hysteria that occurred among female dormitory students. This report described the psychological aspects of the epidemic in sufficient detail to allow us to elaborate on the cultural and group dynamics associated with the occurrence of epidemic hysteria.

The dormitory, located in a small town not far from Kuala Lumpur, accommodated 50 adolescent Malay girls. It was initially supervised by a woman teacher, who later resigned because the headmaster constantly interfered with her job. After she resigned, the headmaster managed the dormitory himself and made no real attempt to find a new supervisor, which annoyed the girls, their parents, and the entire community.

Based on their Muslim beliefs, the Malay have rigid social taboos against a man's entering the living quarters of a Malay female, and the sexes are separated at an early age. Thus, the community felt strongly that it was improper for the headmaster to manage the girls' dormitory. However, the headmaster appeared in the girls' rooms unannounced, day and night. He pampered and "fussed over" the girls, even telling the younger ones how to wear their sanitary napkins. As a headmaster, he held a key position in the community and no one dared oppose him directly.

This situation set the stage for an epidemic of hysteria. First, a 15-year-old girl suddenly appeared depressed, complained of difficulty in breathing, and experienced hyperventilation and a tetanic spasm. She groaned in severe pain and complained that someone was calling her from the vicinity of the toilets. Several days later, two of her dormitory mates developed similar symptoms. Screaming and shouting, one claimed that students had thrown soiled sanitary napkins around the dormitory and had polluted the territory of the local gods. This girl made it clear that she felt a strong attraction for the headmaster and jealousies resulted among the girls.

The girls were sent home to rest, but when they returned the symptoms recurred. More girls then developed attacks. When the chief education officer of the state investigated, he found five girls running around, screaming, hyperventilating, and fainting as the outbreak reached a climax. During the attack, one of the girls demanded a human sacrifice. The terrified headmaster bargained with her, and she settled for the sacrifice of a goat. A traditional local healer was called and the sacrificial ceremony was performed. The outbreak of hysteria finally forced the community to publicly express dissatisfaction with the headmaster and to pressure him into either changing his behavior or being transferred. The headmaster agreed to appoint a new dormitory mistress and also promised to improve physical conditions at the school.

It is obvious that this outbreak centered around the headmaster's behavior, primarily his intrusion into the girls' private lives. However, because this culture provided no appropriate way to oppose his authority, mass hysteria became the only way to force him to recognize and change the source of the problem. As pointed out by Murphy (1959), Malayan children, traditionally reared in a relatively anxiety-free environment and protected against frustration, were not prepared to handle the anxieties and general stresses of life when they reached adolescence. Hysteria could easily be utilized by a group of relatively innocent girls in reaction to a stressful situation. Clearly, the epidemic was also greatly colored by psychosexual issues: the intrusion of the schoolmaster into the dormitory and some of the girls' attraction to and jealousy over him. This supports the psychodynamic theory of the etiology of hysteria, which maintains that early psychosexual development is arrested at the Oedipus level, and the incestuous tie to the loved parent of the opposite sex is not relinquished. This leads to conflict in adult life over sexual involvement because love retains a forbidden, incestuous quality (Nemiah, 1975).

5. Collective Dissociation Outburst in a Chinese-Malaysian Family

Psychiatric literature has shown that occasionally more than one member of a family may become mentally ill through a process of contagion — forming so-called "double insanity" or "family insanity" (*folie á deu or folie á familie* in French). The psychiatric condition may take the form of dissociation, conversion, delusion, or abnormal behavior. Although the phenomenon of *folie á familie* is considered rare, sporadic occurrences have been reported in the Philippines (Goduco-Angular & Wintrob, 1964), Malaysia (Woon, 1976), and Taiwan (Tseng, 1969). (For the latter case, see Section III,D,1.)

The case reported by Woon (1976) concerned a Chinese-Malasian family whose two young adult brothers and one sister simultaneously developed dissociated conditions, creating sensational turmoil in a rural village in Malaysia. The situation occurred after their aged father, a village shaman, suffered a stroke, making it necessary to choose a successor from among his adult children. Affected by intense feelings of competition and unable to handle these emotions, the siblings one after another developed dissociated conditions (see Fig. 14-5).

Reviewing this contagious family mental disorder, it is apparent that in addition to the existing premorbid personalities of the family members, a strong emotional bond between them facilitated the occurrence of the condition, particularly when they faced a stressful situation together. To share and to be involved by having a similar psychiatric condition appeared to be an alternative way for the siblings to deal with the common crisis they encountered. It is speculated that such an unusual contagious reaction tends to be observed in societies where family ties are stressed.

C. ENDEMIC ANXIETY OR FEAR REACTION

1. Phantom Anesthetist of Matton, Illinois

The sudden development of a communitywide fear reaction in the small city of Matton, Illinois, was reported by Johnson (1945). One evening in September 1944, a woman reported to the police that someone had opened her bedroom window and sprayed her with a sickly sweet-smelling gas that partially paralyzed her legs and made her ill. The police found no sign of an intruder, but the next day the local newspaper carried a front-page story on the "gas attack," with the headline: Anesthetist Prowler on Loose. The following day, a man reported to the police that he and his wife had had a similar occurrence. This "incident" was also reported in the newspaper. It created an atmosphere of fear and anxiety in the community. Two new attacks were reported after the second news report. Following this, within a period of 12 days, a total of 22 cases were reported of similar attacks by the phantom anesthetist — with victims claiming that they smelled the gas, became sick with various somatic symptoms of nausea, vomiting, palpitations, paralysis of the legs, dryness of the mouth and throat, and so on. After analyzing the records and interviewing most of the victims, Johnson concluded that the case of the "phantom anesthetist" was entirely psychogenic. It was his assessment that the news media, by printing exciting, uncritical stories, created anxiety and a fear reaction that snowballed.

2. Slashing Phobia in Taipei, Taiwan

A similar mass phobic reaction that occurred in Taipei, Taiwan, in 1956, was witnessed and reported by American psychiatrist Jacobs (1965). According to Jacobs, in early May of that year, a local newspaper reported that a number of children had been the victims of slashings with what appeared to be razor blades or similar weapons. Various explanations were offered in the newspaper, namely sex sadism, facilitating theft by drawing attention, and blood ritual — the old local superstition that the drawing of blood from a given number of small children brings good luck.

Clearly the message caught the attention of many people. The next day, an 11-year-old boy reported receiving a cut on his arm without knowing how or when it had been inflicted. In addition, a 2-year-old boy also reported being cut in the leg while playing in front of his house. Slashings were reported at a number of girls' primary schools. Parents became more and more nervous about the safety of their children. The smaller ones increasingly were being kept indoors, while those of school age were being accompanied to and from school by adults.

The police were visibly annoyed at what they referred to as "unfounded rumors and absurd stories" built upon the superstitions of ignorant people. However, the police service was secretly increased with the dispatch of a number of plainclothes detectives to marketplaces, theaters, schools, and other areas where people congregated, and which might conceivably be tempting to the slashers. The mayor appropriated extra funds for the city police to investigate the situation. Finally, after careful investigation of more than 20 reported cases, the chief of police announced that a number of alleged cases were due to accident, innocent misrepresentation, or deliberate hoax.

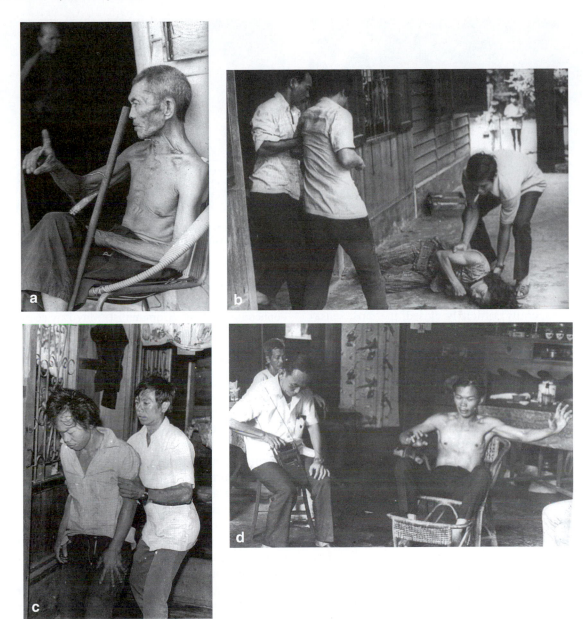

FIGURE 14-5   Collective family dissociation outburst in Malaysia. (a) An aged village shaman suffered a stroke in a rural area, necessitating the choice of a successor from among his three children. (b) The outburst started when the daughter fell on the ground in a dissociated state. (c) The younger son soon fell into a dissociated state. (d) He was followed by the elder son, who also fell into a possessed state. (*Figure continues*)

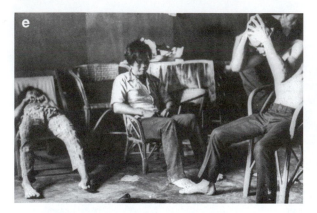
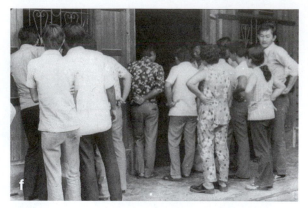

FIGURE 14-5 (continued)   (e) While the three of them were sitting in the living room, they all fell simultaneously into dissociated or possessed states. (f) Villagers watched what was happening in this household. [Courtesy of Woon Tai-Hwang, M.D.].

However, on the very day that the razor blade case was being clarified by the police and the affair was being (hopefully) officially closed, the most sensational incident occurred. A mysterious "woman in red" was chased and caught in the street after she was found trying to slash a baby. The baby was carried by its mother, who saw the woman grabbing her baby's arm. The mother shouted for help, and people in the street chased the woman and caught her. A razor blade was found in her purse, which she tried to throw away while she was running. The woman claimed that her umbrella happened to catch the baby's arm and, as she happened to have a razor in her bag, she panicked and ran away from the scene when the baby's mother shouted to the crowd to catch the "slasher." After this incident, the phantom razor slasher(s) never appeared again on the streets of Taipei, and the 2 weeks of fear reactions shared by the community subsided.

Jacobs offered a social explanation of this event. Rumor mongering carried out by gossiping and the press, which reported the news uncritically and in a highly suggestive way, played a vital part in spreading the hysterical atmosphere. There was constant social and political tension in Taiwan at that time with the communists on the mainland. People's nerves were on edge in the political game of confrontation with the "enemy." Even the police commissioner hinted that perhaps communist agents were trying to create an atmosphere of confusion and uneasiness in connection with the (Communist) May Day season.

D. COLLECTIVE DELUSIONS

The difference between ordinary beliefs and delusions is a matter of degree, with a thin boundary. Particularly if a belief is shared by a mass population, in the form of a political, religious, or folk belief, it may become a matter of judgment to decide whether the belief is "normal" or "pathological." When a group of people face a common enemy or a dangerous situation, collective suspicion is a common reaction. It may take an outsider or a third party to get an objective view of the belief shared by society. It may take time — perhaps one or two decades — to obtain insight into the pathology of a delusion shared collectively by a society. The Nazis' attempt to exterminate the Jewish people in Hitler's era and the Chinese attempt to destroy the established culture and exterminate the intelligent people during the cultural revolution in Mao's era are two examples of political delusions passionately believed by mass populations in recent history.

Paranoia, like depression, can spread from person to person. The French term folie a deux refers to two persons sharing a similar psychopathology through mental contagion. In English, it is called associated psychoses. The people involved are usually members of the same family or emotionally close partners. As extensions of the folie a deux (psychoses of two), a folie a trois (psychoses of three) or folie a famile (psychoses of a family) may develop. These usually take the form of psychosis, hysteria, or delusion.

1. A Paranoid Family in Taiwan

A family of three adults and five children in Taiwan developed a shared political delusion (Tseng, 1969). This family's paranoia was not considered an "endemic mental disorder" in a strict sense. However, reviewing this case as a prototype of collective delusional disorders might help us understand how the delusional system can spread and become contagious (Tseng, 1969).

Time and place were significant in the occurrence of paranoia in this family. It was 1961, only a few years after the National government had retreated from mainland China to Taiwan. Political and social conditions were unstable, and the infiltration of the communists was probable. Among many mainland Chinese who migrated to Taiwan, memories of the communist threat were still fresh.

The key figure, Mr. Chong, developed the delusion that he was being persecuted by the communists. He transmitted his delusion to his sister and her husband (Mr. and Mrs. Wang), and later to the couple's five children, forming a paranoid family.

Mr. Chong, 36, was the youngest son of a successful, strong-willed father, a Protestant lay preacher. Mr. Chong and his sister, Mrs. Wang, had been very close since childhood. As a child, Mr. Chong loved stories of intrigue and fighting. As a young adult, pursuing a desire for authority and superiority, he became a policeman. In 1949, when their hometown on the mainland was taken over by the communists, their father was imprisoned. Chong rescued him and brought his parents and sister to Taiwan, where he married a local Taiwanese woman. There, as a policeman, he frequently criticized his superiors and co-workers for their "incorrect" behavior, until finally his superiors fired him. He then became a lay preacher and lived in the church compound. Soon he was publicly criticizing the church elders, and personality conflicts resulted. Mr. Chong told his sister that the elders were "looking at him" and "talking about him." The sister, remembering the mainland China days, warned him that the elders might have a communist sympathizer or agent in their ranks. Mr. Chong's paranoia increased. His house was burglarized, and he accused the elders. With this, his church employment ended. He viewed this as "enemy persecution." With his church quarters gone, he went to live with his sister and her family. (Due to her work, his wife lived in another town.)

Soon both Mr. Chong and his sister believed that they were being watched and harmed by the communists, the family maid, the church elders, neighbors, and even strangers. They quarreled with their neighbors, who they thought were saying that they had an "abnormal relationship."

The brother-in-law, Mr. Wang, was, uncomfortably, in the middle of this situation. It was no wonder that he was uneasy; his neighbors were also his business colleagues. Mr. Wang had also known danger and intrigue. During World War II, he had been in the Chinese underground. There he learned to poison the (Japanese) enemy. At first, Mr. Wang refused to believe his wife's and Chong's suspicions. Later, when his colleague–neighbors grew unfriendly, he, too, became suspicious. The situation reached a climax when he drank some tea in his office and then felt ill. "My colleagues are poisoning me," he thought. "My wife, brother-in-law, and I really are being persecuted."

One by one, four of the Wang's five children succumbed to the contagion of fear, suspicion, and delusion. Only Sen, 19, the eldest son, held out. It is interesting that Sen was a rigid, rebellious youth, a poor student, and not as bright as his siblings. Long, the timid and obedient 10-year-old son, was the first to accept the family delusion. He found some candy on the street, ate it, and became ill. Father and son then decided that the "enemy" had poisoned them. Half-sisters Mei, 13, and Hwai, 15, followed suit within a month. They decided that strangers were talking about and making fun of them. At their father's order, both girls quit school. Ten, the 17-year-old boy, was allowed to stay in school because his father believed he could cope with the "enemy." Ten, intelligent and curious, fond of arguing and desirous of power, had even anticipated his father's conclusion that communists were the persecutors. Eventually, even the rebellious Sen yielded to pressure and quit school. The four young persons were now home every day, cut off from their companions. Daily the family discussed the "enemy," watched for "suspicious-acting" persons, believed the water was poisoned, and quarreled with the neighbors.

Mrs. Chong, the only adult born in Taiwan, had formerly agreed with her husband that all things conspired against him. However, listening to the repeated stories of persecution, she began to be skeptical. At this point, her husband asked her to give up her job and live with him and the brother-in-law's family to fight against the enemy. She refused. Mr. Chong then believed that even his wife was being persuaded to side with the enemy. The next move was dramatic. Mr. Chong, Mr. and Mrs. Wang, and the children all went to the president's residence to seek protection against their "enemies." This brought the paranoid family to psychiatric attention.

The case meets almost classically the diagnostic criteria for psychosis of association: evidence that participants are in close contact; that the delusional content of everyone concerned is similar; and that the partners support, accept, and share each other's paranoid ideas. Under the stress of unemployment, burglary, and sickness, a crisis for this family occurred that necessitated externalization of their anger. The environment was the most crucial factor in the development of the group political–persecutor delusion. The sociopolitical situation in Taiwan at that time made it easy to label the enemy "communists." Such an invisible enemy was so available, plausible, and probable that anyone might easily believe in it and thus succumb to a collective paranoid formation within a family.

2. Collective Delusion of Windshield Pitting in Seattle, Washington

While individuals, or a family member, may at times lose touch with reality as their culture defines it, whole communities ordinarily do not. However, Medalia and Larsen (1958) reported a community-wide delusional windshield-pitting epidemic that broke out in Seattle, Washington, in the spring of 1954. Beginning on March 23, a Seattle newspaper carried intermittent reports of damage to automobile windshields in a city located to the north of Seattle. On April 14, newspapers reported windshield damage in a town near Seattle. Initially, police suspected vandalism, but failed to gather proof. Conjecture as to the cause ranged from meteoric dust to sandflea eggs hatching in the glass, but centered on possible radioactive fallout from the Eniwetok H-bomb tests conducted earlier that year. Then an epidemic occurred in Seattle itself between April 14 and 15 — a total of 242 persons telephoned the Seattle Police Department reporting damage to over 3000 automobiles. Most commonly, the damage reported consisted of pitting marks that grew into bubbles in the glass of about the size of a thumbnail. On the evening of the 15th, the mayor of Seattle declared the damage was no longer a police matter and made an emergency appeal to the governor and to President Dwight Eisenhower for help. The newspaper mentioned the possibility that the community's collective concern with pitting might have sprung largely from mass hysteria. On April 16, calls to police dropped to 46; to 10 on the 17th; and there were no more calls after the 18th, ending this short-lived collective delusional reaction that was stirred up by mass communication — the newspaper.

3. Collective Delusion of Cargo Cult in Melanesia

When the Europeans arrived in many parts of Melanesia, the indigenous people developed a pidgin word, "cargo," to refer to the manufactured goods that were brought by the Europeans (usually by airplane). The cargo often included canned foods and weapons, which were greatly desired by the indigenous people. Without knowing how the "cargo" was manufactured (in the home countries of Europe), the local folk interpretation was that the cargo was given to the white people by their powerful ancestors through the performance of proper rituals.

A cultural psychiatrist who practiced in Papua New Guinea, B. G. Burton-Bradley (1975, 1982), presented the phenomenon of the "cargo-cult syndrome," referring to the people's belief in the cargo cult and their possession by the magical, grandiose idea that they could communicate with and eventually receive cargo from the gods. In order to achieve their goal, they practiced various odd rituals, usually following white people's behavior, such as building a cross on the seashore, or clearing their back yards as if building an airstrip, hoping that the "big bird" (airplane) would land with their cargo. In some instances, this behavior was individual; in others, it involved a group of followers who gave up their regular lives and work for religious ritual, waiting for the arrival of the cargo not only for several months, but for many years. Led by a cult leader, they became collectively deluded (cross-reference to Chapter 13: Culture-Related Specific Syndromes).

E. Endemic Depression

A whole society may suffer from a depressive mood, such as in the Great Depression experienced by the American people in the 1930s for more than a decade. A group of war prisoners or criminal inmates subjected to long-term torture or maltreatment may collectively suffer from a depressive mood. However, the collective occurrence of a depressive disorder within a short period of time is rather rare. The occurrence of an endemic depressive disturbance in a Japanese leprosarium has been reported by Ikeda (1966). The episode, which occurred in 1960, involved 11 nurses in a leprosarium with a staff of 67 nurses, and about 1200 patients.

According to Ikeda's report, a new head nurse, inexperienced in leprosy nursing, began duty on the ward. In the same month, a young male patient killed an older, female patient with whom he had been having a love affair. Two months later, a patient beat a ward housekeeper. Soon after this, another patient attempted suicide. In connection with the suicide attempt, the patients' governing body accused a staff nurse of negligence, and the new head nurse severely reprimanded her. Several days later, a patient attempted to escape, and the same staff nurse was again criticized by the patient group. This nurse then began to suffer from sleeplessness, loss of appetite, and headaches. She feared that the patients might persecute her or attack her sexually, and became so depressed that she was hospitalized for psychiatric treatment. Very soon, a second nurse, a close friend, complained of similar symptoms and attempted suicide. Within a short time, 11 nurses, one after another, suffered various kinds of emotional disturbances, with symptoms of somatic complaints, depression, fear of persecution, and visual hallucinations. Several nurses attempted suicide by drug overdose. When the public learned of this, an official investigation resulted.

In Ikeda's analysis, the collective emotional disturbances were due to several factors: The sanatorium was an isolated and closed society; the nurses' daily lives were monotonous and unrewarding; and there were almost no social gatherings or recreational activities for the nurses, even those who lived in the same dormitory. An important element was the significant changes in the relationships between the nurses and the patients after World War II. The patients had developed a community government, were encouraged to protest for their rights, and made more demands of the nursing staff.

In this particular leprosarium, the nurses were understaffed, and morale was low. The new head nurse constantly criticized the nurses and gave them little support. In this setting of low morale, insufficient staff, and militant patients, the traditional, conservative nurses, faced with constant frustration, found no other alternative except a rampant outbreak of fear and depression.

F. COLLECTIVE SUICIDE

It is well known that some individuals or a group of people might collectively commit suicide in war time. For instance, in medieval times in India, the rite of *Jauhar* was practiced, in which women would commit mass suicide by self-immolation to avoid capture and dishonor at the hands of the Muslim invaders (Adityanjee, 1994). According to the rite of *Jauhar,* when defeat threatened and there was no other way, as a last resort, it was better for the men to go out and die in the fields of battle and for the women to burn themselves on a pyre. Death was considered preferable to slavery and degradation. At this century, at the end of World War II, a number of Japanese soldiers and citizens committed group suicide on Saipan and Okinawa [cross-reference to Chapter 8: Stress and Coping Patterns (Section III,B,2)]. However, collective suicidal actions have also occurred in non-wartime situations in various societies for one reason or another. It is commonly known that psychiatric patients in hospitals might kill themselves in an endemic fashion. For instance, Taiminen, Salmenpera, and Lehtinen (1992) reported that six inpatients committed suicide in a psychiatric hospital in Finland over a short period of time. Suggestion and identification were considered the precipitating factors of this suicide endemic.

Religious belief-related, ceremonial, mysterious, group suicidal acts have been heard of occasionally in Europe or Canada among members of the Sun cult. The Japanese psychiatrist Takahashi (1989) reported an incident in which seven female members (between 25 and 67 years of age) of a local religious cult (the Truth Church) committed suicide one after another following the leader's death in Japan in 1986. The collective suicidal action of 914 cult members at Jonestown in 1978 is still fresh in our memories (see Fig. 14-6). Many explanations have been offered in efforts

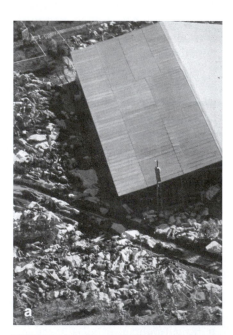 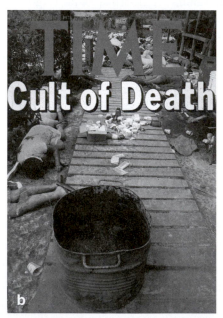

FIGURE 14-6   Mass suicide in Jonestown, Guyana, in 1978. (a) More than 900 American citizens, members of the People's Temple, followed their leader to a jungle settlement in South America and committed suicide together by swallowing poison, either voluntarily or by threat. (b) They died from cyanide that was put into their drinks. [From the *Times,* 1978].

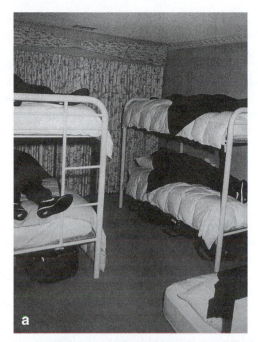

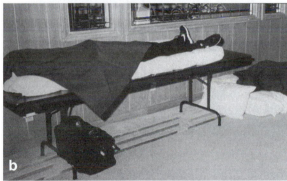

FIGURE 14-7 Planned group suicide of Heaven's Gate members, 1997. (a) In order to ascend to the next levels of their lives, 39 members of the Heaven's Gate cult journeyed together to their deaths. (b) The members packed their suitcases, covered their bodies with purple cloths, and took poison. [From *Newsweek*, April, 1997. Courtesy of Associated Press].

was founded on a pattern of interaction characterized by the leader's sadistic demand for mirrored grandiosity and the followers' masochistic surrender in the hopes of merging with an idealized and omnipotent self-object. The religious vision of death as the ultimate beauty was the base for the group undertaking collective suicide. The occurrence of mass suicide by self-immolation in Waco, Texas, in the United States is another example of mass suicidal behavior related to a cult movement (Adityanjee, 1994). The recent episode of the Heaven's Gate mass suicide surprised many of us. As Comet Hale-Bopp grew bright — reaching its closest proximity to earth on March 22, 1997 — the 39 members of Heaven's Gate committed a planned group suicide, orchestrated by their director. In a rich suburban California mansion, they quietly packed their suitcases with clothes and spiral notebooks, swallowed phenobarbital, and died in waves over the next 3 days (see Fig. 14-7). The members followed their leader in what they believed was an ascension to the next level of their lives ("Special Report," 1997).

IV. OVERVIEW AND SUGGESTIONS

A. TERMINOLOGY

Several different terms have been used by clinicians or behavior scientists to refer to epidemic mental disorders. These include mass hysteria, collective mental disorder, mass psychogenic illness, and epidemic mental disorder. There is a need for clarification and unification of the terminology.

Perhaps because many epidemic mental disorders — nearly two-thirds of them — manifest themselves as mass conversion, the term "mass hysteria" has been loosely used by clinicians as well as laymen as synonymous for epidemic mental disorder. However, as has been mentioned previously, emotional disorders can become collective or epidemic in many forms of pathology other than hysterical conversion. Examples are group panic over the fear of sexual impotence (Ngui, 1969); collective anxiety or fear with hysterical

to understand this rather unusual mass madness. The concept of collective pathological regression within a charismatically led mass movement was suggested by Ulman and Abse (1983). It was speculated that the psychic stability of both the leader and the followers

attribution of accidental cuts or bleeding scratches to a "razor slasher" (Jacobs, 1965); morbid fear of being gassed by a "phantom anesthetist" (Johnson, 1945); collective delusions (Medalia and Larsen, 1958); endemic depression (Ikeda, 1966); massive or collective suicides (Anonymous, 1977; Takahashi, 1989); and even collective group behavior disorders, such as an outbreak of connected arson episodes (Boling & Brotman, 1975). Therefore, hysterical "conversion" is merely one of the psychopathologies manifested. The term "massive hysteria" only emphasizes one of the qualities of the phenomena; that the epidemic usually occurs in a dramatic way in an intense emotional atmosphere.

The term "collective mental disorder" is also used by some clinicians; however, such a term simply means that a group of patients has developed more or less similar mental disorders within a short period of time. The term does not convey the contagious process involved in the development of such unique phenomena in an epidemic fashion. Therefore, the term "epidemic mental disorder" is preferable.

The term "mass psychogenic illness" has been used by some behavior scientists (R.E. Bartholomew, 1994). It is intended to emphasize that the disturbance manifested is not necessarily a "mental disease," but can be merely a culturally comprehensible emotional reaction or illness. The term correctly stresses that the disturbance is induced by psychological factors. However, from a psychiatric perspective, clinicians prefer to use the term "mental disorder" in a broad sense rather than substituting it with the term "psychogenic illness." This is because certain psychopathologies, such as delusion, depression, and suicidal behaviors, cannot simply be regarded as "psychological illnesses."

Occasionally the term "epidemicity" is used by some scholars or clinicians to address the prevalent occurrence of certain mental disorders or problems over a relatively long period of time, such as an epidemic occurrence of suicide (Rubinstein, 1983) or running away behavior (Justice & Duncan, 1976) among adolescents, or *amok* (massive homicidal attacks) among adults (Westermeyer, 1973). It means that the behavior problems occurred significantly within a period of several years or decades. It may imply that such problems occurred in a fashionable way. However, unless the problems developed within a relatively short period of time — several days, weeks, or months — with evidence that they occurred as the result of "direct," "contagious" transmission, it is better not to refer to them as "epidemic mental disorders" in a strict sense.

B. The Matter of Frequency

News about the occurrence of epidemic mental disorders may appear in local newspapers, yet such events may or may not always be reported in scientific literature. Thus, information from literature is usually limited and occurrences are underreported.

Sirois (1974) found 78 episodes of epidemic hysteria outbreaks in literature from around the world during a 100-year period (1872–1972). However, according to Teoh and associates (1975), in Malaysia alone, 29 episodes involving school students were reported in the 10-year period between 1962 and 1971.

In a computer search of English literature for the period 1985 to 1996, 30 citations were revealed, with case reports of 23 incidences from Medline and 19 citations from Clinpsyc. This supports the fact that epidemic mental disorders are frequently elaborated academic topics and that the occurrence of epidemics is not as rare as one may think. In past literature, reports of incidences were found from many societies. Following are some examples: America (Helvie, 1968; Knight, Friedman, & Sulianti, 1965; Levine, 1977; Small, Propper, Randolph, & Eth, 1991), Australia (Hall & Morrow, 1988), Canada (B.W. Taylor & Werbicki, 1993), China (Tseng et al., 1988), England (McEvedy & Beard, 1970), Ghana (Adomakoh, 1973), Greece (Boulougouris, Rabavilas, Stefanis, Vaidakis, & Tabouratzis, 1981), Hong Kong (Tam, Tsoi-Mona, Kwong, & Wong, 1982; Wong, Kwong, Tam, & Tsoi-Mona, 1982), India (Chowdhury, Nath, & Chakraborty, 1993; Dutta et al., 1982), Japan (Ikeda, 1966; Takahashi, 1989), Malaysia (Tan, 1963),

Singapore (Chew, Phoon Mae-Lim, 1976), Sweden (R.E. Bartholomew, 1993), Taiwan (Jacobs, 1965), Tanganyika (Rankin & Philip, 1963), Thailand (Swanlert & Chouwanachinda, 1996; Suwanlert et al., 1978), Uganda (Kagwa, 1964; Muhangi, 1973), and Zambia (Dhadphale & Shaikh, 1983).

It may be concluded that collective mental disorders are observed around the world, whether the society is developing or developed, in the East or in the West. Such disorders are not that rare, but are a part of our common daily lives. As pointed out by Kumasaka (1966), most standard textbooks of psychiatry either do not mention the subject or at best devote a few lines to it under the heading of epidemic hysteria or mass hysteria. However, based on the rather frequent occurrence of these disorders and the need to know how to manage them from the standpoints of social and public health, psychiatrists must be fully aware of their nature and characteristics.

C. COMMON FEATURE AND ELEMENTS

Several common elements are observed among the collective mental disorders reported. First, they are more likely to take place in institutional settings, such as schools, factories, or hospitals, where a group of people are interrelated and associated in a very special manner, rather than in a group or crowd with no special affiliation. In most outbreaks of hysteria, those affected are predominantly young females (Sirois, 1974), although some forms of disorder, such as koro, by definition involve mainly (young) men (Tseng et al., 1988).

The first person affected in an outbreak usually has an ordinary onset of mental disorder. Soon, others manifest similar symptoms until eventually a large-scale incident is triggered. Occasionally, the initial sufferer has a special status in the group and thus functions as a model of identification for others (F.K. Taylor & Hunter, 1958). Sometimes it is a special event that attracts attention, especially one imbued with shock and horror, kindling a kind of emotional storm that precipitates subsequent episodes. A more impor-

tant condition seems to be the presence of some preexisting stress or group apprehension caused by a variety of sources, such as an authority-submission conflict (Teoh et al., 1975), academic or achievement stress (Muhangi, 1973), fear of enemy infiltration (Suwanlert et al., 1978), or sociocultural or interethnic tension associated with ethnic migration, refugees, or socioeconomic change (Jilek, 1986; Tseng et al., 1988). In other words, some unusual tension, fear, or anger among the group becomes a fertile ground for such outbreaks.

D. SOCIAL MECHANISMS AND GROUP DYNAMICS

From a sociological point of view, several mechanisms, including group influence, social isolation, or crowd response, should be considered in group contagion (Kerckhoff & Back, 1965). Today, mass communication by newspaper or radio, especially television, may facilitate the rapid spread of information and help create an atmosphere of excitement, frenzy, or fear. In this way, a whole community may become involved very quickly and deeply (Hefez, 1985; Johnson, 1945).

However, it is important to note that the precipitating ideas, beliefs, or false beliefs (delusions) transmitted or shared by members of the group must seem so true and/or familiar that the group readily accepts or adopts them. For example, the koro epidemics that occurred in Hainan Island in China illustrated that even though suoyang (koro) attacks have recurred again and again during the past several decades, the epidemic victims only involve Han nationals living in the coastal areas of the island and have never involved the Li or Miao nationals living in the central mountain areas of the same island. The Li or Miao nationals, as minority groups, did not share the concept of suoyang and, in addition, they seldom identified with the majority Han nationals. These factors made them immune from the suoyang epidemic (Tseng et al., 1988). In other words, the illness-belief or collective misperception has to be shared by the people in the community. Group members then transform these ideas into conflicts to which they are already vulnerable, or which are latent in them. Conflicts are then expressed as disabling symptoms or as a culturally rational attempt at problem-solving (R.E. Bartholomew, 1994).

It does not matter whether the information concerns a "scientific" explanation, such as gas intoxication or radiation from H-bomb tests as the cause of "pitting marks" on car windshields (Medalia & Larsen, 1958); a "religious" one, such as believing the end of the world will arrive on a certain day, causing a community's collective panic over the predicted disaster (as observed on many occasions, and recently in Korea, in 1995); or a supernatural explanation, such as obeying the spirits of dead ancestors as the cause of agitated behavior (Ebrahim, 1968) or the famous witch hunting that occurred in 1692 in Salem, Massachusetts, in the United States. The important factor is that the reaction is expressed within a social context to which people collectively respond and react. Based on the *koro* epidemic observed in China, Cheng (1996) took the view that it is a social malady maintained by cultural beliefs that affect the whole community.

For the purpose of understanding the psychological mechanism involved in the occurrence of epidemic mental disorder, Hefez (1985) has summarized several theoretical explanations proposed by various scholars or clinicians. The contagion theory proposes that the members of the crowd lose their rationality and become highly suggestible. Imitation, identification, and circular emotional reactions are the assumed psychological mechanisms. The convergence theory takes the view that the shared but concealed characteristics of the members become manifest in the crowd setting. The emergent-norm theory contends that transactions in the group are the source of new norms to which the members eventually conform.

From a dynamic point of view, the occurrence of such epidemics may serve as a coping defense that helps the group deal with problems they are facing. The epidemic may develop as a "group protest" against authority, as in the case of the girl students angered by the rumor that school officials would force them to submit to pregnancy tests to check for sexual promiscuity (Knight et al., 1965). The epidemic may provide a channel to express a complaint when no other alternative exists (Adomakoh, 1973). However, it may also be merely a collective reaction to the emotional frustration or helplessness of losing a school football game (Levine, 1977).

E. SUGGESTIONS FOR MANAGEMENT

1. Prompt Differential Diagnosis

From a public health standpoint, when any collective mental disorder begins, it is important to establish a diagnosis quickly so that an organic cause, such as infection or intoxication, can be ruled out. It is quite possible that the leakage of gas from a nearby factory may cause intoxication, fainting, headaches, nausea, or other symptoms, making it difficult for clinicians to make a differential diagnosis. Food poisoning should be ruled out if there are predominant digestive symptoms. A diagnosis of mass hysteria should not be made loosely simply because there is no substantial evidence to support medical etiology. There have been several incidences in which massive hysteria was initially suspected, but, after careful public health investigation, chemical intoxication was disclosed as the cause for the endemic occurrence of illness (Aldons, Ellam, Murray, & Pike, 1994; Baker & Selvey, 1992). However, in the collective occurrence of unique symptoms, such as "pseudo-seizure" or "peculiar panic attack" (such as a *koro* panic) or "laughing" (Rankin & Philip, 1963), it is much easier to see that such disorders are not organic in nature, a psychological diagnosis can be made, and proper management undertaken.

A review of literature shows that under the diagnosis of mass hysteria (conversion), various symptoms have been listed, including fainting or syncope (Levine, 1977), shortness of breath, crying and laughing (Helvie, 1968), screaming (Chew et al., 1976), or dissociation (Chowdhury et al., 1993), and numerous somatic complaints. Mass hysteria, depression, anxiety and fear reaction, delusion, and even suicidal behavior were reported as cardinal symptoms of epidemics. If the symptomatology or complaints are multiple and complex, organicity should be suspected and ruled out first. However, if there are more similar patterns suggesting imitation of symptoms, a diagnosis of psychogenic transmission may be favored.

In addition to the type of symptomatology, gender is another fact that may be helpful in making a diagnosis. A more prominent occurrence of female subjects in the same setting favors the consideration of an illness of a hysterical nature rather than one that is organic.

2. Immediate Formal Reaction to Counteract a Stressful Atmosphere

When the nature of an epidemic occurrence is known to be psychological, it is desirable that an explanation of the real cause be given publicly as soon as possible. It is suggested that official action be taken and administrative authority exercised to lessen the panic atmosphere that usually occurs in response to alarming phenomena. For instance, in a *koro* epidemic in Thailand, the government quickly formed a mobile public health team, which visited the affected areas by car, using megaphones to announce that the occurrence was emotional rather than medical, and asking the people to calm down. Such government measures seem to work well in these circumstances (S. Suwanlert, personal communication, 1977). In a *koro* epidemic in India, after official reassurance through mass media communication, the almost 3-months-long panic epidemic was ended (Dutta et al., 1982).

3. Management of Secondary Gain

If the episode appears "hysterical" in nature, the principle for treating individual cases should be applied to the group situation. Attention given to the victims should be kept to a minimum to reduce any secondary gain from the illness. Detailed public reports of the victims through mass media, particularly the primary victim, should be limited so that they do not aggravate the possibility of group identification. Special care from teachers, parents, or authority figures should be regulated carefully so that no excessive attention is given to satisfy the needs of the victims.

4. Appropriate Control of Mass Media

Closely associated with the management of potential secondary gain, it is important to pay attention to the effects of mass media on the community (Small & Borus, 1987). Any unfounded news should be discouraged and dramatic reports by the media should be minimized to reduce the unnecessary arousal of emotional tension or excitement in the community. In many societies, the freedom of mass media must be respected, and official authorities are limited in their ability to restrict the media, as may be done in autocratic societies. However, suitable advice and suggestions can be communicated to the news reporters so that not only can the harmful effects of mass media be avoided, but mass communications can be utilized in a positive and healthy way to calm the hysterical atmosphere — one of the major strategies used to control epidemics.

5. Resolution of Primary Stress

Once the underlying cause of a tension or conflict is detected, an effort should be made to focus on the problem and resolve it as soon as possible. This is especially true if the situation involves a local institution and the cause can be identified quickly. A good example was the Malay schoolgirls' problem with the schoolmaster's intrusion into their dormitory (Teoh et al., 1975). Another was the Japanese leprosarium case in which there was a real need to replace the inexperienced head nurse and resolve the tension with the patients (Ikeda, 1966). Otherwise, the endemics might have continued.

F. SUGGESTIONS FOR FUTURE INVESTIGATION

A public health-style demographic survey is not enough to understand the nature of an epidemic if the epidemic is psychogenic in nature. It has been shown in the past that a psychometric study of individual victims or a demographic description of the occurrence is not helpful in comprehending this unique social, cultural phenomena. It is suggested that more dynamic and socioculturally oriented investigations are needed in the future. If a questionnaire survey is to be conducted, the design should start with working hypotheses. The survey should be aimed at testing specific hypotheses for the elaboration of the cause of the occurrence. Comparison with nonvictims (as a control group) from the epidemic area is one effective way of testing the working hypotheses.

In summary, from community, social, and cultural points of view, epidemic psychiatric disorders are fascinating phenomena that deserve more careful attention and investigation. They provide opportunities to examine how social and cultural factors may contribute significantly to the formation and spreading of psychopathologies. They also call attention to the need to understand such unique phenomena and to be ready to take professional action when they occur, including making a prompt assessment, an appropriate diagnosis, dealing with the social media, and controlling and ending the psychologically contagious epidemic.

REFERENCES

Adityanjee (1994). Mass suicide by self-immolation in Waco, Texa. *Journal of Nervous and Mental Disease, 182*(12), 727–728.

Adomakoh, C.G. (1973). The pattern of epidemic hysteria in a girls' school in Ghana. *Ghana Medical Journal, 12,* 407–411.

Aldous, J.C., Ellam, G.A., Murray, V., & Pike, G. (1994). An outbreak of illness among schoolchildren in London: Toxic poisoning not mass hysteria. *Journal of Epidemiology and Community Health, 48*(1), 41–45.

Amin, Y., Hamdi, E., & Eapen, V. (1997). Mass hysteria in an Arab culture. *International Journal of Social Psychiatry, 43*(4), 303–306.

Anonymous. (1977). A suicide epidemic in a psychiatric hospital. *Diseases of the Nervous System, 38,* 327–331.

Baker, P., & Selvey, D. (1992). Malathion-induced epidemic hysteria in an elementary school. *Veterinary and Human Toxicology, 34*(2), 156–160.

Bartholomew, R.E. (1993). Redefining epidemic hysteria: An example from Sweden. *Acta Psychiatrica Scandinavica, 88*(3), 178–182.

Bartholomew, R.E. (1994). Tarantism, dancing mania and demonopathy: The anthro-political aspects of "mass psychogenic illness." *Psychological Medicine, 24*(2), 281–306.

Bartholomew, R.E., & Gregory, J. (1996). "A strange epidemic": Notes on the first detailed documented case of epidemic koro. *Transcultural Psychiatric Research Review, 33,* 365–366.

Boling, L. & Brotman, C. (1975). A fire setting epidemic in a state mental health center. *American Journal of Psychiatry, 132,* 946–950.

Boulougouris, J.C., Rabavilas, A.D., Stefanis, C.N., Vaidakis, N., & Tabouratzis, D.G. (1981). Epidemic faintness: A psychophysiologic investigation. *Psychiatria Clinica, 14*(4), 215–225.

Burton, R. (1961). *Anatomy of melancholy.* In H. Jackson (Ed.), Everyman's Library London: J.M. Dent and Sons. (Original were published 1628)

Burton-Bradley, B.G. (1975). Cargo cult. In B.G. Burton-Bradley *Stone age crisis: A psychiatric appraisal* (pp. 10–31). Nashville, TN: Vanderbilt University Press.

Burton-Bradley, B.G. (1982). Cargo cult syndromes. In C.T.H. Friedman & R.A. Faguet (Eds.), *Extraordinary disorders of human behavior.* New York: Plenum Press.

Cantril, H. (1940). *The invasion from Mars: A study in the psychology of panic.* Princeton, NJ: Princeton University Press.

Chakraborty, A. (1982, December). *Koro makes an epidemic appearance in India. Transcultural Psychiatric Newsletter, 3,* (3 & 4).

Chakraborty, A. (1984). An epidemic of *koro* in West Bengal (India). *Transcultural Psychiatric Research Review, 21*(1), 59–61 [Abstracted by W.G. Jilek].

Cheng, S.T. (1996). A critical review of Chinese *koro. Culture, Medicine and Psychiatry, 20,* 67–82.

Chew, P.K., Phoon, W.H., & Mae-Lim, H.A. (1976). Epidemic hysteria among some factory workers in Singapore. *Singapore Medical Journal, 17,* 10–15.

Chowdhury, A.N., Nath, A.K., & Chakraborty, J. (1993). An atypical hysteria epidemic in Tripura, India. *Transcultural Psychiatric Research Review, 30*(2), 143–151.

Dhadphale, M., & Shaikh, S.P. (1983). Epidemic hysteria in a Zambian school: "The mysterious madness of Mwinilunga." *British Journal of Psychiatry, 142,* 85–88.

Dutta, D., Phookan, H.R., & Das, P.D. (1982). The *koro* epidemic in Lower Assam. *Indian Journal of Psychiatry, 24*(4), 370–374. (Reviewed in *Transcultural Psychiatry Research Review, 21*(1), 59–61 [1984].)

Ebrahim, G.J. (1968). Mass hysteria in schoolchildren: Notes on three outbreaks in East Africa. *Clinical Pediatrics, 7,* 437–448.

Goduco-Angular, C., & Wintrob, R. (1964). Folie á famille in the Philippines. *Psychiatric Quarterly, 38,* 278–291.

Hall, W., & Morrow, L. (1988). "Repetition strain injury": An Australian epidemic of upper limb pain. *Social Science Medicine, 27*(6), 645–649.

Hefez, A. (1985). The role of the press and the medical community in the epidemic of "mysterious gas poisoning' in the Jordan West Bank. *American Journal of Psychiatry, 142*(7), 833–837.

Helvie, C.O. (1968). An epidemic of hysteria in a high school. *Journal of School Health, 38,* 505–509.

Ikeda, Y. (1966). An epidemic of emotional disturbance among leprosarium nurses in a setting of low morale and social change. *Psychiatry, 23,* 152–164.

Ivanova, A. (1970). *The dance in Spain.* New York: Praeger.

Jacobs, N. (1965). The phantom slasher of Taipei: Mass hysteria in a non-Western society. *Social Problems, 12,* 318–328.

Jilek, W. (1986). Epidemic of "genital shrinking" (koro): Historical review and report of a recent outbreak in Southern China. *Curare, 9,* 269–282.

Johnson, D.M. (1945). The "phantom anesthetist" of Mattoon: A field study of mass hysteria. *Journal of Abnormal and Social Psychology, 40,* 175–186.

Justice, B., & Duncan, D.F. (1976). Running away: An epidemic problem of adolescence. *Adolescence, 11*(43), 363–371.

Kagwa, B.H. (1964). The problem of mass hysteria in East Africa. *East African Medical Journal, 41,* 560–565.

Kerckhoff, A.C., & Back, K.W. (1965). Sociometric patterns in hysterial contagion. *Sociometry, 28,* 2–15.

Knight, J.A., Friedman, T.I., & Sulianti, J. (1965). Epidemic hysteria. A field study. *American Journal of Public Health, 55,* 858–865.

Kumasaka, Y. (1966). Collective mental illness within the framework of cultural psychiatry and group dynamics. *Psychiatric Quarterly, 40*(2), 333–347.

Levine, R.J. (1977). Epidemic faintness and syncope in a school marching band. *Journal of American Medical Association, 238,* 2373–2378.

McEvedy, C.P., & Beard, A.W. (1970). Royal Free epidemic of 1955: A reconsideration. *British Medical Journal, 1,* 7–11.

Medalia, N.Z., & Larsen, O.N. (1958). Diffusion and belief in a collective delusion: The Seattle windshield pitting epidemic. *American Sociology Review, 23,* 180–186.

Mo, G.M., Chen, G.Q., Li, L.X., & Tseng, W.S. (1995). *Koro* epidemic in Southern China. In T.-Y. Lin, W.S. Tseng, & E.K. Yeh (Eds.), *Chinese societies and mental health* (pp. 231–243). Hong Kong: Oxford University Press.

Moss, P.D., & McEvedy, C.P. (1966). An epidemic of overbreathing among school girls. *British Medical Journal, 2,* 1295–1300.

Muhangi, J.R. (1973). A preliminary report on "mass hysteria" in an Akole school in Uganda. *East African Medical Journal, 50,* 304–309.

Murphy, H.B.M. (1959). Cultural factors in the mental health of Malayan students. In D.M. Funkenstein (Ed.), *The student and mental health: An international view.* Cambridge, MA: Mass Riverside Press.

Nemiah, J.C. (1975). Hysterical neurosis, conversion type. In A.M. Freedman, H.I. Kaplan, & B.J. Sadock (Eds.), *Comprehensive textbook of psychiatry-II* (Vol. 1). Baltimore: Williams & Wilkins.

Ngui, P.W. (1969). The koro epidemic in Singapore [Special issue], *Australian New Zealand Journal of Psychiatry, 3,* 263–266.

Rankin, A.M., & Philip, P.J. (1963). An epidemic of laughing in the Bukoba District of Tanganyika. *Transcultural Psychiatric Research Review, 2,* 128.

Robbins, R.H. (1959). *The encyclopedia of witchcraft and demonology.* New York: Crown.

Rubinstein, D.H. (1983). Epidemic suicide among Micronesian adolescents. *Social Science Medicine, 17*(10), 657–665.

Schuler, E.A., & Parenton, V.J. (1943). A recent epidemic of hysteria in a Louisiana high school. *Journal of Social Psychology, 17,* 221–235.

Sirois, F. (1974). Epidemic hysteria. *Acta Psychiatrica Scandinavica, Supplementum, 252,* 1–46.

Small, G.W., & Borus, J.F. (1987). The influence of newspaper reports on outbreaks of mass hysteria. *Psychiatric Quarterly, 58*(4), 269–278.

Small, G.W., Propper, M.W., Randolph, E.T., & Eth, S. (1991). Mass hysteria among student performers: Social relationship as a symptom predictor. *American Journal of Psychiatry, 148*(9), 1200–1205.

Special report: UFO's comets and cuts—'Follow me': Inside the Heaven's Gate mass suicide. (1997; April 7). *News week.* pp. 26–49.

Suwanlert, S. (1983, July 11–16). *The second koro epidemic in northeast Thailand.* Post presentation at the Seventh World Congress of Psychiatry, Vienna.

Suwanlert, S., & Chouwanachinda, P. (1996). *Cultural study of mass hysteria in Thailand.* Presented at the sixth Congress of Asian Federation and Mental Health and the 10th Asian forum on Child and Adolescent Psychiatry.

Suwanlert, S., & Coates, D. (1979). Epidemic koro in Thailand—Clinical and social aspects. *Transcultural Psychiatric Research Review, 15,* 64–66.

Suwanlert, S., Sugondhabhirom, A., Pimpanit, S., & Chaiyasit, W. (1978, October 15–20). *The koro epidemic in northeast Thailand.* Presented at the 15th annual Congress Asian meeting of the Royal Australian and New Zealand College of Psychiatrists, Singapore.

Taiminen, T., Salmenpera, T., & Lehtinen, K. (1992). A suicide epidemic in a psychiatric hospital. *Suicide and Life-Threatening Behavior, 22*(3), 350–363.

Takahashi, Y. (1989). Mass suicide by members of the Japanese friend of Truth Church. *Suicide and Life-Threatening Behavior, 19*(3), 289–296.

Tam, Y.K., Tsoi-Mona, M., Kwong, B., & Wong, S.W. (1982). Psychological epidemic in Hong Kong: II. Psychological and physiological characteristics of children who were affected. *Acta Psychiatrica Scandinavica, 65*(5), 421–436.

Tan, E.S. (1963). Epidemic hysteria. *Medical Journal of Malaya, 18,* 72–76.

Taylor, B.W., & Werbicki, J.E. (1993). Pseudodisaster: A case of mass hysteria involving 19 schoolchildren. *Pediatric Emergency Care, 9*(4), 216–217.

Taylor, F.K., & Hunter, R.C.A. (1958). Observation of a hysterical epidemic in a hospital ward. *Psychiatric Quarterly, 32,* 821–839.

Teoh, J.-I., Soewondo, S., & Sidharta, M. (1975). Epidemic hysteria in Malaysian schools: An illustrative episode. *Psychiatry, 38,* 258–268.

Tseng, W.S. (1969). A paranoid family in Taiwan: A dynamic study of *folie à famille. Archives of General Psychiatry, 21,* 55–65.

Tseng, W.S., Mo, G.M., Chen, K.C., Li, L.S., Wen, J.K., & Liu, T.S. (1993). Social psychiatry and *koro* epidemic, (4): Regional comparison of *SuoYang* belief. *Chinese Mental Health Journal, 7,* 38–40 (in Chinese).

Tseng, W.S., Mo, K.M., Hsu, J., Li, L.S., Chen, G.Q., Ou, L.W., & Zheng, H.B. (1992). Koro epidemics in Guandong, China: A questionnare survey. *Journal of Nervous and Mental Disease, 180*(2), 117–123.

Tseng, W.S., Mo, K.M., Hsu, J., Li, L.S., Ou, L.W., Chen, G.Q., & Jiang, D.W. (1988). A sociocultural study of koro epidemics in Guandong, China. *American Journal of Psychiatry, 145*(12), 1538–1543.

Ulman, R.B., & Abse, D.W. (1983). The group psychology of mass madness, Jonestown. *Political Psychology, 4*(4), 637–661.

Westermeyer, J. (1973). On the epidemicity of *amok* violence. *Archives of General Psychiatry, 28,* 873–876.

Wong, S.W., Kwong, B., Tam, Y.K., & Tsoi-Mona, M. (1982). Psychological epidemic in Hong Kong: I. Epidemiological study. *Acta Psychiatrica Scandinavica, 65*(5), 421–436.

Woon, T.H. (1976). Epidemic hysteria in a Malaysian Chinese extended family. *Medical Journal of Malaysia, 31,* 108–112.

15

Anxiety Disorders

I. INTRODUCTION

In this chapter, under the heading "anxiety" disorders, numerous minor psychiatric disorders will be examined, mainly from a cultural perspective. In *Diagnostic and Statistical Manual of Mental Disorders,* 4th Edition (DSM-IV) these disorders are formally categorized as general anxiety disorders, specific phobias, social phobias, panic disorders, obsessive-compulsive disorders (OCD), and posttraumatic stress disorders (PTSD). All of them, even though they may be attributed to biological factors, are understood to occur psychologically in reaction to external stress or internal psychic conflict. They share the common core problem of "anxiety," even though they may manifest distinctly different or mixed clinical pictures.

These disorders are nonpsychotic and, together with others, such as dissociation, somatoform, and adjustment disorders, are labeled "minor," in contrast to "major" (psychotic), psychiatric disorders. In the past, they were also called neurotic disorders, as they are still referred to in many parts of the world outside of America. This is reflected in the presence of the generic term "neurotic" disorders in the latest version of *International Statistical Classification of Diseases*

and Related Health Problems, 10th Revision (ICD-10), published in 1992. However, the generic term was eliminated from the American classification system of DSM-III in 1980 due to changed attitudes of American psychiatrists with regard to the professional orientation of the classification system.

It is worth mentioning that the term "psychoneuroses" was originally coined by Sigmund Freud early in his career, in the late 19th century. He wanted to stress his view (as a neurologist and psychiatrist) that this group of disorders (including phobia and obsessive-compulsive disorders) was induced predominantly by psychological factors; therefore, they were grouped as "psycho-neuroses" (nervous system disorders caused by psychic factors), whereas the "true" neuroses ("actual" disorders of the nerve system, including neurasthenia, anxiety disorder, and hypochondriasis) were nerve disorders caused by an organic disturbance. Such a distinction was later abandoned and "neuroses," as a generic term, was used to address all of these disorders. It has been a landmark of psychiatry to recognize the importance of psychological factors in causing these disorders and to emphasize psychotherapy as the primary approach with which to treat them.

Interestingly, associated with recent advancements in psychiatric knowledge, particularly in the areas of genetics, neurochemistry, and psychopharmacology, clinicians have begun to reconsider and claim that some of these "neuroses" are predominantly caused by biological factors, including genetics, and that drug therapy is the best choice of treatment. Thus, there is a trend to revert to the pre-Freudian organic orientation of these disorders. However, there is still room to examine how psychological, social, and cultural factors may contribute concomitantly to these disorders. Such an examination will be attempted in this chapter, based on information obtained from cross-cultural perspectives. Anxiety disorders strongly related to culture — recognized as culture-related specific syndromes — will be also be briefly elaborated in order to demonstrate the role of culture in such specific psychopathology.

II. CULTURE, EMOTION, AND STRESS

The cultural dimensions of minor psychiatric disorders should be studied first in terms of culture and emotion. To do this, one needs to know how people express emotion from a developmental point of view. As pointed out by Werner (1948), in terms of the comparative psychology of mental development, primitive emotions are characterized by syncretism, i.e., affective excitement is closely bound up with physical response. Later, in higher mental life, "emotion" is gradually differentiated from "somatic" response. Following this view, it has been suggested that, clinically, certain individuals who are organically vulnerable to the physiological concomitants of affect may develop psychophysiological (or psychosomatic) disorders as a result of emotional arousal. Individuals who have an underdeveloped ability to communicate by verbal symbols may utilize a primitive body language to communicate their problems (Kaplan & Kaplan, 1967).

However, these views ignored the cultural contribution to the expression of affect at both normal and abnormal levels. As elaborated previously [cross-ref-erence to Chapter 6: Psychology, Customary Behavior, and Ethnic Identity (Section II,A)], culture has a significant influence on the expression of emotional reaction. People in different cultures reveal their emotions differently, in words, gestures, and facial expressions. Instead of differentiating emotional reactions into psychological and somatic, some cultures encourage a combination of the two, whereas others place more emphasis on expression through the body than through psychological words. Some cultures have highly elaborate cultural ways of expressing "emotion" through "somato-organ-language" for affectional expression. For instance, *fa pi qi* (lost spleen spirit, meaning losing one's temper) and *gan fuo da* (elevated liver fire, meaning emotionally irritated) in Chinese are equivalent to organ language expressions used in English, such as "butterflies in the stomach" or "a pain in the neck."

Furthermore, clinical experience shows that patients seldom present clearly and specifically about anxiety, depression, fear, or worry. Their complaints are often combined and undifferentiated. Thus, clinically, diagnoses that are a mixture of anxiety and depression are more prevalent. This is truer in societies in which the distressful condition is viewed as a holistic experience rather than a specifically categorized emotional reaction.

Finally, it must be remembered that psychological disorders, such as anxiety or depression disorders, cannot be approached merely from a phenomenological perspective. The nature and origin of the distress need to be included. This is true, at least from the standpoint of culture, because the nature of stress varies greatly according to cultural background [cross-reference to Chapter 8: Stress and Coping Patterns (Section I,A–D)]. It is neceesary to elaborate on how people of different culture backgrounds perceive and react to certain stresses and how they manifest different kinds of emotion in response to distressful situations. Further, the whole picture needs to be understood not merely from a "disease" aspect, but also from an "illness" perspective, including how the distress is communicated by the patient and his or her family through folk idioms (Good & Kleinman,

1985). Examining these issues comprehensively from individual, social, and cultural perspectives will enable clinicians to offer culturally oriented care for their patients. This is the basic orientation that a clinician should have before exploring the nature of anxiety disorders further.

III. DIAGNOSTIC DISTRIBUTION OF ANXIETY DISORDERS

A. INFORMATION FROM PSYCHIATRIC OUTPATIENT SURVEYS

Numerous reports are available on the diagnostic distribution of minor psychiatric disorders from outpatient surveys. However, probably very much influenced by the professional pattern of diagnostic practice, the prevalence of anxiety disorders varies greatly among different societies. Only a few will be mentioned here for the sake of discussion.

For instance, one of the earlier reports was made in the 1960s by Saenger (1968), who compared psychiatric patients in selected outpatient facilities in the Netherlands and the United States. According to him, regarding neuroses, the most common diagnoses among Dutch patients were hysterical reaction (19.5%), conversion reaction (16.0%), and depressive reaction (14.2%); among American patients, depressive reaction (36.6%), anxiety reaction (13.8%), other neurotic reactions (7.6%), and obsessive-compulsive reaction (6.9%). Due to methodological limitations, Saenger warned that these findings needed to be seen as suggestions rather than conclusions. However, they do illustrate the wide gap in the distribution of diagnostic categories, even among a sample of Euro-Americans.

Tseng, Xu, Ebata, Hsu, and Cui (1986) reported that according to data from a university clinic in Bejing, China, the most common diagnoses were unclassifed neuroses (37.5%), neurasthenia (18.6%), hysteria (16.7%), and obsessive-compulsive disorder (10.6%). In Japan, one psychiatric institute (Iwai, 1982) reported diagnoses in the following order: hypochondriasis (16.7%), unclassified neuroses (10.8%), phobia (10.1%), and other unspecified disorders (23.5%). In contrast, in Hawaii, the most common diagnostic categories were adjustment disorder (46.9%), depression (37.5%), and anxiety disorder (10.8%).

These data illustrate that the diagnostic criteria of minor psychiatric disorders are so subjectively defined and loosely constructed that they tend to vary according to practitioners' patterns of practice. It also points out that the nature of minor psychiatric disorders is closely related to a person's cognitive conceptions, emotional reactions, and life experiences and therefore varies widely, depending on individual as well as environmental factors.

B. DATA FROM GENERAL HEALTH CARE

As described previously [cross-reference to Chapter 12: Culture and Psychiatric Epidemiology (Section II,D,4)], a large-scale international, multisite comparative investigation was carried out by WHO — the Collaborative Study of Psychological Problems in General Health Care (Üstün & Sartorius, 1995) — involving 14 countries around the world. The investigation focused on (medical) patients visiting general health care facilities. In addition to the prevalence of minor psychiatric disorders, other clinical issues were examined.

As illustrated in Table 12-1, patients' presenting complaints were subdivided into four categories for comparison: psychological, fatigue/sleeping disturbance, pain, and other somatic complaints. Interestingly, it was revealed that the proportion of psychological complaints made to the treating physicians varied a great deal. The percentages were high in most European centers investigated: 12.8% in Groninge (Netherlands), 11.0% in Paris (France), and 9.4% in Manchester (UK). They were also high in some South American centers: 13.2% in Santiego de Chile (Chile) and 7.6% in Rio de Janeiro (Brazil). In European centers, it was interpreted that medical patients with minor psychiaric disorders were accustomed to presenting their psychological problems to their physicians even in general health care facilities. In South American centers, the reasons are not clear. They may relate to that psychiatric service is a specialty that is not widely available to patients with emotional problems, who thus have no choice but to attend general care facilities. In contrast, the percentages of patients making psychological complaints were rather low in Asian centers: 0.2% in Shanghai (China) and 1.3% in Nagasaki (Japan). They were also quite low in certain other centers: 1.3% in Bangalore (India), 2.2% in Arthen (Greek), 2.3% in Ibadan (Nigeria), or 2.6% in Ankara (Turkey). It may be speculated that, in these cultural areas, people do not perceive having emotional problems as a reason to visit physicians of general medicine, who mainly treat physical illness.

It is understandable that patterns of problem presentation are affected by multiple factors, including the patient's help-seeking behavior, his or her orientation to the care system, the function of the facilities, and the customary manner of complaining. It seems to be based on these various factors that the proportion of patients presenting psychological problems varies among European and Asian centers.

The mental disorders investigated in this WHO study included general anxiety disorder, panic disorder, agoraphobia, depression, dysthymia, somatization disorder, hypochondriasis, and neurasthenia, as defined by ICD-10. The results showed that there are certain degrees of variation in terms of the prevalence of these disorders (Table 12-1). For example, the prevalence of general anxiety disorder is relatively high in South America: 22.6% in Rio de Janirio (Brazil) and 18.7% in Santigo de Chile (Chile). In contrast, it is only 0.9% in Ankara (Turkey) and 1.9% in Shanghai (China), paralleling the trend that patients visiting general health facilities there seldom present psychological problems. Given the information obtained from this study, it is unclear what cardinal factors influence these results.

This investigation also examined to what extent the treating physicians recognized the psychological cases that attended the general health care facilities.

Again, it was revealed that the estimated proportions varied remarkably. In Santigo de Chile (Chile), 58% of the cases were recognized by the physicians as psychological. In Verona (Italy), it was 47.3%. In contrast, in Nagasaki (Japan), it was merely 4.8%, and in Shanghai (China), it was 5.4%.

It seems probable that, in some countries, such as Japan and China, patients with psychological problems seldom attend general health care facilities, are less likely to present psychological problems, and are infrequently recognized by their physicians as psychological cases. In contrast, in Brazil and Chile, patients with psychological problems do attend general health care facilities and are often recognized by their physicians as having anxiety disorders or other psychological problems.

C. REPORTS FROM COMMUNITY SURVEYS

It is useful to have cross-cultural information about the nature and pattern of problems presented by patients attending general health care facilities; however, such data are limited because it is not clear to what extent it reflects the actual situation in the community. Several community survey studies have shed some light for us, even though their data are difficult to compare with data obtained from different cultural areas because no standardized methodology was applied.

1. China: Twelve-Region Epidemiological Study of Neuroses

In order to comprehend the prevalence of various neuroses in the community, China undertook a national survey in 1982, involving 12 geographic areas around the country, both rural and urban (Cooper & Sartorius, 1996; Psychiatric Epidemiological Collaboration Team, 1986). Through mechanical random-sample selection in each selected region, a total of 6754 subjects, aged 15 to 59, of both genders, were included in the study. After a questionnaire screening (such as Psychiatric State Examination, PSE), a clinical interview was conducted for case identification and diagnosis according to Chinese Classification of Mental Diseases (CCMD) — the Chinese formal classification system for mental disorders, which recognizes the generic term neuroses. Results revealed that 150 neurotic patients were identified with a prevalence rate of 22.21 per 1000 population investigated. In terms of the total prevalence rate, there were no significant differences between the rural and the urban areas investigated. However, significant differences were noted between genders: the total prevalence rate per 1000 population was 4.71 for males and 39.93 for females (the much higher rate for females was found in both rural and urban areas).

As for different categories of neurotic disoders, as a whole, the total prevalence rates per 1000 population, in declining order, were 13.0 for neurasthenia, 3.55 for hysteria, 3.11 for neurotic depression, 1.48 for anxiety disorder, 0.59 for phobic disoder, 0.30 for obsessive-compulsive disorder, and 0.15 for hypochondriasis. It should be noticed that neurasthenia was the most frequently diagnosed category, with a prevalence rate of 13.0, far higher than any other kind of neurosis disorder. Anxiety disorders, including phobic and obsessive-compulsive disorders, had a prevalence rate of only 2.37 altogether.

2. United States: Catchment Area Study

The Epidemiological Catchment Area (ECA) Study carried out in the United States in 1980s by design was not primarily for cross-cultural study. Still, cross-ethnic comparison was made among three ethnic groups: Caucasian-American, African-American, and Hispanic-American, depending on the number of subjects investigated available in the selected catchment area for statistical comparison.

Regarding anxiety disorders, there were several findings concerning these three ethnic groups. The lifetime prevalence of panic disorder was found to be 1.62, 1.31, and 0.87%, respectively, in the three ethnic groups. Caucasian-Americans had a relatively higher prevalence, Hispanic-Americans lower, while

African-American were in between (Eaton, Dryman, & Weissman, 1991, p. 159). The 1-year prevalence rates of general anxiety disorder were 1.64, 2.74, and 0.86%, respectively, for the three groups, with African-Americans being relatively higher and Hispanic-Americans lower (Blazer, Hughes, George, Swartz, & Boyer, 1991, p. 187). Regarding obsessive compulsive disorder, the lifetime prevalence was 2.63, 2.31, and 1.82%, respectively, with Caucasian-Americans relatively higher and Hispanic-Americans lower (Karno & Golding, 1991, p. 211). Thus, there were different variations among the three ethnic groups examined for each different category of anxiety disorder surveyed.

3. Cross-Societal Comparison of Catchment Area Surveys

In order to avoid the problem of diagnostic patterns applied in different settings, it is desirable to use the same (standardized) diagnostic criteria to carry out comparative studies among different societies, particularly in investigations of populations from communities rather than from clinics. By adopting the same methodology and instrument, namely the Diagnostic Interview Schedule (DIS) used in ECA studies in the United States, several studies have been undertaken in other societies. Their results concerning anxiety disorders are as follows.

a. United States–Taiwan (China) Comparison

The Chinese version of the DIS was adopted in the Psychiatric Epidemiological Project in Taiwan, China, from 1981 to 1986 (Yeh, Hwu, & Lin, 1995). Data were analyzed according to three different geographical communities investigated: metropolis, townships, and rural villages. The findings from the project were compared with those obtained from the USA–Catchment Area Project (Comptom et al., 1991; Yeh et al., 1995). It was revealed by Comtom and colleagues (1991) that the lifetime prevalence rate of generalized anxiety disorder in Taiwan was lower in the metropolis (4.72%) and higher in townships (11.64%) than in every site in the United States; whereas in rural villages (8.42%), it was well within the range of the United States. Rates of total phobic disorders (4.56, 5.90, 3.50%), panic disorders (0.30, 0.57, 0.27%), and obsessive-compulsive disorders (1.02, 0.70, 0.30%) in the three geographic sites in Taiwan, respectively, were all significantly lower than in every area in the United States.

b. United States–Korea Comparison

In a psychiatric epidemiological study carried out in Korea (C.K. Lee et al., 1990a, 1990b), the areas selected for study were Seoul (as city area) and scattered rural locations over the country. The results revealed lifetime prevalence rates for overall general anxiety disorders of 9.19 and 9.85% for Seoul and rural Korea, respectively. These were lower than the rate for St. Louis in the United States, namely 11.0%. The differences were much greater for phobias. Those percentages were 5.89 for Seoul and 5.97 for rural Korea, in contrast to 9.4 for St. Louis. However, there was a tendency for general anxiety disorder rates to be higher in Korea (3.56 and 2.89% for Seoul and rural Korea, respectively) than in St. Louis (0.0%). No specific interpretation was given for these findings.

IV. CULTURAL ASPECTS OF VARIOUS TYPES OF ANXIETY DISORDERS

The studies just described reflect methodological improvements in cross-societal epidemiological comparison. However, from a cultural perspective, the meaning and validity of data obtained in such cross-cultural studies using standardized instruments still remain in considerable question. This is particularly true when a study examines minor psychiatric disorders, which are shaped by subjective personal experiences and cultural value systems. A cautious interpretation is still needed for this kind of cross-cultural study.

From a cultural point of view, anxiety disorders, which differ from culture to culture, are characterized

not according to frequency of occurrence (namely, prevalence rate), but more according to the factors that contribute to their occurrence and the way the anxieties are manifested. These aspects will be elaborated further by reviewing each of the following disorders.

A. (SIMPLE) ANXIETY DISORDERS

The adjective "simple" is added here to the term "anxiety disorder" to imply that, unlike a general anxiety disorder (as defined by DSM-IV), it can occur as a brief episode, in reaction to external distress or intrapsychic conflict, and may be manifested primarily as an anxiety picture. The DSM-IV included in the definition of a general anxiety disorder the arbitrary requirement that the anxiety state lasts more than 6 months.

As already elaborated in Chapter 8, in addition to individual factors, the source and nature of stress are subjected greatly to the sociocultural environment. Briefly, culture itself produces stress, influences the perception of stress, shapes the way people cope with the distress encountered, and affects supporting resources for managing stress. Anxiety can be created by cultural beliefs, such as penis shrinkage anxiety (koro cases), semen leakage anxiety (daht and shenkui syndromes), taboo-breaking anxiety (causing voodoo death or malgri attacks) [cross-reference to Chapter 13: Culture-Related Specific Syndromes (Section II,A,1–5)]. Anxiety can also be produced by cultural demands. Bearing a son to succeed the family line, academic achievement, the regulated choice of a mate, or the restricted life of a widow are some examples. Family conflicts associated with widening generational gaps among immigrants, severe discrimination by a majority group, rapid change and confusion of value systems, and family separation due to war or social disaster are additional examples of sources of anxiety that are closely related to sociocultural situations. In many societies, cultural dictates on how to secure food, how to find money to pay debts or mortgages, and how to obtain medicine for sicknesses are some causes of daily anxiety.

From a clinical point of view, it should be mentioned that the reaction to distress does not necessarily take the "pure" or "typical" form of an anxiety state. The reaction often manifests as a mixture of anxiety, depression, and various somatic symptoms.

B. Social Phobia

The diagnostic consideration of social phobia has increased considerably in the United States in the past decade. Whether this is due to an increase in such cases (doubtful) or an increase in diagnostic attention by clinicians (likely) deserves examination. It should be pointed out that the diagnostic category of social phobia was not listed among international classification systems, not even ICD-8 (1968) or ICD-9 (1977), and only recently appeared in ICD-10 (1992). In the American system of DSM, there was no such category in DSM-II (1968); it did not appear until 1980, when the DSM-III was revised. Therefore, social phobia was referred to as a neglected anxiety disorder (Liebowitz, Gorman, Fyer, Klein, 1985). In contrast, Japanese psychiatrists coined the diagnostic term *taijin-kyofu-sho* (disorder of fear of interpersonal relations, also translated as "anthrophobia" in English) at the beginning of the 20th century, and it has been used widely since [cross-reference to Chapter 13: Culture-Related Specific Syndromes (Section II, C,1)]. Study revealed that Japanese psychiatrists are familiar with this disorder clinically and diagnose it easily (Tseng, Asai, Kitanish, McLaughlin, & Kyomen, 1992). A special mode of therapy has even been invented for treating this disorder.

By definition (according to DSM), social phobia refers to a marked and persistent fear of social performance situations in which the person is exposed to unfamiliar people or to possible scrutiny by others. This suggests that the disorder will tend to occur in a society in which social performance is crucial. It also hints that a person will experience it when he encounters and must perform in front of unfamiliar persons. Theoretically, if an individual lives in a small society, where the environment (such as a village) is filled with familiar people and there is no pressure to perform in front of them, the possibility of suffering from a social phobia is potentially low. However, if an individual is living in a large setting, relating to many strangers in school, the workplace, or in social settings and there is a hidden but high pressure to compete and perform in mate selection and other psychosexual activities and relationships, the potential for social anxiety will increase.

From a developmental perspective, socialization is a developmental task. When an individual who is excessively protected or indulged by his or her caregivers (parents or grandparents) in childhood grows into adolescence or young adulthood, with expectations suddenly involving social relations outside of the family, he or she mayl feel unprepared for socialization with peers or others, unsure about him- or herself, and embarrassed when relating with schoolmates, colleagues, or superiors. This is the underlying cause given by Japanese psychiatrist Kenji Kitanish (personal communication, 1990), who specializes in the treatment of this disorder with the Morita therapy for the dynamic development of *taijinkyofusho*. Kitanish's view is in line with the findings obtained by Australian psychiatrist Gordon Parker (1979), which indicated that higher agoraphobic scores were associated with less maternal care and less maternal overprotection, whereas higher social phobic scores were associated with greater maternal care and greater maternal overprotection. Canadian cultural psychiatrist Laurence J. Kirmayer (1991) pointed out that *taijinkyofusho* can be understood as a pathological amplification of culture-specific concerns about the social presentation of self and the impact of improper conduct on the well-being of others.

Although Western psychiatrists are eager to include *taijinkyofusho* as social phobia in a broad sense, Japanese psychiatrists insist that the disorder is different from Western social phobias. They (Kasahara, 1974; Kimura, 1982) have pointed out that Japanese patients with *taijinkyofusho* are more concerned with self (in others' views), associated with feelings of embarrassment, and many dysmorphobic concerns. The patients are eager to socialize with others and have no problems relating with strangers, but are concerned with how to properly relate to friends, colleagues, or superiors (to make a good impression on them). As indicated by Kimura (1982) and Uchinuma (1990), if the subjects of social relations are divided into three groups — intimate (family, close friends), intermediately familiar, or acquainted with (neighbors, classmates, or co-workers), and strangers (nonacquainted persons) — Japanese *taijinkyofusho* patients have difficulty mainly with the intermediately familiar group in semiprivate/public circumstances. Western social phobic patients defined by DSM-IV, however, are those who have problems mostly with strangers in open public settings [cross-reference to Chapter 13: Culture-Related Specific Syndromes (Section II,C,1)].

This point is echoed by Korean psychiatrist Si-Hyung Lee (1998), who claimed (1987) that patients with *taijinkyofusho*-like syndromes (*tae-in-kongpo* in Korean) are frequently observed in Korea and that their problems, similarly, involve difficulties with the acquainted group. Thus, according to this concept, two kinds of social phobia could be recognized based on different cultural settings in which different kinds of problems arise. Comparing the Japanese "interpersonal relations fear disorder" and the American "social phobia," Cousins (1990) pointed out that they differ in the cultural percepts of the self and vary clinically in situations in which the phobias occur and the symptomatology is manifested. Japanese *taijinkyofusho* patients are more intensely concerned with their own bodily signs, which reveal their inner anxieties and cause humiliation; American social phobic patients are greatly concerned with their performance in public settings.

Stimulated by the claim that *taijinkyofusho*-like syndromes are commonly observed in Korea as well (S.-H. Lee, 1987), Kitanish, Miyake, Kim, and Liu (1995) carried out a questionnaire survey of *taijinkyofusho* tendencies among college students in Japan, Korea, and China. Although the selection and size of the sample for study was not ideal methodologically (only about 100 students from one selected university in each country), the results were interesting. Japanese

and Korean college students showed a considerable frequency of *taijinkuofusho*-related fears in interpersonal situations. Such fears were much less frequent among Chinese college students. Further, among the Japanese students, the focus of worry was others' opinions of oneself, not being part of the group, and eye contact with strangers; among the Korean students, the focus was fear of rejection by others and extreme sensitivity to shame. This illustrated that, in Asian countries, not only was there a difference in prevalence, but also a different focus in interpersonal relations.

C. Obsessive-Compulsive Disorders

Although OCD have relatively clear and unique clinical manifestations and are easy to diagnose, only a handful of works address their cultural aspects. In the United States, based on discharge diagnostic data collected from the McLean Hospital from 1969 to 1990, Stoll, Tohen, and Baldessarini (1992) reported that the proportion of patients discharged with this diagnosis increased almost fourfold. They speculated that the increase was associated with advances in the clinical study and treatment of these disorders. There is no comparable information from other countries. However, by reviewing epidemiological literature, Staley and Wand (1995) reported that OCD is generally similar in prevalence, sociodemographic characteristics, and clinical features in adult populations in Western and non-Western societies. Associated with the improvements in the psychopharmacological treatment of this disorder, biological causes for this disorder are becoming more prevalent among psychiatrists at the present time.

D. Posttraumatic Stress Disorders

It is common knowledge, even among laymen, that humans will react mentally to severe stress, including acute trauma, severe disaster, sexual or violent assault, and chronic, intense tension. This includes war situations in which people encounter extreme danger with the possibility of death. By reviewing the literature, concerning epidemiology of PTSD, de Girolamo and McFarlane (1996) pointed out that the 1-year victimization rates (by percentage of population) for physical/threats and for sexual assaults in industrial societies range between the lower one: 0.6 (for Japan) or 0.8 (for Italy) to the higher one: 5.7 (for New Zealand) or 5.0 (for USA), with average of 3.0 for all 20 countries reviewed. In addition to the frequency of occurrence and the nature of trauma, Chemtob (1996) pointed out that cultural factors will influence the perception and interpretation of trauma, and modify the core process of trauma reaction and the expression of trauma symptoms.

Historically, different diagnostic labels have been used for war-related stress disorders in different wars, such as "nostalgia" during the American Civil War, "shell shock" in World War I, "combat neuroses" in World War II, and "combat exhaustion" in the Korean War. It has been the practice of Army psychiatrists to manage psychiatric casualties in a war zone according to the three basic principles of immediacy, proximity, and expectancy (Block, 1969).

PTSD are newly recognized and frequently diagnosed disorders in the United States, particularly among Vietnam War veterans, during the last several decades. In contrast to the traditional wars of the past, the Vietnam War was different in many respects for American soldiers. There was no clear distinction between civilians and the "enemy." The battles often took place in the jungle. There was no clear front, or combat zone, or base to which to retreat. The goal of the war was unclear. Many civilians were killed by the soldiers, and many soldiers were severely tortured when captured by the enemy. In other words, it was a "terrible" war. After losing the war, the returning veterans were not welcomed by their fellow countrymen. Those were the primarily different experiences of Vietnam veterans. However, most interesting is that after the so-called posttraumatic stress disorder was "discovered," identified, and labeled, and a welfare system was established to deal with it, the number of

patients claiming this disorder increased rapidly. It was estimated that among the veterans, the prevalence of this disorder ranged from 20 to 60% (Friedman, 1981). This may be because, after official recognition of the disorder and the establishment of a treatment program for it, many patients became more comfortable with admitting their suffering and seeking help. However, people could not help but wonder, beyond the actual occurrence of the trauma-related mental disorder and the increased tendency to recognize and seek treatment for it, to what extent it was magnified by fashionable prevalence, associated with the welfare system that was provided by the veterans administration.

This speculation is provoked by available information from other countries. Relatively few reports of war-related PTSD appeared in literature — some from Israel (Solomon, 1989) and a few from Europe (Bell, Key, Loughrey, Roddy, & Curran, 1988), but almost no reports from Japan, relating to the Pacific War, or from China, relating to the 4-year China–Japan War, followed by another 4-year Pacific War and the Civil War between the communist and the nationalist governments. Was it that the war-related traumatic disorders did not occur, or that they did occur, but never caught the attention of clinicians and the government? This is an interesting question awaiting future investigation and clarification.

Based on a small sample, Davidson, Kudler, Saunders, and Smith (1990) compared American World War II veterans and Vietnam veterans who suffered from posttraumatic stress disorder. They found that Vietnam veterans, in contrast to World Ware II veterans, exhibited more severe PTSD symptoms, had more survivor guilt, had a greater lifetime frequency of panic disorder, and an earlier onset age for alcoholism. They speculated that the variations may be attributed to the different nature of the war experiences the subjects encountered.

From a cross-cultural point of view, Marsella, Friedman, Gerrity, and Scurfield (1996) have raised an interesting question. Do people (from non-Western societies) living with the philosophical attitude that one must accept events in life regardless of their impact, adjust, and react to traumatic events differently than people in Western societies? This an academic challenge for cross-cultural study.

V. CULTURE-RELATED SPECIFIC ANXIETY DISORDERS

Another way to study the impact of culture on minor psychiatric disorders is to examine culture-related specific syndromes characterized with anxiety features, as such disorders are heavily colored by cultural elements. Many such disorders have been elaborated previously in Chapter 13 with regard to their clinical pictures and how they are influenced by culture. Those with cardinal pictures of anxiety associated with somatic symptoms (*dhat* syndrome and malignant anxiety) will be reviewed here briefly, whereas others, manifested primarily with somatic symptoms (neurasthenia), will be discussed in Chapter 16.

A. *DHAT* SYNDROME IN INDIA

Dhat syndrome is a culture-related specific anxiety disorder. Based on the cultural belief that excessive semen loss will result in illness, the patient is morbidly concerned about the excessive loss of semen from an "improper way of leaking," such as nocturnal emissions, masturbation, or leaking through urination [cross-reference to Chapter 13: Culture-Related Specific Syndromes (Section II,A,2)].

Patients, mainly of young males, often present vague, multiple somatic symptoms, such as fatigue, weakness, anxiety, or feelings of guilt (for having indulged in certain sexual actions, such as masturbation or prostitution). Some may complain of sexual dysfunction (impotence or premature ejaculation) or concern about the leaking of semen in the urine. As a result, a patient will often ask the physician to examine his urine to determine whether there is leaking of semen. From a clinical perspective, the patient is char-

acterized as anxious or hypochondriac, associated with multiple somatic complaints.

This disorder is mainly observed in India and is known by the folk term of the disorder (Akhtar, 1988). However, the syndrome is also observed, with different folk names, in Nepal and Sri Lanka (where it is referred to as *prameha* disease) (Bhatia & Malik, 1991), Bangladesh, and Pakistan (Malhotra & Wig, 1975). In Taiwan, it is known as the disorder *shenkui* (a term from traditional medicine, meaning "kidney deficiency," or insufficient vitality due to excessive loss of semen) (Wen, 1995). Thus, there are several counterparts of the *dhat* syndrome observed among the people of Asian and south Asia.

Whether it is labeled *dhat* syndrome in India, *prameha* in Sri Lanka, or *shenkui* in China, there is a common characteristic among these syndromes; the core of the anxiety is derived from the folk belief that excessive loss of semen will result in illness.

B. MALIGNANT ANXIETY IN AFRICA

In 1960, Nigerian psychiatrist T. Adeoye Lambo described a special form of anxiety disorder that he claimed was widespread in Africa. The condition was characterized by intense anxiety, extreme irritability, restlessness, and intense fear. It was associated with a complex disturbance of a patient's feelings of reality, without deterioration or disintegration of the personality. Thus, Lambo insisted that patients suffering from this disorder were not psychotic. They often suffered from intense feelings of anger leading to homocidal behavior. Therefore, it was named "malignant anxiety."

According to Lambo (1962), the occurrence of the disorder was associated with adaptation to new and stressful life situations. Often, the patients were "marginal" Africans who were in the process of renouncing their age-old culture, but had failed to assimilate the new. At the time of the report, their criminal conduct had become the source of the most common capital crimes in Africa.

VI. CLOSING COMMENTS

Minor psychiatric disorders, including anxiety disorders, are very different from major psychiatric disorders and vary greatly in terms of their diagnostic distribution among societies with different cultural settings. This shows that the identification and diagnosis of minor psychiatric disorders are subject to a great many factors, including a patient's subjective perception of the suffering or problems, his or her style of complaint presentation, the clinician's orientation and sensitivity to comprehending and diagnosing the disorders, and the classification system utilized to categorize the disorders. Beyond these clinical factors, there is good reason to suspect that the stress encountered and the coping pattern utilized by the patient to deal with problems, as well as his or her illness behavior (including help-seeking pattern), vary at both individual and sociocultural levels, which further complicates the situation.

Nevertheless, it is clear that anxiety and other minor psychiatric disorders are greatly subject to sociocultural factors and cannot be understood or approached without cultural considerations. This includes understanding the nature of the problem, making a clinical assessment and diagnosis, and offering treatment for the patient.

REFERENCES

Akhtar, S. (1988). Four culture-bound psychiatric syndromes in India. *International Journal of Social Psychiatry, 34,* 70–74.

Bell, P., Kee, M., Loughrey G.C., Roddy, R.J., & Curran, P.S. (1988). Posttraumatic stress in Northern Ireland. *Acta Psychiatrica Scandinavica, 77,* 166–169.

Bhatia, M.S., & Malik, S.C. (1991). Dhat syndrome—A useful diagnostic entity in Indian culture. *British Journal of Psychiatry, 159,* 691–695.

Blazer, D.G., Hughes, D., George, L.K., Swartz, M., & Boyer, R. (1991). General anxiety disorder. In L.N. Robins & D.A. Regier (Eds.), *Psychiatric disorder in America: The Epidemiologic Catchment Area Study.* New York: Free Press.

Block, H.S. (1969). Army clinical psychiatry in the combat zone—1967–1968. *American Journal of Psychiatry, 126*(3), 289–298.

Chemtob, C.M. (1996). Posttraumatic stress disorder, trauma, and culture. In F. Lih Mak & C.C. Nadelson (Eds.), *International review of psychiatry* (Vol. 2) ((pp. 257–292). Washington, DC: London.

Compton, W.M., III, Helzer, J.E., Hwu, H.G., Yeh, E.K., McEvoy, L., Topp, J.E., & Spitznagel, E.L. (1991). New methods in cross-cultural psychiatry: Psychiatric illness in Taiwan and the United States. *American Journal of Psychiatry, 148,* 1697–16704.

Cooper, J.E., & Sartorius, N. (Eds.). (1996). *Mental disorders in China.* London: Gaskell.

Cousins, S.D. (1990). *Culture and social phobia in Japan and the United States.* Ann Arbor: University of Michigan (Dissertation Information Service).

Davidson, J.R.T., Kudler, H.S., Saunders, W.B., & Smith, R.D. (1990). Symptom and comorbidity patterns in World War II and Vietnam veterans with posttraumatic stress disorder. *Comprehensive Psychiatry, 31*(2), 162–170.

de Girolamo, G., & McFarlane, A.C. (1996). The epidemiology of PTSD: A comprehensive review of the international literature. In A.J. Marsella, M.J. Friedman, E.T. Gerrity, & R.M. Scurfield (Eds.), *Ethnocultural aspects of posttraumatic stress disorder: Issues, research, and clinical applications* (pp. 33–85). Washington, DC: American Psychological Association.

Eaton, W.W., Dryman, A., & Weissman, M.M. (1991). Panic and phobia. In L.N. Robins & D.A. Regier (Eds.), *Psychiatric disorder in America: The Epidemiologic Catchment Area Study.* New York: Free Press.

Friedman, M.J. (1981). Post-Vietnam syndrome: Recognition and management. *Psychosomatics, 22*(11), 931–943.

Good, B., & Kleinman, A. (1985). Culture and anxiety: Cross-cultural evidence for the patterning of anxiety disorders. In A.H. Tuam & J. Master (Eds.), *Anxiety and the anxiety disorders.* Hillsdale, NJ: Erlbaum.

Iwai, H. (1982). *Shinkeisho [Neuroses]* (in Japanese). Tokyo: Nihonbunka Kagakusha.

Kaplan, H.S., & Kaplan, H.I. (1967). Current concepts of psychosomatic medicine. In A.M. Freedman & H.I. Kaplan (Eds.), *Comprehensive textbook of psychiatry.* Baltimore: Willams & Wilkins.

Karno, M., & Golding, J.M. (1991). Obsessive compulsive disorder. In L.N. Robins & D.A. Regier (Eds.), *Psychiatric disorder in America: The Epidemiologic Catchment Area Study.* New York: Free Press.

Kasahara, Y. (1974). Fear of eye-to-eye confrontation among neurotic patients in Japan. In T.S. Lebra & W.P. Lebra (Eds.), *Japanese culture and behavior: Selected readings* (pp. 396–406). Honolulu: University Press of Hawaii.

Kimura, S. (1982). *Nihonjin-no taijinkuofu [Japanese anthrophobia].* Tokyo: Keiso Book Co.

Kirmayer, L.J. (1991). The place of culture in psychiatric nosology: Taijin kyofusho and DSM-III-R. *Journal of Nervous and Mental Disease, 179*(1), 19–28.

Kitanish, K., Miyake, Y., Kim, K.I., & Liu, X.H. (1995). A comparative study of *taijinkyofusho* (TSK) tendencies among college students in Japan, Korea, and the People's Republic of China. *Jikeikai Medical Journal, 42*(3), 231–243.

Lambo, T.A. (1960, December 10). Further neuropsychiatric observations in Nigeria: With comments on the need for epidemiological study in Africa. *British Medical Journal,* pp. 1696–1704.

Lambo, T.A. (1962). Malignant anxiety: A syndrome associated with criminal conduct in Africans. *Journal of Mental Science, 108,* 256–264.

Lee, C.K., Kwak, Y.S., Yamamoto, J., Rhee, H., Kim, Y.S., Han, J.H., Choi, J.O., & Lee, Y.H. (1990a). Psychiatric epidemiology in Korea. Part I. Gender and age differences in Seoul. *Journal of Nervous and Mental Disease, 178*(4), 242–246.

Lee, C.K., Kwak, Y.S., Yamamoto, J., Rhee, H., Kim, Y.S., Han, J.H., Choi, J.O., & Lee, Y.H. (1990b). Psychiatric epidemiology in Korea. Part II. Urban and rural differences. *Journal of Nervous and Mental Disease, 178*(4), 247–252.

Lee, S.-H. (1987). Social phobia in Korea. *Proceeding of the First Cultural Psychiatry Symposium between Japan and Korea.* Seoul, Korea: East Asian Academy of Cultural Psychiatry.

Lee, S.-H. (1998). *Offensive type of social phobia: Cross-cultural perspectives.* Paper presented at the annual meeting of the American Psychiatric Association, Toronto, Canada.

Liebowitz, M.R., Gorman, J.M., Fyer, A.J., & Klein, D.F. (1985). Social phobia: Review of a neglected anxiety disorder. *Archives of General Psychiatry, 42,* 729–736.

Malhotra, H.K., & Wig, N.N. (1975). Dhat syndrome: A culture-bound sex neurosis of the Orient. *Archives of Sexual Behavior, 4*(5), 519–528.

Marsella, A.J., Friedman, M.J., Gerrity, E.T., & Scurfield, R.M. (1996). Ethnocultural aspects of PTSD: some closing thoughts. In A.J. Marsella, M.J. Friedman, E.T. Gerrity, & R.M. Scurfield (Eds.), *Ethnocultural aspects of posttraumatic stress disorder: Issues, research, and clinical applications* (pp. 529–538). Washington, DC: American Psychological Association.

Parker, G. (1979). Reported parental characteristics of agoraphobics and social phobics. *British Journal of Psychiatry, 135,* 555–560.

Psychiatric Epidemiological Collaboration Team. (1986). Epidemiological survey of neuroses in 12 geographic regions. *Chinese Neuropsychiatric Journal, 19*(2), 87–91 (in Chinese).

Saenger, G. (1968). Psychiatric outpatients in America and the Netherlands: A transcultural comparison. *Social Psychiatry, 3*(4), 149–164.

Solomon, Z. (1989). Psychological sequelae of war: A 3-year perspective study of Israeli combat stress reaction casualties. *Journal of Nervous and Mental Disease, 177*(6), 342–346.

Staley, D., & Wand, R.R. (1995). Obsessive-compulsive disorder: A review of the cross-cultural epidemiological literature. *Transcultural Psychiatric Research Review, 32*(2), 103–136.

Stoll, A.L. Tohen, M., & Baldessarini, R.J. (1992). Increasing frequency of the diagnosis of obsessive-compulsive disorder. *American Journal of Psychiatry, 149*(5), 638–640.

Tseng, W.S., Asai, M.H., Kitanish, K.J., McLaughlin, D., & Kyomen, H. (1992). Diagnostic pattern of social phobia: Comparison in Tokyo and Hawaii. *Journal of Nervous and Mental Disease, 180,* 380–385.

Tseng, W.S., Xu, D., Ebata, K., Hsu, J., & Cui, Y.H. (1986). Diagnostic pattern for neuroses in China, Japan, and the United States. *American Journal of Psychiatry, 143*(8), 1010–1014.

Uchinuma, Y. (1990). *Taijinkyofusho [Disorder of interpersonal relations fear]* (in Japanese). Tokyo: Kodansha.

Üstün, T.B., & Sartorius, N. (Eds.). (1995). *Mental illness in general health care: An international study.* Chichester: Wiley (on behalf of WHO).

Wen, J.K. (1995). Sexual beliefs and problems in contemporary Taiwan. In T.-Y. Lin, W.S. Tseng, & E.K. Yeh (Eds.), *Chinese societies and mental health.* (pp. 219–230). Hong Kong: Oxford University Press.

Werner, H. (1948). *Comparative psychology of mental development.* New York: International University Press.

Yeh, E.K., Hwu, H.G., & Lin, T.-Y. (1995). Mental disorders in Taiwan: Epidemiological studies of community population. In T.-Y. Lin, W.S. Tseng, & E.K. Yeh (Eds.), *Chinese societies and mental health* (pp. 247–265). Hong Kong: Oxford University Press.

16

Somatoform Disorders, Including Neurasthenia

I. INTRODUCTION

A. HISTORICAL PATH OF CONCEPT AND DEFINITION

Along with the evolution of professional knowledge, as well as the viscidity of psychiatric disorders relating to sociocultural change, there has been considerable revision of formal classification systems for certain psychiatric disorders. This is particularly true regarding the nosology of conversion, neurasthenia, chronic fatigue syndrome, and somatoform disorders — a cluster of medical terms centering around the clinical condition manifested primarily by somatic symptoms or characterized by somatic complaints.

Historically, the term *somatization* was used in psychoanalysis to indicate that despite the existence of psychological stress, the distress was not verbalized through emotional channels but expressed through bodily symptoms. That is, due to emotional difficulty, hesitation, or resistance, the psychological component was manifested by its transformation into a somatic component; thus, it was referred to as "somati-zation." The manifestation of somatization is often insidious

and chronic in nature. If the occurrence of somatic dysfunction develops rather acutely, in a dramatic way, it is referred to as *conversion,* one of the major manifestations of hysteria.

The terms *psychosomatic disorders* and *psychophysiological disorders* were used in the past (around the 1950s and 1960s) to indicate that certain psychological distresses directly impact the occurrence of particular forms of physiological disorders. Hypertension, peptic ulcers, asthma, skin rashes, irritable colon, migraine, coronary heart disease, and so on were referred to by these old terms. These concepts were abandoned when it was realized that such disorders were primarily due to biological–medical factors, whereas emotional factors had merely an indirect impact, if any. Now, the term *psychosomatic medicine* is used, reflecting the medical orientation toward the mutual impact between body and mind. Clinically, this emphasizes the need to regard the patient as a whole in treatment — caring for him or her from both psychic and somatic perspectives.

In order to make a distinction from the term somatization, which originated from the psychoanalytic concept, the terms *somatic complaint syndrome* (Prince, 1990) and *functional somatic syndrome* (Canino, Rubio-Stipec, Canino, & Escobar, 1992) have been used by some scholars to clarify that the disorders are not necessarily related to the transformation of psychological conflict, nor are they expressions of underlying affect. They are, rather, merely patterns of psychiatric disorders responding to stress with somatic presentation.

Clinically, the presentation of somatic symptoms may have multiple implications. As pointed out by Kirmayer and Young (1998), it can be seen as an index of a disorder, an indication of a psychopathology, a symbolic condensation of intrapsychic conflict, a culturally coded expression of distress, a medium for expressing social discontent, and a mechanism through which patients attempt to reposition themselves within their local worlds. Thus, it broadly covers biological, psychological, and sociocultural dimensions and needs to be approached dynamically (Tseng, 1975).

In *Diagnostic and Statistical Manual of Mental Disorders* (DSM), published by the American Psychiatric Association (APA), the diagnostic term *somatoform disorder* appeared in DSM-IV (1994). It was invented as the result of the revitalization of the descriptive approach in psychiatric classification, which tried to categorize disorders based primarily on their cardinal clinical manifestations. It refers to psychiatric conditions characterized primarily by multiple and chronic somatic symptoms, which cannot be fully explained by the patient's general medical condition or the existing medical disorders. It is based on the unspoken assumption that a psychiatric disorder is usually manifested with "psychic" symptoms or complaints, namely "psychicform" disorder. If the psychiatric disorder is presented mainly with symptoms of somatic nature, the disorder is regarded as a "somatoform" disorder.

Associated with the radical change of medical concepts relating to the classification of disorders in the American classification system, the nosology of neurasthenia, although included in DSM-II (1968), was excluded from DSM-III (1980) and the disorder of hysteria (which was previously recognized as having subtypes of conversion and dissociation) was split into conversion disorders (categorized as one kind of somatoform disorders) and dissociative disorders. The generic term "neuroses" was abandoned, abolishing the traditional distinction between psychoses and neuroses. Psychophysiological disorders (or psychosomatic disorders) were eliminated entirely.

The formal international classification system, *International Statistical Classification of Diseases and Related Health Problems* (ICD), published by the World Health Organization (WHO), is another story. The ICD-9 (revised in 1977) continued to recognize the disorder of neurasthenia and the term hysteria was still used. However, in the ICD-10 (revised in 1992), under the influence of the American DSM classification system, the diagnostic terms of hysteria and neurasthenia were also removed. Now, "undifferentiated somatoform disorder" is used to refer to the condition that was previously labeled "neurasthenia." In contrast, the classification system officially used in China, the Chinese Classification of Mental Disorder-2 (CCMD-2, revised in 1989), retains the diagnostic categories of hysteria and neurasthenia, as these medical terms are used prevalently by professionals. It is an academic challenge for psychiatrists to ignore certain diagnostic terms, such as hysteria or neurasthenia, in "official" international classification systems, while such terms are widely used in many geographic areas for a large portion of the world's population.

From practical and cultural perspectives, conversion disorder and neurasthenia are elaborated here because they are still rather prevalent in many societies and the diagnostic terms are still commonly used, a fact that cannot simply be ignored.

B. CHALLENGE TO THE DICHOTOMY OF BODY AND MIND

As pointed out by Kirmayer (1984, 1988), *somatization* (as well as *somatoform disorders*) is a concept born of Western mind–body dualism. Even though the concept of psychological impact on the health of the body is clearly recognized in many traditional medical systems, such as the Chinese or Ayurveda medicine (practiced in India), there is no sharp dichotomization between mind and body, and a psychological orientation to problems is not considered "superior" to — or more "developed," from an evolutionary perspective

— than a somatic one [cross-reference to Chapter 30: Culture and Psychiatric Service (Section II,C,1–3)].

One explanation given by some Western scholars is that, simply borrowing a concept from comparative developmental psychology, primitive or undeveloped people, due to their limited cognitive concepts and semantic ability, tend to manifest stress in body symptoms, whereas more sophisticated and developed people, equipped with improved language and psychology, tend to express distress through psychological symptoms. This explanation has been criticized for its lack of anthropological knowledge and experience and its overgeneralization of the developmental theory of humankind, without validation.

This evolutional view also lacks cultural insight into the meaning of somatic complaining from the perspective of help-seeking behavior as a part of patient's illness–behavior. *Somatic complaining* or *somatic presentation* refers to the clinical situation in which the patient tends to make a presentation (or complaint) of a somatic nature, an entirely different matter from the narrow view of *somatization*. As the patient's illness–behavior, it involves the patient's understanding of the medical system, the purpose of the visit, and the socioculturally patterned problem presentation. It does not necessarily mean that the patient is unable to present emotional problems or does not know how to make psychological complaints. It simply indicates that the patient presents somatic symptoms for numerous reasons, including that he or she is following a culturally molded pattern of problem presentation (Racy, 1980; Raguram, Weiss, Channabasavanna, & Devins, 1996; Tseng, 1975).

C. CULTURAL IMPACT ON PATHOSELECTIVE EFFECTS OF SOMATIC PRESENTATION

How cultural factors will shape patients' illness–behavior and guide them to make somatic presentations during their visits to a psychiatric clinic is well illustrated by Racy (1980) in a study of Muslim women in Saudi Arabia. As an American-trained, Arabic-speaking psychiatrist, Racy observed that during his consultantship to Saudi Arabia, the women patients would often make predictable and stereotyped complaints to the psychiatrists, mainly of a somatic nature.

He elaborated that Saudi women were taught and reminded repeatedly that they were "inferior" to man and subject to their rule and whim. When a woman failed to bear a male child, it caused her almost as much difficulty as if she were sterile. With polygamy still practiced, the common concern for married women was being neglected or rejected by their husbands in favor of a younger and prettier wife. In such a cultural setting, negative feelings, unhappiness, and conflicts within herself, and between her and members of her family, readily translate into somatic terms, as physical symptoms in such a culture are safe, morally acceptable, and generally lead to some form of help-seeking. In other words, as Racy pointed out, for women in strictly controlled, socially inferior positions, somatic complaints can express emotional problems that have no other outlets.

In Taiwan, Tseng (1975) examined psychiatric patients who visited psychiatric clinics. In their initial visits, more than 80% of them, if skillfully guided in the process of evaluation, were ready to describe the psychological problems that brought them to see the psychiatrists. Tseng pointed out that making a somatic presentation initially is merely a culturally sanctioned "prologue" for the occasion. Thus, the nature of somatic presentation needs to be understood and grasped dynamically rather than merely given the label of somatization or somatoform disorders.

In a clinical study in Montreal, Canada, Kirmayer, and Robbins (1996) reported that patients who "somatize" in primary care can be divided into three groups — initial, facultative, and true somatizers — based on their willingness to offer or endorse a psychosocial cause for their symptoms. Initial somatizers readily acknowledge their psychological distress, despite their initial somatic presentation; true somatizers tend to reject psychosocial explanations; facultative somatizers are in between. Kirmayer and Robbins pointed out that patients with somatic symptoms exist hetero-geneously in the spectrum, acknowledging a range of degrees a psychosocial contribution to their distress.

Among Hispanic groups, Koss (1990) pointed out that the process of somatization could have three meanings. Namely, the use of the body as a channel of communication; the result of attention focused on the body; and an idiom of distress or a way of making sense out of suffering. She indicated that somatic complaint syndromes are not necessarily indicative of severe psychological distress or psychiatric disorder. Furthermore, she pointed out that although Western culture values the mind (and person) who dominates and controls his or her body and distances him/herself from body feelings, popular Hispanic culture's priori-ties lie on opposite sides of the objective/subjective, rational/irrational, monistic/holistic continuum.

Comparing Mexican-Americans born in the United States, Mexican-Americans born in Mexico, non-His-panic whites — all living in East Los Angels areas, with Puerto Rican in Puerto Rico — Canino and asso-ciates (1992) reported that the mean number of func-tional somatic symptoms was significantly greater among Puerto Rican respondents than the other three groups studied. As for the symptom configuration, it was found that Puerto Ricans were more similar to the Mexican-American groups (whether born in the United States or Mexico) than the non-Hispanic whites examined.

African psychiatrist Olatawura (1973) described typical somatic symptoms of psychiatric patients in Africa: heat sensation from inside the head or body, peppery and crawling sensations in various parts of the body, baffling muscular fasciculation, feelings of heaviness, soreness, numbness, and localized aches. Thus, somatic symptoms in Nigerian Africans have been described as "paresthesia" (Ayonrinde, 1977). For psychiatric screening of adult patients seeking help from primary health care facilities in rural set-tings in Nigeria, Ohaeri and Odejide (1994) included somatic symptoms of feelings of heat, peppery and crawling sensations, and numbness in questions (such as in the General Health Questionnaire or WHO's Self-Reporting Questionnaire). They claimed that

screening questionnaires that include culture-pat-terned somatic symptoms can become reliable indexes of psychiatric distress.

In Asia, Tseng et al. (1991) carried out a ques-tionnaire survey of psychiatric outpatients suffering from minor psychiatric disorders (including neu-roses, situational adjustment, and acute emotional reaction) in five research cities: Chiang-Mai, Thai-land; Bali, Indonesia; Kao-Hsiung, Taiwan, China; Shanghai, China, and Tokyo, Japan. The Mental Symptom Questionnaire (for Asian populations) was developed by the collaborators from the five sites, composed of the frequent psychic and somatic com-plaints presented by the patients in each place. Nine symptom clusters were identified through factor analysis: conversion, neurasthenia, temper, anxiety, phobic, depression, and three somatics (head, chest, and abdomen, respectively). The results indicated that, in Asia, minor psychiatric patients who visited psychiatric clinics tend to manifest many somatic symptoms so that, among a total of nine clusters of symptoms, there are three somatic subgroups, in addition to conversion and neurasthenia. The somatic symptoms are not only frequently present, but also elaborate that they are differentiated and distributed into three clusters.

II. CULTURAL PERSPECTIVES OF SOME FORMS OF DISORDERS

A. CONVERSION DISORDER

As mentioned previously, historically, conversion disorder and dissociation disorder were grouped under the diagnostic category of "hysterical disorder." They were thought to share the same basic nature they tended to occur abruptly, were often precipitated by emotional stress, could manifest clinically in a theatri-cal way, and subsided when the stress was eliminated. The historical path regarding the concept of hysteria, as well as the frequency of hysterical disorders observed in non-Western societies, will be reviewed in detail later [cross-reference to Chapter 17: Dissociation, Possession, and Hysteria (Section I,B)]. It will be pointed out here merely that, associated with the movement of descriptively oriented classification, the hysterical disorder lost its role as a generic term. Starting from DSM-III (1980), conversion disorder was separated from dissociation disorder and categorized into one kind of somatoform disorder. The unique nature of such a disorder is entirely ignored in such classification.

From an epidemiological perspective, conversion disorder as a pathological condition disappeared almost, if not completely, from many developed societies. However, it is still commonly observed in many other societies. It is thought to occur primarily in societies with relatively strict social systems, in which people cannot express their feelings or desires toward others directly, particularly when they encounter conflict or distress. The society is still required to observe traditional ways of life, and many behaviors, including sexual ones, cannot be manifested freely. Temporary somatic dysfunction is one mode of communication available to people, particularly for a suppressed gender or less privileged group of people. Furthermore, people in the society tend to give considerable attention to the dramatic occurrence of such phenomena so that the clinical condition serves certain social functions for patients who develop such disorders.

However, once people become more psychologically minded and begin to understand such morbid conditions as emotional disorders, with rather negative attitudes toward them, the disorders tend to fade away. This is rather similar to the fate of "fainting," which was often "practiced" by females in Western societies in the past.

B. NEURASTHENIA

1. Historical Perspective

The term "neurasthenia" was originally applied in 1869 by an American neuropsychiatrist, George M. Beard, to describe a clinical syndrome with core symptoms of mental fatigue, associated with poor memory, poor concentration, irritability, headaches, tinnitus, insomnia, and other vague somatic complaints. Beard believed that the disorder derived from an exhaustion of the victim's nervous system. It was interpreted that the condition occurred as the result of overstimulation and the sufferer's mind refusing to take on new stresses. As mentioned in Chapter 15, Sigmund Freud, in an early stage of his career (1894), categorized neurasthenia together with anxiety neuroses and hypochondriasis "actual neurosis," conceptualizing that such a disorder has a neurological base in the nervous system (therefore, "actual"); in contrast to hysteria, phobia, and obsessional neuroses, which are psychological in nature and regarded as "psychoneuroses" (implying that they originated from a "psychic" cause) (Gabbard, 1995, p.453). According to Gelder, Gath, Mayou and (1983, pp. 136–37), Janet, in 1909, introduced the term "psychasthenia" to emphasize that the neurasthenia was psychological and not neurological. The search for biological factors for the occurrence of neurasthenia has not been entirely abandoned by scholars (Corrigan, MacDonald, Brown, Armstrong, & Armstrong, 1994; Orbaek & Nise, 1989; van Vliet et al., 1989; Wang, 1989). At the same time, exploration of the sociocultural attributions for the disorder is still prevalent (Abbey & Garfinkel, 1991; Cheung & Lin, 1997; Starcevic, 1991).

In the formal classification system in the United States, neurasthenia was not included in DSM-I (established in 1952), but was included in DSM-II (a revision made in 1968). Later, in 1980, when there was a radical change in the classification system, it was removed from DSM-III. Thus, the diagnosis eventually fell into disuse in its country of origin. However, the term caught on in the rest of the world. As pointed out by Sartorius (1997), the neurasthenic syndrome was probably seen frequently in Europe in the late 19th century, and Beard's neurasthenia quickly found acceptance first in Germany and France and then in other European countries. In Russia, the concept was readily incorporated into Pavlovian theory and was prevalent clinically in Stalin's time.

2. The Situation in China

In Asia, associated with the introduction of modern psychiatry into China in the late 19th century, the medical term neurasthenia was introduced and translated literally as *shenjing-suairuo* (nerve-weakened disorder). It became widely known as a mild mind–body disorder related to nerve exhaustion — a concept compatible with the traditional Chinese concept of *shen-kui* (kidney deficiency disorder), and easily understood and accepted by laymen. In the 1960s, during the period of the Great Leap Forward movement, a grand-scale national campaign was initiated against neurasthenia — "the number one mental problem" identified. A special treatment program, named rapid comprehensive treatment, was even designed to eradicate this socially concerned mental problem [cross-reference to Chapter 33: Culture-Influenced Unique Psychotherapy (Section II,D)]

After China opened its doors to outsiders, several years after the Culture Revolution, in 1982, American cultural psychiatrist Arthur Kleinman (1982), in collaboration with Chinese colleagues, carried out a clinical study of patients diagnosed with neurasthenia in Hunan, China. He claimed that 87% of 100 patients he examined could be "rediagnosed" as having depressive disorders. However, his report created controversy among psychiatrists in and outside of China (Lin, 1989). Many prominent Chinese psychiatrists insisted that neurasthenia was a distinctly recognized psychiatric disorder, not to be rediagnosed and categorized as a depressive disorder according to some Western psychiatrists (Yan, 1989; Young, 1989; Zhang, 1989).

In 1982, an extensive epidemiological study of psychiatric disorders was carried out in China (Psychiatric Epidemiological Collaboration Team, 1986). The survey involved 12 selected sample areas around the nation, with subjects aged between 15 and 59. The total population surveyed was 6754 (Cooper & Sartorius, 1996). The prevalence rate for neurasthenia at the time of the survey was found to be 13.03 per 1000. (Rates for hysteria, depressive neurosis, anxiety, phobia, obsessive disorder, and hypochondriasis were 3.55, 3.11, 1.48, 0.59, 0.30, and 0.15 per 1000, respectively.) Thus, neurasthenia was found to comprise 58.7% of the total neurotic disorders identified at the time of the survey. On the whole, the rate was slightly higher in urban (14.02 per 1000) than in rural areas (12.05 per 1000). In general, the rate was much higher among females than among males, with a ratio of 6.86/1 (X.H. Liu, 1994).

Reviewing hospital records, it was found that, in China, almost 80% of psychiatric outpatients were diagnosed with neurasthenia by the clinicians in provincial (rural) areas, with the percentage of diagnosed neurasthenia relatively much lower, or becoming less, in university-affiliated clinics in city areas. For instance, according to Tseng, Xu, Ebata, Hsu, and Cui (1986), Xiu and Cui from the Institute of Mental Health, Beijing Medical University in Beijing, an institute staffed with more professionally sophisticated clinicians, gave data that diagnoses of neurasthenia were given to 18.6% of all outpatients with minor disorders (*N*=360 within a 6 month period in 1985), whereas diagnoses of depression and anxiety were 8.0 and 6.7%, respectively, and unclassified neuroses, 37.5%. This showed that, even in China, the distribution of diagnosed neurasthenia disorder varied in different locations and was influenced by the backgrounds of clinicians and patterns of practice.

In order to clarify how ordinary Chinese people conceptualize neurasthenia, S. Lee and Wong (1995) carried out a self-reporting questionnaire for undergraduate students in Hong Kong. They revealed that the college students conceived neurasthenia as a disorder composed of symptoms of anxiety, insomnia, depression, and fright. They pointed out that after adopting medical terminology originally derived from the West, categorizing neurasthenia as a disorder of mental fatigue, the concept of neurasthenia was transformed and acquired distinctive local meanings for Chinese laymen (college students) in Hong Kong. It comprised a much broader psychopathology (including psychological symptomatology), beyond somatoform symptoms, almost equivalent to "neurosis," as it was referred to in the past.

A psychologist from Hong Kong, Cheung (1989), has pointed out that despite its origin in Western psychiatry, literally referring to an "asthenic state of nerves," *shenjing-suairuo* (neurasthenia) has become a popular concept in Chinese folk medicine, referring to a variety of somatic and psychological symptoms. Popular Chinese books on neurasthenia suggest that it might be attributed to an unhealthy lifestyle, psychological factors, and physical health problems. Change of lifestyle and attitude, relaxation, and application of tonics are recommended treatments. As a broad term used loosely by professionals and the lay public in Hong Kong, *shenjing-suairuo* serves the important function of destigmatizing psychiatric disorders. Cheung emphasized that the indigenization of neurasthenia exemplifies how an originally Western concept has acquired cultural meaning.

3. Situation in Japan and Korea

In Japan, as in China, the concept of neurasthenia *(shinkei-suijaku)* was adopted from the West in the late 19th century and was rather commonly used. The condition was also known among clinicians by the German term *erschöpfungsneurasthenie* (exhaustive neurasthenia). Nevertheless, by the late 20th century, these diagnoses were almost discarded. They were replaced by the term neuroses after World War II (Suzuki, 1989). According to Iwa (1982), among outpatients seen in his clinic (*N*=102), no case was given the diagnosis of neurasthenia, whereas 16.7% were diagnosed with hypochondriasis. A similar report was made by Mori and Kitanishi (1984) from an institute specializing in treating Morita-*shinkei-shitsu* (Morita nervous temperament disorders). Among all outpatients with minor disorders (*N*=370), none received a diagnosis of neurasthenia, whereas 34.2% were given a diagnosis of *taijinkuofusho* (anthrophobia or, more correctly, interpersonal relationship phobia). The Japanese psychiatrists adopted the American psychiatric classification system immediately after World War II, and the term neurasthenia evaporated from practice, as it was not recognized in the American classification system (Kitanishi & Kondo, 1994).

According to the Japanese psychiatrist Machizawa (1992), due to the persistent stigma toward psychotic disorders, nearly 70% of Japanese psychiatrists tend not to reveal the diagnosis of schizophrenia to patients in their daily practice. The diagnosis of neurasthenia is conveniently used as a substitute for such severe mental disorders. A tragic incident occurred in Japan in 1982 when a pilot for Japan Airlines, who had been experiencing auditory hallucinations and delusions, caused the crash-landing of a large airliner into the seaside near Narita International Airport. His psychotic symptoms had developed over years, but only received a diagnosis of neurasthenia for the sake of diagnostic disguise (Munakata, 1989).

In Korea, when psychiatric epidemiology was carried out (C. K. Lee et al., 1990), the instrument of DIS-III from NIMH of the United States was applied. Therefore, no diagnostic category of neurasthenia was used. As a result, unfortunately, no information was available for the situation in Korea regarding the prevalence of this disorder. However, according to Korean cultural psychiatrist K.I. Kim (personal communication, 1990), the diagnostic term neurasthenia is still used frequently by contemporary clinicians.

Thus, even in Asia, due to patterns of professional practice and orientation, as well as other social and cultural factors, there are wide differences in how often the diagnosis of neurasthenia is given in a society.

4. Worldwide Perspectives

It is important to point out that, according to Üstün and Sartorius (1995), a worldwide epidemiological study of ICD-10 defined psychological studies, including neurasthenia, revealed that the estimated prevalence of neurasthenia syndrome was frequently seen (though not always recognized) in both economically advantaged and less advantaged countries. According to the study, the prevalence of neurasthenia was 10.5% in both Groningen (Netherlands) and Santiago (Chile); 9.7% in Manchester (UK); 9.3% in Paris (France); 7.7% in Mainz and 7.4% in Berlin (Germany); 4.6% in Athens (Greece); 4.1% in Ankara (Turkey); 3.4% in Nagasaki (Japan); 2.1% in Veronia

(Italy); and 2.0% in Shanghai (China). It is surprising to note that the prevalence of the disorder, according to this study, is relatively low in Shanghai, China. In a separate study (Zheng et al., 1997), it was revealed that the prevalence of neurasthenia was 6.4% among Chinese-Americans in Los Angeles, California.

As pointed out by Starcevic (1994), neurasthenia has been a frequent diagnosis in Europe, particularly in some Eastern European countries, even though there are considerable cross-national differences in the way the disorder is conceptualized. According to Starcevic, in the former Soviet Union, approximately 60% of neurotic patients were given a diagnosis of neurasthenia in one study (Saveleva et al., 1982), and in former Yugoslavia, more than 30% of neurotic patients was reported in one article (Katanec, 1976).

It should be mentioned that, beyond commonly referred neurasthenia, there are several culture-variative neurasthenia-like syndromes reported in different societies. A relatively well-known example is brain-fag syndrome, originally reported by Prince (1960) and reviewed by Jegede (1983). According to Prince, while he was working in Nigeria, Africa, he noticed that many young patients, mostly students, visited the clinic with somatic complaints — mostly of pain or a burning sensation in the head and neck. The student–patients also complained that they had problems concentrating, reading, grasping what they were reading, or recalling what they had just read. Prince described the patients as mostly students in secondary school or the university, or teachers or government clerks who were studying in their spare time to raise their educational levels. The patients generally attributed their illness to fatigue of the brain due to excessive mental work. Prince suggested using the term "brain fag" to describe the condition, characterized with subjective complaints of intellectual impairment, (visual) sensory impairment, and somatic complaints.

In Euro-American societies, patients with complaints primarily of tiredness have been given the diagnosis of chronic fatigue syndrome, a disorder characterized by fatigue lasting months to years (Ware & Kleinman, 1992; Wessely, 1994). According to Goldberg and Huxley (1980), investigation has shown that complaints of fatigue and irritability commonly accompany anxiety and mild depression.

5. Interpretations and Integration

It is becoming a challenge for clinicians and scholars to examine to what extent neurasthenia is a nosological entity or merely a by-product of symptom interpretation (Chung & Singer, 1995) or diagnostic issues (Farmer et al., 1995; S.X. Liu, 1989; P. White, 1989; Zheng et al., 1994). Based on information obtained from an international study of patients with neurasthenic syndrome contacting general health care facilities (Üstün & Sartorius, 1995), Sartorius (1997) pointed out that it seems to be a ubiquitous morbid state; it is frequent and it produces disability. This explains why neurasthenia has been retained in the classification system of ICD-10.

Theoretical questions are raised as to why neurasthenia, as a diagnostic entity, is frequently used in some parts of world, such as China, but not necessarily in others. Besides the change in professional views about the disorder, there are several possible explanations.

First of all, it is closely related to professional practice and diagnostic patterns. This has been illustrated by cross-cultural studies of diagnosis making (Tseng et al., 1986, 1992) [cross-reference to Chapter 27: Clinical Assessment and Diagnosis (Section III,B)].

Second, there is a cultural meaning to the concept of nosology. It is commonly acknowledged that the labeling of a disorder is not merely to meet the need of medical practice, but also to fulfill a social function. For the Chinese, it is more acceptable to have a "weakened and/or exhausted nerve" than to have emotional problems — either anxiety or depression. Anxiety and depression are considered daily-life phenomena that a person has to endure and with which he must cope. If a person complains excessively of anxiety or depression, he will be perceived as a person who has a weak mind. One does not receive proper attention and support from the family, co-workers, or others when one presents and is labeled as suffering from such emotional problems. In contrast, being labeled as having a weakened or exhausted nerve brings no blame to the victim, and his problem is accepted as a justifiable disorder that has its root in a physical condition rather than an emotional one.

Third, there is a cultural affinity or compatibility with the term weakened or exhausted nerve, with the concept of such a morbid condition being rather close to the medical concept of "weakened kidney" or related disorders that have been described in traditional medicine. Thus, people are familiar with the concept and terminology. In contrast, anxiety and depression are newly introduced psychiatric terms that have less meaning for them. As pointed out by S. Lee (1997), the official term "undifferentiated somatoform disorder" does not appeal to clinicians in their daily clinical practice, as it is difficult for them to explain to the majority of their patients. It does not make any sense to the patients to force them to adopt such an unfamiliar diagnostic term.

Fourth, neurasthenia was speculated during Freud's time to occur in association with the excessive practice of masturbation. Freud even hypothesized that certain chemical substances, tentatively labeled X, as the product of excessive masturbation, may weaken the nervous system. Sexual exhaustion is still believed to be the cause of nervous weakness in many societies even at the present time. This is illustrated by the existence of *dhat* syndrome (a disorder believed to occur as the result of excessive loss of semen) observed in India.

Fifth, there is still the possibility that, in some societies, people's lives are full of persistent and monotonous stresses. To work long hours in a factory or elsewhere to make a living or to be forced to study and compete for academic performance are still a part of daily life in many societies and may contribute to the occurrence of a disorder due to mental exhaustion. In poor economic conditions, people often have to work excessively. Many work day and night without adequate rest, not to mention proper food. A combination of physical and mental exhaustion can lead to neurasthenia-like symptoms.

Finally, there is also the possibility that people living in relatively less desirable environmental settings — from a physical health perspective — are more vulnerable to various undesirable physical conditions or illnesses that may manifest numerous neurasthenia-like somatic conditions. Malnutrition, anemia, parasites, tuberculosis, hepatitis, and chemical intoxication are some examples of physical conditions or disorders that tend to be associated with a general malaise, lack of energy, or fatigue, the core symptoms of conceptualized neurasthenia. Thus, for people living in less desirable physical environments, neurasthenia-like somatic complaints are frequently observed, not due to emotional problems, but to physical illness or poor physical conditions.

Thus, many factors may contribute to the occurrence, labeling, and official usage of diagnostic terms relating to neurasthenia. This issue deserves further investigation and clarification.

C. HYPOCHONDRIASIS

As pointed out by Barsky and Klerman (1983), hypochondriasis can be conceptualized in different ways: clinically, as a unique psychiatric syndrome composed of "functional" somatic symptoms, bodily preoccupation, fear of disease, and the persistent pursuit of medical care; psychodynamically, as a derivative of aggressive or oral drives, defending against psychological problems; psychologically, characterized by a perceptual amplification of bodily sensations and their cognitive misinterpretation; and socioculturally, as a learned illness behavior eliciting interpersonal rewards for attention and care from others. Based on the last view, it is reasonable to speculate that hypochondriacal behavior is closely related socioculturally to illness behavior.

Cross-cultural differences among people of different cultural groups have been commented on by numerous scholars. For instance, regarding clinical study, a Jewish psychiatrist from Jerusalem (Hes, 1958) did a comparative study of Jewish immigrants to Israel. Based on clinical data, he reported that, in comparison to an Occidental group (from west, central, or east Europe), Oriental Jewish immigrants (from Iraq, North Africa, Yemen, etc.) showed a greater incidence of hypochondriacal symptoms.

D. Pain Disorder

As pointed out by Streltzer (1997), relief of pain has been a critical part of the practice of medicine throughout history, yet the pain disorder as a diagnostic nosology has not been clearly held by psychiatrists until very recently. The complaint of pain is a subjective experience for which there is no objective measurement. There is a good reason to suspect that pain-related experience, including complaining behavior and care for it, is subject to cultural influences.

The most well-known and earliest study relating culture to pain was carried out by Zborowski (1952) in New York. He studied veterans with chronic pain and divided them into ethnic groups. He reported that the patients with white Anglo-Saxon Protestant backgrounds, whose families had lived in the United States for several generations, labeled the "old Americans" group, were characterized as stoic in response to pain — in marked contrast to two other ethnic groups studied: Jewish people and Italians. Both groups did not hesitate to complain about pain, being quite expressive and emotional. However, they were different from each other in certain ways: The Italians were eager for pain relief, whereas the Jewish people were fearful of medication that would take away their pain.

A more objective study with a larger number of subjects was carried out by Woodrow, Friedman, Siegelaub, Collen and in 1972, through the Kaiser Foundation Health Plan in California, on experimental pain. As a test, a certain apparatus was used to give pressure to the Achilles tendon to evaluate the threshold for pain. It was found out that Caucasians tolerated more pain than African-Americans, who in turn tolerated more pain than Asians.

Regarding chronic pain, there have been relatively few studies carried out from a cross-ethnic perspective. Bates and Edwards (1992) used a structured questionnaire to study patients attending a chronic pain clinic. Among the ethnic groups of old Ameri-

cans, Irish, Italians, French Canadians, Poles, and Hispanics, it was found that the Hispanics showed the clearest differences of all the groups. They complained of more pain than the other groups and were less likely to be working. It was not clear whether the phenomena was related to educational background, as the Hispanics were substantially less educated than the other groups included in the study. It was also noted that the Hispanics were somewhat more likely to be on workers' compensation, a social factor that would have a potential impact on how the pain was complained about for compensation.

Streltzer and Wade (1981) carried out a comparative study of acute clinical pain in the multiethnic society of Hawaii. Surgery patients receiving elective gall bladder removal were examined in terms of the medication received for pain at the stage of postoperative care in the hosptial. It was found that Caucasian patients received the most pain medication. Filipinos, Japanese, and Chinese received the least, whereas Hawaiians were intermediate. Multiple regression analysis revealed that all the factors studied accounted for only 15% of the variance in the amount of pain medication received. It is presumed that individual factors accounted for the bulk of the variance. Of the factors examined, however, ethnic groups accounted for the largest proportion, about 6% of the variance. Thus, it was concluded that a very real difference existed in the way patients were treated clinically for pain, according to their ethnic group. In trying to explain the results, the ethnicities of the surgeons were examined. It was revealed that the surgeon's orders were almost identical, irrespective of their ethnic backgrounds. The investigators interpreted that the differences appeared to be at the level of nurse–patient interaction. It was speculated that the Asian patients were less vocal and allowed themselves to be more undertreated for pain. It may also be speculated that Asian patients, in general, are concerned about receiving pain medication, which they often associate with addiction-forming narcotics.

These findings are related to the study of the pain experience or pain management rather than the disorders themselves. However, they give us a glance at how ethnic factors may influence the pain experience in either experimental or clinical situations.

E. Body Dysmorphic Disorder

From a cross-cultural perspective, there are few studies about body dysmorphic disorder. It is commonly known that Japanese patients diagnosed with *taijinkyofusho* often presented symptoms concerning their dysmorphic condition; however, they were not diagnosed primarily with body dsymorphic disorder.

It is known from social experience that some Asian women receive cosmetic surgery to create double eyelids so that they look like Westerners, but not as many Asian women receive cosmetic surgery for their breasts as women in European-American societies. This suggests that, based on cultural attitudes, there are different parts of body with which people are not satisfied, leading them to want surgical "improvement." It also suggests that there are culturally different emphases on body parts for self-image and beauty, as well as for sexual attraction. To what extent the differences in emphasis on various parts of the body may relate to dysmorphobic concern is a question awaiting future investigation.

F. Some "Psychosomatic Disorders"

During the 1950s and 1960s, psychiatrists categorized certain medical conditions as "psychosomatic disorders." These included hypertension, myocardiac infarction, peptic ulcer, asthma, and others. It was conceived that these disorders were closely related to psychological conditions and were influenced heavily by the patient's emotional state. Psychological factors were regarded as causative factors, not merely precipitating or aggravating factors. These views are no longer held by psychiatrists, and the category of psychophysiological disorders was eliminated from the formal classification system when the DSM-III was revised in 1980.

Some of these so-called psychosomatic disorders are reviewed here briefly to examine how certain medical disorders may be influenced by culture in the perception of, and reactions to, them.

1. Premenstrual Syndrome

Stout and colleagues (1986) noticed that almost all of the women seeking treatment from the Premenstrual Syndrome Clinic at Duke University Medical Center were white, although 40% of the population in there were African-American. They carried out an evaluation of premenstrual symptoms in a representative community-based sample and found no difference in the prevalence or severity of premenstral symptoms reported by African-Americans and Caucasian-Americans. Their interpretation was that social and cultural factors contribute to the help-seeking behavior of women for premenstrual complaints.

2. Menopause Syndrome

Although the perception and experiences of menopause vary cross-culturally, Beyene (1986) and Charney (1996) pointed out that this developmental event needs biocultural investigation of factors such as diet, fertility patterns, and genetic difference in addition to cultural attitudes. It has been observed that Asian women tend to suffer less menopause symptoms than Caucasian women. According to Lock (1998), in a comparative study of postmenopausal experiences and symptoms reporting among women in Japan, Canada, and America, the reporting of hot flashes and nights sweats was significantly lower in Japan. From an anthropological perspective, she speculated that these findings may be related to the lifestyle and role of women in Japanese society. However, from a biological study, it is now realized that Asian people, including the Japanese, consume a lot of *tofu* in their daily diet. Tofu (bean curd) is rich in vegetable estrogen, which minimizes menopausal symptoms, including flushing and other discomforts. Thus, cultural factors, such as patterns of food consumption, *indirectly* influence the severity of the menopause syndrome.

III. FINAL INTEGRATION

A cross-cultural study supports the view that there is a spectrum of symptoms and complaints between "psychological" and "somatic" dimensions. The extent to which somatic symptoms will be focused on and presented varies among patients of different sociocultural backgrounds and is subject to cultural orientations toward the distinction between body and mind, as well as other factors (G.M. White, 1982).

As pointed out by Kirmayer and Young (1998), historically the tendency of somatization among psychiatric patients was regarded by cultural psychiatrists as a culture-related specific clinical feature of some ethnic groups (including many Asian and Hispanic ethnic groups). Associated with the increase of cross-cultural information and knowledge, it is no longer viewed as an ethnic-related unique clinical feature. While the prevalence and specific features of somatic complaining syndromes vary considerably across cultures, clinically presenting somatic distress is universal, and somatic symptoms are probably the most common clinical expressions of emotional distress worldwide (Isaac, Janca, & Orley, 1996).

Some scholars in the past attributed the tendency to manifest somatic symptoms to psychological underdevelopment and, therefore, believed it was observed more frequently among undereducated people. However, it has been learned that this is not necessarily true. Somatic complaining has been observed broadly, regardless of educational level. After studying the phenomenon of somatization in 14 countires around the world, Guerje, Simon, Üstün, and Goldberg (1997) reported that somatization was a common problem in primary care across cultures, and the association with low education was only modest. It is a mistake to theorize about the distinction between body and mind simply from an evolutionary or developmental point of view. It is not necessarily better, from a psychotherapeutic point of view, for patients to present more psychological symptoms than for patients to focus more on somatic symptoms. Somatic presentation may be closely related to and influenced by cultural views and customs, but is not necessarily related to the extent to which patients are willing to work on their distress or problems they encounter in their lives.

The concept and category of "somatoform disorder" is a product of the contemporary professional orientation (mainly shared by Euro-American scholars) that dichotomatizes the body and mind and categorizes disorders simply by the nature of symptomatic manifestation.

Although sufficient and adequate epidemiological information is not available for meaningful cross-cultural comparisons clinically, it is clear that the frequency of somatoform disorders varies considerably among different societies. It is influenced greatly by professional habits of making diagnoses, the psychological implications of using certain suitable diagnostic terms, culturally patterned problem-presenting styles, and perhaps, reflects that the frequency of such disorders varies among different societies for reasons still not fully explored.

REFERENCES

Abbey, S.E., & Garfinkel, P.E. (1991). Neurasthenia and chronic fatigue syndrome: The role of culture in the making of a diagnosis. *American Journal of Psychiatry, 148*(12), 1638–1646.

American Psychiatric Association (APA) (1994). *Diagnostic and Statistical Manual of Mental Disorders* (4th Rev.). (DSM-ID) Washington DC: APA.

Ayonrinde A.O. (1977). Heat in the head or body—a semantic confusion? *African Journal of Psychiatry, 1,* 59–63.

Barsky, A.J., & Klerman, G.L. (1983). Overview: Hypochondriasis, bodily complaints, and somatic styles. *American Journal of Psychiatry, 140*(3), 273–283.

Bates, M.S., & Edwards, W.T. (1992). Ethnic variations in the chronic pain experience. *Ethnicity and Disease, 2,* 63–83.

Beyene, Y. (1986). Cultural significance and psychological manifestations of menopause: A biocultural analysis. *Culture, Medicine and Psychiatry, 10,* 47–71.

Canino, I.A., Rubio-Stipec, M., Canino, G., & Escobar, J.I. (1992). Functional somatic symptoms: A cross-ethnic comparison. *American Journal of Orthopsychiatry, 62,* 605–612.

Charney, D.D. (1996). The psychoendocrinology of menopause in cross-cultural perspective. *Transcultural Psychiatric Research Review, 33*(4), 413–434.

Cheung, F.M. (1989). The indigenization of neurasthenia in Hong Kong. *Culture, Medicine and Psychiatry, 13*(2), 227–241.

Cheung, F.M., & Lin, K.M. (1997). Neurasthenia, depression and somatoform disorder in a Chinese-Vietnamese woman migrant. *Culture, Medicine and Psychiatry, 21*(2), 247–258.

Chung, R.C., & Singer, M.K. (1995). Interpretation of symptom presentation and distress. A Southeast Asian refugee example. *Journal of Nervous and Mental Disease, 183*(10), 639–648.

Cooper, J.E., & Sartorius, N. (Eds.). (1996). *Mental disorders in China.* London: Gaskell.

Corrigan, F.M., MacDonald, S., Brown, A., Armstrong, K., & Armstrong, E.M. (1994). Neurasthenic fatigue, chemical sensitivity and GABAa receptor toxins. *Medical Hypotheses, 43*(4), 195–200.

Farmer, A., Jones, I., Hiller, J., Llewelyn, M., Borysiewicz, L., & Smith, A. (1995). Neurasthenia revisited: ICD-10 and DSM-III-R psychiatric syndromes in chronic fatigue patients and comparison subjects. *British Journal of Psychiatry, 167*(4), 503–506.

Gabbard, G.O. (1995). Psychoanalysis. In H.I. Kaplan & B.J. Sadock (Eds.), *Comprehensive textbook of psychiatry/VI,* (Vol.1). Baltimore: Williams & Wilkins.

Gelder, M., Gath, D., & Mayou, R. (1983). Neurosis: Part I. In M. Gelder, D. Gath, & R. Mayou *Oxford textbooks of psychiatry* (pp. 136–137). Oxford: Oxford University Press.

Goldberg, D., & Huxley, P. (1980). *Mental illness in the community.* London: Tavistock.

Gureje, O., Simon, G.E., Üstün, T.B., & Goldberg, D.P. (1997). Somatization in cross-cultural perspective: A World Health Organization study in primary care. *American Journal of Psychiatry, 154*(7), 989–995.

Hes, J.P. (1958). Hypochondriasis in Oriental Jewish immigrants: A preliminary report. *International Journal of Social Psychiatry, 44,* 18–23.

Isaac, M., Janca, A., & Orley, J. (1996). Somatization—a culture-bound or universal syndrome? *Journal of Mental Health, 5,* 219–222.

Iwa, H. (1982). *Shinkeisho [Neuroses].* Tokyo: Nihonbunka Kagakusha.

Jegede, R.O. (1983). Psychiatric illness in African students: "Brain fag" syndrome revisited. *Canadian Journal of Psychiatry, 28,* 188–192.

Kirmayer, L.J. (1984). Culture, affect and somatization. *Transcultural Psychiatric Research Review, 21,* 159–188.

Kirmayer, L.J. (1988). Mind and body as metaphors: Hidden values in biomedicine. In M. Lock & D.R. Gordon (Eds.), *Biomedicine examined.* Boston: Kluwer Academic Publishers.

Kirmayer, L.J., & Robbins, J.M. (1996). Patients who somatize in primary care: A longitudinal study of cognitive and social characteristics. *Psychological Medicine, 26,* 937–951.

Kirmayer, L.J., & Young, A. (1998). Culture and somatization: Clinical, epidemiological and ethnographic perspectives. *Psychosomatic Medicine, 60,* 420–430.

Kitanishi, K., & Kondo, K. (1994). The rise and fall of neurasthenia in Japanese psychiatry. *Transcultural Psychiatric Research Review, 31*(2), 137–152.

Kleinman, A. (1982). Neurasthenia and depression: A study of somatization and culture in China. *Culture, Medicine and Psychiatry, 6,* 117–190.

Koss, J.D. (1990). Somatization and somatic complaint syndromes among Hispanics: Overview and ethnopsychological perspectives. *Transcultural Psychiatric Research Review, 27*(1), 5–29.

Lee, C.K., Kwak, Y.S., Yamamoto, J., Rhee, H., Kim, Y.S., Han, J.H., Choi, J.O., & Lee, Y.G. (1990). Psychiatric epidemiology in Korea. Part I: Gender and age differences in Seoul. *Journal of Nervous and Mental Disease, 178,* 242–246.

Lee, S. (1997). A Chinese perspective of somatoform disorders [Editorial]. *Journal of Psychosomatic Research, 43*(2), 115–119.

Lee, S., & Wong, K.C. (1995). Rethinking neurasthenia: The illness concepts of *shenjing shuairuo* among Chinese undergraduates in Hong Kong. *Culture, Medicine and Psychiatry, 19*(1), 91–111.

Lin, T.Y. (1989). Neurasthenia revisted: Its place in modern psychiatry. *Culture, Medicine and Psychiatry, 13*(2), 105–129.

Liu, S.X. (1989). Neurasthenia in China: Modern and traditional criteria for its diagnosis. *Culture, Medicine and Psychiatry, 13*(2), 163–186.

Liu, X.H. (1994). Neurasthenia. In Y.C. Shen (Ed.), *Psychiatry* (3rd ed., pp. 696–704). Beijing: People's Health Publisher (in Chinese).

Lock, M. (1998). Menopuase: Lessons from anthropology. *Psychosomatic Medicine, 60,* 410–419.

Machizawa, S. (1992). Neurasthenia in Japan. *Psychiatric Annals, 22*(4), 190–191.

Mori, W., & Kitanishi, K. (1984). *Morita-shinkeishitsu to* DSM-III [Morita nervous temperament disorders and DSM-III]. *Rinsho-seishinigaku (Clinical Psychiatry), 13,* 911–920.

Munakata, T. (1989). The socio-cultural significance of the diagnostic label "neurasthenia" in Japan's mental health care system. *Culture, Medicine and Psychiatry, 13*(2), 203–213.

Ohaeri, J.U., & Odejide, O.A. (1994). Somatization symptoms among patients using primary health care facilities in a rural community in Nigeria. *American Journal of Psychiatry, 151*(5), 728–731.

Olatawura, M.O. (1973). The problem of diagnosing depression in Africa. *Psychopathologie Africaine, 9,* 389–403.

Orbaek, P., & Nise, G. (1989). Neurasthenic complaints and psychometric function of toluene-exposed rotogravure printers. *American Journal of Industrial Medicine, 16*(1), 67–77.

Prince, R. (1960). The brain fag syndrome in Nigerian students. *Journal of Mental Science, 106,* 559–570.

Prince, R. (1990). *Somatic complaint syndromes and depression: The problems of cultural effects on symptomatology*. Paper presented to the Spring Convention of the Korean Neuropsychiatric Association, Seoul, Korea, 1989 (Reviewed in *Transcultural Psychiatric Research Review, 27*(1), 31–36. 1990.)

Psychiatric Epidemiological Collaboration Team. (1986). Epidemiological survey of neuroses in 12 geographic regions. *Chinese Neuropsychiatric Journal, 19*(2), 87–91 (in Chinese).

Racy, J. (1980). Somatization in Saudi women: A therapeutic challenge. *British Journal of Psychiatry, 137,* 212–216.

Raguram, R., Weiss, M.G., Channabasavanna, S.M., & Devins, G.M. (1996). Stigma, depression, and somatization in South India. *American Journal of Psychiatry, 153*(8), 1043–1049.

Sartorius, N. (1997). Diagnosis and classification of neurasthenia. In L.L. Jud, B. Saletu, & V. Filip (Eds.), *Basic and clinical science of mental and addictive disorders* (Bibl. Psychiatr. No. 167, pp. 1–5). Basel: Kargero.

Starcevic, V. (1991). Neurasthenia: A paradigm of social psychopathology in a transitional society. *American Journal of Psychiatry, 45*(4), 544–553.

Starcevic, V. (1994). Neurasthenia in European psychiatric literature. *Transcultrual Psychiatric Research Review, 31*(2), 125–136.

Stout, A.L., Grady, T.A., Steege, J.F., Blazer, D.G., George, L.K., & Melville, M.L. (1986). Premenstrual symptoms in Black and White community samples. *American Journal of Psychiatry, 143*(11), 1436–1439.

Streltzer, J. (1997). Pain. In W.S. Tseng, & J. Streltzer, Eds)., *Culture and psychopathology* (pp. 87–100). New York: Brunner/Mazel.

Streltzer, J., & Wade, T.C. (1981). The influence of cultural group in the undertreatment of postoperative pain. *Psychosomatic Medicine, 43,* 397–403.

Suzuki, T. (1989). The concept of neurasthenia and its treatment in Japan. *Culture, Medicine and Psychiatry, 13*(2), 187–202.

Tseng, W.S. (1975). The nature of somatic complaints among psychiatric patients: The Chinese case. *Comprehensive Psychiatry, 16*(3), 237–245.

Tseng, W.S., Asai, M.H., Kitanish, K.J., McLaughlin, D., & Kyomen, H. (1992). Diagnostic pattern of social phobia: Comparison in Tokyo and Hawaii. *Journal of Nervous and Mental Diseases, 180,* 380–385.

Tseng, W.S., Asai, M.H., Liu, J., Pismai, W., Suryani, L.K., Wen, J.K., Brennan, J., & Heiby, E. (1991). Multi-cultural study of minor psychiatric disorders in Asia: Symptom manifestation. *International Journal of Social Psychiatry, 36,* 252–264.

Tseng, W.S., Xu, D., Ebata, K., Hsu, J., & Cui, Y.H. (1986). Diagnostic pattern for neuroses in China, Japan, and the United States. *American Journal of Psychiatry, 143*(8), 1010–1014.

Üstün, T.B., & Sartorius, N. (Eds.). (1995). *Mental illness in general health care: An international study.* Chichester: Wiley.

van Vliet, C., Swaen, G.M., Meijers, J.M., Slangen, J., de Boorder, T., & Sturmans, F. (1989). Prenarcotic and neurasthenic symptoms among Dutch workers exposed to organic solvents. *British Journal of Industrial Medicine, 46*(8), 586–590.

Wang, H.L. (1989). Preliminary investigation of neurasthenic syndrome induced by occupational hazards. *Zhonghua Shenjing Jingshenko Zaji (Journal of Chinese Neuropsychiatry), 22*(5), 278–282, 317–318.

Ware, N.C., & Kleinman, A. (1992). Culture and somatic experience: The social course of illness in neurasthenia and chronic fatigue syndrome. *Psychosomatic Medicine, 54*(5), 546–560.

Wessely, S. (1994). Neurasthenia and chronic fatigue: Theory and practice in Britain and America. *Transcultural Psychiatric Research Review, 31*(2), 173–209.

White, G.M. (1982). The role of cultural explanations in "somatization" and "psychologization." *Social Science and Medicine, 16,* 1519–1530.

White, P. (1989). Fatigue syndrome: Neurasthenia revived. *British Medical Journal, 298,* 1199–1200.

Woodrow, K.M., Friedman, G.D., Siegelaub, A.B., & Collen, M.F. (1972). Pain tolerance: Differences according to age, sex and race. *Psychosomatic Medicine, 34*(6), 548–556.

World Health Organization (WHO) (1992). *International Statistical Classification of Diseases and Related Health Problems,* (10th Rev.) (ICD-IO). Geneva: WHO.

Yan, H.Q. (1989). The necessity of retaining the diagnostic concept of neurasthenia. *Culture, Medicine and Psychiatry, 13*(2), 139–145.

Young, D.S. (1989). Neurasthenia and related problems. *Culture, Medicine and Psychiatry, 13*(2), 131–138.

Zborowski, M. (1952). Cultural components in responses to pain. *Journal of Social Issues, 8,* 16–30.

Zhang, M.Y. (1989). The diagnosis and phenomenology of neurasthenia: A Shanghai study. *Culture, Medicine and Psychiatry, 13*(2), 147–161.

Zheng, Y.P., Lin, K.M., Takeuchi, D., Kurasaki, K.S., Wang, Y., & Cheung, F. (1997). An epidemiological study of neurasthenia in Chinese-American in Los Angeles. *Comprehensive Psychiatry, 38*(5), 249–259.

Zheng, Y.P., Lin, K.M., Zhao, J.P., Zhang, M.Y., & Yong, D. (1994). Comparative study of diagnostic systems: Chinese Classification of Mental Disorders—Second Edition versus DSM-III-R. *Comparative Psychiatry, 35*(6), 441–449.

17

Dissociation, Possession, and Hysteria

I. INTRODUCTION AND BASIC CLARIFICATIONS

Among all mental phenomena and psychopathology, the related mental states of trance, dissociation, possession, and altered personality have fascinated clinicians and scholars for a long time (Bourguignon, 1973; Prince, 1968; Ward, 1989). These unique mental conditions are characterized by their dramatic, puzzling, and mysterious nature. The description and understanding of the phenomena have changed a great deal along the developmental path of psychiatry. They have caught the interest of scholars from the perspectives of medical history and cultural anthropology. Because various impacts of culture on mental conditions can be studied explicitly by examining this particular set of mental phenomena, it has also attracted great attention among cultural psychiatrists.

A. THE CORE OF PHENOMENA: ALTERED CONSCIOUSNESS

Although trance, dissociation, possession, and altered personality states differ in certain ways, they share several common characteristics. As mental conditions, they are related to some extent to the basic mechanism of the alteration of the state of consciousness and the awareness of self-identification. They are related to the verification of mental integration and involve change of personality and awareness and identity of selfness. Based on these mental mechanisms, different mental conditions emerge that may occur as normal life conditions, on special daily life occasions, or as morbid states. Thus, they are found on a spectrum ranging between the normal and the pathological (Fig. 17–1). Another unique feature of these mental conditions is that they can be induced by the self, can occur rather suddenly, and the individual experiencing them can return to his or her original state within a certain time. These conditions can occur in ordinary daily life situations, such as meditation and daydreaming, or as part of a religious or healing ceremony or professional practice, such as hypnosis. They can also occur in reaction to emotional stress. If they occur as pathological disorders, psychological therapy becomes the main approach for treatment.

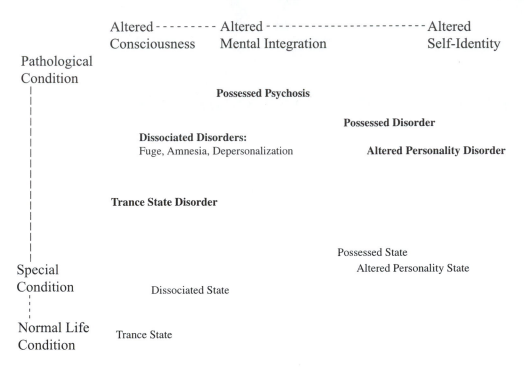

FIGURE 17-1   Spectrum of various altered consciousness states.

B. Phenomenological Distinction

1. Trance State

This is characterized by a dream-like, stunned mental condition that is often induced by intense concentration, monotonous external stimulation, or tranquilizing settings. The consciousness is altered in such a way that a person becomes less sensitive in responding to external stimuli while still maintaining a relatively narrowed but partially alert sense of awareness.

The trance state can occur often in one's ordinary daily life. For instance, when a person is calmly listening to a monotonous sound, or an enchanting musical rhythm; sitting in a rhythmically moving car or train, watching monotonously changing scenery; indulging in a daydream, or fantasy, a person may fall into a momentary trance state. Through practices such as meditation or concentrated praying, a person can induce a deeper trance state. These are practiced routinely followed as part of self-training or religious activities. A well-known dance performed in Bali, Indonesia, for entertainment is often performed gracefully while the dancers are in a trance state. In India, during religious ceremonies, selected faithful believers will cut their tongues with a knife, put long needles through their cheeks, or hook the skin on their chests or backs with metal hooks and pull heavy objects by them. These acts take place during trance states in which they claim they feel no pain. These are public demonstrations to illustrate that they are blessed by a supernatural power.

Trances can be "morbid" conditions (trance state disorders). When a person encounters severe mental stress or emotional trauma, he may fall into a trance state to ward off the emotional pain or stress. The condition may be brief or last for a prolonged period of time. When a person behaves differently for a while, his behavior may be interpreted as the result of a "loss of soul," a common illness behavior around the world, but found more frequently among people with Latin backgrounds. This state can be observed as a part of posttraumatic stress disorder in which a trance state occurs repeatedly when a traumatic situation is reencountered (Bremner et al., 1992). Trance states are the basis for developing other forms of altered consciousness disorders.

2. Dissociated State

The dissociated state is characterized by the disconnection and disintegration of various mental functions. The level of alternation of consciousness may vary For some, consciousness becomes cloudy, whereas for others, the experience may be only slight — thus, they are still in full consciousness. Normal dissociated states can be observed in religious or healing ceremonies. After the occurrence of a transient trance state, the subject does not have any recollection of what happened.

Clinically various subforms of morbid dissociated conditions can be identified. For instance, when a person encounters an unbearable stressful event, the memory relating to it will temporarily be dissociated from the sphere of conscious mental activity, manifested as temporary memory loss (labeled dissociated amnesia). The purpose of action and behavior may be dissociated from the consciousness transiently, with the person wondering around as if in a dream state, becoming a fugitive for a time without retrospective recollection (dissociated fugue). If a person loses his sense of self, perceiving and observing himself as an outsider, this is called a depersonalized state.

3. Altered Personality State

This refers to the situation in which a person temporarily changes his personality as a whole, behaving as if he is a different person — manifested by a different tone and style of speech (speaking in a different tone or even an unfamiliar language), a different behavior pattern and character. After recovering from this altered personality state, the person resumes his original personality, often claiming no recollection of what happened.

This condition is well exemplified by the *latah* phenomena observed among Malaysian people. Typically, a woman, startled by sudden stimulation (hearing an unexpected noise or seeing snake-like subjects) or being startled purposely by others for amusement, the person goes into a trance state. During this state, she will talk eroticaly, touch people around her, including men (which is forbidden by Malay culture), and manifest other strange behavior. After recovering from the state, she will often be embarrassed to learn what she did in the *latah* episode [cross-reference to Chapter 13: Culture-Related Specific Syndromes (Section II,D,1)].

The altered personality state can occur as a morbid condition. After encountering psychological stress, the person will alter "other" personal identities so the original self does not have to face the psychological pain of the stress. In the meantime, while in this altered personality state, the person can communicate his wishes or desires or perform certain behaviors to gratify unfilled needs. After the recovery of the original self, the person does not admit what has happened. The novel story of *Dr. Jekyl and Mr. Hyde,* about a doctor who shifts between a kind, civilized doctor and a cruel, savage person, is a good example of a double personality disorder. If a person has more than one other personality, he is suffering from a multiple personality disorder.

4. Possessed State

If the altered personal state is so dramatically different from the original self, it may be interpreted by other (or occasionally claimed by the person himself) to be the result of being possessed by "others." Then, it is addressed as a possessed state. In other words, a possessed state is the same as an altered personality state except that the person behaves so differently from his original self that he is interpreted as being possessed. That is, there is the replacement of the customary personal identity by a new identity. The new identity can be of various beings, which may include the spirit of an animal (such as the fox spirit in Japan) (Eguchi, 1991), the spirit of deceased family members or ancestors (as often observed among Chinese), or a special god (such as Zar in the Zar cult ceremony performed by Muslim people in mideastern areas). In many folk-healing practices, such as shamanistic performances, the healer goes into a trance state and is possessed by an identified god(s). In this possessed state, by utilizing the supernatural power, the healer tries to offer a healing service to clients. Alternatively, clients may be possessed during the healing ceremony, as was observed in the Salvation Cult healing practice described in Japan (Lebra, 1976) or the Zar ceremony observed in the Mideast [cross-reference to Chapter 32: Culture-Embedded Indigenous Healing Practices (Section II,A,1–3)].

In summary, it should be pointed out that the various mental conditions outlined here can occur as "normal" behavior in ordinary daily life or during special activities, such as religious ceremonies, as art performances (such as in the Balian trance dance), or as healing practices. It is clear that there are several kinds of mental conditions that stemmed from the most fundamental state of trance and evolved into other conditions. From a psychological point of view, a possessed state is a much more complicated psychic function than a simple trance state, as it takes mental work to play a person other than one's self. This view is supported by anthropological field work.

C. ANTHROPOLOGICAL STUDIES OF PHENOMENA

Concerning the trance and possession state, as observed in the ordinary life of society, cultural anthropologist Erika Bourguignon (1968) carried out statistical studies by drawing a worldwide sample of 488 societies (mostly of traditional one) from Murdock's *Ethnographic Atlas*. She reported that 437 (or 90%) of these societies have institutionalized some form of altered state of consciousness. Furthermore,

she pointed out that there is a relationship between types of altered states manifested by the members of society and societal characteristics reflecting variations in complexity. Social complexity is defined sociologically by matters such as size of population or community, the complexity of jurisdictional hierarchy, stratification of the social structure, and so on. She pointed out that the less complex a society, the more likely it is to have only a trance state, whereas a more complex society is more likely to have a possession trance.

Bourguignon (1976) interpreted trance as an intrapersonal psychic event. In contrast, possession involves the impersonation of another being on an occasion when there are witnesses. As such it is an interpersonal event because the witnesses and the audience play a crucial role in the event. In other words, a possession state, in contrast to a simple trance state, involves much more complex psychic function.

Based on her studies of sub-Saharan Africa, another anthropologist, Lenora Greenbaum (1973), speculated that a mediumistic possession trance is more likely to exist in rigid societies than in more flexible ones. She interpreted the medium acting as the spirit may make it possible for the individual, for the client, to be provided with solutions for some of his/her problems in ways that circumvent the rigid demands of the society. The client follows the social constraints in that he/she relies on an external authority, a spirit speaking through the medium, to get authorization for his actions.

In order to make a clear distinction between an institutionalized possessed state and a morbid possessed disorder, anthropologist C.A. Ward (1980) suggested using the term ritual possession for the former and pathological possession for the latter. He elaborated further that ritual possession tends to occur to persons who are respected by society, serve as religious persons or healers, or persons who are "central" members of society, whereas pathological possession often occurs to those who are "peripheral" members of society.

The distinction between "central" and "peripheral" members in terms of ritual and morbid possession is valid only in societies where folk healers are highly regarded. In some societies, they are not. For instance, it was found that in Japan and Taiwan there are several pathways for a person to take to become a professional shaman: through formal selection and training of suitable candidates or the self-conversion of a formal mentally ill person into a healer after self-training (Sasaki, 1969; Tseng, 1972).

D. Psychological Nature of the Conditions

From a psychological point of view, there are several issues that need to be pointed out. Besides the fact that the state of trance, dissociation, or possession, including an altered personality state, can occur as normal phenomena to an individual, it is important for psychiatrists to realize that such a mental condition is often institutionalized for various purposes, including fortune-telling, religion, and healing activities for many societies — in both the East and the West. It is based on the fact that, during a trance state, a person's perception may become less disturbed by complex factors, more focused and sharp, relying more on basic emotion and instinct for action. Thus, it provides a different level of mental function with the insight to deal with the reality. It is culturally patterned and utilized in specific ways.

If these conditions occur as morbid reactions toward psychological stress, it is characterized defensive. The mechanisms of repression, denial, avoidance, and dissociation operate to cope with the emotional difficulty and stress. Phenomenologically it occurs reactively and abruptly, and will resume to the original condition dramatically without any mental sequel if the disturbing stress is removed or resolved. This is the basic nature of the disorder labeled "hysteria." As the disorder of hysteria clinically contains the manifestations of trance, dissociation, possession, or altered personalization, it is relevant to discuss it here.

II. THE UNIQUE DISORDER OF HYSTERIA

A. Historical Path

As pointed out by medical historian Ilza Vieth (1965), hysteria has undergone many and radical changes historically in terms of the concept of its nature, its manifestation, and its management. Thus, of all mental disorders, hysteria has occupied the most interest among scholars for illustrating how time and knowledge shape and modify the view and understanding of disease.

1. Ancient Concept: Wandering of Uterus and Running Pig

a. Illness as Recognized in the West

In the ancient Egyptian document, the *Kahun Papyrus,* dating back to about 1900 B.C., a description was found stating that the conduct of certain unstable females was attributed to displacement of a discontented womb. As a remedy, the parts were fumigated with precious and sweet-smelling substances to lure or drive the organ back to its position. A specific appellation for the condition was not given yet. This step was taken by the Greeks. In the Hippocratic writings (about 6th century B.C.) the nosological term "hysteria" first appeared, referring to this morbid condition (Vieth, 1965, p.10). Certain forms of respiratory difficulty with a choking sensation were believed to be due to the pressure of the displaced uterus. The Hippocratic physicians were aware of the importance of a careful differentiation between hysterical symptoms and those of organic disease. If digital pressure was applied to the patient's abdomen and the patient could feel and respond to it, it was hysteria; if not, it was epilepsy.

According to Vieth (1965, p.94), the explanation of the disorder of the uterus changed in the Middle Ages. For instance, according to Aetius of Amida (about the 5th century), the uterus remains in its normal position during a hysterical attack, but is seized with violent contractions, which then similarly affect the other organs. Aetius observed that the disorder occurred most frequently in the winter and spring and generally in young women. He believed that the disorder was caused by a cooling of the uterus during menstruation.

By the 16th century, Edward Jorden, a physician in England, transferred the seat of all hysterical manifestations from the uterus to the brain, marking a major turning point in the history of hysteria. At that time, based on the Platonic idea, it was believed that the soul was tripartite and seated in separate organs: the brain the animal faculty; the heart the vital faculty; and the liver the natural faculty. Involvement of the brain disturbed the animal faculty governing reason, memory, the five senses, and motor control. Jorden explained that the cardinal symptoms of hysteria, such as sudden loss of hearing or sight, as well as convulsions or paralysis, were due to the brain (Vieth, 1965, pp.122–123).

It wasn't until the late 17th century that Italian physician Giorgio Baglivi began to consider the emotions to be the cause of hysteria. In the early 19th century, the French physician Jean-Martin Charcot was assigned to serve a group of inmates — mainly of epilepsy and hysteria — from the Salpetriere Hospital. Through this accidental arrangement, he was given the opportunity to study hysteria. He divided the hysterical symptomatology into three categories: the disturbance of the sensory system, the special senses, and the motor system. He also made observations about the role of suggestion in creating as well as removing hysterical symptoms. He utilized hypnosis as a diagnostic procedure for hysteria and also attributed a major significance to psychic trauma in the production of hysterical attacks. This was soon followed by the famous story that the Viennese internist, Josef Breuer, and Austrian neurologist, Sigmund Freud, used hypnosis as a tool to treat a well-known hysterical patient (Miss Anna O). This led to the development of the psychoanalytic theory of repression and psychic trauma. Thus, in a way, hysteria as a unique mental disorder became a gateway through which clinicians could examine the deep psychology of the human being and played a significant role in the evolution of psychoanalysis.

b. Illness Described in the East

In contrast to the West, in China there is an ancient medical document, *Classic of Internal Medicine,* written in 7th century B.C., shortly before Hippocrates' writings. It included descriptions of febrile delirium, falling sickness, or excited insanity, but no record of a disorder similar to hysteria. However, in the *Golden Box Summary* (written about the 1st century), there was a description of a "hurrying-pig sickness" and a "sickness of the hasty organ" (Tseng, 1973). Symptoms of the hurrying-pig sickness were discomfort that started from the abdomen and moved up to the throat. The patient felt as if he or she was going to die, but the symptoms soon subsided. The disorder was induced by fear and being frightened. During the attack, the person would run around wildly and aimlessly like a hurrying pig, but after a while, the condition subsided as if nothing had happened. The psychological cause of the disorder was recognized. Chinese traditional medicine is founded on the theories of yin and yang, the five elements, and the visceral organ-related microcosm–macrocosm concepts. The "sickness of the hasty organ" (either the heart or the uterus) was described according to these theories. The woman who suffered from this sickness felt sad wanted to cry, and behaved as if possessed by a spirit. Herb medicine, as well as acupuncture, was prescribed for treatment.

Psychological treatment for hysteria was suggested in *Chin-Yue's Medical Book* written in the 17th century. In the book, the term "deceiving sickness" was used to describe a woman manifesting somatic symptoms after having quarrelled with others. The physician, knowing the psychological nature of the illness, purposely made an announcement to the family members in front of the patient, "explaining" that the illness was a serious one, needing more drastic treatment by burning herb medicine on the patient's abdomen if the patient failed to recover from the medicine prescribed. After hearing this, the patient's illness subsided soon after taking the medicine. The Chinese term for hysteria is *yi-zheng,* which literally means "sickness of mind."

It is interesting to note that, in both the East and the West, associated with developments in medical knowledge, the disorder was initially conceived as the disorder of an organ, the "uterus," and was thought to occur predominantly in women. It was later thought to be a disorder of the brain. The psychological nature of the disorder was revealed early in the first century in the East, but not until the 17th century in the West (Leff, 1981; Tseng, 1973).

2. Disorder of Hysteria

In ancient times, the disorder, "hysteria" (literally meaning: uterus disorder), was believed to occur as the result of displacement of the uterus. This explanation has long been abandoned and the diagnostic term hysteria, or hysterical neurosis, is used by contemporary clinicians merely in a symbolic way. From a psychiatric standpoint, it is understood as an emotional disorder that tends to occur rather abruptly in response to psychological stress or conflict. Clinically the symptoms may include simple emotional turmoil; psychic manifestation of trance, dissociation, depersonalization, or possession state; or converted somatic symptoms involving sensory organs or the motor system. Based on this, the disorder was subdivided into two subtypes: conversion type and dissociation type. As a clinical course, the disorder is also characterized by the fact that the symptoms may subside and the patient recovers rather quickly after the emotional stress is resolved. Thus, the occurrence of trance, dissociation, or possession, as well as the conversion of somatic symptoms, is understood as defenses against stress. As a whole, the hysteria is characterized as a "reaction" toward psychological difficulty, which may occur suddenly and subside quickly.

3. Elimination of "Hysterical Disorders"

Influenced by shifting orientations in the American psychiatric classification system to classification by clinical phenomenology rather than by the presumed underlying etiology, the nosological concept of "neuroses" has been abandoned and the term "hysterical

neurosis" was eliminated from the third edition of the American psychiatric classification system of the *Diagnostic and Statistical Manual of Mental Disorders* (DSM-III) published by APA in 1980. The subtype phenomena of hysterical disorder, the dissociation and conversion subtypes, were split into "dissociation disorders" and "conversion disorders." The former maintained its own category with further elaboration into dissociative amnesia, fugue, or depersonalization, whereas the latter was categorized into a subtype of somatoform disorders. This revision was made as a result of the revision of the basic classification orientation adopted by the DSM system. It also reflected that conversion disorder is no longer observed frequently in American society. Therefore, for practical purposes, the disorder was demoted from its own category and subcategorized as merely one of a number of somatoform disorders.

The International Classification of Disease, 10th revision (ICD-10), published by the World Health Organization (WHO) in 1992 still retains the generic diagnostic term "neurotic" disorder. However, following the American DSM system, it eliminated "hysteria" as an individual disorder. Instead, the disorder was recategorized into "dissociative (conversion) disorder," which includes dissociative disorders as well as conversion disorders of various kinds. Thus, it reflects the professional confusion and transition that is still going on surrounding the issue of hysteria.

Despite this revision in formal classification, in practice, in many parts of the world, the concept and term of "hysteria" are still used prevalently for diagnosis and to guide clinicians in treating this unique disorder.

B. FREQUENCY OF HYSTERICAL DISORDERS

Although the phenomenon of hysterical disorder is unique, dramatic, and fascinating, epidemiological studies and reports of the disorder are scarce. This is because the condition often occurs rather abruptly and briefly, and the patient (as well as his family) tends to "forget" about the episode afterward so that formal retrospective epidemic surveys often fail to catch most cases. The best information should perhaps rely on clinical data derived from emergency clinics where patients are often sent for service. Another limitation on the study of the frequency of hysteria is that the diagnosis of the disorder is often made by clinical judgement without any solid means of confirmation. Further, the situation is complicated by the fact that various diagnostic terms and criteria have been used in the past, particularly since the dramatic change in the diagnostic classifications of the DSM system in its third version. The disorders are studied and reported either by hysteria globally in its original concept, or by its specific forms of dissociation disorder, conversion disorder, or possession disorder. Despite these difficulties in study, the fragmented information will be presented here to shed some light on the cross-cultural perspectives of this disorder.

A large-scale psychiatric epidemic study of minor psychiatric disorders was carried out in China in 1982, involving 12 geographic areas and nearly 7000 people. From this study, it was reported (Epidemic Survey Collaboratory Teams, 1986) that the overall prevalence rate for hysteria was 3.55 per 1000 population of adults between the ages of 15 and 59. Among all neurotic disorders, hysteria was second only to neurasthenia; thus, it was a commonly observed minor psychiatric disorder. In rural areas, the rate was 5.00, whereas in urban areas, it was 2.09, indicating that the disorder was much more prevalent in rural areas. The disorder occurred much more frequently among females than males. For instance, in the area of Shangtong Province, the rate for women was 14.2, whereas that for men was merely 0.85.

Luo and Zhou (1984) investigated the diagnostic distribution of psychiatric patients who made visits to the emergency room. They reported that during the period of 1972 to 1982 there were a total of 1622 cases who made emergency visits to the Institute of Mental Health of Beijing Medical School, one of the major teaching institutes in Beijing. Among them, besides schizophrenia (15.5%), organic psychoses (7.1%), and other disorders, 820 cases (50.6%) were diagnosed as neuroses. Among these neurotic cases, almost all of them (781 cases, 95.2%) were diagnosed as hysteria. In these cases, the cardinal symptoms were convulsion (40.6%), emotional turmoil (31.1%), trance state (4.2%), and others. In other words, among the psychiatric patients who visited the emergency clinic, nearly half of them were diagnosed with hysteria, with major symptoms of convulsion or emotional turmoil.

In India, a report was made by Dube (1970) based on an epidemiological study carried out by home visits in a census survey in the Agra region of Uttar Pradesh, northern India. Among 29,468 residents, they found 261 cases of conversion symptoms in the form of hysterical fits, with a prevalence rate of 8.9 per 1000 population. They reported that females (mostly ages 15 to 24) constituted 96.1% of all cases. The roles of caste, marital status, and educational level were found to be associated with the occurrence of hysteria.

Another report was made by Srinath, Bharat, Girimaji, and Seshadri (1993) concerning childhood hysteria observed in inpatient and outpatient psychiatric populations. They reviewed the case records for a 1 year interval of inpatients admitted (n=143) and outpatients visited (n=640) at the Child and Adolescent Psychiatric Unit of the National Institute of Mental Health and Neuroscience, Bangalore, in south India. They found that among these clinical cases, 30.8% (n=44) of the inpatient and 14.8% (n=95) of the outpatients were diagnosed with hysteria. The inpatient cases were mostly postpubertal and, interestingly enough, their gender distribution was approximately even. Clinically, psudoseizure was the most frequent presentation.

C. WANING OF THE DISORDER?

In addition to the fact that the prevalence of hysteria differs remarkably among various societies — being more prevalent in traditional and culturally restricted societies and less in culturally liberal and modernized societies — there is another trend that has been noticed by clinicians. That is, based on historical observation and clinical impression, the occurrence of hysteria is waning around the world in both traditional and modern societies. There was one follow-up epidemiological study carried out in rural areas of India supporting the declining trend of hysteria there.

Indian psychiatrists Nandi, Banerjee, Nadi, and Nandi (1992) reported data that derived from their follow-up epidemiological studies carried out in two rural communities: Gambhirgachi and Paharpur, in West Bengal. The former was surveyed in 1972 and, 10 years later, in 1982; the latter was studied in 1972 and, 15 years later, in 1987. The total population of Gambhiragachi grew from 1060 to 1539 within 10 years. Over 90% of the villagers were Muslim and the rest Hindu. The total population of Paharpur increased from 1114 to 1464 within 15 years. The villagers were divided almost equally between Hindu and Muslim. The results of the surveys indicated that the prevalence of hysteria declined considerably in these two villages, from 16.9 to 4.6 per 1000 population and 32.3 to 2.05 per 1000 population in Gambhirgachi and Paharpur, respectively. It is interesting that, associated with this remarkable decline in the prevalence of hysteria, there was a moderate increase in depression: from 37.7 to 53.3 per 1000 population and 61.9 to 77.2 per 1000 population in the two villages, respectively.

Nandi and associates reported that, between these two surveys, besides the increase in population, there was a clearly visible change in the quality of life of the people. In 1972 most of the villagers had no work in the fields for a major part of the year. After the introduction of multiple crops and increased input in farming, people had work throughout the year and were paid a higher wage. Along with this economic improvement, there was an increase in educational and health care facilities. Nandi and associates attribute the improvement in social status of women to the fall of the prevalence of hysteria.

A retrospective study was carried out by Stefanis, Markidis, and Christodoulou (1976) in Athens regarding the prevalence of hysteria. They reviewed the medical records of more than 17,000 psychiatric patients who attended the outpatient department of Eginition Hospital in Athens during three periods; 1948–1950, 1958–1960, and 1969–1971. They revealed that the percentage of patients diagnosed with hysteria was 6.0, 3.0, and 3.1%, respectively, indicating a trend of decreasing of hysterical disorders among outpatients.

D. Diagnostic Consideration

Because the clinical picture presented by most of the hysteria patients in India is so different from that described in ICD-10 as well as DSM-IV, psychiatrists from Manipal, India, Alexander, Joseph, and Das (1997), claimed that their own proposed category of "brief dissociative stupor" needs clinical work. Several studies from India (Das & Saxena, 1991; Saxena & Prasad, 1989) have revealed that up to 90% of the patients with dissociative disorders treated in the outpatient psychiatric clinic were classified as being in the "unspecified" or "atypical" categories of dissociative disorders of the DSM-III or DSM-III-R. Das and Saxena (1991) reported that 81% of their patients with dissociative disorders met the criteria for "simple" dissociative disorders, which are characterized simply by transient episodes of alternations in consciousness (manifested by a relative lack of responsiveness to the external environment), namely trance states. The states may be associated with some bizarre or convulsion-like motor movements or crying, shouting, or verbalizing thoughts. Based on their clinical experiences with psychiatric in-patients in a general hospital, Alexander and associates (1997) reported that a significant number of the patients with dissociative disorders experienced recurrent episodes of unresponsiveness lasting for a short period (without convulsions, motor movements, or verbalization). Therefore, they suggested using the term "brief dissociative stupor" to describe their hysterical patients.

It seems that if we rely on worldwide clinical observation, it would be fair to say that there is a great variety of clinical manifestations of hysteria. The majority of cases exhibit the clinical syndrome of a simple trance state disorder, which may be associated with stupor, motor excitement, or emotional outburst. Beyond that, some cases manifest more specialized forms of disorders, including dissociated amnesia, depersonalization, or possession. Clearly there is a wide range of altered mental conditions relating to the function of consciousness, mental integration, and self-identity within normal life conditions, special conditions, and pathological conditions. Thus, within the spectrum of pathology, there is a need for more diagnostic subgroups to capture the whole perspective of this group of disorders. This is particularly true from a cross-cultural perspective.

III. DISSOCIATION AND DISSOCIATION DISORDER

A. Between Normal and Abnormal: *Latah* Condition

Between normal and pathological conditions there is a unique phenomenon called *latah,* mainly observed among people in Malaysia. The person, after being startled, will suddenly fall into a trance state and behave like a different person, i.e., an altered personality. In this condition the person will talk, act, and behave as if he/she is a different person, ignoring socioculture restrictions, and manifesting uninhibited and usually erotic behavior. As usual, the person will claim no recollection of what happeed during the episode. Because neither the person nor others claim that he/she was possessed by an "other" being, this is not categorized as a "possessed state." However, the audience gives the explanation that the person is not him/herself during the attack and, therefore, any behavior of an obscene but amusing nature during the episode is socially excused. Furthermore, on most such occasions, the *latah* episode occurs to a person who is not facing recognizable stress. The phenomenon tends to be provoked by others for the social function of amusement, with the person acting as a clown on social occasions. Thus, by nature, the majority of

latah attacks are accepted as "ordinary" behavior by local people. The only exception is when the person manifests harmful behavior toward him/herself or others during the attack. Then the episode is labeled "malignant *latah,*" implying that it is a morbid condition [cross-reference to Chapter 13: Culture-Related Specific Syndrome (Section II,D,1)].

B. Possession and Possession Disorder

1. From a "Normal" Possession State to "Morbid" Possession Disorders

As mentioned in Section I,A and B, there is a range of possession states, from normal to morbid (see Fig. 18-1). Normal possession is observed in two circumstances: when healers are possessed by a guardian god(s) during a healing ceremony so that, in the name of the supernatural power, they can perform healing practices. This includes finding and explaining the causes of problems and making suggestions to remedy them. This is observed in many folk-healing practices around the world, which are described under the generic term shamanism. The other circumstance is when the client(s) becomes possessed during the healing ceremony. In this condition, the individual client will complain about his/her problems and request a way to remove or resolve them. More than one client can fall into a possessed state during the ceremony. This is known to occur in Zar cult ceremonies observed in Arabian societies or in Salvation cult ceremonies in Japan [cross-reference to Chapter 32: Culture-Embedded Indigenous Healing Practices (Section II,A)].

The common features of these (normal) possessed states are that, under particular circumstances, with certain methods of induction, the person can enter into the possessed state by his/her own will, and can also at will reverse the state of being possessed and resume his/her ordinary condition. In other words, the state can be invoked for the needed period of time under the voluntary control of the person involved. Possessed states can also fulfill certain social functions, or healing practices. However, this is not necessarily true all the time. Occasionally, some possessed subjects may lose control, fall into a possessed state at any time, or have difficulty resuming their normal condition. Thus, the boundary between normal and morbid is not absolutely maintained. Some shamans may become vulnerable and manifest morbid mental conditions (Tseng, 1972).

2. Possession Disorders in Some Cultures

Possession disorders are believed to occur in many parts of the world. As mentioned previously, according to the medical anthropologist Bourguignon (1976), trance states tend to occur more in simple societies and possession states in more complicated societies. This suggests the possible relation between the level of complexity of a society and the mental condition of being possessed by another being. Possession and possession disorder tend to be reported more in psychiatric literature from Asian regions. This may reflect that such phenomena are still prevalent there and have therefore caught the interest of cultural psychiatrists for investigation and report.

a. Japan

Besides the orthodox religion of *Sin-do,* traditionally Japanese are pantheists, believing animals (such as foxs, raccoons, dogs, snakes), trees, mountains, stones, and other subjects are all associated with spirits. In Japanese folk legend, animal spirits, particularly the fox spirit, are commonly described. The spirit of the cunning fox can disguise itself into any human form, often a young lady, and play tricks on you. The Japanese commonly say *kitsune-ni-bakasareru,* literally meaning to be fooled by the spirit of a fox *(kitsune).* Perhaps related to this, when a person is possessed, people tend to interpret him as being possessed by an animal spirit, mostly a fox, and occasionally a dog or a cat. According to Kitanish (1993), after studying possession phenomena in Japan, possession by the spirit of a fox is widespread geograph-

ically in Japan, whereas possession by the spirits of dogs and snakes only occurs in the southern part of Japan (such as Shikoku and Kushiu Islands), indicating that there are geographical differences. Furthermore, Kitanish mentioned that the spirit of the animal that tends to possess people is believed to stay in certain households. The household with *tsukinomo-suji* (spirit lineage) tends to be looked down upon by others and is kept at a distance socially. It is speculated that such households may have originally been those of migrated families that wandered into the established village. Another explanation is that the possessing spirit was brought by a shaman to inhabit the designated household. It is generally believed that such animal spirits will be transmitted through marriage and kept within a family.

b. Korea

Perhaps due to the fact that Korea is close to Siberia geographically, the practice of shamanism in Korea is believed by scholars to exist from early history. Anthropological investigations of shamans and shamanism are well documented (Harvey, 1979; Kendall, 1985). Possession by animal spirits, deceased ancestors, or ghosts is still observed in the country.

c. Thailand

In Thailand, although most possessing beings are the spirits of animals or deceased persons, as elsewhere, there is a unique phenomenon by which a person can be possessed by the spirit of a living person. According to a cultural psychiatrist from Thailand, Sangun Suwanlert (1976), Thai people believe that *phii pob* is the soul of a living person that may come and go among people. When *phii pob* possesses you, you take the role of that living person. Such possession by a living person's soul is observed mainly in northern Thailand.

Suwanlert described the following interesting case from among his reports. A 16-year-old girl was sent to live with her grandmother at age 2, when her father died. Many years later, when her mother remarried, she came back to live with her mother and her stepfather. One day, when she witnessed her drunken stepfather slap her mother during an argument, she suddenly acted differently, as if she was one of her stepfather's male friends who lived in the next village. It was clear to others that she was possessed by *phii pob*. In a male voice, she warned her stepfather that if he did not behave, the ancestor's spirit would punish him by breaking his neck. After the stepfather, in front of relatives, promised that he would behave, the *phii pob,* the soul of the stepfather's friend, departed via the patient's mouth.

The case illustrates beautifully how a young girl, faced with a fearful situation, and without knowing how to deal with her drunken, abusive stepfather, turned herself (via a possession state) into a socially more powerful person and borrowed the authority of an ancestor to control her stepfather.

d. Taiwan

Despite governmental suppression during the Japanese occupation, the shamanistic practice become popular again after World War II, when Taiwan was returned to China. Associated with this, the phenomena of possession disorders became more visible than in the past. Cultural psychiatrist Jung-Kuang Wen (1996) conducted a community survey of a selected area in the south of Taiwan and estimated that the people who had possession experiences (both ordinary and morbid conditions) were not less than 1% of the adult population. He pointed out that the traditional belief of pantheism and ancestor worship — belief in close relations and interaction with deceased ancestors — serves as the common ground for the frequent occurrence of possessed states. However, it is speculated that, in contrast to Japan, the belief in the possibility of interference from an ancestor spirit is more intense for people in Taiwan. This is reflected in concepts of fortune-telling, shamanism, and daily-life language, such as "if you disgraced your ancestor, their spirit will come to punish you," or "if you are in trouble, you may ask your ancestor's spirit to protect you."

Through his investigation, Wen (1996) described that, in both normal possession and possession disorders, a person can be possessed by spirits of at least 12 different ranks, according to the hierarchy of deities. This ranking goes from the lowest wandering, wild spirit to a deceased infant's spirit, a deceased ancestor's spirit, the sprit of various historically recognized heros or generals, then to Guanyin, Buddha, and finally, the Jade Emperor — the highest deity recognized in Chinese folklore. Thus, theoretically, a shaman needs to identify the kind of deity that possesses the client and then try to be possessed by a higher ranking deity himself in order to overpower the client's spirit.

e. China

According to the available literature, possession disorders are reported more frequently in the northeastern region of China, including the areas previously called Manchuria and internal Mongolia. These areas are geographically close to Siberia, where anthropologists believe the practice of shamanism (in a narrow sense) originated.

According to Zhang (1992), a psychiatrist from Liaoning Province Mental Hospital, there were a total of 4714 forensic cases brought to the hospital for psychiatric evaluation. Of those cases, 52 (1.1%) had committed murder under possession disorders. Interestingly, among them, there were six groups of patients (with more than four people in each group) who carried out murder together. Most of them were family membes or relatives who had developed a collective trance state or a "shared" possession state. In these conditions, they killed their victims with the conviction that the person was possessed by an evil that needed to be exorcized.

Following is a group murder case reported by Zhang (1992). Mr. and Mrs. Wang were a middle-aged couple in their fifties. They had two sons. Mrs. Wang had a past history of possessed episodes, claiming that she was often possessed by the spirit of her deceased mother-in-law. Their 24-year-old eldest son, after illegally cohabiting with his girlfriend, began to behave seclusively and strangely, claiming that he was a "headless evil" and intended to kill all of his family members. One night, hearing a noise on the roof, the mother suddenly fell into a possessed state, claiming that she was possessed by a shaman who had come to expel the headless evil from her son. She induced her husband, Mr. Wang, and her 18-year-old son to fall into trance states. In these states, together they pounded 43 nails into the eldest son's body and stabbed his abdomen with a knife. As a result, the eldest son died. After the event, Mrs. Wang remained in a trance state for 10 days, claiming that she had expelled and killed the dangerous headless evil. After she recovered from her trance state and learned that she had killed her son, she began to cry loudly.

Dynamically, a tempting interpretation is that the mother who psychologically lost her son to his girlfriend reacted with the belief that her son was evil. Her possessed state gave her an excuse to act out her wish to punish the unfilial (or emotionally betraying) son. Clinically, it is a case of associated or collective mental disorders, which take place among the members of a family. The common belief in the possibility of a person being possessed by evil and the need to conduct an exorcism was the basis for this family group of psychiatric disorders.

3. Boundary between Possession Disorders and Possession Psychoses

From the case just described, it becomes immediately clear that the distinction between possession disorder (of a hysterical nature) and possession psychoses is not merely a clinical matter, but also a forensic challenge, if the patient is involved in a crime.

The term "invocation psychosis" is still used by psychiatrists in some societies, including Japan. It refers to a psychotic condition characterized by the delusion of being possessed, in addition to other psychotic pictures, including hallucination, bizarre behavior, and thought disorder. This condition, even though manifested as a possession state, is different from possession disorder of a hysterical nature in that

its onset is not necessarily sudden or in reaction to external stress, it may last a relatively long time, more than several weeks or months, and it does not respond favorably to any psychological treatment for underlying psychological stress. From a forensic point of view, the patient suffering from this condition is considered less responsible for criminal acts that he or she may commit.

Invocation psychosis should not be confused with "hysterical psychosis," which has been misused by some medical anthropologists to include all mental disorders in different cultures that are of a hysterical nature, i.e., that have an acute onset and a brief and benign course. The culture-related specific disorders of *latah,* arctic hysteria, *amok,* and others have been included in this ill-defined term. In an entirely different way, some psychiatrists still use the term hysterical psychosis to refer to the clinical condition characterized by a brief and acute psychotic state, often occurring as a reaction to stress, associated with symptoms of a theatrical nature, and from which the patient tends to recover with a good prognosis, without mental sequels.

C. Altered Personality Disorder

Characteristically different from possession disorder is the altered personality. In the latter there is no interpretation by either the patient him/herself or other people that the patient is possessed by "others." It is understood that the person alternates between (or among) different personalities either in a trance state or without it. In other words, there is a psychological and not a supernatural interpretation of the phenomena. Therefore, it is observed mainly in "modernized" societies where folk beliefs of a supernatural nature have more or less diminished.

It is a common notion among psychiatrists that, in traditional societies, where trance and possession states are more frequent, the phenomena of altered personality and multiple personality disorders are seldom found. In contrast, in modern societies, possessed disorders are rare or diminishing, and double or multiple personality disorders are becoming more prevalent.

According to Ross (1991), the frequency of diagnosed multiple personality disorder in clinical populations increased exponentially during the 1980s. Reviewing the entire world literature, Greaves (1980) pointed out that not more than a couple of hundred cases (mainly in Western societies) have been reported since the beginning of this century. However, according to Ross, P. Coons in 1986 estimated that 6000 cases of multiple personality disorders had been diagnosed in North America.

In contrast to this, Adityanjee, Raju, and Khandelwal (1989) in India reported that only two cases of multiple personality disorder had been reported in India in the past. They reported encountering three more cases over a period of 3 years at a psychiatric clinic in New Delhi. Based on their clinical experience, Adityanjee and colleagues estimated that the frequency of this disorder was about 0.15 per 1000 psychiatric outpatients per year in their clinic. They claimed that there was a frequent diagnosis of possession disorder, but the diagnosis of multiple personality disorder was rare.

A similar situation has been observed in Japan. In order to confirm the clinical impression of Japanese psychiatrists, Takahashi (1990) conducted a review of 489 psychiatric inpatients who were hospitalized during a 5-year period (1983–1988) in the psychiatric ward of the College General Hospital of Yamahashi Medical College where he worked. He reported that seven cases were diagnosed as dissociative disorders, but none were multiple personality disorders. It may be criticized that he used psychiatric inpatients rather than outpatients for the study, but he claimed that his findings reflected the situation in Japan: that multiple personality disorders are rare and, instead, there are cases of dissociation and possession disorder.

Beyond the influence of diagnostic practice patterns in different societies, there is good reason to speculate that, in association with the level of modernization or the degree of belief about folk supernatural powers, there is a trend away from the possessed state to the altered personality state.

If we think carefully, we will realize that the possession state and the altered personality state are similar, except that the former is interpreted as the takeover of the self by an "external (supernatural) being," whereas the latter is the taking over of the self by an "internal (psychological) being," or another part of the self. Both offer mechanisms for avoiding taking responsibility for one's actions, but in different ways, based on the common beliefs shared by the people in the society.

D. Possession without Alterations

Finally, one unique phenomenon — Zar sickness — needs to be mentioned here. According to Modarressi (1968), Zar is a possession cult found in Ethiopia, the Sudan, Egypt, and some parts of Arabia. It is based on the belief that a person is "possessed" (or inhabited) permanently by a spiritual being, Zar, who may cause illness if he is not satisfied. Thus, the Zar cult is devoted to healing, with the person going into a trance-possessed state in which the Zar spirit expresses the demands to be met. As pointed out by Bourguignon (1968), possession (by Zar) is seen as the cause of illness, and a possession–trance is induced in the healing ceremony in order to question the spirit as to its demands. However, the spirit is not exorcized or dispatched during the healing ceremony. Rather, attempts are made to meet its demands through certain manipulations of the patient's social environment. It is interesting that although a person is believed to be "possessed" by Zar for life, he does not manifest any unusual mental phenomena or personality alterations in his regular life, beyond the transient trance–possession state induced during the Zar ceremony. Zar possession is merely a concept and belief of being possessed.

IV. FINAL INTEGRATION

A. Vicissitude Fate of the Disorders

Although there are no statistical data to confirm this directly, based on clinical observations that have been made through time, it is the consensus among clinicians that there has been an obvious change in the frequency of hysteria from both historical and geographic perspectives. Generally, it has been noted that hysterical disorders, whether in simple, trance, possessed, or conversion forms, are gradually fading away in many societies in which they used to be prevalent. The reasons are unclear, but several possibilities are offered in the following discussion.

B. Cultural Aspects of Hysteria-Related Disorders

1. Multiple Levels of Cultural Impact

As has been elaborated previously [cross-reference to Chapter 11: Culture and Psychopathology (Section II,A–F)], there are basically five ways that culture impacts psychopathology: through psycho-pathogenic, -plastic, -selective, -facilitating, and -reactive effects. This is not only true of hysteria but in every way.

Based on contemporary psychiatric knowledge, hysteria is understood as a reaction to psychological stress. However, the nature of stress varies according to cultural background. In some societies, insoluble stress for a young person may be created by parental authority, which does not permit him to date someone who is not approved by the parents, or forces him to obey his parents and marry someone without affection. Severe stress might also be experienced by a submissive wife who has no way of handling her husband's unfaithful behavior, or of dealing with a constantly overpowering and abusive mother-in-law. It is not uncommon for a person to develop a hysterical disorder when such socioculturally created stresses go beyond their threshold for endurance. However, these stresses may not be important in other societies. Instead, breaking off a romantic relationship, the traumatic loss of a family member, loneliness associated aging, and so on may constitute major problems in life, which may cause a hysterical reaction. Becoming depressed or indulging in excessive drinking or sub-

stance abuse may be other choices. Thus, culture has a **pathogenic** as well as a **pathoselective** effect with regard to hysteria.

Centered around the core issue of altered consciousness, there are many ways to manifest hysteria-related disorders: as a simple emotional outburst, a simple trance, a specific dissociated condition, or a more complicated possessed state or altered personality. Thus, culture has a **pathoplastic** effect. Even with the possessed state, there are many "other beings" that can possess the person, depending on the kind of animal spirits or deities that are familiar to him and to others in the community. Thus, there are variations of Zar possession, fox spirit possession, and *phii pob* possession observed in different cultures.

The most important characteristics of hysteria are its dramatic reaction to stress and the theatrical quality of its response to audiences — family members, friends, and people surrounding the patient, including care deliverers. The outcome of the disorder will vary depending on how these people conceive and understand the disorder, how they react toward the illness-event, and how they deal with the patient during the hysterical attack. A person claiming that he is possessed by the spirit of his deceased ancestor, for instance, needs to be believed by the people around him, or the morbid condition, unreinforced, will not last long. It is like an actor who cannot give a performance without an interested audience. Thus, culture contributes significantly to both the **pathoreactive** and the **pathofacilitating** effects. If family members, friends, and other people in the community regard the hysteria as a sign of weakness in the patient's personality, his inability to handle stress, and an unconscious calling for attention and help-seeking, then the severity of the disorder will be reduced and the morbid condition will not last long. This may explain why hysteria-related disorders occur less in modern societies, where people are more or less psychologically educated and value surviving independently, without seeking help and attention from others.

Thus, hysteria is a psychological disorder very much bound by cultural settings. The vicissitude of the disorder is directly determined by the views, attitudes, and reactions shared by the culture toward the phenomenon. During Victorian times in Europe, it was almost fashionable for a lady to "faint" in public if she encountered a stressful situation or heard bad news. Even in the movie *Gone with the Wind,* written about the mid-19th century, Scarlett fainted to got attention from gentlemen. Can you imagine what would happen if a contemporary American woman habitually fainted? Most likely she would receive negative comments from others and, certainly, she would be less likely to receive kind treatment from men.

2. Cultural Implication of Altered Consciousness States

After elaborating on the vicissitude of hysteria from the perspective of time, it is pertinent to ask what the function of hysteria has been in traditional cultures. The answer is clear and simple: hysterical episodes offer patients a socially acceptable relief from stress and a culturally relevant outlet from repression. It gives a social signal to family, friends and others that the person concerned is on the verge of a breakdown and needs special attention. Because it is not the patient him/herself who exhibits the behavior during the episode of altered consciousness and/or personality, whatever he or she says, complains about, or requests is attributed to others. Thus, a hysterical attack serves as a safety valve for an individual.

3. Alternative Outlets in Modern Life

What happens in modern societies in which people feel that the person is responsible for his or her behavior even during the altered consciousness state, and the person thus loses the privilege of this socioculturally sanctioned time-out or safety valve?

The answer is also simple: Instead of a hysterically induced trance, dissociation, or possession state, people in contemporary modern societies experience trance or dissociation induced by other means. These include individual trances through the practice of meditation, group trances through rock music performances or religious ceremonies in ordinary daily life, or, morbidly, trances induced by chemical substance abuse. In other words, modern men still need alternative conscious states, but find them in different ways.

As the privilege of being possessed by "(supernatural) others" is removed from the modern scientific world, the contemporary person is also left with the choice of being possessed by other parts of the "self," with or without an altered consciousness state, i.e., through double or multiple personalities.

D. CLINICAL CRITICS: CONTEMPORARY IGNORANCE (IN THE WEST)

From a world perspective, it is obvious that due to their current clinical situations and experiences, there is professional ignorance of hysteria-related mental conditions among psychiatrists in European and North American societies. The academic ignorance can be described in several areas.

Due to the descriptive orientation in the present DSM system, the hysterical disorder is split into the different compartments of dissociated and conversion disorder. This diverts attention from the basic element of the disorder, its reactive and defensive nature. The symbolic meaning and protective function of the disorder are disconnected from the sociocultural setting in which it takes place. Phenomenologically, only the specific forms of the disorder, such as dissociative amnesia, depersonalization or identity disorder, or conversion disorder, are concerned, whereas the basic type of the hysterical disorder, such as emotional turmoil, simple trance, or stupor state (most commonly observed in non-Western societies), is almost neglected.

Associated with this is the neglect of possession disorder, which is still observed frequently in many non-Western societies. Instead, only the altered personality disorder is included in the classification system. The epidemic occurrence of hysteria, or mass hysteria, which is still not observed infrequently in developing as well as developed societies, is not included in the classification system.

The ignorance described earlier is primarily due to the rarity of trance, dissociation, and possession in modern Western societies. However, it needs to be recognized that in non-Western societies, which comprise more than three-quarters of the world's population, these phenomena are still prevalent and require continued clinical attention and consideration.

Trance, dissociation, and possession are various mental conditions experienced by human beings, whether ordinary, special, or morbid. They are predominantly psychologically related and culturally attributed mental conditions that are unique, interesting, and still mysterious, and deserving of greater attention.

REFERENCES

Adityanjee, Raju, G.S.P., & Khandelwal, S.K. (1989). Current status of multiple personality disorder in India. *American Journal of Psychiatry, 146*(12), 1607–1610.

Alexander, P.J., Joseph, S., & Das, A. (1997). Limited utility of ICD-10 and DSM-IV classification of dissociative and conversion disorders in India. *Acta Psychiatrica Scandinavica, 95*, 177–182.

American Psychiatric Association (APA). (1980). *Diagnostic and Statistical Manual of Mental Disorders,* (3rd rev.) (DSM-III). Washington DC: APA.

Bourguignon, E. (1968). World distribution and patterns of possession states. In R. Prince (Ed.), *Trance and possession states* (Proceedings of Second Annual Conference). Montreal: R.M. Bucke Memorial Society.

Bourguignon, E. (Ed.). (1973). *Religion, altered states of consciousness, and social change.* Columbus: Ohio State University Press.

Bourguignon, E. (1976). Possession and trance in cross-cultural studies of mental health. In W.P. Lebra (Ed.), *Culture-bound syndromes, ethnopsychiatry, and alternate therapies* (pp. 47–55). Honolulu: University Press of Hawaii.

Bremner, J.D., Southwick, S., Brett, E., Fontana, A., Rosenheck, R., & Charney, D.S. (1992). Dissociation and posttraumtic stress disorder in Vietnam combat veterans. *American Journal of Psychiatry, 149*(3), 328–332.

Das, P.S., & Saxena, S. (1991). Classification of dissociative states in DSM-III-R and ICD-10 (1989 draft). *British Journal of Psychiatry, 159*, 425–427.

Dube, K.C. (1970). A study of prevalence and biosocial variables in mental illness in a rural and an urban community in Uttar Pradesh, India. *Acta Psychiatrica Scandinavica, 46*, 327–359.

Eguchi, S.Y. (1991). Between folk concepts of illness and psychiatric diagnosis: Kitsune-tuski (folk possession) in a mountain village of western Japan. *Culture, Medicine and Psychiatry, 15*(4), 421–452.

Epidemic Survey Collaboratory Teams. (1986). Epidemic survey of neurotic disorders in 12 geographic areas. *Chinese Neuropsychatric Journal, 19,* 87–91.

Greaves, G.B. (1980). Multiple personality disorder: 165 years after Mary Reynolds. *Journal of Nervous and Mental Disease, 168,* 577–596.

Greenbaum, L. (1973). Possession trance in Sub-Saharan Africa: A descriptive analysis of fourteen societies. In E. Bougguignon (Ed.), *Religion, altered states of consciousness, and social change* (pp. 58–87). Columbus: Ohio State University Press.

Harvey, Y.S.K. (1979). *Six Korean women: The socialization of shamans.* New York: West Publishing.

Kendall, L. (1985). *Shamans, housewives and other restless spirits: Women in Korean ritual life.* Honolulu: University of Hawaii Press.

Kitanish, K. (1993). Possession phenomena in Japan. In *The Proceedings of the Fourth Cultural Psychiatry Symposium: Possession phenomena in East Asia* (pp. 34–50). Seoul: East Asian Academy of Cultural Psychiatry.

Lebra, T.S. (1976). Taking the role of supernatural "other": Spirit possession in a Japanese healing cult. In W.P. Lebra (Ed.), *Culture-bound syndromes, ethnopsychiatry, and alternate therapies* (pp. 88–100). Honolulu: University Press of Hawaii.

Leff, J. (1981). The history and geography of hysteria. In J, Leff. *Psychiatry around the globe.* New York: Dekker.

Luo, H.C., & Zhou, C.S. (1984). Clinical analysis of 1,622 psychiatric emergency cases. *Chinese Neuropsychiatric Journal, 17*(3), 137–138.

Modarressi, T. (1968). The Zar cult in South Iran. In R. Prince (Ed.), *Trance and possession states* (Proceedings of Second Annual Conference). Montreal: R.M. Bucke Memorial Society.

Nandi, D.N., Banerjee, G., Nadi, S., & Nandi, P. (1992). Is hysteria on the wane? *British Journal of Psychiatry, 160,* 87–91.

Prince, R. (Ed.) (1968). *Trance and possession states* (Proceedings of Second Annual Conference). Montreal: R.M. Bucke Memorial Society.

Ross, C.A. (1991). Epidemiology of multiple personality disorder and dissociation. *Psychiatric Clinics of North American, 14*(3), 503–517.

Sasaki, Y. (1969). Psychiatric study of the shaman in Japan. In W. Caudill & T.Y. Lin (Eds.), *Mental health research in Asia and the Pacific* (pp. 223–241). Honolulu: East-West Center Press.

Saxena, S., & Prasad, K.V.S.R. (1989). DSM-III subclassification of dissociative disorder applied to psychiatric outpatients in India. *American Journal of Psychiatry, 146*(2), 261–262.

Srinath, S., Bharat, S., Girimaji, S., & Seshadri, S. (1993). Characteristics of a child inpatient population with hysteria in India. *Journal of the American Academic Child and Adolescent Psychiatry, 32*(4), 822–825.

Stefanis, C., Markidis, M., & Christodoulou, G. (1976). Observations on the evolution of the hysterical symptomatology. *British Journal of Psychiatry, 128,* 269–275.

Suwanlert, S. (1976). *Phii pob:* Spirit possession in rural Thailand. In W.P. Lebra (Ed.), *Culture-bound syndromes, ethnopsychiatry, and alternate therapies* (pp. 68–87). Honolulu: University Press of Hawaii.

Takahashi, Y. (1990). Is multiple personality really rare in Japan? *Dissociation, 3*(2), 57–59.

Tseng, W.S. (1972). Psychiatric study of shaminism in Taiwan. *Archives of General Psychiatry, 26,* 561–565.

Tseng, W.S. (1973). The development of psychiatric concepts in traditional Chinese medicine. *Archives of General Psychiatry, 29,* 569–575.

Vieth, I. (1965). *Hysteria: The history of a disease.* Chicago: University of Chicago Press.

Ward, C.A. (1980). Spirit possession and mental health: A psycho-anthropological perspective. *Human Relations, 33*(3), 146–163.

Ward, C.A. (Ed.). (1989). *Culture and altered states of consciousness.* Beverly Hills, CA: Sage.

Wen, J.-K. (1996). Possession phenomena and psychothreapy. In W.S. Tseng (Ed.), *Chinese mind and therapy* (pp. 295–330). Taipei: Laureate Publisher (in Chinese).

World Health Organization (WHO). (1992). *International classification of Disease* (10th rev.) (ICD-10). Geneva: WHO.

Zhang, X.F. (1992). A report of 32 cases with hysteria involved in homicide. *Chinese Mental Health Journal, 6*(4), 175–176 (in Chinese).

18

Disorders of Depression

I. INTRODUCTION

The cultural aspects of depression have created keen interest among cultural psychiatrists since the 1960s. This coincided with the availability of antidepressants for treatment, but was motivated by the discovery that, despite a sharply increasing clinical trend in Euro-American societies of diagnosing depression, there was a low prevalence of it in non-Western societies. Instead of investigating why there were fewer depressive cases observed in non-Western societies, many Western clinicians and investigators turned their attention to the examination and exploration of the possibility that depression might be masked in its manifestation (as an emotional expression of depression) in non-Western societies.

In the early stages, in order to explore the cross-cultural aspects of depression, cultural psychiatrists from McGill University, Murphy, Wittkower, and Chance (1967), asked psychiatrists around the world for their "impressions" of the symptomatology of depression in their cultural areas. The replies to the question indicate that there is a basic depressive disorder, which, in all cultures, exhibits certain primary symptoms: a depressive mood, diurnal mood change,

insomnia with early morning wakening, and diminution of interest in one's social environment. Other (secondary) symptoms, such as thought retardation and self-depreciation, appear to be shaped culturally. This "instant research" was criticized by scholars for its methodology. Nevertheless, it was an initial attempt to use the concept of primary and secondary symptoms to explore possible cultural variations of depressive manifestations. From psychological and social perspectives, the theory has been proposed that the level of social cohesion contributes to the psychological life of people, which in turn might relate to the occurrence of depression within a society (Chance, 1964).

With an increase in clinical knowledge, psychiatrists now take the view that depression, particularly of a severe or endogenous type, is closely related to biological factors. However, as pointed out by Marsella, Sartorius, Jablensky, and Fenton (1985), even if some types of depression are shown to have primary biological causes, cultural factors could still exert pathoplastic effects (modifying the behavioral expression of the biological factors) and pathoreactive effects (interpreting abnormal experiences and responding to the social reactions to that behavior).

Even though the manifestation of depression is rather straightforward and uncomplicated, there are difficulties in cross-cultural studies of depression, simply from the standpoint of the basic issues of diagnostic concepts and categorization (Horwath & Weissman, 1995). Depressive mood disorders include various disorders centering around the disturbance of the mood. Historically, attempts have been made to categorize them by various diagnostic terms, e.g., endogenous versus reactive depression, psychotic versus neurotic depression, and major depression versus (minor) dysthymic disorder. Such diverse diagnostic categories make it difficult, if not impossible, to meaningfully compare data obtained from different periods and across cultures. Further, because the reaction to loss or frustration is not always evidenced as a depressive mood disorder, but could be manifested as a somatoform disorder, substance abuse, drinking problems, or violent or suicidal behavior, an investigation from cross-cultural perspectives is complicated. It is clear, however, that in order to pursue the cultural aspects of depression, it is better to focus on minor depression with a reactive nature (in contrast to major depression with an endogenous nature), which is characterized primarily by psychological dimensions and whose cultural attributes are easier to examine.

Associated with the improvement of epidemiological study in the community, more information is becoming available about different ethnic groups in a society. Reviewing data from the National Comorbidity Survey, Blazer, Kessler, McGonagle, and Swartz (1994) have indicated that major depression is a frequent and disabling psychiatric disorder in the United States. Concerning African-Americans, Brown, Ahmed, Gary, and Milburn (1995) examined a probability sample of urban African adults, 20 years of age and older, by the National Institute of Mental Health Diagnostic Interview Schedule, and found a 1-year prevalence of 3.1% for major depression. They reported that young age and fair to poor physical health appear to be more powerful risk factors for major depression among African-Americans than other variables. Golding, Karne, and Rutter (1990)

carried out a survey of selected Mexican-Americans. They reported that the lifetime prevalence of symptoms of a major depressive episode for Mexican-Americans born in the United States resembled that of non-Hispanic Caucasian-Americans born in the United States; however, the rates for Mexican-Americans born in Mexico were lower in eight of nine symptoms clusters. In their study of Jews, Levav, Kohn, Golding, and Weissman (1997) analyzed data from the National Institute of Mental Health Epidemiologic Catchment Area (ECA) study regarding Jews, Catholics, Protestants, individuals in other religious groups, and individuals with no religious affiliation from the Los Angeles and New Haven catchment areas. They revealed that while no differences were found among females, Jewish males had significantly higher rates of major depression than the other groups. They pointed out that the results support in part the earlier speculation that Jews have higher rates of major depression.

II. EMOTIONAL EXPERIENCE OF DEPRESSION

A. QUESTIONS ABOUT DIFFERENT QUALITIES OF DEPRESSION

As with anxiety, elaborated previously (in Chapter 15: Anxiety Disorders), there is a great breadth of issues raised by a cross-cultural study of depression, including: Do all people, regardless of their cultures, experience emotions in similar ways? Does the description of the experience of an emotion change from culture to culture, or is it the same?

In order to explore cross-cultural variations in the meaning and subjective experience of depression, Tanaka-Matsumi and Marsella (1976) asked Japanese, Japanese-American, and Caucasian-American college students to associate a word with "depression." According to them, of the Japanese students in Japan, 44% gave "rain" and "cloud" and 22% gave "dark" and "gray" — relating depression to external environment (weather) or objective terms (color). Nearly 19% supplied words related to somatic problems and illness, namely: "disease," "tiredness," "headache," or "fatigue." In contrast to this, among Japanese-American students in Hawaii, about 56% gave "sadness" and 25% "loneliness" — reflecting internal moods. The Japanese-American associations were very similar to those given by Caucasian-American students on the United States mainland. Tanaka-Matsumi and Marsella concluded that Japanese do not experience depression in the same way as Americans. Nor do they express feelings in the same way. For the Japanese, concrete images from nature allow personal emotions to be expressed impersonally. As this particular study utilized normal college students as subjects, a basic question still remained: Are the tendencies revealed applicable to clinically depressed groups?

B. INQUIRIES ABOUT THE MASKING OF DEPRESSION

Another clinical concept used by psychiatrists in the past was "masked depression," which takes the view that certain individuals, in reacting to loss or frustration, instead of manifesting the emotional reaction of depression, show other clinical pictures, such as somatization or behavior problems. This view is founded on the basic assumption that when a person encounters the psychological trauma of loss or frustration, he or she responds primarily with the mood disorder of "depression." If, for some reason, the person is not able to respond with depression, and the trauma is manifested by another mental condition, it is considered to be masked depression. This clinical assumption is not useful, and is even misleading, in cross-cultural applications. It assumes that human beings are allowed to react emotionally only in a defined way, ignoring that there are rich variations in the emotional and behavioral reactions of human beings in different cultural environments. It is biased in identifying one reaction as primary and others as masked.

C. PATTERNS OF CLINICAL PRESENTATION: DEPRESSION AND SOMATIC SYMPTOMS

From a cultural perspective, it is more useful to understand the problem–presentation styles (or patterns) manifested by patients. As elaborated subsequently in Chapter 26 [Therapist and Patient (Section II,A–D)], the information and problems presented by patients to physicians are subject to various factors, including patient–therapist relations, culturally molded patterns of making complaints, and the clinical setting in which the interactions take place. This also applies to depression. The meaning of complaining about depression versus somatic symptoms deserves careful evaluation and consideration. Simon, von Korff, Piccinelli, Fullerton, and Ormel, (1999) used data from the World Health Organization study of psychological problems in general healthcare to examine the relation between somatic symptoms and depression. They found out that among patients studied at 15 primary care centers in 14 countries on five continents, about 10% who presented somatic symptoms to the primary caretaker met the criteria for major depression. Further, they revealed that a somatic presentation was more common at centers where patients lacked an ongoing relationship with a primary care physician than at centers where most patients had a personal physician. This supports indirectly the view that the nature of complaints made by the patients is closely related to patient–doctor relations.

III. VARIATIONS IN CLINICAL PICTURES

A. VARIATIONS OF DEPRESSION AS A CLINICAL CONDITION

Even focusing merely on clinically recognized conditions of "depression," cultural variations are recognized. In the late 1970s, German cultural psychiatrist Wolfgang Pfeiffer (1968) reviewed many works on depression in non-European cultures. As already pointed out, the "core" symptoms of depression (i.e., change of mood, disruption of physiological functions, such as sleep and appetite, and hypochondriacal symptoms) in these cultures were the same as in Europe. However, other symptoms, such as feelings of guilt and suicidal tendencies, showed variations of frequency and intensity among cultures. This view was later supported by other investigators (Binitie, 1975; Sartorius, 1975).

1. Individual Scholars' Reports

There are many clinical reports that back up the view just given. For instance, based on clinical observation of depressive illness in Afghanistan, Waziri (1973) reported that while the biological symptoms of depression were similar to other ethnic groups, the majority of depressed patients expressed "death wishes" instead of suicidal intentions or thoughts. In Afghanistan, with their Muslim religious backgrounds, people believe suicide is a sin. Waziri said that 54% of the depressed patients who were asked how they viewed life answered that they "wished they were dead" or that they had "prayed to God to take their life away." Actually, the suicide rate among the general population is very low, namely 0.25 per 100,000 population (Gobar, 1970). This illustrates that even though a suicidal tendency is associated with depression, cultural attitudes either sanctioning or forbidding self-destruction can modify the expression of suicidal ideas.

The presence or absence of self-depreciation, self-blame in the form of feeling ashamed or guilty, is another aspect that has gained attention and been debated from cross-cultural perspectives. According to Prince (1968), in Africa, mental–emotional self-castigation is rare or absent in the early stages of depressed patients. Earlier, Murphy and associates (1967) had proposed that the higher incidence of guilt feelings in Western cultures was perhaps due to the influence of Christian religion. However, after examining depressed Christian and Muslim patients in Cairo, El-Islam (1969) reported that the presence or absence of guilt feelings was often associated with the level of education or literacy and the degree of depression and not to religious background. He concluded that guilt and Christianity are not necessarily closely linked.

In Iraq, it was noted that open, hostile aggression is often a part of depression. From there, Bazzoui (1970) reported that aggressive behavior and paranoid ideas were relatively common in depressed patients. In his interpretation, this was because the primitive mechanisms of defense in the forms of attack and escape were not deeply suppressed in Iraqi culture. He pointed out that, in affective illness, there are numerous mechanisms (escape or attack, denial or project, for instance) that are open to people from many cultures. The *amok* syndrome [elaborated previously in Chapter 13: Culture-Related Specific Syndromes (Section II,A,1)] provides an extreme example, i.e., becoming homicidal, even en masse and nonselectively, to deal with psychological frustration or insult.

Manson, shore, and Bloom (1985) pointed out problems of cross-cultural application in the use of officially existing classification criteria to diagnose depression. Based on their clinical experiences with Native Americans, they pointed out that the duration of depression for Native Americans is relatively shorter (often only a few weeks) than the duration arbitrarily defined by the Diagnostic and Statistical Manual for Mental Disorders (DSM).

2. WHO's International Survey of Depressive Symptomatology

The possibility of cultural variations of depressive symptomatology was investigated systematically by WHO, using standardized methods, beginning in 1972 (Sartorius et al., 1983). Five study centers in four countries were involved: Basel (Switzerland), Montreal (Canada), Nagasaki (Japan), Teheran (Iran), and Tokyo (Japan). The WHO Schedule for Standardized Assessment of Depressive Disorders (SADD) was used for clinical assessment by trained clinicians in each study center. Specified diagnostic criteria of the International Statistical Classification of Diseases and

Related Health Problems, 9th Version (ICD-9), was included in the study of depressive patients. A total of 573 patients from the five centers were examined. The results revealed similar patterns of depressive disorders in all settings. Patients in all the sites were found to have high frequencies of sadness, joylessness, anxiety, tension, lack of energy, loss of interest, concentration difficulties, and feelings of inadequacy, but there were also considerable variations in the frequencies with which certain symptoms appeared across the study centers. For example, guilt feelings were present in 68% of the Swiss patients, but in only 32% of the Iranian patients; somatic symptoms were present in 57% of the Iranian patients, but in only 27% of the Canadian patients. Suicidal ideas were present in 70% of the Canadian patients, but in only 40% of the Japanese patients. There were different levels of severity of depression in the different study centers — patients in Nagasaki, Montreal, and Basel were more anergic and retarded than patients in Tokyo and Teheran. It is not clear whether the differences in frequencies of certain symptoms were due to those levels of severity or to ethnocultural variations.

A 10-year follow-up of the cohorts of these depressed patients was carried out. Available data from Basle, Nagasaki, and Tokyo revealed interesting findings. Despite the differences in countries, the best clinical course (one or two reasonably short episodes of depression with complete remission between episodes) was experienced twice as frequently in patients diagnosed with endogenous depression than in those diagnosed with psychogenic depression (Thornicroft & Sartorius, 1993).

B. MIXED ANXIETY–DEPRESSION–SOMATIC STATE

Closely associated with what has been discussed, it is important for clinicians to be aware that the clearly defined and sharply distinguished depressive state is not necessarily a rule. Rather, it is often mixed with anxiety and a somatic state. This is true for patients from our society and, even more so, from societies with different cultures. The disorders of depression include various clinical conditions on a spectrum that ranges from primarily biologically determined depressive "disorders" (exemplified by endogenous, periodically occurring depression) to predominantly psychologically related depressive "reactions." The human mind does not respond to an internal or external situation purely according to a defined "disorder." This is particularly true when a person is reacting to psychological distress. The response is often a combination of anxiety, depression, anger, a feeling of frustration, and many concomitant physiological symptoms. This is very important for cross-cultural applications. Diagnostically mixed types of disorders can be more the rule than the exception. Sometimes, when a classification system that originated from one culture is applied to another, an "atypical" type is a more typical occurrence, while a "typical" type is more atypical.

C. ALTERED PSYCHIATRIC CONDITIONS

Following this view, we would discover that many diagnostic categories identified by official diagnostic classification systems could be closely related to and centered around the same problems, only manifested differently from a phenomenological perspective. It is clear to clinicians that depressive disorders are often associated with the clinical problems of alcoholism, substance abuse, violence, or homicidal or suicidal behavior as peripherally associated disorders. This would become much clearer if examined from a cross-cultural perspective; it would be found that many psychiatric conditions occur, not as peripherally "associated" disorders, but as "alternative" disorders.

Reviewing clinical studies from non-Western cultures, Marsella and colleagues (1985) explained that all of the studies allude to the reduced frequency or absence of psychological components of depression and the dominance of somatic aspects in non-Western cultures. Kleinman (1982) even tried to rediagnose neurasthenia observed in China as a depressive disorder rather than recognizing neurasthenia as an alternative clinical entity that exists in China and is recognized by Chinese psychiatrists.

IV. THE STUDY OF FREQUENCY OF DEPRESSION

Although many investigators have reported the frequency of depression in different societies, a meaningful cross-cultural comparison is limited. As mentioned at the beginning of this chapter, the clinical manifestation of depression is more straightforward and uncomplicated than other psychopathologies. However, there are difficulties in the cross-cultural study of depression, particularly regarding frequency of occurrence, that stem its diagnostic categorization. Historically, psychiatrists have used various diagnostic categories for depression such as endogenous depression, reactive depression, depressive psychosis, neurotic depression, major depression, and dysthymic disorder. These categories make it difficult to compare cross-cultural data obtained in the past from different cultures. What is needed is a cross-cultural epidemiological study that uses standardized methods and uniform diagnostic criteria. However, even then, clinical problems would remain. In reality, there are not only different kinds of depressive nosological entities, but often different degrees of depression of the same diagnostic entity. Thus, it becomes necessary to deal with the different levels of severity of depression. Theoretically, the situation is complicated because the reaction to loss or frustration is not always evidenced as the mood disorder of depression, but could be manifested as alternative psychiatric disorders, such as substance abuse, drinking problems, or violent or suicidal behavior, complicating a cross-cultural investigation.

It is clear that in order to make meaningful comparisons, there is a need to specify particular diagnostic entities for evaluation rather than comparing "depression" as a whole. From a cultural perspective, it is better to focus on minor depression, with its reactive nature (in contrast to major depression, with its endogenous nature), because it is characterized more by psychological dimensions and is easier to examine from a cultural standpoint.

V. CULTURAL CONTRIBUTIONS TO CAUSES OF DEPRESSION

Perhaps, from a cultural psychiatric point of view, one of the most useful areas of study is the psychological causes of depression from a cross-cultural perspective because it offers a rich resource of examples of how human beings experience psychological trauma or distress and react to loss or frustration in various ways. Of course, it would need to focus on the study of "reactive" rather than "endogenous" depression. Dynamic psychiatrists view depression as a reaction to loss, deprivation, frustration, injury to self-esteem, conflict over the aggressive drive, or as a threat to a personality structure marked by narcissism or dependency. In addition to these clinical theories, the psychological causes for depression can also include social–cultural determinants.

Many clinicians speculate that childhood separation produces a vulnerability to depression that can be triggered by separation in adult life. Not only a parent's death during one's childhood can precipitate later depression, but separation, divorce, or prolonged absence of parents may cause the same delayed result. It is not always the loss itself that plants the seed of later depression. The circumstances of the original loss and the provision or lack of alternative relationships or supportive figures also influence the emotional impact of the initial trauma. From a sociocultural viewpoint, family structure (such as the nuclear or extended family), child-rearing practices (e.g., child rearing with or without care), and the presence or absence of parental substitutes (e.g., grandparents or aunts who live nearby) all must be considered as causes or deterrents to later depression. In societies that discourage divorce or parental separation, and in those that provide a satisfactory substitute for a dead parent, perhaps a future depressive episode may not occur. In such cases, when a child is reared with care, support, and concern, the early separation experience carries less potential for emotional trouble later on.

How a community views death and ritualizes mourning may also affect the occurrence of depression. In Samoa, death is seen as a natural event in life experience. Behavior patterns in the Samoan family and community provide effective support when someone dies (Ablon, 1971). In Fiji, Indian people still hold the traditional view that when a woman's husband passes away, she is no longer allowed to participate in any social activities or to have any social contact with men other than her father-in-law and brothers-in-law. Remarriage is unthinkable, even if she is still young. She is expected to devote herself to the care of her own children and to observe her widowhood for the rest of her life. Consequently, many widows suffer from depression. This phenomenon is not observed among the Fijian women living on the same island, as the indigenous Fijians have no such views of or practices for widows.

A social, occupational, or economically deprived status can also help weave the fabric of depression. In fact, the minority status of an ethnic group may outweigh ethnic characteristics as a contributing cause of depressive illness. Fernando (1975) compared Jewish and Protestant depressive patients in the East End of London. He studied familial and social factors and found that increasing paternal inadequacy and weakening ethnic links and religious faith were related to depressive ills among Jews, but not among Protestants. He suggested that mental stress arose from the marginal position of Jews in British society rather than from specific traits or customs within Jewish culture.

Depression is not necessarily caused by psychological factors, but can be attributed to stress in life. For Indians, Rao (1966) listed occupational or daily-living stress, such as retirement, or business or financial difficulties, as precipitating depression. These contrast with the loss of a mate or the failure of an affair, which are frequently described as precipitants in Western society.

VI. INTEGRATION

Like anxiety or anger, depression is part of the emotional phenomena that all men have exhibited through history. It is clear that in different lifestyles, individuals react in different degrees and manners to the loss, loneliness, or frustration that may lead to depression. It is also obvious that different societies offer different support systems for coping with the problems and minimizing the severity of depression. It is, therefore, reasonable to assume that different severities and frequencies of depression exist in different sociocultural settings. However, due to the difficulty of defining depression clinically for cross-cultural comparison, epidemiological data obtained are not easily interpreted cross-culturally in a meaningful way.

Even though the situation may improve by establishing standard and international criteria for depression and uniform methods of investigation, such an approach will encounter the problem of the "netting effect" — many alternative ways of reacting to loss or frustration, manifested by other clinical conditions, will be screened out from the "standardized" criteria, and data obtained will no longer be meaningful for comparison from a cross-cultural perspective.

It is suggested that instead of studying "depressive disorders" broadly or inclusively, attention should be focused on psychologically induced depression, which is more culturally related. There is clearly room for meaningful examination of the causes of the disorders of depression.

REFERENCES

Ablon, J. (1971). Bereavement in a Samoan community. *British Journal of Psychology, 44,* 329–337.

Bazzoui, W. (1970). Affective disorders in Iraq. *British Journal of Psychiatry, 117,* 195–203.

Binitie, A. (1975). A factor-analytical study of depression across cultures (African and European). *British Journal of Psychiatry, 127,* 559–563.

Blazer, D.G., Kessler, R.C., McGonagle, K.A., & Swartz, M.S. (1994). The prevalence and distribution of major depression in a national community sample: The National Comorbidity Survey. *American Journal of Psychiatry, 151*(7), 979–986.

Brown, D.R., Ahmed, F., Gary, L.E., & Milburn, N.G. (1995). Major depression in a community sample of African Americans. *American Journal of Psychiatry, 152*(3), 373–378.

Chance, N.A. (1964). A cross-cultural study of social cohesion and depression. *Transcultural Psychiatric Research Review, 1,* 19–24.

El-Islam, M.F. (1969). Depression and guilt: A study at an Arab psychiatric clinic. *Social Psychiatry, 4,* 56–58.

Fernando, S.J.M. (1975). A cross-cultural study of some familial and social factors in depressive illness. *British Journal of Psychiatry, 127,* 46–53.

Gobar, A.H. (1970). Suicide in Afghanistan. *British Journal of Psychiatry, 116,* 493–496

Golding, J.M., Karno, M., & Rutter, C.M. (1990). Symptoms of major depression among Mexican-Americans and non-Hispanic Whites. *American Journal of Psychiatry, 147*(7), 861–866.

Horwath, E., & Weissman, M.M. (1995). Epidemiology of depression and anxiety disorders. In M.T. Tsuang, M. Tohen, & G.E.P. Zahner (Eds.); *Textbook in psychiatric epidemiology.* (pp. 317–344). New York: Wiley-Liss.

Kleinman, A. (1982). Neurasthenia and depression: A study of somatization and culture in China. *Culture, Medicine and Psychiatry, 6,* 117–190.

Levav, I., Kohn, R., Golding, J.M., & Weissman, M.M. (1997). Vulnerability of Jews to affective disorders. *American Journal of Psychiatry, 154*(7), 941–947.

Manson, S.M., Shore, J.H., & Bloom, J.D. (1985). The depressive experience in American Indian communities: A challenge for psychiatric theory and diagnosis. In A. Kleinman & B. Good (Eds.), *Culture and depression: Studies in the anthropology and cross-cultural psychiatry of affect and disorder.* (pp. 331–368). Berkeley: University of California Press.

Marsella, A.J., Sartorius, N., Jablensky, A., & Fenton, F.R. (1985). Cross-cultural studies of depressive disorders: An overview. In

A. Kleinman & B. Good (Eds.), *Culture and depression: Studies in the anthropology and cross-cultural psychiatry of affect and disorder.* Berkeley: University of California Press.

Murphy, H.B.M., Wittkower, E.D., & Chance, N. (1967). Crosscultural inquiry into the symptomatology of depression: A preliminary report. *International Journal of Psychiatry, 3*(1), 6–22.

Pfeiffer, W. (1968). The symptomatology of depression viewed transculturally. *Transcultural Psychiatric Research Review, 5,* 121–124.

Prince, R. (1968). The changing picture of depressive syndromes in Africa: Is it fact or diagnostic fashion? *Canadian Journal of African Studies, 1,* 177–192.

Rao, A.V. (1966). Depression: A psychiatric analysis of thirty cases. *Indian Journal of Psychiatry, 8,* 143–154.

Sartorius, N. (1975). Epidemiology of depression. *WHO Chronicle, 29,* 423–427.

Sartorius, N., Davidian, H., Ernberg, G., Fenton, F.R., Jujii, I., Gastpar, M., Guibinat, W., Jablensky, A., Kielholz, P., Lehmann, H.E., Naraghi, M., Shimizu, M., Shinfuku, N., & Takahashi, R. (1983). *Depressive disorders in different cultures: Report on the WHO collaborative study on standardized assessment of depressive disorders.* Geneva: World Health Organization.

Simon, G.E., von Korff, M., Piccinelli, M., Fullerton, C., & Ormel, J. (1999). An international study of the relation between somatic symptoms and depression. *New England Journal of Medicine, 341*(18), 1329–1335.

Tanaka-Matsumi, J., & Marsella, A.J. (1976). Cross-cultural variations in the phenomenological experiences of depression: I. Word association studies. *Journal of Cross-Cultural Psychology, 7,* 379–396.

Thornicroft, G., & Sartorius, N. (1993). The course and outcome of depression in different cultures: 10 year follow-up of the WHO collaborative study on the assessment of depressive disorders. *Psychological Medicine, 23,* 1023–1032.

Waziri, R. (1973). Symptomatology of depressive illness in Afghanistan. *American Journal of Psychiatry, 130,* 213–217.

19

Schizophrenic Disorder

I. INTRODUCTION

Among all major psychiatric disorders, schizophrenia has been of greatest concern to clinicians and scholars since the very beginning of the history of psychiatry because it is one of the most severe and prevalent mental disorders of humankind. Many approaches have been taken in the past to understand the nature of this disorder, including social and cultural investigations. Although most scholars now view schizophrenia as predominantly attributed to biological, including hereditary, factors, past attempts to investigate the disorder from social and cultural perspectives have made certain contributions that deserve to be reviewed here.

II. CROSS-ETHNIC COMPARISON OF CLINICAL MANIFESTATIONS

A. PIONEER INVESTIGATION

Before Eugen Bleuler renamed the disorder with the nosological term schizophrenia in the early 20th century, it was originally known as dementia precox (a deteriorating disorder occurring in adolescence and ending with dementia, in contrast to dementia senile). It is well known that Emil Kraepelin, the founder of modern (descriptive) psychiatry, based on his organic orientation and descriptive approach, established a classification system for psychiatric disorders in the late 19th century. He was curious as to how his classification system, which was based on the clinical observation of patients in Germany, could be applied to patients in other societies with diverse cultures. He traveled to southeast Asia, including Indonesia, in the 1890s to make field observations and to test his classification system. Through his pioneering interest in comparative psychiatry, he was relieved to learn that dementia precox of a basically similar clinical picture was found in other cultures, such as Indonesia. If there was any difference, it was in the variation of subtypes, e.g., catatonic cases were found more in Indonesia than in Germany.

B. EARLY-STAGE CROSS-ETHNIC COMPARISONS

A pioneer in the field of culture and mental health, American anthropologist and sociologist Marvin K.

Opler (1959) carried out a cross-ethnic comparison of the symptomatology of schizophrenia between Italian- and Irish-American patients. Examining hospitalized schizophrenic patients of different ethnic backgrounds in New York City, he reported that seven variables (homosexual type, sin and guilt preoccupation, behavior disorder, attitude toward authority, fixity in the delusional system, somatic complaints, and chronic alcoholism) among a total of 10 showed significant differences between the Italian-American and the Irish-American schizophrenic patients compared. He reported that there were more Italian patients than Irish patients manifesting overt homosexual tendencies during psychotic conditions, behavior problems, and attitudes of rejecting authority. In contrast, more Irish patients than Italian patients were preoccupied with sin and guilt ideation, manifested chronic alcoholism, and had fixed delusional thoughts. Opler's study opened the door to the study of schizophrenic symptomatology cross-ethnically. However, it was later criticized by scholars that the findings revealed ethnic personality differences rather than differences in the schizophrenic disorders themselves. In other words, the differences had nothing to do with the core of the schizophrenic condition, but merely represented secondary symptoms or behavior problems associated with such psychotic conditions.

Another early-stage cross-cultural investigation was attempted by pioneer Murphy, Wittkower, Fried, and Ellenberger (1963) from McGill University, Montreal, Canada. By utilizing an international network that they had established around the world, they distributed a questionnaire containing a list of 26 symptoms or signs of schizophrenia to psychiatrists in different cultures and regions. The psychiatrists were asked to rate the frequency of symptoms they observed in their clinical practices. Based on the analysis of data they provided, the distribution of schizophrenic symptoms appears to vary according to social and cultural factors, as well as to observational and conceptual factors of the psychiatrists. The investigators were aware of the limitations of such surveys of their clinical impressions. However, it was an early attempt to examine the possible impact of social and

cultural factors on severe mental disorders. An interesting by-product of the survey was the finding of some Asian psychiatrists that there was a relatively high percentage of the simple and catatonic subtypes and a low percentage of the paranoid subtype of schizophrenia in their clinical settings. This stimulated the question of whether the delusional systems that are the most familiar feature of chronic schizophrenia in Euro-American hospitals are an essential part of the disease process.

C. Multicenter Comparison: International Study of Symptoms

More than a decade later, a systematic study on a larger scale was launched by the World Health Organization, the International Pilot Study of Schizophrenia (IPSS), involving nine study centers around the world: Aarhus (Denmark), Agra (India), Cali (Colombia), Ibadan (Nigeria), London (UK), Moscow (USSR), Prague (Chechoslovakia), Taipei (Taiwan, China), and Washington (USA) (World Health Organization, [WHO], 1973). It was the first formal comparative study involving multiple culture sites using standardized methods to collect information and to compare the clinical picture of schizophrenia from different societies of divergent ethnic/culture backgrounds [for methodological detail, cross-reference to Chapter 12: Culture and Psychiatric Epidemiology (Section II,D,1)].

The results revealed first that the average percentage scores were very similar across all the centers. All had high scores on lack of insight, predelusional signs, flatness of affect, auditory hallucinations (except the Washington center), and experiences of control. This indicated that schizophrenic patients from diverse cultural settings share basically similar symptomatology.

It was also revealed that among all the patients studied from all the centers (811 cases in total), the largest distribution of subtype was paranoid schizophrenia, comprising a total of 323 cases (39.8%). This was also the largest single diagnostic subgroup in most of the individual centers, except Agra, Cali, and

Moscow. The subtype accounted for 75% of all schizophrenic patients in London, 53% in Aarhus and Washington, and 40% or more in Ibadan and Taipei. The second largest single subgroup was the schizoaffective, comprising a total of 107 cases (13.2%). There were only 54 cases of the catatonic subtype (6.7%): 22 from Agra (India), 13 from Cali (Colombia), and 10 from Ibadan (Nigeria). This shows that the distribution of the catatonic subtype was rather uneven among the nine study centers, found mainly in three centers in developing societies. These findings support the clinical impression held by clinicians that catatonic schizophrenia is diminishing and that paranoid schizophrenia is rising in developed societies.

III. EPIDEMIOLOGICAL STUDY WITH SOCIAL VARIABLES

In the past, many investigations have been carried out around the world regarding the nature of schizophrenia. Many of these studies have been reviewed from epidemiological perspectives [cross-reference to Chapter 12: Culture and Psychiatric Epidemiology (Section II,A–E)]. Some of the unique findings will be reviewed briefly here to shed light on the nature of the disorder, mainly in terms of social aspects.

A. MIGRATION STUDY

Numerous investigations have been based on the early clinical impression that more immigrants than others in a community were hospitalized (as schizophrenic patients) in mental hospitals. It was even speculated that life stress associated with transcultural immigration caused or, at least, provoked the occurrence of severe mental disorders. An alternative speculation was that people with psychotic tendencies were already not stable in their lives and might more often choose to migrate to foreign societies. Later, however, scholars pointed out that the process of migration is a complex phenomenon, and there is no simple relation between it and the occurrence of

severe mental disorders such as schizophrenia [cross-reference to Chapter 44: Migration Refuge, and Adjustment (Section II,A and B)].

B. SOCIAL CLASS STUDY

There have been several investigations on the possible effects of social class on the occurrence of mental disorders, including severe disorders such as schizophrenia. For instance, Hollingshead and Redlich (1958) carried out an epidemiological investigation in late 1950s in the Great New Haven area in the United States. The subjects were grouped into five classes according to the ecological area of residence, occupation, and education. Results revealed that the patients diagnosed as psychotic (mainly with schizophrenia) were found more in the lower social classes. This has generated several hypotheses regarding this phenomena, namely social drifting or social attraction. Subsequent studies support the speculation that severe mental patients, due to the general deterioration of their lives, tend to drift into social settings characterized as lower class [cross-reference to Chapter 12: Culture and Psychiatric Epidemiology (Section II,C,1)].

C. LONGITUDINAL FOLLOW-UP STUDY ASSOCIATED WITH SOCIAL CHANGE

Only a few studies have involved longitudinal follow-up investigations of the prevalence of mental disorders. The 15-year follow-up study by Lin, Rin, Yeh, Hsu, and Chu (1969) in Taiwan was one such investigation. The study of the prevalence of mental disorders was carried out in selected three communities in 1946–1948. Fifteen years later, after significant socioeconomic-cultural changes in the society, a follow-up survey was conducted by the same chief investigators, using similar methods. It was revealed that although the prevalence rate of neurotic disorders increased remarkably (almost seven times), the rate of psychoses had not changed. This indicated that rapid sociocultural change occurring in the community over one and a half decades did not affect the prevalence of psychotic disorders (mainly schizophrenia) [cross-reference to Chapter 12: Culture and Psychiatric Epidemiology (Section II,B,1)].

D. International Study of Incidence Rates in Multiple Societies

Stimulated by the success of the IPSS international study of the clinical picture of schizophrenia, described earlier, several years later, in the late 1970s, the World Health Organization launched another multisociety investigation, the WHO Collaborative Study on the Determinants of Outcomes of Severe Mental Disorders (DOS) (Jablensky et al., 1991). This time, 12 study centers were selected: Asrhus (Denmark), Agra and Chandigarh (India), Cali (Columbia), Dublin (Ireland), Honolulu and Rochester (USA), Ibadan (Nigeria), Moscow (USSR), Nagasaki (Japan), Nottingham (UK), and Prague (Czechoslovakia). [For methodological issues, cross-reference to Chapter 12: Culture and Psychiatric Epidemiology (Section II,D,2).]

The goal of the study (mainly concerned with schizophrenia) was twofold: to investigate the incidence and prognosis of the disorders. Methodologically, to achieve the former goal, all individuals from a defined catchment area making a first contact with a psychiatric or other service agency due to symptoms of a possible schizophrenic illness were identified, assessed, and examined for incidence rate.

The results revealed that (Jablensky et al., 1991, pp.45–52) if a broad definition of schizophrenia was used, incident rates were found to be different in the different centers investigated. However, the annual incidence rates ranged merely from 1.5 to 4.2 per 10,000 population at risk, ages 15–54. If a stricter research definition of schizophrenia was used, the incidence rates did not differ among the centers with a range of 0.7 to 1.4 per 10,000 population aged 15–54.

This finding of incidence rates was compatible with the findings of other epidemiological studies carried out in the past in several different countries, although each investigation used its own methods. For example, according to Jablensky et al. (1991 p.53), from Norway, Ödegaard (1946) reported an incidence rate of 2.4; from the United Kingdom, Norris (1950) revealed a rate of 1.7; from Germany, Häfner and Reimann (1970) gave a rate of 5.4; and from China, Shen et al. (1981) disclosed a rate of 1.1 — all incidence rates per 10,000 for the geographically defined population.

E. Prevalence among Different Ethnic Groups within a Society

In the 1980s, an intensive epidemiological study organized by the National Institute of Mental Health, the Epidemiological Catchment Area (ECA) Study, was carried out in the United States (Regier et al., 1984) [cross-reference to Chapter 12: Culture and Psychiatric Epidemiology (Section II,E).] This study involved several catchment areas in the nation and produced much useful information about the prevalence of mental disorders in the United States. Due to the limitation of sample selection, only African-Americans, Hispanic-Americans, and Caucasian-Americans were compared for prevalence of any disorders in their ethnic groups (Regier & Kaelber, 1995, pp. 142–143).

Based on ECA data obtained from the Los Angeles site, Karno, Hough, et al. (1987) were able to compare the lifetime prevalence of specific psychiatric disorders among Mexian-Americans and non-Hispanic whites in Los Angeles, the only site where there was a sufficient sample size to compare these two ethnic groups. The analysis showed that the overall rates for any diagnosed disorder were similar for the two groups. There was a significant difference for only two disorders: drug abuse/dependence and major depression, which were more prevalent among non-Hispanic whites. The lifetime prevalence rate for schizophrenia was 0.4 for Mexican-Americans and 0.8 for non-Hispanice whites, not a significant difference.

F. Variable Prevalence Rates within Island Societies in Micronesia

Although on a small scale, interesting data were derived from Micronesia that deserve attention from a biosocio-cultural point of view. Geographically, Micronesia is composed of more than 2000 tiny islands (actual number, 2203) scattered in clusters east to west in the middle of the Pacific Ocean between Hawaii and the Philippines. It is distributed in an ocean area almost equal to the size of the continental United States. However, the total land area is only 530 square miles and is inhabited by little more than 60,000 local residents. Politically, Micronesia was occupied by the Germans and later the Japanese before World War II and was a United States Trust Territory for several decades after the war. They now belong to several political districts (such as the Republic of Belau and Federated Micronesia). With the exception of two southern islands inhabited by Polynesians, the people of Micronesia are of the same Micronesian race, even though they are recognized as several subgroups belonging to the islands of Truk, the Marshalls, Ponape, Belau, Yap, C. Caroline, and Kosrare. Because of the vast distance between the island districts, these subgroups were almost completely isolated from each other in the past, seldom communicating and, thus, developing their own languages and maintaining their own subcultures. However, from an anthropological point of view, they live similar island lifestyles and share common racial ancesters.

Clinical experience suggests that there are considerable differences in the number of schizophrenic patients observed in the different island areas. In order to validate this observation, an epidemiological survey was undertaken by American psychiatrist Pale Dale after he had served there for many years. Dale (1981) reported that there were remarkable differences in the prevalence rates among the islands. Prevalence rates

per 1000 persons over age 15 ranged from 9.7 for Yap, 7.6 for Belau (previously know as Palau), 3.4 for C. Caroline, 2.2 for Truk, 1.4 for Ponape, and 0.8 for the Marshalls.

In this naturally occurring, unique setting, it was demonstrated that due to the centuries-old separation of these island districts, even though the people were of the same racial stock, there were marked differences in the prevalence of schizophrenia. Heredity was considered a contributing factor to the uneven distribution of this biologically determined disorder. The endogamy of an island people for generations could have created gene pools on some islands, such as Yap or Belau, that resulted in world-record-high prevalence rates for schizophrenia. A genetic study has been launched that may validate the genetic hypothesis for this phenomenon.

IV. FOLLOW-UP STUDIES FOR CLINICAL PROGNOSIS

A. From the International Pilot Study of Schizophrenia

As described previously, as the second phase of WHO's International Pilot Study of Schizophrenia, a 2-year follow-up study was carried out to examine the outcomes of the schizophrenic patients in the different sites investigated. On the average, over 75% of those patients investigated in the nine collaborating centers around the world were traced 2 years after the initial examination (Sartorius, Jablensky, & Shapiro, 1977). Surprisingly, results revealed that the level of social development has a certain relation to the short-term prognosis of schizophrenia, i.e., cases in developing societies, in contrast to more developed societies, have more favorable outcomes. It has been speculated that the family, social, and cultural factors may have psychopathoreactive effects on functional psychoses, such as schizophrenia, resulting in different prognoses. An accommodating community, supportive family, and relatively simple lifestyle may favor the recovery of the psychotic condition (Sartorius, Jablensky, & Shapiro, 1978).

Later, a 5-year follow-up of the patients initially included in the IPSS was conducted in eight of the nine centers (Leff, Sartorius, Jablensky, Korten, & Ernberg, 1992). Adequate information was obtained concerning clinical and social outcomes. Results indicated that both clinical and social outcomes were significantly better for patients in Agra (India) and Ibandan (Nigeria) than for those in the centers in developed countries. In Cali (Columbia), only social outcome was significantly better.

B. From the Determinants of Outcomes of Severe Mental Disorders

As described in Section III,D, in order to validate the reverse relation between the level of social development and the prognosis for schizophrenia found in the IPSS, a few years later, the World Health Organization undertook a second study, the DOS. In addition to the frequency of occurrence, this study aimed to focus more sharply than the IPSS on the natural history of schizophrenic illness and the factors associated with differences in course and outcome.

A 2-year follow-up study was carried out among schizophrenic patients in the 12 study sites, which had different levels of social development. The outcomes of the disorder were defined in terms of the frequency of relapse and the length of remission. Results reconfirmed the previous findings that the outcomes of schizophrenic patients were better in developing societies than in developed ones. It was also revelated that the difference could not be fully explained by the higher frequency of acute onsets among the developing countries — a speculation that had been made after the IPSS (Sartorius et al., 1986).

Although much more social and family information was collected in this study than in the IPSS, no fundamentally different findings emerged to clarify the kind of factors that contributed to the favorable prognosis of the disorder. It was speculated that it was

a mixture of numerous factors, including biological, individual, and social, that contributed compoundly to the clinical course of this severe mental disorder. This speculation is still awaiting further investigation and clarification. A long-term follow-up study (15 and 25 years after initial examination) of schizophrenia by WHO in 16 countries is currently under way to gather even more information in addition to the short-term follow-up studies that have been conducted so far (Sartorius, Gulbinat, Harrison, Laska, & Siegel, 1996).

C. Possible Attribution of Expressed Emotion within Family

Based heavily on their clinical experiences and on the results of the surveys on the prognoses of schizophrenia in different settings, scholars have proposed that the course of schizophrenia is highly influenced by the family atmosphere (Vaughn & Leff, 1976a). Based on the concept of expressed emotion (EE), studies have been conducted to explore the attitudes of close relatives toward a mentally ill family member, especially measuring critical and hostile comments and evidence of emotional overinvolvement, such as exaggerated affect and overly self-sacrifycing behavior (Vaughn & Leff, 1976b). Such investigations have been carried out cross-culturally among Mexican-Americans (Jenkins, 1992; Karno, Jenkins, et al., 1987; Weisman, Lópes, Karno, & Jenk, 1993) and Australians (Vaughn et al., 1992), for example. Most of the studies have indicated that patients who returned from the hospital to live with relatives who reacted with high expressed emotions toward them relapsed more often than patients whose relatives did not express negative attitudes (Hooley, 1987; Weisman et al., 1993). Associated with this was a study (Penn & Mueser, 1996) illustrating that family intervention in the form of family psychoeducation and/or behavioral family therapy were highly effective in reducing families' expressed emotions and improving patients' relapse rates and outcomes. All this information led to the speculation that cultural factors possibly contributed to the outcomes of severe mental patients, such as schizophrenics, based on the attitudes toward mental patients and the reactions toward patients in home settings.

V. INTEGRATION

It has been a long, difficult challenge for clinicans and scholars to understand the nature of schizophrenia, one of the most severe and prevalent of existing mental disorders. It may be observed in any society, despite diverse sociocultural environments. Formal, multisite epidemiological studies using standardized methods have indicated that schizophrenia (if a "broader" definition is applied) occurs in many of the societies investigated with rather similar annual incident rates (about 1.5 and 4.2 per 100,000 population at risk ages 15–54) (Jablensky et al., 1991). The range of the rates was relatively small (less than three times) compared with other mental disorders (such as suicide and alcohol-related problems), which may have a range of variations of 10 or 20 times in different societies. These findings indicate that humankind is closely associated in this mental disorder and that biological, including hereditary, factors contribute predominantly to it.

From a clinical perspective, in studies using standardized methods of collecting information from multiple study sites in different cultural settings, it has been disclosed that the symptomatology of schizophrenia is basically similar. However, there is a difference in subtypes observed — the catatonic subtype is observed mainly in developing societies, whereas the paranoid and affective types are found more in developed societies.

From a sociological point of view, schizophrenia was observed more often among people of lower socioeconomic class, probably due to social drifting. It was also found that the prognosis of this disorder was relatively more favorable in developing than in developed societies. Although it has been speculated that a simple life in a rural setting with a close family may contribute to a relatively better outcome, there are no substantial data available from the investigations carried out so far to validate this speculation.

Most of the findings regarding schizophrenia are derived from epidemiological studies carried out primarily from a social perspective. Very few investigations have been attempted thus far from a strictly cultural standpoint. Nevertheless, it is suspected that cultural factors, in a narrow sense, such as beliefs and attitudes toward such a disorder, have little direct impact on its occurrence.

REFERENCES

Dale, P.W. (1981). Prevalence of schizophrenia in the Pacific island populations of Micronesia. *Journal of Psychiatric Research, 16*(2), 103–111.

Hollingshead, A.B., & Redlich, F.C. (1958). *Social class and mental illness: A community study.* New York: Wiley.

Hooley, J.M. (1987). The nature and origins of expressed emotion. In K. Hahlweg & M. Goldstein (Eds.), *Understanding major mental disorder: The contribution of family interaction research.* New York: Family Process.

Jablensky, A., Sartorius, N., Ernberg, G., Anker, M., Korten, A., Cooper, J.E., Day, R., & Bertelsen. (1991). *Schizophrenia: Manifestations, incidence and course in different cultures: A World Health Organization Ten-Country Study* (Psychological Medicine, Monograph Supplement No. 20). Cambridge, UK: Cambridge University Press.

Jenkins, J.H. (1992). Too close for comfort: Schizophrenia and emotional overinvolvement among Mexicano families. In A.D. Gaines (Ed.), *Ethnopsychiatry: The cultural construction of professional and folk psychiatries* (pp. 203–221). Albany: State University of New York Press.

Karno, M., Hough, R.L., Burman, A., Escobar, J.I., Timbers, D.M., Santana, F., & Boyd, J.H. (1987). Lifetime prevalence of specific psychiatric disorders among Mexican Americans and non-Hispanic Whites in Los Angeles. *Archives of General Psychiatry, 44,* 695–701.

Karno, M., Jenkins, J.H., De La Selva, A., Santana, F., Telles, C., Lopes, S., & Mintz, J. (1987). Expressed emotion and schizophrenia outcome among Mexican-American families. *Journal of Nervous and Mental Disease, 175*(3), 143–151.

Leff, J., Sartorius, N., Jablensky, A., Korten, A., & Ernberg, G. (1992). The International Pilot Study of Schizophrenia: Five-year follow-up findings. *Psychological Medicine, 22,* 131–145.

Lin, T.-Y., Rin, H., Yeh, E.K., Hsu, C.C., & Chu, H.M. (1969). Mental disorders in Taiwan, fifteen years later: A preliminary report. In W. Caudil & T.Y. Lin (Eds.), *Mental health research in Asia and the Pacific* (pp. 66–91). Honolulu: East-West Center Press.

Murphy, H.B.M., Wittkower, E.D., Fried, J., & Ellenberger, H.F. (1963). A cross-cultural survey of schizophrenic symptomatology. *International Journal of Social Psychiatry, 9,* 237–249.

Opler, M.K. (1959). Cultural differences in mental disorders: An Italian and Irish contrast in the schizophrenia—U.S.A. In M.K. Opler (Ed.), *Culture and mental health: Cross-cultural studies* (pp. 425–442). New York: Macmillan.

Penn, D.L., & Mueser, K.T. (1996). Research update on the psychosocial treatment of schizophrenia. *American Journal of Psychiatry, 153*(5), 607–617.

Regier, D.A., & Kaelber, C.T. (1995). The Epidemiologic Catchment Area (ECA) Program: Studying the prevalence and incidence of psychopathology. In M.T. Tsung, M. Tohen, & G.E.P. Zahner (Eds.), *Textbook in psychiatric epidemiology* (pp. 135–155). New York: Wiley.

Regier, D.A., Myers, J.K., Kramer, M., Robins, L.N., Blazer, D.G., Hough, R.L., Eaton, W.W., & Locke, B.Z. (1984). The NIMH Epidemiologic Catchment Area Program: Historical context, major objectives, and study population characteristics. *Archives of General Psychiatry, 41,* 934–941.

Sartorius, N., Gulbinat, W., Harrison, G., Laska, E., & Siegel, C. (1996). Long-term follow-up of schizophrenia in 16 countries: A description of the International Study of Schizophrenia conducted by the World Health Organization. *Social Psychiatry and Psychiatric Epidemiology, 31,* 249–258.

Sartorius, N., Jablensky, A., Korten, A., Ernberg, G., Anker, M., Cooper, J.E., & Day, R. (1986). Early manifestation and first-contact incidence of schizophrenia in different cultures: A preliminary report on the initial evaluation phase of the WHO Collaborative Study on Determinants of Outcome of Severe Mental Disorders. *Psychological Medicine, 16,* 909–928.

Sartorius, N., Jablensky, A., & Shapiro, R. (1977). Two-year follow-up of the patients included in the WHO International Pilot Study of Schizophrenia. *Psychological Medicine, 7,* 529–541.

Sartorius, N., Jablensky, A., & Shapiro, R. (1978). Cross-cultural differences in the short-term prognosis of schizophrenic psychoses. *Schizophrenia Bulletin, 4,* 102–113.

Vaughn, C., Doyle, M., McConaghy, N., Blaszczynski, A., Fox, A., & Tarrier, N. (1992). The relationship between relatives' expressed emotion and schizophrenic relapse: An Australian replication. *Social Psychiatry and Psychiatric Epidemiology, 27,* 10–15.

Vaughn, C.E., & Leff, J.P. (1976a). The influence of family and social factors on the course of psychiatric illness. *British Journal of Psychiatry, 129,* 125–137.

Vaughn, C.E., & Leff, J.P. (1976b). The measurement of expressed emotion in the families of psychiatric patients. *British Journal of Social and Clinical Psychology, 15,* 157–165.

Weisman, A., Lópes, S.R., Karno, M., & Jenkins, J. (1993). An attributional analysis of expressed emotion in Mexican-American families with schizophrenia. *Journal of Abnormal Psychology, 102*(4), 601–606.

World Health Organization (WHO). (1973). *The international study of schizophrenia.* Geneva: WHO.

20

Alcohol-Related Problems

I. INTRODUCTION

Abuse and dependence on alcohol or other chemical substances, including drugs, are biologically related phenomena as far as the clinical conditions of intoxication, dependence, and withdrawal are concerned. However, psychological factors are associated with the indulgence in and control of substance abuse. Furthermore, sociocultural factors contribute to the prevalence and viscidity of alcohol problems or substance abuse. Thus, basically, the three dimensions of biology, psychology, and socioculture need to be considered simultaneously — none of them can be ignored. However, in this chapter, the focus will be more on the sociocultural dimensions of these problems.

There are many substances that are abused by people and lead to intoxication or dependence. These include alcohol, drugs, tobacco, volatile paint, and many others. Alcohol has been used by humans for many centuries and is accepted as a part of daily life in many societies. Also, differences in attitude toward drinking associated with religious, ethnic, and cultural background are obvious. Thus, it will be examined separately from the abuse of drugs or other substances. Alcohol-related problems will be the focus of this chapter, and drugs or other substance abuse and dependence will be addressed in Chapter 21: Substance-Related Problems Other Than Alcohol.

II. FACTORS AND PROBLEMS RELATED TO DRINKING

A. ATTITUDES TOWARD DRINKING AND VARIATION OF DRINKING PATTERNS

People learned to use alcohol even in prehistoric times (Westermeyer, 1988). It is easy to produce alcohol by simply fermenting fruits, rice, wheat, or other plant products. In many societies, it has been a part of daily drinking, or has been used for special celebrations, or only for religious ceremonies. However, distinctly different attitudes toward drinking have developed in different societies.

1. Different Attitudes

An anthropologist distinguishes four different types of attitudes represented in various cultural groups that seem to have different effects on the rate of alcoholism (Bales, 1949).

a. Complete Abstinence

For various reasons, often religious, drinking alcohol is not allowed for any purpose. Muslims are an outstanding example. They take the view that it is wrong to influence the soul by chemical substance, so it is considered a taboo to drink, although in practice the taboo has been unevenly observed.

b. A Ritual Attitude

In this case, alcoholic beverages are used only as part of religious ceremonies. The beverages may be regarded as sacred; drinking them as a ritual act of communion with sacred powers. This is a chracteristic attitude toward drinking among many aboriginal people and also among Orthodox Jews.

c. A Convivial Attitude

Drinking is a "social" ritual; it symbolizes social unity or solidarity and releases emotions that further social ease and good will. The American attitude toward drinking belongs to this type.

d. A Utilitarian Attitude

This includes drinking for medicinal reasons and drinking designed to further self-interest or gain personal satisfaction. It is often, though not necessarily, "solitary" drinking. Because there is no counter-anxiety attached, the individual is apt to adopt drinking as the means of dealing with his particular maladjustment.

2. Variations of Drinking Patterns

Besides the attitude toward drinking, the pattern of drinking also varies among different societies. For instance, in the wine-drinking society of France, people drink wine as part of their daily lives, at lunch and/or dinner. Although they consume a large amount,

they carefully regulate the manner of their drinking. This may increase the prevalence for liver complications, but is seldom associated with intoxicated behavior or alcohol abuse.

Among the Chinese, if anyone drinks daily, he is looked down on as a "drinking person" by family members or others in the society. On special occasions, however, such as weddings, birthdays, or festivals, people are expected to drink during a banquet. As a matter of fact, a hand game is often played to provoke drinking, making the person who loses the game drink more. As a result, acute intoxication may happen occasionally. In China, Japan, and Korea, as well as Lao, he who could drink more was considered more "manly."

In Japan, women were traditionally sanctioned from drinking. However, recently, the alcohol consumption of women has increased tremendously. Liberated young women drink in bars and other public places with others, but middle-aged women, still under the influence of traditional views, drink within their private households by themselves, even in the daytime, and are described by the Japanese as "kitchen drunks."

In Micronesia, drinking was strictly prohibited by the previous rulers (Germans and Japanese). The Micronesians were forbidden to drink, for the reason that "savage people will become wild after drinking." However, after World War II, when Micronesia became an American Trust Territory, the people were relieved of this prohibition. They started to drink American-imported beer daily, almost in the same way as drinking Coca Cola, Seven Up, or other kinds of soft drinks. Even children, in the company of adults, drink beer without any prohibition. As a result, empty beer cans are piled up in the front of almost every household, as if to show off how much they have consumed. Furthermore, as with most Pacific Islanders, whenever alcohol is available, groups of friends tend to drink excessively on weekends and holidays until they become drunk or all the drink is gone. There is no concept or habit of regulating the amount of drink. Among teenagers, such drinking often results in violent behavior, involving fighting and injuring others. Thus, there are different patterns of drinking among different cultures (see Fig. 13-13 and 13-14 in Chapter 13).

B. ALCOHOL CONSUMPTION IN VARIOUS SOCIETIES

Closely associated with the attitude toward drinking, the amount of alcohol consumed varies remarkably among different societies. As shown in Table 20-1 (based on data prior to 1992, gathered by Mackay, 1993), regarding the annual consumption of alcohol as defined by the total amount of alcohol (liter by 100% alcohol) consumed by a person per year, there is a very wide range: from 16.2 liters in France (or 18.3 liters in Luxembourg) to 0.1 liter in Libya and Egypt (or even less than 0.1 liter in India). If the drinking is arbitrarily subdivided into high (above 6 liters), moderate (between 1 to 6

liters), and low (less than 1 liter) consumption, it can be said that most of the high consumption is observed among Euro-American societies, with the exception of Japan and South Korea. Most societies in Asia and some in northern Europe and South America have moderate to low consumption. Obviously, societies with Muslim backgrounds all have low consumption.

In general, religious beliefs and attitudes toward drinking affect the amount of consumption. This is particularly true for Muslim societies, in which drinking is strictly prohibited. This applies also to Orthodox Jewish people in Israel and, even more so, in Ethiopia. However, this does not apply to people of Christian religions in European or North American societies. As for Buddhism, despite the fact that monks are inhibited from drinking, no explicit rule applied to the ordinary people so that the pattern of drinking varies greatly among Buddhist societies, as illustrated by South Korea and Japan being high and Thailand low.

TABLE 20-1 Annual Alcohol Consumption Around the World (Unit by Liter)[*]

High consumption		Moderate consumption		Low consumption	
France	16.2	Ireland	6.0	Thailand	0.9
Argentina	12.6	South Africa	5.9	Turkey	0.9
Italy	12.6	Sweden	5.6	Angola	0.8
Spain	11.9	Norway	4.2	Ethiopia	0.8
Germany	11.6	North Korea	3.7	Albania	0.6
Portugal	11.6	Nigeria	3.6	Cambodia	0.6
Belgium	11.3	Iceland	3.3	Iraq	0.4
Switzerland	11.0	Panama	3.1	Indonesia	0.4
Czechoslovakia	10.3	Israel	2.9	Vietnam	0.4
Australia	10.1	Bolivia	2.9	Iran	0.3
Austria	9.7	Philippines	2.8	Jordan	0.3
Denmark	9.7	Colombia	2.7	Nepal	0.2
New Zealand	9.1	Congo	2.7	Libya	0.1
Netherlands	8.9	Brazil	2.6	Egypt	0.1
United States	8.4	Mexico	2.6	India	0.1
South Korea	8.1	Peru	2.4		
Poland	7.4	Cuba	2.3		
Greece	7.3	Hong Kong	2.2		
United Kingdom	6.9	Singapore	1.6		
Japan	6.8	Kenya	1.6		
Chile	6.7	China	1.2		

[*]Based on data from *The state of health atlas,* by J. Mackay (1993).

TABLE 20-2 Chronological Trends of Alcohol Consumption (100% Alcohol Liters per Adult) in Some Societies[*]

Society	1950	1955	1960	1965	1970	1975	1980	1985	1990	1995
Japan[a]				5.9	6.9	7.6	8.1	8.6	8.8	8.7
Korea[b]			1.0			8.3	8.7	9.1	9.8	11.0
Taiwan[c]				3.4			4.2		4.4	4.8
New Zealand[d]			5.4						8.7	9.1
United States[e,f]		9.1	9.5	10.0	11.4	12.3	12.5	10.8	10.5	9.5
Finland[g]	1.9	2.0	2.0	2.3	4.2	6.5	6.2	6.3	8.0	

[*] From W.S. Tseng et al., *International Journal of Social Psychiatry,* (in press).

[a] *Annual Report of Mental Health,* Ministry of Health & Welfare, Japan (1996).

[b] *Annual Statistics of Health and Welfare,* Ministry of Health and Welfare, Korea (1997).

[c] *Statistics of Taiwan Tobacco and Wine Monopoly Bureau,* Taipei (1997).

[d] Shen, Y.C. (1987). *Chinese Mental Health Journal, 1*(5).

[e] *Statistical Abstract of the United States,* 1997. Washington, DC: Bureau of the Census (1997)

[f] *U.S. Alcohol Epidemiologic Data Reference Manual.* Washington, DC: U.S. Govt. (1998)

[g] Osterberg, E. (1993). *Alcohol Health and Research World, 17*(3).

Based on chronological data available from some societies regarding the amount consumed over the past several decades, trends are shown in Table 20-2. In these societies, namely Japan, South Korea, and Taiwan in Asia, Finland in Europe, and the United States in North America, as well as New Zealand in the South Pacific, the amount of consumption has been steadily increasing during the past several decades. The only exception is that United States has decreased to the lower level in the last few decades. This invites people to speculate that there is a worldwide trend that, associated with economic improvement, coupled with a change to favorable attitudes toward drinking, there will be an increase in alcohol consumption even within the same society. This is particularly observed in urban settings, associated with industrialization and modernization.

C. Difference by Gender and Age

Closely related to the various amounts of alcohol consumed in different societies, there is a need to elaborate on any differences that are observed in association with the factors of gender and age in alcohol consumption and alcohol problems.

1. Between Male and Female

Very much related to cultural attitudes toward gender difference and the socially defined roles and statuses of men and women, there are wide differences in drinking patterns and prevalence of alcohol problems between males and females cross-culturally. Generally speaking, in societies that value the equality of role and status between male and female, such as many Euro-American societies, the gap between male and female drinking behavior and alcoholism is relatively less. In societies that traditionally emphasize the difference between male and female, and tend to assign a conservative role for the female, as most Asian and Muslim societies, the gap between male and female in the amount of consumption and degree of alcohol problems is very wide. This is merely a general trend. Even in the same cultural system, or within the same society, associated with social factors or cultural change, variations can be observed.

As for the prevalence of alcohol problems, the difference by gender in different cultures is well demonstrated by the comparison made of five societies studied: St. Louis, Missouri, in the United States; Edmonton, Alberta, in Canada; Puerto Rico; Taiwan; and South Korea (Helzer et al., 1990). Through collaboration, and using the same instrument, the Diagnostic Interview Schedule (DIS) used for the Epidemiologic Catchment Area (ECA) study, community surveys were carried out in these societies. Results indicated that the lifetime prevalence rates of males and females were 31 and 7%, with a male/female ratio of 4.4/1 for Canadians in Edmonton; 29 and 4% with a ratio of 7.3/1 for Americans in St. Louis; 25 and 2% with a ratio of 12.5/1 for people in Puerto Rico; 43 and 3% with a ratio of 14.3/1 for people in South Korea; and 13 and 0.7% with a ratio of 185.7/1 for the Chinese in Taiwan.

In mainland China, an epidemiological research team (Shen et al., 1992) carried out a nation-wide community investigation in 1989. A total of 44,920 subjects from nine cities, from four different occupations, were surveyed. Results revealed that the prevalence rate for alcoholism was 5.79% for 28,877 male subjects surveyed and 0.09% for 16,043 female subjects examined. The male/female ratio was 304/1. This showed that, associated with a negative cultural attitude toward drinking for females, alcoholic problems were very rare among women in mainland China.

The just-mentioned studies clearly support the findings that the ratios between male and female vary widely among different societies, indicating that social and cultural factors have a strong impact on the occurrence of such problems.

2. Among Different Age Groups

For cross-cultural comparison, the possible connection between age group and drinking behavior deserves attention, as people of different age groups may manifest drinking behavior and problems differently in different societies.

Again, from the just-mentioned five-society collaborative study (Helzer et al., 1990), epidemiological data were used to compare the lifetime prevalence rate of DSM-III-defined alcohol abuse and dependence. According to Helzer and collaborators, the differences in the age groups involved in alcoholism were quite different. As illustrated in Fig. 20-1, of the five societies studied among the populations of St. Louis (American), Edmonton (Canadian), and Taiwan (Chinese), the curve reached its peak with the age group between 25 and 44 and than gradually declined. This shows that alcoholism decreases after aging in these three societies. In contrast, for the people of South Korean and Puerto Rico, the curve did not fall after the age of 45 — actually it continued rising — showing that the problems of alcoholism did not decrease with age in the latter two societies. Helzer and coauthors raised the issue of whether older respondents in some cultures might show a decreased willingness to admit drinking prob-

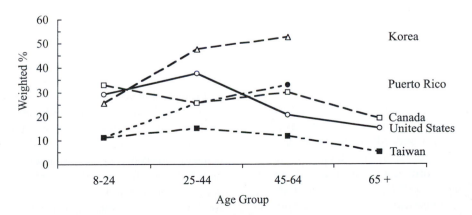

FIGURE 20-1 Lifetime prevalence of alcoholism by age: Comparison of five societies. [Revised from J.E. Helzer et al., *Archives of Geneneral Psychiatry*, 1990].

lems. Thus, the differences might be a result of the research method. Besides, in Korean and Puerto Rican studies, subjects aged 65 years or older were not included in the survey, so information after age 65 was not available to determine the whole life pattern.

Clinical observation in Micronesia revealed that drinking was often not observed among middle-aged or older persons, as they were forbidden to drink when they were young. After the removal of prohibition, the abuse of drinking was mainly observed among the younger generation. Teenagers as a group had the the most drinking-related problems (see Fig. 13-13, 13-14 in Chapter 13).

D. Boundary between Drinking and Alcoholism

Bennett, Janca, Grant, and Sartorius (1993) reported the Cross-Cultural Application Research (CAR) study that was jointly carried out in 1991 by the World Health Organization (WHO), the National Institute on Alcohol Abuse and Alcoholism (NIAAA), and the National Institute on Drug Abuse (NIDA). The investigation involved the collaboration of nine centers around the world, and was primarily concerned with the future design of internationally valid diagnostic criteria for alcoholism. This worldwide study resulted in valuable knowledge, namely, that wide cross-cultural differences exist in how people describe the amount of alcohol they consume, how they defined heavy drinkers, and the signs of alcohol effects on them. Gureje, Mavreas, Vazquez-Barquero, and Janca (1997) pointed out that a number of core concepts underpinning diagnosis of disorders relating to the use of alcohol have no equivalence in the local languages of the various cultures, whereas some others lacked cultural applicability because of their relative "distance" from cultural and ethnic norms of drinking. This distance often relates to the difficulties of adapting descriptions of drinking norms in a "wet" culture to one that is decidedly "dry." Overall, the study suggests that the boundaries between "socially normal" and "socially abnormal" drinking need to be defined carefully for cross-cultural application.

E. Difference between Abuse and Dependence

From a clinical point of view, scholars have realize that it is necessary to recognize alcohol problems as two kinds of disorders; alcohol abuse and alcohol dependence. Alcohol abuse is defined by the presence of both maladaptive (pathological) drinking patterns and impairment of social functions, whereas alcohol dependence is defined by, in addition to the presence of either pathological drinking patterns or impaired social functions, the presence of increased tolerance for or withdrawal symptoms when alcohol drinking is discontinued. This distinction is useful because dependence involves more biological factors, whereas abuse may involve more psychosocial factors. This is particularly helpful for cross-cultural examination.

In the five-site study of alcohol (Helzer et al., 1990), it was found that for the Americans in St. Louis, the Canadians in Edmonton, and the Puerto Ricans, the lifetime prevalence of alcohol abuse was less than that of alcohol dependence: 8% versus 9%, 7% versus 12%, and 4% versus 8%, respectively, whereas the reverse was true for the Chinese people in Taiwan and the Koreans, i.e., abuse was more prevalent than dependence: 5% versus 2% and 14% versus 9%, respectively. This suggests indirectly that, in the former group, alcohol withdrawal may contribute more to their drinking problems, whereas the latter group is not influenced as much by alcohol withdrawal.

F. Alcohol-Related Serious Complications

From a clinical perspective, it is well known that excessive drinking or chronic consumption of alcohol tends to result in many kind of complications. These include the medical disorder of liver cirrhosis and behavior problems, including violence and accidents, particularly traffic accidents. Those variations of complications offer an indirect index of drinking problems for cross-societal comparison, as data of such complications can be obtained more easily. However, caution is necessary in such a comparison, as complications merely reflect certain aspects of the consequences of drinking and do not necessarily represent the whole picture of the problems.

1. Mortality from Liver Cirrhosis

It is medically known that chronic consumption of large amounts of alcohol tends to result in liver cirrhosis. Thus, the mortality rate from liver cirrhosis has been used by scholars for cross-society comparisons of alcoholism, as the cause of death due to such a pathology can be obtained more accurately from most developed or developing countries. Based on data available from the WHO, Murphy (1982) has reviewed the mortality rate per 100,000 adults aged 45–64 by sex as illustrated in Fig. 20-2. Comparing the information illustrated in Figs 20-1 and 20-2, it can be said that, in general, there is a close relation between the amount of alcohol consumed and the prevalence of mortality from liver cirrhosis. However, there are some exceptions. For instance, in Chile, the consumption amount was not very high, but the mortality rate for liver cirrhosis was the highest. In Egypt, the consumption was very low, but the mortality rate

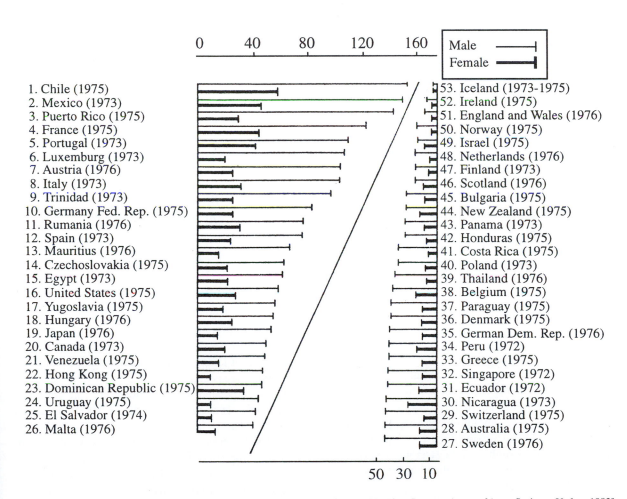

FIGURE 20-2 **Mortality from liver cirrhosis in 53 Countries.** [From H.B.M. Murphy, *Comparative psychiatry.* Springer-Verlag, 1982].

for cirrhosis was relatively high. Therefore, it needs to be pointed out that high mortality from liver cirrhosis is not entirely attributed to the amount of alcohol consumed.

2. Drinking-Related Violence

The effect of alcohol on behavior varies by factors such as the amount consumed, the pattern in which it is consumed, and who consumes it, in what circumstances. It is the general impression that when a person drinks a large amount of alcohol in a relatively short period of time and becomes intoxicated, he tends to manifest violent behavior toward others, expressing an unsatisfied emotional condition in an explosive way. This is especially true for males, and young people, in particular. Violent behavior associated with drinking is commonly observed among some minority groups — those suffering from an underprivileged lifestyle.

As mentioned previously, in Micronesia, there has been a sudden increase in alcohol consumption among teenage males. They always gather together on weekends or holidays, consuming all the beer or liquor they can obtain. After such a large amount of consumption, many youngsters are involved in physical fights. Many are brought into hospital emergency rooms for injuries they received during the fights. As it has become a pattern, the physicians in the hospital have learned to be prepared for the visits of these "weekend warriors" — as they have been labeled by the local people. This is a good example of how drinking leads to the occurrence of violent behavior.

3. Drunken Traffic Accidents

Traffic accidents associated with drunk drivers are a familiar theme in most societies. Traffic crashes are the leading cause of death in developed societies, such as the United States, among teenage and young adult populations. Alcohol involvement in these deaths is estimated to be as high as 45% (Defour, 1995). This illustrates another serious complication that can occur as a result of drinking.

G. THE EFFECT OF ALCOHOL CONTROL

The possible effects of official prohibition in a society on the amount of alcohol consumption and the occurrence of drinking problems have gained attention from a public health perspective. According to Österberg (1993), Bruun and associates (1975) described the extreme examples of alcohol control observed in Canada, Finland, Norway, and the United States. It was found that after Prohibition went into effect, alcohol consumption and problems reached the lowest levels ever achieved in any previous period. However, in later years, as the illegal alcohol trade became well established, consumption returned to pre-Prohibition levels.

In Finland, as reported by Österberg, medium beer has been sold in state monopoly stores since the repeal of Prohibition in 1932. The sale of medium beer in grocery stores started in 1969 as part of a total revision of alcohol legislation. As a result, alcohol consumption increased by 46% in the same year. This supports the view that availability of alcohol encourages drinking in Finland.

III. DRINKING AND PROBLEMS IN VARIOUS SOCIETIES

A. EAST ASIA

1. Chinese Ethnic Group

The ethnic Chinese have been understood to have a traditionally low prevalence of alcoholism. In mainland China, in 1982, an epidemiological study of psychiatric disorders was undertaken that involved 12 geographic areas and a total of 38,136 Han nationals. The study revealed that the morbidity rate for alcoholism was very low, only 0.19 per 1000 population (Shen, 1987).

In 1989, another national survey was conducted. This time the survey examined only urban areas — nine selected cities — and only a particular group of people in four different kinds of occupations (technical professional, administrative, light labor, and heavy labor), using the Chinese version of the Screening Interview for Alcohol Dependence (SIAD) that was developed by St. Louis University (Shen et al., 1992). A total of 44,920 subjects were surveyed. It was revealed that the prevalence rate was 3.7% for all the subjects investigated. As mentioned before, there was a wide gap between males and females. The rate was 5.8% for males and 0.09% for females. The male/female ratio was 64.4/1, indicating that it was mostly a male problem.

An epidemiological survey carried out in 1948 in Taiwan, involving a total population of 19,931, disclosed the prevalence of alcoholism was merely 0.1 per 1000 population (Lin, 1953). However, a more recent epidemiological survey, carried out in 1990 with a total of about 11,000 subjects from the selected sample areas of a metropolitan city, a small town, and a rural village, revealed lifetime prevalence rates for alcohol abuse of 3.4, 8.0, and 6.3% and, for alcohol dependence, 1.5, 1.8, and 1.2%, respectively (Hwu, Chen, & Yeh, 1995). The 1-year prevalence rates were about half of the lifetime prevalence rates for both abuse and dependence. It was noted that a different methodology was applied in the survey in the 1950s and the 1990s. The previous study used key informants' reports and a field census survey revealing the point prevalence at the time of the survey, whereas the latter standardized case-identification tool was used for lifetime prevalence, including those who had recovered or had only mild social impairment due to alcoholism. Still, Hwu and associates concluded that there had been a significant increase in alcohol problems in Taiwan during the past three decades.

2. Japan

In Japan, a small bottle of *sake* has long accompanied the festivity of weddings and the gravity of mourning. Social drinking is a Japanese tradition, but drinking as a real problem is a post-World War II development. Before the war, per capita consumption was 2.3 liters of alcohol (Yamamuro, 1973). However, according to the Ministry of Health and Welfare

(1996), in 1965, it had increased to 5.9 liters and in 1990 it had reached 8.9 liters. Surprisingly, the increase in consumption was attributed mainly to the increase in drinking by women. The amount of consumption by females increased almost seven times after the war. Alcoholism was estimated roughly at 3% of the population in 1963 by Moore (1964).

Kawakami, Haratani, Hemmi, and Araki (1992) carried out a questionnaire survey of employees of a computer factory in suburb of Tokyo (*N*=2581). They found that 15% of the male and 6% of the female subjects were classified as having alcohol-related problems on the basis of the (KAST) score they used. It was quite alarming to Japanee mental health workers that drinking problems among females was higher than in the past.

3. Korea

The situation in South Korea is similar to that in Japan, but worse in terms of the amount consumed annually. As pointed out by Kim (1990, 1993), most Korean psychiatrists had the impression that there was no serious alcoholic problem in Korea because of an an extremely low admission rate of alcoholics to hospitals, and they attributed it to racial sensitivity to alcohol. However, epidemiological surveys indicated that the occurrence of alcoholic disorder was very high. According to the Ministry of Health and Welfare (1997) in Seoul, the alcohol consumption rate was only 1.0 liter in 1960, but it increased rapidly to 8.3 liters in 1975 and reached a peak of 11.0 liters in 1995, the highest consumption among Asian societies (see Table 20-2). Associated with rapid economic development and improvement of the quality of life, the habit of drinking has increased among Korean people in South (Kim, 1990). This is quite a contrast to North Korea — with much different economic conditions and style of life due to the political system, the alcohol consumption was only 3.7 liters in 1990 (Mackay, 1993). This shows that even the same group of people, divided politically into north and south and living in remarkably different social systems, have very different patterns of alcohol consumption.

An epidemiological study conducted in South Korea by C.K. Lee and his research team (1990a) utilizing DIS/DSM-III criteria revealed that the lifetime prevalence rate for alcohol abuse was 12.95%, and dependence, 8.76%. By gender, alcohol abuse was 25.63% for males and 1.59% for females; alcohol dependence was 17.23% for males and 1.04% for females, indicating that the rate of alcoholism is very high and predominantly among males. This is considered to be due to the traditional Confucian teaching that sanctions drinking only for males.

Lee and associates (1990b) also analyzed their data for urban and rural differences. It was found that the rate for alcohol abuse was 12.95% in Seoul and 10.65% in rural areas; that of alcohol dependence was 8.76% in Seoul but 11.74% in rural areas, illustrating that there is an obvious difference between the city and the country: abuse is higher in the city, but dependence is higher in the country.

Lee and his team compared data obtained from Seoul in Korea and St. Louis in the United States, indicating that the total rate of alcohol abuse and dependence was 21.71% for people in South Korea, much higher than the rate of 15.7% for Americans in St. Louis. As the studies both used the same methodology and diagnostic criteria, they considered data comparable. They recognized the prevalence of the aldehyde dehydrogenase isoenzyme 1 deficit (ALDH) was about 20–50% for Asian people. However, they explained that cultural encouragement for males to drink with others in social groups has so powerful an effect on drinking that it overpowered the negative biological effects due to ALDH problems on drinking.

B. North America

1. The United States

A comprehensive review of the trends of alcohol problems in the United States has been made by M. C. Defour (1995) and the Group for the Advancement of Psychiatry (GAP) (1996). Concerning the historical trend, based on resources from Doernberg and Stinson (1985), Defour reported that after Prohibition — when alcohol was illegal from 1925 to 1933 — the per capital alcohol consumption of Americans increased through the 1960s (about 9.5 liters) and 1970s (about 11.5 liters), peaking in 1980 (about 12.5 liters) (see Table 20-2). According to the Statistical Abstract of the United States (1997), the annual consumption, after the peak in 1980, gradually declined to 9.5 liters in 1995.

Defour (1995) continued to describe that the alcohol-related cirrhosis rate per 100,000 population has been declining gradually from about 6 in 1974 to about 4 in 1990. Alcohol-related traffic fatality rates per 100 million vehicles miles traveled (VMT) have decreased slightly from about 1.4 in 1980 to 1.0 in 1990. This suggests that American people are becoming more careful about drinking, and drinking-related traffic accidents have declined slightly in this decade, in contrast to the 1970s and 1980s.

As for ethnic group differences, based on data from the ECA study, Helzer, Burnam, and McEvoy (1991, pp. 7–89) summarized that the ethnic groups show strikingly different patterns of age-related lifetime rates of alcoholism. When the age groups are subdivided into young adults (18–29), adults (30–44), middle-age adults (45–64), and aged adults (65+), it was found that the lifetime rates (by percentage) for the Caucasian-American male are high for young adults, but gradually decrease with age. In contrast, African-American males show a relatively low rate for young adults, increasing remarkably among adults and middle-age adults, with rates higher than the other two groups at middle-age. As for Hispanic-American males, the rate starts high for young adults, reaching a peak at the adult level, and then declining with age.

Female are generally lower than males. Regarding lifetime rates, in general, the ratios are lower when they are younger, but increase in the older groups. This is particularly true for aged Hispanic-American adults who are still under the influence of past tradition.

Because the lifetime rates are relatively lower for females, changes over the life cycle are not so obvious than among the males. In general, the rate tends to decrease with age, but for African-American females, the rate does not decline among middle-age adults, remaining the same as that for adults, only declining among aged adults. Thus, among African-Americans, both males and females, the highest prevalence was found in the middle-age groups, between 45 and 64, where the rate was 32.99 for males and 7.33 for females.

2. The Native American

Although there is a general impression that alcohol has a disruptive effect on North American Indians, there are no systematic data to indicate the nature and extent of the problem. There is only some indirect information. For instance, Brod (1975) cited studies documenting several phenomena. For Native Americans, the alcohol-related arrest rate is 12 times the national average; the alcoholism-related death rate is 4.3 to 5.5 times the United States rate for all races. It is generally considered that the rates of alcohol problems differ among different tribes, and overall generalization should be avoided.

Westermeyer (1972) reported that the Native American Chippewa of Minnesota recognize and practice two types of drinking, which they themselves call "white" and "Indian." The "white" type refers to drinking with restrained behavior, often observed among white people. The "Indian" type means drinking which, after one or two drinks, results in noisy behavior, often precedes fighting, or leads to heavy drinking and a stupor. Indian drinking is an accepted, expected way to maintain in-group relationships and tribal or familiar loyalties. The Chippewa, who must ordinarily behave according to majority white mores, can restate his Chippewa values by "Indian" drinking.

C. SOUTH AMERICA

South America is a large continent composed of 12 countries and two geopolitical units. In each country, the population is composed of different proportions of indigenous people and outside migrants (mostly Latin American). For instance, in Argentina, Brazil, Chile, Uruguay, and Venezuela, the indigenous populations are relatively small compared with the white and mixed-race populations. In contrast, in Bolivia, Ecuador, and Peru, indigenous people may constitute up to nearly half of the country's population. By and large, Latin American drinking customs are highly liberal. Alcoholic beverages can be obtained easily in all kinds of stores and public places. Cultural pressure toward drinking is particularly high for males. In some areas, a heavy drinking habit is considered a manifestation of virility, and men who exhibit an ability to "hold their liquor" carry a fair amount of social prestige (Negrete, 1976).

Caetano and Carlini-Cotrim (1993) reviewed the alcohol epidemiology in South America. They pointed out that alcohol consumption was present in almost all aspects of daily life, but that drinking patterns and types of alcohol beverages consumed varied substantially from country to country. They pointed out that the annual consumption by liter per capita was 7.5 for Argentina, 6.4 for Uruguay and Chile, 3.4 for Brazil, 3.3 for Venezuela, 3.0 for Colombia, 1.4 for Peru, and 1.2 for Paraguay. These figures are comparable with data reported by Mackay (1993) in *The State of Health Atlas* (Table 20-1), indicating that most of the consumption in South American countries was in the moderate range and was lower than in the United States. In general, the social norms in South America governing alcohol consumption were less restrictive for men than for women. Caetano (1984) described that in some areas of South America, the young drank more than the old, but elsewhere, middle-age men have the highest consumption rates.

Regarding the prevalence of alcoholism (broadly and variously defined as cases with some degree of psychological and physiological dependence) among men varied from 5% in Argentina to 10% in Colombia (Caetano & Carlini-Cotrim, 1993). As for alcohol-related problems, the range was from 12% in Chile to 28% in Argentina (Caetano, 1984). There was also considerable variation within countries, especially in large countries such as Brazil, where rates of alcohol abuse and dependence in three metropolitan areas ranged from 7.5 to 9.2% (Almeida Filho et al., 1992).

Yamamoto, Silva, Sasao, Wang, and Nguyen (1993) carried out a study in Peru. A population sample (*N*=815) from Lima was chosen for interviews with a revised from of the Spanish translation of the Diagnostic Interview Schedule (DIS). Results revealed that according to DSM-III diagnostic criteria, the prevalence of alcohol abuse or dependence was 34.8% for men and 2.5% for women. The male/female ratio was 14.1/1. Compared with data derived from United States studies concerning the Hispanic population, Yamamoto and colleagues pointed out that the prevalence for Peruvian men was higher than the prevalence for Hispanic men in the United States, but that the prevalence among Peruvian women was much lower than that of their counterparts in the United States. Yamamoto and colleagues interpreted the high prevalence among men in Peru as likely due to cultural mores, which allowed men to drink due to the *machismo* attitude, but also possibly linked to the stresses encountered by men in impoverished societies undergoing rapid social, cultural, and economic change.

D. EUROPE

1. Italy

In Italy, drinking wine with meals is taken for granted. The average Italian may drink a significant amount of alcohol every day, yet he is not often, or seriously, drunk. Even the Italian who, at times, may show signs of intoxication is not considered to be an alcoholic. Drinking is, and always has been, a part of Italian culture. Acceptance of the wine-with-food kind of drinking is complete. Attitudes are also tolerant toward alcoholism, a condition recognized in Rome before the time of Christ.

However, Bonfiglio, Falli, and Pacini (1977) found that this traditional Mediterranean wine drinking is now being overshadowed by alcoholism of the northern European and Anglo-Saxon type. Drinking wine is supplemented or replaced by drinking hard liquor.

Between 1941 and 1972, Italy's wine consumption increased almost 100%, beer consumption increased by more than 600%, and drinking spirits jumped by approximately 700%. During this same period, deaths from cirrhosis of the liver increased from 9.32 to 29.90 per 100,000 population. The government has used mass media to try to reduce per capital intake.

2. France

In France, similarly to Italy, drinking patterns have also changed in recent years. In the 1960s, alcoholic intake was 95% wine. In the 1980s, wine accounted for only 6% of the total consumption; whiskey, vodka, and gin consumption have doubled in a decade, and beer drinking has risen. Today, *la défonce du samedi soir,* "the Saturday night bender," drinking oneself into a stupor on hard liquor, has entered the French way of life.

3. Russia

As described by Dorman and Towle (1991), official concerns about alcohol consumption in Russia have been evident since at least the beginning of the century, when the Czarist regime implemented prohibition in 1914. Prohibition was imposed by Stalin in the late 1920s, by Khrushchey in 1958, and by Brezhnev in 1972 and 1979. The campaigns against drinking were seen as fragmented and ineffective, and heavy drinking and alcohol-related problems continued to increase into the early 1980s. It was reported that, between 1960 and 1980, annual consumption had doubled from 3.9 liters to 8.7 liters even by a conservative estimate. However, it needs to be noted that alcohol consumption patterns differed according to region and ethnicity. According to Dorman and Towle, *The Economist* (1989) reported that a decrease in life expectancy for Soviet males, from 66 years in 1965 to 62 years in 1984, was largely attributed to heavy alcohol consumption. Studies from the West suggested that alcoholism was the third leading cause of death in the former Soviet Union, after heart disease and cancer.

E. AFRICA

It has been described that traditionally alcohol played a very important social function in sub-Saharan, non-Muslim African cultures. Alcohol was always present in meetings when elders settled disputes, after a successful hunt or harvest, and when marriages were arranged. In contrast to other parts of the world, as stressed by Haworth (1993), one of the most important patterns in Africa was the high rate of consumption of homemade, often illegal, alcoholic beverages; home brews were assumed to have a high alcohol content and to be potentially toxic.

A psychiatrist from Nairobi, Kenya, Acuda (1985) reviewed past research and publications on alcohol consumption and problems from east Africa. For instance, the first Western psychiatrist to work in Kenya, Carothers, reported that of the total 558 patients admitted to the hospital in Nairobi between 1939 and 1943, only four cases (0.7%) were admitted with alcohol psychosis, despite the heavy consumption of drinks with a high alcohol content by the Africans in the reserves. In contrast, concerning Uganda, Wood found alcohol psychoses was an important cause of admission to the mental hospital in Butabiak during the 1960s, constituting 13% of all admissions.

According to Acuda, in the 1980s, following a general concern about alcoholism and drug abuse among Kenyan youth, several investigations were carried out. Bittah, Owola, and Oduor (1979) surveyed 200 randomly selected households in a rural district and reported that up to 27% of the males and 24% of the females interviewed could be classified as alcoholics using the 1952 WHO definition of alcoholism, which was not the same as the definition in DSM-IV in terms of either dependence or abuse, but similar to both. According to Acuda, another study by Wanjiru (1979) was carried out in an overpopulated slum area of Nairobi. He reported that up to 46% of the male and 24% of the female heads of households interviewed were classified as alcoholics using the same WHO criteria. Acuda also mentioned a more sophisticated study carried out by Yambo and Acuda (1983) in

Kenya covering Nairobi city and a rural district. A total of 563 youths aged 10 to 29 years old were interviewed in a household survey using a questionnaire. Results disclosed that only 11% of the boys and 4.1% of the girls could be classified as abusers or regular users of alcohol. It was found that the situation was not as bad as it was feared to be by the news media.

Although these studies reviewed by Acuda were related to east Africa, and mostly Kenya, and the studies involved relatively small community samples, they offer us a glimpse into the drinking situation in east Africa. As summarized by Acuda, in a region where so much alcohol is produced both traditionally and commercially and drinking, sometimes quite heavily, is more or less a normal part of life, alcohol problems are bound to arise in various proportions. It should be mentioned that the problems involve both males and females.

IV. CLOSING COMMENTS

Problems related to drinking are good examples of the close interaction of biological, psychological, and sociocultural factors in the manifestation of psychopathology. Wide differences in attitudes toward drinking, patterns of drinking, and amounts consumed all indicate the strong sociocultural impact on drinking behavior, which, in turn, coupled with biological predisposition and psychological vulnerability, contribute to the development of physiologically related psychopathology. The sociocultural input into this disorder is evidenced by the wide range of the amount consumed, the prevalence of alcohol problems among societies with different cultures, and the obvious fluctuation of the prevalence of the disorder observed even within the same society in association with changes occurring in the society.

Alcoholism serves as one of the social indexes of mental health conditions. There is also the potential of regulating drinking problems through social and cultural approaches. Among the trends observed around the world, there are two common threads. First, among culturally uprooted, economically unprivileged minority groups, drinking problems tend to be prevalent. This suggests that when people are trapped in a situation characterized by chronic frustration, without hope for the future, they tend to indulge in drinking as one way to cope with the stress. The second thread is that, associated with the improvement of economic conditions, drinking tends to increase. It has been observed that drinking and problems, after reaching their peak, tend to level off in some developed societies; however, in many developing societies, drinking is increasing and complications from drinking are becoming serious, calling for urgent attention.

Although cultural differences in alcohol consumption and the impact of culture on the occurrence of alcohol problems have been widely studied (Day, 1995; Heath, 1986; Helzer, Canino, & Chen, 1998), very little attention has been given to cultural perspectives in the treatment of alcoholism. In European-American societies, although about half or more of alcoholics refuse Alcoholics Anonymous (AA), the number of such AA groups is great. With a structured stage for treatment, and through intense group support, AA tries to enhance the process of recovery. However, such a self-help method for drinking problems has not been widely accepted in other parts of the world. Cultural incompatability of this approach has been raised [cross-reference to Chapter 33: Culture-Influenced Unique Psychotherapy (Section II,C)]. Few studies have examined culturally relevant approaches to treating drinking problems in diverse cultural settings. This is an area awaiting future exploration.

REFERENCES

Acuda, S.W. (1985). International review series: Alcohol and alcohol problem research. I: East Africa. *British Journal of Addiction, 80*(2), 121–126.

Almeida Filho, N., Mari, J.J., Coutinho, E., Franca, F.F., Fernandes, J.G., Andreoli, S.B., & Busnello, E.D. (1992). Estudo multicentrico de morbidade psyquiátrica em areas unbans brasileiras (Brasilia, São Paulo, Porto Alegre). *Revista de ABP-APAL, 14,* 93–104.

Bales, R.F. (1949). Cultural differences in rates of alcoholism. *Quarterly Journal of Studies on Alcohol, 6,* 480–499.

Bennett, L.A., Janca, A., Grant, B.F., & Sartorius, N. (1993). Boundaries between normal and pathological drinking: A cross-cultural comparison. *Alcohol Health & Research World, 17*(3), 190–195.

Bittah, O., Owola, J.A., & Oduor, P. (1979). A study of alcoholism in a rural setting in Kenya. *East African Medical Journal, 56,* 665–670.

Bonfiglio, G., Falli, S., & Pacini, A. (1977). Alcoholism in Italy: An outline highlighting some special features. *British Journal of Addiction, 72,* 3–12.

Brod, T.M. (1975). Alcoholism as a mental health problem of Native Americans: A review of the literature. *Archives of General Psychiatry, 32,* 1385–1391.

Caetano, R. (1984). Manifestations of alcohol problems in Latin America: A review. *Bulletin of the Pan American Health Organization, 18*(3), 258–280.

Caetano, R., & Carliini-Cotrim, B. (1993). Perspectives on alcohol epidemiology research in South America. *Alcohol Health & Research World, 17*(3), 244–250.

Day, N.L. (1995). Epidemiology of alcohol use, abuse, and dependence. In M.T. Tsuang, M. Tohen, & G.E.P. Zahner (Eds.), *Textbook in psychiatric epidemiology* (pp. 345–360). New York: Wiley-Liss.

Defour, M.C. (1995). Twenty-five years of alcohol epidemiology: Trends, technique, and transitions. *Alcohol Health & Research World, 19*(1), 77–84.

Doernberg, D., & Stinson, F.S. (1985). *U.S. Alcohol Epidemiological Data Reference Manual: Vol. 1. U.S. apparent consumption of alcohol beverages based on state sales, taxation or receipt data.* Washington, DC: U.S. Government Printing Office.

Dorman, N.D., & Towle, L. (1991). Initiatives to curb alcohol abuse and alcoholism in the former Soviet Union. *Alcohol Health & Research World, 15*(4), 303–306.

Group for the Advancement of Psychiatry (GAP). (1996). *Alcoholism in the United States.* (Formulated by the Committee on Cultural Psychiatry) (Rep. No. 141). Washington, DC: American Psychiatric Press.

Gureje, O., Mavreas, V., Vazquez-Barquero, J.L., & Janca, A. (1997). Problems related to alcohol use: A cross-cultural perspective. *Culture, Medicine and Psychiatry, 21,* 199–211.

Haworth, A. (1993). A perspective on alcohol studies in Africa. *Alcohol Health & Research World, 17*(3), 242–243.

Heath, D.B. (1986). Concluding remarks. *Annals of the New York Academy of Sciences, 472,* 234–237.

Helzer, J.E., Burnam, A., & McEvoy, L.T. (1991). Alcohol abuse and dependence. In L.N. Robins & D.A. Regier (Eds.), *Psychiatric disorders in America: The Epidemiologic Catchment Area Study.* New York: Free Press.

Helzer, J., Canino, G., & Chen, C.N. (1998). *Cross-national studies of alcoholism.* New York: Oxford University Press.

Helzer, J.E., Canino, G.J., Yeh, E.K., Bland, R.C., Lee, C.K. Hwu, H.G., & Newman, S. (1990). Alcoholism—North America and Asia: Comparison of population surveys with the diagnostic interview schedule. *Archives of General Psychiatry, 47,* 313–319.

Hwu, H.G., Chen, C.C., & Yeh, E.K. (1995). Alcoholism in Taiwan: The Chinese and aborigines. In T.-Y. Lin, W.S. Tseng, & E.K. Yeh (Eds.), *Chinese societies and mental health* (pp. 181–146). Hong Kong: Oxford University Press.

Kawakami, N., Haratani, T., Hemmi, T., & Araki, S. (1992). Prevalence and demographic correlates of alcohol-related problems in Japanese employees. *Social Psychiatry and Psychiatric Epidemiology, 27*(4), 198–202.

Kim, K.I. (1990). Alcoholic disorder in Korea. *Mental Health Research, 9,* 131–147.

Kim, K.I. (1993). Drinking behavior in Korea. In *Culture and alcoholism, Proceeding of the Seminar on the Prevention and Treatment of Alcoholism.* Seoul, Korea: Yonsei University Department of Psychiatry and World Health Organization.

Lee, C.K., Kwak, Y.S., Yamamoto, J., Rhee, H., Kim, Y.S., Han, J.H., Choi, J.K., & Lee, Y.H. (1990a). Psychiatric epidemiology in Korea. Part I. Gender and age differences in Seoul. *Journal of Nervous and Mental Disease, 178*(4), 242–246.

Lee, C.K., Kwak, Y.S., Yamamoto, J., Rhee, H., Kim, Y.S., Han, J.H., Choi, J.K., & Lee, Y.H. (1990b). Psychiatric epidemiology in Korea. Part II. Urban and rural differences. *Journal of Nervous and Mental Disease, 178*(4), 247–252.

Lin, T.-Y. (1953). An epidemiological study of the incidence of mental disorder in Chinese and other cultures. *Psychiatry, 16,* 313–336.

Mackay, J. (1993). *The state of health atlas.* New York: Simon & Schuster.

Ministry of Health and Welfare. (1996). *Annual report of mental health.* Tokyo: Ministry of Health and Welfare.

Ministry of Health and Welfare. (1997). *Annual statistics of health and welfare.* Seoul, Korea: Ministry of Health and Welfare.

Moore, R.A. (1964). Alcoholism in Japan. *Quarterly Journal of Studies on Alcohol, 25,* 142–150.

Murphy, H.B.M. (1982). Disorders associated with alcohol and other drugs. In H.B.M. Murphy *Comparative psychiatry: The international and intercultural distribution of mental illness* (Chap. 8) Berlin: Springer-Verlag.

Negrete, J.C. (1976). Alcoholism in Latin America. *Annals of the New York Academy of Sciences, 273,* 9–23.

Österberg, E. (1993). Global status of alcohol control research. *Alcohol Health & Research World, 17*(3), 1993.

Shen, Y.C. (1987). Recent epidemiological data of alcoholism in China. *Chinese Mental Health Journal, 6,* 251–256.

Shen, Y.C., Zhang, W.X., Lu, Q.Y., Wong, Z., Duang, C.F., Gau, H., Zhau, L.Z., Zhu, H.F., Li, Q.S., Wang, J.Y., Zhang, Z.Q., & Shi, M.J. (1992). Epidemiological survey on alcohol dependence in populations of four occupations in nine cities of China. (I): Method and prevalence. *Chinese Mental Health Journal, 6*(3), 112–115.

Tseng, W.S., Ebata, K., Kim, K.I., Krahl, W., Kua, E.K., Lu, Q.Y., Shen, Y.C., Tan, E.S., & Yang, M.J. (in press). Mental health in Asia: Social improvement and challenges. *International Journal of Social Psychiatry.*

Wanjiru, F. (1979). *Alcoholism, the man and his integration into society.* B.A. dissertation, University of Nairobi.

Westermeyer, J. (1972). Chippewa and majority alcoholism in the Twin Cities: A comparison. *Journal of Nervous and Mental Disease, 155,* 322–327.

Westermeyer, J. (1988). The pursuit of intoxication: Our 100 century-old romance with psychoactive substances. *American Journal of Drug and Alcohol Abuse, 14,* 175–187.

Yamamoto, J., Silva, J.A., Sasao, T., Wang, C., & Nguyen, L. (1993). Alcoholism in Peru. *American Journal of Psychiatry, 150*(7), 1059–1062.

Yamamuro, B. (1973). Alcoholism in Tokyo. *Quaterly Journal of Studies on Alcohol, 34,* 950–954.

21

Substance-Related Problems Other Than Alcohol

I. INTRODUCTION

After examining alcohol-related problems in Chapter 20, the abuse of substances other than alcohol will be elaborated in this chapter. It will focus mainly on drug abuse, even though many nondrug chemical substances can be abused, such as paint, for example. Substance abuse as one kind of psychopathology is characterized, on the one hand, as strongly related to biological factors in its occurrence and manifestation and, on the other, as heavily influenced by psychological and sociocultural factors in its development and spread. It is a particular kind of psychiatric disorder that shows remarkable vicissitude subject to social and cultural factors.

The usage of psychoactive substances by human beings started in prehistory. The people of Africa, Asia, and Europe, in addition to preparing alcohol, also grew opium, cannabis, and some stimulant plant compounds (Westermeyer, 1999). The chemical substances that have been abused have varied in different societies and at different times in the same societies. Abuse depends on the availability of a substance, as well as economic aspects, social control, and cultural fashions. Pro-

scribed or taboo use of certain chemical substances exists in many societies. Some substances are totally forbidden under any circumstances. Alcohol in Saudi Arabia, coffee among Mormons, and heroin in the United States are examples (Westermeyer, 1987). Substances take on symbolic meaning, in some instances — representing certain values, attitudes, and identities related to ethnicity. For instance, alcoholism or drunkenness is considered by many Jewish people as non-Jewish behavior and sinful by many Muslims. In China, as a result of the Opium War, opium was regarded as a substance of national shame.

When substance abuse is illegal, it is difficult to conduct formal community surveys because abusers tend to deny abusive behavior. Therefore, it is extremely difficult to obtain epidemiological data (Anthony & Helzer, 1995). At best, studies rely on indirect information, such as number of people arrested by police. However, even such data are subject to the nature of the law and the way it is carried out. An alternative way to collect data is to examine the rate of treatment service utilization. However, as most of abusers may not utilize treatment services, data are incomplete.

In order to help countries seeking to implement prevention programs, a World Health Organization (WHO) project was established: the Development of Strategies and Guidelines for the Prevention of Drug-Related Problems. Smart, Murray, and Arif (1988) reviewed the reports that countries around the world prepared for this WHO project. They pointed out that while the pattern and degree of drug abuse varied from country to country, some general findings were noticed. Clearly the typical abuser of most illegal drugs was a young male, unemployed, relatively unskilled, and living in lower-class circumstances. This pattern fit nearly all 29 countries that submitted the reports. Exceptions were noted in Hong Kong (where 64% of addicts were aged 30 and over) and Burma and Pakistan (where most opim addicts were middle-aged). Judging from the reports, the attitudes toward drug abuse also varied among countries. In several, such as India, Kenya, Mauritius, Nigeria, and Togo, drug abuse was not considered an important problem. In others, such as Canada, Finland, France, Ireland, and the United Kingdom, drug abuse was dwarfed by concerns with more serious alcohol problems. Experts from several countries saw drug abuse as an important problem that could not be addressed because more pressing concerns took priority. Examples were economic concerns in Bangladesh and Peru, for instance. Many countries, at the government level, clearly saw drug abuse as a major national concern that demanded action. Those countries were Australia, Germany, Hong Kong, Indonesia, Japan, Malaysia, Mexicao, Pakistan, the Phillipines, Singapore, and the United States. Thus, it was a worldwide concern.

It is almost impossible to describe in detail the phenomena of substance abuse around the world on a cross-cultural comparative base. Here, some historical episodes or unique situations observed in some societies will be reviewed first to illustrate the social and cultural contributions to the phenomena. Then epidemiological data available from some regions will be elaborated, with the intention of highlighting the sociocultural impact of the problems.

II. UNIQUE EPISODES OR SITUATIONS IN SOME SOCIETIES

A. POSTWAR EPIDEMIC OF AMPHETAMINES IN JAPAN

Immediately after World War II, the Japanese were faced with grave problems of social reconstruction. Most of the cities of manufacturers were severely damaged from the bombing. Everyone was forced to work long and hard for food, clothing, housing, and to rebuild the industries. During this period, the central nervous stimulant amphetamine appeared on the market. Amphetamines were widely used by the Army during World War II to promote a fighting spirit among soldiers (Kato, 1990). Later, many Japanese learned that the *kamikaze* pilots had used the drugs in their suicide attacks. Now, it was being sold commercially with advertising that advised, "Get rid of slumber and be full of energy." At first, only night workers, such as waitresses, bartenders, and entertainers, took amphetamines. Later, use of the drug spread to the general population. College students used it for late night study, laborers for extended work hours. Very soon society reacted against the mass abuse of the drug and restrictions to control it went into effect. Soon, use of the drug virtually ceased; only runaways and juvenile delinquents took amphetamines (Hemmi, 1974). Thus, the phenomenon was a transient one that reflected the social atmosphere at the time.

According to Tamura (1989), the stimulant epidemic started in 1945 and ended around 1956. However, beginning in the mid-1950s, associated with rapid industrialization and remarkable improvement in the standard of living, opiates, particularly heroin, replaced amphetamines in popularity among the drug-abusing population (Kato Price, wada, & Murray, 1995). Later, between the 1960s and mid-1970s, when economic growth reached its peak, for some reason, paint thinner became popular among adolescents, whereas amphetamine abuse began to reemerge rapidly among adults, entering a second epidemic phase

(Kato Price et al., 1995; Tamura, 1989). Thus, associated with changes in social-economic condition, lifestyle, and social atmosphere, there was change and fluctuation in the substances abused.

B. RADICAL ERADICATION OF OPIUM ABUSE IN CHINA

Toward the end of the Chin dynasty, when China was under the influence of Western imperialism, opium addiction had become a serious social problem in China. For economic benefit, the British East India Company imported and sold opium to China. This provoked the Chinese–British Opium War when the Chinese people tried to burn the imported "poison" at the harbor of Guangzhou. The Chinese lost the war, and the British government was allowed to conduct its opium business for many decades. It was estimated that, by the turn of the 20th century, many millions of Chinese were addicted to opium (Fields & Tararin, 1970; Lowinger, 1973).

When the communists took over China in 1949, the new government immediately tried to eradicate the problem through political action. Premier Chou En-Lai signed an official order prohibiting opium in 1950. A massive campaign was undertaken, labeling opium abuse as an offense against the country. The major thrust was to change the ideology of the young and prevent new addicts, whereas those already addicted were treated medically and socially for rehabilitation. Associated with the distribution of the land from landlords to peasants, all poppy fields were replaced by food crops. As the country's door toward the outside was closed, there was no way to sneak the "poison" into the country again. Local communist cadres serving each household in the neighborhood were used to detect any person abusing opium. Heavy penalties, including execution, were imposed for those responsible for growing, manufacturing, and selling opium. Thus, almost a century of opium abuse had been relegated to history within just 3 years.

Substance abuse was strictly controlled for more than three decades, until the 1980s, when China again opened her doors to the outside world. Many substances were then smuggled into the border areas near southeast Asia, as well as over the Silk Road.

C. POST-VIETNAM WAR EPIDEMIC IN THE UNITED STATES

Most Americans witnessed the rapid rise of substance abuse around the era of the Vietnam War. Associated with the Hippie movement, as a cultural reaction against the establishment and conservative tradition, many young people lived lifestyles characterized by informality. Marijuana was widely used. When the Vietnam War started, many young people were concerned about the purpose of the war and were afraid of being drafted and involved in it. An antigovernment and antiwar movement arose, which contributed to the tension within the society. It accelerated drug abuse as well. In the meantime, soldiers fighting in Vietnam, under severe stress, began to indulge in substance abuse. When they returned to American soil, many continued abuse of various kinds. As a result, there was a substance-abuse epidemic in the United States for more than a decade (Trimble, Bolek, & Niemcryk, 1992).

D. UNIQUE SITUATION OBSERVED IN LAOS

The opium use among the Meo people of Laos is rather unique. As described by the American cultural psychiatrist Joseph Westermeyer (1971, 1974), who did field work there for many years, for most of these tribal people, the primary value of opium was economic; nearly every household grew opium to trade for silver and iron. Although some Meo smoked opium occasionally and some were addicted, the majority did not abuse it. Westermeyer found that most addicts were farmers living in rural areas, women addicts far outnumbered men, and addiction was not associated with criminality or related to decreasing social competency. This was very different from other places, where opium addiction was primarily a city phenomenon associated with criminality and low social competency. Because the Meo raised their own opium, no one was driven to crime or violence to obtain it. Addiction was not considered socially desirable, but no great social opprobrium descended on the addicted person.

E. Dilemma in the Islamic World

It is widely known that alcohol is strictly prohibited in the Islamic world. As Baasher explained (1981), even though the brewing of alcohol from dates, grapes, and honey was generally popular among pre-Islamic communities living on the Arabian peninsula, the drinking of wine was clearly identified as a disruptive social evil, and alcohol abstention was practiced for religious reasons from the beginning of the Islamic era to the present. In contrast, the situation concerning drug abuse is different. Baasher reported that opium and cannabis have been used as therapeutic remedies since pre-Islamic times and have gradually come to be abused by laymen. Despite early attempts by various governments and rulers to ban the use of cannabis, hashish smoking became endemic in some Arab countries. It was not unusual to come across a patient with cannabis dependence in the

Sudan or opium dependence in Egypt. In Egypt, there is a current movement away from traditional opium and cannabis use to synthetic drugs. Those people dependent on drugs are firmly convinced that it is not wrong to indulge in the use of these drugs, "because they have not been prohibited by God and, anyway, they are not mentioned in the Quran." Thus, while the condemnation of alcohol generally continues in the Islamic world, the history of the use of dependence-producing drugs in the various Islamic countries is somewhat varied and complex.

III. EPIDEMIOLOGICAL DATA FROM VARIOUS SOCIETIES

A. Comparison among Asian Societies

As shown in Table 21-1, there are considerable data available from most Asian societies for cross-societal comparison and longitudinal comparison within the same society (Tseng et al., in press). Data are the recorded number of people arrested for substance abuse, mainly for defined illegal substances. It needs to be cautioned that such figures are heavily influenced by political attitudes toward abusive behavior and the pattern of law enforcement. These go beyond the general social contributions to substance abuse, including social stability, economic conditions, avail-

TABLE 21-1   Substance Abuse in Some Asian Societies: Annual Number of People Arrested per 100,000 Population[*]

Society	1980	1982	1984	1986	1988	1990	1992	1994	1996
Taiwan, China[a]	0.1	0.9	1.1	1.1	1.4	2.6	16.0	41.7	
Japan[b]	19.2	20.1	20.4	19.4	17.0	12.5	12.4	12.0	15.9
Korea[c]		1.8	1.8	2.3	4.1	4.1	4.2	5.3	5.2
Malaysia[d]	75.2		66.5	46.5		38.7			35.0

[*] From W.S. Tseng et al., *International Journal of Social Psychiatry,* (in press).
[a] *Statistics of the Department of Police,* Taiwan Provincial Government, Vol. 31, Taiwan, China (1996)
[b] *Annual Report of Crime,* Ministry of Law, Japan (1997)
[c] *Annual Statistics of Police,* Department of Police, Seoul, Korea (1997)
[d] *National Drug Monitoring System,* Malaysia (1991) and Tseng et al. (1998)

ability of the substances, and people's attitudes toward the abuse of certain substances. Thus, there are limitations for direct cross-societal comparisons based on the number of people arrested for abuse. However, comparisons made within the same society are relatively meaningful from a chronological standpoint.

It is clear that the figures may fluctuate differently in different societies. For instance, in Japan, the number of arrest cases was high in the 1980s and became lower in the 1990s. In South Korea, the rate increased steadily from the 1980s to the 1990s. Singapore seemed to have the same tendency. Beginning in the mid-1970s, heroin abuse in Malaysia became such a rampant problem that, in 1984, it was declared "public enemy No. 1" by the prime minister.

As mentioned previously, after it was established, the communist regime in China became known for its remarkable, radical elimination of the opium addiction problem that had existed for nearly a century. However, the problems of substance abuse have been rising again, particularly in the south border area, since China opened her doors to the rest of the world.

In 1993, in order to understand the extent of this rising problem, a collaborative research team was formed to conduct a community survey in China (Xiao et al., 1996). Five high-risk areas were chosen for the study: Langzho and Xian, located on the so-called Silk Road connecting China to the Western border countries, and Anshun, Wenshan, and Guangzhou, which have access to southeast Asia. It was revealed that most of the cases started their abuse after 1988, when an international crime group established the so-called China Channel for importing illicit drugs into China. It was found that the overall lifetime prevalence for these five areas surveyed ranged between 0.69 and 1.60%, with an average of 1.08%. The highest rates were found in the country of Anshun in Gueizhou Province (1.60%) and in Guangzhou City (1.41%). Anshun was used by the international criminal group as its main station for importing illicit drugs into China.

It is fair to say that substance abuse, in general, is not as serious in most Asian societies as it is in European and American societies. However, there are some exceptions. No figures are available, but it is suspected that the problems of substance abuse are becoming rather severe in Thailand.

B. DATA FROM THE UNITED STATES

In the early 1960s, the number of opiate addicts in the United States started to rise, reaching a peak in the late 1970s. According to Kaplan (1983), the estimated number of heroin addicts ranged between 387,000 and 453,000 at the peak of usage. Meanwhile, other drugs became popular and drug problems became more widespread. According to the U.S. Department of Health and Human Services (USDHHS) (1991), over one-fifth of adolescents (ages 12 to 17) and over half of young adults (ages 18 to 25) reported trying illicit drugs by 1974. The lifetime rate of marijuana use among college students doubled between 1970 and 1984, whereas cocaine use increased 10-fold in that same period, from 2.7 to 30% (Rouse, 1991).

Data available from the Drug Abuse Warning Network in 1993 showed different patterns among three ethnic groups compared in the manner of drug-related deaths (National Institute on Drug Abuse, 1995, p. 85). It was revealed that the percentage of death associated with accident or suicide was 62.9% vs 7.8% among African-Americans (with a ratio of 8.1/1), 80.5% vs 11.1% for Hispanic-Americans (with a ratio of 7.3/1), and 51.8% vs 26.7% for Caucasian-Americans (with a ratio of 1.9/1). In other words, African-American and Hispanic-American drug abusers tended to end their lives through drug-related accidents, Caucasian-Americans by suicide.

As illustrated in Table 21-2, it is interesting to note that, in the United States, data available from the USDHHS (1997) concerning the percentage of users in a community show a national trend of steady decline for all substances from the 1980s to the 1990s. This is true for marijuana, cocaine, and cigarettes, respectively. This indicates that, associated with an increased concern for health, as well as changes in the social situation, there has been considerable improvement from the peak of substance abuse observed in the

TABLE 21-2 **Substance Abuse in the United States by Percentage**[a]

	1979	1982	1985	1988	1990	1992	1994
Marijuana	16.6	15.9	13.6	9.8	9.4	7.9	8.5
Cocaine	4.8	5.6	5.1	3.6	2.7	2.1	1.7
Cigarettes			40.5	38.5	36.1	35.2	31.7

[a] From *National Household Survey on Drug Abuse: Main Findings 1995,* U.S. Department of Health and Human Services (1997)

post-Vietnam era. Associated with the recent increased awareness of the health hazards of smoking, cigarette use has been declining slowly but significantly over the past two decades.

C. INFORMATION FROM EUROPE

From Italy, Davoli and associates (1997) reported that there was a persistent rise in mortality among injection drug users in Rome between 1980 and 1992. They reviewed a total of 4200 injection drug users attending the three largest drug treatment centers in Rome between 1980 and 1988. The cohort of subjects was followed up in December 1992. Results revealed that the age-adjusted mortality rate of this cohort reached a minimum of 7.8/1000 persons/year in 1985/86 and rose steadily to 27.7/1000 in 1991 to 1992. The major cause of death was overdose in 1987/88; thereafter, AIDS became the first cause of death.

D. FRAGMENTED INFORMATION FROM AFRICA

Comprehensive epidemiological information about substance abuse in Africa is scarce. Abiodun (1991) reviewed drug abuse with special reference to Nigeria. He pointed out that in addition to alcohol, other substances abuse had become a major public health problem in Nigeria. Among all substances, cannabis was

the most widely abused illicit drug in the country. It was introduced into the country and other parts of west Africa during and after World War II by soldiers and sailors returning from the Middle East, the Far East, and north Africa. Bensodiazepines are the most widely abused therapeutic agents. The widespread use of this group of drugs results partly from the overprescribing habits of medical practicners and the freedom of patients to purchase drugs without prescription from chemists' shops and medicine stores. These drugs were found to be more abused by females and older persons. Psychostimulants, such as proplus (a caffeine concentrate) and amphetamines, were mainly abused by students, long-distance drivers, and soldiers. Stimulants are taken not for their pleasurable effects, but to improve intellectual performance and to postpone inattentiveness and sleepiness. Organic solvents and hallucinogens remain uncommon, but hard drugs, such as cocaine and heroin, appear to be on the increase in big cities.

IV. SUMMARY

It is clear that substance abuse needs to be understood as a pathology attributed to different biological, psychological, and sociocultural factors. Cultural factors, functioning closely with social ones, contribute to the basic attitudes toward the abuse of substances, the choice of chemical indulgence as a coping mechanism for stress, and efforts to deal with social problems. There is a general tendency, when a society as a whole is facing certain stresses, whether socioeconomic crisis, social instability, or cultural disintegration, for the problems of substance abuse and other associated social pathologies (such as suicidal, violent, or criminal behavior) to rise. The emerging of substance abuse, in turn, accelerates the process of social and cultural disintegration in a vicious way. Thus, substance abuse serves as one of the indexes for social stability. As pointed out by Westermeyer (1999), there are consequences of addiction on ethnicity. For instance, a decline in ethnic affiliation among addicted individuals accompanies reduced activities (such as religious rituals and ethnic celebrations) that reinforce ethnic identity and support ethnic organizations. Addicted individuals often become alienated and isolated from their ethnic groups.

From the examples reviewed, several issues have become clear regarding the unique nature of substance abuse. The situation in Laos, for instance, illustrates that the availability of a substance plays a role in determining whether criminal behavior will be associated with its abuse. The example from China shows that even a serious and chronic abuse problem can be eradicated within a short period of time, providing the society has a dictatorial political system, with strong social motivation and firm policies to enforce it, and that there are effective ways to control the supply of the substance being abused. In other words, the effectiveness of actions taken to eradicate the abuse of a certain substance depends on the social structure and cultural attitudes. In general, if a society is healthy enough, the problems of abuse will fade away naturally (as happened in postwar Japan). Otherwise, substance abuse will add to the speed of sociocultural deterioration.

The actual therapy for substance abuse needs to be carried out at a microscopic level, relying on individual and group therapy and a social rehabilitation program; however, it is useful to understand the nature of the problem in its sociocultural dimensions and to develop a general policy for treatment as well as social prevention at the macroscopic level (Smart et al., 1988).

REFERENCES

Abiodun, O.A. (1991). Drug abuse and its clinical implications with reference to Nigeria. *Central African Journal of Medicine, 37,* 24–30.

Anthony, J.C., & Helzer, J.E. (1995). Epidemiology of drug dependence. In M.T. Tsuang, M. Tohen, & G.E.P. Zahner (Eds.), *Textbook in psychiatric epidemiology* (pp. 361–406). New York: Wiley-Liss.

Baasher, T. (1981). The use of drugs in the Islamic world. *British Journal of Addiction, 76,* 233–243.

Davoli, M., Perucci, C.A., Rapiti E., Bargagli, A.M., D'lppoliti, D., Forastiere, F., & Abeni, D. (1997). A persistent rise in mortality among injection drug users in Rome, 1980 through 1992. *American Journal of Public Health, 87,* 851–853.

Fields, A., & Tararin, P.A. (1970). Opium in China. *British Journal of Addiction, 64,* 371–382.

Hemmi, T. (1974). Sociopsychiatric study of drug abuse in Japan. In *Proceedings of the fifth World Congress of Psychiatry, Mexico, D.F.:* World Psychiatric Association.

Kaplan, J. (1983). *The hardest drug: Heroin and public policy.* Chicago: University of Chicago Press.

Kato, M. (1990). Brief history of control, prevention and treatment of drug dependence in Japan. *Drug and Alcohol Dependence, 25,* 213–214.

Kato Price, R., Wada, K., & Murray, K.S. (1995). Protective factors for drug abuse: A prospectus for a Japanese-U.S. epidemiological study. In R., Kato Price, B.M., Shea, & H.N. Mookherjee, (Eds.), *Social psychiatry across cultures: Studies from North American, Asia, Europe, and Africa.* New York: Plenum Press.

Lowinger, P. (1973). How the People's Republic of China solve the drug abuse problem. *American Journal of Chinese Medicine, 1*(2), 275–282.

National Institute on Drug Abuse. (1995). *Drug use among racial/ethnic minorities.* Rockville, MD: National Institute of Health.

Rouse, B.A. (1991). Trends in cocaine use in the general population. *NIDA Research Monograph, 110* (DHHS Publication No. ADM 91-1787).

Smart, R., Murray, G.F., & Arif, A. (1988). Drug abuse and prevention programs in 29 countries. *International Journal of the Addictions, 23,* 1–17.

Tamura, M. (1989). Japan: Stimulant epidemics past and present. *United Nations Bulletin of Narcotics, 41,* 81–93.

Trimble, J.E., Bolek, C.S., & Niemcryk, S.J. (Eds.). (1992). *Ethnic and multicultural drug abuse: Perspective on current research.* New York: Harrington Park Press.

Tseng, W.S., Ebata, K., Kim, K.I., Krahl, W., Kua, E.K., Lu, Q.Y., Shen, Y.C., Tan, E.S., & Yang, M.J. (in press). Mental health in Asia: Social improvement and challenges. *International Journal of Social Psychiatry.*

U.S. Department of Health and Human Services (USDHHS). (1991). *Drug abuse and drug abuse research. The third triennial report to Congress from the Secretary, Department of Health and Human Services* (DHHS Publication No. ADM 91-1704). Rockville, MD: U.S. Department of Health and Human Services

U.S. Department of Health and Human Services (USDHHS). (1997). *National household survey on drug abuse: Main findings 1995.* Washington, DC: USDHHS.

Westermeyer, J. (1971). Use of alcohol and opium by the Meo of Laos. *American Journal of Psychiatry, 127,* 1019–1023.

Westermeyer, J. (1974). Opium smoking in Laos: A survey of 40 addicts. *American Journal of Psychiatry, 131,* 165–170.

Westermeyer, J. (1987). Cultural patterns of drug and alcohol use: An analysis of host and agent in the cultural environment. *United Nations Bulletin of Narcotics, 39,* 11–27.

Westermeyer, J. (1999). Cross-cultural aspects of substance abuse. In M. Galanter & H.D. Kleber (Eds.), *Textbook of substance abuse treatment* (pp. 25–85). Washington, DC: American Psychiatric Press.

Xiao, S.Y., Hao, W., Young, D.S., & National Collaborating Research Teams. (1996). Epidemiological study on illicit drug use in five high-risk areas of China. Part I: Lifetime prevalence of illicit drug use. *Chinese Mental Health Journal, 10*(5), 234–238 (in Chinese).

22

Suicidal Behavior

I. INTRODUCTION

Suicidal behavior is relatively more suited to cross-cultural comparative study than any other kind of psychopathology. This is because it is well-defined behavior about which official data is often available. Thus, studies of suicidal behavior present fewer problems in terms of diagnostic criteria than studies of other psychiatric conditions. Physicians, police, or even laymen can identify suicidal behavior without psychiatric knowledge and experience. Further, suicidal behavior is predominantly related to psychological factors and can therefore be analyzed and understood as an emotion-related disturbance whose sociocultural aspects can be examined (Farberow, 1975; Kok & Tseng, 1992; Tseng et al., in press).

However, there are some problems inherent in the cross-cultural study of suicide. Strictly speaking, from the standpoint of cause, suicide is not a homogeneous clinical phenomenon. Some suicide behaviors occur as complications of severe psychiatric disorders, such as delusion or hallucination, or are associated with major depression. They may occur as a secondary reaction to stigmatized mental disorders that are chronic or untreatable. Suicide is often associated

with substance abuse or dependence. Thus, some suicide behaviors are directly related to psychiatric disorders. Many other suicide behaviors occur as daily life reactions to emotional turmoil or frustration and, as psychologically related, very much reflect the distress that exists in a society or cultural system. The different natures of suicide behavior are generally not distinguished in statistical data of suicide, but are lumped together, which influences the interpretation of the information from a sociocultural perspective. Depending on their religious backgrounds, social attitudes toward suicide vary greatly in different societies and may affect medical and official willingness to report suicide occurrences. These factors need to be taken into consideration in cross-cultural comparisons of epidemiological data.

Finally, the distinction between "committed suicide" or "completed suicide" (normally referred to simply as "suicide") and "suicidal attempt" (or "para-suicide," in the British system) is arbitrary and depends on whether the suicidal behavior is successful or not. However, clinicians generally believe that the two have some different features. The age of the population, male/female ratio, motivation for action, and associated psychiatric disorders, for instance, are relatively different in committed and attempted suicides. Following professional custom, the two will be reviewed separately in this chapter.

II. SUICIDE

A. COMPARISON OF FREQUENCIES OF SUICIDE

1. Total Suicide Rate

Based on the World Health Organization's (WHO) special report on suicide (1973) for the period between 1950 and 1969, official annual data from the World Health Statistics Annuals (WHO, 1976–1996), available for the period of 1970–1994, supplemented by information from individual investigators (mostly from underdeveloped and developing countries), the total suicide rates (per 100,000 population) of different countries (or societies) in different world regions are compiled in Table 22-1. Although in most of the countries there were considerable differences in rates between males and females, for the sake of convenience, they are combined as total suicide rates. Differences in male/female suicide rates will be discussed separately later.

There are several findings regarding the total suicide rates of various countries. First, there is a rather wide range of rates among the different countries. They can be subdivided arbitrarily into groups of "high," "moderate," and "low." The "high" group has total suicide rates above 20 per 100,000 population. Hungary, Finland, Denmark, South Korea, Austria, and Switzerland belong to this group. Many countries, including Czechoslovia, Japan, France, and Belgium, belong to the "moderate" group, which has total suicide rates between 10 and 20 per 100,000 population. The "low" group, with total suicide rates below 10 per 100,000 population, includes the United Kingdom the Netherlands, Italy, Israel, and Spain. Several countries, such as Greece, Mexico, Malaysia, and the Philippines, have noticiablly very low suicide rates: below 5 per 100,000 population.

There is a difference of almost 30 to 40 times between the very high rate countries, such as Hungary (36.2–41.9) and Finland (21.8–28.2) and the very low rate countries, such as Mexico (0.7–3.0), the Philippines (0.6–1.2), or Malaysia (0.6–1.6). This range of differences in rates is in very wide contrast to other psychiatric disorders, such as schizophrenia, which has a difference of merely several times. There are no particular geographic distribution patterns noted among the groups. Actually, considerable differences have been found among neighboring countries, such as Denmark, Sweden, and Norway in Scandinavia, a phenomenon that has attracted the interest and speculation of scholars. Many of the very low rate countries are Muslim or Catholic societies that have prohibitive religious attitudes toward self-killing.

Another valuable finding derived from Table 22-1 is that the suicide rates for many countries are generally stable even over several decades. However, if there is dramatic sociocultural change or political turmoil, there are relatively obvious vicissitudes of suicide rates. Based on detailed information available, this latter situation will be elaborated later, as exemplified in societies such as Japan, Taiwan, and Micronesia.

After reviewing international data derived from the WHO data bank, other resources, and available literature, Diekstra and Garnefski (1995) concluded that there has been a true increase in suicide mortality and morbidity over the last three decades among the white urban populations of North America and Europe, particularly among male adolescents and young adults. Among the possible causal mechanisms they listed are the corresponding increase in the prevalence of depressive disorders and substance abuse; psychobiological changes, in particular, the dramatic lowering of the age of puberty; an increase in the number of social stressors; and changes in attitudes toward suicidal behavior and the related increase of availability of suicidal models.

Examining the WHO mortality database for the period 1955 to 1989, La Vecchia, Lucchini, and Levi (1994) pointed out that, with respect to trends over time, the figures for suicide rates were relatively

TABLE 22-1 Worldwide Suicide Rates: Chronological Trends from 1950 to 1994[a]

Country	50–54	55–59	60–64	65–69	70–74	75–79	80–84	85–89	90–94
Hungary					36.9	38.4		41.9	36.2
Finland					24.0	25.1	21.8	28.2	27.2
Denmark		22.0	19.2	19.2	23.9	24.1	23.9	28.0	22.6
South Korea[b]				29.8	27.0	31.9	26.0	21.0	17.0
Austria					23.4	24.1	22.5	25.0	23.1
Switzerland	22.1	20.9	18.0	17.8	19.5	20.6		22.7	21.6
Czechoslovakia					24.6		18.5	19.2	18.8
Japan	20.0	24.5	18.0		16.8	18.0	14.5	18.9	17.0
France		16.6	15.5	15.4	16.1	15.6	15.5	22.1	21.6
Belgium		14.2	14.2	15.0	15.4	14.9	17.1	22.5	18.0
Sweden					20.3	19.4	15.5	18.5	15.2
Germany		18.8	19.1	20.6	19.9	21.0		17.9	15.8
Australia	10.2	11.3	13.4	13.7		11.7	10.3	13.8	11.6
USA			10.7	10.9	11.5	12.1	10.4	12.9	12.4
Taiwan, China[c]	10.0	14.0	16.0	19.0	13.0	10.0	11.0	12.0	
Canada	7.4	7.4	7.6	9.4	12.2	12.9	12.9	12.3	12.8
Poland					12.0	11.3		12.4	14.9
Singapore[d]	13.1	12.2	10.4	9.4	9.8	10.9	10.7	9.9	12.7
Norway			7.3	7.6	9.0	10.4	14.5	15.6	14.5
New Zealand	9.6	9.2	8.8	9.6	8.8	9.0	10.3	11.0	12.9
UK	10.5	11.6	11.7	9.8	7.7	7.9	8.7	10.3	7.6
Netherlands	6.1	6.4	6.5	6.8	8.2	8.9	9.0	11.4	10.5
Italy			5.5	5.3	5.8	5.4	5.7	8.3	8.1
Israel					7.5	5.5		7.8	7.1
Spain					4.4	4.0	4.5	6.6	7.9
Chile					5.5	5.5	6.3	5.4	5.8
Greece					27		2.9		3.5
Mexico					0.7	2.1		2.2	3.0
Malaysia[e]						0.6	1.5	1.6	
Philippines					0.6	1.2			

[a] Based on World Health Statistics, WHO, 1976–1996, and other sources.
[b] The Bureau of Statistics (1998) *Annual Statistics of Death and Its Cause 1998*. Seoul Korea.
[c] M.Y. Chong et al. (1992).
[d] L.P. Kok (1992).
[e] S. Ong and Y.K. Leng (1992).

favorable in less developed areas of the world, including Latin America and several countries in Asia. (In the WHO database, no data were available from most of the African countries, so comment was not possible about that region.) In contrast, there was an upward trend, particularly among elderly men, in Canada, the United States, Australia, and New Zealand.

The popular belief in the past was that suicide was a product of civilization and development and was rare in preliterate cultures (Zilboorg, 1936). More current reports show considerable variation. Hoskin, Friedman, and Cawte (1969) reported that although New Guinea reputedly had a very low suicide rate, one area of New Guinea, namely the Kandrian district of southwest New Britain, a "preliterate-primitive" society, had a high incidence of suicide, estimated to be 23 per 100,000 population—almost double the rates reported in Western countries. A disruption of cooperative interpersonal relationships was speculated to be the main reason for the high rate of suicide.

Another stereotypical view was that suicide rates were high among culturally uprooted indigenous people. This may have beeen true in many cases, but, as pointed out by Shore (1975), concerning Native Americans in the United States, there is a need to distinguish between fact and fantasy. High suicide rates among tribes with relatively small population bases have received widespread publicity and have been generalized to include all Native Americans. However, lower suicide rates in larger tribes have received little or no emphasis. Shore reported that, in fact, there are considerable differences among different tribes, with suicide rates varying between 8 and 120 per 100,000 population. He warned that tribal differences should be recognized and overgeneralization should be avoided.

In terms of socioeconomic development, some scholars have indicated that the rate of suicide is generally low in less developed cultural areas. For example, Asuni (1962) estimated that the suicide rate in Western Nigeria (from 1957 to 1960) was extremely low, less than 1 per 100,000 population. Fallers and Fallers (1960) reported that the suicide rate for Busoga in Uganda (from 1952 to 1954) was 7.0 per 100,000 population.

2. Age Distribution of Suicide

Even within the same society, suicide behavior is subject to different variables, such as age and gender, which provide valuable information regarding the nature of suicide behavior in the society concerned. Based on information available regarding age distribution of suicide rates, WHO (Ruzicka, 1976) has recognized three types of suicide curves: the "Czechoslovakian," "Finnish," and "Japanese." (The "Berlin" type was also described, but, as it was not found in many other societies, it was omitted here.) The "Micronesian" type was added by Tseng and Kok (1992) to describe the particular pattern observed in Micronesia, Hawaii, and other island societies in the Pacific. These are illustrated in Fig. 22-1.

The perception and experience of stress and reactions to distress are not necessarily the same among different age groups, even within the same society. As a result, the frequency of suicide among different age groups differs, manifesting different age-related suicide curves.

a. Czechoslovakian Type

This type of suicide curve is characterized by a continuous increase in rate associated with an increase in age. The reason for this age distribution is not clear. It is suspected that it is related to the stress encountered in old age or attitudes toward life held by the elderly, as well as the society in general. This is a subject that awaits future investigation. Elderly suicide was most notable in Czechoslovakia and Hungary. The extremely high rates of suicide in old age (e.g., 75.7 for 65 to 74 years and 108.7 for 75 years and above in Hungary in 1975; and 45.0 and 65.5, respectively, in Czechoslovakia in 1972) contributed to the very high total rates. France and Austria also had this type of curve.

b. Finnish Type

Basically similar to the Czechoslovakian type, the suicide rate of this group gradually increases with age, peaking around 50 or 60 years and declining thereafter. This suggests that life is full of distress around late middle age and early old age, but not in very old age. Again, future study is necessary to confirm this speculation. Besides Finland, this type is found in Canada, Sweden, Poland, and elsewhere. According to Robins and Kulbok (1988), suicide rates for older men in the United States declined between 1950 and 1980; therefore, the age-related suicide curve was becoming the Finnish type.

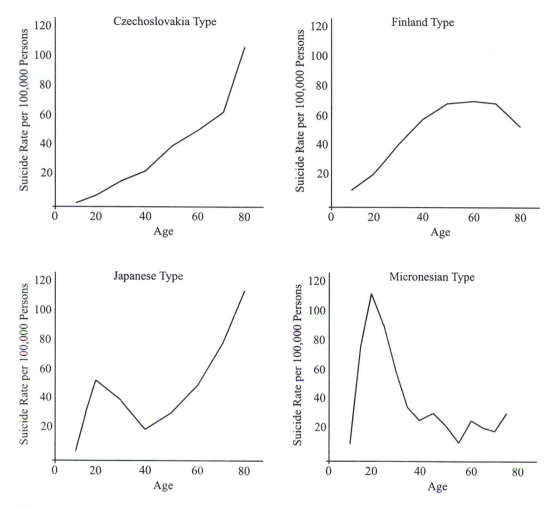

FIGURE 22-1 **Various types of age-related suicide curves.** (From WHO, 1988; and W.S. Tseng and L.P. Kok, in *Suicide behavior in the Asia-Pacific Region,* Singapore University Press, 1992).

c. *Japanese Type*

This type is characterized by a bimodal curve, peaking in youth, declining in middle age, then rising again thereafter. This is related to the considerable social restrictions on and expectations of youth that tend to make their lives stressful, leading some to take suicidal action. While this type reflected the charac-

teristic suicide pattern in Japan three decades ago (and was accordingly), the suicide curve in contemporary Japan has changed. With the lives of young people becoming more favorable after World War II, the peak that originally existed in the 20- to 30-year-old age group disappeared. As a result, the total suicide curve for the Japanese gradually changed into the Czecho-

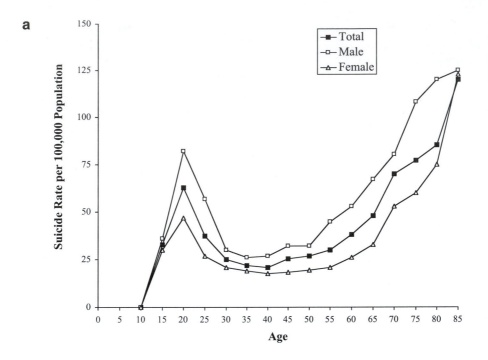

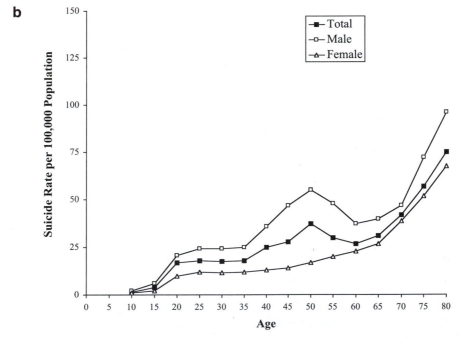

FIGURE 22-2 Conversion of age-related suicide curves in Japan from 1955 to 1986. (a) 1955 and (b) 1986. (From K. Yoshimatsu, in *Suicide behavior in the Asia-Pacific Region,* Singapore University Press, 1992).

slovakian type over the past three decades (see Fig. 22-2). A similar phenomenon was observed in Taiwan: the peak that was previously observed in the 20- to 30-year age group disappeared between 1964 and 1988, and the bimodal curve converted into the Czechoslovakian type (Chong, Yeh, & Wen, 1992, p. 74). However, the Japanese type of suicide curve is still found among many countries in Asia, such as Thailand and China, and in Central and South American countries, such as Mexico and Chile.

d. Micronesian Type

This unique suicidal curve is found in societies where suicide among adults is traditionally relatively rare. However, associated with a rapid increase in the young population, and socioeconomical changes and cultural uprooting that result in considerable distress, confusion, or frustration among the young, there is a rapid rise in suicidal behavior among teenagers and young adults (Tseng & Kok, 1992). The suicide is often associated with other psychiatric disturbances, such as substance abuse, drinking problems, and violent behavior. The suicide curve is characterized by a high peak around the 15- to 30-year age group. The rate declines gradually from adulthood to the aged (Rubinstein, 1992). This type of curve is found mainly among male subjects. Besides Micronesia, this curve is observed in other parts of the Pacific, including Hawaii and Samoa, as well as among many native or aboriginal tribes on the American and other continents that have encountered cultural uprooting.

3. Male/Female Suicide Ratios

In contrast to suicide attempts, which are more prevalent among female subjects, the rate of committed suicide is generally higher for males than females in most countries around the world. The male/female ratios vary considerably. For instance, data from WHO (1993) showed that the rate (or ratio) of male/female was 19.9/4.8 (4.15/1) for the United States; 20.4/5.2 (3.92/1) for Canada; 34.6/11.6 (2.98/1) for Austria; and 30.0/15.1 (1.99/1) for Den-

mark. Thus, disregarding the actual rates, the ratios are always higher for male than for female completed suicides (Canetto & Lester, 1998). Scholars in the past have interpreted this as due to the use of more lethal methods by male than female subjects, ending more often in successful suicides. However, this view needs to be revised. Newly available data from mainland China, which comprises nearly a quarter of the world's population, has shown that the committed suicide rate is considerably higher for females than males, with a male/female ratio of 0.77/1 (Pritchard, 1996). This is particularly true in rural areas and among young females. For the 15- to 24-year age group, the male/female ratio is 0.52/1 for the whole country, meaning the rate for young females is almost twice that of young males (Pritchard, 1996). This reflects that, as in the past, the role of women is still less favorable than that of men, especially in rural traditional society, and the lives of young females, as unmarried women, young wives, or daughters-in-law, are still more full of distress. Ending their own lives remains one of the choices available to them for dealing with difficulties they encounter.

4. Vicissitude of Suicide Rates within the Same Society

As mentioned previously, although the total suicide rate for a society may tend to be stable over many decades, a considerable fluctuation may be noticed in association with dramatic social changes occurring within a decade or so. This situation occurred in the following three societies.

a. Japan

According to Yoshimatsu (1992), the total suicide rate for the Japanese was rather consistent from 1890 to 1935 — mostly in the range of 15 to 20 per 100,000 population. However, after 1935, when Japan went to war with China and later was involved in the Pacific War with America and its allies, the suicide rate declined considerably, reaching a bottom of 12 in 1943, shortly before World War II ended.

After the war, while the Japanese were trying to reconstruct their country, the suicide rate increased gradually but steadily, reaching a peak of 25 around 1958, when reconstruction was completed and people started to enjoy affluent lives again. After this, the rate declined and returned almost to its previous baseline (see Fig. 22-3). This supports the view that suicide tends to decline when a society is at war with an external enemy. Yoshimatsu pointed out that the increase in the suicide rate between 1955 and 1960 was attributed to the increase in suicide among the elderly. He called this a cohort phenomenon, explaining that this cohort of the population went through hard times as children and teenagers during the war, worked very hard for socioeconomic recovery during adulthood, but, when they reached old age, lost their life goals and had difficulty adjusting to the cultural changes in their society.

b. Taiwan

Vicissitudes in the total suicide rates associated with rapid sociocultural change have been reported in Taiwan as well (Chong et al., 1992; Yeh, 1985). The total suicide rate was around 10 per 100,000 population in 1948, rising sharply and reaching a peak of 18 in 1963, then declining gradually to a level of 10 after 1975 (see Fig. 22-4). The change in suicide rates was associated with the rapid sociocultural change that occurred in Taiwan during that period of time. After mainland China was taken over by the Communists in 1948, the Nationalist government retreated to Taiwan with a couple of million soldiers and civilians. This massive internal migration, along with the military tension that remained in the China Strait, produced dramatic social, political, and cultural changes. After two decades, when the society was stabilized, the total suicide rate returned to its original level. It deserves

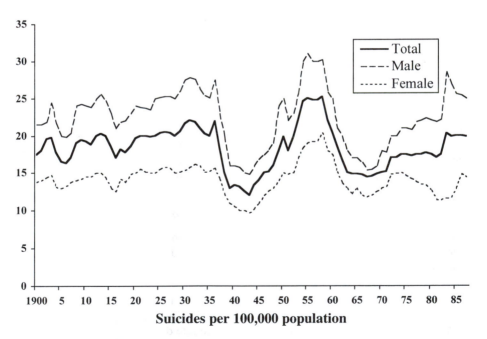

FIGURE 22-3 Suicide rates in Japan from 1890 to 1987. (From K. Yoshimatsu, in *Suicide behavior in the Asia-Pacific Region,* Singapore University Press, 1992).

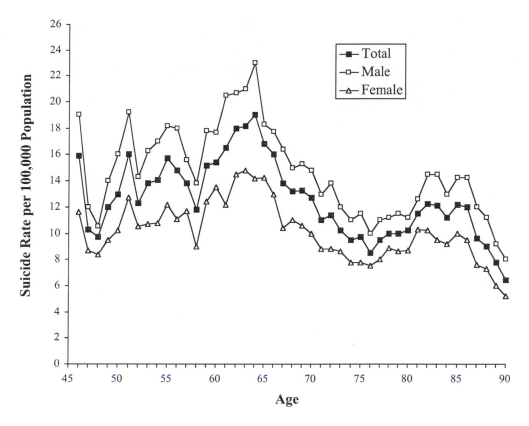

FIGURE 22-4   Suicide rates in Taiwan between 1946 and 1990. (From M.Y. Chong & T.A. Cheng, in *Chinese societies and mental health,* Hong Kong: Oxford University Press, 1995).

mentioning that a 15-year follow-up epidemiological study carried out during this period of social change (Lin, Rin, Yeh, Hsu, & Chu, 1969) revealed that there was a considerable increase in minor psychiatric disorders as well [cross-reference to Chapter 12: Culture and Psychiatric Epidemiology (Section II,B,1)].

c. Micronesia

After its occupation by Germany and Japan, Micronesia became part of the American Trust Territories after World War II. There was an improvement in health systems, resulting in a decline in the infant mortality rate, leading to a sudden increase in population, particularly the youth. More than half of the pop-

ulation was under 18. There were radical changes in education and political structure, and the society changed from a subsistence economy to a cash-employment system. Many youngsters, after finishing their formal school education, were unable to find jobs. Previously, during the era of colonialism, alcohol was forbidden to local inhabitants. After their liberation by the Americans, restrictions on drinking were removed and great quantities of beer and liquor were imported. It was not the adults but the youngsters who soon indulged in drinking. Excessive drinking, substance abuse, and violent behavior became common daily phenomena among young people. Suicidal behavior became common among them, too. In the past, suicidal behavior had seldom been observed among the islanders. In 1960, the total rate was 3.9 per 100,000. Among females, it was less than 5. However, among young males, it became almost epidemic, with a sharp increase that reached an extremely high peak of 50 around 1980, bringing the total rate to 29.9 (Rubinstein, 1992, pp. 203–205). Clearly, the high suicide rate was a manifestation of the difficulties young males were having in adjusting to the rapidly changing island society (see Fig. 22-5).

5. The Same Ethnic Group in Different Societies

Although there has been no systematic collection of data for the comparison of the same ethnic groups in different social settings, there is some information that allows us to make inferences on how suicide rates may change within the same ethnic groups after they migrate to other cultures.

For instance, after three or four generations, the suicidal behavior of Japanese who migrated to Hawaii changed in frequency and method of suicide from that of Japanese Nationals in Japan. The rate for Japanese-Americans in Hawaii was 14.1 per 100,000 from 1973 to 1987 (Tseng, Hsu, Omori, & McLaughlin, 1992). This was relatively lower than the 16.0 to 19.0 per 100,000 for Japanese Nationals in the same period (Takahashi, Hirasawa, Koyama, Senzaki, Sensaki, 1998; Yoshimatsu, 1992). Further, family suicide (or parents–children group suicide), a special form of suicide that was still observed in Japan, was not observed among Japanese-Americans in Hawaii.

Suicide rates were found to vary considerably among ethnic Chinese living in different political–economic and subcultural settings. In mainland China in 1994, the rates per 100,000 population were 27.1 in some selected rural areas and 6.8 in some urban areas (WHO, 1995), 9.0 in Hong Kong (Lo, 1992), 12.0 in Taiwan (Chong et al., 1992), 9.9 in Singapore (Kok, 1992), and 57.1 in Malaysia (Ong & Leng, 1992). Because data were derived from different sources, the limitations of direct comparisons should be considered. However, broad differences were clearly observed between rural and urban regions, even within China, whereas differences were less in Hong Kong, Singapore, and Taiwan. However,

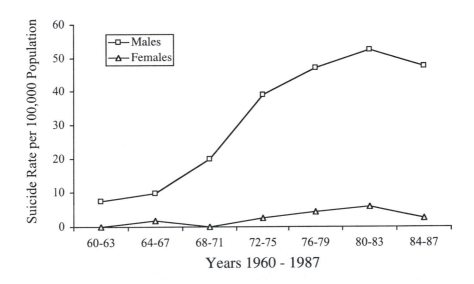

FIGURE 22-5   Suicide rates in Micronesia between 1960 and 1987. (From D.H. Rubinstein, in *Suicide behavior in Asia and Pacific Regions,* Singapore University Press, 1992).

the rate among Chinese in Malaysia was comparatively very high. This shows that the rate of suicide can change remarkably among groups of the same ethnic origin living in different societies with different socioeconomic–cultural environments.

6. Different Ethnic Groups within the Same Society

In addition to comparing the suicide rates of the same ethnic group living in different social environments, it is equally valuable to compare suicide patterns of different ethnic groups residing in the same society, as factors that may affect the patterns of reporting suicides are minimized and cross-ethnic comparisons can be made more reliably.

In Singapore, there are three ethnic groups living in the same city/country: Chinese, Malays, and Indians. The composition of these groups is 76, 15, and 6%, respectively. An analysis of coroners' cases showed that, in 1986, the suicide rates per 100,000 population (ages 10 and above) were 24.2 for the Indians, 17.4 for the Chinese, and only 2.5 for the Malays (Kok, 1992). Malays have less materialistic concerns and philosophical attitudes that lead to relatively high thresholds for life stress. In addition, they have strong negative sanctions against self-injurious behavior because of their Muslim background. These factors contribute to an extremely low rate of suicide among Malays, in contrast to the other ethnic groups residing in Singapore.

In peninsular Malaysia, the population is composed of the same three ethnic groups: Malays, Chinese, and Indians. Their composition, however, is proportionately different: Malays make up about 57%, Chinese 33%, and Indians 10%. However, in 1985 to 1986, the suicide rate per 100,000 population was 57.1 for the Chinese, 29.9 for the Indians, and only 3.9 for the Malays (Ong & Leng, 1992). Again, this showed that suicidal behavior was much less common among the Malays.

In the multiethnic society of Hawaii, the rate of suicide varies considerably among different ethnic groups. This is reflected more in the male population. In the years 1978 to 1982, the rate per 100,000 population was relatively higher in the Hawaiian (29.2) and Korean-American (24.4) groups, relatively lower among the Filipino-Americans (8.7) and the Chinese-Americans (7.1), with the Caucasian-Americans (18.5) and Japanese-Americans (11.7) in between (Tseng et al., 1992). This illustrated greater differences than similarities among different ethnic–cultural groups, even though they shared the same geographical and social environment over a period of time.

B. Comparison of Suicidal Behavior

1. Method of Suicide

Cross-ethnic comparisons of methods used to commit suicide reveal considerable differences. After members of the same ethnic group have moved to a different social environment and associated with the length of time they have been there, their method of suicide will change. In general, this illustrates that availability of method is a major determining factor in the one that is chosen for suicide, while familiarity of method also contributes to the choice. Mostly, there is no strong belief or attitude attached to the method of ending one's life. This will be illustrated by some examples.

A comparison of Japanese in Japan and Japanese-Americans in Hawaii revealed that drug overdose was used more frequently by Japanese Nationals, whereas the traditional method of hanging and the newer method of shooting were used by Japanese-Americans in Hawaii. People in Japan could buy drugs without a physician's prescription, but could not purchase guns; in Hawaii, civilians could possess guns, but could not buy lethal drugs without a doctor's prescription. Thus, social conditions shaped the choice of suicide method even among members of the same ethnic group.

Among ethnic Chinese, it was found that the ingestion of chemicals was a frequent method in rural areas of mainland China, using agricultural insecticides often used by farmers. Jumping from high rises was common in Hong Kong (more than 50% of those who were younger than 39 years, and 30 to 40% of those older than 40) (Hau, 1993) and Singapore, both urban societies with concentrations of high rises.

2. Motives for Suicide

Because information on possible motives for suicide is often the result of speculation by family members or others after the occurrence of the event, it is not adequate or reliable. However, available information can be used to discuss general trends and to illustrate that cultural factors may contribute strongly to the motives for suicide. Instead of reviewing in detail all the possible causes for suicide examined in various studies, only some characteristic trends will be summarized here to show how culture can contribute to suicide.

In a society where mental illness still carries a strong stigma, a relatively high percentage of people may commit suicide due to mental illness. For instance, in Hong Kong, 401% of suicides were attributed to mental disorders (Lo and Leung, 1985), whereas in Beijing, China, they accounted for 25.1% (Zhang, 1996). In Hawaii, among females, 11.1% Caucasian-American, 14.3% Hawaiian, and 20.0% Japanese-American, the stated reason for suicide was mental illness (Tseng et al., 1992). A report from Nigeria by Asuni (1962) indicated that, among all precipitating factors, 54 cases out of 110 cases (49.1%) were attributed to psychoses. Chia and Tsoi (1972) revealed that, in Singapore, 35.5% of suicides were related to psychiatric illness.

Suffering from a serious physical illness is another cause of suicide, particularly for males in cultures where men are considered the key financial support of the family. In Hawaii, 20.5% of Japanese-American male suicides were committed because of health problems, whereas only 11.8% of Caucasian-American male and 3.0% of Hawaiian male suicides were due to physical illness. According to Chia and Tsoi (1972), 28.8% of suicides in Singapore were caused by physical illness.

Suicide is often attributed to family conflict in societies in which family relationships are highly valued and there is still a strong emphasis on hierarchy within the family system. Hidden tensions or open conflicts exist in such family systems, often between in-laws, and suicide becomes one of the choices for resolving the conflict when few alternatives are available. Family conflict as a cause of suicide is often found in Eastern societies, such as the Philippines (79.3% of suicides were attributed to individual plus family stress by Ladrido-Ignacio and Gensaya, 1992), China (18.2% cited in Beijing by Zhang, 1996), and India (Ganapathi & Rao, 1966).

Relationship problems are common reasons for suicide in societies in which romantic relations are highly valued and the man–woman relationship is a predominant axis in interpersonal relations. A failure in man–woman relations can cause serious emotional frustration and become a cause for ending one's life. This is often observed in many Western societies.

Poverty, financial debt, or unemployment as causes for killing oneself are relatively rare in economically developed societies; however, financial difficulty can be a serious life threat and, as a motive for suicide, it is still common in undeveloped or developing societies. In India, Ganapathi and Rao (1996) reported that unemployment and poverty were common reasons for suicide, particularly among older individuals. In Thailand, socioeconomic factors were identified among the major causes of suicide. This was particularly true for males. According to Eungprabhanth (1975), among 177 males who committed suicide, 43 (24.3%) did so because of socioeconomic problems. In contrast, in the neighboring country of Singapore, economic factors comprised merely 9.9% of the causes for suicide (Chia & Tsoi, 1972).

It is obvious that many different reasons can lead to the same phenomenon of self-killing. Culture has a strong impact on people's perception and experience of and reaction to stress. The reasons for choosing suicide as a way of solving life problems are elaborated further in the following section, which addresses some unique forms of suicide.

III. SPECIAL FORMS OF SUICIDE

A. MULTIPLE SUICIDE

Ordinarily, suicide occurs as an individual self-killing behavior. However, it may sometimes involve more than one person, such as a couple, a family, or a group collectively. There is usually a strong cultural element in cases of multiple suicide. Following are different forms of suicide involving more than a single person.

1. Double Suicide

This is also called couple suicide and refers to the situation in which two people commit suicide together. It usually involves two people who are in love, but, due to social restrictions or parental disapproval, are not permitted to be together or get married. As a result, they decide to die together. This form of suicide is still observed in some societies that have certain social taboos or restrictions that young couples must observe. For instance, in China or Korea, cultural forbids a man and woman with the same surname to marry. It is believed that, theoretically, having the same surname, they are descendants of the same ancestors, even though in reality they are not blood "relatives." Defining incestuous relations broadly, marriage between two persons with the same surname is considered a cultural taboo. Unfortunately, there is a rather limited number of family names in China and Korea, in particular. In Korea, there are no more than a dozen common surnames, such as Kim, Pak, Lee, and Chong. Thus, there is a good chance that a young person might fall in love with someone with the surname. This becomes a serious matter if they do not want to give up their relationship. Dying together is one of the choices they can make.

In many traditional societies, a young couple still needs parental permission to marry. The parents may oppose their union if one partner does not have a properly matched family background or is not of an equivalent social caste (as in India). In some soci-eties, it is considered unacceptable for a man with a respected status (such as the son of a well-known family) to marry a woman who was married before or has children from a previous marriage. It is considered improper for such a man to marry such a woman. This was actually the theme of a popular novel, *Aizenkatsura,* written in Japan several decades ago. Facing such an unresolvable situation, some couples may commit double suicide, wanting to be united in another world after their deaths. According to Ohara (1963), in the 1960s and 1970s, double suicides accounted for about 4% of all suicides in Japan.

Occasionally, a husband and wife may plan to die together. For instance, if one of them is suffering from a terminal illness and the spouse does not want to survive alone, they may seek to die together as a couple. In Japan, when the Meiji emperor died, General Nogi, who led the army against Russia during the Japanese–Russian War and lost many soldiers in battle, in order to show his regret and loyalty toward the emperor, decided to commit suicide. Knowing of his decision, his wife joined him on his journey of death. The couple suicide of General Nogi and his wife was regarded as an example of loyalty in prewar Japan.

2. Family Suicide

As described previously [cross-reference to Chapter 13: Culture-Related Specific Syndrome (Section II,B,2)] this describes a culture-related unique phenomenon observed in Japan in which a whole family jointly commits suicide. It is called *ikka-shinju* in Japanese. One of the parents suggests suicide because of an unbearable personal situation, such as severe debt, an incurable disease, or other problems that seem insurmountable. The spouse then consents to die with his or her mate. Together the parents kill their young children and finally kill themselves, or plan to die by taking poison or drowning together. Thus, this suicide actually occurs as the double suicide of the parents combined with the homicide of the children

(Ohara, 1963). This form of family suicide is still observed in Japan. More than 100 cases are reported in Japanese newspapers annually.

Family suicide sounds like a great tragedy, but there are several motives behind it. First, it is a Japanese cultural belief that death is one way to resolve problems in life. If you are willing to take your life, all the debts or problems that you leave behind will be resolved—your responsibility is carried no further. Second, it is a cultural belief that "blood is thicker than water." It is assumed that no one will care for the children if they become orphans after the parents commit suicide. Family suicide occurs in a society that greatly values the ties between parents and their own children; it is believed that it is better to die together as a family than to leave behind a member of a broken family. Legally, it has long been forbidden in Japan for parents to carry out family suicide, but the phenomenon is still observed. The society reacts to family suicide with sympathy rather than criticism. Clearly, this form of suicide is closely related to cultural beliefs and attitudes. In a sense, it could be considered a culture-related specific syndrome based on culture-patterned stress-coping reactions.

3. Group Suicide

This occurs when members of a large group commit suicide together. It is also referred to as mass suicide or collective suicidel. This rather unusual phenomenon is often associated with a strong, underlying sense of patriotism or a unique communal spirit. Prompted by a shared experience and a common belief system, the group decides it is better to die together than to confront the disgrace and mistreatment of a surrender (if it is associated with war) than to suffer from the loneliness and grief that follow the death of a revered leader (if it is a tightly connected group) or to pursue together the truth of life or happiness in another world (if it is related to religion). Although this is not a commonly observed behavior, there is no shortage of examples.

Shortly before the end of World War II, many Japanese civilians committed collective mass suicide in Okinawa, Saipan, and Manchuria (China). When Russian soldiers took over Manchuria from the Japanese, the Japanese soldiers retreated to the border between China and Korea, leaving many civilians unprotected. Some of them took refuge, whereas others, members of a whole village, following military command, took cyanide together to end their lives. In Okinawa, civilians, including young students, hiding in caves from the American army used grenades distributed by the Japanese army to kill themselves. The most tragic story, however, happened in Saipan. Many hundreds of Japanese civilians (mostly Okinawans) were asked to commit mass suicide by jumping from the cliff at Parpi Point to the knife-edged rocks below (Crow, 1960). They were instructed by the military slogan of "preferring to be broken jade rather than to remain as a whole brick." The American Army used microphones to try and persuade them to surrender rather than kill themselves, assuring them that they would be properly treated, but they continued jumping from the cliff, shouting *"banzai"* (wishing the emperor 10,000 years of life!). Thus, afterward, the cliff was named *Banzai* cliff.

Mass suicides have also occurred in other parts of the world, mainly related to religion. The mass suicide in Jonestown, Guyana, in 1978, was one of the most shocking examples. In this tragedy, approximately 900 United States citizens, members of the People's Temple, swallowed potassium cyanide at the command of their cult leader, Jim Jones. In April 1997, near San Diego, California, 39 members of the Heaven's Gate cult carefully planned their death journeys when a comet appeared in the sky. They followed their cult leader to a higher level of life in outer space. Occasionally, newspapers will report a mysterious religious-group suicide in some part of Europe or Canada, performed by members of a Sun cult. Again, such group suicides are a part of cult behavior [cross-reference to Chapter 14: Epidemic Mental Disorders (Section III,F)].

B. Suicide to Serve a Certain Social Purpose

Suicide may be committed by a person not simply as a reaction to emotional frustration, but to serve a certain social purpose. The latter is the more prominent reason for committing suicide, and the self-killing action is undertaken in a certain way to communicate a significant message to others or to the society at large — expressing anger, resentment, revenge, protest, warning, or advice. When Vietnam monks burned themselves in the street to protest the government during the Vietnam War or a general killed himself to warm the emperor of his wrongdoing in dynasties in the past, the suicide actions were taken mainly to communicate a political message. When a woman kills herself to "preserve her chastity" or a soldier commits suicide to avoid being captured, they die willingly rather than face disgrace. A person who is accused unfairly or treated maliciously, without other ways to deal with such misfortune, might commit suicide, leaving the message that he will come back as a ghost to take revenge. In many societies, suicide is one way to expiate mistakes; the belief is that, legally and morally, one is pardoned for errors by killing oneself.

C. Socially Codified Suicidal Action

When it is demanded by an institution, follows cultural expectation, or fulfills a social purpose, some self-killing behavior is undertaken in a codified manner. This is distinctly different from personal-psychiatric suicide.

The best example is the practice of *suttee,* the old Hindu custom in which a widow cremates herself upon her husband's funeral pyre. In this obligatory self-killing, rules govern the place, the day, and the specific manner in which the suicide should take place. An individual's decision may be voluntary or virtually forced, but it is determined by a sense of responsibility to the established cultural system. Usually, the person who performs such a suicide does not suffer from any psychological disorder, but acts in a predetermined situation in a prescribed manner (Carstairs, 1956–1957).

In Japanese *kamikaze* missions during World War II, many — but not all — of the pilots committed suicide in an attempt to prevent their country's defeat. However, some *kamikaze* pilots went to their deaths unwillingly, shackled into their planes. The *kamikaze* actions near the end of the war were desperate military attempts to save the nation; however, at the beginning of the Pacific War, the Japanese navy carried out a suicidal minisubmarine attack on Pearl Harbor to win the war—a perfect example of suicidal action that is rooted in cultural thought and taken for a social purpose.

IV. SUICIDE ATTEMPTS

A. General Cautions for Comparisons

As mentioned previously, suicide attempts (also called parasuicides by the British) are arbitrarily distinguished from successful suicides. The distinction depends on whether a serious method of suicide was used or if the person attempting suicide was found and rescued in time. From the standpoint of frequency, in contrast to suicides, attempted suicides are often underestimated. This is because the former generally require medical–legal attention, so figures are closer to reality, whereas figures for the latter depend on the extent to which those who attempted suicide are referred for medical attention. If there is a negative attitude toward suicide in the society, such as in India, where, until recently, suicidal behavior was regarded as "a punishable legal offense" (Latha, Bhati, & D'Souza, 1996), suicide attempts tend to be concealed by the community.

Thus, if suicide attempts are to be examined cross-culturally, several issues need special attention. It is necessary to consider cultural attitudes that may influence or even lead to the concealment of the medical diagnosis and recording of attempted suicides. Customary patterns of referring attempted suicide cases for psychiatric examination and treatment need to be clarified. Also, a distinction needs to be made as to whether data are based on community surveys versus records of service utilization. The latter tends to reflect far less than the actual number of suicide attempts.

B. Reports from Different Societies

1. Europe

Perhaps the best study of attempted suicides in Europe is the WHO/EURO Multicentre Study on Parasuicide, which was implemented as a WHO program. The investigation was carried out in 16 centers in 13 European countries between 1989 and 1992, and produced a great deal of information. According to Schmidtke and colleagues (1996), the highest male age-standardized rate of suicide attempts was found in Helsinki, Finland (314/100,000), and the lowest in Guipuzcoa, Spain (45/100,000), representing a seven-fold difference. The highest average female age-standardized rate was found in Cergy-Pontoise, France (462/100,000), and the lowest, again, in Guipuzcoa, Spain (69/100,000). (It is also noted that there was a parallel between attempted suicide and committed suicide rates, with both very high for Finland and France and very low for Spain.) Further, it was found that, with only one exception (Helsinki), the suicide attempt rates were higher among women than among men. According to Bille-Brahe and associates (1997), the male/female sex ratio ranged from 0.41 to 0.85; and the mean age range for men was 33–45 years, for women, 29–45 years. In the majority of centers studied, the highest rates were found in the younger age groups. Schmidtke and colleagues (1996) indicated that compared with the general population, suicide attempters more often belonged to social categories associated with destabilization and poverty.

2. America

The lifetime prevalence of thoughts of death, wanting to die, and suicide attempts was examined by the NIMH Epidemiologic Catchment Area Study. In this community survey, 10.2% said that they had thought about committing suicide and 2.9% had attempted it at some time in their lives.

Concerning ethnic/racial differences, Pederson, Awad, and Kindler (1973) investigated the epidemiological differences between white and nonwhite suicide attempters. They examined 1,345 cases of attempted suicide, who were consecutively treated in the emergency department of a general hospital in Rochester, New York, during the period 1964 to 1967. According to hospital registration records, the ethnic backgrounds were recorded as either white or nonwhite. The white group included all Caucasians and most Puerto Rican and American Indian ethnic groups; the nonwhite group was almost exclusively African-American. They reported that, in the white group, 73% were women and 27% were men, a ratio of approximately 3:1. In contrast, in the nonwhite group, 86% were women and only 14% were men, a ratio of 6:1—significantly more women among the nonwhites. Regarding socioeconomic levels in the white group, persons from lower social classes, identified as IV and V, represented only 27%, whereas in the nonwhite group, 84%, a majority, were from these two social classes. This illustrated that there were considerable differences between the two groups in terms of gender distribution and socioeconomic levels.

3. India

There are sporadic reports from India regarding suicide attempts that give us a glimpse into the characteristics of such behavior there. First, it must be remembered that, until recently, suicidal behavior in India was considered a "legally punishable offense," therefore, there was a tendency to conceal such attempts by covering them up or labeling them "accidents" in order to avoid social stigma and legal consequences (Latha et al., 1996). Venkoba (1971), who investigated the attempts reported in Maduai between 1967 and 1969, estimated the rate of attempts to be 43/100,000 for New Delhi, which is much lower than the rate reported for most European and American societies.

An interesting point is that according to Latha and colleagues (1996), who examined 73 consecutive patients who had attempted suicide and had been admitted to an emergency medical unit, 62% were men and 38% were women. The male/female ratio was the reverse of what had been reported by most other societies. The interpretation of Latha and colleagues was that India continued to be a male-dominated society and the culturally accepted "stereotype" of the man's roles made him more vulnerable to stress. However, we may wonder if, in such a male-dominated society, and one in which suicide attempts were considered illegal, there was a possibility that male subjects were more often brought into emergency units to be saved, whereas females tended to be neglected, or if it was actually that there were more attempted suicides by males than females in India. This subject deserves future investigation, perhaps by community, rather than medical service surveys.

4. China

There are only a handful of reports available in China regarding clinical findings of attempted suicide. For instance, M.Z. Fan, Li, Wang, and Zhang (1992) reported that among 100 patients who were treated consecutively in the emergency department of the Third Hospital of Beijing Medical University at Beijing between 1987 and 1988, the women/men ratio was 2.03/1. From an occupational point of view, 49 were laborers, 7 were farmers, 7 were intellectuals, 18 were students, and the remaining 19 were unemployed or other. Regarding the method of the attempts, 65 cases were by drug overdoses, 29 by insecticides, and the small remaining number by

knife or jumping. As for the precipitating causes identified, failed romance (23 cases) and marital conflict (23 cases) were two of the most frequently identified reasons. In Nanjing, J., Fan and Zhai (1994) carried out a similar study of hospital cases. They revealed that the female/male ratio was 2.33/1, and from an occupational point of view, the majority were laborers and farmers, the same as data from Beijing. It needs to be pointed out that these reports relied on cases that came to the emergency facility for treatment. There were no community studies. Furthermore, the number of subjects studied was relatively small. Thus, generalization from those data needs to be very cautious.

C. OVERALL VIEWS ABOUT SUICIDE ATTEMPTS

Despite limited data on suicide attempts available internationally, some trends have been observed through cross-cultural comparisons among various countries. Weissman (1974) reviewed investigations of annual incidence rates of suicide attempts in several countries between 1960 and 1971, noting several common trends. In contrast to the relatively stable rate for committed suicide, there was a marked increase in the rates of suicide attempts. This was particularly noted in many Western societies, with an almost twofold increase in Great Britain, Australia, and the United States in the decade investigated.

Regardless of place or time, there is no exception to the observation that suicide attempts tend to be among the young, between the ages of 20 and 30 years, with the peak from 20 to 24. In terms of gender, the preponderance of female over male attempters was noted in all countries in the time period studied—most of the studies reported a ratio of about 2:1. The only exception was the report from India, with a ratio of .83/1. Data were based on one hospital in New Delhi. It was not clear whether it reflected the actual situation or whether, due to sexual discrimination, female attempters were ignored and were not sent to hospitals for treatment.

Weissman speculated that the increase in suicide attempts worldwide reflected the problems of the youth culture. The strong family life and religion that at one time served to integrate the person within a social group were no longer effective resources for young people. The changing roles of women may also have had an impact, with young women facing the conflicts and challenges of traditional and contemporary lifestyles.

V. OVERVIEW

In this chapter, ordinary and special forms of suicide, as well as socially codified suicides, have been examined. Suicide is a heterogeneous phenomenon that ranges from psychiatric-related personal suicide to culture-influenced or culture-embedded suicide. Personal suicide can occur as the result of psychiatric illness or emotional frustration; special forms of suicide are heavily influenced by culture; and socially codified suicide is culture-embedded behavior without emotional problems.

A. WORLD TRENDS IN SUICIDAL BEHAVIOR

Based on this review, some general observations can be made on world trends of ordinary individual suicides. A remarkable range of difference in total suicide rates has been noticed among different societies around the world (nearly 30-fold in some instances). It has also been noted that when a society is stable, the total suicide rate tends to remain stable; however, the sudden social turmoil associated with war, massive migration, revolution, or sociopolitical–economical change may cause the total suicide rate to fluctuate within a remarkable range.

Furthermore, considerable variations have been found in suicidal behavior. Even though, males tend to commit suicide more often than females in many societies, the reverse is true in other societies, such as in rural areas of China, indicating that suicidal behavior

is related to the roles and lives of males and females within the society. Although different types of age-related suicidal curves are described, indicating that the experience of distress tends to occur more in certain age groups, such curves are not necessarily fixed within a particular society. The curves may change over a period of time, when the distress of a particular age group changes.

Finally, the motives for suicide also vary considerably among different societies. In some, suicide is commonly related to negative reactions toward mental disease or physical illness, family disputes, pressure, or conflict, or financial problems, whereas in others it may be closely related to relationship problems or substance abuse. It is notable that special forms of suicide exist in certain societies, such as double suicide, family suicide, or collective suicide, illustrating that people may choose certain forms of suicide according to their beliefs and attitudes and their familiarity with those forms as ways of dealing with their distress.

All of these findings indicate that suicide, even though it is a personal act, is very much socioculturally shaped and susceptible to sociocultural factors. Although some suicides are the result of severe mental disorders, suicide overall can be seen as socioculturally related emotional problem that serves as one of the indexes of the mental health of a society. As indicated by Diekstra (1989), suicide, on the one hand, appears to be the most personal action an individual can take; on the other, social and cultural factors play an important, if not decisive, role in its causation.

B. CULTURAL CONTRIBUTIONS TO SUICIDE: REINTEGRATION

Although the cultural contribution to suicidal behavior has been elaborated throughout this chapter, it deserves reintegration here. It has been pointed out that the impact of culture on psychopathology can occur on different levels, in the form of pathogenetic, pathoselective, pathoplastic, pathoelaborating, pathofacilitative, and pathoreactive effects [cross-reference to Chapter 11: Culture and Psychopathology (Section II, A–F)]. These different ways in which culture can affect psychopathology are all observed in regard to suicidal behavior. Let us review the following.

1. Impact on Stress That Causes Suicide

Although some suicidal behavior occurs as the result of mental disorders, most, particularly personal suicide, is related to the psychological stress a person suffers. Culture contributes to the nature and severity of the distress that people may suffer, which in turn may contribute to the occurrence of their suicidal behavior. Thus, culture demonstrates the **pathogenetic effects** of suicidal behavior. This is illustrated by cultural systems, such as those of China and Korea, that prohibit the union of certain couples, even when they love each other, and thereby tend to facilitate the occurrence of double suicide.

2. Impact on the Choice of Suicide as a Coping Method

Even when one person encounters severe emotional distress in his life, he does not have to choose to end his life as a way of dealing with his problems. However, culture plays a significant role in the making of such a choice. In many Western societies, when faced with terrible financial debt, people are given the opportunity to claim bankruptcy as a way of solving the problem. However, in other cultures, particularly interpersonally oriented societies, such as Japan, it is considered so disgraceful to claim bankruptcy — shaming the family for many generations — that people may rather end their lives to resolve their debts. Clearly culture demonstrates **pathoselective effects** in a person's choice of suicide over other possible solutions to his problems.

3. Impact on the Forms of Suicidal Behavior

The **pathoplastic effect** of culture on suicide is well illustrated by the manifestation of special forms of suicidal behavior in addition to individual personal suicide. Among the special forms of suicide are double suicide, family suicide, and mass suicide. Further, there are socially expected codified suicidal actions, such as *seppuku* (as observed traditionally in Japan) and *suttee* (practiced in India in the past).

4. Impact on the Elaboration of Suicidal Action

The behavior of self-killing is not only prevalent but is also such a concern of the people that it may be elaborated by the society as a whole. This may be reflected in the various terminologies that have evolved to recognize various forms of suicide. Such a **pathoelabortaing effect** is well illustrated by the situation in Japan, where many terms are used by laymen in their daily language to refer to different kinds of suicide. Relating to methods of suicide, the terms *dokuyaku jisatsu* (suicide by poison), *jusui jisatsu* (drowning), *tooshin jisatsu* (jumping from a height), *harakiri* or *seppuku* (self-disembowelment) are used; concerning motive, the terms *jun-shi* (suicide following the master's death), *gisei-shi* (sacrificial suicide), *fun-shi* (suicide for indignation), *kashitsu-shi* (suicide for expiating mistakes), and *kan-shi* (suicide for remonstration) are used. Regarding special modes of suicide, *oyako-shinju* (parent–child suicide) or *ikka-shinju* (family suicide) are used (Iga & Tatai, 1975).

5. Impact on the Frequency of Suicidal Behavior

Data reviewed in this chapter have shown that the frequency of suicide varies greatly in different societies and, in many cases, the difference in rates can be attributed to the cultural system of the society. Even within the same society, rapid sociocultural change will have a significant impact on the frequency of suicidal behavior during the period of change. The **pathofacilitative effects** of culture on suicide are so significant that they support the view of suicide as a socioculturally related psychopathology, at the macroscopic level.

6. Impact of Social Reaction toward Suicidal Behavior

It is clear that many societies have very negative attitudes toward suicidal behavior. Muslims, who believe that the body is given by god, consider injuring one's body a sin. In India, suicidal behavior is socioculturally considered a crime that should be punished by law. In contrast, suicidal behavior is viewed much more sympathetically in other societies. In Japan, people believe that if a person is willing to take his own life, he should be excused from any wrong action or debt. This shows apparent **pathoreactive effects** of culture on suicidal behavior.

C. Clinical Implications and Suggestions

A certain "personal profile" has been identified clinically for individuals who are considered to be potentially at high risk for committing suicide, such as aged widowers with physical illnesses or drinking problems who are living alone (among male Caucasians, for instance). However, knowledge of such a personal profile is not useful in dealing with an individual patient in a clinical setting. Each person needs to be assessed and dealt with according to his own individual situation. This is also true of a "cultural profile" for suicide that has been recognized in an ethnic or cultural group. Even knowing about the cultural profile, including the ethnic or cultural group's shared attitudes toward death or the likelihood of its members choosing suicide as a way of solving life problems, will not give us a concrete guide on how to deal with an individual patient of that ethnic–cultural background. Although suicidal behavior as a whole is very much colored by sociocultural factors, each person needs to be evaluated and approached clinically on an individual basis, considering many variables.

However, from a cultural point of view, several issues can be recommended for consideration in clinical situations. First, it should be kept in mind that there are different cultural attitudes toward the com-munication of suicidal ideas. People in some cultures consider having suicidal ideas very disgraceful or a private matter that should not be readily revealed to others, including physicians or psychiatrists. Even when asked directly, they tend to deny having them. In contrast, people in other cultures may feel comfortable disclosing such ideas. In some societies, people have even learned that expressing suicidal ideas is a powerful way of getting professional attention and care, even if, in reality, they are not seriously occupied with such depressive thoughts. In other words, there are cultural differences in the disclosure of suicidal ideas.

It is necessary to recognize that culture influences people's consideration of self-killing as one of their choices in dealing with their problems. In cultures, such as the Muslim, with strong religious beliefs that the body should not be damaged intentionally, self-injury is less likely. Societies with statistically relatively low suicide rates belong to this category. In ethnic groups where self-killing is a traditionally accepted way of dealing with distress, suicide is a relatively easier action to undertake. People with statistically relatively high suicide rates belong to this category.

Finally, it is useful to be aware of common causes of suicide among different ethnic groups so that suitable management can be given accordingly. For instance, a person from a group with a strong stigma toward mental illness, when diagnosed with a mental disorder with a poor prognosis, has a relatively high chance of choosing to end his life. When a man who culturally believes that it is important to be physically healthy and support his family discovers that he has a serious physical illness and cannot fulfill his culture's image of a man, he might become vulnerable to suicide. When a young woman in a traditional family with close relationships suffers from frequent conflicts with in-laws, her chances of committing suicide may be higher than someone from a different family system.

In summary, knowledge of the cultural profiles for suicide of different ethnic groups will be helpful to the clinician in many ways: assisting him in determining culturally sensitive ways to approach the subject of suicide, making culturally accurate clinical assessments of suicidality, and undertaking culturally relevant actions in dealing with matters relating to suicidal behavior.

REFERENCES

Asuni, T. (1962, October). Suicide in Western Nigeria. *British Medical Journal,* 1091–1097.

Bille-Brahe, U., Kerkhof, A., De Leo, D., Schmidtke, A., Crepet, P., Lonnqvist, J., Michel, K., Salander-Renberg, E., Stiles, T.C., Wasserman, D., Aagaard, B., Egebo, H., & Jensen, B. (1997). A repetition-prediction study of European parasuicide populations: A summary of the first report from Part II of the WHO/EURO Multicentre Study on Parasuicide in co-operation with the EC Concerted Action on Attempted Suicide. *Acta Psychiatrica Scandinavica, 95,* 81–86.

Canetto, S.S., & Lester, D. (1998). Gender, culture, and suicidal behavior. *Transcultural Psychiatry, 35*(2), 163–190.

Carstairs, G.M. (1956–1957). Attitude toward death and suicide in an Indian cultural setting. *International Journal of Social Psychiatry, 1–2,* 33–41.

Chia, B.H., & Tsoi, W.F. (1972). Suicide in Singapore. *Singapore Medical Journal, 13*(2), 91–97.

Chong, M.Y., Yeh, E.K., & Wen, J.K. (1992). Suicidal behaviour in Taiwan. In L.P. Kok & W.S. Tseng (Eds.), *Suicidal behavior in the Asia-Pacific region.* (pp. 69–82). Singapore: Singapore University.

Crow, P.A. (1960). *Campaign in the Marianas: Vol. 9. The War in the Pacific.* Washington, DC: Department of the Army, Office of the Chief of Military History.

Diekstra, R.F.W. (1989). Suicide and the attempted suicide: An international perspective. *Acta Psychiatrica Scandinavica, 80* (Suppl. 354), 1–24.

Diekstra, R.F.W., & Garnefski, N. (1995). On the nature, magnitude, and causality of suicidal behaviors: An international perspective. *Suicide and Life-Threatening Behavior, 25*(1), 36–57.

Eungprabhanth, V. (1975). Suicide in Thailand. *Forensic Science, 5,* 43–51.

Fallers, L.A., & Fallers, M.C. (1960). Homicide and suicide in Busoga. In P. Bohannan (Ed.), *African homicide and suicide.* Princeton, NJ: Princeton University Press.

Fan, J.X., & Zhai, S.T. (1994). Analysis of 71 cases of suicide attempters treated at a general hospital. *Chinese Neuropsychiatry Journal, 20*(4), 227–228 (in Chinese).

Fan, M.Z., Li, C.P., Wang, J.J., & Zhang, E.Y. (1992). Suicidal behavior in China. In L.P. Kok, & W.S. Tseng (Eds.), *Suicidal behavior in the Asia-Pacific region* (pp. 58–68). Singapore: Singapore University Press.

Farberow, N.L. (Ed.). (1975). *Suicide in different cultures.* Baltimore: University Park Press.

Ganapathi, M.N., & Rao, A.V. (1966). A study on suicide in Madurai. *Journal of Indian Medical Association, 46*(1), 18–23.

Hau, K.T. (1993). Suicide in Hong Kong 1971–1990: Age trend, sex ratio, and method of suicide. *Social Psychiatry and Psychiatric Epidemiology, 28,* 23–27.

Hoskin, J.O., Friedman, M.I., & Cawte, J.E. (1969). A high incidence of suicide in a preliterate-primitive society. *Psychiatry, 32,* 199–210.

Iga, M., & Tatai, K. (1975). Characteristics of suicides and attitudes toward suicide in Japan. In N.L. Farberow (Ed.), *Suicide in different cultures.* (pp. 255–280). Baltimore: University Park Press.

Kok, L.P. (1992). Suicidal behaviour in Singapore. In L.P. Kok & W.S. Tseng (Eds.), *Suicidal behavior in the Asia-Pacific region* (pp. 176–198). Singapore: Singapore University.

Kok, L.P., & Tseng, W.S. (Eds.). (1992). *Suicidal behavior in the Asia-Pacific region.* Singapore: Singapore University.

Ladrido-Ignacio, L., & Gensaya, J.P. (1992). Suicidal behaviour in Manila, Philippines. In L.P. Kok & W.S. Tseng (Eds.), *Suicidal behavior in the Asia-Pacific region* (pp. 112–126). Singapore: Singapore University.

Latha, K.S., Bhat, S.M., & D'Souza, P. (1996). Suicide attempters in a general hospital unit in India: Their socio-demographic and clinical profile—emphasis on cross-cultural aspects. *Acta Psychiatrica Scandinavica, 94,* 26–30.

La Vecchia, C., Lucchini, F., & Levi, F. (1994). Worldwide trends in suicide mortality, 1955–1989. *Acta Psychiatrica Scandinavica, 90,* 53–64.

Lin, T.-Y., Rin, H., Yeh, E.K., Hsu, C.C., & Chu, H.M. (1969). Mental disorders in Taiwan, fifteen years later: A preliminary report. In W. Caudil & T.Y. Lin (Eds.), *Mental health research in Asia and the Pacific.* Honolulu: East-West Center Press.

Lo, W.H. (1992). Suicidal behaviour in Hong Kong. In L.P. Kok & W.S. Tseng (Eds.), *Suicidal behavior in the Asia-Pacific region* (pp. 83–111). Singapore: Singapore University.

Lo, W.H., & Leung, T.H. (1985). Suicide in Hong Kong. *Australian and New Zealand Journal of Psychiatry, 19,* 287–292.

Ohara, K (1963). Characteristics of suicides in Japan, especially of parent-child double suicide. *American Journal of Psychiatry, 120*(4), 382–385.

Ong, S., & Leng, Y.K. (1992). Suicidal behaviour in Kuala Lumpur, Malaysia. In L.P. Kok & W.S. Tseng (Eds.), *Suicidal behavior in the Asia-Pacific region* (pp. 144–175). Singapore: Singapore University.

Pederson, A.M., Awad, G.A., & Kindler, A.R. (1973). Epidemiological differences between white and nonwhite suicide attempters. *American Journal of Psychiatry, 130*(10), 1071–1076.

Pritchard, C. (1996). Suicide in the People's Republic of China categorized by age and gender: Evidence of the influence of culture on suicide. *Acta Psychiatrica Scandinavica, 93,* 362–367.

Robins, L.N., & Kulbok, P.A. (1988). Epidemiological studies in suicide. *Psychiatric Annals, 18*(11), 619–627.

Rubinstein, D.H. (1992). Suicidal behaviour in micronesia. In L.P. Kok & W.S. Tseng (Eds.), *Suicidal behavior in the Asia-Pacific region* (pp. 199–230). Singapore: Singapore University.

Ruzicka, L.T. (1976). II. Special subject: Suicide, 1950 to 1971. *World Health Statistic Report, 29*(7), 396–413.

Schmidtke, A., Bille-Brahe, U., De Leo, D., Kerkhof, A., Bjerke, T., Crepet, P., Haring, C., Hawton, K., Lonnqvist, J., Michel, K., Pommereau, X., Querejeta, I., Phillipe, I., Salander-Renberg, E., Temesvary, B., Wasserman, D., Fricke, S., Weinacker, B., & Sampaio-Faria, J.G. (1996). Attempted suicide in Europe: Rates, trends and sociodemographic characteristics of suicide attempters during the period 1989-1992. Result of the WHO/EURO Multicentre Study on Parasuicide. *Acta Psychiatrica Scandinavica, 93,* 327–338.

Shore, J.H. (1975). American Indian suicide: Fact and fantasy. *Psychiatry, 38,* 87–91.

Takahashi, Y., Hirasawa, H., Koyama, K., Senzaki, A., & Senzaki, K. (1998). Suicide in Japan: Present state and future directions for prevention. *Transcultural Psychiatry, 35*(2), 271–289.

Tseng, W.S., Ebata, K., Kim, K.I., Karahl, W., Kua, E.H., Lu, Q.Y., Shen, Y.C., Tan, E.S., & Yang, M.J. (in press). Mental health in Asia: Social improvement and challenges. *International Journal of Social Psychiatry.*

Tseng, W.S., Hsu, J., Omori, A., & McLaughlin, D.G. (1992). Suicidal behavior in Hawaii. In W.S. Tseng & L.P. Kok (Eds.), *Suicidal behavior in the Asia-Pacific region* (pp. 238–248). Singapore: Singapore University.

Tseng, W.S., & Kok, L.P. (1992). Conclusion: Comparison of reports from Asia and the Pacific. In L.P. Kok & W.S. Tseng (Eds.), *Suicidal behavior in the Asia-Pacific region* (pp. 249–265). Singapore: Singapore University.

Venkoba, R.A. (1971). Suicide attempters in Madurai. *Journal of the Indian Medical Association, 57,* 278–284.

Weissman, M.M. (1974). The epidemiology of suicide attempts 1960 to 1971. *Archives of General Psychiatry, 30,* 737–746.

World Health Organization (WHO). (1973). *Epidemiological and vital statistics report: Mortality from suicide 1950–1969.* Geneva: WHO.

World Health Organization (WHO). (1976–1996). *World health statistic annual.* Geneva: WHO.

World Health Organization (WHO). (1993). *1992 World Health Statistic Annual.* Geneva: WHO.

World Health Organization (WHO). (1995). *World health statistic annual* (pp. B-706–B-713). Geneva: WHO.

Yeh, E.K. (1985). Sociocultural changes and prevalence of mental disorders in Taiwan. In W.S. Tseng & D.Y.H. Wu, (Eds.), *Chinese culture and mental health* (pp. 15–40). Orlando, FL: Academic Press.

Yoshimatsu, K. (1992). Suicidal behaviour in Japan. In L.P. Kok & W.S. Tseng (Eds.), *Suicidal behavior in the Asia-Pacific region* (pp. 15–40). Singapore: Singapore University.

Zhang, J. (1996). Suicides in Beijing, China, 1992–93. *Suicide and Life-Threatening Behavior, 26*(2), 175–180.

Zilboorg, G. (1936). Suicide among civilized and primitive races. *American Journal of Psychiatry, 92,* 1347–1369.

23

Eating Disorders

I. INTRODUCTION: ISSUES NEEDING CLARIFICATION

Eating disorders, such as anorexia nervosa, bulimia nervosa, and other eating-related behavior problems, have become a new concern recently, particularly among societies in western Europe and North America, due to the relative increase in their prevalence in the past several decades. Associated with the increased sociocultural emphasis on slimness in Western societies, eating disorders are considered closely related to such cultural concerns over body weight and image. Some cultural psychiatrists have even speculated that eating disorders are Western culture-related specific psychiatric syndromes (DiNichola, 1990; Littlewood & Lipsedge, 1987).

Before discussing the possible impact of culture on the occurrence of clinically recognized eating disorders, it is necessary to discuss various issues related to body weight, image, and eating behavior that are observed among people of different ethnic backgrounds, which may directly or indirectly impact clinically observed eating disorders.

A. CROSS-ETHNIC DIFFERENCES CONCERNING BODY IMAGE AND EATING HABITS

From a cross-racial or cross-ethnic point of view, it is obvious that, as with body height, there are considerable differences in the (average or mean) body weight of people of different racial or ethnic groups. For instance, people in Polynesia, such as Hawaiians and Samoans, are well known for their relatively heavy body weight. There is no shortage of examples of people weighing over 300 pounds, and 600 or 700 pounds in some extreme cases. In contrast, Asian people, particularly Filipinos, Vietnamese, Thais, and Indians, are commonly known for their light body weights, usually not much above 100 pounds, even among adults.

Although many reasons have been considered for overweight, biological elements are major predisposing factors that cannot be denied. Twin studies have shown that the similarity of body weight between identical twins, in contrast to nonidentical twins, is very high, even when they are raised apart. People living in an island environment for many centuries, such as Hawaiians or Samoans, because of environmental restrictions, tend to intermarry. Thus, they may keep the genes for heavy body weight among their own ethnic group. However, even though body weight is closely related to hereditary factors, culture can contribute to it secondarily in many ways.

Attitudes toward a certain body image are psychological phenomena that can contribute to body weight from a cultural point of view. Hawaiians and Samoans both hold the cultural attitude that heavy men and women are beautiful, healthy, and desirable for mates. People in Asia used to consider "being fat" as a sign of wealth and fortune. The happy Buddha is portrayed as having an extended belly. A "skinny" person is interpreted as possibly suffering from poverty or being sick. To the Asian eye, a tall, skinny contemporary (Western) fashion model is "terribly" skinny. Thus, there are clearly culture-biased perceptions, definitions, and attitudes toward "desirable" body weight and body image.

There is no doubt that a sexually attractive or appealing body will change over time even in the same societies. Women in Western paintings of several centuries ago tended to be "fat" according to contemporary Western standards. This is true even for Asians. The "pretty" women portrayed in ancient paintings were generally characterized by round faces and plump figures.

Associated with increased medical knowledge and the realization that overweight tends to be related to numerous medical disorders (such as diabetes mellitus, hypertension, heart problems, cancer), it seems to be a general trend for most modern people to make an effort to keep their bodies in good shape, linking slimness with health, youth, and vitality, as well as beauty and sexual appeal. At the same time, people living in affluent, developed societies tend to enjoy ample nutritious foods (often full of fat and high in calories) and, at the same time, due to technological improvements, they have fewer opportunities for physical exercise in their daily lives to work off the calories they consume. Thus coupled with high calorie intake, there is decreased activity and people become overweight easily.

Based on the National Health Examination Survey and the National Health and Nutrition Examination Surveys at different stages between 1960 and 1994, Flegal, Carroll, Kuczmarski, and Johnson (1998) reviewed data obtained for prevalence and trends of overweight and obesity in the United States. Body mass index (BMI) was calculated from measured weight and height. Using standardized international definitions, "overweight" (BMI equal or above 25), "preobese" (BMI between 25 and 29.9), and "obesity" (BMI above 40) were defined in the study. They found that during the survey periods of 1960–1962, 1971–1974, 1976–1980, and 1988–1994, the age-adjusted prevalence of "preobese" showed little or no increase over time (ranging from 30.5, 32.0, 31.5, and 32.0%, respectively). However, the prevalence of "obesity" showed a large increase (12.8, 14.1, 14.5, and 22.5%, respectively). There was a large increase between 1976–1980 and 1988–1994. It was also reported that these trends were generally similar for all ages, genders, and race–ethnic groups. The race–ethnic groups were divided into non-Hispanic white, black, and Mexican-American. It was pointed out that the remarkable increase in the prevalence of obesity during the past two decades in the United States was in agreement with trends seen elsewhere in the world, mostly in developed societies where life was characterized by an abundance of food and diminished physical exercise.

It is common knowledge that culture has a direct and indirect influence on eating habits. The kinds of food people favor, how much they consume, and to what extent they emphasize eating in their daily lives are all culture-related issues that have a strong impact on diet, which, in turn, contributes to body-weight issues. Again, coming back to the example of Hawaiian people, in the past they enjoyed traditional foods such as taro and (luau) pigs — all high-calorie foods. After the arrival of Westerners to the Islands, Hawaiians became fond of canned meat foods — also high-fat and high in calories. In contrast, people in the Philippines, Thailand, and Vietnam generally enjoyed fish, vegetables, and rice, and many were vegetarians, who avoided consuming meats — either for religious reasons or simply because of childhood-patterned eating styles. It is also well known that people with Muslim backgrounds consider it taboo to eat pork, whereas Asian farmers dislike the meat of cows or buffalo, believing that it is not fair to kill them and eat their meat because they work hard for the farmer in the field. Thus, there are many examples of how various cultural attitudes influence people's eating habits, which contribute to their body weight to some extent.

B. From Ordinary Eating Behavior to Intensified Eating Concerns to Clinical Eating Disorders

Thus, it is clear that cultural factors contribute to body image and eating habits, which, in turn, interact with biological factors to influence body weight. However, to what extent such culture-related eating behaviors are related to clinically identified, morbid eating disorders, such as anorexia nervous and bulimia nervosa, is not yet clarified. From cultural and clinical perspectives, it seems necessary to distinguish eating-related behavior at three levels: (1) "ordinary" eating-related attitudes and behavior — observed in daily life as anxiety-free life patterns, subject to cultural variations, which tend to last for life and may be transmitted through generations; (2) "intensified" (or "alerted") eating-concerned attitudes or behavior — manifesting extra concern with diet, being overcareful in choices of food and calorie intake, or engaging in excessive physical exercise to control body weight, and a conscious concern with body image, which tends to occur as a time-limited fashion phenomenon; and (3) "morbid" eating behavior, which is clinically identified and categorized as anorexia nervosa or bulimia nervosa, has a recognized onset, and runs a certain clinical course. It is very clear that cultural factors will have a direct impact on the former two conditions, shaping "ordinary daily eating behavior" and creating "excessive" concern over eating and body-weight control. However, no substantial evidence to date supports the notion that culture has a direct

impact (as an etiological factor through "pathogenetic effects") on the occurrence of clinically identified "morbid" eating disorders. Culture might indirectly promote (through "pathofacilitative effects") the occurrence of such disorders, at most [cross-reference to Chapter 11: Culture and Psychopathology (Section II,A–F)].

C. Methodological Problems of Cross-Cultural Study of Eating Disorders

There are several methodological problems at present that limit relevant cross-cultural comparisons of eating disorders and the study of eating disorders from cultural dimensions. Some of the methodological handicaps are listed here.

First, eating disorders, as clinical entities, are new concerns among clinicians mainly in western Europe and North America, and most of the literature is derived from those geographic areas, with relevance to Caucasian groups. There is scarce clinical information from other ethnic and racial groups in other geographic regions, limiting meaningful cross-cultural comparisons. It is unclear whether eating disorders are rare in other cultures or whether they are neglected and underreported. This is a question awaiting future clarification. Even in Europe, as pointed out by Habermas (1991), there were national differences in reports of anorexia nervosa in France, Germany, and Italy for the period 1973–1918, basically due to different medical orientations toward the disorder.

Second, many of the reports, particularly from other geographic regions, are clinical case reports, which are often colored by subjective interpretations. When quantitative investigations were performed by questionnaire surveys there were some basic problems. If the investigators used their own idiomatic questionnaires, it made cross-comparisons almost impossible. If Western-derived questionnaires were used, there were problems of content equivalence, as the eating-related behavior could be heavily subject to cultural factors. A good example from India (King & Bhugra, 1989) will be elaborated later (Section II,B,7).

Third, there are problems with criteria used in defining eating disorders. Although clinically recognized morbid eating disorders (anorexia nervosa and bulimic nervosa) are characterized by rather homogeneous clinical manifestations (in contrast to other psychiatric disorders), some investigators tend to use their own criteria in defining cases, making comparisons with data from other investigations limited.

The presently used clinical criteria for eating disorders in the American classification system of DSM-IV are rather strict, making many of the clinical cases that seek professional treatment "atypical" even for American patients. Actually, "atypical" cases outnumber "typical" ones. As pointed out by Walsh (1997), many clinical cases of anorexia nervosa may not involve the cessation of menstruation as defined by DSM-IV. Binge-eating cases may not be followed by self-induced vomiting with twice-a-week frequency; it is often less than this arbitrarily defined frequency. Thus, the nature of the problems becomes uncertain when the clinical picture for patients from other ethnic groups differs from the description in the American classification system. Whether it is a problem of diagnostic criteria defining a "typical" case or the reflection of cultural variations due to "pathoplastic effects" on the manifestation of eating disorders are questions that require further investigation.

II. CLINICAL EATING DISORDERS

A. GENERAL KNOWLEDGE ABOUT ANOREXIA AND BULIMIA

Although anorexia nervosa and bulimia nervosa have different clinical pictures, they are customarily considered to be of the same clinical nature. Following this professional view, they are discussed together here.

According to Walsh (1997, p. 1202) the syndrome of anorexia nervosa was already recognized and named in the late 19th century, almost simultaneously by Sir William Gull in England and Charles Lasegue in France. The clinical features described more than a century ago were remarkably similar to those presented by patients in the late 20th century. Although current prejudice against obesity is strong and the idealization of thinness is high among Western societies, as pointed out by Garfinkel (1995, p. 1364), the disorders were well described clinically long before thinness achieved its current high social desirability.

After reviewing modern history (in the West), Russell and Treasure (1989) pointed out that a phenomenon comparable to fashionable thinness in the 1960s was found in the 1920s in the wake of the "flapper fashion." They quoted B. Silverstein and his associates' article, which stated that although it was not possible to quantify the extent of eating disorders over the era, nevertheless the 1909 to 1925 noncurvaceous trend in fashion was associated with a fall in weight among college students, and an increase in literary references to self-starvation among schoolgirls, college girls, and office workers. This supports the view that culture influences the fashionable view and perception of body image, which impact eating patterns.

Russell and Treasure (1989) pointed out that professional views and theories about anorexia nervosa have changed over time. At the end of the 19th century, it was regarded as a disorder of a hysterical nature. Until the mid-1960s, the recurring theme in the literature was that anorexia nervosa represented a defense against sexuality. No mention was made of a "disturbance of body image" until 1962. By 1970, the patients seen in clinical practice directly expressed an exaggerated fear of becoming fat. It was then that "a morbid dread of fatness" was viewed as characteristic of the psychopathology and was included as one of its necessary diagnostic criteria.

Strictly speaking, the medical term of anorexia nervosa (nervousness-induced anorexia) is a misnomer for the clinical condition. Patients seldom complain of "anorexic" (lack of appetite), while the clinical picture is characterized by a willful, fanatically accomplished abstinence from food, or a dramatic self-starvation, resulting in excessive underweight. Psychogenic hypophagia (undereating) has been suggested for contrast with psychogenic hyperphagia (bulimia, or overeating).

Based on clinical experiences, American psychiatrist Hilde Bruch (1978) pointed out that anorexia nervosa tended to affect girls from well-to-do families. She speculated that there were several sociological factors that contributed to the increasing occurrence of this disorder in the past several decades. There was the enormous fashion emphasis on slimness; mass communication gave the message that one could be loved and respected only when one was slender. There was an increased trend for women to have greater freedom to use their talents and abilities, but some growing girls experienced this liberation as a demand or pressure. There was greater sexual freedom, and girls were expected to begin dating or to have heterosexual experiences at a much earlier age than before. In other words, Bruch attributed the eating disorders to social factors associated with "modern" Western values and lifestyle.

Garner and Garfinkel (1980) studied and compared a population of professional dance and modeling students, who, because of their career choices, had to focus increased attention and control over their body shapes, with normal female university students, music students, and patients with anorexia nervosa. When the results of the Eating Attitudes Test (EAT) were compared among those groups, it was revealed that anorexia nervosa and excessive concern with dieting (as indicated by the EAT score above the cutting point) were overpresented in the dance and modeling students. Furthermore, it was also revealed that within the dance group, those from the most competitive environments had the greatest frequency of anorexia nervosa. Based on these findings, it was suggested that both the pressure to be slim and achievement expectations increased the risk for the development of anorexia nervosa.

B. INVESTIGATIONS FROM DIFFERENT SOCIOCULTURAL SETTINGS

1. The United States

Heatherton, Nicholas, Mahamedi, and Keel (1995) carried out a follow-up investigation regarding body weight, eating habits, dieting tendencies, and eating disorder symptoms among college students in 1982 and 1992. In 1982, randomly selected women and men students at Radcliffe College were studied by questionnaire survey. Ten years later, a nearly identical survey was carried out at the same college. They reported that on almost all measures, there were significant reductions in problematic eating behaviors and disordered attitudes about body, weight, and shape from 1982 to 1992. The estimated prevalence of bulimia nervosa dropped from 7.2 to 5.1% for women and from 1.1 to 0.4% for men. Subjects in 1992, in contrast to those in 1998, reported healthier eating habits in terms of dietary intake and meal regularity; however, women in 1992 were on average 5 pounds heavier than their 1982 counterparts. Based on these findings, Heatherton and colleagues interpreted the prevalence of problematic eating behaviors and eating disorder symptoms as apparently abating (among college students). However, these behaviors remained a significant problem that affected a substantial segment of this population.

Although traditionally it was believed by clinicians and researchers that eating disturbances were confined primarily to white, upper-middle-class, college-age women, J.E. Smith and Krejci (1991) investigated high school minority populations and obtained unpredicted findings. They used the Eating Disorder Inventory (EDI, by Garner, Olmsted, & Polivy, 1983) and Bulimia Test (BULT, by M. Smith & Thelen, 1984) for questionnaire surveys of three public high schools in the southeast United States. The student–subjects were composed of 60% Hispanics, 23.7% Native Americans, and 16.3% (non-Hispanic) Caucasians. The results revealed that the Native Americans consistently scored highest on each of seven items representing disturbed eating behaviors and attitudes. For instance, in the responses to binge eating (greater than once per month), the response rates were 14.2% for Native Americans, 13.1% for Hispanics, and 10.1% for non-Hispanic Caucasians. From these results, the researchers felt it was safe to conclude that the rates of disturbed eating patterns among Native Americans and Hispanic youth were at least comparable to those of Caucasian adolescents.

2. Scotland

In order to determine whether there had been an increase in the incidence of anorexia nervosa in the female population, a study was conducted by Eagles, Johnston, Hunter, Lobban, and Millar (1995) in northeast Scotland. They reviewed case records since the 1960s. Age-standardized annual incidence rates were calculated on the basis of the female population aged 5 to 44 years. They found that over the years 1965 to 1992, the mean annual increase in incidence was 5.3%, which was highly significant.

3. Denmark

Joergensen (1992) investigated the epidemiology of eating disorders in Fyn County in Denmark from 1977 to 1986. He reported that the incidence of anorexia nervosa among females 10 to 24 years of age was 11.0 per 100,000 per year, representing a significant rise compared with studies carried out 20 years before. The incidence of bulimia was 5.5 per 100,000 per year. Joergensen also reported that 60% of the anorexia nervosa patients were admitted to hospitals, compared to only 30% of the bulimia patients.

Pagsberg and Wang (1994) also carried out an epidemiological study in Denmark, but in a different location, on the island of Bornholm County. A total of 42 cases were found in a population of 47,000 from 1970 to 1989. They reported that the incidence rates for anorexia nervosa for the total population were stable from 1970 to 1984 (with a mean value of 1.6 per 100,000), yet a significant increase had occurred from 1985 to 1989 (the mean value increased to 6.8 per

100,000). A similar phenomenon was observed for bulimia nervosa. The average annual incidence rate for the total population was relatively constant from 1970 to 1984 (with a mean value of 0.7 per 100,000). However, from 1985 to 1989, there was an obvious increase (the mean value was 3.0 per 100,000).

Pagsberg and Wang pointed out that the maximal incidence rate occurred in the last year of the study, 1989, when the rate of the high-risk group of females (10 to 24 years of age) was 136 per 100,000 for anorexia nervosa and 45 per 100,000 for bulimia nervosa.

4. France

As part of an epidemiological study concerning young people and their health, Ledoux, Choquet, and Flament (1991) conducted a questionnaire survey of adolescents between the ages of 12 and 19 in the Haute-Marne area of France. The 15-item questionnaire designed by the research team concerned the students' eating behavior. As a result, they identified the incidence of bulimia (according to DSM-III-R diagnostic criteria) to be 0.2% for boys, 1.1% for girls, and 0.7% for both. Their results suggested that the prevalence of bulimia among French adolescents was not as high as rates reported for the population in North America.

5. Switzerland

Willi and Grossman (1983) conducted a retrospective study of the anorexia nervosa cases admitted to hospitals in the industrialized canton of Zurich during three randomly selected sampling periods between 1956 and 1975. They found that the incidence of first-time admitted cases per 100,000 population increased significantly from 0.38 in 1956–1958 to 0.55 in 1963–1965 to 1.12 in 1973–1975. They explained that this increase reflected that anorexic patients were now being hospitalized for less severe illnesses. Later, Willi, Giacometti, and Limacher (1990) did a follow-up study for the period 1983–1985. They reported that the incidence of anorexia nervosa did not increase from the previously studied period of 1973–1975. However, they commented that there was more frequent use of vomiting and abuse of laxatives in 1983–1985, which may have indicated an increase in cases with mixed features of anorexia and bulimia.

6. Russia

There is one article in English literature that discusses anorexia nervosa as it is conceptualized and diagnosed in Russia. The article was written by Russian psychiatrists Korkina, Tsyvilko, Marilov, and Kareva (1992) in Moscow. Based on their clinical experiences, they reported that three-quarters of the patients exhibited anorexia nervosa linked with a borderline state, and one-quarter associated with schizophrenia. American psychologist G.R. Leon (1992), who had the opportunity of working in Moscow for several years and visited M.V. Korkina there, commented that bulimia nervosa was not diagnosed often in Russia. Leon also pointed out that, in Russia, the conceptualization of anorexia nervosa was different. In contrast to western European and American diagnostic systems, Russian psychiatrists viewed anorexia as part of a clinical manifestation that was often associated with a borderline personality disorder and schizophrenia.

7. India

In order to test the general clinical impression that the prevalence of eating disorders was very low in Third World populations, psychiatrists from London, King and Bhugra (1989), carried out a field survey in India. Five-hundred-eighty schoolgirls living in a small north Indian industrial town were screened, using the EAT. EAT is a 26-item questionnaire that was developed by Garner et al. (1983) for the evaluation of abnormal eating attitudes and has been used widely in Western societies as a screening inventory for eating disorders. Surprisingly, the results revealed that among 574 students who completed the questionnaire and were included in the analysis, 167 girls (29%) scored above the recom-

mended cutoff for the EAT — opposite findings from what had been believed on the basis of clinical impressions.

In order to solve this puzzle, a detailed study was made of the responding pattern. By comparing the responses to individual items made by the Indian subjects with those by English subjects (M.B. King, unpublished data, 1986), the investigators disclosed that there were consistent patterns of response for the whole population on five items, which appeared to have been due to sociocultural influences. The five items to which the Indian girls often responded "always," contributing to the high total scores, were questions 5, 17, 18, 19, and 23. The investigators interpreted question 5 (cut my food into small pieces) and question 19 (display self-control around food) as addressing culturally desirable behaviors for Indians and many of the girls therefore answered affirmatively. Question 17 (eat diet foods) and question 23 (engaged in dieting behavior) were related to Hindu religious fasting concepts, whereas question 18 (feel that food controls my life) appeared to have been interpreted literally by the girls.

If examined carefully, these questions are not "specific" (or "pathognomic") to eating disorders and are very much subject to cultural situations. For instance, cutting food into small pieces is a regular way of preparing food in societies where the fingers (India) or chopsticks (most of Asia) are used for eating; this is different from societies that use a knife and fork. In many societies where food is often potentially scarce, it is common to value food, feeling that "food controls one's life."

The investigators revealed that in contrast to these five culture-biased questions, other questions concerning "core" characteristics of abnormal eating attitudes, such as "find myself preoccupied with food," "have gone on eating binges when I felt that I may not be able to stop," and "think about burning up calories whenever I exercise," were answered affirmatively only by 45 (7.8%), 16 (2.8%), and 28 (4.9%) subjects, respectively. This information indicated that the number of subjects with abnormal eating attitudes was low.

Indian psychiatrists Khandelwal, Sharan, and Saxena (1995), after intensive review of the literature, presented their Indian perspective of eating disorders. They described five clinical cases and pointed out that they did not show the overactivity or disturbances in body image characteristically seen in (Western) anorexia nervosa — thus, their cases tended to be "atypical" in terms of Western criteria. According to them, possible reasons for the seeming rarity of anorexia nervosa in India were lack of sensitivity about the diagnosis among clinicians; the use of Western diagnostic criteria, which possibly missed the diagnosis of "atypical" cases commonly seen in India; and the absence of pressure on a majority of young women to be thin or to restrain their eating, which may have protected vulnerable individuals from the principal route of entry into a clinical morbid condition.

8. Pakistan

After studying the eating disorders of Asian schoolgirls (mostly children of immigrants from Pakistan) in Bradford, United Kingdom (Mumford et al., 1991), Mumford, Whitehouse, and Choudry (1992) carried out a survey of 369 schoolgirls studying in English medium schools in Lahore, Pakistan. They used the EAT and Body Shape Questionnaire (BSQ), in English, for the initial screening. Girls who scored highly on either questionnaire were invited for interviews. As a result, they reported that one girl met DSM-III-R criteria for bulimia nervosa (and five girls a partial syndrome of bulimia), but no girls were found to be suffering from anorexia nervosa. They estimated a prevalence rate of 0.3% for bulimia nervosa among the Pakistan schoolgirls they investigated.

The investigators were aware of the potential problems of using a Western questionnaire for investigating non-Western subjects. However, they compared the factor structure of the EAT and BSQ between data obtained from subjects surveyed in Lahore and Western subjects. They found a similarity in the factor structures and claimed cross-cultural validity for using the questionnaire.

Mumford and Whitehouse (1988) conducted a survey among Asian and Caucasian schoolgirls in Bradford, United Kingdom. They described the prevalence of bulimia nervosa among ethnic Asians schoolgirls in Bradford (mostly of Pakistani backgrounds) as 3.4%, somewhat higher than the rates of 0.3% for schoolgirls in Lahore, Pakistan, and 0.6% for Caucasian schoolgirls in Bradford.

From the investigation in Lahore (Mumford, whitehouse, & Choudry, 1992) it was found that girls with the highest "Westernization" scores (measured by the consumption of Western food and the speaking of English in the home) had the highest mean EAT and BSQ scores. In contrast, in Bradford, the risk of eating disorders was found to be greatest among girls from the most traditional families. In order to explain these almost contradictory findings among subjects with the same ethnic background in different settings, Mumford and colleagues pointed out that the multifactorial model of the etiology of eating disorders might be useful. In Lahore, Western influence, associated with more concern about food intake and weight, was more significant, whereas in Bradford, it might have been intrafamilial stresses associated with traditional emphases that most strongly determined the risk of eating disorders.

Because most of the Asian schoolgirls studied in Bradford were children of immigrants from an underdeveloped region of Pakistan, the Mirpur district, about 100 miles north of Lahore, another investigation was carried out there (Choudry & Mumford, 1992). The results revealed that only one case of bulimia nervosa (as defined by DSM-III-R) was identified among 271 schoolgirls investigated. The estimated frequency of bulimia nervosa among Mirpur subjects was 0.4%, similar to the 0.3% for Lahore subjects, and much lower than the 3.4% for Asian subjects (mainly of Pakistani backgrounds, who migrated originally from the Mirpur area), described previously. This supported the view that after migrating to Western society (Bradford in the United Kingdom, in this case), the frequency of bulimia among youngsters of immigrants increased remarkably and was even higher than for local youngsters of Caucasian background, which was estimated at 0.6%.

9. Egypt

Nasser (1986) investigated matched samples of Arab female college students attending Cairo University in Cairo and several colleges in London universities, as well as independent colleges in London. He applied the Eating Attitude Test to the two groups of subjects, the Cairo group and the London group. Using the cutoff score of 30 on the EAT [as originally designed and validated on Canadian subjects by Garner and Garfinkel (1979)], Nasser reported that 22% of the London sample scored as positive cases, compared to only 12% of the Cairo sample. Furthermore, Nasser conducted clinical interviews of the high scorers in both groups and reported that, in the London group, 6 out of 11 EAT-positive cases fulfilled diagnostic criteria of bulimia nervosa and none for anorexia nervosa. In contrast, no cases of anorexia or bulimia nervosa were identified in the Cairo group.

Regarding the differences found between the Arab female colleges students in Cairo and those in London, Nasser felt that because the latter group went to London as family members, selective factors associated with migration were unlikely. He interpreted the differences as related to the degree of exposure and contact with the Western style of life. The Arab students in London were similar to European students in dress and social behavior, whereas the Cairo students were generally more traditional in their dress, some of them still even wearing veils. However, there was an influx of Western clothes into Cairo, which fit only slim figures. New concepts of beauty and femininity were constantly being transmitted through television so that there was no immunity from the Western emphasis on slimness. Nassar concluded that abnormal eating attitudes did occur among non-Western populations, but were influenced by the degree of Westernization and the degree of adherence to traditional religious beliefs and conservative rules.

Later, Dolan and Ford (1991) performed a questionnaire study of Arab students attending American University in Cairo regarding binge eating and dietary restraint. The instruments used were the nine-item Binge Scale Questionnaire (Hawkins & Clement, 1980) and 10-item Restraint Scale. The latter was designed by Polivy, Herman, and Warsh (1978) and was used by Wardle (1986) to measure British subjects.

Results showed that the Binge Scale mean score was 6.8 for Arab women, which did not differ significantly from the mean score of 5.6 for British women reported by Hawkins and Clement (1980) in their original development sample. The mean score for the Restraint Scale was 10.1 for the Arab women, significantly lower than the 13.5 reported by Wardle (1986) for British women.

10. Israel

Using the Eating Attitudes Test (EAT-26) and body image scale, Apter and colleagues (1994) conducted a questionnaire survey in Israel to assess eating attitudes and body images among different subpopulations. This included Jewish female high school populations in five distinct residential settings (kibbutz, moshav, city, and two different boarding schools) and five ethnically distinct Arab female high school populations (Muslim, Christian, Druze, Circassian, and Bedouin). In addition to these 10 healthy subgroups, a group of hospitalized adolescent girls with anorexia nervosa was included for comparison. Results showed that the anorexic group scored highest, and in most cases significantly so, among all the subgroups studied, indicating the usefulness of EAT-26 for the detection of anorexia. Among all 10 healthy subpopulations studied, the (Jewish) kibbutz adolescents had the highest scores for total eating pathology, EAT-26, and most subscales, whereas (Arabic) Circassian adolescents had the lowest scores, respectively.

Apter and colleagues explained that Circassian adolescents lived in small, relatively selfcontained, endogenous communities. The Circassians most often maintained the traditional female nurturing roles and were relatively unconcerned with dieting and thinness. In contrast, kibbutz adolescents were under the most severe role stress, being expected to succeed at work, as homemakers, and as attractive, sexually desirable objects. They were exposed to conflict between the traditional female and the self-disciplined, controlled, and sexually liberated "new women." Thus, even among the students living in Israel, there were distinctly different ethnic–culture subgroups with different attitudes towards the expected female role, which in turn led to different eating attitudes and body images.

11. Japan

Japanese psychiatrist Nogami and Yabana (1977) used the Japanese term *kibarashi-gui* to describe the binge-eating behavior observed in Japan. *Kibarashi-gui* (literally, diversion overeating), also called *yake-gui* (desperate overeating) by the Japanese, referred to excessive eating for the sake of relaxing, diversion, and amusement. They used the word to distinguish "hyperorexia" (excessive appetite). They emphasized that cases labeled *kibarashi-gui* (diversion overeating), in addition to episodes of pathological overeating, tended to be associated with clinical symptoms of depression or behavior problems of aggression, dependency, and acting out.

Suematsu, Ishikawa, Kuboki, and Ito (1985) sent questionnaires to physicians at 1030 representative institutions throughout Japan, asking for information about anorexia nervosa cases that had been under their care. Data were collected from 315 institutions, and a total of 940 outpatients and 372 inpatients were identified. It was found that the number of patients under care in 1981 was twice as high as the number in 1976.

12. China

Questionnaire surveys were administered to 509 college freshman (males and females) in two cities, Chongqing and Shanghai, in China by Zhang and colleagues (1992). The 100-item questionnaire, designed by the investigators, was used to elicit attitudes about weight and food, weight control behavior, and information needed to diagnosis anorexia nervosa and bulimia according to the criteria of the Chinese classification system and DSM-III-R. They reported that 1.1% of the students investigated (1.1% of females)

met both Chinese classification and DSM-III-R criteria for bulimia; however, none were binge eating and purging on a regular basis. None met the diagnostic criteria for anorexia nervosa.

Although Lee, Ho, and Hsu (1993) reported that 58.6% of the anorexic patients reviewed in Hong Kong did not exhibit any fear of fatness through their course of illness and were thus labeled as "nonfat phobic anorexia," the finding was not the same in Beijing. Psychiatrists from Beijing, Song and Fang (1990), reported nine anorexic patients who had visited the Institute of Mental Health of Beijing Medical University between 1982 and 1988. They reported that all of these patients were female, aged 13 to 25, most were concerned about "being fat," and they started diet control after their friends commented that they were overweight.

An interesting report was given by psychiatrists from the Fujien area regarding child anorexia cases. Chen, Cheng, and Wang (1993) reported 200 cases of children, between 8 months and 9 years old, who were brought by their parents to visit a children's eating disorder clinic from December 1988 to December 1990. They were diagnosed as child anorexics with criteria of eating habit disturbance, body weight 15% less than average body weight, and no evidence of medical illness. Surprisingly, among these 200 cases, 112 cases were boys and 88 were girls. They explained that, associated with the single-child family-planning policy, many single children were spoiled by their parents and allowed to pick at their food, have an unbalanced diet, or develop unhealthy eating habits, which contributed to their underweight.

13. Malaysia

A study was carried out by Buhrich (1981) by approaching 18 psychiatrists who were currently practicing in Peninsula Malaysia. Among them, 11 responded to a questionnaire survey and 6 were interviewed or contacted by telephone. It was estimated that these 17 psychiatrists had seen a total of approximately 60,000 new psychiatric referrals in their practices. Of these, 28 females and 2 males were reported to have had primary anorexia nervosa. Among the 28 females, 19 were Chinese, 7 Indians, 1 Malay, and 1 Eurasian. As the racial distribution of the general population was 53% Malay, 36% Chinese, and 11% Indian, the Malay cases of anorexia were comparatively scarce. The investigator was aware of the limitation of this method of study and pointed out that most of the Malay patients preferred to seek help from traditional medicine men (Bomoh) rather than modern physicians, not to mention psychiatrists. Thus, the figures may have been affected by the service utilization patterns. However, he claimed that data supported the general impression that anorexia nervosa was relatively rare among Malaysians.

14. Africa and Others

No English survey reports were found from Africa, except one clinical report (Buchan & Gregory, 1984). However, there was one report regarding the estimated incidence from the Caribbean island of Curacao (with African descendants) by Hock, van Harten, van Hoeken, and Susser (1998). They reviewed the medical records of all inpatients of the Curacao General Hospital as well as the Curacao Psychiatric Case Register for the period 1987 through 1989 for cases of an eating disorder. They disclosed six cases of anorexia nervosa. Based on this, they estimated the yearly incidence of anorexia nervosa on Curacao was 2.6 per 100,000 women. They reported that even though being overweight was socially acceptable in Curacao, anorexia cases were still found, with the rate within the range of rates reported in Western societies.

III. INTEGRATION AND COMMENTS

A. CONSOLIDATION OF CROSS-CULTURAL FINDINGS

From these findings of eating disorder studies carried out in various sociocultural settings, several issues may be summarized as follows.

1. Increased Prevalence

It is commonly noted by clinicians in various parts of the world that there has been an increased prevalence of eating disorders in Western societies recently, which is simply attributed to the influence of Western culture (Iancu, Spivak, Ratzoni, Apter, & Weizman, 1994). A review of several investigations carried out between 1931 and 1986, in different locations in Europe (south Sweden; Switzerland; Northeast Scotland; London, UK; Assen, Holland) and the United States (Monroe County, New York), Hock (1993) indicated that the registered incident rates of anorexia nervosa have increased sharply, but it is still unclear whether the rates in the community have increased. Eagles and associates (1995) have also reviewed the reports concerning any changes over time in the incidence of anorexia nervosa from multiple societies. According to them, there are some reports indicating the increase, such as those from New York State (Jones et al.); Zurich, Switzerland (Willi & Grossmann); Grampian, Scotland (Szmukler et al.); England (Williams & King); and Denmark (Moller-Madsen & Nystrup), but there are also reports remarking that there has been no change, such as those from Denmark (Nielsen); Zurich, Switzerland (Willi et al.); Fyn County, Denmark (Jorgensen); and Wellington, New Zealand (Hall & Hay). After examining the investigations that have been carried out in the past regarding the epidemiology of anorexia nervosa, Szmukler (1985) commented that there were basic methodological problems regarding the definition as well as the detection of cases. Apparently, different times and settings, different methods of investigation, and the use of the same or different investigators led to different conclusions about the increase of anorexia nervosa among western European and North American societies.

It is not only in western European and North American societies that eating disorders are considered prevalent at present. There are also notions that eating disorders are rising in some non-Western regions and that the increased prevalence is beginning to attract attention. For instance, Nogami and Yabana (1977) mentioned that eating disorders, particularly bulimia, were seldom diagnosed by Japanese psychiatrists until the early 1980s, when Nogami published a paper about bulimia and aroused attention among his Japanese colleagues. Similar comments have been made in India (Khandelwal et al., 1995), Hong Kong (Hsu & Lee, 1993), and Pakistan (Mumford et al., 1992).

After visiting Russian for several years, Leon (1992) also commented that in Russia, eating disorders were seldom diagnosed as a sole psychiatric entity, and if they were, they were associated with borderline personality disorders or schizophrenia (Korkina et al., 1992). The same point has been made by Nogami that, from a nosological point of view, eating disorders were distributed in a wide-ranging spectrum of psychiatric disorders: from neuroses to schizophrenia. It seems that in societies where the prevalence rate (or reported rate) is low, the eating disorder tends to be considered a part of other psychiatric disorders (or a dual diagnosis).

If it is true, as many investigators have commented, that eating disorders are increasing, not only among Western societies but among non-Western societies as well, what is the reason for this phenomena? Several explanations have been given. Some have speculated that it is a matter of diagnostic pattern. Associated with the increased awareness of such disease entities, there is a rising tendency to disclose and diagnose eating disorders. (This is also suspected to be the situation with depression, social phobias, and for borderline personality disorders.) Another explanation is the genuine increase of such disorders due to the tendency to improve one's health, changes in food consumption, a decrease in physical work, and a resulting increase in body weight, which are observed rather universally in association with modernization. Another frequent explanation is the influence of the Western cultural attitudes toward exposing the body and an emphasis on body image and sexual attraction, and the view that slimness is beautiful, sexually attractive, and healthy.

2. "Typical" and "Atypical"

Several investigators, based on their clinical experiences with different ethnic populations — such as

Hsu and Lee (1993) and Lee and colleagues (1993) and the ethnic Chinese in Hong Kong and Khandelwal and associates (1995) and the people of India — have pointed out that eating disorders have an "atypical" clinical syndrome complex compared with "typical" diagnostic criteria set up in American classification criteria. More specifically, Hsu and Lee (1993) raised the question of whether weight phobia was necessary for a diagnosis of anorexia nervosa. Their experiences with ethnic Chinese anorexic patients in Hong Kong indicated that nearly half seldom showed a concern with being overweight. Khandelwal and associates (1995) also claimed that the eating disorder cases in India lacked a fear of becoming fat — body-image distortion.

These views raised the question: What do we mean by "typical" cases and "atypical" cases or "variations?" As mentioned previously, Walsh (1997, p. 1202) pointed out that (even among American patients) "atypical" eating disorders outnumbered "typical" eating disorders. There seems to be a need to clarify and reexamine the diagnostic categories of eating disorders, particularly from cross-cultural perspectives. According to Hsu and Sobkiewicz (1991), the general assumption that perceptual body width distortion was pathognomic for eating disorders deserves reexamination and clarification.

3. "Culture-Bound" and "Biologically Predisposed"

Although many investigations have pointed out that eating disorders are more prevalent among young females in western Europe and North America, with an increased prevalence during the past several decades, we should not jump to the conclusion that this is a result of Western cultural factors and describe eating disorders as Western culture-bound syndromes. As pointed out by Prince (1985), the concept of "culture-bound syndromes" (or culture-related specific psychiatric syndromes) should be used in a more careful and restricted way. More empirical evidence is required to assure that illnesses are confined to or closely related to Western cultures. If we found a high prevalence of a certain psychiatric disorder among certain ethnic groups, as medical professionals, the first thing we would consider would be the possible biological factors contributing to the phenomena. It is not unusual in the field of medicine for an ethnic or racial group to carry a certain gene pool that predisposes it to develop a particular medical illness. The same is possible for psychiatric disorders. For instance, the high prevalence of schizophrenia among Belau islanders in Micronesia should be explored from the standpoint of a possible gene pool accumulated through endogamy over many centuries rather than as a result of their culture-related lifestyle. As Banks (1992) warned, the designation of anorexia nervosa as a syndrome limited to Western cultures or to those cultures influenced by them may reflect an unexamined assumption on the part of researchers that dieting and secular ideals of slimness are "primarily" involved in the disorder as causative factors.

Those subjects who tend to eat Western food and speak English (such as the schoolgirls in Lahore, Pakistan, studied by Mumford et al., 1992) should not be interpreted right away as influenced by "Westernization." Having Western food more often merely implies a change in eating habits, which may modify the patterns of food consumption, calorie intake, resulting body weight, and so on. Culture is a unique life pattern based on certain belief and values. Westernization needs to be treated as such rather than simply as a change of food intake patterns or language used.

After reviewing various reports, Davis and Yager (1992) stated that among the at-risk population in Western societies, the rate for anorexia nervosa ranged from 0.25 to 6.0%, and for bulimia nervosa from 2 to 19%. However, no study has been done to examine why there is a difference in rate even among Western societies. What is the degree of variation of so-called "Western cultures" in terms of concern with body weight, emphasis on slimness, and body-related sexual attraction among different Western societies and is there any correlation among the different degrees of body weight concern and emphasis on slimness with the frequency of eating disorders observed in different Western societies? These are issues that deserve future investigation.

B. Comments and Suggestions

1. Distinction among Western Cultures, Modernization, and Migration Effects

An increase in body weight and excessive concern with health and body weight are common phenomena observed around the world. As pointed out by Littlewood (1995), they are related to the phenomenon of "modernization" rather than "Westernization."

Modernization associated with industrialization, urbanization, and improvement of health always brings changes to the living environment. Abandoning traditional food resources and consuming high-calorie food are common. Together with technological improvements, resulting in decreased physical activity and diminished physical work in daily life, these factors make it easier to increase body weight than in the past. An increase in average body weight and height has been observed in many non-Western societies. A need has developed for the establishment of children's overweight clinics in many societies, including Singapore, Hong Kong, China, Japan, and Korea in Asia, which were categorized as "developing" societies where people were still struggling to get enough to eat only a few decades ago. Clearly, modernization, or contemporary modern life, contributes to an increase in problems related to being overweight.

In contrast to the modernization that is observed in many societies around the world, the impact of "Western culture" should be defined in a more restricted way. Attitudes encouraging exposure of the body and even nudity (such as on nude beaches) and the emphasis on the whole-body figure for sexual attraction (rather than the partial-body figure, such as the face) may be considered Western-related attitudes and values. An emphasis on sexual gratification, concern with heterosexual relationships, and an earlier start of heterosexual activities are unique features of modern Western culture. These attitudes are coupled with an emphasis on equality between man and woman and the liberation of woman from the protected domestic environment to the competitive social environment. There is both conflict and challenge associated with women's rights to perform and to be successful.

In addition to the influences of modernization and Western culture, the impact of "migration" should be considered. Several studies have indicated that immigrants' adolescent children, who migrated to Western societies from non-Western societies, tended to have a relatively higher prevalence of eating disorders — higher than the adolescents of the hosting society or the immigrants' home country. This suggests that transcultural migration induces certain changes in the family value systems and in living styles, which, in some way, make immigrant adolescents vulnerable to eating disorders. The disorders may be simply related to the change in food-intake patterns, or they may involve stress from the process of acculturation. These are issues needing further investigation. However, it is clear that, in addition to the influence of Western culture, there are multiple factors that can contribute to the occurrence of eating disorders.

2. Clarification of the Scope and Nature of Cultural Impact

Even though there is substantial evidence to support the notion that eating disorders are closely related to (Western) culture, there still is a need to clarify the ways in which culture contributes to the psychopathology of eating disorders. It is highly possible that the emphasis on slimness and body-related sexual attraction may *intensify* (or facilitate) an excessive concern with food-intake behavior and induce a fear of being overweight, but it does not necessarily *cause* clinical eating disorders such as anorexia nervosa or bulimia nervosa. The biophysiological pathology of eating centers is an area that is still reserved for future study.

From the clinical information available at present, it may be summarized that although culture may contribute to the "pathofacilitative effect" or the "pathoplastic effect" of anorexia nervosa, there is no suffi-

cient evidence to indicate that culture contributes to the "pathogenic effect" of the disorder. The desire for slimness may give the anorexic patient a cognitive excuse for (pathological) hypophagia and intensify the preoccupation with and fear of becoming fat. However, this is merely a pathofacilitative plastic effect. As pointed out by Wilfley and Rodin (1995), despite the social obsession with thinness in the 1990s, with unrealistic societal ideals, many adolescent girls and women experienced discontent with their weight and shape; nevertheless, only a small percentage developed full-blown eating disorders. The sociocultural milieu may facilitate and potentiate the risk, but additional factors beyond culture need to be explored.

3. Improving Cultural Investigations

There is much room for improvement in the investigation of the possible cultural effects on the occurrence of eating disorders. First, there is a need for cross-culturally useful and universally applicable definitions of eating disorders. There is also a need for the retesting, revision, and development of culturally valid instruments for measuring disorders.

There are not enough surveys of the frequency of eating disorders in different cultural settings. There is a need to first survey the eating attitudes among general populations in the community. Based on this baseline, the eating attitudes of the targeted population (the patient group) can be measured and meaningfully interpreted. From a cross-cultural perspective, it would be desirable to select cultural samples that illustrate wide differences in the perception of body image, attitudes toward obesity, and eating habits for cross-comparison. Through such well-designed cross-cultural comparisons, the dimensions of culture could be highlighted for examination.

Because the definitions and boundaries of different eating disorders are not yet well established, at least in terms of cross-cultural application, following the suggestions made by Firburn and Beglin (1990), it is worth considering a study of the whole spectrum of eating disturbances that exists in the community rather than merely identifying and selecting restrictively defined, particular kinds of disorders. Otherwise, we may be influenced by the "netting effect" and catch only certain fish from the sea [cross-reference to Chapter 29: Clinical Assessment and Diagnosis (Section II,D)].

Because several investigations have indicated that children of immigrants from non-Western backgrounds to Western societies tend to have an increased risk of eating disorders, there is a need to clarify whether this is simply due to the pressures of acculturation or to the influence of the (Western) host culture. As suggested by Dolan (1991), it would be useful to study longitudinally any changes in frequency and patterns of eating disorders among immigrants from non-Western to Western cultures. Monitoring changes in manifestation and prevalence of eating disorders over time in women from the same immigrant ethnic groups in a Western culture may show more clearly the outcomes of any impact of the acculturation process on the occurrence of eating disorders. Immigrants to non-Western societies could be studied for control and comparison. Because such a longitudinal study would be time-consuming, a cross-sectional approach to the study of immigrants at different stages of assimilation into a Western host society may be a short-term solution. It is clear that a great deal of improvement in investigations is needed before any conclusive remarks can be made about the relation between culture and eating disorders.

REFERENCES

Apter, A., Abu Shah, M., Iancu, I., Abramovitch, H., Weizman, A., & Tyano, S. (1994). Cultural effects on eating attitudes in Israeli subpopulations and hospitalized anorectics. *Genetics, Social and General Psychology Monographs, 120*(1), 83–99.

Banks, C.G. (1992). "Culture" in culture-bound syndromes: The case of anorexia nervosa. *Social Science and Medicine, 34*, 867–884.

Bruch, H. (1978). *The golden cage: The enigma of anorexia nervosa.* Cambridge, MA: Harvard University Press.

Buchan, T., & Gregory, L.D. (1984). Anorexia nervosa in a Black Zimbabwean. *British Journal of Psychiatry, 145*, 326–330.

Buhrich, N. (1981). Frequency of presentation of anorexia nervosa in Malaysia. *Australian and New Zealand Journal of Psychiatry, 15*, 153–155.

Chen, D.G., Cheng, X.F., & Wang, L.L. (1993). Clinical analysis of 200 cases of child anorexia. *Chinese Mental Health Journal, 7*(1), 5–6 (in Chinese).

Choudry, I.Y., & Mumford, D.B. (1992). A pilot study of eating disorders in Mirpur (Pakistan) using an Urdu version of the Eating Attitudes Test. *International Journal of Eating Disorders, 11*(3), 243–251.

Davis, C., & Yager, J. (1992). Transcultural aspects of eating disorders: A critical literature review. *Culture, Medicine and Psychiatry, 16*(3), 377–394.

DiNichola, V.F. (1990). Anorexia multiform: Self-starvation in historical and cultural context. Part II: Anorexia nervosa as a culture-reactive syndrome. *Transcultural Psychiatric Research Review, 27*, 245–286.

Dolan, B. (1991). Cross-cultural aspects of anorexia nervosa and bulimia: A review. *International Journal of Eating Disorders, 10*(1), 67–78.

Dolan, B., & Ford, K. (1991). Binge eating and dietary restraint: A cross-cultural analysis. *International Journal of Eating Disorders, 10*(3), 345–353.

Eagles, J.M., Johnston, M.I., Hunter, D., Lobban, M., & Millar, H. (1995). Increasing incidence of anorexia nervosa in the female population of northeast Scotland. *American Journal of Psychiatry, 152*, 1266–1278.

Firburn, C.G., & Beglin, S.J. (1990). Studies of the epidemiology of bulimia nervosa. *American Journal of Psychiatry, 147*, 401–408.

Flegal, K.M., Carroll, M.D., Kuczmarski, R.J., & Johnson, C.L. (1998). Overweight and obesity in the United States: Prevalence and trends, 1960–1994. *International Journal of Obesity, 22*, 39–47.

Garfinkel, P.E. (1995). Eating disorder. In H.I. Kaplan & B.J. Sadock (Eds.), *Comprehensive textbook of psychiatry/IV*, (6th ed., Vol. 2, chap. 22). Baltimore: Williams & Wilkins.

Garner, D.M., & Garfinkel, P.E. (1979). The eating attitude test: An index of the symptoms of anorexia nervosa. *Psychological Medicine, 9*, 273–279.

Garner, D.M., & Garfinkel, P.E. (1980). Socio-cultural factors in the development of anorexia nervosa. *Psychological Medicine, 10*, 647–656.

Garner, D.M., Olmsted, M.P., & Polivy, J. (1983). Development and validation of a multitimensional eating disorder inventory for anorexia nervosa and bulimia. *International Journal of Eating Disorders, 2*, 15–34.

Habermas, T. (1991). The role of psychiatric and medical traditions in the discovery and description of anorexia nervosa in France, Germany, and Italy, 1873–1918. *Journal of Nervous and Mental Disease, 179*(6), 360–365.

Hawkins, R.C., & Clement, P.F. (1980). Development and construct validation of a self-report measure of binge eating tendencies. *Addictive Behaviours, 5*, 219–226.

Heatherton, T.F., Nicholas, P., Mahamedi, F., & Keel, P. (1995). Body weight, dieting, and eating disorder symptoms among college students, 1982 to 1992. *American Journal of Psychiatry, 152,* 1623–29.

Hock, H.W. (1993). Review of the epidemiological studies of eating disorders. *International Review of Psychiatry, 5,* 61–74.

Hock, H.W., van Harten, P.N., van Hoeken, D., & Susser, E. (1998). Lack of relation between culture and anorexia nervosa — Results of an incidence study on Curacao. *New England Journal of Medicine, 338*(17), 1231–32.

Hsu, L.K.G., & Lee, S. (1993). Is weight phobia always necessary for a diagnosis of anorexia nervosa? *American Journal of Psychiatry, 150*(10), 1466–1471.

Hsu, L.K.G., & Sobkiewicz, T.A. (1991). Body image disturbance: Time to abandon the concept for eating disorder? *International Journal of Eating Disorders, 10*(1), 15–30.

Iancu, I., Spivak, B., Ratzoni, G., Apter, A., & Weizman, A. (1994). The sociocultural theory in the development of anorexia nervosa. *Psychopathology, 27,* 29–36.

Joergensen, J. (1992). The epidemiology of eating disorders in Fyn County, Denmark, 1977–1986. *Acta Psychiatrica Scandinavica, 85,* 30–34.

Khandelwal, S.K., Sharan, P., & Saxena, S. (1995). Eating disorders: An Indian perspective. *International Journal of Social Psychiatry, 41*(2), 132–146.

King, M.B., & Bhugra, D. (1989). Eating disorders: Lessons from a cross-cultural study. *Psychological Medicine, 19,* 955–958.

Korkina, M.V., Tsyvilko, M.A., Marilov, V.V., & Kareva, M.A. (1992). Anorexia nervosa as manifested in Russia. *International Journal of Psychosomatics, 39*(1–4), 35–40.

Ledoux, S., Choquet, M., & Flament, M. (1991). Eating disorders among adolescents in an unselected French population. *International Journal of Eating Disorders, 10*(1), 81–89.

Lee, S., Ho, T.P., and Hsu, L.K.G. (1993). Fat phobic and non-fat phobic anorexia nervosa — A comparative study of 70 Chinese patients in Hong Kong. *Psychological Medicine, 23,* 999–1017.

Leon, G.R. (1992). Commentary: Korkina, Tsyvilko, Marilov, and Kareva's "Anorexia nervosa as manifested in Russia." *International Journal of Psychosomatics, 39*(1–4), 35–40.

Littlewood, R. (1995). Psychopathology and personal agency: Modernity, culture change and eating disorders in South Asian societies. *British Journal of Medical Psychology, 68,* 45–63.

Littlewood, R., & Lipsedge, M. (1987). The butterfly and the serpent: Culture, psychopathology and biomedicine. *Culture, Medicine and Psychiatry, 11*(3), 289–335.

Mumford, D.B., & Whitehouse, A.M. (1988). Increased prevalence of bulimia nervosa among Asian schoolgirls. *British Medical Journal, 297,* 718.

Mumford, D.B. Whitehouse, A.M., & Choudry, I.Y. (1992). Survey of eating disorders in English-medium schools in Lahore, Pakistan. *International Journal of Eating Disorders, 11*(2), 173–184.

Mumford, D.B., Whitehouse, A.M., & Platts, M. (1991). Socio-cultural correlates of eating disorders among Asian schoolgirls in Bradford. *British Journal of Psychiatry, 158,* 222–228.

Nasser, M. (1986). Comparative study of the prevalence of abnormal eating attitudes among Arab female students of both London and Cairo Universities. *Psychological Medicine, 16,* 621–625.

Nogami, Y., & Yabana, F. (1977). On *kibarashi-gui* (binge eating). *Folia Psychiatrica et Neurologica Japonica, 31*(2), 159–166.

Pagsberg, A.K., & Wang, A.R. (1994). Epidemiology of anorexia nervosa and bulimia nervosa in Bornholm County, Denmark, 1970–1989. *Acta Psychiatrica Scandinavica, 90,* 259–265.

Polivy, J., Herman, P., & Warsh, S. (1978). Internal and external components of emotionality in restrained and unrestrained eaters. *Journal of Abnormal Psychology, 92,* 497–504.

Prince, R. (1985). The concept of culture-bound syndromes: Anorexia nervosa and brain-fag. *Social Science and Medicine, 21*(2), 197–203.

Russell, G.F.M., & Treasure, J. (1989). The modern history of anorexia nervosa: An interpretation of why the illness has changed. *Annals of the New York Academy of Sciences, 575* 13–27.

Smith, J.E., & Krejci, J. (1991). Minorities join the majority: Eating disturbances among Hispanic and native American youth. *International Journal of Eating Disorders, 10*(2), 179–186.

Smith, M., & Thelen, M.H. (1984). Development and validation of a test for bulimia. *Journal of Consulting and Clinical Psychology, 52,* 863–872.

Song, Y.H., & Fang, Y.Q. (1990). Clinical report on nine anorexia nervosa cases. *Chinese Mental Health Journal, 4*(1), 24–25 (in Chinese).

Suematsu, H., Ishikawa, H., Kuboki, T., & Ito, T. (1985). Statistical studies on anorexia nervosa in Japan: Detailed clinical data on 1,011 patients. *Psychotherapy and Psychosomatics, 43*(2), 96–103.

Szmukler, G.I. (1985). The epidemiology of anorexia nervosa and bulimia. *Journal of Psychiatric Research, 19,* 143–153.

Walsh, B.T. (1997). Chapter 63: Eating disorders. In A. Tasman, J. Kay, & J.A. Lieberman (Eds.), *Psychiatry,* (Vol. 2) (pp. 1202–1290). Philadelphia: Saunders.

Wardle, J. (1986). The assessment of restrained eating. *Behaviour Research and Therapy, 24,* 213–215.

Wilfley, D.W., & Rodin, J. (1995). Cultural influences on eating disorders. In K.D. Brownell & C.G. Fairburn (Eds.), *Eating disorders and obesity: A comprehensive textbook.* New York: Guilford Press.

Willi, J., Giacometti, G., & Limacher, B. (1990). Update on the epidemiology of anorexia nervosa in a defined region of Switzerland. *American Journal of Psychiatry, 147* (11), 1514–1517.

Willi, J., & Grossman, S. (1983). Epidemiology of anorexia nervosa in a defined region of Switzerland. *American Journal of Psychiatry, 140,* 564–567.

Zhang, F.C., Mitchell, J.E., Kuang, L., Wang, M.Y., Yang, D.L., Zheng, J., Zhau, Y.R., Zhang, Z.H., Filice, G.A., Pomeroy, C., & Pyle, R.L. (1992). The prevalence of anorexia nervosa and bulimia nervosa among freshman medical college students in China. *International Journal of Eating Disorders, 12*(2), 209–214.

24

Personality Disorders

I. GENERAL DEBATES ABOUT PERSONALITY DISORDERS

Of the various kinds of psychopathologies, personality disorders have been the least subject to empirical research. There have been many debates among clinicians regarding the nature, diagnosis, and categorization of personality disorders. Further, knowledge about how to treat such disorders is still very scant. From a cross-cultural point of view, although the relation between culture and personality stirred up keen interest among scholars several decades ago [cross-reference to Chapter 5: Personality and Depth Psychology (Section I,C)], attention to disorders of the personality has only been recent (Alarcón, Foulks, & Vakkur, 1998). Cross-cultural information about personality disorders is nearly vacant, awaiting further investigation.

A. SPECTRUM OR CATEGORIES

There is a basic debate among clinicians about the nature of personality disorders. One group takes the spectrum view and regards personality disorders as the extreme of normal personality (Paris, 1997). Others maintain that personality disorders belong to a distinct category of disorders. For instance, as pointed out by Haslam (1997), substantial evidence, shows that antisocial, schizotypal, and probably borderline personality disorders correspond to discrete categories rather than continua.

Gunderson and Philips (1995) made a comprehensive proposal to resolve these dichotomized views. They distinguished three subgroups of personality disorders: "trait disorders," "self-disorders," and "spectrum disorders," located between the spectrum of normality and the category of psychoses. Obsessive, histrionic, avoidant, or dependent are categorized as trait disorders and are at the end of the spectrum, close to normality. Schizoid, antisocial, and borderline, categorized as self-disorders, are in the middle of the spectrum, between normality and psychoses. Schizotypal, paranoid, hyperthymic, or depression, as spectrum disorders, are at the end of the spectrum close to the category of psychosis. This indicates that there are different subgroups of personality disorders with different natures ranging from deviation from the spectrum of normality to discrete categories of psychiatric disorders.

B. Hereditary or Environmental

Associated with the debate between spectrum and category, there has been another argument as to whether hereditary or environment cause personality disorders. At present, many scholars attribute personality disorders, closely related to the personality, to both hereditary and environmental factors. For instance, Paris (1997) presented the view that the form of personality pathology largely depends on underlying traits, which are subject to strong genetic influence, and that different social structures tend to reinforce some traits and discourage others. He also pointed out that genetically influenced personality traits determine the specificity of personality disorders, whereas psychological and social factors only affect the threshold at which personality traits become maladaptive.

The issue of genetic and environmental contributions to personality disorders was elaborated by twin studies conducted by Livesley, Lang, Jackson, and Vernon (1993), who compared volunteer pairs of twins — monozygotic and dizygotic — from the general population. The twins were asked to complete the Dimensional Assessment of Personality Pathology, a questionnaire that assesses 18 dimensions of personality disorders. Comparing data obtained from monozygotic and dizygotic twins, the estimates of broad heritability ranged from 0% (for conduct problems) to 64% (for narcissism). Behavior associated with submissiveness and attachment problems had low heritability. They pointed out that these results were similar to those reported for normal personalities. In their interpretation, the results suggested a continuity between normal and disordered personality.

II. CULTURAL INFLUENCE ON PERSONALITY DISORDERS

A. Diagnosing the Disorder

The identification of personality disorders is based on the general diagnostic criteria of "an enduring pat-tern of inner experience and behavior that deviates markedly from the expectations of the individual's *culture*" and "the enduring pattern leads to clinically significant distress or impairment in *social,* occupational, or other important areas of functioning" (DSM-IV). This means that the diagnostic decision relies on how the society views and tolerates the behavior concerned. It is subjective, relative, and culturally defined. Naturally, there is ample room for cross-cultural bias and differences in making diagnoses and identifying the disorders. As stressed by Foulks (1996), different cultures have tended to emphasize different traits of personality as ideal. From a cultural perspective, defining or labeling deviances from "normal personality" is clearly a culture-relative exercise, and its boundaries are reflective of the specific values, ideas, worldview, resources, and social structure of the society.

The International Personality Disorder Examination (IPDE) was carried out (Loranger et al., 1994) as a joint project of the World Health Organization and the U.S. Alcohol, Drug Abuse, and Mental Health Administration. Fourteen participating centers in 11 countries in North America, Europe, Africa, and Asia were involved. The results proved that the IPDE was acceptable to clinicians with satisfactory interrator reliability in different nations, languages, and cultures by using the semistructured clinical interview. This finding was quite challenging to cultural psychiatrists, who still view the assessment of personality disorders as very much influenced by cultural factors.

Responding to the greater likelihood of more men being diagnosed as "antisocial" than women, and of more women being diagnosed as "histrionic" than men, Nuckolls (1992) pointed out that such diagnostic patterns are rooted in cultural histories, representing (in extreme their forms) values strongly congruent with cultural stereotypes, i.e., the "independent" male and the "dependent" female.

B. Frequency of Disorder

The frequency of a personality disorder is relatively difficult to study through epidemiological surveys because they are one-time studies and do not examine a person's life thoroughly or objectively enough to make it possible to diagnose a "personality disorder." Unless a survey was carried out with intensive psychological assessment, most kinds of personality disorders would be difficult to diagnose. Of all the recognized personality disorders, antisocial personality disorder is the most relatively possible to identify due to its nature. In the Epidemiologic Catchment Area (ECA) study carried out in the United States, only data for antisocial personality were examined among three ethnic groups surveyed. It was revealed that the lifetime prevalence rates were 2, 2.3, and 3.4%, respectively, for Caucasian-American, African-American, and Hispanic-American ethnic groups (Robins, Tippi & Pryzbeck, 1991, p. 265). These data contrasted with the ethnic distribution of inmates diagnosed with antisocial personality disorder. That is, the African-American group had a relatively higher percentage distribution than the Caucasian-American group. This was interpreted as the result of bias against African-Americans in law enforcement situations and in making diagnoses.

There are scant epidemiological data about personality disorders examined across societies for cross-cultural comparison. Unless a similar methodology and criteria is used, there is no point in making cross-cultural comparisons. However, without knowing the cultural impact and implication of the method and criteria used, data obtained becomes meaningless. This is exemplified by the cross-cultural comparison of personality disorders between America and Taiwan. The same method and questionnaire used in the ECA study in the United States was applied in an epidemiological study in Taiwan (Hwu, Yeh, & Chang, 1989). Results revealed that the prevalence of antisocial personality disorders was 0.2% in Taiwan and 3% in the United States (Compton et al., 1991). Even though similar rating instruments and sampling populations were involved in both studies, it was not clear whether obtained data reflected true differences in the prevalence rates or other more subtle things — like the tendency to give socially acceptable answers in Taiwan due to cultural attitudes toward antisocial disorders.

Tang and Huang (1995) pointed out that the reported rate of personality disorders in (mainland) China seemed exceptionally low when compared with that reported from Western societies. While this could be due to underreporting or differences in official classification used regarding professional criteria of personality disorders (Lee, 1996; Zheng, Lin, Zhao, Zhang, & Yong, 1994), Tang and Huang indicated that there was also a major conceptual difference between Chinese and Western cultures regarding personality and personality disorders.

C. SOCIAL PATTERNS AND TYPES OF PERSONALITY DISORDERS

A hypothesis was proposed by Paris (1997) regarding the matching of social patterns and types of personality problems observed. He speculated that in societies that provided relatively secure and predictable roles for every individual and in which conformity with the expectations of family and community was normative (and intense), social structures would promote individual behaviors characterized by emotional inhibition and constriction. If we extended this assumption, it would be possible to expect that personality disorders of cluster C — avoidant, dependent, or obsessive-compulsive — would be more likely to be observed. In contrast, societies that demanded a high level of autonomy, where individuals were expected to create their own roles, the social structure would tend to reward behaviors associated with a more active and expressive personality style. It would be possible to anticipate that personality disorders of cluster B — characterized by antisocial, borderline, histrionic, and narcisstic behavior — would tend to occur.

D. PROTECTION OR EXPOSURE BY CULTURE

Paris (1996) tried to explain that culture has the function of protecting its members from manifesting certain personality disorders or exposing them, particularly in the case of borderline personality disorders. Presenting clinical cases, he explained that when a person migrated to a different cultural setting, the protective function of the original society was removed and the person's vulnerability was exposed in the host society, manifesting character problems. For instance, a person with a relatively reserved personality may have functioned all right in his conservative home society, but when he moved to an aggressive host society, his reserved personality may have been exposed and manifested as inadequate or displaying passive personality problems.

Examining the personality traits of hardiness and type A behavior observed in a Japanese male sample, Nakano (1990) commented that Japanese social structure encourages competitiveness, but, at the same time, values self-discipline, attentiveness to others, and a sense of personal and group identity. Therefore, the personality trait of hardiness seemed to be a good resource in the complex society, which expected both competitiveness and harmony with others. A type A personality seemed to be more maladaptive in Japanese than in American society. Type A behavior is characterized by hard-driving competitiveness, time consciousness, impatience, and striving for achievement, and is also associated with hostility and aggression. Hostile and aggressive behaviors are not likely to be accepted in Japanese society.

E. Cultural Reaction to Personality Disorders

The extreme of sociocultural reaction toward personality disorders is exemplified by the way in which a political system shapes the categories of those disorders. In Russia, during the Soviet era, it was believed that, within the community-oriented communist society, there was no room for self-centered, narcisstic people. Therefore, the category of narcisstic personality disorder was removed from the official classification system (C. Korolenko, personal communication, 1997).

The identification and labeling of personality disorders are not only colored by political ideology, but are also influenced by clinicians in their practice. As indicated by Zheng and colleagues (1994), Chinese psychiatrists are in general reluctant to accept and use the diagnoses of most personality disorders in their clinical practice, and tend to reject some of the Western-based concepts and categories, including borderline, avoidant, dependent, schizoid, and narcissistic personality disorders.

III. SPECIFIC CATEGORIES OF PERSONALITY DISORDERS

A. Antisocial Personality Disorder

As mentioned in Section II,B, based on the findings obtained from the ECA study, Robins and colleagues (1991) reported that there were no racial differences whatever in the prevalence of antisocial personality in the United States. However, at the same time, it was also commonly known that the percentage of racial distribution among inmates in prisons was remarkably influenced by racial factors. Kosson, Smith, and Newman (1990) reported that 45% of the prisoners in the United States were African-American (while their percentage in the general population was less than 13%).

Lopez (1989) suggested that there was an overpathologizing bias toward African-Americans and lower-class individuals relative to Caucasian-American and female subjects in the diagnosis of antisocial personality disorder. Alarcón and Foulks (1995) pointed out that as many as half of inner city youth may have this diagnosis misapplied, as the criteria are inappropriate for settings in which value systems and behavioral rules make learning to be violent a protective and survival strategy.

B. Histrionic Personality Disorder

It is a well-known trend that clinically the diagnosis of hysterical personality disorder is especially prone to gender bias from the point of view of the examiner: more females than males are diagnosed with this order by (male) clinicians. A male might be labeled as antisocial, instead. This shows that the diagnosis of histrionic personality disorder relies heavily on the view of the examiner and is subjective. In transcultural practice, if there is a wide gap between the patient and the clinician in terms of how they express emotion, due to cultural factors, there is a high possibility of a misdiagnosis in the category of personality disorder. This is particularly true if the clinician, according to his or her cultural background, emphasizes the control of emotional expression, whereas the patient, following his or her cultural experience, values the free and dramatic expression of emotion.

C. NARCISSTIC PERSONALITY DISORDER

It is speculated that narcissistic personality disorder may be misapplied more commonly to minorities, especially those that are more alienated from the mainstream and those that hold "machismo" as a cultural value, such as younger people of Latin descent.

D. BORDERLINE PERSONALITY DISORDER

The frequency of clinical diagnoses of borderline personality disorder has increased significantly in North America during the past three decades, associated with the clarification of the concept of nosology and the increased awareness of such a disorder among clinicians. In contrast, in many other societies, particularly in Asia, while attention to the disorder is increasing, the number of cases actually diagnosed is not necessarily rising accordingly. To what extent the increased prevalence of the disorder is related to diagnostic patterns or to the actual increase of such cases is not clear.

An unstable early childhood, increased history of abuse, unstable family environment, and other life fac-

tors have been hypothesized as the precipitating factors for developing borderline personality disorder when the youngster reaches adulthood. Thus, there is good reason to speculate that such a disorder may be less prevalent in certain societies where people go through a relatively less traumatic early childhood and live in a stable family environment. Examining those who had developed borderline disorder after migrating to developed societies, Paris (1996) considered that the social protective factors (that existed in traditional socities) may have suppressed the development of the borderline traits into diagnosable personality disorders. Certainly, this speculation is awaiting cross-ethnic or cross-cultural validation.

In the United States, Castaneda and Franco (1985) examined inpatient samples who were admitted to a city hospital in New York City. Among 1583 patients, 101 cases were given the diagnosis of borderline personalty disorder. The distribution of this disorder among Caucasians, African-Americans, and Hispanics was similar to the distribution of these three ethnic groups among all psychiatric inpatients. The only difference noted was that in the Caucasian and African-American groups, fewer men than women were diagnosed as having this personality disorder; this was not true in the Hispanic group. The reason for this was not clear.

There is little literature from other societies regarding borderline personality disorder. The validity of the borderline concept is still challenged (Kroll, Carley, & Sines, 1982). From Japan, Moriya, Miyake, Minakawa, Ikuta, and Nishizono-Maher (1993) have reported that, comparing their data with data obtained from literature on American patients, Japanese borderline patients tended to show fewer symptoms of substance abuse, but had higher scores for depersonalization and derealization. Japanese patients were more likely to have intense masochistic-dependent relationships, were less likely to be socially isolated, and were more likely to be living at home rather than being homeless.

Paris (1992) pointed out that the most characteristic symptoms of borderline personality disorder, i.e., repeated suicide attempts in the form of overdoses or self-mutilation, were not seen by psychiatrists in many traditional societies. Recurrent overdoses or self-injury could be a sign of underlying personality vulnerability, but could also reflect a unique help-seeking behavior that may be effective, depending on the nature of the medical system and the professional as well as social attitudes toward such behavior. Thus, borderline personality disorder could be influenced by culture through pathoreactive effects in addition to possible pathofacilitative effects.

E. DEPENDENT PERSONALITY DISORDER

The concept of "dependent" or "avoidant" is based very heavily on social relationships. As pointed out clearly by Lin (1997) in (Western) societies, where individual independence and autonomy are emphasized greatly, a person who tends to depend on others will stand out as a deviant of that social norm and be labeled as having a dependent personality disorder. In contrast, in societies where it is considered a virtue to be mutually dependent, to rely heavily on the group, and to act collectively rather than individually, such as Japanese society (Doi, 1973), to be "dependent" is not a problem. On the contrary, as pointed out by some Japanese psychiatrists, to be "independent" is a disorder — requiring the category of "(excessively) independent personality disorder" in the Japanese cultural context.

The official psychiatric classification in China does not entirely follow the International Statistical Classification of Disease and Related Health Problems (ICD) of the World Health Organization or the Diagnostic and Statistical Manual of Mental Disorders (DSM) developed by the American Psychiatric Association. Chinese psychiatrists maintain their country's national classifications with their uniqueness suitable for actual clinical application. Regarding personality disorders, for instance, the Chinese do not include the dependent or passive-aggressive personality disorders that are listed in ICD-10 (Lee, 1996). Perhaps such personality tratis are more tolerated and even accepted in Chinese culture.

Alarcón and Foulks (1995) indicated that in Asian and Arctic societies, passivity, politeness, deferential treatment, and acceptance of others' opinions are normative. Self-blame and self-depreciation may exist as conventionally acceptable means for gain in the larger social context. Based on such cultural attitudes, certain personality traits that are considered "disorders" in Western culture are not viewed as such in other countries.

F. AVOIDANT PERSONALITY DISORDER

If a society stresses the importance of social interaction in daily life, avoiding such relations may be recognized as avoidant. In a society that has a high tolerance for withdrawn behavior, people (such as hermits) may be considered "saints" for periodically going on long retreats for the purposes of self-training. No one in those social circumstances would label such people as having "avoidant" or "schizotypal" personality disorders.

As pointed out by Foulks (1996), many individuals in severely oppressed, minority groups are reluctant to participate in social situations because of a fear of saying something inappropriate; they show anxiety in front of others, are unwilling to get involved with people, and avoid social activities involving oppressive majority groups. These characteristics are related to acculturation problems and are not to be labeled as avoidant behavior.

G. OBSESSIVE PERSONALITY DISORDER

We should not confuse obsessive personality traits and obsessive personality disorder. From daily life observations, it has been noted that certain ethnic groups are characterized by obsessive-compulsive traits in their social behavior. For instance, British people in Western societies and Japanese people in Eastern societies tend to value orderliness as well as cleanliness in their daily lives. They prefer to do things in an orderly manner, with a plan and in a precise way. Emotionally, control is emphasized in public settings. However, whether, and to what extent, there is more obsessive personalty disorder among them is a challenging question.

IV. CLOSING REMARKS

There is no argument that in each society there are a certain number of people who manifest enduring patterns of behavior that "deviate markedly from the expectations of their culture" and result in a disturbance in social functioning. However, there is a need to clarify the threshold for such deviation and impairment according to each society. It is most likely that, depending on its culture, each society tends to show a different tolerance for different kinds of behavior deviation. Therefore, the identification and labeling of personality disorders are very much subject to cultural definition and social recognition. According to Offer and Sabshin (1974), normality and abnormality could be determined by various ways: by professional definition, by deviation from the mean, according to the nature and level of function, and by social definition. Personality disorders rely heavily on the last approach, which is subject to social and cultural views, attitudes, tolerance, and judgement.

Thus, clinically there is a need for cross-cultural validation of diagnostic categories as well as the method and standard for evaluation and identification of clinically dysfunctional cases. In transcultural practice, when the patient and clinician have divergent cultural backgrounds as well as different modal personalities, the assessment and diagnosis of personality must be made very carefully. They need to be culturally sensitive and relevant. Otherwise, they may result in serious mistakes in clinical practice.

One of the major bases for making a diagnosis of personality disorder is that the enduring pattern of behavior is inflexible and pervasive across a broad range of personal and social situations for a long time into adulthood. It is essential to have a longitudinal history to support this. However, in transcultural practice, it often becomes a problem to obtain a compre-

hensive lifetime personal history, particularly if there is a language obstacle as well as limited knowledge about the social and cultural situation in which the behavior pattern occurred. Unless there is sufficient information to support that the problem is not only inflexible but also pervasive over a long period of time, the diagnosis of personality disorder needs to be made with caution and reservation.

From an academic point of view, there is a need for more cross-cultural epidemiological studies of personality disorders. It would be meaningless to compare the number of cases or prevalence rates cross-culturally without knowing how to make cultural adjustments. However, cross-societal comparisons of the distribution of subtypes of personality disorders within a society would certainly offer valuable information about the relationship among the social structure, the cultural system, and the kinds of personality disorders the society recognized. The comparisons would increase our insight into the nature and implication of such disorders from both social and cultural perspectives greatly.

REFERENCES

Alarcón, R., & Foulks, E. (1995). Personality disorders and culture: Contemporary clinical views, Part A. *Cultural Diversity and Mental Health, 1,* 3–17.

Alarcón, R.D., Foulks, E.F., & Vakkur, M. (1998). *Personality disorders and culture: Clinical and conceptual interactions.* New York: Wiley.

Castaneda, R., & Franco, H. (1985). Sex and ethnic distribution of borderline personality disorder in an inpatient sample. *American Journal of Psychiatry, 142*(10), 1202–1203.

Compton, W., Helzer, J., Hwu, H.G., Yeh, E.K., McEvoy, M., Topp, M., & Spitznagel, E. (1991). New methods in cross-cultural psychiatry: Psychiatric illness in Taiwan and the U.S. *American Journal of Psychiatry, 148,* 1697–1704.

Doi, T (1973). *The anatomy of dependence: The key analysis of Japanese behavior.* Tokyo: Kodansha International.

Foulks, E.F. (1996). Culture and personality disorders. In J.E. Mezzich, A. Kleinman, H. Fabrega, Jr., & D.L. Parron (Eds.), *Culture and psychiatric diagnosis: A DSM-IV perspective* (pp. 243–252). Washington, DC: American Psychiatric Press.

Gunderson, J.G., & Philips, K.A. (1995). Personality disorders. In H.I. Kaplan & B.J. Sadock (Eds.), *Comprehensive textbook of psychiatry/VI,* (6th ed., Vol. 2, chap. 25) Baltimore: Williams & Wilkins.

Haslam, N. (1997). Personality disorders as social categories. *Transcultural Psychiatry, 34*(4), 473–479.

Hwu, H.G., Yeh, E.K., & Chang, L.Y. (1989). Prevalence of psychiatric disorders in Taiwan defined by the Chinese Diagnostic Interview Schedule. *Acta Psychiatrica Scandinavica, 79,* 136–147.

Kosson, D.S., Smith, S.S., & Newman, J.P. (1990). Evaluating the construct validity of psychopathy in Black and White male inmates: Three preliminary studies. *Journal of Abnormal Psychology, 99*(3), 250–259.

Kroll, J., Carley, K., & Sines, L. (1982). Are there borderlines in Britain? *Archives of General Psychiatry, 39,* 60–63.

Lee, S. (1996). Cultures in psychiatric nosology: The CCMD-2-R and international classification of mental disorders. *Culture, Medicine and Psychiatry, 20,* 421–472.

Lin, K.M. (1997). Personality and personality disorder in the context of culture. *Transcultural Psychiatry, 34*(4), 480–488.

Livesley, W.J., Lang, K.L., Jackson, D.N., & Vernon, P.A. (1993). Genetic and environmental contributions to dimensions of personality disorder. *American Journal of Psychiatry, 150,* 1826–1831.

Lopez, S.R. (1989). Patient variable biases in clinical judgement: Conceptual overview and methodological considerations. *Psychological Bulletin, 106,* 184–203.

Loranger, A.W., Sartori, N., Andreoli, A., Berger, P., Bucheim, P., Channabasavanna, S.M., Coid, B., Dahl, A., Diekstra, R.F.W., Ferguson, B., Jacobsberg, L.B., Mombour, W., Pull, C., Ono, Y., & Regier, D.A. (1994). The international personality disorder examination. *Archives of General Psychiatry, 51,* 215–224.

Moriya, N., Miyake, Y., Minakawa, K., Ikuta, N., & Nishizono-Maher, A. (1993). Diagnosis and clinical features of borderline personality disorder in the East and West: A preliminary report. *Comprehensive Psychiatry, 34,* 418–423.

Nakano, K. (1990). Hardiness, type A behavior, and physical symptoms in a Japanese sample. *Journal of Nervous and Mental Disease, 178*(1), 52–56.

Nuckolls, C.W. (1992). Toward a cultural history of the personality disorders. *Social Science and Medicine (Medical Anthropology), 35*(1), 37–47.

Offer, D., & Sabshin, M. (1974). *Normality: Theoretical and clinical concepts of mental health* (2nd ed.), New York: Basic Books.

Paris, J. (1992). Social factors in borderline personality disorder: A review and hypothesis. *Canadian Journal of Psychiatry, 37,* 480–486.

Paris, J. (1996). Cultural factors in the emergence of borderline pathology. *Psychiatry, 59,* 185–192.

Paris, J. (1997). Social factors in personality disorders. *Transcultural Psychiatry, 34*(4), 421–452.

Robins, L.N., Tipp, J., & Pryzbeck, T. (1991). Antisocial personality. In L.N. Robins & D.A. Rogers (Eds.), *Psychiatric disorders in America: The Epidemiologic Catchment Area Study.* New York: Free Press.

Tang, S.W., & Huang, Y. (1995). Diagnosing personality disorders in China. *International Medical Journal, 2,* 291–297.

Zheng, Y.P., Lin, K.M., Zhao, J.P., Zhang, M.Y., & Yong, D.S. (1994). Comparative study of diagnostic systems: Chinese Classification of Mental Disorders — Second Edition versus DSM-III-R. *Comprehensive Psychiatry, 35,* 441–449.

25

Childhood-Related Disorders

I. INTRODUCTORY REMARKS

Although a vast amount of work has been done in the area of child development from cross-cultural perspectives, very little cross-cultural investigation has been carried out in clinical areas. Thus, the literature is rather scanty on the cultural aspects of childhood-related mental disorders.

There is good reason to believe that, beyond the basic stages of development that every child goes through, the lives of youngsters are shaped differently by culture in different societies [cross-reference to Chapter 4: Child Development and Enculturation (Section III, A–E)]. As an extension of this, there is enough evidence to speculate that children's mental health problems, beyond mental disorders that are determined predominantly by biological factors (such as mental retardation and autisim), will be different in different cultures. This is truer of mental health problems that are predominantly attributed to psychological factors and are more subject to sociocultural impact. There is a need for cultural considerations in the assessment and diagnosis of childhood disorders (Canino, Canino, & Arroyo, 1998).

Child psychiatry, as a branch of psychiatry, is still in the early stages of development. There are not many specialists in the field, even in developed societies such as the United States. There are only a handful in many developing societies (Nikapota, 1991). Thus, there is no sufficient clinical information available for cross-cultural study (Minde & Nikapota, 1993). Many childhood-related disorders are still in the stages of speculation. The cultural aspects of child mental health problems are seldom elaborated in literature (Ensink & Robertson, 1996).

Only some childhood psychiatric disorders or mental health problems are closely related to cultural factors primarily in the formation of pathology; there is also the issue of how clinical assessment or management is influenced by culture secondarily. This chapter attempts to review childhood-related mental disorders within cross-cultural contexts. The issue of how to work with children and adolescents from a cross-cultural perspective will be elaborated in Chapter 38.

II. SOME EPIDEMIOLOGICAL COMPARISONS

As pointed out by Bird (1996), a sizable number of epidemiological studies have been carried out in different parts of the world during the past two decades.

However, methodological problems have limited meaningful cross-cultural comparsions. The studies have involved two principal approaches, each reflecting a different way of conceptualizing and classifying childhood disorders. One approach used an empirically based quantitative taxonomy that aimed to detect patterns of occurring problems. For this approach, behavior checklists, such as the Child Behavior Checklist (CBCL) and its parallel instruments for teachers (TRF) and youth self-rating (YSR), are commonly used. The other approach used classification systems to survey the disorders, which tended to have problems with defining disorders and cross-cultural methods of assessment.

Bird (1996), who reviewed the epidemiological research on childhood psychopathology that had been carried out in different cultural settings in the previous 15 years, reported that national differences were observed in mean CBCL scores ranging from a low of 20.0 on the U.S. east coast sample to a high of 35.4 in Greece. Data from teachers' ratings (TRF), available from six nations (the United States, Jamaica, the Netherlands, Puerto Rico, Thailand, and rural/urban areas in China), showed that the mean score ranged from a low of 17.6 for the Dutch sample to a high of 39.0 for the Chinese rural sample. Bird summarized that there were great similarities in the characteristics of psychopathology manifested in different settings, despite the differences that existed in the rates of symptomatology.

A WHO collaborative study in the western Pacific region of the emotional and behavioral problems of primary schoolchildren in metropolitan areas was initiated in 1986 in Tokyo (Japan), Beijing (China), and Seoul (Korea) (Matsuura et al., 1993). Rutter's questionnaire was used as an instrument for assessment in this cross-national prevalence study. Children's behavior at school was scored by the teachers and at home by the parents. Results revealed that the prevalence rates of children with deviant scores were 3.9, 8.3, and 14.1%, respectively, for children in Japan, China, and Korea, as reported by a teacher, and 12.0, 7.0, & 19.1%, respectively, as rated by the parents.

The investigators pointed out that the prevalence of deviance was scored higher at home (12.0%) than at school (3.9%) in Japan. The situation in China was different. The prevalence of deviance was higher in school (8.3%) than at home (7.0%). In China and Korea, the prevalence of deviance was higher in children from one-parent families than in those from two-parents families; however, for some unknown reason, this was not the case in Japan.

Bengi-Arslan, Verhulst, van der Ende, and Erol from the Netherlands (1997) conducted a cross-cultural comparative survey of children's behavior problems based on their parents' responses to Achenbach's CBCL. It concerned 2081 Dutch children in the Netherlands, 3127 Turkish children in Ankara, Turkey, and 833 Turkish immigrant children living in the Netherlands. They reported that immigrant Turkish children scored higher than Dutch children on 6 of the 11 CBCL scales, most markedly anxiety/depression. Immigrant Turkish children scored higher than Turkish children in Ankara on five scales. However, these differences were much smaller than those between immigrant Turkish children and Dutch children. The total problem scores did not differ between Turkish children who had migrated to the Netherlands and those in Turkey.

Concerning major diagnosis-based epidemiological studies, Bird (1996) reported that in three studies using ICD-9 criteria, the rates of major disorders ranged from 12.4% in France to 51.3% in Mannheim, Germany, with an average of approximately 28% across the three studies. In six studies that used DSM-III or DSM-III-R criteria (without taking severity of impairment into account), the rate ranged from 17.6% in the Dunedin study to 49.5% in the Puerto Rico study with an average of approximately 29% across all six studies. Based on these studies, Bird commented that the field of child psychiatric epidemiology had yet to develop a widely accepted methodology for surveys of mental disorders of children and adolescents that could be used systematically with different cultural groups and applied in different cultural settings.

III. SPECIFIC MENTAL HEALTH PROBLEMS

A. CHILD ABUSE OR CHILD INDULGENCE PROBLEMS

Of all the different kinds of childhood psychopathology, child abuse is relatively easy to compare and discuss cross-culturally because the concept of abuse is rather explicit, even though its actual definition and clinical recognition are subject to cultural variations. It is generally considered that child abuse and neglect are worldwide problems (Krugman, 1996).

The subject of child abuse and neglect has been reviewed extensively in a book edited by Jill E. Korbin (1981) to make up for the lack of knowledge beyond the Euro-American situation. It helps greatly to understand child abuse from a cross-cultural perspective. LeVine and Levine (1981, pp. 35–55) made several remarks on the situation in sub-Saharan Africa, where the sexual molestation of girls is a known phenomenon. For instance, they encountered cases of rape of prepubescent girls by adult Gusii men, who, in many instances, were closely related to members of their victims' parents' generation. Actual father–daughter incest occurred occasionally. In addition, the seduction of pubescent girls by male schoolteachers was the occasion for recurrent scandals in Nigeria and Kenya. LeVine and Levine also reported that "marginal" children — the residue of casual unions or of marital breakups — constituted a rapidly increasing high-risk population for abuse or neglect because they tended to receive inferior care. They reported that in their study of the Gusii, those marginal children, while constituting only 2.5% of the study population, amounted to 25% of the malnourished children in the area. Infanticide, formerly practiced for religious purposes in certain African societies, would seem to have been eliminated in the contemporary period. Finally, LeVine and LeVine commented that the use of child labor, like many other aspects of African child-rearing practices that have evolved in response to the exigencies of

an agricultural economy, might seem harsh or neglectful by Western standards.

Johnson (1981, pp. 56–70) found that despite a wide range of caretaking practices found in most areas of lowland South America, it was widely acknowledged that throughout Amazonia, mothers attended to infants with scrupulous care, nursing them on demand and providing close physical contact. It was only when a child reached the crawling or walking stages that parents in some cultures became indifferent to its needs. Children were left for long periods of time without food and were denied emotional reassurance. Johnson went further to explain that, similarly to other societies, undesirable social and economic conditions, such as insecure resources, social isolation, and lack of support, tended to be associated with the occurrence of child neglect. Mothers lacking support from their husbands and extended kinmen were more likely to find their children frustrating, were less inclined to consider their needs, and were more harsh and punitive with them.

Concerning child-rearing practices in rural areas of India, Poffenberger (1981, pp. 71–95) reported the differential treatment of boys and girls within this cultural framework. Young girls had to be obedient and learn to conform both in their own homes and in the homes of their in-laws. Because the difficulty in adjusting to a new family required strength of personality, the kind of emotional dependence on the mother that was desirable in sons was not encouraged in daughters. Poffenberger described discipline as common in India, but not battering abuse and neglect. He commented that the very social structure in India that required conformity provided parents with a support system of other adults and older children. The presence of others in the household restrained parental temper and reduced the likelihood that frustration would lead to uncontrolled violence toward young children.

Different forms of child abuse observed in Japan were reported by Wagatsuma (1981, pp. 120–138). He described the phenomenon of child abandonment, leaving an infant in a hospital, a clinic, or another public place, such as a railway station or a department store. The reasons for deserting infants were unwed pregnancy, financial problems, or family conflict. In Japan, to give one's baby to an orphanage was associated with feelings of shame, as it was necessary to publicly expose the parents' identity. The secret abandonment of their babies became the choice for young mothers who had difficulty keeping them. Wagatsuma further said that according to the ministry survey, cases of abandonment were much more frequent than cases of child abuse or neglect. During the years 1973 to 1974, there were 26 cases of abuse or neglect, but 139 cases of abandonment reported officially nationwide. A similar figure was found (137 cases) for murder–abandonment. Murder–abandonment included cases in which the death of the baby was not originally intended, but in which the baby died before being found. Because most of them were neonates, it was difficult for them to survive if they were not found by others soon, particularly in unfavorable conditions, such as cold weather. The causes of abandonment or infanticide were mostly related to the mothers being unwed or having serious marital problems with the possibility of divorce. In Japan, to be an unwed mother and to have an illegitimate child was considered very shameful. Having a child from a previous marriage made remarriage very unlikely for a woman. Therefore, it was cultural attitudes toward the status and the fates of these women that led to child abandonment.

Another form of child abuse pointed out by Wagatsuma was associated with the unique phenomenon of children–murder/parents–suicide acts known as "family suicide." When parents decided to commit joint suicide, they involved their children in their journey to death. The children were killed before their parents killed themselves or were forced to commit suicide with their parents by taking poison or other methods. This unique pattern of family suicide was based on the cultural belief that it was better for children to die with their parents than to become orphans and be neglected by nonblood-related others [cross-reference to Chapter 13: Culture-Related Specific Syndromes (Section II, B, 2)].

Based on clinical observations, the Japanese child psychiatrist Yoshiko Ikeda (1987) reported case material regarding child abuse in Japan. She pointed out that the physical abuse of children does exist in Japan, despite the notion that Japanese parents in general are fond of their children. She pointed out that when a nuclear family is isolated from extended family ties, because of frequent moves, living in urban settings, and particularly when the father had drinking problems, child abuse tended to occur. If the child was young, abuse was by the biological parents, whereas older children often suffered abuse by stepparents, particularly stepmothers. The image of the mean and cruel stepmother is common among laymen in Japan and frequently a fact.

Chinese-American anthropologiest David Y.H. Wu (1981, pp. 139–165) indicated that, in Taiwan, filial piety was one of the oldest moral codes. Extensions of traditional filial piety toward parents are certain extraordinary expectations of children, as described in old books or classic children's stories (Tseng & Hsu, 1972). These have many themes, such as sacrificing a child's life for the parents' sake; a child accomplishing an impossible task or suffering self-inflicted pain to fulfill a parent's wishes or demands; or a child supporting his parents despite difficult circumstances or self-sacrifice. Wu pointed out that such filial concepts and codes express fundamental values in parent–child relations, and child abuse-like behavior is practiced within this cultural context. Institutionalized child abuse against adopted daughters was mentioned by Wu as well. In the past, when a poor family had difficulty supporting itself, one solution was to sell its young daughters to an affluent family. They were called adopted daughters, but, in fact, the girls served as young live-in maids. Very often, these "adopted daughters" were subjected to harsh treatment by their masters or "foster parents."

In Hong Kong, Tang (1998) conducted a telephone survey of nearly 1000 randomly selected households to gain information on child abuse. The Chinese version of the Conflict Tactics Scale (by Straus) was used for assessment. Tang reported that physical abuse was 526 per 1000 children for minor violence and 461 per

1000 children for severe violence. Comparing this with data from United States families, he concluded that Chinese families in Hong Kong showed slightly lower rates of minor violence, but higher rates of severe violence toward children as defined by the scale.

Regarding contemporary mainland China, Korbin (1981, pp. 166–185) commented that there were very few cases of child abuse or neglect acknowledged officially. There is good reason to believe that this more or less reflects the actual situation. Associated with the national family policy of "one child per couple" to prevent a potential population explosion, most young couples in urban settings have only one child, whereas nearly half of young parents in rural areas have a second child. A child is viewed as a "treasure" of the parents and is often indulged by the grandparents. Thus, instead of abuse or neglect, child psychiatrists have witnessed problems associated with child indulgence syndrome. According to a 10-year follow-up survey of the same cohort in Nanjing (Tao, Qiu, Li, Tseng, Hsu, & Goebert, 1999), it was found that there were certain differences between single and nonsingle children among both boys and girls, the former tending toward more introverted and the latter more extroverted behavior. This was true statistically when the children were young. However, when they reached adolescence, after exposure to socialization opportunities with their peers in school, the differences between single and nonsingle children tended to disappear among the boys, but not among the girls, who retained certain introverted or neurotic traits (Tseng, Tao, Hsu, Qiu, & Goebert, 2000). It was suspected that the single girls were more protected by their parents and prevented from having adequate socialization experiences.

Based on the cross-cultural information available, Korbin (1981, pp. 1–12, 205–210) remarked on the cultural aspects of child abuse. He indicated that certain facts in the cultural context can act either to increase the incidence of child abuse and neglect or to diminish the likelihood of their occurrence. The factors were the cultural value of children (whether children were viewed as valuable for future generations), beliefs about the categories of children (whether chil-dren were considered inadequate or unacceptable categories by cultural standards), beliefs about child capabilities and developmental stages of children (expecting children to behave in certain way at certain ages in terms of competence and humanness), embeddedness of child rearing in kin and community networks (the existence of a network of concerned individuals beyond the biological parents — a crucial element in the etiology of child abuse). Finally, Korbin pointed out that while children in general might be highly valued by a cultural group, there were categories of children that were more vulnerable to maltreatment. These included illegitimate, adopted, deformed, retarded, high birth order, and female children. Vulnerability depended to a large degree on the cultural context. In summary, child abuse as a childhood-related problem is shown to be subject to various cultural influences in the nature of pathoplastic, pathoselective, and pathofacilitating effects [cross-reference to Chapter 11: Culture and Psychopathology (Section II, A–F)].

From a clinical point of view, Maitra (1996) raised the question about a universal diagnostic category for child abuse. Based on his work with south Asian families in Britain, Maitra pointed out that based on cultural beliefs about the self, subjective experience and interpersonal connections, and child-rearing patterns, child abuse could be viewed and defined differently in different societies. Special caution and careful assessment are thus necessary in transcultural practice.

B. SEXUAL ABUSE

It is not easy to obtain epidemiological data from communities regarding the prevalence of sexual abuse for cross-cultural comparison. This is primarily because the actual occurrence of abuse is often concealed. Instead, many studies rely on retrospective data, examining childhood histories of the sexual abuse of adult subjects, particularly college students, even though they often represent a special subpopulation from an epidemiological perspective.

Pope, Mangweth, Negrao, Hudson, and Cordas (1994) examined bulimic university students in the United States, Australia, and Brazil to determine the possible relation of sexual abuse in childhood to occurrences of bulimia nervosa in young adulthood. Childhood histories of sexual abuse were examined retrospectively. It was revealed that, in these particular populations, there were no significant differences between rates of sexual abuse, supporting the notion that there was no direct relation between past experience of sexual abuse and the occurrence of bulimia nervosa in adulthood.

Meston, Heiman, Trapnell, and Carlin from Austin, Texas (1999), examined university students of Asian and European ancestry regarding their past histories of childhood abuse. Results showed that male and female students of Asian ancestry reported higher levels of physical and emotional abuse and neglect than their European counterparts. However, in contrast, female students of European ancestry reported a higher incidence of sexual abuse than female students of Asian ancestry.

Moghal, Nota, and Hobbs (1995) from the United Kingdom also carried out a retrospective study concerning Asian ethnic minority populations. They reviewed cases referred to two teaching hospitals in Leeds, United Kingdom, over the 8-year period between 1985 and 1993. A total of 37 cases were identified. Among them, 25 were girls and 12 boys, with ages ranging from 1 to 15 years (mean 7 years). The perpetrators were identified in 16 of the 37 cases. All of them were male: 7 were fathers, 3 were mothers' partners, 1 was an uncle, 1 a grandfather, 1 a brother, and the remaining 3 were strangers. Moghal and colleagues pointed out that, in the United Kingdom, professionals as well as lay people tended to deny the existence of the sexual abuse of children among Asian ethnic minority populations based on assumptions about the Asian family structure, its culture, and its religion. However, they commented that Asian family members were less likely to initiate concerns and that professionals need to be more open to the possibility of sexual abuse.

C. Parent-Abuse Syndrome

A unique form of child and adolescent psychopathology is observed in some Asian societies, including Japan and mainland China. It is called parent-abuse syndrome, and refers to the physical violence of an older child or adolescent toward his parents, mostly his mother. It has been the opinion of Japanese psychiatrists that this problem occurs as the result of overindulgence of the child. When he was small, he was overindulged by his mother for various reasons, mostly because his father was busy at work and not involved in domestic matters, leaving the emotionally lonely mother to cling to her children (particularly her son). A boy growing up in such a situation, overprotected and exposed infrequently to a father figure for needed discipline, tended to become bullying, if not tyrannical. When he reached adolescence, he tended to exhibit violent behavior toward his parents if his needs were not satisfied, or when his parents tried to set limits on his behavior. Being physically strong at that age, he could hurt or even injure his parents rather seriously when he became violent. Thus, this phenomenon is referred to as parent-abuse syndrome, the opposite of child abuse. This unique problem may be understood from a developmental perspective as part of the rebelliousness of adolescence, when a child wants to distance himself from his parents, only it is manifested in a pathological way.

D. Behavior Disorders

Canino and colleagues (1998) pointed out that of all childhood psychiatric disorders, conduct disorder is perhaps the most highly influenced by cultural and other contextual variables. For clinical diagnosis, it is recommended in DSM-IV (American Psychiatric Association, 1994, p. 88) that conduct disorder should be applied only when the behavior in question is symptomatic of an underlying dysfunction within the individual and not simply a reaction to the immediate social context.

Cross-cultural comparison of children's behavior disorders is difficult because the identification of behavior disorders is subject to sociocultural definition. There is no universal standard for defining such disorders. Furthermore, unless a community survey is carried out, clinical data are subject to the influence factor of illness behavior, depending on the reasons and mechanisms for seeking professional help.

E. SUBSTANCE ABUSE

Although was pointed out that substance abusers worldwide are generally young males (Smart, Murray, & Arif 1988), it was not clarified to what extent their problems were shared by other children and what would become of them. Data available from the National Institute on Drug Abuse (1995, pp. 46–49) were used, concerning students during the period 1977–1994, which showed that there were considerable differences in prevalence, depending on the nature of the substance abused, among the three ethnic groups (African-Americans, Caucasian-Americans, and Hispanic-Americans) surveyed. For instance, in the prevalence for daily cigarette usage, Caucasian-American students were consistently and relatively higher than the other two ethnic minority group students during the nearly two decades surveyed. Caucasian-American students and Hispanic-American students shared almost identical patterns of prevalence for cocaine, which were obviously higher than those of the African-American students. Regarding LSD and stimulants, respectively, Caucasian-American students were always higher, African-American students lower, and Hispanic-American students in between during the period surveyed. The prevalence for marijuana was rather similar among the three ethnic group students surveyed. This indicated that, within the same society, among different ethnic groups, the prevalence rates were different or similar depending on the substances abused. Economic factors and availability of substances, as well as fashions among them, appeared to work together to shape the pattern of abuse. Abuse of paint inhalants by yongsters in developing societies was clearly determined by such factors.

F. CHILD SUICIDAL BEHAVIOR

Adolescent suicidal behavior, particularly attempted suicide (or parasuicide), is rather commonly observed in many societies and has been elaborated previously [cross-reference to Chapter 22: Suicidal Behavior (Section IV, A–C)]. In most instances, suicide is rarely attempted by young children. In Japan, at where self-killing is a commonly acknowledged and practiced method for coping with problems, it has been reported that children undertake life-ending behavior starting as early as the age of 5 or 6.

G. CHILD OBESITY

Excessive body weight is attributed to multiple factors, including genetic predisposition, food intake patterns, physical exercise, and attitudes toward excessive body weight. It covers a wide spectrum of factors: biological, psychological, and cultural. There has been an increase in child obesity in Asian societies, such as mainland China, Hong Kong, Japan, Korea, Singapore, and Taiwan. People in these societies, including children, tend to have slim physical statures. However, along with economic improvement and sociocultural changes after World War II, the number of overweight children has increased so remarkably that clinics for overweight children have been set up — a new phenomenon that was unheard of in those societies in the past.

Several factors contribute to the new phenomenon of child obesity problems in these societies. Associated with economic improvements, there have been remarkable changes in food intake. More nutritious food has become available and more meat is consumed than before. This has resulted in a higher calorie intake. This is in contrast to the lives of children before and during the war, when they often suffered from malnutrition due to a shortage of food.

In contrast, physical exercise among children has decreased markedly. Slated with improvements in transportation, children seldom walk to school, as they did in the past, often for many miles. It was not unusual to walk for nearly an hour. Now, school buses and private cars are so available that children hardly ever walk to school. After school, children used to participate in sports and outdoor games, or join their parents in doing household chores. Now, children are busy watching TV, engaged in electronic games, or studying for school assignments because of heavy educational pressure. They hardly move their bodies or exhaust their energy. It is becoming common to see obese children. Overweight clinics and body-weight control programs are being advocated. Things have changed greatly from several decades ago, and parents are facing new problems associated with changes in the lifestyles of their children.

Opposite to overweight problems are eating disorders, such as anorexia nervosa. There is currently insufficient information available for cross-cultural comparisons. However, certain issues are being examined, such as how cultural factors may contribute to the assessment and judgment of eating disorders from a cultural perspective, and that such disorders are not considered prevalent in some societies, such as India and Egypt [cross-reference to Chapter 23: Eating Disorders (Section II, B)].

H. Narrow-Gate Syndrome

This is a culture-related specific mental health problem observed in some societies, particularly east Asian, that places great emphasis on the importance of education and academic study, creating mental health stress for youngsters in the process of development.

This phenomenon is typically observed in Japan, where the educational system is closely related to career development. In order to be hired by a good company (usually for lifelong employment), it is critical to enter and graduate from universities from which companies recruit future employees. In order to enter these prestigious universities, it is important to

go to prestigious high schools and junior high schools that prepare students to pass the college entrance examinations. To be successful, it is essential to go to good grade schools, and even good kindergartens before that. In other words, there are preset stages of education that must be completed to ensure a future career. This creates the narrow-gate syndrome, meaning that opportunities are limited and competition is very high. This sense of competition and success is stressed from kindergarten on.

In order to cope with this situation, mothers usually stay at home to devote themselves to the supervision of their children's education. The majority of housewives in Japan quit their jobs when they marry (in the cultural belief that it is not proper for married women to work outside of the household, and that it is their primary role to serve their husbands and take care of their children). When the children reach kindergarten age, the mother, called "educational mother," devotes considerable time to supervising her children's academic work. Children are often expected to cut their play time, are allowed only a certain number of hours of TV, and spend a lot of time studying. When they reach senior grade school, the pressure of academic study becomes very intense. They are often expected to skip lunch, study while eating, skip weekend pleasures to do homework assignments, skip summer vacations for extra study, and work with private tutors hired by their parents. There is constant pressure to study throughout the stages of development from childhood to young adulthood. This contributes to various mental health problems, such as the narrow-gate syndrome, which is one kind of culture-related specific mental health problem observed in Korea, Taiwan, and mainland China, as well in other areas where children's education is highly valued and academic achievement is stressed (see Fig. 8-1 in Chapter 8: Stress and Coping Pattern).

I. Hyperactive Behavior

From a clinical point of view, hyperactive disorder, or attention deficit disorder, is basically understood as a mental disorder that occurs as the result of minor (and multiple) lesions in the brain. It may be attributed to brain injury, intoxication, or other organic, biological causes during early childhood. However, the behavior problems associated with the disorder may be perceived, tolerated, and reacted to differently in different cultures, demonstrating a "pathoreactive effect" [cross-reference to Chapter 11: Culture and Psychopathology (Section II, F)].

In order to study how a child is perceived and assessed as "hyperactive," Mann and colleagues (1992) carried out a cross-cultural study involving mental health professionals from China, Japan, Indonesia, and the United States. Children considered "hyperactive" by clinicians in their own countries were videotaped in individual and group activities. Videotaped vignettes of four cases were edited and shown to child mental health professionals in these countries. They were asked to rate the degree of hyperactivity based on rating scales. Results showed that Chinese and Indonesian clinicians gave significantly higher scores for hyperactive-disruptive behavior than their Japanese and American counterparts.

This study demonstrated clearly that the perception of socially tolerated hyperactive behavior varied greatly among different cultures and that the boundaries between normal and hyperactive behavior were defined differently by specialists in different societies. In other words, the recognition and diagnosis of hyperactive behavior among children were not absolute. It was relative, depending on the attitudes and tolerance of such behavior in the sociocultural context.

How such a disorder is perceived and reacted to by society was clearly demonstrated by a situation that occurred in China around the early 1980s (Yang, 1985). In order to promote concern for child mental health, a news release was sent to a newspaper announcing that medication was available for children who would not sit still and study. In response to this, many parents brought their youngsters to the child mental health center for medication. Many of the children were diagnosed as hyperactive children and medication (Ritalin) was prescribed for them. Hospital sta-

tistics showed that the percentage of hyperactive disorder increased sharply during this period. This interesting phenomena was closely related to the sociocultural situation. That is, in accordance with the one child-per-couple policy, the majority of families in urban areas had only one children. The parents were very concerned about their only children and invested considerable energy in raising them. In addition, as in other Asian countries, as described earlier, education was considered very important in China as the way to assure future success in a professional career. When parents learned that there was medication for children who would not sit and "study," they rushed to the clinic to get it for their children who had problems in academic performance. This created a "hyperactive child sensation" in the society.

J. Reading Disability

Originally, some child psychiatrists (such as Makita, 1968) claimed that Japanese and Chinese children who were trained to use the logographic system of writing (Chinese characters) from childhood tended to have a lower possibility of developing a reading disability than European and American children who were taught to use the alphabet. It was speculated that Chinese characters were graphic in nature, and left–right reverse seldom occurred. However, a Chinese child psychiatrist in Taiwan, Hsu, Yang, Yeh, Chen, and Luo (1995) carried out an intesive study of Chinese children, reporting that reading disabilities did exist among children who learned to read in the Chinese logographic system, and that the prevalence rates were by no means lower than those among children who learned alphabetic writing systems. The pattern of reading disabilities was not manifested by mirror writing (as shown in children reading alphabetic writing systems), but was also associated with Chinese writing, illustrated by the displacement, rotation, or addition or substitution of a basic unit in the Chinese character. In other words, while the manifestation of reading disabilities may vary in association with the writing system, the prevalence was similar cross-racially, supporting the biological–neurological nature of such a disorder.

IV. SUMMARY

It is obvious that no cross-cultural study has been done in the area of child psychiatry that is sufficient for meaningful comparison. Nevertheless, available data suggest that, as is the case for adults, those disorders that are attributed predominantly to biological factors (such as reading disability, mental retardation, attention deficient disorder) could occur in any culture due to environmental and possibly genetic factors. Disorders that are attributed more to sociopsychological factors (such as child abuse, sexual abuse, parent-abuse by children, or emotional problems associated with sociocultural expectations, such as the so-called narraw-gate syndrome) vary greatly cross-culturally in prevalence and variations in the nature of the problems.

It is believed that there is rich information awaiting future investigations. Available data presented earlier, although limited, clearly point out that culture has a strong impact on children's mental health problems. It indicates the necessity of considering cultural factors in order to understand those problems and make clinical assessments and diagnoses, and, most importantly, treat the disorders. This will be elaborated further in Chapter 38: Working with Children and Adolescents.

REFERENCES

Americal Psychiatric Association. (1994). *Diagnostic and statistical manual of mental disorders,* (4th ed.). Washington, DC: American Psychiatric Association.

Bengi-Arslan, L., Verhulst, F.C., van der Ende, J., & Erol, N. (1997). Understanding childhood (problem) behaviors from a cultural perspective: Comparison of problem behaviors and competencies in Turkish immigrant, Turkish and Dutch children. *Social Psychiatry and Psychiatric Epidemiology, 32*(8), 477–484.

Bird, H.R. (1996). Epidemiology of childhood disorders in a cross-cultural context. *Journal of Child Psychology and Psychiatry and Allied Disciplines, 37*(1), 35–49.

Canino, I., Canino, G., & Arroyo, W. (1998). Cultural considerations for childhood disorders: How much was included in DSM-IV? *Transcultural Psychiatry, 35*(3), 343–355.

Ensink, K., & Robertson, B. (1996). Indigenous categories of distress and dysfunction in South African Zhosa children and adolescents as described by indigenous healers. *Transcultural Psychiatric Research Review, 33*(2), 137–172.

Hsu, C.-C., Yang, Y.K., Yeh, T.L., Chen, S.J., & Luo, J.M. (1995). Reading success and failure in logographic writing systems: Children learning to read Chinese do evidence reading disabilities. In T.-Y. Lin, W.S. Tseng, & Y.K. Yeh (Eds.), *Chinese societies and mental health.* Hong Kong: Oxford University Press.

Ikeda, Y. (1987). *Child abuse — Dysfunctional parent-child relation (in Japanese)* (pp. 93–105). Tokyo: Chu-O Koron-Sha.

Johnson, R.O. (1981). The socioeconomic context of child abuse and neglect in native South America. In J.E. Korbin (Ed.), *Child abuse and neglect: Cross-cultural perspectives* (pp. 56–707). Berkeley: University of California Press.

Korbin, J.E. (Ed.). (1981). *Child abuse and neglect: Cross-cultural perspectives.* Berkeley: University of California Press.

Krugman, R.D. (1996). Child abuse and neglect: A worlwide problem. In F. Lih Mak & C.C. Nadelson (Eds.), *International Review of Psychiatry,* (Vol. 2.) (pp. 367–377). Washington, DC: London.

LeVine, S., & Levine, R. (1981). Child abuse and neglect in Sub-Saharan Africa. In J.E. Kobin (Ed.), *Child abuse and neglect: Cross-cultural perspectives* (pp. 35–55). Berkeley: University of California Press.

Maitra, B. (1996). Child abuse: A universal 'diagnostic' category? The implication of culture in definition and assessment. *International Journal of Social Psychiatry, 42*(4), 287–304.

Makita, K. (1968). The rarity of reading disability in Japanese children. *American Journal of Orthopsychiatry, 38,* 599–614.

Mann, E.M., Ikeda, Y., Mueller, C.W., Takahashi, A.H., Tao, K.T., Humris, E., Li, B.L., & Chin, D. (1992). Cross-cultural differences in rating hyperactive-disruptive behaviors in children. *American Journal of Psychiatry, 149*(11), 1539–1542.

Matsuura, M., Okubo, Y., Kojima, T., Takahashi, R., Wang, Y., Shen, Y.C., & Lee, C.K. (1993). A cross-national prevalence study of children with emotional and behavioral problems — A WHO collaborative study in the Western Pacific Region. *Journal of Child Psychology and Psychiatry, 34,* 307–315.

Meston, C.M., Heiman, J.R., Trapnell, P.D., & Carlin, A.S. (1999). Ethnicity, desirable responding, and self-reports of abuse: A comparison of European- and Asian-ancestry undergraduates. *Journal of Consulting and Clinical Psychology, 67*(1), 139–144.

Minde, K., & Nikapota, A.D. (1993). Child psychiatry in the developing world: Recent development. *Transcultural Psychiatric Research Review, 30*(4), 315–346.

Moghal, N.E., Nota, I.K., & Hobbs, C.J. (1995). A study of sexual abuse in an Asian community. *Archives of Diseases in Childhood, 72*(4), 346–347.

National Institute on Drug Abuse. (1995). *Drug use among racial/ethnic minorities.* Rockville, MD: National Institute of Health.

Nikapota, A.D. (1991). Child psychiatry in developing countries. *British Journal of Psychiatry, 158,* 743–751.

Poffenberger, T. (1981). Child rearing and social structure in rural India: Toward a cross-cultural definition of child abuse and neglect. In J.E. Korbin (Ed.), *Child abuse and neglect: Cross-cultural perspectives* (pp.71–95). Berkeley: University of California Press.

Pope, H.G., Jr., Mangweth, B., Negrao, A.B., Hudson, J.I., & Cordas, T.A. (1994). Childhood sexual abuse and bulimia nervosa: A comparison of American, Australian, and Brazilian women. *American Journal of Psychiatry, 151*(5), 732–737.

Smart, R., Murray, G.F., & Arif, A. (1988). Drug abuse and prevention programs in 29 countries. *International Journal of the Addictions, 23,* 1–17.

Tang, C.S. (1998). The rate of physical child abuse in Chinese families: A community survey in Hong Kong. *Child Abuse and Neglect, 22*(5), 381–391.

Tao, K.T., Qui, J.H., Li, B., Tseng, W.S., Hsu, J., & Goebert, D. (1999). Longitudinal study of psychological development of single and non-single children in the family—A 10 year follow-up study in Nanjing. *Chinese Mental Health Journal. 13* (4), 210–212. (In Chinese).

Tseng, W.S., & Hsu, J. (1972). The Chinese attitude toward parental authority as expressed in Chinese children's stories. *Archives of General Psychiatry, 26,* 28–34.

Tseng, W.S., Tao, K.T., Hsu, J., Qiu, J.H., Li, B., & Goebert, D. (2000). Longitudinal analysis of development among single- and non-single children in Nanjing, China: Ten-year follow-up study. *Journal of Nervous and Mental Disease, 188* (10), 701–707.

Wagatsuma, H. (1981). Child abandonment and infanticide: A Japanese case. In J.E. Kobin (Ed.), *Child abuse and neglect: Cross-cultural perspectives* (pp. 120–138). Berkeley: University of California Press.

Wu, D.Y.H. (1981). Child abuse in Taiwan. In J.E. Korbin (Ed.), *Child abuse and neglect: Cross-cultural perspectives* (pp. 139–165). Berkeley: University of California Press.

Yang, X.L. (1985). An investigation of minimal brain disorders among primary school students in the Beijing area. In W.S. Tseng, & D.Y.H. Wu (Eds.); *Chinese culture and mental health* (pp. 315–323). Orlando, FL: Academic Press.

Section E

Culture and Clinical Practice

Associated with improvements in the field and in response to clinical demand, the focus of cultural psychiatry has expanded from an exploration of the influence of culture on psychopathology to clinical practice. This includes performing culture-relevant assessment, diagnosis, and treatment for patients of diversified ethnic and cultural backgrounds.

In this section, six chapters are devoted to the cultural perspectives of psychiatric practice. Chapter 26 addresses how cultural factors influence relationships, communication, and the interaction between therapist and patient — a crucial issue in the clinical process. Chapter 27 focuses on how cultural factors, in addition to other variables, impact the process and the results of clinical assessment and diagnosis in transcultural situations. Chapter 28 examines the classification of mental disorders from social and cultural perspectives.

As a part of clinical evaluation and mental health practice, many psychological tests and measure-ments have been developed. The ways in which cultural factors influence the validity and application of instruments of measurement and the process of formal psychological testing are elaborated in Chapter 29.

Following this, in Chapter 30, various social and cultural factors that influence the practice of psychiatric service in general are discussed. These include folk beliefs, knowledge derived from traditional medicine, issues of minorities and racism, sociomedical systems, and medical culture.

Drug therapy is a major aspect of psychiatric practice. Drug treatments for patients are elaborated in Chapter 31, not only from a psychophamarcological perspective, regarding cross-ethnic or -racial differences, but also from a psychological perspective, elaborating how culture plays a role in the psychology of giving and receiving medication.

26

Therapist and Patient: Relations and Communication

I. THERAPIST–PATIENT RELATIONSHIP

From a clinical point of view, it is crucial to understand and pay attention to the therapist–patient relationship, as it represents the requisite condition for rendering effective health care (Fisher & Leigh, 1989). This is particularly true in psychiatric practice, which relies heavily on the face-to-face interaction and relationship between the therapist and the patient. The relationship is itself a therapeutic tool and the outcome of treatment may vary significantly depending on the quality of the relationship. This is particularly true and requires special attention and adjustment when a therapist is going to offer services to a patient with a different cultural background because the relationship between healer and client may vary according to differing cultural attributes.

A. BASIC PARAMETERS OF INTERPERSONAL RELATIONSHIPS

Sociologically speaking, a relationship between two people can be examined from the standpoint of multiple parameters. These may include status

assignment, role division, power structure, communication, affections, bond, and commitment. Based on the relationship of the people involved, such as husband–wife, parent–child, employer and employee, colleague and colleague, the nature of the diad relationship varies. The relationship between healer and client, physician and patient, or psychotherapist and patient tends to form a special kind of diad relationship.

In general, the therapist–patient relationship is an open one. The therapist and the patient come into contact and establish a temporary relationship based on the need for professional care. By definition, the status assigned is unsymmetrical — with one person offering service and the other receiving care. As for the roles played, the therapist is expected to have special knowledge and experience, while the patient is expected to follow the treatment suggested as well as he can in order to benefit from it. Beyond this, there are many variations due to cultural expectations and medical–professional rules.

For instance, the status and power between therapist and patient can be hierarchical or egalitarian. The communication between them can be asymmetrical or symmetrical — namely, the therapist offers explanations and instructions unilaterally and the patient listens and follows passively — or they can communicate by mutual questions and elaboration, even negotiating. The commitment can be explicitly expressed and agreed upon or subtle and flexible. The patient may be expected to comply or may be free to make his own choices and decisions, without adhering to the prescribed treatment. The reward or payment for the therapist can be formally predetermined or carried out in an informal way, based on his contribution and the patient's appreciation.

In psychotherapy, the feeling and affection between therapist and patient is crucial, as it affects the course of treatment. What kind of relationship is more "therapeutic" is carefully examined and constantly manipulated by the therapist from a "profes-sional" perspective. However, his professional rules may or may not be understood and agreed upon by the patient. Bridging the gap of understanding between actual therapy and the expectations of therapy is a challenge for the therapist, especially from a cultural perspective (see Fig. 26-1).

B. Cultural Differences in Therapist–Patient Relations

Reviewing the cultural aspects of the physician–patient relationship, Nilchaikovit, Hill, and Holland (1993) explained the possible differences that may be observed among Asians and Americans. They pointed out that, in America, the predominant form of

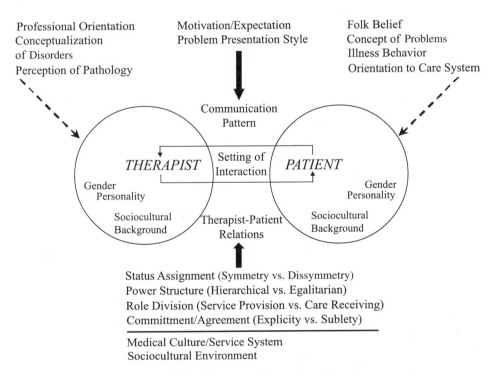

Professional Orientation
Conceptualization
of Disorders
Perception of Pathology

Motivation/Expectation
Problem Presentation Style

Folk Belief
Concept of Problems
Illness Behavior
Orientation to Care System

Communication
Pattern

THERAPIST   Setting of
Interaction   *PATIENT*

Gender
Personality

Gender
Personality

Sociocultural
Background

Therapist-Patient
Relations

Sociocultural
Background

Status Assignment (Symmetry vs. Dissymmetry)
Power Structure (Hierarchical vs. Egalitarian)
Role Division (Service Provision vs. Care Receiving)
Committment/Agreement (Explicity vs. Sublety)

Medical Culture/Service System
Sociocultural Environment

FIGURE 26-1   Cultural factors that influence therapist–patient interaction.

physician–patient relationship is egalitarian, based on a contractual agreement between the two, influenced heavily by an ideological emphasis on individualism, autonomy, and consumerism. In contrast, in many Asian cultures, the relationship is modeled after the ideal form of hierarchical relationship. The physician is seen as an authority figure who is endowed with knowledge and experience. An ideal doctor should have great virtue and be concerned, caring, and conscientiously responsible for the patient's welfare. In return, the patient must show respect and deference for the physician's authority and suggestions.

Although their comments refer to idealized situations with some overgeneralizations, for the sake of reference, it is useful for therapists to be aware that such differences exist. As pointed out by Nilchaikovit and colleagues, when an Asian patient is seen by an American physician, some intercultural problems may occur. Particularly when expectations are not fulfilled, the patient does not usually express his or her feelings and communicate his or her frustrations. In return, the patient is seen as passive-aggressive and noncompliant by the physician. The treatment is often terminated prematurely and the patient goes "doctor shopping."

C. THERAPIST–PATIENT MATCHING

Associated with the increase in the number of female psychiatrists, new attention is being paid to the effect of therapist–patient matching by gender. It has been a clinical impression that, with some exceptions, female patients, in general, feel more comfortable seeking help from female psychiatrists. They feel that a therapist of the same gender is more likely to have understanding and empathy for their lives and problems. Besides, there are fewer of the relational complications that are often noticed between male therapists and female patients, including sexual involvement. It has been pointed out that ethical complaints against female psychiatrists by female patients are relatively fewer than those against male psychiatrists by female patients (Mogul, 1992).

As an extension of this, there is considerable concern among mental health workers for the need of therapist–patient matching by ethnicity, race, and cultural background. This concern is very much stimulated by the human rights movement. Although the matching of therapist and patient by ethnicity, race, or cultural background sounds reasonable and desirable, it is not a simple matter. Such matching may not only be impractical, but, clinically, it does not necessarily guarantee successful therapy. Successful therapy relies on professional competence reflected in knowledge and experience. It also depends on the therapist's personal ability to establish a positive relationship with and show empathy toward the patient. In other words, while the matching of ethnic or cultural background might be beneficial, without clinical competence, it will not necessarily bring about desirable therapy outcomes. In addition, therapists with the same ethnic or racial backgrounds as their patients may sometimes bring about ill effects. This is particularly true if the patient does not want to reveal his personal background to a therapist with the same background or the therapist does not offer a proper figure for ethnic identification. Ethnic and cultural transference and countertransference need to be considered as well. These issues will be elaborated further in a later chapter (cross-reference to Chapter 36: Intercultural Psychotherapy).

II. COMMUNICATION BETWEEN PATIENT AND THERAPIST

Communication is one of the major aspects of therapist–patient interaction. How the patient presents complaints and informs the therapist of his or her problems and how the therapist, reciprocally, listens and provides relevant explanations to the patient are key areas of patient–therapist communication that closely relate to the achievement of meaningful, satisfactory, and effective therapy (Francis, Korsch, & Morris, 1969).

A. Patient's Mode of Presenting Initial Complaints

Similarly to medical practice, in psychiatric practice, it is generally expected that the patient will present his (chief) complaint(s) to the therapist. How a patient presents his cardinal complaints in the initial encounter with the therapist is an interesting subject that deserves attention. The symptoms or problems presented initially may be the patient's major concerns. They may be merely excuses for the presentation of problems that is expected as part of the initial meeting with the therapist or the patient may simply be following a certain custom (or fashion) of complaint presentation. In other words, his may be a socioculturally patterned or stylized presentation of complaints.

Tseng (1975) has elaborated this point with regard to the nature of somatic complaints among Chinese psychiatric patients. Even though nearly 70% of the neurotic psychiatric outpatients presented somatic complaints to their psychiatrists during their first visits, careful clinical examination revealed several explanations for this: the influence of the patient's knowledge and concepts about "problems"; the socially recognized and accepted signs of illness; reluctance and resistance to explore emotional problems; and, finally, a hypochondriacal cultural trait among the Chinese. Thus, the patient's mode of complaint presentation needs careful evaluation and understanding, including from a cultural perspective.

B. Patient's Style of Communicating Information about Illness

Although it is desirable for a patient to communicate freely his personal background, history of illness, and other related information to the therapist, this is not always true in clinical situations. The patient's ability to describe things and willingness to communicate are often influenced by his clinical condition and his motivation and understanding of the purpose of doing so. In addition, there is a cultural impact on the process of problem–communication.

Emotional problems and personal feelings are generally considered highly private matters. As pointed out by Nilchaikovit and colleagues (1993), for people in many cultures, talking about one's inner feelings is about as discreet and commendable as parading nude in public. Family conflicts are often regarded as "inside" problems that should not be revealed to an outsider (Hsu, 1983).

Sex life and sexual problems are often difficult areas to explore. For instance, with the Chinese, the anatomical terms for "penis" or "vagina" should be avoided. They should instead be referred to indirectly as the "yang part" and the "yin part." The Japanese refer to them as "private parts" or "shameful parts" of the body. It is considered blunt to refer explicitly to sexual intercourse between husband and wife. Depending on the culture, many different terms, such as "intimacy between a couple," "business in the (bed) room," and "making a baby," are used by physicians as delicate and sophisticated ways of inferring sexual intercourse.

Further, clinicians should be aware that in some cultures, it is "taboo" to reveal certain things to others. Inquiring about a lady's age may be socially impolite in Western society, as it is considered embarrassing for a lady to disclose her age, while asking about the cause of a parent's death is a breach of a taboo in Micronesia that will invite fear of punishment.

It may be all right for a friend to ask an Asian person how much it cost him to buy a new house or a new car, how much he spent for his children's wedding, and so on, but for Westerners, in general, these are considered private matters. Even when asked by a close friend, such questions would be viewed as impolite intrusions into a person's confidential matters.

C. Therapist's Format and Skill for Inquiring about Needed Information

In modern medical practice, it is common, and even required, for the therapist to inquire into the patient's past, his present illness, his family history, and so on. Physicians are trained to conduct interviews with the patient or his family following certain formats in order to gather the needed medical information systematically, comprehensively, and effectively within a limited time so that a hypothesis of the nature of the disorder can be made (Elstein, Kagan, Shulman, Jasen, & Loupe, 1972). This information gathering is considered a professional skill, and includes examining the patient's mental status by asking a particular set of questions, involving mathematical calculations, memory, and judgment. A set of standardized proverbs are used to examine the thought process as well as social judgement. "A rolling stone does not gather moss," "do not keep all your eggs in one basket," or "who were the last three presidents of the United States?" are examples of sayings and questions trainees are taught to use.

In contrast, a herb doctor may simply ask about a patient's appetite and the color of his urine, examine the patient's tongue, and take his pulse. It is expected that a skillful herb doctor does not need to ask too many questions, but can make a good diagnosis simply by taking the patient's pulse. It is a reflection of a fortune-teller's mastery and skill that he does not need the client to tell him any more information than his name and date of birth. Thus, modern professional therapists, traditional physicians, and folk therapists (such as fortune-tellers) all have different formats for approaching their clients or patients and their patients learn what modes of inquiry to expect from them. This explains why a patient feels frustrated when a modern psychiatrist asks him to answer questions about how he was raised as a small child or "what is the similarity between an orange and an apple?" when he is consulting the therapist for a headache, insomnia, or low spirits.

D. THERAPIST'S LISTENING SKILL

In contrast to ordinary psychiatric practice, we all know that, knowing how to listen to patients is an important, specialized skill in psychotherapy. The psychotherapist listens not so much to gather information for making a scientific assessment and establishing a professional diagnosis as in general psychiatric clinical practice, rather he listen with concern and empathy in a humanistic mode to facilitate the healing of the patient (Jackson, 1992). Listening with empathy involves not only professional knowledge, experience, and general sensitivity to the patient's situation, but also cultural knowledge and sensitivity. This point will be elaborated again in a later chapter (cross-reference to Chapter 36: Intercultural Psychotherapy).

E. THERAPIST'S MODE OF COMMUNICATING INFORMATION ABOUT DISEASE

Finally, it is considered a professional necessity for the therapist to offer a certain explanation to the patient and his family about the diagnosis, the nature of the disease from which the patient is suffering, and the therapist's plan for dealing with the sickness. Several matters are involved in the skill of explanation giving (Waitzkin & Stoeckle, 1972). Naturally, there needs to be concern over factors such as the patient's age, level of education, ability to understand, and psychological condition with respect to hearing the information, and so on. Beyond this, it is necessary to consider the orientation, terms, and language that should be used to make the patient understand and also to be meaningful to him. In this process, a knowledge of folk concepts of illness and the culture-patterned explanation modes become important variables that need consideration. How to inform the patient of the nature of a serious illness, how to communicate the possibility of a terminal illness, to whom the information should be communicated, and who should not be informed are among several issues that need careful consideration from a cultural point of view. What information about the illness will mean to the patient and his family and what the possible impact will be need to be considered. For instance, "epilepsy" may be a sickness that makes the patient unsuitable for driving a car in some societies, while it may be a sickness that should be hidden because it is considered a stigma and may interfere with marriage arrangements in other cultures. "Neurasthenia" may be a diagnosis preferred over "depression" for people in some cultures because "weakness of nerve" is acceptable whereas "depression" is seen as the result of weakness of will. A skillful clinician will approach the subject carefully by exploring the probable reactions of the patient, his family, and other people surrounding the patient.

F. COMMUNICATION THROUGH INTERPRETERS

The problems of communication between therapist and patient are highlighted when the therapist and the patient do not share the same language and have to rely on the assistance of interpreters to communicate. Who serves as the interpreter — whether a close family member, a friend, a member of the same ethnic group, or a trained interpreter with mental health knowledge and experience — will affect the process and quality of interpretation significantly. There will be problems of how to translate properly, relevantly, and meaningfully for clinical purposes. How to select a proper interpreter and utilize the interpreter for the goal of communication with the patient is a matter of clinical skill that will be elaborated in detail in a later chapter [cross-reference to Chapter 36: Intercultural Psychotherapy (Section II,B,8)].

III. ORIENTATION, EXPECTATION, AND VALUES

Besides the matter of communication, many other issues affect the operation of therapy between patient and therapist. These include orientation toward and expectations of therapy and the value systems held by the patient and the therapist regarding life in general and matters relating to solving problems in particular.

A. ORIENTATION TOWARD AND EXPECTATIONS OF THERAPY

A person can have several orientations toward therapy. For instance, therapy can be seen as a practice through which a therapist is going to offer treatment for the patient and cure the patient's sickness or problems. In this orientation, the patient is expected to play a passive role, allowing the therapist to actively treat him. The patient believes that a competent therapist should know how to treat him and a good patient needs only to comply with his therapeutic maneuvers. In its extreme form, this mode of therapy is observed in surgical treatment, but is seldom applied in psychiatry, particularly in modern psychotherapy. At the other extreme, the patient is supposed to take a very active role in solving his own problems; the therapist only offers assistance in his efforts to improve. This mode of therapy is generally expected in modern Western psychotherapy, but not necessarily by people who are unfamiliar with it or perceive the therapist–patient role quite differently. In other words, based on their cultural backgrounds, different patients may have different orientations toward therapy.

Also based on cultural background, the mode of service delivery can be seen differently and operate in various ways. For instance, it is generally understood in the American medical system that a person has a family doctor, who refers him to a specialist when necessary, and, once the special consultation and/or treatment is completed, the patient returns to his family doctor. Thus, a person is always under the care of his family doctor, unless he is not satisfied and chooses to change doctors. In contrast, in many parts of world, this is not the case. A person may shop around for physicians, consult several, changing them as he wishes, and see specialists without referral from a primary physician. There is no contract between the patient and therapist to carry out therapy on an ongoing basis. There is a "take it or leave it" kind of working relationship. Thus, theoretically, the patient and therapist might have different orientations and expectations regarding therapy, unless these matters are clarified from the very beginning and both agree to share the same orientation. Otherwise, dissatisfaction will occur.

B. Congruence of Values between Therapist and Patient

In addition to the orientation toward therapy, there are the matters of how the patient and therapist see things and the values they hold. "Values" refer to a way of viewing things with strong conviction. Value systems can be discussed in various dimensions, including how an individual views a person, interpersonal relations, and things that happen in life, as well as the nature of mankind, the world, or life. Here, we are concerned with value systems that may have a direct impact on illness: for instance, whether it is a good idea for children to raise opinions against their parents, a wife to insist on her own rights against her husband, a husband and wife to get divorced if there is emotional conflict, a woman to have an abortion if she prefers not to have a baby, a person to end his own life, and so on. These are values held by the patient and the therapist as well. Clinical experience indicates that values held by the patient and the therapist — either congruently or incongruently — will affect the relationship between them, the process and direction of therapy, and the outcome of their therapeutic involvement.

Investigation has proven that the degree of congruence of values held between the therapist and the patient, particularly regarding beliefs about the illness that the patient is suffering, will affect the therapy as manifested by the degree of adherence to the therapy (Foulks, Persons, & Merkel, 1986). The clinician should examine the value systems held by him and his patient and deal with any great dissimilarities that exist due to differences in their medical, social, and cultural backgrounds.

IV. INTERACTION INVOLVING THE PATIENT AND HIS FAMILY

A. The Need for Involving the Family in Therapeutic Situations

Although it is a common practice for a pediatrician to involve the parents when he is treating a small child, or for a geriatrician to include adult children or a spouse when he is treating an elderly person, when treating ordinary adults, modern therapists with Western backgrounds seldom consider the need to involve family members, such as spouse, children, or other relatives. This stems from the Western therapist's basic philosophical attitude that a person should handle his own problems.

However, this is not necessarily true from a theoretical or cultural perspective. General system theory has indicated that we are living in a system that involves others all the time. Even our own inner thoughts, fantasies, and daydreams cannot take place in a vacuum. They are always related to other people, including family members, friends, colleagues, neighbors, or strangers. Further, from a cultural point of view, it has been shown that, for many cultures, family ties and interpersonal relationships are so tight that an individual seldom exists by himself or herself. If a person becomes sick, he may be accompanied by his parents, spouse, children, and visited by a group of relatives or friends. This is a culture-derived custom. A therapist should take the opportunity to involve family members whenever they are available and to offer family-oriented therapy (Tseng & Hsu, 1991).

B. The Role of Family in Therapeutic Interaction

It needs to be recognized that family members — whether parent(s), spouse, sibling(s), or children — can play different roles when one member becomes sick. A family member can play the role of spokesperson, making statements for the patient as well as the rest of the family. He can play the role of negotiator, trying to communicate with the therapist through indirect channels and to advocate on the patient's behalf. He can provide important assistance to the patient, offering a resource for support, or assist the therapist in supervising the patient's behavior to assure that the patient complies with the prescribed therapy. Conversely, a family member can become an oppositional person, resisting the treatment and becoming a major obstacle to improvement.

Thus, recognizing the role played by a family member(s) and managing the family for the sake of therapy and improvement are among the tasks a competent therapist must master (Hsu, 1983). This is quite true when a therapist is dealing with a patient who, according to his culture, is very closely related to his family. Knowing how to deal with the patient alone, without knowing how to relate to his family, is not enough for a therapist — at least from a cultural perspective.

REFERENCES

Elstein, A.S., Kagan, N., Shulman, L.S., Jasen, H., & Loupe, M.J. (1972). Methods and theory in the study of medical inquiry. *Journal of Medical Education, 47,* 85–92.

Fisher, F.D., & Leigh, H. (1989). Models of the doctor-patient relationship. In R. Michels (Ed.), *Psychiatry,* (Vol. 2). Philadelphia: Lippincott.

Foulks, E.F., Persons, J.B., & Merkel, R.L. (1986). The effect of patient's beliefs about their illnesses on compliance in psychotherapy. *American Journal of Psychiatry, 143*(3), 340–344.

Francis, V., Korsch, B.M., & Morris, M.J. (1969). Gaps in doctor-patient communication. *New England Journal of Medicine, 280*(10), 535–540.

Hsu, J. (1983). Asian family interaction patterns and their therapeutic implications. *International Journal of Family Psychiatry, 4*(4), 307–320.

Jackson, S.W. (1992). The listening healer in the history of psychological healing. *American Journal of Psychiatry, 149*(12), 1623–1632.

Mogul, K.M. (1992). Ethic complaints against female psychiatrists. *American Journal of Psychiatry, 149*(5), 651–653.

Nilchaikovit, T., Hill, J.M., & Holland, J.C. (1993). The effects of culture on illness behavior and medical care: Asian and American differences. *General Hospital Psychiatry, 15,* 41–50.

Tseng, W.S. (1975). The nature of somatic complaints among psychiatric patients: The Chinese case. *Comprehensive Psychiatry, 16,* 237–245.

Tseng, W.S., & Hsu, J. (1991). *Culture and family: Problems and therapy.* New York: Haworth.

Waitzkin, H., & Stoeckle, J.D. (1972). The communication of information bout illness. *Advances in Psychosomatic Medicine, 8,* 180–215.

27

Clinical Assessment and Diagnosis

I. ASSESSMENT AND DIAGNOSIS: INTRODUCTION

In contrast to medical practice, psychiatric work relies heavily on clinical skill to solicit information from the patient for assessment and diagnosis. Soliciting information involves interaction between the clinician and the patient. This interaction is subject to personal factors of the patient (such as communication skill, understanding of problems, motivation for making complaints) and the psychopathology involved (such as its severity and nature). It is also very much influenced by the clinician–patient relationship and the perception and skill of the evaluator. Naturally, the process of clinical assessment is subject to cultural impact (Fabrega, 1987; Rogler, 1993).

In order to understand the impact of culture on clinical assessment, several basic issues need to be clarified and understood. The clinician needs to comprehend how normality versus pathology is determined in the clinical setting, the difference between making an "assessment" and a "diagnosis," and how the process of clinical assessment takes place in clinical situations with dynamic natures.

A. DEFINITION OF NORMALITY AND PATHOLOGY

In order to assess the influence of culture on psychopathology, one must first take into account the operating definition of normality versus pathology, as the distinction between normal and abnormal where certain psychopathologies are concerned may vary greatly in different cultures. Clinically, as pointed out by Offer and Sabshin (1974), there are four ways to distinguish normality from pathology.

1. By Professional Definition

This approach takes the view that normality or pathology can be differentiated clearly by the nature of the phenomenon itself and a judgment made on it by professionals. In medicine, bleeding or a bone fracture, by its nature, is judged without doubt to be pathological and requiring medical care. In psychiatry, if a person talks to nonexistent people, claims to hear the voice of a spaceman, or eats his own feces, he or she will professionally be considered to be suffering from a pathological mental condition. This approach

443

maintains that certain conditions (manifested as signs or symptoms) are absolutely pathological in nature. A diagnosis can be made on such conditions that is applicable universally, beyond cultural boundaries. Gross organic brain disorders, such as severe dementia, a delirious state, or a severe psychotic condition with pathological thought disorders or disorganized behavior, tend to be easily and without too much doubt diagnosed by experts, even cross-culturally.

2. By Deviation from the Mean

This approach relies on mathematical measurement and uses a range of deviations from the mean to distinguish between normal and abnormal. For example, hypertension and underweight are medical conditions defined as normal according to certain scales and measurements; a pathological condition is diagnosed when the measurement goes beyond the average range. In psychiatry, the measurement of IQ serves to distinguish normal or subnormal intelligence. The concept of mean is universal, yet the range of mean often needs to be adjusted for different populations. This is quite true when personality is assessed by questionnaires cross-culturally. The cutting point for defining behavior disorders as measured by questionnaires is another area that requires careful cross-cultural adjustment. Determining what amount of drinking is excessive requires biological, social, and cultural adjustments.

3. By Assessment of Function

This approach considers the effect of thoughts, feelings, or behavior on function. Whether the condition provides (healthy) function or (unhealthy) dysfunction in the individual is the basis for the judgment. Memory disturbance is determined by the extent to which a person can retain information and reproduce it through recollection. If a person living in an urban setting cannot recall the street number of his house or the name of the street where he lives, and, thus, does not know how to return home, he is clearly suffering from memory dysfunction. In contrast, if a person living in a remote rural area, where a street number is not significant, does not recall it, he may not be considered "dysfunctional" unless he forgets where his village is located, how it looks, and loses his way returning to it. Thus, it is the purpose and function of memory that need to be considered rather than the information that needs to be recollected (Thompson, Donegan, & Lavond, 1986). Regarding outward behavior, generally, openly aggressive behavior that frequently disturbs family, neighbors, or society will be perceived by the family or community as dysfunctional and, therefore, pathological. However, quiet, seclusive, and asocial behavior, if it does not cause any problems to other people, may not be considered dysfunctional and thus may not be labeled pathological. Studies have shown that clinicians' evaluations of hyperactive children vary greatly in different cultures (Mann et al., 1992). In other words, behavior tends to be judged primarily by its impact on the individual, others, and the environment, from a functional point of view.

4. By Social Definition

This approach utilizes social and cultural judgment in deciding if behavior is normal or pathological. The decision is subject to the social knowledge and cultural attitudes found among the members of a society. Thus, the conclusion is subjective and collectively made. For instance, walking half-naked in a public area may be considered "normal" behavior in one situation (such as on Waikiki Beach in Honolulu), "unusual" in another (such as on Fifth Avenue in New York), and "obscene" in a third (such as at the Meiji Shrine in Tokyo), depending on how each society defines such behavior and its cultural tolerance of it. When a man continues to live with his parents after age 25 he may be considered "dependent" in America, but "ordinary" in Filipino society. Speaking out against authority figures (such as parents, teachers, or the police) may be regarded as "brave" behavior in a democratic society, but "antisocial" in an autocratic one. The judgments made by a society may vary greatly, depending on its customs, beliefs, and values.

In general, social behavior tends to be assessed and defined by sociocultural judgment.

It is important for a clinician to be aware of which of the approaches just given is being utilized in making a clinical judgment, to recognize the limitations of each, and to make whatever adjustments are necessary in making the final assessment.

B. DIFFERENCES BETWEEN "DIAGNOSIS" AND "ASSESSMENT"

1. Making a "Diagnosis"

In the field of medicine, it is general practice to gather the medical information necessary to make a medical "diagnosis." The sources of medical information can be a patient's description of his symptoms, the course of the illness, signs observed or detected in a physical examination (by a physician), or laboratory data obtained through the examination. Thus, the patient contributes only part of the information needed for making a diagnosis. Furthermore, a medical diagnosis is based on the assumption that there are certain disease entities which are characterized by particular clusters of manifestations and can be categorized according to certain diagnostic criteria. The information gathered is fitted to diagnostic criteria for any disease entity recognized or classified. In other words, making a medical diagnosis involves trying to put information into existing pigeon holes. Once the diagnosis is made, a treatment plan can be carried out and the course of the disease can be predicted, including the patient's response to the medicine prescribed. Cultural impact on the process of medical diagnosis is only partial. It is related mainly to how the patient makes complaints and how he describes his symptoms.

These medical traditions in making diagnoses are adopted in descriptive (or biomedically oriented) psychiatry, which holds that there are certain groups of mental disorders. The art of diagnosis is to determine the disorder from which the patient is suffering. Once a diagnosis is made, the prognosis becomes pre-

dictable and epidemiological data can be presented. Again, cultural influence on such a medically oriented diagnostic procedure is only partial. Making "diagnoses" works well when the clinician is dealing with certain psychiatric disorders, such as organic brain disorders, psychoses, or others that are determined predominantly by biological factors. However, the diagnostic process is limited, from a cross-cultural point of view, when it comes to minor psychiatric disorders that are determined predominantly by psychological or social factors.

2. Making an "Assessment"

Because of the dynamic nature of psychiatry and psychotherapeutic practice, a psychiatrist needs to know in detail the background of a patient, not only how his problems started and how he copes with them, but also his personal life, family, personality, and behavior patterns. Needless to say, this includes how he perceives things and interprets, understands, and believes in them. In other words, it is a process of understanding the patient from a broader perspective, including past and present, individual and family, intrapsychic and interpersonal, conscious and unconscious. It is not a process focused merely on the patient's symptom complaints, but on the context within which his problems were encountered and developed. Even the symptoms need to be evaluated according to the patient's understanding, motivation, implications, and functioning in making such complaints — thus, assessment involves a very comprehensive evaluation. It is understood that the assessment process is carried out as the result of a personal process (within the patient as well as the evaluator) and interpersonal interaction (between the patient and the evaluator). There is a lot of room for cultural influence in behavior-determined clinical assessment.

In summary, a medically oriented, mechanical diagnosis is less influenced by cultural factors than a dynamically oriented, behavior assessment, which is very heavily impacted by them. Let us examine in detail the dynamic nature of psychiatric evaluation.

C. THE DYNAMIC NATURE OF PSYCHIATRIC EVALUATION

As emphasized by Mezzich, Kleinman, Fabrega, and Parron (1996b), culture is involved in psychiatric assessment in different ways, including shaping the phenomenology of clinical manifestations; providing the matrix for the interpersonal situation of the diagnostic interview, including the transcultural process between clinicians and patient; influencing diagnostic rationales and practices that group symptoms; and impacting the overall conceptualization of the diagnostic system.

Psychiatric assessment results from a dynamic process that involves multiple levels of interaction between the patient (and sometimes the patient's fam-

ily) and the clinician (Tseng, 1997). This process involves a series of steps, as illustrated in Fig. 27-1. It starts with the distress or problems experienced and perceived by the patient and proceeds to the presentation of complaints made by the patient to the clinician. These are perceived and understood as specific types of problems by the clinician. Finally, an assessment, which includes categorization and diagnosis, is made by the clinician of the disorder in question. Thus, it is a process involving different steps or compartments.

1. Experience of Problems or Distress (by the Patient)

This refers to the distress the patient experiences inside of himself. A person experiences "pain" when

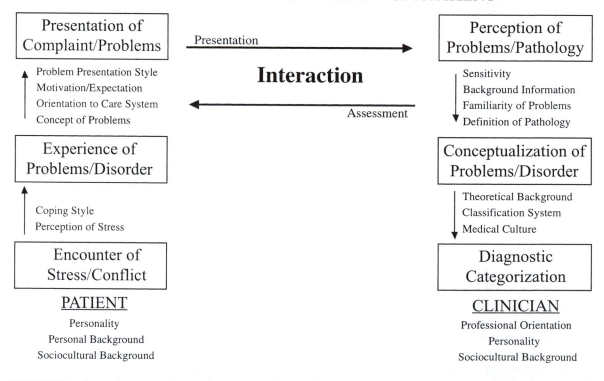

FIGURE 27-1 Dynamic process of clinical assessment. (From W.S. Tseng, in *Culture and Psychopathology,* Brunner/Mazel, 1997).

he is hit; feels "anxious" if he is worried about something; becomes "paranoid" if he suspects that he is being persecuted by others; or has the feeling of going "downhill" if he has lost something significant to him. All these reactions to distress, which may be manifested as symptoms or signs, are subjective, experiential phenomena. They cannot be precisely measured from the outside. It is thus impossible to know to what extent the actual "experience" of distress is influenced by cultural factors.

However, it is clear that the forerunner of the distress, namely, the stress itself, can be impacted by sociocultural factors. Stress can be produced by culture in numerous ways. One is by culturally demanded performance. For example, a culture that demands a woman produce a male child blames her, and the woman feels guilty, if she fails to have a boy. Many societies expect children to achieve high academic performance; if the child fails to meet such parental expectations, he is shamed. Stress can be created by culturally maintained beliefs. For instance, if a person believes that it is very important to define the territory between sea and land, and he breaks a culturally held taboo and brings food across the land–sea territory, he may develop severe anxiety and associated somatic complaints, described as *Malgri* reaction (Hippler & Cawte, 1978). If a person believes that it is fatal if his penis shrinks into his abdomen, he may become fearful that his penis is "shrinking" and develop a panic attack, known as *koro* reaction (Tseng et al., 1988). Stress can be generated by cultural restrictions of behavior, culture-supported attitudes, or other culture-related factors, all of which may provoke distress in the individual [cross-reference to Chapter 8: Stress and Coping Patterns (Section II, A–C)].

2. Perception of Problems or Disorders by the Patient

Following the experience of distress and symptom manifestation, the next step is for the patient to perceive and interpret his distressful experience. How he does this is a psychological phenomenon that is subject to the influence of cultural factors, in addition to other variables, such as the patient's personality, knowledge, and psychological needs.

Based on how the problem is understood and perceived by the patient, he will show a secondary process of various reactions to the distress. For instance, if a person interprets the chest pain he is having as nothing but a chest pain, he will react to it lightly; if he perceives and interprets it as a sign of an impending heart attack, he may become very anxious and even panic, further complicating the primary symptom of the chest pain. In a similar way, if a person believes that shrinking of the penis into the abdomen is fatal, he will react severely to any sign of penis shrinkage, even if his penis never shrinks into his abdomen. If a person does not adhere to such beliefs, he will be impervious to normal changes in his body. In other words, the patient's perception of and reaction to the primary symptoms will add secondary symptoms that compound the clinical picture. The process of forming secondary symptoms is usually subject to cultural influences.

3. Presentation of Complaints or Illness by the Patient or His or Her Family

The next step is the presentation of the complaints or illness by the patient to others: the process and art of "complaining." Analysis of this process has shown that the way the problem, symptom, or illness is presented or communicated to the clinician is based on the patient's (or his or her family's) orientation to illness, the meaning of the symptoms, motivation for help-seeking, and culturally expected or sanctioned "problem-presenting style." It is a combination of the results of these factors that affects the process of complaining. However, culture definitely plays a clear role in this complaining process.

For instance, patients of certain ethnic groups tend to make somatic complaints to their clinicians in their initial sessions at mental health clinics. This tendency needs careful understanding. There may be several alternative implications, namely, a physical condition is the patient's primary concern; somatic symptoms are being used as socially recognized signals of illness; a culturally sanctioned prelude to revealing psychological problems; or a reflection of hypochondriacal traits that are shared by the group (Tseng, 1975). Thus, the nature of the somatic complaint needs to be carefully evaluated and understood, rather than simply dealt with or labeled a somatoform disorder.

In the reverse of this situation, a patient from another ethnic background may present many psychological problems to the therapist in the initial session, complaining that, as a small child, he was abused by some adult, never adequately loved by his parents, and is now confused about his own identity, unclear about the meaning of life, and so on. It is necessary for the clinician to determine how much of this psychologized complaint may merely reflect the patient's learned behavior from public communication about patienthood, and how much of it is really his primary concern.

It has been clinically observed that many war veterans in the United States, who are applying for social financial compensation on the basis of posttraumatic stress disorder, tend to present a set of rather stereotyped, textbook symptoms, such as nightmares, impulsivity, anger, flashbacks, and so on. This raises the question of whether this disorder, in contrast to other psychiatric disorders, is actually associated with a very limited range of psychopathologies and, as a result, manifests a very similar cluster of symptoms or whether the patients, through their mutual social experience and interaction with peer-veterans, have learned how to present their DSM-IV-defined symptoms so they are classified as such in order to qualify for social welfare.

That is, the performance of complaining or problem presentation is an art that does not directly reflect the distress or problem from which the patient is suffering. A dynamic interpretation and understanding are very necessary (Westermeyer, 1985).

4. Perception and Understanding of the Disorder by the Clinician

A clinician, as a human being, a cultural person, and a professional has his own ways of perceiving and understanding the complaints that are presented by his patients. His psychological sensitivity, cultural awareness, and professional orientation and experience, as well as medical competence, will all act together to influence his assessment of the problems a patient has presented. The cultural background of the clinician is a significant factor and deserves special attention, particularly when he is examining a patient with a different culture background or one with which the clinician is unfamiliar.

How the clinician's own cultural background affects the clinical assessment was shown in a study of the assessment of parent–child behavior by Japanese and American psychiatrists (Tseng, McDermott, Ogino, & Ebata, 1982). A series of videotaped family interaction patterns was shown to child psychiatrists in Tokyo and Honolulu. The clinicians in the two cultures reached remarkably different assessment conclusions. In one videotape, a father did not interact with his daughter, leaving this role to his wife. Japanese child psychiatrists tended to view this as "adequate" and "all right" parenting behavior, whereas their American counterparts viewed it as "not involved" and "inadequate" parenting behavior. The main reason for these different assessments was the clinicians' cultural expectations of a father's behavior. For Americans, it is culturally expected that the father, like the mother, interact and be involved with all of his children, whereas the Japanese consider it the mother's job to interact and be involved with the children and not appropriate for the father. If a father interacts directly and too much with his daughter, it is considered "inappropriate behavior" in Japanese culture. This clearly demonstrates that a clinician's value system and cultural beliefs affect his way of making assessments.

It is well recognized that the clinician's style of interviewing, perception of and sensitivity toward pathology, and familiarity with the disorder under examination all influence the interaction between the patient and the clinician, which, in turn, influences the outcome of the clinician's understanding of the disorder.

For example, an Asian patient's elaborate idiomatic complaints of suffering due to "weakness of the kidney" (psychosexual problem), "elevated fire in the body or liver" (anger or anxious), "loss of soul" (depression or dissociated), "disturbance from a deceased aunt's spirit," and so on may not be fully comprehended with cultural empathy by an Occidental clinician; and the problems of polysubstance abuse or psychosexual problems presented by an Occidental patient may be unfamiliar to an Asian clinician, who is at a loss as to how to relevantly explore and understand the problems.

A clinical study supports the idea that how familiar a clinician is with a patient's pathology will shape the result of his clinical assessment. A group of case vignettes of social phobia was presented to clinicians in Tokyo and Honolulu for their clinical diagnosis. More than 90% of the Japanese psychiatrists recognized the diagnosis of social phobia, compared to only a small percentage of the American psychiatrists. This illustrates that Japanese psychiatrists, who commonly see social phobia in their clinical work, will give congruent diagnoses of social phobia when such cases are presented to them, whereas American psychiatrists, who are relatively unfamiliar with this condition, will not — they tend to give diagnoses of anxiety disorder, avoidant personality disorder, or others (Tseng, Asai, Kitanish, McLaughlin, & Kyomen, 1992).

5. Diagnosis and Categorization of the Disorder by the Clinician

The final step in the process of evaluation is making a clinical diagnosis. Finding the appropriate clinical category for diagnosis is influenced by the professional orientation of the clinician, the classification system used, and the purpose of making the diagnosis (Cooper, Kendall, Gurland, Sartorius, & Farkas, 1969; Tseng et al., 1992). In many societies, a clinician needs to take into consideration the social impact of diagnostic labeling on the patient and his family when making a clinical diagnosis.

In order to understand why most of the psychotic inpatients in the United States were diagnosed with schizophrenia, while a much higher percentage of those in the United Kingdom were diagnosed with affective disorders, a clinical investigation was conducted. A videotaped record of a group of (psychotic) patients was presented to psychiatrists in both New York and London. Despite equivalent recognition of symptoms by both British and American psychiatrists, their diagnoses were different. British psychiatrists tended to diagnose affective psychoses in the same patients that American psychiatrists diagnosed schizophrenia. At the time of the investigation, American psychiatrists had a broad concept of schizophrenia, whereas British psychiatrists had a more restrictive view.

In sum, making a clinical assessment and diagnosis is a complex matter involving a dynamic process between the help seeker and the help provider. This assessment and diagnostic process is influenced in a variety of ways by the cultural background of the **patient,** as well as that of the **clinician.** The clinician should be aware of how cultural factors will affect each step in the process of interaction between him or her and the patient.

II. SOME THEORETICAL CONSIDERATIONS

A. CONCEPTUAL DISTINCTION BETWEEN "DISEASE" AND "ILLNESS"

As elaborated previously [Chapter 9: Mental Illness: Folk Categories and Explanation (Section V, A)], in medical anthropology a conceptual distinction is made between the concepts of "disease" and "illness" (Eisenberg, 1977). The term "disease" refers to the pathological or malfunctioning condition that is diagnosed by a doctor or folk healer. It is the clinician's conceptualization of the patient's problem that derives from the paradigm of disease in which the clinician was trained. For example, a biomedically oriented psychiatrist is trained to diagnose brain disease; a psychoanalyst is trained to diagnose psychodynamic problems; and a folk healer might be trained to conceptualize and interpret such things as spirit possession or sorcery. For a medically oriented psychiatrist, a mental "disease" is used to describe a pathological condition that can be grasped and comprehended from a medical point of view — it provides an objective and professional perspective on how the sickness may occur, how it is manifested, how it progresses, and how it ends.

In contrast, the term "illness" refers to the sickness that is experienced and perceived by the patient: his subjective perception, experience, and interpretation of his suffering. Although these two terms, "disease" and "illness," are linguistically almost synonymous, they are purposely used differently to refer to two separate conditions. It is intended to illustrate that "disease" as perceived by the healer or doctor may be similar to "illness" as perceived and experienced by the person in suffering. This artificial distinction is useful from a cultural perspective because it illustrates a potential gap between the healer (or doctor) and the help seeker (or patient) in viewing the problems. Although the biomedically oriented physician tends to assume that "disease" is a universal and medical entity, from a medical anthropological point of view, all clinicians' diagnoses, as well as patients' illness experiences, are congnitive constructions based on cultural schema.

The potential gap between disease and illness is an area that deserves the clinician's attention and management in making the clinical assessment meaningful and useful, particularly in a cross-cultural situation.

B. RANGE OF THE PHENOMENOLOGY OF PSYCHOPATHOLOGY

Language reflects the concerns of the cultural group. For example, Eskimo people, who are surrounded by snow year-round, recognize many different kinds of snow, which they refer to with different words. Likewise, Micronesian people living on small islands in the middle of the ocean have different terms to distinguish many types of clouds, rather than referring simply to clouds in general. This helps them predict weather conditions for survival in sailing. Asian people use many different terms to express their concern with the delicate hierarchy of relations among family members. For instance, the Chinese use two terms, *gege* and *didi,* to address elder brother and younger brother, respectively, rather than simply referring to them both as "brothers"; three terms, *bobo, shushu,* and *jiujiu,* refer to paternal elder uncle, paternal younger uncle, and maternal uncle, respectively, rather than addressing them all by the single term "uncle," as in English. In contrast, the Chinese are familiar with only one or two kinds of wine (mostly rice wine), whereas Westerners are familiar with endless varieties. In the Japanese language, many vocabulary words exist to refer to the intimate dependency that exists in an interpersonal relationship, such as *amai, amaeru, amanzuru,* and *suneru, higamu, hinekureru, uramu,* referring to various states of mind when dependency needs are not satisfied. These linguistic phenomena reflect a characteristic of the Japanese people and their culture, in which dependence is valued, permitted, elaborated, and expected (Doi, 1973).

All the examples just described indicate that, beyond a universal base, there are variations in human thought or concern, which are reflected in a peoples' use of language. In a similar way, it can be expected that human beings experience or manifest different spectrums, fields, or ranges of mental conditions based on their life context or sociocultural background — certain areas are elaborated greatly, whereas others are less defined. Further, it may be speculated that this phenomenon applies to pathological mental conditions. In addition to the basic, core, or universal pathologies, people with different cultural backgrounds will experience and manifest different ranges of psychopathology. This is particularly true in the case of minor psychiatric disorders, which are influenced more predominantly by psychological and social factors [cross-reference to Chapter 11: Culture and Psychopathology (Section III, A–E)].

This speculation can be illustrated by the study of folk terms used by people in different societies in describing their normal and pathological mental conditions. Beiser, Benfari, Collomb, and Ravel, (1976) investigated stress-related mental symptoms described by the people of Senegal in western Africa. Instead of using existing symptom questionnaires designed for Western populations, they constructed an indigenous questionnaire based on local ways of expressing disturbance. This helped investigators avoid the danger of forcing data into categories or scales that exist in their minds. Collected data were factor analyzed and four clear-cut factors emerged: physiological anxiety, topical depression, health preoccupation, and episodic anxiety. These four groups represented the spectrum of mental disturbance that was described and presented by the local people, which was different from the mental spectrum presented by other cultural groups.

Similarly, a group of psychiatrists collaborated on a multicultural study of minor psychiatric disorders in Asia (Tseng et al., 1990). The psychiatrists, from China, Indonesia, Japan, and Thailand, were asked, based on their clinical experiences, to list the most commonly presented neurotic or emotional symptoms in their own cultural settings. Based on the compiled list of symptoms, a mental symptom questionnaire (for Asian populations) was constructed and applied to the nonpsychotic psychiatric outpatient populations in Bali (Indonesia), Chiang-Mai (Thailand), Kao-hsiung (Taiwan), and Shanghai (mainland China). When all collected data were put together for factor analysis, nine clusters emerged. Among them, in addition to anxiety, depression, phobia, conversion, neurasthenia, and temper, *three* clusters were **somatic** in nature and could be recognized as somatic symptoms related to the head, chest, and abdomen. This illustrated that somatic symtoms for the Asian populations studied were not only prevalent, but greatly elaborated and differentiated. When the symptom profiles of these five sites were compared, it was found that the subjects from Kao-hsiung and Shanghai — the same Chinese groups living in different sociopolitical settings — were almost identical, whereas those from Chiang-Mai — a group from a different ethnic and cultural background — were distinctively different from the rest. The findings supported the notion that people from different cultural backgrounds have different ranges or spectrums of commonly presented mental symptoms.

C. "MAJOR" VERSUS "MINOR" PSYCHIATRIC DISORDERS

In the past, clinicians distinguished between psychoses and neuroses. Among psychiatric disorders, the more severe disturbances, characterized by gross distortion from reality, were labeled psychoses, and those with a lesser degree of impairment, as neuroses. Although the concepts and terminology of psychoses and neuroses as used by psychoanalysts have been abandoned by the present American classification system, the distinction between "major" and "minor" psychiatric disorders still can be made, substituting for the previous distinctions between "psychoses" and "neuroses."

"Major psychiatric disorders" include severe organic mental disturbances and functional psychoses (such as schizophrenia or delusional disorders), which are etiologically attributed predominantly to biological factors, manifested by severe distortions of reality and gross functional impairment. In contrast, "minor psychiatric disorders" (such as anxiety disorders or adjustment disorders) are less severe, attributed predominantly to psychological factors in their formation, and characterized by partial impairment in relation to reality, while still maintaining a reasonable level of functioning.

This conceptual distinction is useful from cross-cultural perspectives. It is considered that, in general, the occurrence and manifestation of major psychiatric disorders are less related to cultural factors. If they are, it is more or less in a secondary way. For instance, an international study of schizophrenia has revealed that the symptomatology does *not* show great variation among different centers investigated (World Health Organization [WHO] 1973) [cross-reference to Chapter 19: Schizophrenia (Section II, C)] whereas there is considerable impact of cultural factors on minor psychiatric disorders — not only on the manifestation of symptomatology, but also on the etiological attribution. An extreme situation is illustrated by the existence of culture-related specific psychiatric syndromes that are characterized by a unique clinical picture, such as *koro* (penis-shrinking fear), *frigophobia* (excessive fear of catching cold), or *dhat* syndrome (obsessive concern with semen leakage), which cannot be categorized into "ordinary" classification systems (cross-reference to Chapter 13: Culture-Related Specific Syndromes). Thus, from a clinical point of view, we need to consider which kind of psychopathology or which group of psychiatric disorders is under consideration when we are discussing cultural influence in the matter of making assessments and diagnoses. When a clinician is dealing with a minor psychiatric disorder, he or she needs to pay attention to the possible cultural variations of the symptomatology.

D. The "Netting Effect" in Assessment

Closely related to the concepts of variation of range of psychic expression and the different nature of cultural impact on psychopathology as described previously is the concept of the "netting effect" on collecting psychic expression. The netting effect is best illustrated by fishing with a net. The results of fishing will be very different, depending on what *kind* of fishing net (e.g., the size or shape of the mesh) is used to catch the fish and *where* the fishing net is cast, as different kinds of fish exist in different areas. These factors will determine the size and kind of fish that will be caught.

Related to this analogy, we need to understand that clinicians in their practices use different "fishing nets" to catch (or gather) information about their patients, and the symptoms or signs manifested. The "fishing net" used by a clinician is composed of his professional knowledge, experience, laboratory instruments, or diagnostic classification system. Based on his professional training, experience, or orientation, a clinician learns to use different ways (or "nets") to gather, organize, and interpret information. The outcome of the clinical assessment is influenced by the process

and method of this "netting." In a cross-cultural setting, the clinician should be aware that his clinical evaluation is very much influenced by the netting effect, depending on how perceptive and sensitive he is and what method and criteria he uses to analyze and categorize data.

E. "Etic" or "Emic" Approach

Finally, one more important matter that needs attention is whether to use an etic or emic approach in making clinical assessments. The terms "etic" and "emic" were originally derived from the linguistic terms "phonetic" (sound for universal language) and "phonemic" (sound for a specific language) **Etic** is used to address things that are considered universal (or culture-common), whereas **emic** is culture specific (Brislin, 2000). In the field of research, the etic strategy holds that investigation can take place anywhere in the world because the characteristics to be studied are universal; the emic approach takes the position that the characteristics are indigenous and distinctive, and only applicable to certain cultural groups (Draguns, 1989). At another level, the etic approach implies that research is conducted by an **outsider;** the emic approach, by an **insider.** Each approach has its own inherent advantages and shortcomings.

Applied to the clinical task of assessment, from a cultural perspective, **etic** evaluation is performed by a clinician who is from outside of the patient's cultural system. An **etic** evaluation may have the advantage of the outsider's fresh and objective perspective, but may be handicapped by the loss of meaning in interpreting the phenomena observed. In contrast, an **emic** evaluation is carried out by a clinician of the same cultural group as the patient. The advantage is that meaningful interpretation may be obtained with cultural insight, but it may be biased by subjectivity. In doing clinical assessment, it is pertinent for the clinician to be aware of his position, whether it is **etic** or **emic,** in making his clinical assessment and interpretation, and to recognize the advantages as well as the shortcomings of his situation.

III. CROSS-CULTURAL PERSPECTIVES OF CLINICAL DIAGNOSIS

A. DIFFERENT CLASSIFICATION SYSTEMS USED IN DIFFERENT SOCIETIES

It is important for clinicians to be aware that, in different societies, different classification systems have been adopted and used in the field of psychiatry. This is still true, even though efforts have been made to unify the classification system at an international level — through the work of the World Health Organization, which suggests the use of **the International Classification of Disease** (ICD system). The expanding influence of the American psychiatric classification system — the **Diagnostic and Statistical Manual** (DSM system) — beyond national boundaries is noticeable. Also, a collaborative effort to reduce the discongruence between ICD and DSM has been undertaken. Nevertheless, there are still considerable differences in the formal classification systems adopted and practiced among various societies around the world. Also, as pointed out by Westermeyer (1985), certain specific psychiatric disorders have been identified in some countries that have been carried over from the past. For instance, French psychiatrists still use the diagnostic term "bouffees delirantes" to refer to a type of acute psychosis; Spanish and German psychiatrists still use the diagnostic term "involutional paraphrenia" to refer to a delusional disorder that occurs in mid-life; and Scandinavian psychiatrists continue to prefer the diagnostic concept of reactive psychosis, as distinct from schizophrenia. These and other specific diagnostic nosologies used in some countries, but not in others, illustrate that the diagnostic categories are rather unique (cross-reference to Chapter 28: Classification of Disorders).

B. IMPACT OF DIFFERENT PROFESSIONAL TRAINING AND HABITS

Beyond the classification systems used, there is good reason to believe that different professional practicing patterns superimpose the ways in which clinical diagnoses are made, particularly for minor psychiatric disorders. This view is illustrated by clinical data obtained from various clinical settings in different locations, including China, Japan, and Hawaii, concerning the distribution of diagnoses given by clinicians for minor psychiatric disorders in outpatient settings (Tseng, Xu, Ebata, Hsu, & Cui, 1986). In a provincial clinic located in a rural area in China, almost 60% were given the diagnosis of neurasthenia, while 30% were unclassified neuroses. In contrast, in a university clinic in Beijing, only 18.6% were labeled as neurasthenia, while 6.7% were anxiety, 8.6% depression, 16.7% hysteria, and 37.5% unclassified neuroses. In Taipei, Taiwan, among the same Chinese population in a different social setting, treated by professionals with different medical training, 49% of the disorders were diagnosed as anxiety and 28.1% as psychophysiological disorders. In a psychiatric clinic in Tokyo, 16.7% were diagnosed as hypochondria, 10.1% as phobic, 9.8% as obsessive-compulsive disorder, only 7.8% as depression, and 4.9% as anxiety disorders. In Hawaii, different from Asian countries as a part of the United States, 37.5% of the disorders were diagnosed as depression and 46.9% as adjustment reaction. It needs to be remembered that these clinical data were taken in the 1990s, when ICD or DSM were not yet commonly adopted in those settings. It was speculated that the patients being from different groups with different clinical pathologies in different societies was only part of the reason for the different diagnostic distributions. The major reason was the different patterns of making diagnosis among professionals in different societies. This point was supported by the results of an investigation of diagnostic patterns that will be elaborated in Section IV, B.

C. SOCIOCULTURAL IMPLICATIONS OF DIAGNOSTIC NOSOLOGY

As a clinician, it is important to raise the questions: What are the clinical implications for making a certain diagnosis and what are the social and cultural implications of the diagnosis? The labeling of a disorder can bring a certain social stigma on the patient and his or her family. Leprosy is a medical disease that is still seen negatively in many societies. Similarly, schizophrenia, a psychosis, is regarded as a terrible disease in many cultural areas. Many efforts are applied to avoid such labeling. Suicide is a negative category in many societies with strong Muslim or Catholic backgrounds. Many alternative labels might be used instead.

In contrast, certain mental disorders give a legitimate excuse for a person to be relieved from social responsibility. This is particularly true if such a disorder is considered to be caused by either internal or external factors, and is not the patient's own fault. Chinese prefer the diagnosis of neurasthenia, as it if attributed to the weakness or exhaustion of the nervous system, rather than the patient's emotional vulnerability. In contrast, American patients prefer the label of adjustment disorder, as it is attributed to a noxious external situation. Labels are not welcome that suggest a person has an inherent vulnerability, such as a weak nervous system.

Thus, a clinician needs to pay attention to the implications for the patient, his family, his friends, and the society when certain diagnostic labeling is given. This consideration is needed not only from a personal level but also from social and cultural levels.

IV. CROSS-CULTURAL INVESTIGATION OF DIAGNOSIS

Although cross-cultural studies on diagnosis have already been mentioned briefly and sporadically, they deserve to be mentioned here again, in more detail, in order to review this subject.

A. THE UNITED STATES–UNITED KINGDOM STUDY OF DIAGNOSTIC PATTERNS OF SCHIZOPHRENIA

It had long been noticed by epidemiologists that there were large and persistent differences between the diagnostic statistics generated by American and British public psychiatric hospitals. Namely, the admission rates for schizophrenia were considerably higher in the United States, and those for affective psychoses were higher in England. These differences could be due to genuine differences in the clinical characteristics of patients entering hospitals in the two countries, or to differences in the diagnostic criteria used by American and British psychiatrists. In order to find an answer, a collaborative research project was carried out (Cooper et al., 1972). Among the investigations, psychiatrists from both countries were asked to review videotaped psychiatric interviews, assess the findings, and make clinical diagnoses (Cooper et al., 1969). As a result, they found that psychiatrists in the two nations tended to observe and describe the patients' psychopathology similarly, but made different clinical diagnoses. The American psychiatrists tended to give diagnoses of schizophrenia, whereas British psychiatrists diagnosed affective disorders. It became clear that the American psychiatrists defined schizophrenia broadly and loosely, while the British psychiatrists did so within more circumscribed limits. This finding took place in the 1970s, when the countries did not share similar classification systems and diagnostic patterns.

B. DIAGNOSTIC PATTERNS OF NEUROSES IN CHINA, JAPAN, AND AMERICA

Very much inspired by the United States–United Kingdom study, an investigation was undertaken with similar methodology. Videotapes of six Chinese cases with brief written case histories were given to clinicians of different cultures (Tseng et al., 1986). The subject was neuroses, or minor psychiatric disorders, rather than psychoses. The study involved colleagues in Beijing, China, Tokyo, Japan, and Honolulu, in the United States. The investigation was carried out because clinical survey data illustrated that there was a remarkable difference in the diagnostic distribution revealed among these sites, as mentioned previously in Section III, B. Namely, in mainland China, a majority of patients were diagnosed with neurasthenia, while in Hawaii, adjustment disorder was the most frequent diagnostic label.

Through this cross-cultural investigation of diagnostic patterns, it was revealed that, in cases with well-distinguished clinical pictures, the diagnoses tended to be congruent in the three countries. Diagnostic disagreement occurred in cases involving symptoms of a decline in mental function, which were overwhelmingly diagnosed as neurasthenia by Chinese clinicians. Cases involving situational stress tended to be diagnosed as adjustment reaction by the Americans. This supported the view that different professional concepts and classification systems are used in different countries that explain, at least partially, the different diagnostic distributions noted in the clinical survey in these three countries.

C. Diagnostic Patterns of Social Phobia in Tokyo and Hawaii

As an extension of the investigation just described, another study was carried out between colleagues in Tokyo and Honolulu. This study focused specifically on social phobia. It was based on the many patients who were diagnosed with *taijinkyofusho* (interpersonal relation phobia) in Japan, where a special treatment program had even been developed for the disorder. Such a diagnosis was not given often by clinicians in America (in the 1990s, when the investigation took place).

Methodologically, a similar method was applied. That is, videotapes of clinical interviews with patients labeled as social phobics from Tokyo and Honolulu as well as their brief written case histories were shown to the psychiatrists from both settings, and they were asked to make clinical diagnoses based on the material provided. Results indicated that Japanese social phobic patients were all diagnosed as *taijinkyofusho* (the Japanese diagnostic term for social phobia) congruently by Japanese psychiatrists, but only by a small portion of American psychiatrists. As for the American social phobic patients, both Japanese and American psychiatrist gave varieties of diagnoses, including anxiety disorder and avoidant personality disorder, in addition to social phobia. These findings were interpreted that it was influenced by two factors. Japanese social phobic patients, with their popularized knowledge of the disorder in Japan, tended to make clinical presentations with certain stereotyped behaviors that became diagnosed easily as such by Japanese clinicians. Americans, however, did not show such behaviors and that made it difficult for clinicians — both Japanese and American psychiatrists — to make diagnoses. The second factor is that Japanese psychiatrists are familiar with such patients *(taijinkyofusho),* but most American psychiatrists were not familiar with the disorder from their clinical experiences. Thus, familiarity with certain disorders will affect the tendency to diagnose them or not.

D. Diagnostic Issues Relating to Neurasthenia in China

Although the diagnostic term neurasthenia was eliminated from American psychiatric classification systems when the DSM-III was revised in 1980, it is still used frequently in many other countries. In fact, neurasthenia is considered one of the most commonly diagnosed, minor psychiatric disorders in China.

In order to investigate the nature of this diagnostic pattern, American cultural psychiatrist Arthur Kleinman (1982), in collaboration with a Chinese colleague, carried out a clinical study of Chinese patients in Hunan, China, diagnosed by local Chinese clinicians as having neurasthenia. He claimed that, according DSM-III criteria, 87% of the 100 patients he examined could be rediagnosed as patients with depressive disorders. His report created controversy among psychiatrists in and out of China (Lin, 1989). His findings were not shared by a Chinese colleague, D.S. Yang (1989), who had collaborated with him. Many prominent Chinese psychiatrists insisted that neurasthenia was a distinctly recognized psychiatric disorder, not to be rediagnosed and categorized as a depressive disorder, as conceived by Western psychiatrists (Yan, 1989). According to Zhang (1989), he conducted a study in Shanghai in which he attempted to rediagnose clinically identified neurasthenic patients according to ICD-9 criteria. Utilizing Western-designed measurements, he reported that the distribution of the results of his rediagnoses ranged widely from mild character disorder to severe affective disorder. He pointed out that in most cases, if they had to be recategorized in different diagnostic systems, they were rediagnosed as either anxiety or depressive illness (due to the absence of the category of neurasthenia in Western classification systems), and that the prominent features were often a combination of anxiety and depression.

E. ASSESSMENT OF HYPERACTIVE CHILDREN IN ASIAN COUNTRIES

Among child psychiatrists, it is well recognized that the diagnosis of hyperactivity in children is subject to the social context within which the behavior is examined. In order to test this, Mann, in collaboration with international colleagues (1992), carried out cross-cultural comparative studies in Asian countries. First, videotaped records were made of hyperactive children identified by local child psychiatrists in China, Japan, Thailand, the Philippines, and Indonesia. Then the videotapes were shown to child psychiatrists from those countries to rate the severity of the hyperactive behavior. The results demonstrated that the children labeled "hyperactive" differed greatly in their degree of hyperactive behavior. Among these countries, hyperactive children identified by child psychiatrists from Thailand were much less hyperactive than those identified in other countries. This supports the notion that the assessment of hyperactive behavior among children is subject heavily to the norms of behavior established by the professionals in each cultural setting. In other words, the degree of hyperactivity is judged very subjectively by the professional and biased heavily by cultural norms.

V. PRACTICAL CONSIDERATIONS IN CLINICAL ASSESSMENT

In actual practice, there are several challenges that need to be overcome by the clinician in order to conduct an appropriate cross-cultural assessment with a patient of different cultural background. Some of these challenges include the following.

A. OVERCOMING THE LANGUAGE BARRIER — THE FUNCTION OF INTERPRETER

The first problem the clinician needs to solve is overcoming any language barrier that may exist with the patient. Clearly, a language problem will affect communication and limit the process and results of the clinician's evaluation. If there is no common language used between the clinician and the patient, an interpreter is needed. Body language is very limited in making comprehensive mental health evaluations. Marcos, Urcuyo, Kesselman, and Alpert, (1973) reported that if Spanish-American patients suffering from schizophrenia were interviewed in English rather than in their native language, they would be evaluated as having more psychopathology, as the patients tended to give briefer responses, with more frequent misunderstanding, illustrating more distorted thought content. Thus, language is certainly a barrier in assessing psychopathology.

There is a skill involved in using an interpreter during a psychiatric assessment (Kinzie, 1985; Marcos, 1979). It is desirable to have an interpreter who has knowledge and experience in mental health work. The interpreter needs orientation, and perhaps training, for the work that is to be done. Basically, there are several different ways to use an interpreter: word-for-word translation is needed for areas that are delicate and significant; summary translation for areas that require abstract interpretation; and meaning interpretation for areas that need elaboration and explanation in addition to translation [cross-reference to Chapter 36: Intercultural Psychotherapy (Section II, B)]. By coaching the interpreter in these different styles of interpretation, the process will be more efficient and useful.

From a clinical point of view, there are three basic different modes in which interpreters can function (Westermeyer, 1990). The interpreter may be asked to function as an assistant to the therapist, in a subordinate position, in carrying out the psychiatric interview, assessment, and therapy. The main interaction between therapist and patient is maintained as the primary channel while the interpreter works alongside the therapist. Another mode is the therapist, the interpreter, and the patient, working together in a triangular, interactional way, with egalitarian manners, to process the clinical work. The interpreter, as a partner, plays rather an active role in the assessment and intervention. Finally, the interpreter may play a primary role in carrying out the clinical assessment and management, while the therapist functions as a supervisor. In this mode, the interpreter is judged to have basic clinical competence to perform the clinical work, needing only to consult with the therapist whenever there is a need to do so.

Beyond the matter of interpreting, it is necessary to consider the role of the interpreter, particularly his (social) relation to the patient and how he feels and identifies with the patient and the patient's culture. For example, if a family member is used as an interpreter, he or she may not only be functioning as a translator, but also attempting to convey the needs of the patient and/or the family. If social class or caste is still distinctly observed in a society, how such a hierarchical background will affect the clinical work needs special attention. For instance, if the interpreter comes from a lower caste and the patient from a higher caste, the therapy will most likely not work well, as the patient will not be willing to reveal his or her own personal matters to a person of lower status. The patient will disclose private issues only to the respected therapist. This and other factors need proper attention and management, as they all will significantly affect the process and results of the interpretation.

Finally, a caution is needed when there is a common language between the clinician and the patient, so that communication is possible, but the common language is not the clinician's primary language. There may be a symbolic cultural meaning behind a word or a phrase that is beyond semantic understanding. Many subtle misunderstandings may occur without the clinician even being aware of them (Hsu & Tseng, 1972).

B. Obtaining Cultural Background Information

Because a mental health worker is unlikely to be a trained anthropologist, it is unreasonable to expect that he will have extensive knowledge about people of various cultural backgrounds. However, in clinical practice, it is very important to have a basic knowledge of the cultural background of a patient in order to have a meaningful understanding of the patient's behavior. A clinician may read an anthropological book or consult with an anthropologist to gain the necessary information or he may consult with people from the same cultural background as the patient. One practical approach is to ask the patient or a member of his or her family to assist the clinician in understanding his or her cultural background. "How do your friends or the people in your community normally behave, think, and react in such a situation?" and "What is their interpretation of such behavior?" are the types of questions to be asked. The aim is to learn the common behavior collectively shared in the patient's society in order to distinguish it from an individual idiosyncratic response.

A caution is needed in how to refer to cultural matters. Sometimes, everything is attributed to ethnic or cultural matters, whereas at other times, the existence of cultural impact is completely denied (Lopez & Hernandez, 1987). The appropriate and objective utilization of cultural matters in interpreting the nature of behavior is in need of careful evaluation. Either overinterpretation or underinterpretation of cultural impact will miss the point.

C. Becoming Culturally Sensitive and Empathetic

Although, practically speaking, it is impossible to expect all clinicians to receive training as cultural psychiatrists or mental health workers, it should be the aim of every clinician or mental health worker to learn to be culturally sensitive. As long as clinicians are aware of the possible effect of culture on psychopathology and mental health practice, they will be more likely to search for and understand human behavior from a cultural dimension, in addition to other dimensions that impact our behavior and psychopathology. This cultural sensitivity should be a basic expectation for every mental health worker. Beyond cultural sensitivity, another desirable quality is the ability for cultural empathy. This refers to the mental ability to understand emotionally and experientially another's perception, experience, and feeling from a cultural point of view. What does it mean to a person to have his infidelity made public, why does he attempt suicide when such a personal matter is exposed to the community; or why does a person become angry enough to try to kill his fellow villagers when he is teased for his unmanly behavior — these are some examples of things a clinician needs to know in order to understand what a person is experiencing and feeling in his own cultural environment.

D. Becoming Familiar with the Cultural Variations of Psychopathology

There is no shortcut to learning about the types of psychopathology that are observed in various cultural groups. Contemporary psychiatry has not reached the point of providing comprehensive knowledge and information about this subject. There are many possible variations, particularly with psychopathology, which is predominantly psychological and sociocultural in nature. It should also be noted that many publications overemphasize or exaggerate the impact of culture on psychopathology. Too many culture-bound syndromes are named and reported, even though they are not necessarily or primarily related to culture in a strict sense (Tseng & McDermott, 1981). Learning objectively and accurately about the possible effects of culture on psychopathology is a major task for clinicians.

E. Dealing Carefully with Certain Diagnostic Dilemmas

Experience has indicated that diagnostic dilemmas in dealing with patients of diversified ethnic or cultural backgrounds occur in certain areas. Following are some of the areas that cause problems in making clinical assessments and diagnoses.

1. Problems in Judging Distortion from Reality

It is often difficult for clinicians to make diagnostic judgments when there is a question as to what extent the patient has lost his sense of reality or his behavior is distorted from reality. This is mainly because the clinician lacks a clear sense of the patient's reality, according to the patient's background, which is necessary in making such a judgment. For instance, if a former inmate complained that he was maltreated by his guards, who forced him to sleep naked on a cement floor, even during the cold winter, how could the clinician tell if his story was true of if he was merely exaggerating or presenting confabulation? If a teenager who stole a car tire and was arrested by police and sent to a clinician for psychiatric assessment told the clinician that the majority of his schoolmates also stole car tires, how would the clinician know whether he was simply behaving like other kids in his (poor and undisciplined) community or was a juvenile delinquent trying to minimize his antisocial behavior? Not having background information with which to verify the reality is, indeed, a dilemma that a clinician must face. Applying this situation cross-culturally, if a person from a faraway foreign country, where the clinician has never been, claimed that he had a half-dozen wives and nearly a hundred children, how would the clinician know if he was describing an actual situation or expressing his own grandiose delusions? If a woman, who lost her son recently, said that she talked to her deceased son often, how would the clinician know if she was manifesting culturally acceptable behavior or demonstrating psychotic self-talking? Delusion or psychotic thought needs to be verified in reality. The clinician needs to gather information about the patient's "reality" in order to make an accurate clinical assessment — something that is always challenging and difficult. Information from the patient's family or friends is often useful, unless they are members of an insane collective sharing the same delusions.

2. Problems in Assessing Unfamiliar Mental Phenomena or Behavior

Another area that is often problematic for clinicians is encountering mental phenomena or behavior with which they are unfamiliar, making a clinical judgment difficult. If the clinician is practicing in a modern Western, urban setting, without experience in the behavior of possession, he or she may have difficultly distinguishing between "normal" possession manifested by ordinary people or a professional person (such as a shaman) and "pathological" possession experienced by a decompensated patient. It will also be difficult to judge between a hermit and a deteriorated schizophrenic patient who does not pay attention to personal hygiene. In contrast, as a clinician practicing in a society where homosexuality is strictly prohibited, you will have difficultly in assessing a person who openly shows intimacy with his/her homosexual partner in public, as such behavior is uncommon in your social environment.

3. Problems in Distinguishing Pathological from Cultural Behavior

Another area that often becomes controversial is that of distinguishing between culturally accepted coping patterns and pathological behavior. Again, referring to the woman mentioned earlier who recently lost her teenage son in a tragic accident: As a part of her grief reaction, she prepared her son's favorite food daily and offered it to him at the family altar, slept on her son's bed at night, and talked to him, comforting him. Such behavior should not be viewed as that of a psychotic mother who is behaving strangely because of the shock of losing her son. Her family and relatives will share with you that she is exhibiting culturally acceptable behavior that is part of the mourning process and that there is no need for alarm. Similarly, if you have never heard of the traditional medical practice of an adult drinking a little boy's early morning urine as a way of treating "kidney deficient disorder," you may, without hesitation, interpret such behavior as "strange" and suspect that the person is psychotic.

These are examples of issues that always challenge the clinician in making assessments and diagnoses. A rule of thumb is not to make a clinical judgment on the basis of a single manifestation. A competent clinician will review all the information gathered and base his assessment on the total picture. If possible, he should obtain information from the patient's family and friends and consult with people from the same ethnic-cultural background. Consultation with a cultural expert is always a good idea.

F. CULTURALLY APPROPRIATE UNDERSTANDING OF BEHAVIOR AND PROBLEMS

Finally, it is important to stress again that making a diagnosis is merely a way of dealing with the clinical task. For the sake of clinical management, or therapy, particularly for a meaningful psychotherapeutic approach, it is more useful to conduct a comprehensive assessment of the patient's problem, and arrive at a culturally relevant understanding of the patient's behavior and the issues presented, rather than categorizing the patient's problems into a diagnostic box that is needed for statistical, legal, or other administrative purposes. The comprehension of the patient's problems needs to be based on professional knowledge, clinical experiences and competence, a humanistic approach, and culture perspectives. It is based on this premise that clinical assessment should be performed. What are the problems that the patient is encountering, what kinds of help he is asking for, what kinds of help can the therapist offer, and what are the most effective ways of helping him — these are questions that go beyond diagnosis that a clinician needs to answer in dealing with a patient, including one with a different ethnic and cultural background than the clinician.

VI. DSM-IV CULTURAL FORMULATION

A considerable improvement has been noted concerning cultural orientation in the official classification system (DSM-IV) that has been revised in the United States (American Psychiatric Association, 1994).

It is suggested that the clinician assess the patient systematically in the following areas:

a. Cultural identity of the individual.
b. Cultural explanation of the individual's illness.
c. Cultural factors related to the psychosocial environment and functioning.
d. Cultural elements of the relationship between the individual and the clinician.
e. Overall cultural assessment for diagnosis and care.

It has been advocated (Lu, Lim, & Mezzich, 1995; Mezzich et al., 1996a) that, from a practical point of view, a systematic evaluation of the cultural background of a patient needs to be performed through such suggested "cultural formulation."

REFERENCES

American Psychiatric Association. (1994). *Diagnostic and statistical manual of mental disorders* (4th ed.). Washington, DC: APA.

Beiser, M., Benfari, R.C., Collomb, H., & Ravel, J. (1976). Measuring psychoneurotic behaviors in cross-cultural surveys. *Journal of Nervous and Mental Disease, 163,* 10–23.

Brislin, R.W. (2000). Some methodological concerns in intercultural and cross-cultural research. In R.W. Brislin (Ed.), *Understanding culture's influence on behavior,* (2nd ed., Chap. 3). Fort Worth, TX: Harcourt.

Cooper, J.E., Kendall, R.E., Gurland, B.J., Sartorius, N., & Farkas, T. (1969). Cross-national study of diagnosis of the mental disorders: Some results from the first comparative investigation. *American Journal of Psychiatry, 125,* (Suppl.), 21–29.

Cooper, J.E., Kendell, R.E., Gurland, B.J., Shaarpe, L., Copeland, J.R.M., & Simon, R. (1972). *Psychiatric diagnosis in New York and London.* London: Oxford University Press.

Doi, T. (1973). *The anatomy of dependence* (pp. 28–32). Tokyo: Kodansha International.

Draguns, J.G. (1989). Dilemmas and choices in cross-cultural counseling: The universal versus the culturally distinctive. In P.B. Pedersen, J.G. Draguns, W.J. Lonner, & J.E. Trimble (Eds.), *Counseling across cultures* (pp. 3–21). Honolulu: University of Hawaii Press.

Eisenberg, L. (1977). Disease and illness: Distinctions between professional and popular ideas of sickness. *Culture, Medicine and Psychiatry, 1*(1), 9–23.

Fabrega, H. (1987). Psychiatric diagnosis: A cultural perspective. *Journal of Nervous and Mental Disease, 175,* 383–394.

Hippler, A., & Cawte, J. (1978). The Malgri territorial anxiety syndrome: Primitive pattern for agoraphobia. *Journal of Operational Psychiatry, 9,* 23–31.

Hsu, J., & Tseng, W.S. (1972). Intercultural psychotherapy. *Archives of General Psychiatry, 26,* 700–705.

Kinzie, D. (1985). Cultural aspects of psychiatric treatment with Indochinese refugees. *American Journal of Social Psychiatry, 5*(1); 47–53.

Kleinman, A. (1982). Neurasthenia and depression: A study of somatization and culture in China. *Culture, Medicine and Psychiatry, 6,* 117–190.

Lin, T.Y. (1989). Neurasthenia revisited: Its place in modern psychiatry. *Culture, Medicine and Psychiatry, 13*(2), 105–129.

Lopez, S., & Hernandez, R. (1987). When culture is considered in the evaluation and treatment of Hispanic patients. *Psychotherapy, 24,* 120–126.

Lu, F.G., Lim, R.F., & Mezzich, J.E. (1995). Issues in the assessment and diagnosis of culturally diverse individuals. In J.M. Oldham & M.B. Riba (Eds.), *American Psychiatric Press review of psychiatry,* (Vol. 14). Washington, DC: American Psychiatric Press.

Mann, E., Ikeda, Y., Mueller, C.W., Takahashi, A., Tao, K.T., Humris, E., Li, B.L., & Chin, D. (1992). Cross-cultural differences in rating hyperactive-disruptive behaviors in children. *American Journal of Psychiatry, 149*(11), 1539–1542.

Marcos, L.R. (1979). Effects of interpreters on the evaluation of psychopathology in non-English-speaking patients. *American Journal of Psychiatry, 136,* 171–174.

Marcos, L.R., Urcuyo, L., Kesselman, M., & Alpert, M. (1973). The language barrier in evaluating Spanish-American patients. *Archives of General Psychiatry, 29,* 655–659.

Mezzich, J.E., Kleinman, A., Fabrega, J., & Parron, D.L. (Eds.). (1996a). *Culture and psychiatric disgnosis: A DSM-IV perspective.* Washington, DC: American Psychiatric Press.

Mezzich, J.E., Kleinman, A., Fabrega, J., & Parron, D.L. (1996b). *Introduction.* In J.E. Mezzich, A. Kleinman, J. Fabrega, & D.L. Parron (Eds.), *Culture and psychiatric diagnosis: A DSM-IV perspective* (pp. xvii–xxiii). Washington, DC: American Psychiatric Press.

Offer, D., & Sabshin, M. (1974). *Normality: Theoretical and clinical concepts of mental health* (2nd ed.). New York: Basic Books.

Rogler, L.H. (1993). Culture in psychiatric diagnosis: An issues of scientifice accuracy. *Psychiatry, 56,* 324–327.

Thompson, R.F., Donegan, N.H., & Lavond, D.G. (1986). The psychobiology of learning and memory. In R.C. Atkinson, R.J. Herrnstein, G. Lindzey, & R.D. Luce (Eds.), *Steven's handbook of experimental psychology,* (2nd ed.), New York: Wiley.

Tseng, W.S. (1975). The nature of somatic complaints among psychiatric patients: The Chinese case. *Comprehensive Psychiatry, 16,* 237–245.

Tseng, W.S. (1997). Overview: Culture and psychopathology. In W.S. Tseng & J. Streltzer (Eds.), *Culture and psychopathology: A guide to clinical assessment.* New York: Brunner/Mazel.

Tseng, W.S., Asai, M.H., Kitanish, K.J., McLaughlin, D., & Kyomen, H. (1992). Diagnostic pattern of social phobia: Comparison in Tokyo and Hawaii. *Journal of Nervous and Mental Disease, 180,* 380–385.

Tseng, W.S., Asai, M.H., Liu, J.Q., Wibulswasdi, P., Suryani, L.K., Wen, J.K., Brennan, J., & Heiby, E. (1990). Multi-cultural study of minor psychiatric disorders in Asia: Symptom manifestations. *International Journal of Social Psychiatry, 36,* 252–264.

Tseng, W.S., & McDermott, J.F., Jr. (1981). *Culture, mind and therapy: An introduction to cultural psychiatry* (pp. 203–221). New York: Brunner/Mazel.

Tseng, W.S., McDermott, J.F., Jr., Ogino, K., & Ebata, K. (1982). Cross-cultural differences in parent-child assessment: U.S.A. and Japan. *International Journal of Social Psychiatry, 28,* 305–317.

Tseng, W.S., Mo, K.M., Hsu, J., Li, L.S., Ou, L.W., Chen, G.Q., & Jiang, D.W. (1988). A sociocultural study of koro epidemics in Guandong, China. *American Journal of Psychiatry, 145*(12), 1538–1543.

Tseng, W.S., Xu, D., Ebata, K., Hsu, J., & Cui, J. (1986). Diagnostic pattern for neuroses in China, Japan and America. *American Journal of Psychiatry, 143,* 1010–1014.

Westermeyer, J. (1985). Psychiatric diagnosis across cultural boundaries. *American Journal of Psychiatry, 142,* 798–805.

Westermeyer, J. (1990). Working with an interpreter in psychiatric assessment and treatment. *Journal of Nervous and Mental Disease, 178,* 745–749.

World Health Organization (WHO). (1973). *The international study of schizophrenia.* Geneva: WHO.

Yan, H.Q. (1989). The necessity of retaining the diagnostic concept of neurasthenia. *Culture, Medicine and Psychiatry, 13*(2), 139–145.

Yang, D.S. (1989). Neurasthenia and related problems. *Culture, Medicine and Psychiatry, 13*(2), 131–138.

Zhang, M.Y. (1989). The diagnosis and phenomenology of neurasthenia: A Shanghai study. *Culture, Medicine and Psychiatry, 13*(2), 147–161.

28

Classification of Disorders

I. PSYCHIATRIC CLASSIFICATION SYSTEM: VARIOUS IMPACTS

Rather than discussing psychiatric classification primarily from the standpoint of clinical aspects and the classification system itself, this chapter focuses on how sociocultural factors impact the classification of psychiatric disorders. It will include how clinicians perceive and categorize mental disorders, their views on nosological terms for certain disorders, and how they respond to the classification of mental disorders (Mezzich, Honda, & Kastrup, 1994; Westermeyer, 1985). These aspects will be discussed from the perspective of clinicians in various societies and in the same society at different times, and will include the following dimensions.

A. HISTORICAL DEVELOPMENT OF THE RECOGNITION OF MENTAL DISORDERS

How human beings have historically perceived, recognized, and understood mental disorders through the progress of civilization and increased intelligence is an interesting subject. A review of the history of psychiatry will give us some insight into this matter. Western psychiatric knowledge about mental disorders can be traced through medical documents that exist from the time of ancient Greece to the present. According to medical historians, the terms for epilepsy (fever-induced), delirium, melancholia, and hysteria (disorder caused by a wandering uterus) were used in Hippocrates' time, around fifth century B.C. The terms phrenities and mania were added later, in Soranus's time, around first century A.D. (Mora, 1967).

In China, there is an important classic medical book, *Huang-di Nei-jing (Yellow Emperor's Internal Medicine),* that has been known since sixth century B.C., although historians suspect that the book was actually written later than this. The book recognized the psychiatric maladies of falling sickness, delirium, and excited insanity (mania). "Hurrying-pig sickness" or "sickness of the hasty organ" (characterized by acute and transient emotional outbursts, referring to hysterical reactions known today) appeared in the medical texts *Treatise on Fevers* and the *Golden Box Summary* written in sixth century A.D. (Tseng, 1973).

In both the East and the West, psychiatric maladies of an acute nature with dramatic clinical pictures were perceived in the early history of medicine. The only difference was that melancholia was recognized early in the West, whereas depression was not identified in China until around the 14th century, when Jing-Yue's medical book was published. Minor psychiatric disorders, such as anxiety, neurasthenia, and so on, were not recognized until very recently, after the 18th century. This illustrates that certain groups of mental conditions were perceived and recognized as disorders according to the level of development of the human mind.

B. Vicissitude of Certain Mental Disorders

Based on clinical experience, psychiatrists have noted that certain neuropsychiatric disorders become prevalent at particular times and then fade away within a century or so. This affects the professional awareness of and familiarity with such disorders as nosological entities. For instance, general paresis (dementia associated with the late stage of syphilis) was one of the most common types of dementia in the past. Today, with advances in medicine (specifically, the use of penicillin in the early stages of syphilis), neurosyphilis has almost disappeared from the field of medicine. Similarly, for some unknown reason, conversion disorder or dissociated disorder is becoming much less frequent in developed societies. Also, there is the clinical impression that catatonia (a subtype of schizophrenia) is almost disappearing, at least in developed societies, whereas paranoid types of schizophrenia are considered to be increasing. It was only a couple of decades ago, when the definition of borderline personality disorder was clarified and accepted, that this diagnostic nosology became widely recognized, and its prevalence seemed to increase considerably, mainly in developed societies. A similar situation exists with posttraumatic stress disorder. After the Vietnam War, this mental disorder was recognized and widely diagnosed in the United States, in association with the welfare system that was developed to handle its treatment. Clearly, the vicissitude of

certain psychiatric disorders will result in changes in the classification system accordingly, even though slowly over a century.

C. Changes in Professional Orientation and Movement

Clearly, the classification system will also be affected by changes in professional knowledge and orientation. Such changes often result in rather rapid revisions of the classification system, sometimes within a decade or so. A good example was the labeling of all mental maladies as "reactions" rather than "disorders" in the official classification system of the 1950s through the mid-1960s. Within little more than a decade, the label was changed back to "disorders" again.

It is also well known that British and American psychiatrists, until recently, used different diagnostic categories to address schizophrenia and affective disorders—even when they were asked to examine the same patient in a diagnostic exercise (Cooper et al., 1972). British psychiatrists tended to place schizophrenia in a relatively stricter diagnostic category, whereas American psychiatrists put it in a broader category [cross-reference to Chapter 27: Clinical Assessment and Diagnosis (Section IV, A)]. After the utilization of the DSM system with more or less well-defined diagnostic criteria, such gaps in diagnostic practice seem to be decreasing.

However, there is a wide gap between the way French and Anglo-American psychiatrists handle the classification of disorders. Based on their philosophical orientation, the French approach is much more abstract in conceptualizing and defining disorders than the Anglo-American, which searches for precise descriptions and concrete criteria. This shows differences in national character as well as professional orientation.

How professional orientation may affect the establishment of a classification system is reflected in the identification of the nature and severity of social stress as a part of the diagnostic exercise. One characteristic of the third version of the DSM is the multiple-axes system in making clinical diagnoses. In the fourth axis the pschiatrist is required to describe the social stress encountered by the patient in developing the disorder. The intention is appreciated in terms of the social contribution to the development of psychopathology; however, as indicated by Kastrup (1994), it is not an easy task to perform, as the stress is perceived subjectively by the patient and is often interpreted subjectively by the clinician. Furthermore, the nature and level of severity of the stress are often related to the sociocultural circumstances in which the situation occurs. There is a need to study to what extent such a diagnostic requirement contributes to clinical work or to academic study.

D. FOLLOWING CHANGES IN THE SOCIAL SITUATION

Beyond factors related to professional knowledge and the habitual use of the diagnostic system, the classification system is also impacted by the actual situation in the society. That is, due to social circumstances in certain periods of time, different psychiatric disorders may become prevalent, and deserve more attention during those times.

This is exemplified by the diagnoses of substance abuse, borderline personality disorder, eating disorders, and posttraumatic stress disorder, which are becoming prevalent enough in some developed societies, particularly America, that relatively heavy concern for them is needed in the classification system.

E. SOCIAL IMPACT ON THE CLASSIFICATION SYSTEM

Finally, it should be pointed out that the psychiatric classification system, which is different from medical classification systems in general, tends to be directly or indirectly impacted by social factors, including political ideology, patterns of clinical practice, and the legal system, as well as the medical system itself, with

particular reference to medical payment. The impact of these social factors will be reviewed briefly here.

1. Political Ideology

In some countries, particularly autocratic ones, the psychiatric classification system may be forced to make modifications to fit the political ideology. The best example was in Russia in the era of the USSR. Very much influenced by the communists' sociological ideology, the psychiatric nosological terms antisocial personality disorder and narcissistic personality disorder were excluded from the official classification system (C. Korolenko, personal communication, 1999). The reason was political. It was conceived by the government that a communist society, with its great emphasis on the collective well-being of the whole society, should "theoretically" not have room for people with disorders such as self-centeredness and antisocial behavior. Therefore, these diagnostic entities were removed from the official classification system. Instead, for the purpose of dealing with political dissidents, the term "vague schizophrenia" was created. The definition and criteria of schizophrenia were expanded to include any "unusual" or "abnormal" thought or behavior that deviated from that of the ordinary citizen of a communist society, and was used to label severe mental disorders requiring "custodial" care. It was used for the purpose of eliminating any person who displeased the administration.

The situation in communist China in its earlier stages had similar tendencies, but was less problematic. Based on the political belief that a successful communist society should not have "socially caused" mental disorders, particularly psychoses, suicidal behavior, or (juvenile) delinquent behavior, the existence of such "social problems" was officially denied. Statistical data about such conditions were handled carefully by the security administration and were not available to the medical field. The situation changed after China opened its doors to outsiders. The government began to admit that mental disorders were observed even in communist society.

2. Clinical Practice, including the Legal System

Stigma toward mental disorders exists in almost all societies, yet the degree of the negative image of and attitude toward the mentally ill differ tremendously among different cultures (cross-reference to Chapter 30: Culture and Psychiatric Service). Associated with such a stigma, there is variation in clinical practices in different societies, particularly in terms of how diagnostic terms are used to label patients. Consequently, this modifies the usage of the classification system. Despite its high level of economic and cultural development, Japan is one society that is still influenced strongly by a stigma toward mental patients, particularly those whose illness is severe. The diagnostic term schizophrenia is avoided, if possible, and a term for a less severe mental disorder, such as anxiety disorder or neurasthenia, is used instead.

In contrast to this, there is a trend to label a person with a medical disorder, often a severe one, to minimize legal responsibility. This is the result of the legal system in many developed societies, which gives special consideration for legal offences committed by those who are mentally ill. Many medical terms, such as dissociation, multiple personality, and transient psychosis, for instance, are used to avoid legal responsibility. Naturally, there is misuse of psychiatric classification in many cases.

3. Payment through Medical Insurance

When medical payment is managed through the insurance system, and the insurance system determines the payability of the service provided in association with the diagnostic nosology, it certainly affects the clinical practice in relation to the usage of the classification system. The most apparent example is in the treatment of marital problems. Even though clinically marital problems are considered by clinicians as mental problems needing psychiatric service, very often this diagnostic category is not "recognized" and accepted by medical insurance companies. As a result, alternative diagnostic nosology is applied by clinicians, such as anxiety or depressive disorder of one of the spouses, for example, to justify payment by the insurance system. Needless to say, the classification system is bent for practical reasons.

II. CLASSIFICATION IN DIFFERENT NATIONS: BRIEF REVIEW

Now, let us turn our attention to how psychiatric classification systems are applied in different countries around the world, and how cultural factors play a role in creating differences among them.

From a world perspective, as pointed out by N.N. Wig (1994), three psychiatric classification systems are recognized at present: the international classification system (e.g., International Statistical Classification of Diseases and Related Health Problems, known as the ICD system), officially developed by the World Health Organization; the American classification system (e.g., Diagnostic and Statistical Manual of Mental Disorder, referred to as the DSM system), which, after its third revision, has demonstrated its significant impact on psychiatry in many parts of the world; and the so-called "private" national classification systems that have existed and been used by psychiatrists in their own countries from the past to the present. It is the latter systems that demonstrate diversity and illustrate how classification systems can be influenced by the professional and sociocultural aspects of psychiatry in various societies (Fabrega, 1994).

From a historical standpoint, as Wig (1994) indicated, in despite considerable differences that may exist among Euro-American countries, it is less difficult for psychiatrists to adopt the international classification system in their daily practice, as the system originated in European countries. However, the situation becomes much more complex in non-Euro-American countries (mainly in Asia and Africa), as there is often a wide gap between what is seen in the actual practice of psychiatry and the international classification system.

In the following, let us review the situation in some countries regarding the use of psychiatric classification systems and the impact of social and cultural factors.

A. FRENCH PSYCHIATRY

It is well known that French psychiatry is rather unique in terms of how heavily it is colored by a philosophical interest and orientation (Kroll, 1979). The French classification system very much reflects the culture, and French-speaking psychiatrists have a strong attachment to their own traditional nosology and the empirical French diagnostic system. As described by Pull and Chaillet (1994), French psychiatrists completely ignore the international classification developed by WHO. In fact, neither the ICD-8 (1965) nor the ICD-9 (1977) has been formally accepted in France. Instead, in 1969, France produced its own official system, INSERM, developed by the Institute National de la Santè et de la Recherche Mèdicale. Attention to classification from outside started in the 1980s, when DSM-III appeared. When ICD-10 was being prepared and field trials were undertaken, the French showed an interest in participating in this international adventure.

From a nosological point of view, French psychiatrists considered schizophrenia a chronic mental disorder, and they differentiated schizophrenia from acute and transient psychotic disorders (called bouffèes dèlirantes). They also recognized chronic delusional states outside of schizophrenia.

B. AMERICAN PSYCHIATRY

As a relatively new country, in contrast to many European and Asian countries, and influenced by American culture itself, American psychiatrists are very active in revising their diagnostic classification system—in radical ways within relatively short periods of time. When the first international psychiatric classification system (ICD-6) appeared in 1948, American psychiatrists were dissatisfied by the proposed international system and created their own

national classification system, DSM-I, in 1952. Very much influenced by Adolf Meyer's concept of psychobiology—stressing pathology as an individual's dynamic reaction to the environment—all the mental disorders were labeled "reactions," such as schizophrenic reaction, manic-depressive reaction, and anxiety reaction. However, 16 years later, in 1968, in the revised DSM-II, the term reaction was abandoned and "disorder" was used instead. The term "disorder" had, in fact, appeared systemwide 3 years earlier, in 1965, in an attempt to make the DSM-II similar to the ICD-8. However, within little more than a decade (12 years), a revelational revision was made in DSM-III (in American Psychiatric Association, 1980), shifting entirely to a descriptive orientation. Among many changes made, the distinction between psychoses and neuroses was discarded. It became atheoretical and removed any nosology related to etiological consideration, with some exceptions, such as posttraumatic stress disorder and adjustment disorder. The entire system was built on clinical phenomenology: the core nature of descriptive psychiatry emphasized in Kraeplin's time. The cultural effort for DSM-IV undertaken by NIMH supported work group (Mezzich, Kleinman, Fabrega, & Parron, 1996), resulted in significant innovations, including an introductory cultural statement, cultural considerations for the use of diagnostic categories and criteria, a glossary of culture-bound syndromes and idioms of distress, and an outline for a cultural formulation (Mezzich et al., 1999).

C. JAPANESE PSYCHIATRY

Historically, when Japanese psychiatry emerged, it was oriented toward German psychiatry. It started in the era of the Meiji Reformation (beginning in 1868), modeling European advancements. Medical students were required to study German, German medical terms were used, and medical charts were written exclusively in German. However, after Japan's defeat by America in World War II, following the social trends of the time, young Japanese psychiatrists were very much interested in American psychiatry and began to adopt the DSM system of classification. The Japanese Society for International Diagnostic Criteria in Psychiatry (JSIDCP) was formed in 1981, with a particular interest in studying the DSM. Later, 3 years after the appearance of ICD-10, the Japanese version of ICD-10 was established for official usage.

This illustrates that, reflecting Japanese culture, Japanese psychiatrists were eager and found it easy to adapt to the "advanced" classification system of "foreign" countries, making the shift rather quickly. At the same time, they maintained their own traditional views and practices. For instance, they still firmly hold the nosological term of *taijin-kyofu-sho* as a unique Japanese-rooted form of social phobia. They also use the clinical term *shinkei-shitsu* (nervous temperament), invented in the Meiji era around the beginning of the 20th century. Those diagnostic terms are not included in DSM or ICD at all.

D. CHINESE PSYCHIATRY

In its beginning in modern history, Chinese psychiatry was influenced by European psychiatry and American psychiatry to some extent. However, during the early stages of the communist regime, when China had close ties with the USSR, its psychiatric orientation was prominently influenced by Soviet psychiatry. It was after the Cultural Revolution, associated with opening its doors to the outside, that China began to be exposed to Euro-American psychiatry again. However, in terms of psychiatric classification, Chinese psychiatrists, with pride in their rich cultural heritage (Shen, 1994), formalized their own classification system, the Chinese Classification of Mental Disorders (CCMD) developed by the Chinese Medical Association in 1981. Later, in 1989, it underwent its second revision.

The Chinese tried to make their classification system (CCMD-II) as close to the ICD system as possible for the purpose of international communication; however, they also gave heavy consideration to the clinical practices they had been applying to their large

population—nearly a fifth of the world's population. Within their system, they maintained the nosology of reactive psychoses that had been used since the 1950s. Also retained was the term neurasthenia, with the claim that it was a unique nosological disorder not to be confused with depression, anxiety, or other disorders, as viewed by some Western psychiatrists (Yan, 1989; Young, 1989).

As a whole, in their national system, they did not follow the ICD or DSM entirely (Lee, 1996), maintaining the uniqueness in their system suitable for actual clinical application (Zheng, Lin, Zhao, Zhang, & Young, 1994). For instance, they did not include certain personality disorders (such as dependent or passive-aggressive personality disorders) that are listed in ICD-10 (perhaps such personality traits are more tolerated and even accepted within their culture), and somatoform disorders that had been proposed by American psychiatrists since DSM-III (it did not make sense to the holistic Chinese mind to distinguish "psychic" and "somatic" disorders from psychiatric disorders; the Chinese found it difficult to recategorize their most popular diagnostic term, neurasthenia, which had been used for their nearly 1.3 billion population as an "atypical" somatoform disorder according to the DSM category). They retained the disorders of neuroses, hysteria, and homosexuality that existed in the past. Interestingly, they added several unique diagnostic categories, such as *qigong,* induced mental disorder—a mostly transient psychotic condition in some people after they practice *qigong* (a traditional form of self-training, including meditation and physical exercise)—to handle a current situation. The practice of *qigong* is becoming popular in China at present and there is an occasional occurrence of this mental complication (Wu, 1997).

E. RUSSIAN PSYCHIATRY

Very little information is available regarding Russian psychiatry, except that it has been very biologically oriented in the past and the present, and there is no uniformly accepted classification system in use.

Regarding psychiatric classification, according to Calloway (1992/1993), the editor of the *Handbook of Psychiatry,* published in Moscow, A.V. Snezhnevsky (1983) writes that most psychiatric disorders can be divided into three major groups. The first group is composed of disorders that are predominantly endogenous in etiology, with exogenous factors playing some role in them. Schizophrenia, manic-depressive psychosis, and some organic mental disorders are in this category. The second group is characterized mainly by exogenous factors, while endogenous factors also play a part. Symptomatic psychoses, alcoholism, or organic mental disorders associated with external factors (such as trauma, tumor, infection, or physical illness) are included in this group. Among these disorders, neuroses and reactive psychoses are identified specifically as psychogenic illnesses. Disorders in the third group are considered to be the results of pathological development. They include oligophrenia and psychopathic personality disorder. It is interesting to note that all psychiatric disorders are classified according to the etiological consideration of being endogenous or exogenous in the first place.

F. LATIN AMERICAN PSYCHIATRY

According to Peruvian psychiatrist Renato D. Alarcón (1983), the psychiatry practiced in Latin America was traditionally oriented toward phenomenological, descriptive psychiatry. Therefore, it was relatively easy for psychiatrists in Peru to adapt to the DSM system that originated in the United States. Nevertheless, Alarcon stressed the importance of considering cultural dimensions in the classification system and recognizing the need to accommodate psychocultural or folkloric syndromes in different parts of the world for relevant application in clinical practice (Alarcón, 1983).

From the description regarding situations in several countries or cultural regions, it can be understood that psychiatric classification systems are not merely determined by professional knowledge, but that changes or revisions in classifications are often influ-

enced by the cultural attitudes held by psychiatrists toward their own system. This is well reflected in the matter of whether to make modifications or revisions of their national classification system to adapt to an international classification system imposed on them from outside of their country.

III. SOCIOCULTURALLY RELATED NOSOLOGY: SOME ELABORATION

A. NEURASTHENIA, BRAIN FAG SYNDROME, AND CHRONIC FATIGUE SYNDROME

The nosological term neurasthenia has disappeared from its country of origin (America); however, it is still used prevalently in many other countries (such as China). Neurasthenia as a diagnostic entity was removed from the American classification system because of its ill-defined clinical picture, with its multiple somatic complaints (which do not fit description- and psychologically oriented clinicians) and its false etiological assumption—weakness of the nervous system.

However, this diagnostic term is welcomed in China, where it fits the traditional medical concept of "weakness" as a cause of illness, as well as the holistic concept of body and mind in traditional Chinese medicine. Besides, clinicians claim that this term is comunicated easily between physician and patient. In Japan, at present, it is often used by clinicians as a substitute diagnosis to cover up more stigmatized, severe disorders, such as psychoses.

According to Prince (1960), brain fag syndrome is observed mostly among students in Nigeria, or other parts of Africa, associated with the social demand for excessive study. It may be considered a special form of neurasthenia related to heavy study.

It is interesting to note that according to a WHO collaboratory study of medical patients attending general healthcare facilities in 15 study centers around the world, including developing and developed societies on different continents and cultural regions, it was revealed that identified neurasthenic patients (according to ICD-10 category) were found in every study center investigated (Üstün & Sartorius, 1995). The prevalence ranged between 2.0 to 10.5% among medical patients seeking care from physicians in medical clinics, and the regions included Seattle, in the United States.

However, it is worth noting that the diagnostic term of burnout syndrome or chronic fatigue syndrome has been used recently by clinicians in some European and American societies. The clinical picture is found to be similar to that of neurasthenia. Is it a new wine in an old bottle? It has been commented by a Chinese psychiatrist, Young (1989), who strongly opposed the idea of abandoning the diagnostic term neurasthenia and rediagnosing it as depression or anxiety, that: "The diagnostic term may change, but the disorder will still be there."

B. *Tajinkyofushio* and Social Phobia

Another dilemma encountered is the diagnostic term *taijin-kyofu-sho* (interpersonal phobic disorder) that has been used by Japanese psychiatrists from the turn of the 20th century. In reaction to an attempt to include this diagnostic category simply as a social phobia in the American DSM classification system, Japanese psychiatrists defended themselves, claiming that the Japanese *taijinkyofusho* differs in nature from social phobia as defined by the DSM. They explained that *taijinkyofusho* patients have interpersonal interactional problems with so-called "intermediately intimate" people (such as classmates, friends, or colleagues) in semipublic settings rather than strangers in public situations. They interpreted the problems of *taijinkyofusho* patients as arising from cultural settings in which proper interpersonal relations and empathy for others are emphasized, whereas American social phobic patients are derived from cultural settings in which performanc and com-

petition are stressed (Kimura, 1982) [cross-reference to Chapter 13: Culture-Related Specific Syndrome (section II, C, 1) and Chapter 15: Anxiety Disorders (Section IV, B)]. Besides, while the patients tend to present their clinical problems in rather unique and stylized ways, making them easily diagnosed by Japanese psychiatrists, they tend to confuse American clinicians, who are unfamiliar with such patients (Tanaka-Matsumi, 1979; Tseng, Asai, Kitanish, McLaughlin, & Kyomen, 1992). This illustrates that the disorder is unique but also that culture influences the diagnosing of certain psychiatric disorders, such as *taijinkyofusho* (Kirmayer, 1991).

C. Subtyping of Dissociation or Substance Abuse

It is a natural law that things are more differentiated if there are more of them. For instance, Eskimo people living in arctic areas learn to recognize different kinds of snow for their survival and Micronesian island people learn to distinguish various kind of clouds to predict weather conditions for sailing.

Dissociation states as a clinical condition have almost disappeared from most industralized societies (perhaps substituted by drug-induced alternate conscious states); however, such clinical phenomena are still prevalently observed in many developing societies. In India, according to psychiatrists Saxena and Prasad (1989), based on their clinical experience, there is a need to recognize subtypes of dissociation into simple and possession types and handle them accordingly [cross-reference to Chapter 17: Dissociation, Possesion, and Hysteria (Section II, D)].

In contrast, in the American classification system, there is detailed subtyping of substance abuse based on the kind of substance abused. This reflects a social situation in which drug abuse is abundant and multiple substances have been abused. Such detailed subcategorization may not be needed in other societies, where substance abuse is not a major problem.

D. Acute, Transient, Psychogenic Psychosis

One of the diagnostic disorders that is not present in the American classification system but is recognized in the classification systems of other countries, such as China, France, Scandinavia, and Africa, is acute or reactive psychosis. This describes a clinical condition that is psychotic, tends to occur as a reaction to external stress, has a brief and transient course, and a relatively benign prognosis. It is commonly observed in many developing countries. It is unclear to what extent such a disorder may be attributed to cultural factors. However, the question is why American psychiatrists ignore or resist entertaining such diagnostic nosology in their national classification system?

E. Culture-Related Specific Syndromes

Finally, it is almost impossible not to discuss culture-related specific syndromes (or culture-bound syndromes) from the perspective of diagnostic classification. Associated with the minority movement, some cultural psychiatrists take the strong position that it is important to give room in the classification system for so-called culture-bound syndromes recognized in many foreign countries outside of developed societies, or among minority groups within Western societies. However, this idea is not supported by the majority of cultural psychiatrists, as it would defeat the purpose of recognizing special syndromes that are closely related to cultural dimensions from the point of view of psychopathogenetic and psychoplastic effects [cross-reference to Chapter 11: Culture and Psychopathology (Section II, A–F)]. Because DSM is phenomenologically based, but not etiologically oriented, there is no room to include psychopathogenetically conceived syndromes [cross-reference to Chapter 13: Culture-Related Specific Syndromes (Section I, C)].

The core purpose for examining culture-related specific syndromes is to understand and acknowledge the existence of such special syndromes in many cultural settings and, through such extreme examples, to understand how culture can contribute to the formation of certain psychopathologies: psychopathogenic effects beyond psychoplastic effects. It is of academic interest and professional importance to study such disorders, but they lose their meaning if we try to categorize them descriptively into certain (Western) diagnostic categories by the nature of their manifestations.

Besides, from a practical point of view, the occurrence of culture-bound syndromes is usually not very prevalent in daily practice in most societies, except those in which certain special syndromes are observed, or when the special syndromes take the form of an epidemic occurrence, such as *koro* epidemic. Therefore, there is no clinical purpose in relabeling them according to the existing official classification system. Such disorders are better understood and recognized as "culture-related specific syndromes," and are simply studied as such (cross-reference to Chapter 13: Culture-Related Specific Syndromes).

IV. INTEGRATION AND SUGGESTIONS

A. Multiple Factors Impacting Classification Systems

From the elaborations in this chapter, it is clear to us that the recognition of psychiatric disorders and the establishment and application of classification systems may be attributed to multiple factors. These include the stages of development of the human mind, the level of professional progress, social factors (including political ones), actual social situation and environment, and last, but not least, cultural factors. Culture impacts the perception and recognition of and attitude toward not only the individual diagnostic nosology, but also the classification system as a whole. It is important for scholars and clinicians to realize this and treat classification systems dynamically and with flexibility. This is particularly true when we are dealing with international and national classification systems, or different national systems originating in different societies.

B. Universality versus Cultural Variations

It is important to develop a classification system of an international nature that can be applied worldwide. This will allow professional communication and sharing of clinical information among clinicians and scholars cross-nationally and -culturally. The World Health Organization has been taking a primary role by consulting professionals from multiple societies and culture regions with the final goal of establishing a classification system that is applicable worldwide (Sartorius, Jablensky, Cooper, & Burke, 1988).

While working toward a classification system with universal application, it also needs to be recognized that there is a need to allow the existence and practice of national classification systems in individual political entities or geographic regions, which reflect the local needs and cultural variations. From a cultural psychiatric point of view, it seems impossible to demand that only a single system be used for diverse cultures. Furthermore, it would be a mistake, academically and clinically, to assume that a classification system that originates in one society or cultural group can be transplanted or imposed on other societies or cultures. This is an ethnic- or nation-centric view that needs to be avoided. Consideration and respect for others are important, even in academic and clinical exercises. It is better to allow the simultaneous existence of international systems for universal communication and national systems for local application in clinical situations.

C. Differences among Different Psychopathologies

As was elaborated previously [cross-reference to Chapter 11: Culture and Psychopathology (Section III, A–E)], from a cultural standpoint, it is useful to recognize various kinds of psychopathology. This is true even when discussing the cultural impact on diagnosis and classification. In general, in more severe mental disorders (or so-called "major" psychiatric disorders), or predominantly biologically influenced psychiatric disorders, there is less confusion in defining the nosological entity. Less severe mental disorders (so-called "minor" psychiatric disorders), or predominantly psychologically determined psychiatric disorders, are more subject to sociocultural factors in their formation and manifestation. Therefore, there is more room for cultural impact on diagnostic labeling, as well as on categorizing the disorders in the classification system. The view that there are different levels of cultural impact on different mental disorders is very important in terms of diagnosis and classification.

D. The Purpose of Diagnosis and Classification

Finally, the purpose of making a diagnosis and establishing a classification system must be remembered. Diagnosis and classification are merely means to assist professional communication, not only for scientific purposes but also clinical use. There is not merely a scientific mission to identify certain pathological entities for the sake of research and treatment, but also a clinical need to identify, label, and communicate with the patient and his or her family so that proper and effective care can be given. For the latter purpose, it is essential to take into consideration the meaning of making diagnoses and classifying categories: how the patient is going to perceive and understand the label for his problems, how the patient as well as his or her family and friends are going to react to the diagnostic labeling, and how to make proper use of it. In this regard, cultural consideration cannot be ignored.

REFERENCES

Alarcón, R.D. (1983). A Latin American perspective on DSM-III. *American Journal of Psychiatry, 140*(1), 102–104.

American Psychiatric Association. (1980). *Diagnostic and statistical manual of mental disorders* (3rd ed.). Washington, DC: APA.

Calloway, P. (1993). *Russian/Soviet and Western psychiatry: A contemporary comparative study.* New York: Wiley.

Cooper, J.E., Kendell, R.E., Gurland, B.J., Shaarpe, L., Copeland, J.R.M., & Simon, R. (1972). *Psychiatric diagnosis in New York and London.* London: Oxford University Press.

Fabrega, H. (1994). International systems of diagnosis in psychiatry. *Journal of Nervous and Mental Disease, 182,* 256–263.

Kastrup, M.C. (1994). Multiaxial diagnosis and environmental factors: Psychosocial stressors and supports. In J.E. Mezzich, Y. Honda, & M.C. Kastrup (Eds.), *Psychiatric diagnosis: A world perspective.* New York: Springer-Verlag.

Kimura, S. (1982). *Nihonjin-no taijinkuofu [Japanese anthrophobia].* Tokyo: Keiso Book Co.

Kirmayer, L.J. (1991). The place of culture in psychiatric nosology: Taijin kyofusho and DSM-III-R. *Journal of Nervous and Mental Disease, 179*(1), 19–28.

Kroll, J. (1979). Philosophical foundations of French and U.S. nosology. *American Journal of Psychiatry, 136*(9), 1135–1138.

Lee, S. (1996). Cultures in psychiatric nosology: The CCMD-2-R and international classification of mental disorders. *Culture, Medicine and Psychiatry, 20,* 421–472.

Mezzich, J.E., Honda, Y., & Kastrup, M.C. (Eds.). (1994). *Psychiatric diagnosis: A world perspective.* New York: Springer-Verlag.

Mezzich, J.E., Kirmayer, L.J., Kleinman, A., Fabrega, H., Parron, D.L., Good, B.J., Lin, K.M., & Manson, S. (1999). The place of culture in DSM-IV. *Journal of Nervous and Mental Disease, 187*(8), 457–464.

Mezzich, J.E., Kleinman, A., Fabrega, H.J., & Parron, D.L. (Eds.). (1996). *Culture and psychiatric diagnosis: A DSM-IV perspective.* Washington, DC: American Psychiatric Press.

Mora, G. (1967). History of psychiatry. In A. Freedman, & H. Kaplan (Eds.), *Comprehensive textbook of psychiatry* (pp. 2–36). Baltimore: Willams & Wilkins.

Prince, R. (1960). The brain fag syndrome in Nigerian students. *Journal of Mental Science, 106,* 559–570.

Pull, C.B., & Chaillet, G. (1994). The nosological views of French-speaking psychiatry. In J.E. Mezzich, Y. Honda, & M.C. Kastrup (Eds.), *Psychiatric diagnosis: A world perspective* (pp. 23–32). New York: Springer-Verlag.

Sartorius, N., Jablensky, A., Cooper, J.E., & Burke, J.D. (1988). Psychiatric classification in an international perspective. *British Journal of Psychiatry, 152* (Suppl. 1). 1–52.

Saxena, S., & Prasad, K.V.S.R. (1989). DSM-III subclassification of dissociative disorder applied to psychiatric outpatients in India. *American Journal of Psychiatry, 146*(2), 261–262.

Shen, Y.C. (1994). On the second edition of the Chinese Classification of Mental Disorders (DDMD-II). In J.E. Mezzich, Y. Honda, & M.C. Kastrup (Eds.), *Psychiatric diagnosis: A world perspective* (pp. 67–74). New York: Springer-Verlag.

Snezhnevsky, A.V. (Ed.). (1983). *Handbook of psychiatry.* Moscow: Meditsina.

Tanaka-Matsumi, J. (1979). *Taijinkyofusho:* Diagnostic and cultural issues in Japanese psychiatry. *Culture, Medicine and Psychiatry, 3,* 232–245.

Tseng, W.S. (1973). The development of psychiatric concepts in traditional Chinese medicine. *Archives of General Psychiatry, 29,* 569–575.

Tseng, W.S., Asai, M.H., Kitanish, K.J., McLaughlin, D., & Kyomen, H. (1992). Diagnostic pattern of social phobia: Comparison in Tokyo and Hawaii. *Journal of Nervous and Mental Disease, 180,* 380–385.

Üstün, T.B., & Sartorius, N. (Eds.). (1995). *Mental illness in general health care: An international study.* Chichester: Wiley (on behalf of WHO).

Westermeyer, J. (1985). Psychiatric diagnosis across cultural boundaries. *American Journal of Psychiatry, 142,* 798–805.

Wig, N.N. (1994). An overview of cross-cultural and national issues in psychiatric classification. In J.E. Mezzich, Y. Honda, & M.C. Kastrup (Eds.), *Psychiatric diagnosis: A world perspective* (pp. 3–10). New York: Springer-Verlag.

Wu, C.Y. (1997). Qigong: Chinese traditional folk therapy. In W.S. Tseng (Ed.); *Chinese mind and therapy* (pp. 372–379). Beijing: Beijing Medical University and Xiehe Medical University United Publisher (in Chinese).

Yan, H.Q. (1989). The necessity of retaining the diagnostic concept of neurasthenia. *Culture, Medicine and Psychiatry, 13*(2), 139–145.

Young, D. (1989). Neurasthenia and related problems. *Culture, Medicine and Psychiatry, 13*(2), 131–138.

Zheng, Y.P., Lin, K.M., Zhao, J.P., Zhang, M.Y., & Young, D. (1994). Comparative study of diagnostic systems: Chinese classification of mental disorders. Second edition versus DSM-III-R. *Comparative Psychiatry, 35,* 441–449.

29

Psychological Testing and Measurement

I. INTRODUCTION

In clinical and research work, psychological testing is often conducted to evaluate a patient's psychological status, personality, psychopathology, the stress encountered, and patterns of adjustment and coping. This provides supplemental objective data in addition to subjective clinical information that will lead to a comprehensive understanding, assessment, and diagnosis of the patient.

Most of the tools of psychological measurement have been designed by Euro-American behavior scientists or clinicians for respondents of Euro-American backgrounds. This raises questions of reliability and usefulness when the tools are applied to respondents of different ethnic–cultural backgrounds living in Euro-American societies or when, after translation and perhaps some modifications, they are applied to respondents or patients in non-Western societies.

As pointed out by Lonner (1990), much of the history of testing and assessment in the field of (Euro-American) psychology has to do with the extent to which techniques developed in the "mainstream" of Euro-America can, or even should, be extended to other cultures or ethnic groups. However, there is a growing recognition that cultural factors cannot be ignored in cross-cultural testing and assessment. This is illustrated by the appearance of a number of books on the subject during the last two decades (Brislin, Lonner, & Thorndike, 1973; Cronbach & Drenth, 1972; Irvin & Berry, 1983; Lonner & Berry, 1986; Ratner, 1997; Segall, Dasen, Berry, & Poortinga, 1990). The transcultural applicability of psychological testing will be addressed and elaborated in this chapter.

II. BASIC ISSUES FOR CONSIDERATION

A. AREA AND SCOPE OF MEASUREMENT

There are numerous basic issues that need to be addressed in testing and assessment in different cultural settings. The first is whether the method and instrument are applied appropriately and adequately cover the scope of the examination: intelligence, personality, psychopathology, or other subjects to be investigated. At the base of this issue is the fundamental question of whether, because we are all human beings, our intelligence performs in the same way, our behavior patterns may be demonstrated within the same categories, or our pathological mental conditions are manifested within the same scope of abnormality.

According to Lonner (1990, p. 59), because people in Euro-American societies assume that "intelligence" means that a person knows many things and can produce responses very quickly, it is measured according to the amount of information and speed of responses. However, among the Baganda people of Uganda, Wober (1974) reported that intelligence *(obugezi)* is associated with wisdom, slow thoughtfulness, and saying the right thing. Given this different concept of intelligence, different areas and qualities need to be considered in measuring it.

Regarding assessment of personality, Chinese psychologists (Song, 1985) have indicated that, using the American Minnesota Multiphasic Personality Inventory (MMPI) to measure personality, the Chinese on average have higher scores on the subscales of schizophrenia and depression, and require radical adjustment of the norm for measurement. Furthermore, Cheung and colleagues (1996) have claimed that the instrument misses (or does not include) areas (or subscales) that are important for measuring Chinese behavior patterns. Therefore, they have developed a new instrument for testing the Chinese.

As elaborated previously [Chapter 27: Clinical Assessment and Diagnosis (Section II,D)], the so-called "netting effect" needs to be considered in the transcultural application of instruments of measurement. Analogous to the situation in fishing — catching different kinds of fish depending on the kind of net used and where the net is cast — the results of psychological measurement will vary depending on the different ways (or "nets") utilized to gather information and different areas or scopes of mental function investigated. The outcome of the clinical assessment will be influenced by the process and method of this "netting effect."

B. Problems of Administration

In the administration of psychological tests in cross-cultural situations, it is important to question the

familiarity of the people with testing. As pointed out by Lonner (1990, pp. 58–59), probably no other country can match the United States in test usage. Most current tests were developed here and are based on the assumptions that individuals can order or rank stimuli along linearly constructed stimuli; can readily produce judgments about social and psychological stimuli; and are capable of self-assessment and self-refection (Trimble, Lonner, & Boucher, 1983). Clearly, such assumptions do not apply to people in many other cultures, even psychologized ones, not to mention those in which people have never heard of, or experienced, testing.

Closely related to this are people's attitudes and reactions to testing, how they feel about revealing to strangers (test administrators) their private selves, their attitudes toward authority (represented by the examiners), and the meaning of being tested. Groups of Japanese and American students were shown movies and a psychophysiological measurement was made of their anxiety responses to the content of the movies. It was found that the Japanese students in general illustrated higher anxiety responses than the American students, regardless of the content of the movies shown to them. The Japanese students responded to the situation of being tested rather than to the content of the movies.

It is common knowledge that people may respond to testing in certain ways, such as agreeing with just about everything (acquiescence), responding in socially approved directions (social desirability), or responding in the middle (positional). Such response styles, in addition to personality, are often shaped by cultural factors and affect the results of measurement greatly.

C. Problems of Sampling

In any study it is essential to consider how the sample to be studied is selected and to what extent the subjects reflect the targeted group as a whole. This is particularly true when the study involves cross-cultural comparison. It must be asked to what extent the subjects are comparable in their backgrounds and are representative of the cultural group to be studied. Most pen-and-paper instruments involve writing, which is a problem if the study is to be carried out in populations that have different literacy rates. Also, there will be an imbalance in volunteer sampling if some members of a society tend to shy away from taking tests, while others do not. For the sake of convenience, many psychological tests are administered to college students. This creates problems in cross-cultural comparisons. College students hardly represent all the members of a society. Also, the status of college students may differ from one culture to another. The sampling needs to take into account not only the range but also the representativeness of the culture and behavior (Berry, 1980).

At another level, in order to examine the influence of culture on the targeted questions in a cross-cultural study adequately, it is important to select cultural units of sufficiently wide range for investigation and comparison. In other words, as stressed by Berry (1980), it is crucial to select a sample of cultures to acquire an adequate range of variation in a variety of interests.

D. Equivalency of Meaning

If cultures are to be meaningfully compared, several kinds of equivalency need to be met. Berry (1980) named functional, conceptual, and metric equivalence; Brislin (2000) indicated translation, conceptual, and metric equivalence; whereas Flaherty and colleagues (1988) were concerned with content, semantic, technical, criterion, and conceptual equivalence.

1. Functional Equivalence

This concerns whether two or more behaviors (in two or more cultural systems) are related to "functionally" similar problems. For example, generosity toward others in one culture might be measured by how much money one donates to a church, in another by how much food one gives to other clan members.

2. Conceptual Equivalence

This demonstrates that our tests and concepts have identical meaning in the cultures being examined. The researchers must find out the local meaning of concepts within the cognitive systems of the people and groups being compared. Only if a common meaning is discovered can comparison legitimately take place (Berry, 1980, p.9). Therefore, it is a precondition of comparison.

3. Semantic or Translation Equivalence

When an instrument designed in one language is to be translated into another for transcultural application, semantic translation becomes an important issue from the standpoint of conceptual equivalence. The use of forward and back translation of words has been suggested (Brislin, 1970, 1976, 2000). This involves an initial translation into a target language by one bilingual person. Then the translated item is translated back into the original language by another bilingual person. For instance, when the English words "I had problems with the police this morning" are translated into another language and translated back as "I committed a crime this morning," this illustrates a conceptual gap in the understanding of "had problems with the police" in the two cultures. Any discrepancies will indicate conceptual nonequivalence. Through back translation, translation equivalence can be assured. In order to operationalize conceptual equivalence, semantic differential analysis should be carried out (Osgood, 1965).

4. Technical Equivalence

The key issue in technical equivalence is whether the method of data collection affects the results differently in different cultures studied (Flaherty et al., 1988). Certain cultures may be uncomfortable and unfamiliar with the technical aspects of testing and data collection methods that are not problems in other cultures.

5. Metric Equivalence

Metric equivalence centers on the analysis of the same concepts across cultures, and its analysis assumes that the same scale (after proper translation procedures) can be used to measure the concept everywhere (Brislin, 2000, p.103). This is important when mean scores between cultures are to be compared. To demonstrate metric equivalence in any two cultures, it is necessary to establish that the statistical behavior of the items in each culture is the same (Kline, 1983). Therefore, a score in one culture can be directly compared with a score in another.

E. VALIDITY OF THE MEASUREMENT

Validity concerns whether a test, questionnaire, or set of observations measures what it is supposed to measure. In the cross-cultural application of testing the most critical matter is the validity of the measurement. What is the value of the results obtained from the testing? Do the results really represent the issues being measured? How do we know that the bases of comparison are equivalent across cultures? These are questions that need to be raised and answered (Rogler, 1999).

F. PROBLEMS OF INTERPRETATION OF DATA

It has been challenged that unless the investigators are very familiar with the culture of the respondents, they may have difficulty interpreting data obtained in cross-cultural settings. Without such knowledge, data cannot be interpreted correctly and meaningfully. Generally speaking, it would be desirable to have a collaboration of investigators from both inside and outside of the culture so that more meaningful and relevant interpretation of the obtained data, both subjectively and objectively, could be made.

III. VARIOUS PSYCHOLOGICAL INVENTORIES

Numerous psychological tests have been developed and used by behavior scientists and clinicians for research and clinical application. Some of the more commonly used measurements are discussed here from the perspective of their transcultural application.

A. PERSONALITY ASSESSMENT

1. Objective Assessment (by Questionnaire)

a. Minnesota Multiphasic Personality Inventory

Perhaps this is one of the most widely used questionnaires for the objective assessment of personality as well as psychopathology. It was originally developed in 1937 by a psychologist, Starke R. Hathaway, and a neurologist and psychiatrist, John C. McKinley. The norm was based on data collected from normal samples (mostly patients' relatives and other visitors to a university hospital) from Minnesota (Hathaway & McKinley, 1940).

However, as pointed out by Colligan and Offord (1985), the MMPI has aged. Since its inception in the 1940s, remarkable changes have taken place in American society. Besides the improvement of living standards, increased levels of education, the impact of the feminist movement, and the liberalizing of religious and moral views, there have been changes in family structure in our technological society. There is a need for revitalization of the MMPI. Based on this, Colligan and Offord carried out a project to develop contemporary norms. From the same geographic area of Minnesota, through random sampling of household residents, they systematically included normal subjects in the survey. They disclosed that MMPI response patterns among normal people have changed. Analysis of data yielded scores and profiles higher than those obtained from the original standardization group in the 1940s. The differences were more apparent for men than for women. The investigators speculated that the response pattern changes were probably due more to changes in social attitudes and perceptions than to a change in mental health status. This illustrates that even within the same society and the same (Caucasian-American) ethnic group, the norm of this instrument needs adjustment to reflect changes that have occurred during the past four decades.

There have been several reports on the application of the MMPI to minority ethnic groups in America. Early in 1970, Gynther (1972) reported that African-American respondents generally obtain higher scores than Caucasian-American respondents on scale *F* (infrequency scale), 8 (schizophrenia), and 9 (hypomania). He interpreted these differences as representing differences in values, perceptions, and expectations rather than levels of adjustment.

Pollack and Shore (1980) reported that Native American respondents from various Pacific northwest tribes all had similar MMPI profiles and, compared to the norm of Caucasian respondents, had significant elevations in scales *Sc* (schizophrenia), *Pd* (psychopathic deviance), and *Pa* (paranoia). The authors believe that the similarity of all subgroup profiles demonstrates a significant cultural influence on the results of the MMPI in the Native American population investigated.

When the MMPI was applied to Chinese in China, Song (1985) reported that, for both for male and female normal respondents, the scores for *D* (depression) and *Sc* (schizophrenia) were elevated in contrast to the norms of American respondents. Song interpreted that the Chinese people have some character traits that are utterly different from those of Americans. The Chinese are emotionally more reserved, introverted, fond of tranquility, overly considerate, socially overcautious, and habitually self-restrained, as manifested in the test results. This indicates the need to use modified norms for the Chinese in measuring personality traits. In other words, if the Chinese norms were applied in the measurement of American respondents, the scores for *D* and *Sc* would be degraded — meaning that, from the Chinese perspective, Americans are more extroverted, freely express emotion, are less considerate in interpersonal relations, and are socially less cautious. This reflects that things are relative, depending on the perspective from which data are measured and interpreted. It also points out that there is definitely a need for adjustment in the transcultural application of the MMPI in terms of

scoring for norms. Based on these findings, Cheung and Song designed a Chinese version of objective personality measurement, including special items for the Chinese, and labeled the instrument the Chinese Personality Assessment Inventory (CPAI) (Cheung et al., 1996). Japanese psychologists also indicated elevations of the scales on *Sc* (schizophrenia) and *D* (depression) when the inventory was applied to Japanese respondents.

b. Personality Research Form (Form E)

This form was developed by D. N. Jackson to measure 29 common personality dimensions. Guthrie, Jackson, Astilla, and Elwood (1983) used this form to compare Filipino and American subjects. They reported that American subjects scored higher than Filipinos on autonomy, endurance, and sentience, whereas Filipinos scored higher on cognitive structure, order, and understanding. It was the investigators' interpretation that two major elements in the lives of the Filipino respondents altered the meanings of many scales: the importance of the extended family and the degree to which Filipinos interpret their world within that context, and their tendency to emphasize the situational determinations of behavior.

2. Projective Assessment

Although many projective tests rely less on written language than objective tests, it is the general opinion that projective testing is subject to problems in cross-cultural application. This is because the mode of testing itself has poor evidence for reliability and validity and is influenced greatly by the variables of attitude and the personal background of the tester, including ethnic or racial background (Holtzman, 1980). Furthermore, there are basic problems regarding the stimulus properties of the items and their cultural relativity. Spain (1972, pp. 286–289) has elaborated in detail on the various nature of problems associated with projective tests for cross-cultural application with regard to the conception, design, and administration of the test and the analysis of the findings.

a. Rorschach Test

The Rorschach test is considered one of the classic projective assessments. The respondents are simply shown a series of arbitrarily designed ink blocks. The respondents are expected to give responses to these figures. Thus, it is considered rather culture free, as there is no language involved and no formalized figures are presented as stimulants. However, even such a supposedly culture-free test is not immune to cultural influences.

It has been pointed out that the large number of scoring categories for the Rorschach, as with other projective tests, leads to the possibility of many different permutations. Even 20 binary indices will yield more than a million types. Thus, an impressive amount of uniformity will have to be present in order to be noticed or else categories defined in more general terms will have to be the focus of the research (Wallace, 1961).

Wallace (1952, 1961) used the Rorschach test to compare personalities in two groups of Native Americans, the Tuscarora and the Ojiba. He arbitrarily but reasonably set a modal range of two standard deviations around the mode, defining as members of the modal class those responses that fell within these limits. Furthermore, individuals whose scores fell within these limits on all 21 variables were to be counted as members of the modal group. As a result, he found that 37% of the Tuscarora were in this group, and only 5% of the Ojibwa. From this study, he suggested that we should look into the "organization of diversity" — the diversity of motives that are related and organized through the medium of shared expectations held by the individuals in an orderly society — rather than the "replication of uniformity" — searching for modal personality characteristics.

Chinese psychologist Kuo-Shu Yang, Su, Hsu, and Huang (1962) reported that they administered the Rorschach test to normal Chinese adults in Taiwan and found that they gave less frequent scores for D than those reported by S.J. Beck in 1950 for American respondents. The authors interpreted the differences as perhaps derived from differences of "habitual inhibi-

tion" manifested by Chinese and American respondents. Associated with child-rearing patterns, Chinese people develop relatively strong habitual inhibitions, which also manifest in testing situations. Therefore, their frequency of selecting the detailed parts of the figures as determinants decreased and their scores for D became relatively lower than those of their American counterparts. The authors concluded that it would be incorrect to use the value of D as reported by the Beck for the American respondents.

b. Thematic Apperception Test (TAT)

TAT is another commonly used projective test. Because human figures are used, even though they, as well as the background settings, are intentionally kept ambiguous, it is greatly subject to sociocultural influences, in contrast to the Rorschach test. For children, the Children Apperception Test (CAT) is used, in which animated figures are substituted. However, even the animals are culture bound. Various kinds of animals have different cultural significance. For instance, pigs raise considerable problems in Muslim or Jewish groups.

Beside such problems, there are several advantages for cross-cultural application. The responses to the TAT are typically more profuse and varied, thus permitting a wider range of inquiries from the same test administration. Further, as pointed out by Spain (1972), the tradition of storytelling is virtually universal, and the user of the TAT can take advantage of this in his field work.

There are few culturally adjusted TATs that are used for people in non-Western societies. The Japanese version of the TAT is one, designed by American cultural anthropologist W. Caudell for study in Japan. According to Kline (1983), S. G. Lee, in 1953, attempted to produce an African TAT, but it proved to be suitable for very few ethnic groups in Africa because the life situation there was so different from that in the West.

As early as the 1950s, there were some reports concerning the comparison of the results obtained for different ethnic groups in the same society. Mussen

(1953) administered the TAT to African-American boys and compared their responses with those of Caucasian-American boys. He reported that, according to the variables expressed in the TAT, there was a considerable number of differences between the two groups. The African-American boys, with their minority background, saw the general environment as more hostile, whereas the Caucasian-American boys saw it as predominantly friendly. More African-American boys told stories in which the hero was hated, scolded, reprimanded, or the victim of physical assault. Interestingly, feelings of rejection, generally by the mother, were less frequent in the stories of the African-American boys than in those of the Caucasian-American boys. This study was done in the 1950s, and it is possible that there would be changes in the findings since then.

Watrous and Hsu (1963) used the TAT to study college students of Chinese, Hindu, and American backgrounds. Surprisingly, the intragroup variability in personality seemed to be very great and the intergroup difference tended to be much smaller. In their interpretation, the test was designed to probe deeply into the psychic structure and content of single individuals, which are shared much less by others than day-to-day levels of personality as manifested by participating members of a particular society.

B. Intellectual Assessment

The presently widely used Binet's Intelligence Quotient (IQ) test was designed by French psychologist Binet. At the request of the board of education of Paris, which felt that the city could not afford to send every child to school, Binet sought to detect in advance children who were unlikely to succeed in the school system. Thus, while Binet's IQ test was developed as a scholastic aptitude test, it is now believed to be an instrument to measure the inborn intellectual capacity of individuals or even whole groups — a false academic assumption, often with dangerous political implications (Segall et al., 1990, p.59).

It is interesting that English psychologist H. Gordon, in the early 1900s, was concerned with children who were raised among the poor canal-boat people in England — members of a subculture who lived on boats that plied the canals of England, were considered lazy and stupid, and failed to behave like middle-class Englishmen due to a basic lack of intelligence. Gordon doubted the validity of this interpretation and set out to discover just how intelligent canal-boat children really were.

Binet's IQ test had just been translated from French into English in an American version. Gordon obtained a copy of it and amended the language to make it conform to "English" English and administered it to a sample of canal-boat children of various ages. According to Segall (1979, pp. 49–51), Gordon found significant results. The average score was equivalent to an IQ of 60, clearly lower than the average of 100 as defined. Furthermore, there was a decline of IQ with age — the older the children, the "less intelligent" they appeared to be — a finding that was against the formal belief that intelligence should be the same through all ages. Gordon concluded that the children's test performances were more a reflection of cultural deprivation due to their environment.

However, from a cross-cultural methodological standpoint, Segall, reviewing this classic study, commented that perhaps the test was influenced by the children's willingness to answer what might have seemed to them very silly questions put to them by a somewhat bizarre stranger or, more importantly, the test was a measure of the familiarity the children had with the content of a culture other than their own.

C. Psychiatric Assessment of Psychopathology

1. Diagnostic Scales for Epidemiological Study

There are several kinds of clinical diagnostic questionnaires designed for epidemiological study. Diagnostic Interview Schedule (DIS) is one that has been chosen in the United States for an Epidemiologic Catchment Area (ECA) study and has been applied in other studies relating to different ethnic groups so that there are more comments from cross-cultural perspectives.

For instance, concerning content validity, Manson, Shore, and Bloom (1985), in their study of Hopi Indians, discovered during pretesting that the concepts of guilt, shame, and sinfulness, which the DIS treated as synonyms, had to be considered as separate concepts.

Guarnaccia, Guevara-Ramos, Gonzales, Canino, and Bird (1992), in their survey of Puerto Ricans, had to modify interpretations of items concerning psychotic experiences. Many features of Puerto Rican culture, because of proclivity to believe in spirits, such as visions, presentiments, and hearing voices, had to be incorporated into mental health assessments to correct for exaggerated attributions of psychotic symptoms.

Egeland, Hostetter, and Eshleman (1983), when they were investigating the Amish people for their bipolar disorders, found that the operationalization of manic symptoms, such as buying sprees, sexual promiscuity, and reckless driving, was not applicable to the old order Amish.

Flaherty and coinvestigators (1988) studied Andean-Indian who migrated from their village to Lima, the capital of Peru. They used the Spanish-language version of DIS but the team eliminated all of the antisocial items, such as: "Have you had at least four traffic tickets in your life for speeding or running lights?" as none of the migrants studied had driven cars in their life. They pointed out that all antisocial items attempted to measure behavior that did not conform to the usual values of society; but such usual values varied from society to society.

2. Scales for Specific Clinical Syndromes

Psychiatric epidemiologist Mollica, Wyshak, de Marneffe, Khuon, and Lavelle (1987) in Boston used the Hopkins Symptom Checklist-25 as a screening instrument for the psychiatric care of refugees from southeast Asia. They claimed that after careful trans-

lation of the instrument for content equivalence, the brief, simple, and reliable instrument was well received by refugee patients and offered an effective screening method for the symptoms of anxiety and depression.

In contrast to this, American cultural psychiatrist J.D. Kinzie and a team of colleagues who had been working with Vietnamese refugees in Oregon for many years found it difficult to use the existing depression scales, such as Zung's (1969), for the assessment of Vietnamese patients under their care. Therefore, they developed a depressive scale in the Vietnamese language that contained culturally consistent items describing the thoughts, feelings, and behaviors of depressed individuals and items describing common clinical characteristics of depressed Vietnamese patients (Kinzie et al., 1982). They claimed that such a specially developed, culturally relevant depressive scale was much more useful for clinical application for this particular group of people.

Concerning the clinical assessment of depression, Zheng and Lin (1991) developed the Chinese Depression Inventory (CDI). They used a sample of 329 currently depressed patients from 24 hospitals across China. They claimed that the CDI was a more culturally sensitive and cross-culturally useful self-report scale for measuring the severity of depression in Chinese than the Beck Depression Inventory designed for Americans in the United States. The inventory was constructed according to culture and verbal styles related to the expression of emotional and physical experiences. For instance, they explained that the words "suicide," "sexual drive," and "sense of failure" were replaced by more euphemistic expressions, namely: "being alive is not interesting," "not interested in the opposite sex," and "a weak person in life." Instead of "depression," the words "being uncomfortable in one's heart" were used. Because suicide is a "bad" behavior and regarded as a shameful thing to talk about in Chinese society, a more culturally appropriate inquiry was considered.

D. Stress and Adjustment Assessment

1. Social Readjustment Rating Questionnaire (SRRQ)

The SRRQ was developed by Holmes and Rahe (1967) for the assessment of stress encountered in daily life. The questionnaire was constructed by sorting events "observed to cluster at the time of disease onset" from the life charts of more than 5000 medical patients. The questionnaire was composed of 43 items of identified life events, such as death of a family member, marital separation, detention in jail, and loss of job. The respondent was asked to use all of his experiences to rate a series of life events as to their relative degree of necessary readjustment.

As described previously [cross-reference to Chapter 8: Stress and Coping Patterns (Section I,D,2)], Masuda and Holmes (1967) used SRRQ to study Japanese in Japan and America. The results indicated that there was a high concordance between the Japanese and the American samples in the manner in which they establishd a relative order of magnitude of life events. However, they reported that it is also evident that from these common bases are derived the cultural variants that distinguish one society from another. For instance, "detention in jail" was ranked second by Japanese and sixth by Americans. "Minor violation of the law" was ranked 28th by Japanese and 43rd by Americans. "Mortgage or loan over $10,000" (a considerably large-size debt at the time of the investigation) was ranked 17th by the Japanese and 28th by Americans. In contrast to these findings, several items, including "marital separation," "marital reconciliation," and "change in number of arguments with spouse," were considered by the Americans to have great meaning, and they ranked them higher than did the Japanese.

Joined by Komaroff, Masuda and Holmes (1968) applied the SRRQ to African-Americans and Mexican-Americans and compared the results with Caucasian-Americans. According to them, in contrast to Caucasian-Americans, Mexican-Americans ranked "marriage" and "marital separation from spouse" as the first and second items of stress, requiring great adjustment in life (the death of a spouse was number one for Caucasian-Americans). Noticeably, "major personal injury or illness" was ranked third, and "mortgage greater than $10,000" was fourth. As for African-Americans, "death of a close family member" was ranked second, "mortgage greater than $10,000" third, and "major personal injury or illness" fourth. Thus, the investigators concluded that in contrast to the differences between Japanese and Caucasian-Americans, who both live in technological societies, one in the East and one in the West, respectively (Masuda & Holmes, 1967), the differences among the three groups studied were much greater, even though they were all living in the same society, America. These reports show that the severity of stress in daily life varies greatly among different ethnic groups, depending on the kinds of lives they have and how they perceive stress, supporting the notion that stress is a matter of perception and the ability to cope with it.

E. Measurement of Daily Life Attitudes and Living Habits

1. Eating Attitude Test (EAT)

EAT is a 26-item questionnaire developed for the evaluation of abnormal eating attitudes (Garner & Garfinkel, 1979). The instrument has been used widely in Western societies as a screening inventory for eating disorders. As mentioned previously [cross-reference to Chapter 23: Eating Disorders (Section II,B,7)], in order to test the general clinical impression that the prevalence of eating disorders is very low in Third World populations, London psychiatrists King and Bhugra (1989) carried out a field survey in India. Surprisingly, results revealed that Indian girl-students scored above the recommended cutoff for the EAT — findings opposite to previous clinical impressions.

In order to solve the puzzle of these findings, a detailed analysis was carried out by the investigators. They disclosed consistent patterns of response for the whole population on five items that appear to have been due to sociocultural influences. The five items (cut my food into small pieces; display self-control around food; eat diet foods; engaged in dieting behavior; and feel that food controls my life) to which the Indian girls often responded "always" contributed to the high total scores. These items addressed culturally desirable behaviors according to Indian and Hindu religious fasting concepts, and many Indian girl respondents answered to them affirmatively.

In contrast to these culture-biased five questions, others concerning "core" characteristics of abnormal eating attitudes (such as find myself preoccupied with food; have gone on eating binges when I feel that I may not be able to stop; think about burning up calories whenever I exercise) were answered affirmatively by only a few subjects among the total subjects analyzed. This indicates that the number of subjects with abnormal eating attitudes is low. It also illustrates that the items constructed for the instrument have transcultural limitations due to different cultural meanings of some of the items included.

IV. INSTRUMENTS DEVELOPED BY WHO

The World Health Organization (WHO), an international organization concerned with the health of the world, has developed a number of assessment instruments over the past three decades that are intended for national and international psychiatric research. These instruments have been tested and used in many collaborative studies involving more than 100 centers in different parts of the world. Based on their primary purposes, the instruments are grouped as instruments for the assessment of psychopathology, disability and burden, quality of life, services, environment and risks, and for qualitative research (Sartorius & Janca, 1996). Only those for assessing psychopathology are listed below, with a brief description of each instrument.

Alcohol Use Disorders Identification Test (AUDIT): A brief structured interview aimed at identifying people whose alcohol consumption has become harmful to their health.

Composite International Diagnostic Interview (CIDI): It was originally designed as a highly standardized diagnostic instrument for the assessment of mental disorders according to the definition and criteria in the ICD-10 (International Statistical Classification of Diseases and Related Health Problems, 10th rev. WHO, 1992) and the revised third edition of the DSM-III-R (American Psychiatric Association [APA], 1987). Revision was made in 1995 to accommodate DSM-IV (APA, 1994) criteria.

ICD-10 Symptom Checklist for Mental Disorders: A semistructured instrument for clinicians' assessment of psychiatric symptoms and syndromes in the F0–F6 categories of ICD-10.

International Personality Disorder Examination (IPDE): A semistructured interview schedule designed for the assessment of personality disorders according to ICD-10 and DSM-III-R criteria. It covers six areas of the respondent's personality and behavior: work, self, interpersonal relationships, affects, reality testing, and impulse control.

Schedules for Clinical Assessment in Neuropsychiatry (SCAN): A semistructured clinical interview schedule designed for clinicians' assessment of the symptoms and course of adult mental disorders. It comprises an interview schedule, the 10th edition of the Present State Examination (PSE), Glossary of Differential Definitions, Item Group Checklist (IGC), and Clinical History Schedule (CHS).

Standardized Assessment of Depressive Disorders (SADD): A structured clinical interview schedule aimed at assessing the symptoms and signs of depressive disorders.

Schedule for Clinical Assessment of Acute Psychotic States (SCAAPS): A semistructured interview schedule for clinicians' recording of information about patients in acute psychotic states.

Self-reporting Questionnaire (SRQ): An instrument designed for screening the presence of psychiatric illness in patients contacting primary healthcare settings. It can be self-administered or administered by an interviewer to illiterate patients.

As discussed by Sartorius and Janca (1996), all the WHO instruments have been developed in the context of collaborative and cross-cultural studies, and special efforts have been made toward transcultural application. For instance, many instruments started from a draft produced by an international group of experts representing several cultural settings and disciplines. Careful steps were taken in the development of equivalent versions of instruments in different languages. These included the examination of the conceptual structure of the instrument by the expert group; translation of items into the target language (or formulation of items in both languages if the instrument was produced anew); examination of the translation by a bilingual group; back translation of the text; and examination of the back translation by a bilingual group. When certain characteristics of patients and their sociocultural settings were so different that it was not possible to assess them using the same instrument, guidelines about the assessment were provided, whereas the formulation of specific items and other measurement tasks were entrusted to groups of experts who were fully acquainted with the circumstances. From the standpoint of language, certain concepts had no natural "home" in other languages and enquiring about them could therefore become very time-consuming and difficult. In such cases, it was usually best to sacrifice an item or section rather than make part of the instrument awkward to use and complicate the training of interviewers. Finally, realizing that cross-cultural differences can best be overcome if the assessments are carried out by individuals who are familiar with the culture and well-trained in the use of the instruments, most of the instruments that WHO has developed are therefore semistructured and have been proposed for application by a well-trained member of the same culture. Those experiences and precautions have been useful to the development and application of instruments for cross-culture research.

V. SUMMARY AND SUGGESTIONS

A. DIFFERENT RANGE OF CULTURAL INFLUENCES

The degree of cultural influence on the results of psychological assessment varies. At one end of the spectrum, the cultural impact is minimal. For instance, the measurement of basic neuropsychological function is relatively culture free. On the other end, cultural influence is apparent. The measurement of life stress encountered in daily life (as shown in the Japanese responses to the Social Readjustment Rating Scale) or assessment of daily life attitudes and living habits (illustrated by the EAT applied to Indian subjects) belongs on this end, showing that such tests are very much subject to cultural bias. Psychopatholgy lies somewhere in between on the spectrum, depending on whether it is a major or a minor psychopathology.

B. MULTIPLE SOURCES OF CULTURAL IMPACT

The impact of culture on psychological assessment is derived from multiple sources. It may simply be related to how the measurement is administered, how the instrument is translated, or whether there are basic problems in the design of the instrument regarding the scope of the areas covered. The problems may be simply a matter of norm and can be resolved by modifying the cutting point. However, they may originate from the validity of the assessment applied.

C. Cultural Limitations of Psychological Assessment

It would be more correct to assume that there are always problems and limitations in the transcultural application of psychological measurement rather than to search for culture-free or universally applicable measurement methods. It would be more useful to examine and disclose in what ways the measurement will be influenced by the cultural factors and how to resolve the problems of transcultural application.

D. Possible Resolution for Transcultural Application

1. Adjustment of Norm or Cutting Point

When the instrument is designed to distinguish between normality and abnormality by a score, the cutting point may need adjustment when the subjects being investigated are from other cultural backgrounds. Clinical validation is needed for such an adjustment.

2. Making Special Efforts in Translation

If the instrument is going to be used in a setting in which the subject uses a language other than that used in the original instrument, extra effort and caution are needed in translating the instrument. This exercise of caution is illustrated in the WHO's work, as reviewed earlier. Problems not merely of language equivalency, but of conceptual equivalency, as well, need to be resolved.

3. Modification of the Test

When items included in the instrument are not relevant or valid for transcultural application, they need

to be removed, modified, or substituted by new items that are more relevant to the culture. If certain areas are not included in the instrument, causing "netting effect" problems, additional items need to be added. Based on these revisions or additions, new factors will be developed for application, even though the basic conceptual structure of the instrument will be maintained.

4. Reconstruction of the Tool

When the existing inventory is found unsuitable for transcultural application in the investigation of a particular cultural group, one final solution is to construct a new, culturally appropriate and valid inventory. This is illustrated by Kinzie's development of the Vietnamese-Language Depression Rating Scale. For different reasons, but with the same purpose, Beiser designed a culturally suitable inventory for the epidemiological study of a particular ethnic group in Africa, with special consideration to include the scope of psychopathology reflected in the indigenous people's knowledge and view.

Finally, a distinction needs to be drawn between culture-free and culture-fair measurement. As pointed out by Segall (1979, p. 52), the culture-free label would be applied to an instrument that actually measures some inherent quality of human capacity equally well in all cultures. Obviously, there can be no such thing as a culture-free test, so defined. Culture-fair instruments aim to contain the same amount of test items with familiarity to the subject of different cultural backgrounds so that it will be fair in making an assessment. Clearly that modification is needed for applications to any cultural group.

It needs to be pointed out that one of the special characteristics and unique functions of psychological measurement is its objectivity for quantitative comparison: its use for comparison of the psychological status of the same person at different times, for comparison of different subgroups (identified either by social demographic factors or by clinical conditions) of the same society, or for comparison of groups of people from different societies. Even though it is difficult to expect universally applicable instruments for pan-cultural use, and there is often a need to modify or even reconstruct the tools, it is still desirable to maintain a certain quality of commonness on the basis of which a certain degree of comparison can be made or at least inferred: the core nature of cultural psychiatry.

REFERENCES

American Psychiatric Association (APA). (1987). *Diagnostic and statistical manual of mental disorders,* (3rd ed.), Washington, DC: APA.

American Psychiatric Association (APA). (1994). *Diagnostic and statistical manual of mental disorders,* (4th ed.), Washington, DC: APA.

Berry, J.W. (1980). Introduction to methodology. In H.C. Triandis & J.W. Berry (Eds.), *Handbook of cross-cultural psychology: Vol. 2. Methodology* (pp. 1–28). Boston: Allyn & Bacon.

Brislin, R. (1970). Back translation for cross-cultural research. *Journal of Cross-Cultural Psychology, 1,* 185–216.

Brislin, R. (1976). *Translation: Applications and research.* New York: Wiley-Halsted.

Brislin, R.W. (2000). Some methodological concerns in intercultural and cross-cultural research. In R.W. Brislin (Ed.), *Understanding culture's influence on behavior,* (2nd ed., chap. 3). Fort Worth, TX: Harcourt.

Brislin, R.W., Lonner, W.J., & Thorndike, R.M. (1973). *Cross-cultural research methods.* New York: Wiley.

Cheung, F.M., Leung, K., Fan, R.M., Song, W.S., Zhang, J.X., & Zhang, J.P. (1996). Development of the Chinese Personality Assessment Inventory. *Journal of Cross-Cultural Psychology, 27*(2), 181–199.

Colligan, R.C., & Offord, K.P. (1985). Revitalizing the MMPI: The development of contemporary norms. *Psychiatric Annals, 15*(9), 558–568.

Cronbach, L.J., & Drenth, P.J.D. (Eds.). (1972). *Mental tests and cultural adaptation.* The Hague, The Netherlands: Mouton.

Egeland, J.A., Hostetter, A.M., & Eshleman, S.K. (1983). Amish study. III. The impact of cultural factors on diagnosis of bipolar illness. *American Journal of Psychiatry, 140,* 67–71.

Flaherty, J.A., Gaviria, M., Pathak, D., Mitchell, T., Wintrob, R., Richman, J., & Birz, S. (1988). Developing instruments for cross-cultural psychiatric research. *Journal of Nervous and Mental Disease, 176*(5), 257–263.

Garner, D.M., & Garfinkel, P.E. (1979). The Eating Attitudes Test: An index of the symptoms of anorexia nervosa. *Psychological Medicine, 9,* 273–279.

Guarnaccia, P.J., Guevara-Ramos, L.M., Gonzales, G., Canino, G.J., & Bird, H. (1992). Cross-cultural aspects of psychotic symptoms in Puerto Rica. *Research in Community and Mental Health, 7,* 99–110.

Guthrie, G.M., Jackson, D.N., Astilla, E., & Elwood, B. (1983). Personality measurement: Do the scales have similar meanings in another culture? In S.H. Irvin & J.W. Berry (Eds.), *Human assessment and cultural factors.* New York: Plenum Press.

Gynther, M.D. (1972). White norms and Black MMPIs: A prescription for discrimination? *Psychological Bulletin, 78*(5), 386–402.

Hathaway, S.R., & McKinley, J.C. (1940). A multiphase personality schedule (Minnesota): I. Construction of the schedule. *Journal of Psychology, 10,* 249–254.

Holmes, T.H., & Rahe, R.H. (1967). The social readjustment rating scale. *Journal of Psychosomatic Research, 11,* 213–218.

Holtzman, W.H. (1980). Projective techniques. In H.C. Triandis & J.W. Berry (Eds.), *Handbook of cross-cultural psychology: Vol. 2: Methodology* (pp. 245–278). Boston: Allyn & Bacon.

Irvin, S.H., & Berry, J.W. (Eds.). (1983). *Human assessment and cultural factors.* New York: Plenum Press.

King, M.B., & Bhugra, D. (1989). Eating disorders: Lessons from a cross-cultural study. *Psychological Medicine, 19,* 955–958.

Kinzie, J.D., Manson, S.M., Vinh, D.T., Tolan, N.T., Anh, B., & Pho, T.N. (1982). Development and validation of a Vietnamese-Language Depression Rating Scale. *American Journal of Psychiatry, 139*(10), 1276–1281.

Kline, P. (1983). The cross-cultural use of personality tests. In S.H. Irvin & J.W. Berry (Eds.), *Human assessment and cultural factors.* New York: Plenum Press.

Komaroff, A.L., Masuda, M., & Holmes, T.H. (1968). The Social Readjustment Rating Scale: A comparative study of Negro, Mexican and White Americans. *Journal of Psychosomatic Research, 12,* 121–128.

Lonner, W.J. (1990). An overview of cross-cultural testing and assessment. In R.W. Brislin (Ed.), *Applied cross-cultural psychology* (pp. 56–76). Newbury Park, CA: Sage.

Lonner, W.J., & Berry, J.W. (Eds.). (1986). *Field methods in cross-cultural research.* Newbury Park, CA: Sage.

Manson, S.M., Shore, J.H., & Bloom, J.D. (1985). The depressive experience in American Indian communities: A challenge for psychiatric theory and diagnosis. In A. Kleinman & B. Good (Eds.), *Culture and depression* (pp. 331–368). Berkeley: University of California Press.

Masuda, M., & Holmes, T.H. (1967). The Social Readjustment Rating Scale: A cross-cultural study of Japanese and Americans. *Journal of Psychosomatic Research, 11,* 227–237.

Mollica, R.F., Wyshak, G., de Marneffe, D., Khuon, F., & Lavelle, J. (1987). Indochinese version of the Hopkins Symptom Checklist-25: A screening instrument for the psychiatric care of refugees. *American Journal of Psychiatry, 144*(4), 497–500.

Mussen, P.H. (1953). Differences between the TAT responses of Negro and White boys. *Journal of Consulting Psychology, 17*(5), 373–376.

Osgood, C. (1965). Cross-cultural comparability in attitude measurement via multilingual semantic differentials. In I. Steiner &

M. Fishbein (Eds.), *Current studies in social psychology.* Chicago: Holt, Rinehart & Winston.

Pollack, D., & Shore, J.H. (1980). Validity of the MMPI with Native Americans. *American Journal of Psychiatry, 137*(8), 946–950.

Ratner, C. (1997). *Cultural psychology and qualitative methodology: Theoretical and empirical considerations.* New York: Plenum Press.

Rogler, L.H. (1999). Implementing cultural sensitivity in mental health reserach: Covergence and new directions. Part I: I. Content validity in the development of instruments from concepts. II. Translation of instrument. *Psychline, 3*(1), 5–11.

Sartorius, N., & Janca, A. (1996). Psychiatric assessment instruments developed by the World Health Organization. *Social Psychiatry and Psychiatric Epidemiology, 31,* 55–69.

Segall, M.H. (1979). *Cross-cultural psychology: Human behavior in global perspective.* Monterey, CA: Brooks/Cole.

Segall, M.H., Dasen, P.R., Berry, J.W., & Poortinga, Y.H. (1990). *Human behavior in global perspective: An introduction to cross-cultural psychology.* New York: Pergamon Press.

Song, W.Z. (1985). A preliminary study of the character traits of the Chinese. In W.S. Tseng & D.Y.H. Wu (Eds.), *Chinese culture and mental health* (pp. 47–55). Orlando; FL: Academic Press.

Spain, D.H. (1972). On the use of projective tests for research in psychological anthropology. In F.L.K. Hsu (Ed.), *Psychological anthropology* (pp. 267–308). Cambridge, MA: Schenkman.

Trimble, J.E., Lonner, W.J., & Boucher, J. (1983). Stalking the wily emic: Alternatives to cross-cultural measurement. In S. Irving &

J.W. Berry (Eds.), *Human assessment and cultural factors.* New York: Plenum Press.

Wallace, A.F.C. (1952). *The modal personality structure of the Tuscarora Indians: As revealed by the Rorschach Test* (Bull. No. 150). Washington, DC: Bureau of American Ethnology.

Wallace, A.F.C. (1961). The psychic unity of human groups. In B. Kaplan (Ed.), *Studying personality cross-culturally.* Evanston, IL: Harper & Row.

Watrous, B., & Hsu, F.L.K. (1963). A Thematice Apperception Test study of Chinese, Hindu and American college students. In F.L.K. Hsu (Ed.), *Clan, cast and club.* Princeton, NJ: Van Nostrand.

Wober, M. (1974). Towards an understanding of the Kiganda concept of intelligence. In J.W. Berry & P.R. Dasen (Eds.), *Culture and cognition.* London: Methuen.

World Health Organization (WHO). (1992). *International statistical classification of diseases and related health problems,* (10th rev.). Geneva: WHO.

Yang, K.-S., Su, C., Hsu, H.H., & Huang, C.H. (1962). Rorschach responses of normal Chinese adults: I. The normal details. *Acta Psychologica Taiwanica, 4,* 78–103 (in Chinese).

Zheng, Y.P., & Lin, K.M. (1991). Comparison of the Chinese Depression Inventory and the Chinese version of the Beck Depression Inventory. *Acta Psychiatrica Scandinavica, 84,* 531–536.

Zung, W. (1969). A cross-cultural survey of symptoms in depression. *American Journal of Psychiatry, 126,* 116–121.

30

Culture and Psychiatric Service

I. INTRODUCTION

The general practice of psychiatry is impacted by various dimensions. It may be influenced by social factors, including economic conditions, medical payment systems, medicine-related legal systems, and so on. Naturally, it is directly affected by the medical system itself, in terms of availability of service and the level of development of psychiatry, its medical knowledge and skill. Certainly, it is shaped by cultural factors, including how people view mental disorders, the attitudes of patients and their families toward psychiatric service, and peoples' help-seeking behavior when they become ill and need professional care. It is relevant for clinicians to grasp this macroscopic level of clinical practice in order to give proper psychiatric service to patients from social and cultural perspectives. As pointed out by Comas-Díaz (1988), given the inevitability of differences between patient and therapist, virtually all clinical practice can be seen as transcultural in nature. A clinician competent in cultural issues is indeed a competent mental health practitioner.

Let us examine first the kind of cultural variables that influence the practice of psychiatry.

II. CULTURAL IMPACT ON PSYCHIATRIC PRACTICE

A. CONCEPT, KNOWLEDGE, AND STIGMA OF MENTAL DISORDERS

Even though modern psychiatry has made significant progress in its scientific understanding of the nature of psychiatric disorders, laypersons still hold various folk concepts about mental illness, usually based on "traditional" medical knowledge. Loss of soul, intrusion of illness objects, the wrongdoing of ancestors, deficiency of vitality, and an imbalance of yin and yang are some examples of folk interpretations of mental illness [cross-reference to Chapter 9: Mental Illness: Folk Categories and Explanation (Section II,A,1–5)]. Such concepts often differ greatly from scientific explanations and seriously affect the practice of psychiatry. For example, instead of taking psychotropic medication, a patient may want to perform religious rituals to regain his lost soul or eat certain foods to correct an imbalance of yin and yang. "Talking therapy" is not considered effective in removing an intruding ill-spirit or correcting deficient vitality.

While increased knowledge and improvements in clinical care for the mentally ill are changing peoples' attitudes toward mental disorders, there are broad differences in attitudes toward mental patients cross-culturally. For instance, in Arabic societies and in India, historically associated with the notion that god sends messages through the mentally ill, people tend to take a no-harm attitude toward them. In contrast, in many societies, there is a general fear of and a strong stigma attached to "insane" people.

In Japan, when matchmaking was still practiced, among the things characteristics checked on in potentital mates were gambling or drinking habits and personal or family medical history of epilepsy, leprosy, and psychosis. This reflects the strong stigma held by society at large, which not only affect marriage arrangements, but also psychiatric practice. This is still true, even though marriage is now by free choice rather than arrangement by parents. Many measures are used to avoid the stigma of pychoses. For example, for the sake of the patient and his family, more serious mental disorders (such as schizophrenia) are rediagnosed by psychiatrists as less severe disorders (such as neurasthenia). Sometimes, a patient may use a false name when seeing a psychiatrist. Institutions are named in such a way that people do not associate them as psychiatric institutions. The metropolitan psychiatric hospital in Tokyo, Japan, is called Matsuzawa Hospital or Asai Hospital, after its founder (such as McLean Hospital in Boston or the Menninger Institute in Rochester). In China, many mental hospitals are given numbers for names, such as the second or third affiliated hospital, or some institutions are simply called "brain" hospitals. This phenomenon is also observed in many other Asian countries as a way of dealing with the stigma attached to mental disorders.

The stigma of mental disorders is derived from a variety of knowledge and concepts about them. Mental illness is viewed as the result of the misbehavior of ancestors. Mental disorders are conceived as hereditary, and therefore should be avoided in a mate. From a functional standpoint, when psychiatric patients behave strangely or violently they disrupt family life and disturb society. In general, patients who are quiet and seclusive, with a tendency to withdraw, are tolerated by family members and neighbors, whereas overtly crazy and violent patients are not.

B. Traditional or Folk Medical Knowledge and Concepts

Another factor that may implicitly or explicitly influence the practice of psychiatry is the folk or traditional medical knowledge of patients. Any medical systems that are outside of formally recognized, modern medicine, which is rooted in Western societies, are labeled "folk," "traditional," or "alternative" medicine (Jilek, 1993). Actually, these nonmodern medicines comprise various kinds of medical systems. Some are well established, with formal, systematic theories, such as Chinese traditional medicine or Indian Ayurvedic medicine, whereas others are less formalized and have no established theories, but are merely based on accumulated experiences of practices related to folk beliefs.

Medical systems, whether modern, traditional, or folk, are always based in "medical knowledge" and are shaped by the cultural system in which they flourish. The concepts or theories behind medicine often reflect cultural ideas and thoughts. Conversely, medical practices often influence life patterns or the cultural system, to some extent. Thus, the systems are mutually influencing.

The practice of general psychiatry, as a part of the medical system, will obviously be influenced by traditional medical systems if they still exist and are powerful in the society, in addition to modern mainstream medicine. Thus, it is useful to examine and understand traditional medicine and its impact on the practice of psychiatry: how its knowledge and concepts impact patients and their families, as well as the physicians and therapists [cross-reference to Chapter 9: Mental Illness: Folk Categories and Explanation (Section II,A–C)].

Information from public psychiatry has indicated that even people from developed societies quite frequently utilize folk medicine or herb medications simultaneously with contemporary medical service. Unless the physician inquires, this information is often not revealed to him. It is important to be aware of and to look into such trends. Whether folk medicine or herb medications supplement contemporary treatments or cause counter effects deserves careful consideration.

C. Ethnicity, Minority, and Racism

It is known from the perspectives of community and sociocultural psychiatrists that people with minority status and different racial backgrounds are often subject to less favorable psychiatric care and treatment. For instance, data collected from the Los Angeles site of the Epidemiologic Catchment Area (ECA) program indicated that Mexican-Americans, especially the less acculturated, had significantly lower rates of use of outpatient psychiatric facilities (Well, Hough, Golding, Burnam, & Karno, 1987). In general, this trend is based on misperceptions and prejudice on the part of psychiatrists and on a lack of knowledge of and misconceptions about mental disorders and the function of psychiatric service on the part of patients.

Concern with the effects of racism on psychiatric practice began in the 1970s in North America (Sabshin, Diesenhaus, & Wilkerson, 1970; Siegel, 1974), and later in western Europe (Burke, 1984; Littlewood, 1992). Clinical studies have illustrated that patients with ethnic minority status or racial backgrounds tend to be given more severe clinical diagnoses. This is the combined effect of various factors, including language barriers, unfamiliarity with clinical settings (on the patients' side), and unfamiliarity with symptom manifestation patterns as well as biased attitudes toward patients of certain ethnic–racial backgrounds (on the psychiatrists' side).

Generally speaking, it is relatively difficult to establish therapeutic relationships between therapists and patients, not only because of communication problems and incongruent views of care delivery, but significantly due to mistrust between them (Neki, Joinet, Hogan, Hauli, Kilonzo, 1985). When the ethnic and racial backgrounds of the therapist and patient are not matched, the treatment sessions tend to be fewer and many patients fail to continue service. It is also a trend for patients of minority status or certain racial backgrounds to more often receive biological or somatic rather than psychological treatment. In other words, simply because they are of a certain ethnic minority or racial background, patients will encounter different clinical care colored by subtle unfairness, if not explicit discrimination. There is a need for therapists to sharpen their sensitivities to some of the racial factors that affect therapeutic relationships (Griffith, 1977).

If patients and psychiatrists have different racial backgrounds and there has historically been a negative relationship between them, there is a potential for racism even in clinical settings. In general, however, little empirical evidence suggests that patients with minority racial backgrounds do better with a therapist of the same rather than the majority racial background, at least concerning African-Americans in the United States prior to the 1970s, when there were few African-American psychiatrists available for service (Siegel, 1974).

Flaskerud and Hu (1992) examined the relationship of racial/ethnic identity to the amount and type of psychiatric treatment received by Caucasian-Americans, African-Americans, Latino-Americans, and Asian-Americans in the Los Angeles County mental health system between 1983 and 1988. Interestingly enough, they reported that race/ethnicity did not have a consistent, significant relationship to the treatment received (regarding number of sessions, treatment modality, treatment setting, and therapist's discipline). However, they found that the diagnosis of psychotic disorders, socioeconomic status, and primary language used by the patients did relate to the variables of treatment received.

Kaplan and Busner (1992) examined the admission of children and adolescents to state mental health facilities in New York. They reported that there were no meaningful differences in population-corrected admission rates among Caucasian-American, African-American, and Hispanic-American children and adolescents. This failed to support an allegation of racial bias in admissions to the mental health system in New York State. However, they described a vast preponderance of African-American children and adolescents admitted to the state juvenile correctional system.

Collins, Dimsdale, and Wilkins (1992) examined the consultation–liaison psychiatric utilization patterns in a university-related general hospital in San Diego. Among the African-Americans, Caucasian-Americans, and Hispanic-Americans compared, they found that the rate of psychiatric referral was lower for Hispanic-Americans. As for the reason for consultation, there were more requests for evaluation of depression and suicide among Hispanic-Americans and grossly abnormal mental status for African-Americans. Thus, clearly, there are different ethnic patterns of psychiatric consultation in liaison service.

D. SOCIAL–MEDICAL FACTORS INFLUENCING THE MODE OF SERVICE

1. Number of Psychiatrists per Population

Having more psychiatrists within a society does not necessarily indicate that better mental health service is available and that people benefit more from qualified psychiatric care. It is, however, one index to measure the quantity of mental health care available in a society.

Some data available from Asia can be compared with data from Western societies in the Pacific Rim, such as the United States and Australia (Tseng et al., in press). As illustrated in Table 30-1, the figures available for Asia for the period 1990–1994 reveal that the number of psychiatrists per 100,000 population was much lower than that for the United States and Australia. In the United States, the number of psychiatrists was 8.0 per 100,000 population. Among Asian societies, Japan had a relatively high number, (5.2), followed by South Korea with 2.4 and Singapore with 2.3. In contrast, the numbers were very low for other Asian countries, including China and Malaysia.

These figures regarding the number of psychiatrists available in a society need thoughtful interpretation. Several issues need to be considered, such as the major function of psychiatrists in their clinical work. In many Asian societies, psychiatrists are primarily involved in the delivery of care to severe psychiatric patients, mainly in inpatient settings, and are less involved in mental health-related work, such as psy-

TABLE 30-1 Number of Psychiatrists per Population in Some Societies[*]

Society	1965	1970	1975	1980	1985	1990[a]	1995
China[b]						0.8	
Taiwan[b]		1.0				2.5	
Japan[b,c]	3.7	4.3	4.3	4.4	4.9	5.2	6.3
S. Korea[d]	0.4	0.8	1.2	1.2	1.6	2.4	3.9
Singapore[e]					2.0	2.3	
Malaysia[b,f]	0.1	0.1	0.2		0.3	0.5	
Australia						7.7	
United States[g]			5.6	7.0	7.8	8.0	8.9

[*] From Tseng et al., *International Journal of Social Psychiatry*, in press.

[a] *Healthcare Handbook, 1994–1995:* Langon, France: F. Faverean & Associates.

[b] Number by estimate.

[c] Member of the Japanese Society of Psychiatry and Neurology (1998), estimated by K. Ebata.

[d] *Annual Statistics of Health and Welfare,* Ministry of Health and Welfare (1972, 1997), Seoul, Korea.

[e] From Kua Ee Heok.

[f] From Wolfgang Krahl.

[g] *Health United States 1996–1997 and Injury Chartbook.* Hyattsville, MD: Department of Health & Human Services (1997).

chological counseling for the less severely ill population, or mental health education and preventive work for the normal population.

2. Distribution and Quality of Services

In addition to the number of psychiatrists available per population, and the function provided for different subgroups of the patient population, there is the matter of the geographic distribution of psychiatrists within a society. In many developed societies, there is a heavy concentration of psychiatrists in urban settings and severe shortages in rural areas, even though the total number of psychiatrists in the society is relatively high.

In many developing societies, the number of psychiatrists is very low, and mainly focused on inpatient care. If psychiatrists provide outpatient service, other problems are encountered. There are only a handful of psychiatrists to provide care for a large number of patients. There is often little time for each patient. In order to take care of 30 or 50 patients in a half-day, providing medication becomes the only pattern of service for a single psychiatrist. Time-consuming psychological counseling becomes an unthinkable luxury. In other words, the number of psychiatrists available shapes the pattern of clinical care.

As pointed out by the World Health Organization (WHO) (1975), in developing countries, about 80 to 85% of the population lives in rural areas, remote from any psychiatric facilities, and the mental ill may never be able to utilize mental health services to regain their social efficiency. In contrast, in rapidly growing urban areas, overcrowding, unemployment, rapid social change, and lack of adequate modern mental health facilities make mental disorders a major problem. It is a challenge for professionals to cope with such situations.

Wig (1986) pointed out that there are serious limitations in the application of modern Western psychiatry in developing societies. According to Wig, the methods of service delivery are largely unsuited to developing or underdeveloped countries, where specialist manpower and material resources are severely

limited. Modern psychiatry has failed to develop a comprehensive model of prevention of mental illness and promotion of mental health, limiting its function from a public health point of view — an approach that is badly needed in developing societies. The roots of modern psychiatry are too deeply embedded in European and North American culture, as reflected in the formulation of its etiological theories, models of classification, and treatment methods. Unless it is changed, modern psychiatry is in danger of becoming a "culture-bound" specialty.

3. Institutional Setting and Care

Medical institutions, namely general or psychiatric hospitals, are built to provide medical or psychiatric service for the patients admitted and are, therefore, designed basically for medical purposes. However, variations are needed to fit the needs of the patients, including the nature of their illnesses, patient populations, socioeconomic conditions, and so on. Cultural considerations should also be incorporated in hospital design. These may include food preparation and various facilities (bed arrangement, bathrooms, recreational facilities), as well as the provision of paramedical personnel services. Different rules are often established to meet the needs of medical care as well, such as family visiting hours, provision of spiritual or religious services, and so on.

In Tokyo, Japan, one of the hospitals specializing in geriatric patients was designed with special facilities that allowed even physically disabled elderly patients to take frequent hot baths in a *furo* tub — an activity enjoyed daily by the Japanese people. In the multiethnic society of Hawaii, most hospitals prepare various ethnic foods to suit the needs of patients. In Urumqi, Xinjiang, at the western end of China, near the border of Pakistan and Afghanistan, a hospital built two kitchens: one for Han-national Chinese, where pork could be cooked, and another for Muslim Chinese, where it could not because their religion prohibits pork. The two kitchens assured that there would be no problems of food contamination for these two groups of patients.

To determine the quality of hospital service, Madhok, Bhopal, and Ramaiah (1992) carried out home interviews with Asian and non-Asian patients who were recently discharged from hospitals in Middlesbrough, United Kingdom. They found that Asian patients (originally from Pakistan, India, and Bangladesh) expressed major dissatisfaction with professional interpreters of minority languages, examination of female patients by male doctors, and the lack of ethnically suitable food in the hospital.

4. Insurance and Payment

Another factor that influences the mode of clinical practice is payment for medical service. Whether public medical insurance is available for the total population or whether patients have to rely on private medical insurance becomes an issue. Each system has its advantages and disadvantages. From a public psychiatric point of view, it is quite alarming to learn that in developed societies such as the United States, only slightly more than half of the people have medical insurance. What is the situation in developing or undeveloped societies where there is no medical insurance at all?

Very closely related to cultural matters are the kinds of medical services for which patients can be charged and how much they can be charged. For instance, in societies where "talking therapy" is not highly valued, it is difficult to charge patients very much for the service. This discourages psychiatrists from performing this time-consuming therapy. In contrast, traditional medical habits and concepts deem it reasonable to charge for prescribing medications. Indirectly, this encourages this kind of medical care. Laboratory examinations using sophisticated scientific instruments usually qualify for high fees. Naturally, this leads to many unnecessary laboratory examinations, such as electric encephalograms (EEGs), or brain scans, for patients with psychological problems who do not need these expensive examinations at all. Payment systems shape the pattern of delivery service, not the medical need.

E. Medical Culture within the Medical System

Closely related to the sociomedical factors mentioned earlier, the practice of general psychiatry is strongly embedded in the medical culture that develops within the medical system. Most physicians and medical staff living within this invisible cultural system, while unaware of it, are influenced and regulated by it. It often takes outsiders to recognize the existence of medical cultures, which may differ among specialities (such as surgery and psychiatry), but share common issues.

For instance, there is the concrete example of wearing white coats. It is believed by medical staff that physicians need to wear white coats. This custom may have started as a need, as with pathologists wearing white coats when performing autopsies, but it has become symbolic for physicians to wear white coats to indicate their status. Influenced by this custom, patients and their families expect physicians to wear white coats. In China, influenced by Russian custom, physicians not only wear white coats, but also white caps. This is also true for psychiatrists, as if there were a fear of contamination even while performing psychotherapy in outpatient clinics. In contrast, psychiatrists in Hawaii do not wear white coats. Following local custom, psychiatrists wear aloha shirts with name tags, even when they are working on psychiatric wards. The idea is to bring physicians close to patients and their families. Even nurses wear *muumuu* — Hawaiian-style long dresses.

How physicians are regarded by nurses and other medical staff varies in different cultural settings. In Japan, reflecting Japanese attitudes toward authority and male figures, physicians are highly respected by medical staff and patients. Nurses are accustomed to bowing to physicians and following orders obediently. As pointed out by Long (1984), nurses often function as intermediaries between the medical world and the patients, who regard physicians as socially distant. Actually, Japanese nurses might be considered the "housewives" of the hospital, not only in terms of their physical duties but also of their caretaking roles. In Japan, patients are expected to bow deeply to physicians when they appear on their ward rounds. Even psychotic patients conform to this expected etiquette. In contrast, in America, the status of nurses is relatively high, and they often take charge of things in ward situations. Physicians may shake hands with patients, but do not expect to receive deep bows from them. Such behavior patterns in medical settings reflect cultural background.

In clinical practice, everybody believes there should be a diagnosis for each patient. Without an illness label on a patient's chart, the practice of medicine is not considered complete, and there can be no treatment. This is a popular medical belief, and patients feel uncomfortable if they are not given a diagnosis and no medication is prescribed.

In psychiatry, there are certain "iron-clad" rules that patients and their families are asked to follow. Psychotherapy patients are supposed to visit their psychiatrists on a weekly basis, for 1 hr per session. This is based on the convenience of the therapist and reflects the spirit of industrialized societies. In many parts of the world, where people are not used to such a medical system, the concept of visiting a clinic for a scheduled appointment does not apply. These peoples' lives are not set up that way. This is not merely a conceptual and habitual matter, but reflects the realities of societies where there are no private cars or public telephones. Patients drop in whenever it is convenient for them and when they feel like it. It is only when they practice in such settings that psychiatrists realize there is no point in trying to force our established medical expectations and culture on these patients.

F. Legal, Ethical, and Humanitarian Aspects

1. Human Rights, Involuntary Admission, and Physical Confinement

Very much influenced by traditional trends, value systems, and political patterns, the basic concern for individual human rights varies greatly among societies. It affects the mode of psychiatric practice both directly and indirectly. For instance, whether patients can be forced to be hospitalized or need voluntary consent, whether patients can be physically constrained when their behavior becomes disturbing, or forced to take medications or receive injections are issues of practice that are dealt with differently in various societies, depending on how the culture, the legal system, and administrative rules regard such practices. Basic attitudes and concepts about human rights, which vary among cultures, shape the practice of service for mentally disordered patients.

It would be a mistake to assume that human beings all place a high value on humanity and have a high regard for basic individual rights. These are culturally related views. In the era of the USSR, it is suspected by Western psychiatrists that psychiatry was abused by the government for political purposes rather than medical aims. The concept and diagnosis of "vague schizophrenia" was developed during the Soviet regime and was applied to any person who manifested certain behaviors. Openly raising opinions against the administration, ignoring the political system and regulations, or demonstrating antigovernment actions could be considered signs of losing psychic control and rationality and lead to a broadly and "vaguely" defined diagnosis of schizophrenia, justifying forced hospitalization and removal from society for custodial care.

2. Ethical Concerns

It is assumed that ethics applies absolutely and universally in medical practice. All physicians should make an effort to care for patients and see that no harm is done to them. However, this assumption may be argued in cross-cultural application. Variations in ethics are observed from a cultural point of view. For instance, is it ethical for a physician to suggest sterilization for psychotic or mentally retarded patients? Is it ethical to regard homosexual persons as disordered patients and to treat them as such, with a punitive approach? What about defining a person as "dead" so that his organs can be removed for transplantation to other people — is he or she brain dead or dead by the cessation of the heartbeat? In Japan, until recently, legal authorities insisted that death, based on cultural belief, was not determined by brain death (as judged by EEG), but only when the heart stopped beating. This is not a matter solely of medical judgement, but involves folk views and ethical concepts that are greatly influenced by culture.

In apartheid South Africa, when there was widespread political conflict between races, Steere and Dowdall (1990) pointed out that a set of ethical guidelines was likely to be plagued by recurrent dilemmas. A comparison of 24 countries regarding psychological ethics codes was made by Leach and Harbin (1997). They reported that Canada's code of ethics was most similar to the U.S. American Psychological Association and that China's was the most dissimilar, indicating the relationship of professional ethical codes to cultural values.

3. Humanistic Concerns Worldwide

Finally, let us look at how mental healthcare is provided for patients with mental problems in low-income societies worldwide. After reviewing mental health in a global context, Desjarlais, Eisenberg, Good, and Kleinman (1995) pointed out that mental illnesses are always experienced and treated in the context of the local healthcare system according to cultural knowledge, local family structures, communities, and systems of popular and folk healing, as well as local medical services. In the so-called Third World, common difficulties are encountered. First, there are extreme shortages of health personnel. For instance, in rural Tanzania, it is estimated that the ratio of physicians to population is 1:20,000, whereas that of traditional doctors is 1:25. Associated with this are critical shortages of psychiatric facilities and mental health personnel in many parts of the world. In addition to the information that was reviewed previously regarding Asia (refer to Table-30-1), Desjarlais and colleagues described some serious situations. For example, there are only 60 psychiatrists for a popula-

tion of 100 million in Nigeria and 10 psychiatrists for 10 million people in Zimbabwe. (In Fiji, in 1980, with a total population of 635,000, there was only 1 psychiatrist in the only mental hospital on the major island.) Coupled with this, mental health fares badly in national budgets. Another problem is the low esteem in which the mentally ill themselves are held. The mad are widely feared as dangerous or held up to ridicule, and the burden and stigma on families are often terrible.

Based on this situation, Desjarlais and colleagues stressed the following: National plans and regional commitment are necessary if mental healthcare is to be made a priority and if limited resources are to be put to their best use; medical treatment should be a basic right for those suffering mental illness, but, in providing treatment, basic human rights must also be protected; the classic insane asylum is not only a blueprint for dehumanizing treatment, but is often associated with involuntary admission, detention, and mistreatment. Economic constraints should not be accepted as a reason for abandoning mental health planning. The development of specialized hospital units in district hospitals instead of continued support for large, central psychiatric hospitals is more appropriate. Due to the extreme shortage of psychiatrists, they need to function as teachers and consultants rather than primarily as front-line mental healthcare providers. Finally, the family needs to be recognized as key to the mental health system, and the benefits of psychoeducational work with families need to be maximized.

Many socioculturally related factors that may influence the clinical practice of psychiatry have been reviewed here. They illustrate how such variables greatly influence the practice of psychiatry in different societies and cultures. This will help clinicians realize the many variables of which they need to be aware, with which they need to be concerned, and which they need to regulate, if possible, in their practice of general psychiatric care. Following this, we will describe some unique modes of psychiatric service that have been developed in some societies or are observed in some areas due to their particular social and medical situations.

III. UNIQUE PSYCHIATRIC SERVICES IN VARIOUS CULTURES

A. COEXISTENCE OF PAST AND PRESENT IN THE MANAGEMENT OF MADNESS IN NIGERIA

Of all the African countries, Nigeria, with an area about four times the size of the United Kingdom, has the largest population, estimated at around 100 million in the 1970s, making it eighth largest in the world. However, at the time, it had only a handful of psychiatrists available. A German cultural psychiatrist, Alexander Boroffka (1995–1996), who served as the first medical superintendent of Yaba Mental Hospital, pointed out that traditional, transitional, and modern mental healthcare were still in existence simultaneously when he left Nigeria in the 1970s.

Boroffka (1973), introducing a documentary film that he produced on the situation, said that "Nowadays it is still possible, in Nigeria, to journey into psychiatry's past. Here one can meet, side by side, a multitude of diagnostic and therapeutic practices at various stages of development. The journey into history starts with the *Babalawo* of the Yoruba. His diagnostic tool is the *Ifa* oracle. Like the *Babalawo,* the *Dibie* of the *ibo* also knows of pharmacologically effective plants, the efficiency of which he seeks to improve with sacrifices. Spiritual sects combine traditional and Christian customs. They attempt to help the mentally disordered through communal prayer and singing. Asylums in the north of Nigeria bear resemblance to those erected at the beginning of the Middle Ages by the Islamic caliphs, and which were the first in Europe. Modern treatment methods, such as drug therapy, are integrated here without any difficulty. There is a widespread belief in witches. A mentally deranged person accusing herself of witchcraft can find shelter in an asylum even nowadays. But to start with, and for long periods of time, the prison was the only place offering this kind of protection in many countries. The lunatic asylum gradually evolved from the 'madhouse and jailhouse' of the past; in recent times, it has gradually developed into a mental home and psychiatric hospital."

Looking at the development of psychiatric care in Nigeria, from the traditional to the transitional and, finally, to the present period, Boroffka (1995–1996) compared it with the development in Western countries, pointing out that the similarities are striking, with two exceptions. First, the total time it has taken from the traditional to the present phase is much shorter in Nigeria, and can be counted in decades rather then in centuries. Furthermore, the stage of large mental hospitals, which has dominated the psychiatric scene in Western countries for a long time, was much shorter or was omitted in Nigeria.

B. ARO VILLAGE INVENTED FOR PSYCHIATRIC CARE

Based on the situation in most parts of Africa, African psychiatrists in Nigeria have experimented with village hospitals (Lambo, 1966). When Lambo, the first Nigerian psychiatrist trained abroad in the United Kingdom, returned to his home country, he realized that psychiatric hospitals were very few and only existed near cities. When someone became mentally ill and needed hospitalization, he was brought to the hospital by his family members, often traveling a far distance. Based on this reality, hospitals were designed to include many houses, as if they were villages. The patients lived in these houses with their family members. Professional treatment was offered by the medical staff within each household in the presence of family members. This offered educational guidance for the family so that continuous care could be provided when the patients left the village hospital and returned with their families to their own villages far away from the cities (Asuni, 1967).

C. RECONSTRUCTION OF HOSPITALS TO ACCOMMODATE CULTURE IN BALI

When a psychiatric hospital was originally built in Bali by the Dutch during their occupation, it was according to modern Western styles imported from Europe. The hospital did not meet the tastes and needs of the local people of Bali. According to Castillo (2001), when Balinese psychiatrist D. Thong (1993) took over the hospital, he reconstructed it according to Bali culture.

For instance, all the beds in the hospital wards were rearranged to have their heads facing toward the north, where the mountain on the island was located. Balinese people are very religion-oriented, and deeply believe that their supernatural being resides in the high mountain. Each household's lot is divided into three sections: the household shrine in the northern section, living quarters in the center section, and the kitchen and restroom in the southern section. In the bedroom, the head of the bed is placed toward the north. Simply rearranging the beds in the hospital ward radically changed the feelings of the local people. A temple was also built in the hospital compound so that patients and their families could visit and worship their god — a daily activity of the people in their ordinary lives. Extra houses were built around the hospital, where patients' families could live, making it convenient for the families, who like to attend to the care of the patients.

D. Religious Institutes Used for Psychiatric Care

In many developing societies there are not enough hospital mental facilities, which creates problems in patient care. In some societies, religious institutions are used for patient care, particularly during the stage of rehabilitation for chronic patients. This is observed in some parts of Taiwan and in many parts of Thailand. Because the facilities and programs are run by religious personnel, there is increased faith for healing among religious patients and their families. Besides, because the settings are not developed for profitable purposes, the charge is often minimal and affordable for families who have already exhausted their financial resources in acute care.

However, such an arrangement does not always bring glorious results. For instance, one particular temple developed an antiprofessional attitude, refusing to cooperate with the medical professional in charge of the patient. It also refused government inspection, even though abuse of patients and mismanagement of funds were suspected (Wen, 1990, personal communication, 1996).

E. Community Psychiatry Mode in the United States

Although it ended in failure, professionals still vividly remember the community psychiatry movement in the United States in the 1960s. Very much influenced by the political idealism and medical views of the time, professionals held that adequate socializing experiences in the community would facilitate the recovery of chronic mental patients. The majority of chronic, severe mentally disordered patients who had been under custodial care for many years were released to live in the community. It was expected that having an ordinary social life and interaction in the community and being cared for in community neighborhood mental health centers the patients would greatly benefit. History has shown that many patients had difficulty rehabilitating in the community and became homeless, wandering the streets without needed and proper care. This movement was started mainly due to culture-related humanistic idealism, without proper professional experimentation and validation of such a mode of care.

F. Three-Level System of Care in Shanghai, China

In China, there is a great shortage of psychiatrists for such a huge population (it is estimated that there are only 0.8 psychiatrists per 100,000 population, as illustrated in Table 30-1). This is due to the delay in the development of psychiatric service and the training of professionals caused by the disruptions of frequent wars since the beginning of this century and, lately, by the cultural revolution. In order to cope with such problems, a three-level system of mental health service has been developed, as illustrated in the example of Shanghai City (Xia, 1985). In order to provide maximal care with a relative shortage of professionals, the service is organized hierarchically at three levels; municipal, district, and grassroots. Psychiatric hospitals at the municipal level provide the most intensive care for difficult patients in inpatient and outpatient settings. Following this, at the district or county level, hospitals are established that provide regular care of ordinary patients either in inpatient or outpatient settings. When there is difficulty treating certain patients, they are transferred to municipal hospitals, which are associated with medical schools with better qualified medical staff. At the grassroots level, factory health stations are set up for outpatient and house-call service — as in Shanghai, an industrial city with numerous manufacturers to support its economy. Further, there are neighborhood health clinics and small communal hospitals at the community level, under which many home-care units or work-therapy stations are established.

While this sounds basically similar to the community psychiatric programs that have been developed in the United States, there are several characteristic differences. At the grassroots level, the clinics, home-care units, and work-therapy stations are closely associated with the neighborhood committee system. In the communist political organization and social system, street or neighborhood committees are established in each neighborhood. People working on the committee serve the multiple functions of political supervision, public health care, and social worker-like service. For instance, the single-child family planning carried out successfully in China basically relies on the street or neighborhood committee members, who work closely with each household to carry out their family plan. The staff takes an active role in referring mental health patients to the neighborhood health clinic or commune hospital and working closely with

the mental staff to provide follow-up care with family members.

After discharge from hospitals for acute and intensive care, severely ill mental patients continue to be cared for by home-care units (involving neighborhood committee members) or are referred to work-therapy stations. The work-therapy stations are established in each neighborhood in association with manufacturers. Simple manual work is programmed for the patients, so they can participate on a daily basis — folding matchboxes, making napkins, and so on. This offers a combination of social rehabilitation service and work therapy. So-called "work therapy" is different from the occupational therapy known in the Western psychiatric system. It is not so much a part of clinical assessment or a means for social rehabilitation as it is real work that requires the patient to participate and perform. It is based on the cultural concept that every person needs to work, that work is an important part of daily life — even for the mentally ill person. Furthermore, it is supported by communist political ideology that requires every member to make a contribution to the society as a whole. In Westerners' eyes, such expectations of work involvement by mentally disordered patients might be misinterpreted as "abuse." It needs to be understood from a different cultural perspective as work-focused therapy.

G. HOME-VISIT SERVICE IN MICRONESIA

The clinical home visit was a mainstay of general medical practice in earlier times, but has been discarded in psychiatry in most developed societies. Instead, patients are cared for only when they visit psychiatric facilities. However, old-style, house-call psychiatric service is still practiced in the island societies of Micronesia. Micronesia is composed of nearly 2000 tiny islands that are scattered between Hawaii and the Philippines, over an area about the size of the United States. There are usually only one or two psychiatrists, or a handful, at most, providing services for these widely scattered islands in the middle of the ocean. The only feasible way for psychiatrists to offer service is to periodically visit villages on one island, or on different — main and outer — islands. American cultural psychiatrist Larry Wilson (1980a), after working in Micronesia for more than a year, came to realize that this home-visit service was not only necessary, but, from a cultural perspective, it provided an opportunity to perform relevant and less biased clinical assessment in a home setting. Wilson (1980b) described the major thrust of the community-focused service as giving clinical consultations, and supervising and teaching local doctors and paraprofessionals about basic concepts of mental health and psychiatric care. Providing psychiatric assistance to courts and jails regarding psychiatrically disturbed people was another significant role for the psychiatrists serving the far-flung and sparsely populated islands of Micronesia.

IV. SUGGESTIONS FOR CLINICAL PRACTICE

A. RECOGNIZING SOCIOCULTURAL IMPACT ON THE PRACTICE OF PSYCHIATRY

Based on the information given earlier, several suggestions may be derived for clinicians in psychiatric practice. First, there is a need for full awareness that clinical work is not performed solely from a medical perspective. It is subject to a significant degree to various social and cultural variables. At a microscopic level, it is influenced by personal variables, including the belief and value systems of the patient, his family, and the therapist. At a macroscopic level, it is impacted by medical, social, and cultural factors. It allows the clinician to choose whether to follow or comply with, regulate, or alter such variables, if possible.

Related to this is that medical practice is not only designed for medical purposes, but also to meet the

needs of the cultural systems of the patient and the therapist. It is useful to know the cultural systems of both so that proper consideration can be given to how to best carry out medical practice, rather than following medical culture rigidly and inflexibly.

B. DEALING WITH AND MINIMIZING ANY NEGATIVE IMPACT OF CULTURAL FACTORS

Coupled with this is the need to know how culture influences psychiatric practice. Sometimes it is in a positive way, helping in the treatment and care of the patient; in other cases, the influence is negative, disrupting or even obstructing needed treatment. For example, a patient might believe strongly in the folk interpretation of soul loss and follow folk practices to regain his soul, refusing to take needed medication for a psychotic condition; or one might believe that his condition is due to a deficiency of vitality and be interested only in regaining his vitality rather than working on existing psychological conflicts. It is quite a challenge for clinicians to revise the concepts of problems and methods of treatment of the patient and his family in order to minimize the negative effects of their cultural beliefs.

C. ACCOMMODATING AND ADJUSTING TO CULTURAL DIFFERENCES

There is often a difference in cultural beliefs between the patient and the therapist, and it is important to resolve this cultural gap. Instead of an "I am right and your are wrong" approach, it is desirable to accommodate the differences, resolving them through reframing and reinterpretation of the issues concerned. For instance, if a patient is excessively or solely interested in regaining vitality, the theme of psychotherapy could be focused on how to regulate lifestyle, behavior patterns, and interpersonal relations so that the patient's "vitality" would not be wasted or lost unnecessarily. For a patient believing in soul loss, therapy could be conducted in such a way that it centered around regaining the lost soul by taking certain medications for the brain, changing certain behaviors, or minimizing certain stresses in life so that the returned soul would not be lost again easily. In other words, the medical goal of therapy could be approached without antagonizing the folk concepts. Folk concepts could be utilized or worked around, adjustments could be made in therapeutic skills by using culturally acceptable terminology, concepts, and views.

At the service level, it is crucial to take into consideration a client's cultural and linguistic characteristics. For instance, the use of a bilingual staff, providing service to walk-ins instead of following the appointment system rigidly, provision of educational and preventive programs, collaborations with traditional or faith healers, gaining cooperation and participation of local political and religious leaders, and so on often prove to be more beneficial to minority groups — as proposed by Abad, Ramos, and Boyce (1974) for delivery of service to Spanish-speaking minorities, for instrance.

D. Balance and Integration of Medical Goals and Cultural Implications

A judgement call is required to balance medical aims and cultural beliefs when there is a wide discrepancy or even antagonistic relations between them. A patient needing an amputation for medical reasons when he and his family oppose disconnecting a part of the body or a patient being forced to comply with an arranged marriage to please his parents when he feels unhappy about marrying a partner for whom he feels no affection are examples of such situations. In the first case, it might be proposed that the amputated extremity be preserved chemically until the patient dies and be buried with his body to satisfy the cultural belief that it is necessary to keep the whole physical body together for the next life. In the case of the arranged marriage, family sessions could be held to facilitate communication between the patient and his parents regarding their expectations and concerns, with the aim of working out a compromise that would satisfy both generations — psychological intervention for encountered problems. There are, in other words, many ways to work out discrepancies between cultural beliefs and practices and the aims of medical practice. With imagination, creativity, and effort, it is possible to resolve problems based on cultural understanding in relation to psychiatric practice.

E. Training of Various Health-Related Personnel for Transcultural Service

Finally, it must be emphasized that there is a need to train vaious health personnel, including physicians, nurses, social workers, clinical psychologists, and other health-related workers, on how to provide culturally sensitive, relevant, and effective medical and mental health service for patients of various ethnic/cultural backgrounds. There is an increased awareness that culture has a significant impact on various forms of healthcare delivery, including nursing (Davis, 1986), social work (Triseliotis, 1986), occupational therapy (Fitzgerald, Mullavey-O'Byrne, & Clemson, 1997), psychological assessment, and psychiatric work. Medical, psychiatric, and mental healthcare need to be delivered collaboratively by multiple personnel. Beginning with medical, nursing, social work, and occupational therapy students and psychological interns, such transcultural education is necessary to enhance the quality of healthcare. Lefley and Bestman (1991) suggested utilizing public–academic linkages to develop and improve culturally sensitive community mental health. Developing and providing adequate mental healthcare around the globe, particularly in the Third World, are challeges for modern mental health professionals (Lin, 1984).

REFERENCES

Abad, V., Ramos, J., & Boyce, E. (1974). A model for delivery of mental health services to Spanish-speaking minorities. *American Journal of Orthopsychiatry, 44*(4), 584–595.

Asuni, T. (1967). Aro Hospital in perspective. *American Journal of Psychiatry, 124*(6), 763–770.

Boroffka, A. (1973). *Management of madness: Past and present.* Film distributed by Kunz und Partner, Germany.

Boroffka, A. (1995–1996). Psychiatric care in Nigeria. *Psychopatholgie Africaine, 27*(1), 27–36.

Burke, A.W. (Ed.). (1984). Transcultural psychiatry: Racism and mental illness. *International Journal of Social Psychiatry, 30*(1&2). (30th anniversary double edition)

Castillo, R.J. (2001). Lessons from folk healings. In W.S. Tseng & J. Streltzer (Eds.), *Culture and psychotherapy: A guide to clinical practice* (pp. 81–101). Washington, DC: American Psychiatric Press.

Collins, D., Dimsdale, J.E., & Wilkins, D. (1992). Consultation-liaison psychiatric utilization patterns in different cultural groups. *Psychosomatic Medicine, 54*(2), 240–245.

Comas-Díaz, L. (1988). Cross-cultural mental health treatment. In L. Comas-Díaz & E. Griffith (Eds.), *Clinical guidelines in cross-cultural mental health* (pp. 335–361). New York: Wiley.

Davis, B.D. (1986). Culture and psychiatric nursing: Implications for training. In J.L. Cox (Ed.), *Transcultural psychiatry* (pp. 218–233). London: Croom Helm.

Desjarlais, R., Eisenberg, L., Good, B., & Kleinman, A. (1995). *World mental health: Problems in low-income countries.* New York: Oxford University Press.

Fitzgerald, M.H., Mullavey-O'Byrne, C., & Clemson, L. (1997). Cultural issues from practice. *Australian Occupational Therapy Journal, 44,* 1–21.

Flaskerud, J.H., & Hu, L.T. (1992). Racial/ethnic identity and amount and type of psychiatric treatment. *American Journal of Psychiatry, 149*(3), 379–384.

Griffith, M.S. (1977). The influences of race on the psychotherapeutic relationship. *Psychiatry, 40,* 27–40.

Jilek, W.G. (1993). Traditional medicine relevant to psychiatry. In N. Sartorius, G. De Girolamo, G. Andrews, & G.A. German (Eds.), *Treatment of mental disorders.* Washington, DC: American Psychiatric Press.

Kaplan, S., & Busner, J. (1992). A note on racial bias in the admission of children and adolescents to state mental health facilities versus correctional facilities in New York. *American Journal of Psychiatry, 149*(6), 768–772.

Lambo, T.A. (1966). The Village of Aro. In M. King (Ed.), *Medical care in developing countries. A symposium from Makerere.* London: Oxford University Press.

Leach, M.M., & Harbin, J.J. (1997). Psychological ethics codes: A comparison of twenty-four countries. *International Journal of Psychology, 32*(3), 181–192.

Lefley, H.P., & Bestman, E.W. (1991). Public-academic linkages for culturally sensitive community mental health. *Community Mental Health Journal, 27*(6), 473–487.

Lin, T.Y. (1984). Mental health and the third world: Challenges and hope. In R.C. Nann, D.S., Butt, & L. Ladrido-Ignacio, (Eds.), *Mental health, cultural values, and social development: A look into the 80s.* Dordrecht; The Netherlands: Reidel.

Littlewood, R. (1992). Psychiatric diagnosis and racial bias: Empirical and interpretative approaches. *Social Science and Medicine, 34,* 141–149.

Long, S.O. (1984). The sociocultural context of nursing in Japan. *Culture, Medicine and Psychiatry, 8*(2), 141–163.

Madhok, R., Bhopal, R.S., & Ramaiah, R.S. (1992). Quality of hospital service: A study comparing "Asian" and "non-Asian" patients in Middlesbrough. *Journal of Public Health Medicine, 14*(3), 271–279.

Neki, J.S., Joinet, B., Hogan, M., Hauli, J.G., & Kilonzo, G. (1985). The cultural perspective of therapeutic relationships: A viewpoint from Africa. *Acta Psychiatrica Scandinavica, 71,* 543–550.

Sabshin, M., Diesenhaus, H., & Wilkerson, R. (1970). Dimensions of institutional racism in psychiatry. *American Journal of Psychiatry, 127*(6), 787–793.

Siegel, J.M. (1974). A brief review of the effects of race in clinical service interactions. *American Journal of Orthopsychiatry, 44*(4), 555–562.

Steere, J., & Dowdall, T. (1990, March/April.). On being ethical in unethical places: The dilemmas of South African clinical psychologists. *Hasting Center Report,* pp. 11–15.

Thong, D. (1993). *A psychiatrist in paradise: Treating mental illness in Bali.* Bankok: White Lotus.

Triseliotis, J. (1986). Transcultural social work. In J.L. Cox (Ed.), *Transcultural psychiatry* (pp. 196–217). London: Croom Helm.

Tseng, W.S., Ebata, K., Kim, K.I., Krahl, W. Kua, E.K., Lu, Q.Y., Shen, Y.C., Tan, E.S., & Yang, M.J. in press. Mental health in Asia: Improvement and challenges. *International Journal of Social Psychiatry*

Well, K., Hough, R.L., Golding, J.M., Burnam, M.A., & Karno, M. (1987). Which Mexican-Americans underutilize health services? *American Journal of Psychiatry, 144*(7), 918–922.

Wen, J.K. (1990). The Hall of Dragon Metamorphoses: A unique indigenous asylum for chronic mental patients in Taiwan. *Culture, Medicine and Psychiatry, 14*(1), 1–19.

Wig, N.N. (1986). Anthropology and mental health: A view from the third world. In R. Rosenberg, F. Schulsinger, & E. Strömgren (Eds.), *Psychiatry and its related disciplines: The next 25 years. Plenary session papers from the World Psychiatric Association, Regional Symposium* (pp. 169–178). Copenhagen: World Psychiatric Association.

Wilson, L.G. (1980a). The clinical home visit in cultural psychiatry. *Journal of Operational Psychiatry, 11*(1), 27–33.

Wilson, L.G. (1980b). Community psychiatry in Oceania: Fifteen months' experience in Micronesia. *Social Psychiatry, 15,* 175–179.

World Health Organization (WHO) (1975). Mental health services in the developing countries. *WHO Chronicle, 29*(6), 231–235.

Xia, Z.Y. (1985). The mental health delivery system in Shanghai. In W.S. Tseng & D.Y.H. Wu (Eds.), *Chinese culture and mental health* (pp. 341–356). Orlando, FL: Academic Press.

31

Culture, Ethnicity, and Drug Therapy

I. INTRODUCTION

One of the most significant developments in the practice of psychiatry during the last half century has been the improvement in psychopharmacology. The availability of many effective drugs for the treatment of various mental disorders, including psychoses, mood disorders, and anxiety disorders, has remarkably changed the pattern of psychiatric care. From an academic point of view, psychiatry has entered the era of psychopharmacological treatment.

While drug therapy for mental disorders involves pharmacology, it also includes the psychology of prescribing and receiving medication. The two aspects exist side by side. The former is seen primarily from a biological perspective, potentially related to race or ethnicity in terms of genetic or biological factors. In contrast, the latter is mainly associated with psychological variables — involving the understanding, attitudes, expectations, and psychological reactions toward medication. It is therefore influenced by customs, beliefs, and values related to taking drugs, with much room for cultural impact. These two aspects are reviewed in this chapter.

II. ETHNICITY/RACE AS BIOLOGICAL VARIABLES

For some time, clinicians who have treated patients in multiethnic societies or in different countries have noticed that patients respond to psychotropic differently to the "formal" recommendations described for Caucasian patients. There has been speculation on the effect of race on drug treatment (Kalow, 1989; Murphy, 1969). This includes the therapeutic dose needed and the severity of side effects manifested by patients. However, it was only a little more than a decade ago that clinicians and researchers began empirical investigations on how people of different ethnic or racial backgrounds may respond differently to psychotropic. There have been remarkable findings revealed on this subject to support clinical experience. One of the pioneers in this field, American cultural psychiatrist K.M. Lin, and colleagues (Lin & Poland, 1995; Lin, Poland & Anderson 1995; Lin & Smith, 2000) have made several comprehensive reviews of psychopharmacotherapy in the context of culture and ethnicity that are very useful for updates on this matter.

In most of the literature that has appeared on this subject, the terms "ethnicity" and "race" have often been used interchangeably, and, customarily, "ethnicity" has been used more frequently. Because most of the studies dealt with interracial comparison (such as Caucasian vs Asian, or "White" vs "Black"), the term "race" was more appropriate, particularly regarding effects related to biological or genetic issues [cross-reference to Chapter 2: Culture and Society (Section I, A, 2 and 3)]. However, following the literature, and for the sake of simplicity, the term "ethnicity" will be used here.

A. Basic Concepts: Pharmacokinetics and Pharmacodynamics

Pharmacokinetics concern factors relating to absorption, distribution, metabolism, and excretion of the medicine administered. These factors together determine the process, fate, and disposition of drugs. Pharmacodynamics refer to how medicines work on target organ receptors to produce pharmacological effects. Through variations in both pharmacokinetics and pharmacodynamics, different drug reactions occur in different persons (interindividual variations) as well as among peoples of different ethnic or racial backgrounds (cross-ethnic/racial variations).

B. Genetic-Related Factors

It is becoming clearer to scholars that in the majority of genes, polymorphism is the rule rather than the exception. It assures the survival of any species and promotes its adaptation to the environment through biodiversity. Further, the frequency and distribution of alleles responsible for polymorphism often vary substantially across ethnic groups. Extensive polymorphism exists in genes governing pharmacokinetics and pharmacodynamics. Therefore, genetic factors may explain not only the interindividual variations but also the cross-ethnic variations in drug responses to a large extent (Lin, Poland, & Nakasaki, 1993).

Most of the drugs are metabolized via phase I and II enzymes. In phase I, mediated by one of more of the cytochrome P450 enzymes (CYPs), oxidation of the substrate takes place. In phase II, mediated by one of the transferases, conjugation occurs. The pharmacokinetics of most psychotropics depend on one or more of the CYP enzymes. The activity of CYP enzymes influences the tissue concentration of drugs significantly. Thus, it determines dose requirements and side effects of their substrates.

Significant genetic polymorphism exists in most of the CYPs, leading to extremely large variations in the activity of these enzymes in any given population as well as across populations of different ethnicities or races (Lin & Poland, 1995). The enzyme CYP2D6, for example, has more than 20 mutations that inactivate, impair, or accelerate its function; most of these mutant alleles are, to a large extent, ethnically specific.

For instance, allele *CYP2D6*4,* which leads to the production of defective proteins, is found in approximately 25% of Caucasians, but is rarely identified in other ethnic groups. This mutation is mainly responsible for the high rate of poor metabolizers in 5–9% of Caucasians, who are extremely sensitive to drugs metabolized by CYP2D6 (Lin & Smith, 2000). Extremely high frequencies of enzyme *CYP2D6*17* are found among people of African origin and of enzyme *CYP2D6*10* among those of Asian origin. Both of these alleles are associated with lower enzyme activities and slower metabolism of CYP2D6 substrates. It is speculated that this is in part responsible for slower pharmacokinetics profiles and lower therapeutic dose ranges observed in African-Americans regarding tricyclic antidepressants, and Asians regarding both antipsychotics and tricyclic antidepressants (Lin & Poland, 1995).

Another example is enzyme CYP2C19, which involves the metabolism of diazepam, tertiary tricyclic antidepressants, and citalopram, the new antidepressant. This enzyme also represents obvious cross-ethnic variations in addition to interindividual variations in drug metabolism. It has been demonstrated that up to 20% of east Asians (Chinese, Japanese, and Koreans) are poor metabolizers, compared to only 3 to 5%

of Caucasians. It has been found that two unique mutations are responsible for the enzyme deficiency: *CYP2C19*2* and *Cyp2C19*3*. The former can be found in all ethnic groups, but the latter appears to be specific to those with eastern Asian origins. The presence of mutation *3, together with a higher rate of *2, is explained as the cause for the higher rate of poor metabolizers among eastern Asians (Goldstein et al., 1997).

Thus, from recent studies, it has become clear to clinicians that genetic factors, associated with individual and ethnic background, contribute greatly to responses to medications. The variations exist as interindividual variations among the same ethnic group and also as variations among different ethnic groups. These two kinds of variations overlap, resulting in the total picture of variations. This is well illustrated by data obtained by Lin, Poland, Lau, and Rubin (1988) regarding the variability of haloperidol concentrations in normal volunteers after the administration of haloperidol (0.5 mg, im) to Caucasian and Asian subjects. As shown on Fig. 31-1, the graph indicates (1) substantial interindividual variability within each of the ethnic groups studied and, at the same time, (2) dramatic differences in the pharmacokinetics of haloperidol between the two ethnic groups examined, illustrating the overall overlap of the pharmacokinetics between the two groups.

C. NONGENETIC BIOLOGICAL FACTORS

It is important to know that numerous nongenetic biological factors significantly influence the expression of genes in the process of drug metabolization. For example, the activity of most cytochrome P450 enzymes declines significantly in the elderly, who are also likely to suffer from a progressive loss of neuron cells and receptors targeted by psychotropics (Salzman, 1984). Thus, the aged person becomes more sensitive to the effects of medication. Steroid hormones, including sex hormones, are known to be the sub-

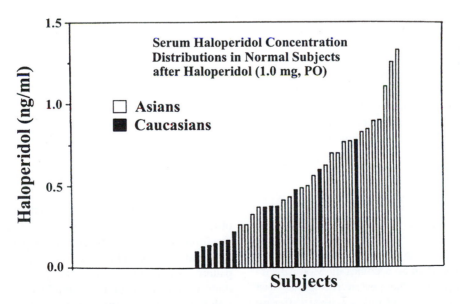

FIGURE 31-1 **Ethnic comparison of serum haloperidol concentration.** (From K.M. Lin et al., *Transcultural Psychiatric Research Review, 32*(1), 1995).

strates of some of the cytochrome P450 enzymes and have the capacity to alter the activity of these enzymes through competitive inhibition. Thus, gender is another biological factor that affects the pharmacodynamics of psychotropics.

Smoking, intake of certain foods, such as grapefruit juice, or high-protein and high-carbohydrate diets are all known to affect the activities of cytochrome P450 enzymes. Coupled with this is the interaction with herb medicines. Many herbs are natural substrates for the drug-metabolizing enzymes. Herb–drug interactions often exert significant impact on drug effects, which brings about clinically significant consequences, frequently unsuspected (Lin & Smith, 2000).

It is important to recognize that among the non-genetic factors, even though they are biological in nature, many are indirectly influenced by lifestyle, which, in turn, is closely related to social and cultural factors. This is particularly true regarding smoking, diet intake, or usage of herb medicines.

III. SOCIETY/CULTURE AS PSYCHOLOGICAL VARIABLES

Although the prescribing and intake of medicine seems primarily a psychopharmacological matter, and can be grasped from a biological perspective, it is actually a combination of biosociocultural phenomena, with are very much influenced by social and cultural dimensions (Smith, Lin, & Mendoza, 1993). This can be elaborated from several perspectives.

A. MEDICINE TAKING AS A PART OF ILLNESS BEHAVIOR

"Illness behavior" simply means how a person reacts and behaves when he becomes ill. More specifically, it includes how the person recognizes and interprets the discomfort and reacts against suffering when illness occurs; how he seeks help, care, or treatment from others; and how he reacts to the therapy

prescribed or treatment offered by healers, including compliance and adherence to therapy (cross-reference to Chapter 10: Illness Behavior: Reaction and Help-Seeking).

Several factors attribute to a patient's illness behavior regarding medicine taking:

1. General Understanding and Customary Behavior of Seeing Doctors

It is common in some societies, such as America, for a person who becomes sick to go to see his "family doctor" first and, unless he is referred to a specialist(s), he continues to see him. There is an unspoken understanding (or even agreement) that a patient sticks to one doctor and takes the medicine prescribed by him. If there is some concern about the medicine prescribed, the patient asks and negotiates with the doctor. In many other societies this is not necessarily the case. It is the patient's choice to shop around among doctors and change doctors if he or she is not satisfied with one; a patient often may see several doctors, either alternatively or simultaneously. In that case, he or she will receive medicine prescribed by these different doctors. It is a patient's own choice which medications he or she will take. There is no concept of only one doctor and drugs prescribed only by him. Neither is there any custom of faithfully taking whatever medicine the doctor prescribes.

2. General Medical Knowledge

Coupled with the choice of seeing multiple therapists and making one's own decisions regarding which medicines to take is the patient's medical knowledge (of his or her sickness) and the function and purpose of the medicine he or she is prescribed. Clearly there are different levels of sophistication in medical knowledge and "understanding" of illness that will shape the pattern of medicine taking. Taking a course of antibiotics to radically treat an infectious agent, or a mood stabilizer to prevent the occurrence of bipolar disorder, is a rather unfamiliar medical concept to people who tend to follow the practical rule of taking medicine only for suffering, and to discontinue it when the suffering disappears.

The etiological conceptions of illness vary greatly in different cultures and include supernatural, nature, biological, and psychological dimensions. The greater the disparity between contemporary scientific concepts of disease and the patient's folk medical beliefs about illness, the greater the likelihood of noncompliance (Ahmed, 2001).

3. Traditional Medicine Concepts and Belief

Laymen's medical knowledge is often influenced by traditional medical concepts and beliefs. This is particularly true if a society has a relatively well-established traditional medical system with a long history. If the traditional medicine holds the hot–cold theory of disease, for example, a layman will be concerned with whether his sickness is due to an excess of heat or cold and, accordingly, the medicine prescribed will be hot or cold in nature. The patient would certainly be reluctant to take medicine that is not compatible with his folk medical beliefs. Based on his traditional medical knowledge, if the patient interprets his sickness as derived from a loss of vitality and believes he needs a tonic or nutritious substance to correct his energy deficiency, he will not welcome medicine that has the side effect of making him feel "weak" rather than "strong" [cross-reference to Chapter 9: Mental Illness: Folk Categories and Explanation (Section III, A–C)].

B. Medicine and Mode of Administration

For various reasons, a patient may hold certain views about the medicine itself and the mode of administering it that it will greatly influence his or her medicine-taking behavior.

1. Medicine Itself

The physical character of medicine, such as its appearance (tablet, capsule, or liquid), color, size, amount, or taste often have different implications to different people concerning its potency or power. For instance, concerning color, white capsules are viewed by Caucasians as analgesics; by African-American as stimulants. However, black capsules are viewed by Caucasians as stimulants, and by African-Americans as analgesics (Buckalew & Caulfied, 1982).

Even the source of medicine — whether it is derived from plants, animals, or is synthetic — can have a psychological impact on a patient's response to it. For example, Muslims may not use alcohol-containing liquid medications; and Muslims and orthodox Jews may not use medications containing porcine products because of their religious proscriptions (Ahmed, 2001).

Associated with past historical experience, in India, "English" medicines may be viewed as being more potent than traditional Ayurvedic ones and, therefore, used only to a limited extent with the very young and the very old, who are considered too weak to tolerate the "English" medicines (Ahmed, in press). The same phenomenon is observed among many Chinese: the feeling that "Western" medicine is strong, but has too many harmful side effects, and should only be used for a short time for very serious illnesses, whereas traditional herb medicine is milder, but safe for long-term use.

2. Mode of Administration

In many societies, it is generally viewed that injectable agents, in contrast to oral, are more potent and have more immediate effects. For patients who need the assurance of immediate effects, injections are the mode of choice. Many hysterical patients respond well to the injection of just vitamins, particularly if a hot sensation occurs immediately after the injection. Fluid therapy satisfies patients and their families who believe that the body is weak and in need of "good" stuff.

C. Meaning of Medication

The giving and receiving of medications is not to be regarded simply as a biological event, but needs to be understood as a psychological interaction between the physician and the patient, with significant psychological meaning and implications. This can be elaborated from several perspectives.

1. From the Physician's Perspective

Beyond the simple reasons for treating a patient with medication, there are often psychological reasons that physicians prescribe medicine. Some of them are subtle, or unconscious, but some occur at the conscious level. Giving medicine usually represents concretely the physician's power to heal a sick person. It can also be the only remedy the physician can use symbolically when there is no alternative or more proper way to help the patient. This is also true when physicians are very much medically and biologically oriented and are not comfortable approaching, or are unable to approach, the patient regarding psychological aspects even when there is a need for such help. Quite commonly, when a physician is not sure of a patient's problem, but feels it is necessary to offer some kind of treatment, medication is the choice of action.

As indicated by Littlewood (1992) from his clinical experience in England and Lopez (1989) in America, African-American psychiatric patients tend to be diagnosed with more severe disorders (such as schizophrenia) compared to their Caucasian counterparts, and, as the clinical picture is often not "comprehendible" to the psychiatrist, more antipsychotics are prescribed. Closely associated with this, when the therapist has negative countertransference toward the patient under treatment, he may, subconsciously or even consciously, prescribe medication (or refuse to prescribe medication) for the patient as a way of expressing his negative feelings. This is particularly observed in cases of substance-abusing patients.

2. From the Patient's Perspective

There are many different psychological implications from the standpoint of the patient. Receiving medication may imply receiving "care" and "concern" from the therapist. It symbolizes love and attention from the caregiver, even though the patient may not actually take it. Sometimes, even when the medicine is stored in the medicine cabinet and never taken, the patient continues to demand a prescription from the physician, simply to assure himself that he is being given something — care and love. This is often observed in hypochondriacal patients or lonely elderly patients.

In other words, the giving and receiving of medication often has many psychological implications that are part of the physician–patient interaction. From this perspective, it needs particularly careful analysis and insightful understanding.

3. From the Health System's Perspective

The situation is often complicated further by the health care system, including service delivery patterns and payment systems. In many societies, there is no appointment system for psychiatric visits. Also, there is often a shortage of psychiatrists for the many patients who visit the clinics daily. In order to deal with many patients that need to be seen within a limited time in the outpatient clinic, sometimes giving only several minutes per patient is the only practical solution. Under such conditions, prescribing medication rather than offering talk therapy becomes the only choice for the psychiatrists. Even before the patient sits down, before he has started making any complaints, the psychiatrist is already filling out a prescription. This is not an unusual situation in developing societies (Nunley, 1996).

Closely related is the existing payment system. In many societies, medical regulation as well as customary expectation is that the physician (or hospital or clinic) may charge the patient for medicine, but not for the time the physician spends talking to the patient. Such a system encourages psychiatrists to prescribe medicine rather than to spend time listening and talking to the patient. This certainly affects the pattern of medical practice, particularly regarding the giving and receiving of medication in psychiatric work.

IV. SUMMARY NOTES

It has been elaborated that in psychiatric practice, the giving and receiving of medication involves various factors, including biological (either genetic or nongenetic related) and psychological ones. These factors together affect the total process and function of medication.

It has been described that even with genetically related biological factors there are multiple variations at the interpersonal as well as the interethnic/racial level. Clearly there are distinct differences among people of different ethnic and/or racial backgrounds, but such diversity has superimposed on it interindividual diversity. This is also true of the psychological aspects of medication. Therefore, as pointed out by Lin and Smith (2000), "stereotypical interpretations of culture and ethnic differences in either psychological or biological characteristics are not only misleading but also potentially divisive and dangerous."

REFERENCES

Ahmed, I. (2001). Psychological aspects of giving and receiving medications. In W.S. Tseng & J. Streltzer (Eds.), *Culture and psychotherapy: A guide for clinical practice* (pp. 123–134). Washington, DC: Amercian Psychiatric Press.

Buckalew, L.W., & Caulfied, K.E. (1982). Drug expectations associated with perceptual characteristics: Ethnic factors. *Perceptual and Motor Skills, 55,* 915–918.

Goldstein, J.A., Ishizaki, T., Chiba, K., de Morais, S.M., Bell, D., Krahn, P., & Evans, D.A. (1997). Frequencies of the defective CYP2C19 alleles responsible for themephenyton poor metabolizer phenotype in various Oriental, Caucasian, Saudi Arabian and American black populations. *Pharmacogenetics, 7,* 59–64.

Kalow, W. (1989). Race and therapeutic drug response. *New England Journal of Medicine, 320,* 588–589.

Lin, K.M., & Poland, R.E. (1995). Ethnicity, culture, and psychopharmacology. In F.E. Bloom & D.I. Kupfer (Eds.), *Psychopharmacology: The fourth generation of progress.* New York: Raven Press.

Lin, K.M., Poland, R.E., & Anderson, D. (1995). Psychopharmacology, ethnicity and culture. *Transcultural Psychiatric Research Review, 32,* 3–40.

Lin, K.M., Poland, R.E., Lau, E.K., & Rubin, R.T. (1988). Haloperidol and prolactin concentrations in Asians and Caucasians. *Journal of Clinical Psychopharmacology, 8,* 195–201.

Lin, K.M., Poland, R.E., & Nakasaki, G. (Eds.). (1993). *Psychopharmacology and psychobiology of ethnicity.* Washington, DC: American Psychiatric Press.

Lin, K.M., & Smith, M.W. (2000). *Psychopharmacotherapy in the context of culture and ethnicity* (Vol. 19). Washington, DC: Amercian Psychiatric Press.

Littlewood, R. (1992). Psychiatric diagnosis and racial bias: Empirical and interpretative approaches. *Social Science and Medicine, 34,* 141–149.

Lopez, S.R. (1989). Patient variable biases in clinical judgement: Conceptual overview and methodological considerations. *Psychological Bulletin, 106,* 184–203.

Murphy, H.B.M. (1969). Ethnic variations in drug responses. *Transcultural Psychiatric Research Review, 6,* 6–23.

Nunley, M. (1996). Why psychiatrists in India prescribe so many drugs. *Culture, Medicine and Psychiatry, 20*(2), 165–197.

Salzman, C. (1984). *Clinical geriatric psychopharmacology.* New York: McGraw-Hill.

Smith, M., Lin, K.M., & Mendoza, R. (1993). "Nonbiological" issues affecting psychopharmacotherapy: Cultural considerations. In K.M. Lin, R.E. Poland, & G. Nakasaki (Eds.), *Psychopharmacology and psychobiology of ethnicity* (pp. 37–58). Washington, DC: American Psychiatric Press.

Section F
Culture and Psychological Therapy

Improvements in cultural psychiatry and an increased awareness of the importance of providing culturally oriented clinical care have led to a concern with how to conduct culturally relevant psychological therapy in accordance with patients' cultural backgrounds.

Thus, in this section, the subject of "culture and psychotherapy" is elaborated in considerable detail. First, various modes of psychotherapy, from indigenous to modern, are reviewed and discussed by dividing them into three subgroups: "culture-embedded" indigenous healing practices (Chapter 32), "culture-influenced" unique psychotherapies (Chapter 33), and "culture-related" common therapies (Chapter 34). Psychotherapy is defined broadly from various cultural perspectives, and different modes of practice, including folk healing, laymen-designed unique therapies, and professional mainstream therapies, are subgrouped according to the nature and degree of the impact of culture upon them. Following this panoramic view of various modes of healing practices

[Note: Part of the material in this section has been published by Tseng (1999), Culture and psychotherapy: Review and practical guidelines. *Transcultural Psychiatry, 36*(2), 131–179.]

is a systematic comparison of their therapeutic orientations, operations, mechanisms, and goals at the end of Chapter 34.

Chapter 35 reviews psychotherapeutic practices in various sociocultural settings in the East and West. It further illustrates how the development of psychotherapy has been influenced by various historical, social, political, economic, and cultural factors in addition to medical knowledge and theories.

Intercultural psychotherapy is reviewed and discussed in Chapter 36. Intercultural psychotherapy refers to therapeutic situations in which the therapist and the patient have significant cultural differences — a practical clinical reality that has become more significant in a modern world characterized by increased interethnic and transcultural contact. It is a clinical situation that demands the detailed examination and elaboration of cultural considerations.

Finally, in Chapter 37, culture-relevant psychotherapy is examined on three levels: operational adjustment, theoretical modification, and philosophical reconsideration. Areas that demand attention in order to carry out culture-effective therapy are examined from a clinical perspective, and requirements for culture-competent psychotherapy are suggested.

32

Culture-Embedded Indigenous Healing Practices

I. WHAT ARE INDIGENOUS HEALING PRACTICES?

Folk healing practices are nonorthodox therapeutic practices based on indigenous cultural traditions and operating outside official health care systems. The practices are often validated by experience, but are not founded on logico-experimental science (Jilek, 1993, 1994). Indigenous healing practices are observed in various societies, particularly so-called "primitive" or "preindustrialized" societies, but they can be observed in modern or developed societies as well. The words "culture embedded" are used in the title of this chapter to indicate that these healing practices are intensely embedded in the cultural systems in which they developed and in which they are practiced. They are, therefore, often difficult to transplant to entirely different cultural settings, where they are viewed differently. The nature and degree of cultural impact on healing practices are further indicated by the adjectives "culture influenced," and "culture related," used in the following two chapters to elaborate unique psychotherapy and common psychotherapy, respectively.

While indigenous healing practices function in general as healing methods for "problems," they are not usually considered by either the healer or the clients to be "psychological therapy" for emotional disorders or psychological problems. Rather, they are recognized as religious ceremonies or healing exercises related to supernatural or natural powers. However, from a mental health point of view, indigenous healing practices often produce psychotherapeutic effects and may be studied as "folk psychotherapy." Originally, anthropologists studied folk healing practices as a part of cultural behavior. Recently, cultural psychiatrists have become interested in examining indigenous healing practices from clinical perspectives. The goals of study are to explore the similarities and differences between folk healing practices and modern psychotherapy, and to disclose the therapeutic mechanisms operating in and being utilized by indigenous healing practices.

Various practices are covered by the loosely defined term, indigenous or folk healing. If a healing practice is closely related to religion, it may be called a "religious healing practice" or a "healing ceremony"; if the healing practice involves the mediumship of spirit, it may be called "spirit mediumship," or "shamanism." Divination or various kinds of fortune-telling, including astrology or physiognomy, may be used to solve psychological problems or to seek answers for life problems and, therefore, can be viewed as folk counseling practices, as well. Further, the practice of meditation, a self-training exercise used to obtain tranquility and growth of mind and to prevent emotional problems, can be considered a folk healing practice if one defines "psychotherapy" very broadly, as not only treating a person's suffering, but also preventing problems and improving the quality of a person's mental life (Prince, 1980). A traditional or herb medical person, often believed to be authorized or empowered by supernatural, magical, or ancestral forces and, in addition to prescribing herb medicine, offers psychologically implicated help to the client, is considered a "medicine man" (Jilek, 1993).

Among magico-religious practitioners, anthropologist Winkelman (1992) distinguishes shamans, shaman/healers, healers, mediums, priests, and sorcerer/witches according to psychological and sociological variables. Shamanism is a particular form of spirit mediumship in which a specialist (the shaman), as a medium, is considered to be possessed by a spirit and to serve as a means of communication between human beings and the spirit world (Firth, 1964). The term shamanism was initially used in a restricted sense, referring to a special kind of religious-healing practice that originated and was prevalent in the northeast region of Asia; today, the term is used broadly, referring to any healing practice that involves spirit mediumship. According to anthropologists (Lessa & Volt, 1965), shamanism tends to predominate in food-gathering cultures, where the shaman most frequently performs a curing rite for the benefit of one or more patients. Thus, shamanistic rites are not calendrical, but are contingent upon mishaps and illness. Priests and priestly cult organizations, however, are characteristically found in the more structurally elaborate food-producing (agricultural) societies, where the common ceremony is a public rite performed for the benefit of a whole village or community. Such rites are often calendrical, or performed at critical points in the ecological cycle (Turner, 1972). As part of the reli-

gious rite, a healing ceremony may be performed by the priest for members of the society who need it. While typology for various practices can be defined for the sake of discussion, in reality, there is always some transition or overlapping among various types of practices.

Although indigenous healing practices are found mainly in preindustrial societies, that does not mean they do not exist in developed societies. In fact, supernaturally oriented folk healing practices abound in industrial societies, no matter what medical or legal attitudes exist toward them. For instance, in the United States, R.C. Ness and Wintrob (1981) have described various folk healing practices utilized by different cultural groups within the society. Jilek (1978, 1982) pointed out that there is recent evidence of the revival of indigenous therapeutic ceremonies among various groups of North American Indians. The reasons are numerous. Indigenous healing ceremonies serve as cultural symbols of a group's ethnic identity and sense of superiority. They point to the inadequacy of Western medicine and health care, not only in terms of quantity, but also in its lack of holistic concepts and practices. Hall and Bourne (1973) reported that in an urban black community in the South, various forms of indigenous therapies, such as faith healing, magic vendors, root doctors, and neighborhood prophets, can be identified. In contemporary communist China, although religion is discouraged and "superstitious" folk healing practices are suppressed, "witch doctors" are still found, particularly in rural areas (Li & Philips, 1990).

No matter what terms are used, "indigenous healing practices" share certain common denotations. They are invented and utilized by local people for the purpose of solving problems or treating suffering — therefore, they are called "indigenous" in contrast to "universal." Because they are distinctly different from modern (Western or orthodox) professional medical approaches, they are called "folk" practices. Most are supernaturally orientated and remote from any "scientific" orientation. These indigenous practices are usually rooted in traditional beliefs and folk interpretations of problems and, thus, are closely related to cultural beliefs.

Most initial studies of indigenous healing practices were carried out by anthropologists as a part of their field work. Since the 1950s, these practices have attracted a great deal of attention among clinicians. Many psychiatrists have shown an interest in studying indigenous healing practices as well. Jerome D. Frank's book, *Persuasion and Healing* (1961), Ari Kiev's *Magic, Faith, and Healing* (1964), and E. Fuller Torrey's *Witchdoctors and Psychiatrists* (1986) are among the well-known publications dealing with this landmark exploration.

Based on their core nature and basic therapeutic orientation, an attempt has been made to subdivide various practices observed in different societies into different categories (Tseng & Hsu, 1979): supernatural orientation (such as spirit mediumship, religious healing ceremonies, and divination), nature orientation (such as fortune-telling, astrology, and meditation), medical–physiological orientation (such as Mesmerism, acupuncture, and herb medicine), and sociopsychological orientation (such as Zen training, Alcoholics Anonymous, est, and most modern psychotherapy). It is recognized that such subdivisions are arbitrary and often overlap. However, they will help us understand various healing practices that exist on a spectrum, which includes the supernatural, natural, physiological, and psychological. This chapter focuses on indigenous healing practices that are basically supernaturally or naturally oriented.

II. SUBDIVISION OF VARIOUS HEALING PRACTICES

A. SPIRIT MEDIUMSHIP (TRANCE-BASED HEALING SYSTEM)

Spirit mediumship broadly refers to a situation in which a healer or a client, or both, experiences altered states of consciousness in the form of dissociation or possession at the time of the healing ritual. Three patterns are recognized, depending on who is dissociated or possessed. In shamanism, it is the healer who experiences the dissociated or possessed state. He is thought to be possessed by a supernatural being and under the influence of a supernatural power, which enables him to provide the service of healing. The proven authority of the healer with supernatural power is the main force of the therapeutic mechanism. In contrast to this, in *zar* ritual, both the healer and the client experience altered states of consciousness. With assistance from the healer, the client, in a dissociated state, expresses his or her desire for fulfillment. Gratification of attention and wish fulfillment are the essential mechanisms for healing. In a special religious healing practice observed in the Salvation Cult in Japan, it is only the client (a cult member) who is trained to experience the altered state of consciousness. With the assistance of the healer, the client explains the cause of his problem and offers a suggestion for its resolution. Thus, from a psychotherapeutic point of view, it is important to distinguish which person is in an altered state of consciousness because the mechanism of therapy differs according to who is dissociated or possessed.

1. The Healer Goes into a Trance or Is Possessed — Shamanism

It is speculated that the geographic heartland of shamanism is central and northern Eurasia, with widespread diffusion to southeast Asia and the Americas (Prince, 1980). Through a religious ceremony, a shaman can work himself or herself into a trance state in which he or she is "possessed" by a god (see Fig. 32-1). Rhythmic singing, dancing, or praying (quiet meditation) seems to assist the self-induction of the trance state. Among native healers in North and South America, a psychedelic substance (such as cactus) is frequently used to induce an altered state of consciousness, and there is a special psychic experience in a peyotism cult (Dobkin, 1968; W. La Barre, 1947). Whether substance- or self-induced, the shaman enters into an ecstatic trance in a healing ceremony. In some cultures, this is not defined as being "possessed" by a supernatural entity; it is merely believed that the shaman is able to link up with the supernatural and work through its pow-

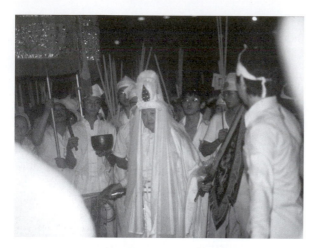

FIGURE 32-1   Chinese-Singaporean woman shaman dressed and behaving as if she were possessed by Guanyin Bhudda (goddess of mercy) for healing practices. [Courtesy of Woon Tai-Hwang, M.D.].

ers (see Figs. 32-2 and 32-3). The client can then consult the supernatural through the shaman for instructions on dealing with his or her problems.

The causes of problems are usually interpreted according to the folk concepts of the culture — involving such things as loss of the soul, sorcery, spirit intrusion, or violation of taboos. The dishar-

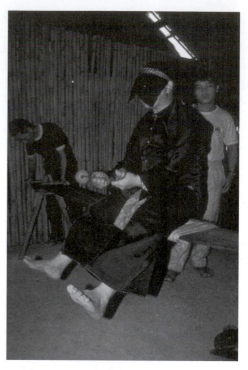

FIGURE 32-2   Hmong shaman in Laos traveling ("riding" a "horse") to the spirit world to retrieve a client's lost soul. [Courtesy of Wolfgang Jilek, M.D.].

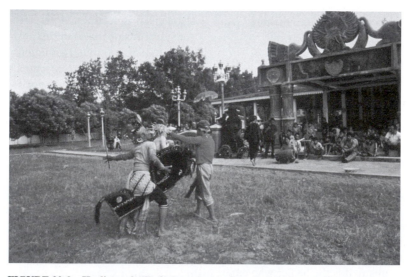

FIGURE 32-3   Healing cult *(Kuda Lumping)* in Java, Indonesia. A participant in a possession-trance state performing a "horse dance." [Courtesy of Wolfgang Jilek, M.D.].

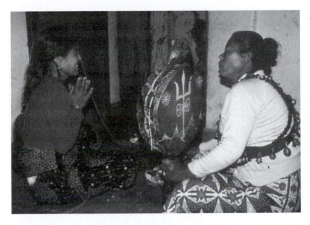

FIGURE 32-4 *Tamang* **shamaness in Nepal.** A shamaness (sitting on the right) treating a depressed patient with suggestive chanting and rhythmic drumming. [Courtesy of Wolfgang Jilek, M.D.].

mony with nature that is the basis of the concept of *feng sui* (geomatic belief) is often interpreted as the cause of problems by Chinese shamans. Coping methods suggested are usually magical in nature, including prayer (see Fig. 32-4), the use of charms, the performance of extraction, exorcism, or other therapeutic ritual ceremonies. The goal of the healing practice is to resolve the client's problems. Utilizing supernatural powers, acting as an authority figure, making suggestions, and providing hope are among the main healing mechanisms provided by the shaman.

The healing ceremony may be performed semiprivately at a shaman's own residence or at a public place so that not only the client and his family may attend and participate, but friends and neighbors (including children) as well (see Figs. 32-5a and 32-5b). In this way, people become more familiar with the service. Also, the therapeutic effects of the ceremony tend to be increased by the direct involvement of family and neighbors. The shaman may conduct a certain ceremony that has a symbolic but significant therapeutic function (see Fig. 32-5c).

The shaman, in the way as other supernaturally oriented indigenous healers, often performs a special ceremony to impress the people in the community that he

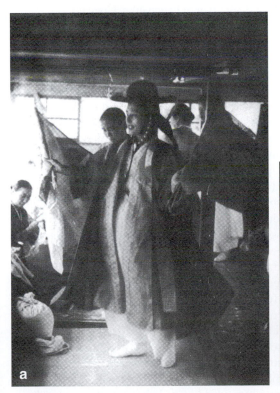

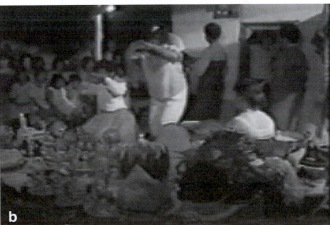

FIGURE 32-5 **Woman shaman in Korea.** (a) A woman shaman performing a healing ceremony during a trance state. From *Six Korean Shamans,* by Y.S. Kim Harvey, Ph.D. St. Paul: West Publishing Company, 1979. (b) Two women clients praying while the ceremony was observed by family members and neighbors. [Courtesy of Kwang-Iel Kim, M.D.]. *(Figure continues)*

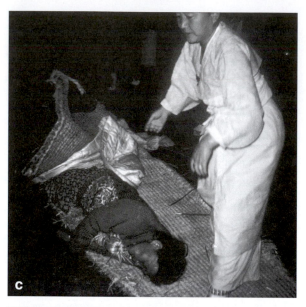

FIGURE 32-5 (continued)   (c) Conducting a "funeral" ceremony as (counter-phobic) therapy for a woman patient preoccupied with the fear that she might die. [Courtesy of Laurel Kendall, Ph.D.].

or she is blessed with supernatural powers. For instance, a shaman may use a specially designed instrument with which to injure his or her body to show that there are no ill-effects or he may undertake a dangerous action to demonstrate that he or she is protected by a supernatural power and comes to no harm (see Figs. 32-6a–32-6c).

In response to the question of whether indigenous healers, or shamans, are psychologically marginal or abnormal, several investigators conducted a study of healers, their personal backgrounds, how they became shamans, and whether they had any special qualities that allowed them to function as healers. For instance, Sasaki (1969), in Japan, studied extensively the way in which shaman candidates achieved their first experiences of spirit possession. He found that their initial experiences occurred in two ways: more than 80% through the process of self-training (shugyo) and the rest as part of a psychopathological breakdown. Tseng (1972) conducted personal interviews with several shamans in Taiwan, elaborating how a shaman's personal psychology and dynamic interplay with society enables him to become a shaman. Korean-American

anthropologist Y.S. Kim Harvey (1979) reported that in earlier times in Korea, shamanism was a male-centered activity. After its official suppression in the Yi dynasty, it was forced underground and the shamanic role was taken over by women. K.I. Kim (1973) pointed out that, according to tradition, certain individuals are predestinated to become shamans, and this destiny is often manifested by "psychiatric" problems, which are regarded as sin-byong (spirit sickness) within the shamanic world. From a psychiatric point of view, sin-byong could be regarded as depression, anxiety, or even hysterical psychoses (Prince, 1992). The only way a potential shaman will recover from this spirit sickness is by beoming a shaman. Based on her field work in Korea, American anthropologist L. Kendall (1985, 1988), reported that the role of a shaman is regarded as a mixed blessing in Korea. Women shamans enjoy considerable prestige and power within the female Korean world and are often quite wealthy. However, a family is often ashamed to have a daughter who is a shaman. Also, women shamans tend to dominate their households and their husbands are sheepish about having shamans as wives.

Anthropologist Ward (1980) observed that dissociation (and/or possession) could be either ritual or pathological from the point of view of normality versus psychopathology. Also, in relation to culture, a distinction can be made between central or peripheral types. The ritual (or central) type occurs to a person (such as a priest) during a religious ritual. The person can induce and terminate the dissociative condition voluntarily; with this control, it is not pathological. The dissociated person is usually a respected member of society who tries to reinforce central cultural values through the ritual. In contrast, the pathological (or peripheral) type is a person without full control whose dissociation is manifested in reaction to an emotional crisis or as part of an illness; therefore, it is labeled pathological. The dissociated person in this case is usually a culturally marginal person, viewed by other members of the society as peripheral. Although this distinction is very useful, caution is needed when saying that the person dissociated for the purpose of healing or ritual is usually a respected person. Depending on how the folk healing

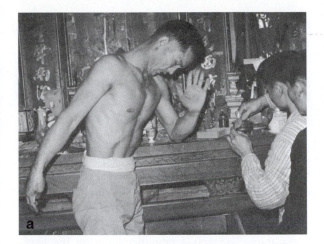

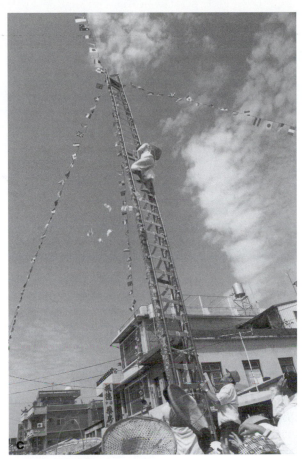

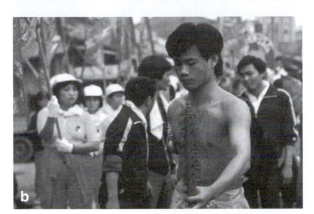

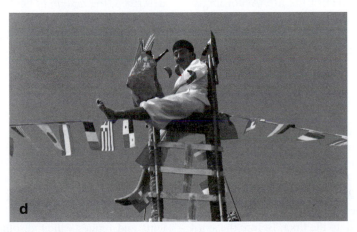

FIGURE 32-6   Chinese indigenous healers in Taiwan. (a) A male shaman performing a healing practice in front of a family altar for many hours while in a trance state. [From *God, Ghosts, and Ancestors,* by David K. Jordan, Ph.D. Los Angeles: University of California Press, 1972.] (b) A shaman hitting his body with a needled club, showing he is blessed because he comes to no harm. [Courtesy of Jung-Kuang Wen, M.D.] (c) A Daoist priest-healer performing a ceremony by climbing up a specially designed "knife ladder," showing he is blessed by not being injured when he steps on the sharp knife blades, which serve as rungs on the ladder. (d) Sitting on top of a four-story-high "knife ladder," the priest is requesting the blessing of the god in the heaven. [From *Chinese Time Post* — photos taken by a reporter, Mr. Gong-Yi Lin. Courtesy of Jung-Kuang Wen, M.D.].

is officially viewed by the society, the healers are sometimes physically or mentally handicapped or marginal members of the society. In those cases, the performance of the healing practice relies greatly on an assistant, who carries out the work of interpretation and makes suggestions, with the shaman playing a merely symbolic role.

2. The Healer and Participant both Fall into Trances — *Zar* Ceremonies

The term *zar* refers to a ceremony as well as a class of spirits. As pointed out by Prince (1980), *zar* rituals are observed primarily in Muslim societies in the Mideast, including Ethiopia, Egypt, Iraq, Kuwait, Sudan, and Somaliland. Modarressi (1968) described the *Zar* cult in south Iran. *Zar* ritual is different from shamanism in that, in addition to the healer, the client also experiences the dissociated or possessed state.

Kennedy (1967) gave a clear picture of the *zar* ceremony practiced by Egyptian Nubians. He pointed out that the ceremony is essentially a means of dealing with the demonic power of evil (*zar* spirit) that may cause an illness. The local people believe that a demon can indeed cause a disorder, and the patient becomes inextricably associated with that particular spirit for the rest of his life. Accordingly, the patient has the responsibility of satisfying the *zar* spirit with a special performance at least once a year and is obligated to attend the *zar* ceremonies of others.

The *zar* ceremony is primarily a female activity. All of those attending wear new or clean clothing to please the spirits. The main patient usually wears a white gown, as much gold jewelry as possible, and is heavily perfumed. The ceremony master (the *shekha,* if female, or *sheikh,* if male) begins the ceremony with a song and drumming. When a spirit associated with some person in the audience is called, that person begins to shake in her seat, dancing and trembling until she falls, exhausted, to the floor. Before the spirit consents to leave, it usually demands special favors, such as jewelry, new clothing, or expensive foods. It is the duty of the relatives and friends to gather around

the prostrate woman and pacify the spirit. The whole tone of the ceremony is one of propitiation and persuasion rather than coercion. The ceremony ends with an animal sacrifice and a feast.

As Kennedy pointed out, the *zar* ceremony is primarily an adult female activity reflecting Nubian social conditions of sex separation, low female status, restriction of women from religious participation, an unbalanced sex ratio, marital insecurity, and relative isolation. The *zar* ceremony provides Nubian women an ideal situation for relief of persistent and regular anxieties and tensions arising from their life conditions. The goods demanded during the ceremony are all things that their husbands should provide. The ceremony fulfills a woman's wish for attention and care. Emotional catharsis, fulfillment of unsatisfied desires, and compensation for the suppressed female role are some of the therapeutic mechanisms working in this kind of therapeutic ritual. Restoring balance in real life is the implict goal of this culture-embedded healing practice (El-Islam, 1967; El Sendiony, 1974).

There are many trance-based healing systems in which both the healer (cult leader) and the participant (client) go into a trance or possession state during the healing practice. In addition to the Zar cult just described, the *umbanda* healing cult in Brazil (Figge, 1975) (see Fig. 32-7) and *voodoo* practice in Haiti (see Fig. 32-8) are some other examples.

3. The Client Goes into a Trance — Salvation Cult

A unique pattern of trance-based healing cults observed in Japan was reported by Lebra (1976). During the healing ceremony, the client (usually female) is the person who goes into a trance or possessed state, taking the role of a supernatural "other." During the altered state of consciousness, with close assistance or suggestions from the healer, the client reveals her problems and requests their resolution. It is interesting to note that it is the client, as a cult member, who is coached by the cult master to perform self-analysis and provide suggestions for the resolution of her problems.

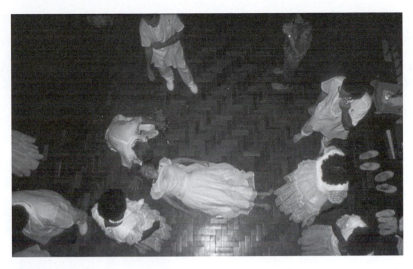

FIGURE 32-7 *Umbanda* healing cult, Rio de Janeiro, Brazil. Participants lying on the floor in a deep trance state. [Courtesy of Wolfgang Jilek, M.D.].

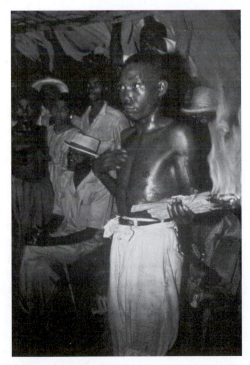

FIGURE 32-8 *Voodoo* healer *(Houngan)* in a trance in Haiti. [Courtesy of Wolfgang Jilek, M.D.].

The opportunity for catharsis, revealing of internal conflict, and gratification of needs are some of the mechanisms operating in this unique form of trance-based healing practice. It should be pointed out that this kind of healing cult (in the same way as the Zar ceremony) works in a society in which the females are suppressed by the males. The goals of the practice are to provide compensatory mechanisms and to restore balance in the client's life through a supernatural system.

B. RELIGIOUS HEALING CEREMONIES

A distinction needs to be made between religion and a religious healing ceremony. Religion refers to a system of belief in a divine or superhuman power or spiritual practice. As part of a religion, some people may perform special ceremonies for the purpose of healing certain problems or disorders. Thus, a religious system and religious healing should not be confused (Ponce, 1995).

There are various kinds of religious healing ceremonies observed in different societies that are considered by mental health workers to serve a therapeutic function for their participants. Leighton and Leighton (1941) studied a religious healing ceremony practiced by the Navahos, the largest Indian tribe in the United States, and pointed out that assurance and suggestions are among the therapeutic mechanisms operating in the ceremony.

Concerning specific healing rituals, Jilek (1974, 1976, 1982) reported on Salish-speaking Indians of the Pacific Coast of North America who practice a unique spirit dancing ceremony. In the initiation process to the spirit dance the novice is expected to experience his/her symbolic death and rebirth into a healthier, culture-congenial life. Physiological and psychological means are utilized to induce altered states of consciousness and achieve personality depatterning and subsequent resynthesis and reorientation. These include surprise shocks, kinetic and sensory overstimulation, especially by loud rhythmic drumming; followed by immobilization and sensory deprivation, fasting and thirst, alternated with dancing, physical training and hardening; and finally cultural indoctrination.

Prince (1975) described a sacrificial ritual observed in Yoruba, Africa. Closely related to divination (called *Ifa*), a person's problems were identified by palm nuts tossed by the diviner. It was usually interpreted that the person or a member of his family had offended the family *orisa* (the lineage deity) or some other spirit. Then, the sacrifice of a certain animal was prescribed for resolution. In the sacrifice, the supplicant passed his bad luck or illness to the animal, and the animal was killed in the supplicant's stead. In his observation, Prince emphasized that the healing power of the ritual was in its reassurance and generation of conviction. The ritual dramatically confirmed the worldview shared by the healer and the patient; the illness was shown to make sense in the context of that culture's particular healing myths; and the ritual demonstrated that proper curative steps were being taken.

In India, during the Hindu Thaipusam ceremonial, selected supplicants will go into a trance state and put needles or hooks over their bodies to show that they are blessed by god and, at the same time, to receive (treatment) benefits through the supernatural power.

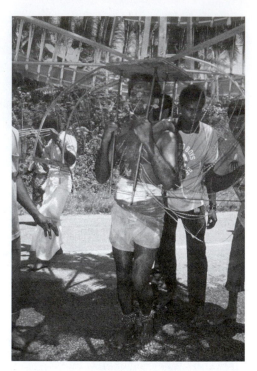

FIGURE 32-9 A Hindu *thaipusam* ceremony in Malaysia. A supplicant undergoing an ordeal in a trance for therapeutic purposes. [Courtesy of Wolfgang Jilek, M.D.].

This religious ceremony is observed among Hindu people living in Malaysia, as well (see Fig. 32-9).

Cultural psychiatrist Sangun Suwanlert (1997) from Thailand described *the phan yak* chanting treatment for the purpose of *sa dor kro* (to let go of bad things). Based on the concept that evil spirits cause any kind of mental disturbances, religious healing ceremonies are occasionally held in temples for exorcism and purification. The treatment ceremony is announced beforehand, and all Buddhists are invited to participate. Often several hundred or even a thousand believers will gather in the temple for the occasion. White sacred threads hang in the courtyard (see Fig. 32-10a). All participants sit and hold the sacred threads as well as a lotus — the symbol of Buddha. The ceremony begins with a spokesman talking about Lord Buddha, the doctrine, and the order. Then several monks together start to chant in a high, eerie tone at a slow speed that can be

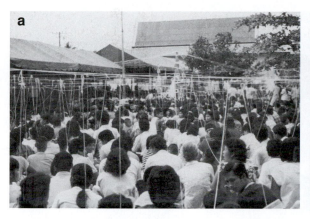

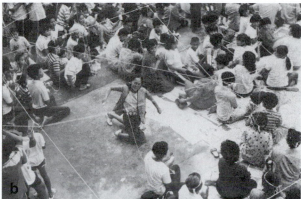

FIGURE 32-10 *Phan Yak* **chanting treatment ceremony in Thailand.** (a) Participants holding a sacred thread in a Buddhist temple to get in touch with a supernatural power for treatment. (b) One of the participants (center) fell into convulsion-like behavior, indicating that her evil spirit was being chased away by the monk's chanting. [Courtesy of Sangun Suwanlert, M.D.].

frightening. Some of the participants begin to fall into trance states, manifesting peculiar behavior, including trembling, jerking, and convulsions (see Fig. 32-10b). This is interpreted as the evil spirit being chased away by the monk's chanting. After a while, the monks pour sacred water over the affected persons so they will regain their normal status.

Traditional opium-detox treatment has been observed in Thailand as well as Laos (Jilek, 1994; Jilek-Aall & Jilek, 1985). Among hill tribes in Laos, where opium was cultivated regularly as a crop, addicted patients were asked to make offerings to the opium goddess and take sacred vows to abstain from opium abuse (see Fig. 32-11). In Thailand, treatment

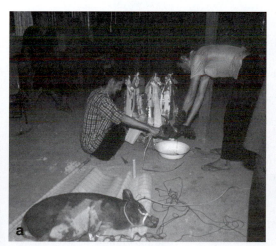

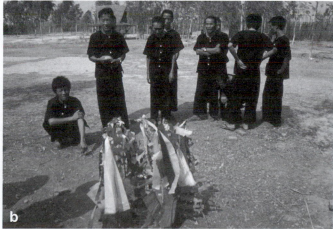

FIGURE 32-11 **Laotian Hill tribe's traditional opium-detox treatment.** (a) A sacrificial offering to the opium goddess. (b) Taking a sacred vow to abstain in front of a model of the palace of the opium goddess. [Courtesy of Wolfgang Jilek, M.D.].

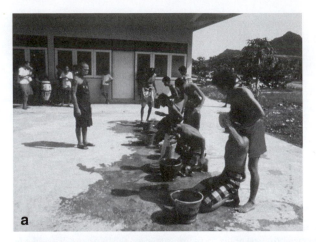

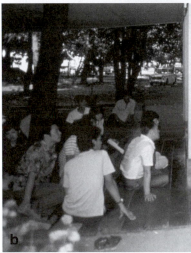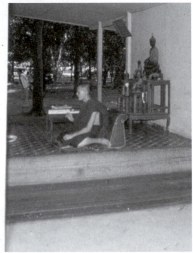

FIGURE 32-12   Treatment of drug addicts at a Buddhist temple in Thailand. (a) Performance of "purification" by herb-induced vomiting. (b) After abstinence is accomplished, a monk instructs patients on how to start new lives. [Courtesy of Wolfgang Jilek, M.D.].

for drug addicts was offered in Buddhist temples. Special herbs were given to the patients to induce vomiting for "purification." After abstinence was achieved, the monks gave formal instruction to the patients, urging them to start new lives (see Fig. 32-12).

Griffith and Mahy (1984) described the religious ceremony of "Mourning" practiced among members of the Spiritual Baptist Church in the West Indies. In a desire for spiritual strength and other benefits,

church members volunteered to participate in the practice. After ceremonial washing and anointing, the mourners were isolated in a small chamber at the back of the church, where they remained for a period of 7 days. During that time, each individual prayed, fasted, and experienced dreams and visions. From their investigation of the participants, Griffith and Mahy reported that the mourners claimed that they obtained the psychological benefit of relief; attained the ability to foresee and avoid danger; improved their decision-making abilities; cured physical illnesses; heightened their facility to communicate with God and to meditate; promoted them within the church hierarchy; and so on.

An extremely different form of religious ritual was a snake-handling cult in the southern United States, described by E.H. La Barre (1962). As part of cult activities, members in trance states handled poisonous snakes as a sign of being blessed by God. Occasionally some of the members died when they were bitten by the snakes. While it is forbidden by the government to perform such cult rituals, these activities still exist. The gratification of emotional excitement was identified as one of the effects sought by cult members — even at the risk of their lives.

It is important to know that religious healing ceremonies are not only observed in primitive societies or among uncivilized populations, but are quite common in many industrialized societies as well (Pattison & Wintrob, 1981). As pointed out by Hufford (1977), religion-related healing systems are increasing rapidly in popularity in the United States. In Christian religious healing, there is a broad spectrum of beliefs and activities, ranging from Christian Science to the fundamentalism of healers such as Oral Roberts to the Roman Catholic rite of anointing of the sick. It is currently very difficult to predict, on the basis of denomination, whether a religious patient is likely to be significantly involved in a religious healing effort. According to Hufford, religious healing systems take two different positions. The first is: "If you fulfill the requirements for healing (that is, sufficient faith, contrition, prayer, etc.), then you will be healed." This position is derived from the basic beliefs that God opposes all suffering, and suffering is the result of sin. Thus, if you are not healed, you did not fulfill the requirements. This position places a great deal of responsibility on the patient. The other position is: "If you do all that lies within your power to carry out the will of God in your life, then what follows is God's will for you." In this position, the final responsibility is removed from the patient. The patient is provided

with the hope for supernatural resources against disease, thus increasing his or her security and sense of well being. As there is a great deal of variation among individual interpretations as well as positions held by different denominations, Hufford suggests that a clinician should not take a stereotypical view in reacting to a patient's religious healing activities. Specific features of a given patient's system must be sought out.

In reviewing Christian religious rituals, Griffith and Young (1988) pointed out that special styles of prayer, testimony, and spirit possession are integral parts of the services in the black church in the United States. These practices serve as a cohesive force binding blacks together. This form of service is particularly effective when conducted by a charismatic black pastor and allows an oppressed minority to externalize its woes and obtain succor from a righteous God.

Thus, in various forms of religious healing ceremonies, the therapeutic operation is carried out through the ritual of prayer, testimony, sacrifice, reliving experience, or even spirit possession. Assurance, suggestions, and the generation of conviction are some of the healing mechanisms utilized in the practices. The aims of therapy are to heal the patient's problems and give a certain perspective to his or her life.

C. DIVINATION

Divination refers to the act or practice of trying to foretell the future or the unknown by occult means. It relies on mysterious, magic, or religious methods. Because the interpretation of divine instruction is usually provided by the diviner himself, or an interpreter, the interaction between the diviner/interpreter and the client becomes an important variable.

There is a range of methods of divination. Some methods are very simple, whereas others are more complicated. For example, in Nigeria, Africa, the divination practiced by the Nsukka Ibo (called *Afa*) is carried out by casting four strings containing half-shells of the seeds of the bush mango (Shelton, 1965); and by the people in Yoruba (known as *Ifa*) by tossing

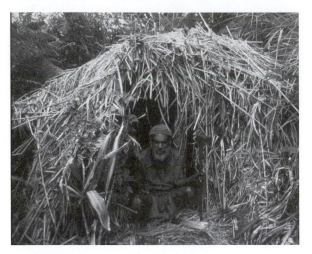

FIGURE 32-13 Diviner's dream house in the southern highlands of Papua New Guinea (for diagnostic dream divination). [Courtesy of Wolfgang Jilek, M.D.].

palm nuts (Prince, 1975). In the divination practiced in other parts of Africa, the diviner simply offers a certain sign himself. For example, divination may occur while his hand is shaking, with the belief that he is guided by a supernatural power to give instructions. In Southern Highland of Papua New Guinea, the diviner performs dream divination, namely taking sleep in specially-built dream house for instruction through dream signs (see Fig. 32-13).

In ancient China, turtle shells or the bones of big animals were burned during divination ceremonies and divine instruction was interpreted through the cracks made from the heat. An elaborate divination system called *chien* was developed in China and a modified version in Japan. To obtain answers to questions about their lives, some Chinese or Japanese visit temples for divination. After a sincere prayer to the god of the temple, the person will ask for divine instruction, which is provided through a fortune stick that the person selects. Corresponding to the number on the stick, there is a fortune paper with an answer written on it. This practice is called *chien* drawing in Chinese (see Fig. 32-14a).

In *chien* drawing, the client will ask for a divine answer to a specific question (such as whether it is

good or bad to move, to change jobs, or to get married to a particular candidate under the present circumstances). There is usually a set of *chien* (which could number 25, 50, or 100, for example) from which a special stick is picked at random by the client. On the *chien* (divine instruction) there are predesigned answers for each category of issues about which clients may inquire, such as moving, changing jobs, family problems, treatment for sickness, interpersonal conflict, and so on (see Fig. 32-14b).

In order to understand the psychological effects operating in divination, Hsu (1976) studied *chien* drawing as practiced by the Chinese in Taiwan. Analyzing the preset answers, she found that they were designed

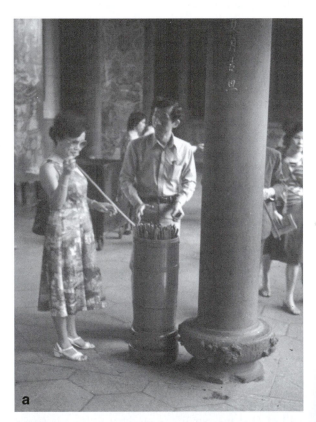

a

FIGURE 32-14 Chinese divination (*Chien* drawing). (a) After a sincere pray, picking up a bamboo stick *(chien)* for divine instruction. [Courtesy of Jing Hsu, M.D.] *(Figure continues)*

Number 1
Good

The creation of the earth sets forth a good fortune. A good and lucky day and everything is perfect.
If you get this divination, it is excellent. If man behaves faithfully and virtuously, the emperor will proclaim his virtues.

Symbolism

The creation of the Earth. Everything is good luck.

Explanation

Very soon by the end of the year, Kuan Yin will deliver the message to you first.

Home:	Pray for Blessings
Health:	Great benefits in Autumn & Winter
Wealth:	Great benefits in Autumn & Winter
Business:	Successful
Marriage:	Successful
Pregnancy:	Boy
Traveller:	Arrive safely
Farm Crops:	Good
Animals:	Good
Missing Person:	Will find
Legal Matters:	Good luck
Lost Items:	Look in the northeast direction
Sickness:	Make offerings
Burial Plot:	Good luck

Number 2
Inauspicious

The whale remains in the river unchanged. It is still too early to have high expectations to leap up. When his body changes, then he can leap over the dragon gate.

Symbolism

The whale has not changed yet, so be patient until the right time comes.

Explanation

You should be patient, you should be patient as patience could be. You must wait for the right time to come. You still have the opportunity to achieve your goals. Your scholarly honor will still endure.

Home:	Not peaceful, disturbed
Health:	Must fulfill a vow
Wealth:	Lacking in benefits
Marriage:	Difficult
Pregnancy:	Make a committment to receive blessings
Traveller:	Safe and sound
Farm Crops:	Good luck
Animals:	Not beneficial
Missing Person:	Will find
Legal Matters:	Peaceful settlement
Lost Items:	Look in the southeast
Sickness:	Pray for protection
Burial Plot:	Good luck

FIGURE 32-14 (continued)   (b) Based on the number on the stick, the corresponding divine paper is obtained, on which the divination is classified, associated with symbolism (described in a poem), and an explanation given along with a set of itemized answers. From *Kuan Yin Bodhisattva: Book of Divination*, English translation by Jinquan Zheng. Honolulu: Typeset Express, Inc., 1991. *(Figure continues)*

to reflect culturally sanctioned resolutions to certain problems. For instance, moving, in an agricultural society, is usually discouraged; in cases of family or marital conflict, the client is often advised to be patient and try to solve the conflict with harmony; lawsuits are discouraged; regarding medical treatment, if the present therapy is not satisfactory, it is suggested the client seek other therapy. In other words, *chien* is designed as an institutional way of reinforcing culturally sanctioned coping methods. As the divine answer is written in the format of an ancient poem or in language that is difficult for laymen to understand, the client needs to consult *chien* interpreters in the temple. The interpreters are usually educated elders. Thus, a "counseling transaction" actually takes place between the interpreters and the divining person (see Fig. 32-14c).

In Japan, similar fortune-telling is practiced, which is called *kujibiki*. The client goes to a temple and, after sincere pray, draws *kuji* (fortune-telling paper) for divine instruction. If the divine instruction fits the client's preference, the client may take the fortune-telling paper with him or her; if not, he or she may leave the *kuji* in the temple by hanging it on a tree to be returned to the god. This means that the client has the choice of accepting the fortune or not, depending

on his or her response to the instruction given. Today, with the mechanization in Japan, fortune-telling machines can be found on the roadside and fortune-telling paper can be obtained simply by putting a coin into the machine.

No matter what method of divination is practiced, the basic therapeutic operation is performed to provide a clear-cut answer for the problems presented. Thus, it is helpful psychologically for a client to find a definite way to address his problems. Naming effects are among the healing mechanisms operating in divination. It is assumed that human life is regulated by the supernatural. It is the basic goal of the person seeking help to find the proper way to comply with the universe through "divine" instruction.

D. FORTUNE-TELLING

The system of reference shifts from the supernatural to the natural in the practice of fortune-telling. Based on the concepts of microcosm and macrocosm, fortune-telling is oriented to the basic belief that human life and behavior are parts of the universe. The nature of the problems is usually explained in terms of an imbalance of vital forces or disharmony with the natural principles that rule the universe. The objective of the practice is to help the client find out how to live compatibly with nature and adjust to the environment more harmoniously.

Based on the sources of information used, fortune-telling can be divided into several groups. In astrology, there is a basic belief that a person's life is correlated to and influenced by the movement of the stars, thus their movement becomes the essential source of information for predicting one's life course. For the Chinese, an ancient record of universal change, the Oracle of Change *(Yi-Jing),* is used for fortune-telling. A person's date and time of birth and the number of strokes in the Chinese character for his or her name are needed to calculate an individual's fortune.

Physiognomy is based on the assumption that there is a close correlation between the mind and the body and that one's character, life, and fortune can be read

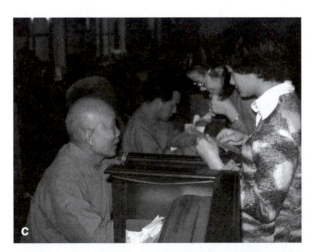

FIGURE 32-14 (continued)   (c) An elderly person in the temple interpretating the fortune and acting as a folk counselor. [Courtesy of Jing Hsu, M.D.].

by examining one's physical features. It is assumed that a person is born with a certain predisposition, which is shown in his physical appearance and will lead him to manifest certain behavior patterns. A physiognomist tries to help a client understand his own character and behavior patterns, learning how to make good use of his talents and, at the same time, make up for his shortcomings.

Although the basic assumption underlying fortune-telling is that every person has a predetermined course in life, this "fate" is not absolutely unchangeable — it may be subject to modification. Thus, it is not a completely passive acceptance of "fate," but allows room for adjustment. Finding a way to adjust your own fortune is the purpose of fortune-telling.

In psychotherapy or counseling, it is important to note that the interaction between the fortune-teller and the client is a significant variable in the effectiveness of the "therapy." Also, it is not so much what fortune is found from the available information, but how the information is interpreted and utilized by the fortune-teller in counseling the individual client that is most critical. Clearly, the fortune-teller can make projective interpretations in order to "counsel" the client. This phenomenon is similar to what is often observed in the practice of divination.

Even though the basic orientation shifts from a supernatural to a natural one and the sources of practice rely on the rules of nature, the therapeutic operation, like divination, is still characterized by offering folk-natured interpretation and providing concrete guidance for a client in making choices. Based on the concepts of microcosm and macrocosm, complying with the fundamental rules of nature is the basic goal of the practice.

E. MEDITATION EXERCISE

The practice of meditation is not psychotherapeutic work in a strict sense. However, many people who practice meditation or meditation-related exercise claim that they obtain considerable benefits from it, such as improving their body–mind condition and promoting mental health. Such practices may therefore be considered a form of folk psychotherapy if we define psychotherapy broadly as an activity to promote a healthy mind.

1. Yoga

Yoga originated in India. Yoga practitioners, or yogis, experience themselves as dual entities. That is, they have two co-conscious selves: a self participating in the world and an uninvolved, observing self. According to the yogis, meditation is the means by which the "participating self" is controlled, allowing the "observing self" to be uncovered or unassimilated from the activities of the participating self. A yogi who has accomplished this split in consciousness on a permanent basis is considered to have achieved liberation (Castillo, 1991). Hindu yoga is becoming popular among some Westerners today as a practice to promote the health of the mind. Probably stimulated by this, some clinicians have begun to pay attention to the study of meditation or transcendence, to examine its relation to psychotherapy, and to explore its sociocultural implications in contemporary industrialized societies (Engler, 1984; Hoehn-Saric, 1974).

2. Qigong

Qigong in Chinese literally means the exercise of "vitality" *(qi)*. It is aimed at regulating the force of vitality through the practice of meditation-related physical exercise. It was practiced by the Chinese in the past and is still practiced today, attracting the interest of some Westerners.

According to German cultural psychiatrist Heise (1999), based on his study in China, *qigong* tries to establish a balanced subtle energetical–functional–bodily system by rhythmic body movement, breathing, and a special hovering awareness. The so-called *qi,* or life energy, can be used as internal energy *(nei-qi)* for regulating psychological and somatical health problems or can be transmitted as external energy *(wai-qi)* by a qigong master for an equal purpose.

According to the clinical observations of Wu (1997), a psychiatrist who is also a *qigong* master, the practice of *qigong* can help a person obtain tranquility of mind, diminish psychosomatic problems, and improve psychological conditions, particularly in the areas of self-image and self-confidence. She speculated that the mechanisms of support, suggestions, and provision of hope all work on the person. However, she also warned that some practitioners, particularly those with a premorbid personality trait of hysteria or a borderline personality disorder, may develop mental complications from the practice of meditation, such as minor or major psychiatric disorders, including various forms of psychoses. Thus, there is a need for careful clinical screening.

Whether it is yoga or *qigong,* the practice of meditation has a somato-natural orientation. Meditation or meditation-related exercise seeks the therapeutic effects of regulating body–mind relations and vitality, and obtaining tranquility. The unspoken goal of the practice is harmony with nature.

III. ELABORATION OF COMMON THERAPEUTIC FACTORS

Reviewing various forms of folk therapy, Frank (1961, p. 62) has pointed out that the core of the effectiveness of different methods of religious and magical healing seems to lie in their ability to arouse hope by capitalizing on the patient's dependency on others.

Comparing the healing practices carried out by witch doctors and psychiatrists, Torrey (1986, pp. 73–74) pointed out that they share a common root. He listed the components of psychotherapy that are shared by traditional and modern healers and contribute to the effects of therapy. Both are able to decrease the client's anxiety by identifying what is wrong with him, i.e., to name the cause of the problems, providing the effect of the Rumpelstiltskin principle; the therapist presents certain personal qualities that are admired by the culture and contribute to the therapy; the client's expectations of therapy, and the emotional arousal that is usually enhanced by the therapeutic setting, the therapist's belief in himself, and his reputation; the emerging sense of learning and mastery that the client obtains through therapy; and, finally, the techniques of therapy that enhance the basic components of psychotherapy. It is clear that folk healing practices and modern psychotherapy share a number of nonspecific therapeutic mechanisms.

Jilek (1994) pointed out that traditional healing practices have several advantages over cosmopolitan modern medicine; cultural congeniality, maximal use of the personality of the healer, a holistic approach, accessibility and availability (particularly for developing areas), effective use of affect and altered states of consciousness, collective therapy management, and cost-effectiveness. Medical anthropologist Richard Castillo (2001) pointed out that folk healing practices often demonstrate certain useful qualitie — comprehensibility, manageability, and meaningfulness — that deserve attention by contemporary clinicians.

It is important to recognize that both folk healing and modern therapy utilize symbols and metaphors for interpretations and suggestions (Kirmayer, 1993). Rhetoric is concerned with the use of language to transform meanings or conceptual positions with perceptions, emotions, and moral convictions, and is of central importance in healing. In contrast to modern psychotherapists, some folk healers make use of symbolic interpretations and suggestions to enhance the effects of healing (Tseng & McDermott, 1975).

Despite the general usefulness of folk therapies, the ill effects of some have not been widely studied and reported. However, clinical observation has disclosed that some folk therapists cause harm to the clients who seek their services. Under the guise of treatment, tricking a client out of his money by deceit or fraud or sexual involvement with a client are examples of disreputable behavior that are occasionally reported. Harming a client by prescribing dangerous substances and physically injuring or even killing a client by accident during the performance of an exorcism are other serious complications that have occurred. Among these negative effects, as Jilek pointed out (1993), a delay in establishing effective modern pharmacological therapy for certain mental disorders, such as schizophrenia or major affective disorders, has been of concern to some modern psychiatrists.

IV. CLINICAL ASSESSMENT OF THERAPEUTIC RESULTS

While there is a great deal of literature analyzing and emphasizing the effects of indigenous healing practices, there have been only a few empirical studies to test their outcomes.

Finkler (1980) conducted follow-up studies of patients who visited a spiritualist temple for treatment of various disorders in a rural region of Mexico. Follow-ups revealed that among 107 subjects who completed the investigation, 38 cases (35.5%) described their disorders as unresponsive to the treatment, whereas 27 cases (25.3%) reported that their disorders improved. Based on these data, Finkler concluded that spiritualist healers failed more than they succeeded in treating their patients. Through further analysis, he indicated that the therapeutic benefits of spiritualist healing tended to occur in four types of disorders: simple diarrheas, simple gynecological disorders, somatized syndromes, and minor psychiatric disorders.

R. Ness (1980) studied two fundamental churches (A and B) in a Newfoundland coastal community of Canada. The Cornell Medical Index (CMI), which includes problems of physical and psychological functioning, was administered to all church members after a year's observation of their religious behavior. The behavior was categorized as glossolalia, testimonials, and seeking possession in church A and as testimonials and attendance in church B. Analyzing data to examine the relationship between religious participation and emotional status, it was found that people who actively participate in religious ritual activities are likely to report fewer symptoms of psychological distress than those who participate less. Based on the differences in the religious activities of the two churches, significant differences were observed among the church members in terms of their reported mental health condition. However, as no assessment was made prior to their participation in religious activities, it was difficult to determine whether the members had benefited by the religious activities. It can be concluded merely that there was a correlation between religious activities and reported mental health conditions.

Kleinman and Gale (1982) compared patients treated by modern physicians and folk healers in Taiwan. Patients with various types of sickness, such as mild acute cases, severe acute cases, somatization cases, and chronic cases, who were treated by local shamans were followed up 3 to 4 weeks after the initial assessment by public health nurses in their home settings. Roughly comparable patients treated by biomedical physicians were also investigated for purposes of comparison. Counter to their hypothesis, a higher proportion of patients, regardless of the kinds of problems they had (either acute, chronic, or somatic), were dissatisfied with shamanistic treatment than with biomedical care by modern physicians. Investigators discuss serious limitations on research design and method associated with such indigenous healing studies, particularly the difficulty of controlling placebo effects and the natural course of sickness, and the problem of criteria for assessment — either to assess improvement of *illness problems* (the psychosocial aspects of sickness) or *disease problems* (clinical symptoms or underlying biological processes). They noted that the study assessed treatment response primarily on physiological and behavioral levels; changes in the social functions and personal and cultural meaning of illness were not evaluated systematically. The evaluators with backgrounds in public health nursing may well have transmitted their professional biases indirectly and inadvertently to the subjects.

By questionnaire survey, Zuroff and Schwarz (1980) conducted a 2-year follow-up of a controlled experiment to measure the outcomes of subjects who had practiced transcendental meditation versus muscle relaxation. From the results, the investigators concluded that although some subjects (about 15 to 20%)

did enjoy and continued to practice transcendental meditation, it was not universally beneficial.

After conducting surveys of the outcomes of folk healing practices, several investigators (Finkler, 1980; Kleinman & Sung, 1976) speculated that while a patient's sociopsychological functioning may not have improved or been restored by traditional techniques, the patient's medical disease was not, in fact, healed. However, Csordas and Lewton (1998) raised the question as to what healing was about in healing practices. Particularly concerning religious healing, they pointed out that it was not only about healing but also about religion. A narrow study of the efficacy of the practice would not suffice.

V. ATTITUDES TOWARD INDIGENOUS HEALING PRACTICES

Scholars, clinicians, and public health workers have different opinions on whether to encourage or discourage indigenous folk healing practices in various societies. Some people (particularly modern medico-surgical clinicians) see folk healing as merely "superstitious" and "primitive," insisting that such "out-of-date" practices should be discouraged or prohibited. Others (such as cultural anthropologists and cultural psychiatrists) consider these folk practices to be interesting subjects for academic study — examining the therapeutic elements that they utilize and why such supernaturally oriented therapeutic exercises are still popular among some groups. Still others (such as some community health workers) believe that due to the shortage of professional personnel available in the community, the existence of "folk" therapies should be supported.

The popular Western opinion and attitude toward traditional healing, as well as its "scientific" evaluation by social science and medical/psychiatric investigators, have changed significantly since the 1950s, from the pathology labeling of folk practitioners, especially shamanic healers, to emphasizing their psychotherapeutic capability (Jilek, 1971). As pointed out by Jilek (1993), the joint declaration on primary health care made in 1978 by the World Health Organization and UNICEF at Alma Ata, Kazakhstan, for the first time gave international recognition to the positive role of traditional indigenous practitioners. The position was taken that any folk healing practice that is proven (or at least considered) to be helpful to the client and useful to the community deserves the support and encouragement of clinicians as well as administrators.

As an extension of this latter view, some have even advocated that the collaboration of indigenous healers and modern clinicians should be encouraged to provide maximal mental health services for the community. In an attempt at such collaboration, several programs have been established to provide educational training for folk healers. A training program in a Navajo school for medicine men was reported by Bergman (1973). Koss (1980) described a project that attempted to integrate two healing systems by providing their practitioners with a means of continuous contact. Spiritual healers, mental health workers, and medical professionals were able to meet on the neutral academic ground provided by the project. As a result, therapists and spiritual healers began to refer patients to each other.

VI. FINAL COMMENTS

In this chapter, various forms of indigenous or folk psychotherapy are divided into subgroups for the purposes of description and discussion. However, it should be recognized that, in reality, the boundaries between different subgroups of folk therapy are not distinct. They always overlap, shifting from one category to another, or combining. From a conceptual point of view, it is useful to recognize how the subgroups are distributed throughout the dimensions of supernatural, natural, or somato-natural orientations. These are part of a total spectrum that includes sociophilosophical and psychological orientations, as represented by culture-influenced unique therapy or culture-related common therapy, which will be elaborated in Chapters 33 and 34, respectively, and systematically compared at the end of Chapter 34 (reference to Table 34-1). Through this comprehensive subgroup comparison, a panoramic view of indigenous and modern therapy can be obtained.

There is academic curiosity among scholars as to whether there is any social reason for the existence and selection of various forms of folk therapy. Studying the Iroquois Indian tribe in the United States, Wallace (1959) noted that the psychotherapeutic needs of individuals tended to center on institutionalized "catharsis" in a highly organized sociocultural system and on "control" (the development of a coherent image of self and the world, and the repression of incongruent motives and beliefs) in a poorly organized system. To what extent such correlations can be observed and generalized in other settings is an interesting subject for further investigation.

The comparative study of indigenous healing practices and modern psychotherapy has revealed the existence of certain universal elements of the healing process that operate as important factors for therapy, whether the therapy is carried out in a primitive or modern form. The universal and nonspecific healing factors identified are the cultivation of hope, the activation of surrounding support, and the enhancement of culturally sanctioned coping mechanisms. The study of indigenous healing practices has also pointed out the existence of supernatural dimensions of healing, which are less intentionally utilized in modern therapy.

One simple fact deserves attention; there is a wide range of "professional" quality among so-called folk healers, and different motivations for practice. Some are benign healers motivated by a desire to serve, while others are not. Some are well trained in their particular professions and know how to practice within its limitations, while others are not — and are liable for malpractice. The major problem is that from a public health point of view, in most societies, there still are no formal guidelines for regulating folk therapy as there are for modern therapy. Folk therapy, whether shamanistic practice or faith healing, should be subject to periodic surveys and reevaluation by professional public health organizations the same as modern clinical work so that its benefits to clients can be protected and any potential malpractice prevented. If any folk therapist refuses to be examined and regulated, he or she should be discouraged or prevented from practicing.

REFERENCES

Bergman, R.L. (1973). A school for medicine men. *American Journal of Psychiatry, 130*(6), 663–666.

Castillo, R.J. (1991). Divided consciousness and enlightenment in Hindu Yogis. *The Anthropology of Consciousness, 2*(3–4), 1–6.

Castillo, R.J. (2001). Lessons from folk healings. In W.S. Tseng & J. Streltzer (Eds.), *Culture and psychotherapy: A guide to clinical practice* (pp. 81–101). Washington, DC: American Psychiatric Press.

Csordas, T.J., & Lewton, E. (1998). Practice, performance, and experience in ritual healing. *Transcultural Psychiatry, 35*(4), 435–512.

Dobkin, M. (1968). Folk curing with a psychedelic cactus in the north coast of Peru. *International Journal of Social Psychiatry, 15*, 23–32.

El-Islam, M.F. (1967). The psychotherapeutic basis of some Arab rituals. *International Journal of Social Psychiatry, 13*, 265–268.

El Sendiony, M.F. (1974). The problems of cultural specificity of mental illness: The Egyptian mental disease and the Zar ceremony. *Australian and New Zealand Journal of Psychiatry, 8*, 103–107.

Engler, J. (1984). Therapeutic aims in psychotherapy and meditation: Developmental stages in the representation of self. *Journal of Transpersonal Psychology, 16*(1), 25–61.

Figge, H. (1975). Spirit posession and healing cult among the Brasilian Umbanda. *Psychotherapy and Psychosomatics, 25*, 246–250.

Finkler, K. (1980). Non-medical treatments and their outcomes. *Culture, Medicine and Psychiatry, 4*(3), 271–310.

Firth, R.W. (1964). Spirit mediumship. In J. Gold & W.L. Kolb (Eds.), *A dictionary of the social sciences* (p. 638). New York: Free Press.

Frank, J.D. (1961). *Persuasion and healing: A comparative study of psychotherapy.* New York: Schocken Books.

Griffith, E.E.H., & Mahy, G.E. (1984). Psychological benefits of spiritual Baptist "mourning." *American Journal of Psychiatry, 141*(6), 769–773.

Griffith, E.E.H., & Young, J.L. (1988). A cross-cultural introduction to the therapeutic aspects of Christian religious ritual. In L. Comas-Díaz & E.E.H. Griffith (Eds.), *Clinical guidelines in cross-cultural mental health* (pp. 69–89). New York: Wiley.

Hall, A.L., & Bourne, P.G. (1973). Indigenous therapists in a Southern Black urban community. *Archives of General Psychiatry, 28*, 137–142.

Harvey, Y.S.K. (1979). *Six Korean women: The socialization of shamans.* New York: West Publishing.

Heise, T. (1999). *Qigong in der VR China: Entwicklung, theorie und praxis [Qigong in China: Development, theory and practice.]* Berlin: Verlag fur Wissenschaft und Bildung.

Hoehn-Saric, R. (1974). Transcendence and psychotherapy. *American Journal of Psychotherapy, 28*(2), 252–254.

Hsu, J. (1976) Counseling in the Chinese Temple: A psychological study of divination by Chien drawing. In W.P. Lebra (Ed.), *Culture-bound syndromes, ethnopsychiatry, and alternate therapies* (pp. 210–221). Honolulu: University Press of Hawaii.

Hufford, D. (1977). Christian religious healing. *Journal of Operational Psychiatry, 8*(2), 22–27.

Jilek, W. (1971). From crazy witch doctor to auxiliary psychotherapist — The changing image of the medicine man. *Psychiatria Clinica, 4,* 200–220.

Jilek, W. (1974). *Salish Indian mental health and cultural change.* Toronto: Holt, Rinehart & Winston.

Jilek, W. (1976). "Brainwashing" as therapeutic technique in contemporary Canadian Indian spirit dancing: A case in theory building. In J. Westermeyer (Ed.), *Anthropology and mental health: Setting a new course.* Paris: Mouton.

Jilek, W. (1978). Native renaissance: The survival and revival of indigenous therapeutic ceremonials among North American Indians. *Transcultural Psychiatric Research Review, 15,* 117–145.

Jilek, W. (1982). *Indian healing: Shamanic ceremonialism in the Pacific Northwest today.* Surrey, BC, Canada: Handcock House.

Jilek, W. (1993). Traditional medicine relevant to psychiatry. In N. Sartorius, G. De Girolamo, G. Andrews, & G.A. German (Eds.), *Treatment of mental disorders: A review of effectiveness.* Washington, DC: American Psychiatric Press.

Jilek, W. (1994). Traditional healing in the prevention and treatment of alcohol and drug abuse. *Transcultural Psychiatric Research Review, 31*(3), 219–258.

Jilek-Aall, L., & Jilek, W.G. (1985). Buddhist temple treatment of narcotic addiction and neurotic-psychosomatic disorders in Thailand. In P. Pichot, P. Berner, & R. Wolf (Eds.), *Psychiatry: The state of the art* (Vol. 8), New York: Plenum Press.

Kendall, L. (1985). *Shamans, housewives and other restless spirits: Women in Korean ritual life.* Honolulu: University of Hawaii Press.

Kendall, L. (1988). *The life and hard times of Korean shaman.* Honolulu: University of Hawaii Press.

Kennedy, J.G. (1967). Nubian *zar* ceremonies as psychotherapy. *Human Organization, 26*(4), 185–194.

Kiev, A. (1964). *Magic, faith, and healing: Studies in primitive psychiatry today.* New York: Free Press.

Kim, K.I. (1973). Psychodynamic study of two cases of shaman in Korea. *Korean Journal of Cultural Anthropology, 6,* 45–65 (in Korean with English summary).

Kirmayer, L.J. (1993). Healing and the invention of metaphor: The effectiveness of symbols revisited. *Culture, Medicine and Psychiatry, 17*(2), 161–195.

Kleinman, A., & Gale, J. (1982). Patients treated by physicians and folk healers: A comparative outcome study in Taiwan. *Culture, Medicine and Psychiatry, 6*(4), 405–423.

Kleinman, A., & Sung, L. (1976). Why do indigenous practitioners successfully heal? *Social Science and Medicine, 13*(B), 7–26.

Koss, J.D. (1980). The therapist-spiritist training project in Puerto Rico: An experiment to relate the traditional healing system to the public health system. *Social Science and Medicine, 14B,* 255–266.

La Barre, E.H. (1962). *They shall take up serpents: Psychology of the Southern snake-handling cult.* Minneapolis: University of Minnesota Press.

La Barre, W. (1947). Primitive psychotherapy in Native American cultures: Peyotism and confession. *Journal of Abnormal and Social Psychology, 42,* 294–309.

Lebra, T.S. (1976). Taking the role of supernatural "other": Spirit possession in a Japanese healing cult. In W.P. Lebra (Ed.), *Culture-bound syndromes, ethnopsychiatry, and alternate therapies* (pp. 88–100). Honolulu: University Press of Hawaii.

Leighton, A.H., & Leighton, D.C. (1941). Elements of psychotherapy in Navaho religion. *Psychiatry, 4,* 515–523.

Lessa, W.A., & Volt, E.Z. (Eds.). (1965). *Reader in comparative religion: An anthropological approach* (2nd ed., p. 410). New York: Harper.

Li, S., and Philips, M.R. (1990). Witch doctors and mental illness in mainland China: A preliminary study. *American Journal of Psychiatry, 147,* 221–224.

Modarressi, T. (1968). The Zar cult in South Iran. In R. Prince (Ed.), *Trance and possession states* (Proceedings of Second Annual Conference). Montreal: R.M. Bucke Memorial Society.

Ness, R.C. (1980). The impact of indigenous healing activity: An empirical study of two fundamental churches. *Social Science and Medicine, 14B,* 107–180.

Ness, R.C., & Wintrob, R. (1981). Folk healing: A description and synthesis. *American Journal of Psychiatry, 138,* 1477–1481.

Pattison, E.M., & Wintrob, R.M. (1981). Possession and exorcism in contemporary America. *Journal of Operational Psychiatry, 12,* 12–30.

Ponce, D.E. (1995, June 3–8). *Is Buddhism psychotherapy?* Presented at the Seventh International Seminar on Buddhism and Leadership for Peace, Honolulu.

Prince, R. (1975). Symbols and psychotherapy: The examples of Yoruba sacrificial ritual. *Journal of the American Academy of Psychoanalysis, 3*(3), 321–338.

Prince, R. (1980). Variations in psychotherapy procedures. In H.C. Triandis & J.G. Draguns (Eds.), *Handbook of cross-cultural psychology: Psychopathology* (Vol. 6) (pp. 291–349). Boston: Allyn & Bacon.

Prince, R. (1992). Religious experience and psychopathology: Cross-cultural perspectives. In J.F. Schumaker (Ed.), *Religion and mental health.* New York: Oxford University Press.

Sasaki, Y. (1969). Psychiatric study of the shaman in Japan. In W. Caudil & T.Y. Lin (Eds.), *Mental health research in Asia and the Pacific* (pp. 223–241). Honolulu: East-West Center Press.

Shelton, A.J. (1965). The meaning and method of Afa divination among the Northern Nsukka Ibo. *American Anthropologist, 67,* 1441–1445.

Suwanlert, S. (1997, October 7–10). Phan yak *traditional chanting treats mental disorders.* Poster display at the regional meeting of the World Psychiatric Association, Beijing, China.

Torrey, E.F. (1986). *Witchdoctors and psychiatrists: The common roots of psychotherapy and its future.* New York: Harper & Row.

Tseng, W.S. (1972). Psychiatric study of shamanism in Taiwan. *Archives of General Psychiatry, 26,* 561–565.

Tseng, W.S., & Hsu, J. (1979). Culture and Psychotherapy. In A.J. Marsella, R.G. Tharp, & T.J. Ciborowski (Eds.), *Perspectives on cross-cultural psychology* (pp. 333–345). New York: Academic Press.

Tseng, W.S., & McDermott, J.F., Jr. (1975). Psychotherapy: Historical roots, universal elements, and cultural variations. *American Journal of Psychiatry, 132,* 378–384.

Turner, V.W. (1972). Religious specialists. In D.L. Sill (Ed.), *International encyclopedia of the social sciences* (pp. 437–44). New York: Crowell Collier & Macmillan.

Wallace, A.E.C. (1959). The institutionalization of cathartic and control strategies in Iroquois religious psychotherapy. In M.K. Opler (Ed.), *Culture and mental health* (pp. 63–96). New York: Macmillan.

Ward, C.A. (1980). Spirit possession and mental health: A psycho-anthropological perspective. *Human Relations, 33*(3), 146–163.

Winkelman, M.J. (1992). *Shamans, priests and witches: A cross-cultural study of magico-religious practitioners.* Tempe: Arizona State University Press.

Wu, C.Y. (1997). Qigong: Chinese traditional psychotherapy. In W.S. Tseng (Ed.), *Chinese mind and therapy* (pp. 372–379). Beijing: Beijing Medical University Press (in Chinese).

Zuroff, D.C., & Schwarz, J.C. (1980). Transcendental meditation versus muscle relaxation: A two-year follow-up of a controlled experiment. *American Journal of Psychiatry, 137*(10), 1229–1231.

33

Culture-Influenced
Unique Psychotherapies

I. WHAT ARE CULTURE-INFLUENCED UNIQUE PSYCHOTHERAPIES?

Culture-influenced unique psychotherapies are therapeutics modes that are very culturally flavored and characteristically "unique," different from the "common" or "mainstream" modes of psychotherapy that are currently practiced in Euro-American societies. Many of the unique therapies were developed in non-Euro-American societies, either by laymen or professionals. Some of them (such as Mesmerism or rest therapy) were invented in Euro-American in the past, but are not applied anymore at present. Although theoretically any form of psychotherapy is more or less influenced by culture, the term "culture influenced" is used here to indicate therapies that are strongly colored by the philosophical concepts or value systems of the societies in which they were created. Therefore, such therapies may be difficult to transplant to other cultures or to practice in the same society in another era if significant cultural change has occurred since they were developed. Because the therapeutic orientations and practices of these therapies are so distinctive, they are referred to as "unique."

In the indigenous healing practices described in the previous chapter, healing is said to occur as a result of the power of a supernatural or natural being rather than the psychological interaction between the healer and the client. In contrast, the psychotherapeutic exercises included in this chapter are recognized by both the healers and the clients as mental practices primarily for the purpose of healing the mind. Thus, they are recognized as practices of "psychotherapy" (or psychological therapy). The modes of therapy may be invented and utilized by laymen, mental health-related workers, or clinicians. The styles of therapy are characterized by a somatic (or biomedical), religious, philosophical, or sociopolitical orientation, in addition to the psychological. Nevertheless, all the practices are aimed directly or indirectly at correcting or treating psychological problems (see Table 34-1). As the impact of cultural factors becomes more explicit, such treatment modes become useful means of examining the cultural aspects of therapy (W.P. Lebra, 1976).

There are seemingly endless numbers of culture-influenced unique psychotherapies that can be identified around the globe. Only some of them have been selected for review and discussion in this chapter. Some modes of therapy have been observed in the past and are now merely a matter of historical record. However, they are included here for the sake of academic exploration and comparison.

II. VARIOUS EXAMPLES OF UNIQUE THERAPIES

A. SOMATO-PSYCHOTHERAPY

This mode of therapy is characterized primarily by a somato-psychological, or biomedical, orientation. Even though the psychological aspects of problems are recognized, it is the intent of this therapy to resolve the problems using a somatic approach — at least from a conceptual point of view. Two examples of this mode are listed here: Mesmerism and rest therapy. Although these therapies are no longer practiced, they deserve to be reviewed for the sake of comparison.

1. Mesmerism

This mode of therapy was invented in the late 18th century by the Austrian physician Franz Anton Mesmer and became popular in Paris (Alexander & Selesnick, 1966). Mesmer subscribed to the theory that planets influence the physiological and psychological phenomena of human beings. He hypothesized that man was endowed with a special magnetic, animal force that, when liberated, could produce amazing healing effects. Based on this assumption, he developed a method for magnetizing neurotic patients to heal them. In treatment sessions, a group of patients was asked to hold hands in a circle around a *baquet,* a tub filled with "magnetized" water. Mesmer, as the therapist, physically touched the patients, or simply gestured with his hands, with the intention of transmitting a magnetic force from his body to the patients, healing them. Thus, conceptually, the therapy was based on the somatic theory of the transmission and supplementing of animal magnetic force. However, in practice, it was the psychological force (i.e., sugges-

tions) produced by the charismatic therapist that affected the patients.

2. Rest Therapy

The rest cure method was designed by a neurologist, Silas Weir Mitchell, in the late 19th century in the United States (Schneck, 1975). It was based on the assumption that a neurotic patient's mental illness was caused by exhaustion of the nervous system, or "anemia of the brain." Thus, rest and recuperation were prescribed for the patient — a logical outgrowth of the concept of neurasthenia, developed by George Beard in 1880. The therapy consisted of rest, proper food, and isolation. The patient was prohibited contact with relatives and was separated completely from the setting in which his illness developed. Mitchell considered rest therapy particularly beneficial in the treatment of neurotic women.

Mesmerism and the rest cure reflected the level of knowledge in the field of medicine at the time. Modern psychiatry was not yet well developed, and mental illness was interpreted from a biological or neurological perspective. Accordingly, somatic therapies were designed in line with such somato-medical interpretations. However, some patients responded fairly well to such therapy, not because of biological influences, but probably due to the psychological effects of the therapy. The therapeutic mechanisms of magical expectation, susceptibility to suggestion, and legitimizing complaints are suspected. Restoration of natural conditions through supplementation or recuperation is the basic aim of this therapeutic maneuver and is shared by the homeopathic approach that is becoming popular among laymen as well as some professionals in the present day.

B. *HO'OPONOPONO* (SETTING TO RIGHT)

Ho'oponopono is a Hawaiian term referring to an indigenous problem-solving practice that was developed and used by native Hawaiians to restore harmonious relations in the family (Shook, 1985). This folk family therapy was used whenever there was a serious conflict among extended family members or other members of the community and a need for setting right the relationships. A meeting was traditionally called of all family or community members involved and was led by a senior family member or a respected outsider, such as a *kahuna* (healer). The meeting was started by asking the members to pray sincerely for help from their god to solve their problems. Then the procedure took the formal steps of statement of the problem, discussion, confession of wrongdoing, restitution when necessary, forgiveness, and release.

Culturally, Hawaiian people are discouraged from expressing negative emotions openly in their ordinary daily life. Concealment of resentment and anger is sanctioned. However, during this traditional problem-solving rite, the member who has a complaint about his family or community life, or a relationship, is permitted to state the problem. After the problem is examined and discussed by the group, the person causing the problem is expected to confess his wrongdoing, and his/her apology will be accepted by the others. It is the rule that after the revealing and confession, all the things disclosed and discussed in the meeting should be returned to the sea, implying that people should forget about the uncomfortable issues explored and repress them back into their minds before they return to their normal lives again. Thus, in a way, the practice of *ho'oponopono* is like a surgical operation on the mind; after exploring of the problem and dealing with it, the wound is sutured. The process starts with prayer, asking the blessing of a supernatural power for guidance in solving the problem. Sincerity is encouraged throughout the process as a condition for the success of the healing rite. *Ho'oponopono* offers a mechanism for setting to right according to the Hawaiian cultural system.

In this socioreligious-psychologically oriented folk practice, a stylized procedure of group revealing and elaboration of conflict is enforced as a cultural time-out process. Public confession and apology are the healing mechanisms utilized in this therapy, reflecting the group emphasis of this island society. Restoring harmonious family and group relationships is the goal of this folk healing rite. The important element in the

tranformation and usefulness of this unique therpay is the maintenance and incorporation of metaphoric understandings about the nature and dynamic of Hawaiian social relations (Ito, 1985).

C. ALCOHOLICS ANONYMOUS

Alcoholics Anonymous (AA) started in the United States in 1935 as a self-help program designed to help alcoholics become sober. AA has since spread to all continents and, in 1990, had an estimated membership of 2 million worldwide. However, as of 1986, more than half of the members (53.8%) were from the United States and Canada, 34.5% from Latin America, and the remaining 11.7% from countries in Europe, indicating that, in terms of member populations, it is prevalent mainly in North America and Latin America. According to Makela (1993), the demographic composition of AA in many countries is a reflection of when and by whom AA was first founded in those countries. There is also considerable variation in the format of AA meetings. For instance, in Austria, most meetings have circular seating arrangements, whereas audience-type seating is common in Mexico. There also are differences in turn-taking rules that impact the flow of discussion. In Finland, AA members usually speak in seating order; in Switzerland, the chair selects the next speaker. There are also differences in interpretations of spirituality. The institutional 12-step treatment program so emphasized in the United States is not necessarily considered important in many other countries, including Austria, Sweden, Finland, and Poland.

It is interesting that the Western-style Alcoholics Anonymous has not been successful among North American Indian populations. However, by omitting certain Western features of philosophy and practice and incorporating important indigenous cultural elements, the transformed "AA" groups have been quite successful in attracting and rehabilitating alcohol-abusing persons among native populations (Jilek-Aall, 1981). The Amerindian AA groups reject the concept of anonymity. Instead, the open identification of participants is practiced and family members, including children, are invited to the meetings. A formal set of rules and procedures, including time frame, is abandoned. Instead, more traditional ways of congregating, without predetermined times of arrival or departure of the participants, are practiced (Jilek, 1994). These culturally transformed "AA" groups are becoming widely accepted among the Amerindian population.

Even though the methods of AA may vary in different societies, the sociopsychological orientation is the backbone of the AA practice. Group confession and testimony are the basic operations, whereas group support and enforcement are some of the healing mechanisms. Restoring an alcohol-free, normal life is the major goal of the activity for this specific population.

D. RAPID INTEGRATED THERAPY

The so-called "rapid integrated therapy" was invented by Chinese psychiatrists as a specific mode of therapy for neurasthenic patients in China during the 1960s. Socioculturally, China at that time was in the middle of vigorously pursuing the so-called "Great Leap Movement." Under Chairman Mao's political ideology, people were encouraged to utilize all means, including traditional or indigenous methods, to obtain rapid economic expansion and improvement. In order to reach the target goal of social achievement, every member of the society was mobilized to participate in economic production. However, in the area of mental health, neurasthenic patients were identified nationally as one of the major patient populations that was not able to participate fully in social production. In response to political demands, in those social–political circumstances, rapid integrated therapy for neurasthenic patients was developed.

The therapy was characterized by a combination of various therapeutic procedures. Educational group therapy was coupled with individual counseling, physical exercise therapy (including *Qigong* exercise), and any needed somatic therapy, such as herb therapy,

acupuncture, or drug therapy. Thus, it was referred to as "integrated" treatment. Patients, in small organized groups, were treated as outpatients in a time-limited, short-term course of therapy (usually 4 weeks). Therefore, it was called "rapid" therapy. It was claimed that the therapy was useful for treating neurasthenic patients, and the program grew throughout the nation.

According to Chinese psychiatrists (Li, 1997), this form of therapy was effective for several reasons. Neurasthenia was originally considered by patients to be a chronic disorder. However, this pessimistic view was corrected through instruction in group therapy — the nature of the disorder was explained and the possibility for improvement was emphasized in the introductory teaching — so that patients were motivated and activated for recovery. Many neurasthenic patients (mostly students and intellectuals) tended in their daily lives to become overinvolved in brain work, lacking adequate physical activities. By participating in the therapy, which emphasizes a balance of mental and physical activities, they normalize their life patterns. Instruction and group activities, integrated with needed somatic therapy, comprised the format of the therapy. Group activation and regulation of the daily life activities of the mentally exhausted person were recognized as the mechanisms for therapy.

However, no matter what mechanism was claimed to be useful, it is clear that this mode of therapy was a product of the time, and the prevailing social atmosphere and political ideology functioned as the main force behind its effectiveness. When the Cultural Revolution started in 1966, creating extensive social turmoil, this therapy was disrupted and discontinued. Somehow, no one was interested in reviving this method of treatment after the Cultural Revolution was over.

E. NAIKAN THERAPY

Naikan therapy was developed by a Japanese monk, Ishin Yoshimoto, in Japan five decades ago for the purpose of treating juvenile delinquency and other problems. *Naikan* in Japanese literally means intrainspection. According to Reynolds (1977), the roots of Naikan lie in the Jodo Shinsu sect of Japanese Buddhism. The founder of the sect, Shinran, promised 10 kinds of profit to those who believed, e.g., "joyful acceptance of any hardship" and "the desire to repay others with a joyful heart." These two benefits are common results of Naikan meditation. Yoshimoto discovered the usefulness of Naikan during his own search for enlightenment. He eased the physical restrictions and modified the procedure somewhat for laymen. Interestingly, as noted by Reynolds, Yoshimoto now maintains that there is no real relationship between Naikan therapy and the Jodo's religious concepts, other than a historical one.

Any person intending to participate in the therapy, which takes place in a temple, needs to sign a formal contract to follow the instruction and vows to respect the master's guidance and discipline. The core of the Naikan practice is the client's self-inspection. Sitting in a corner of a room, facing toward the wall to conduct a self-examination of his own life in the past, with a particular focus on the kind of relationships he or she has had with significant persons, usually his parents. The client is instructed to review the kinds of things his parents did for him and what he did in return. Through the process of self-inspection, the client may obtain insight about his attitudes and learn not to complain and cause trouble for others, but to repay others with appreciation and a joyful heart. The change in the patient's attitude toward others and his view of life are the core of the therapy (Murase, 1976).

Although Naikan therapy was invented by a Buddhist monk, the Japanese cultural psychologist Murase (1984) commented that the goal of Naikan therapy is to assist the client in obtaining the psychological state of *sunao,* a unique Japanese term and value system. *Sunao* is derived from the Japanese character meaning "things in their original state without any transformation." It implies the harmonious and natural state of mind directly associated with honesty, humility, docility, and simplicity. Murase pointed out that the concept of *sunao* does not belong to the

"imported" religions of Buddha, but is essentially derived from ancient Shintoism — a value system that remains a strong undercurrent of Japanese culture. Thus, in his analysis, the emphasis of Naikan therapy is to search for the culturally sanctioned state of mind of *sunao.*

From a psychotherapeutic point of view, Naikan therapy is oriented to philosophical and psychological perspectives of life. Under the therapist's formal but simple guidance, performing preprogrammed self-examination is the therapeutic operation. Reappraising the primary interpersonal relationships within the family and discouraging a narcissistic view of the world by learning to appreciate others, rather than making demands for the self, are the basic therapeutic mechanisms utilized. Making use of culture-sanctioned value systems relating to parent–child relationships to restore family or group relations is the aim of the practice.

In the very beginning, the spread of the practice of Naikan therapy was supported by a millionaire who offered its benefits to prisoners. Other than a major center in Nara, there are only a few religious institutions that offer this therapy. The practice is gradually fading away. However, due to its uniqueness, it has historically attracted the attention of scholars. It has also attracted the interest of some Westerners. An American psychologist, Reynolds, who himself participated in a Naikan therapy experience in Japan, has reported that the few Americans who tried Naikan therapy in Japan shared some characteristic difficulties. According to Reynolds (1983), culturally, the Japanese tend to believe that if they receive some kind of benefit or favor from others, it is their moral duty to repay at least as much as they received. However, Americans tend to see social relations as relations among equals, with shared responsibilities and faults. Thus, because of its culturally patterned view of the world and interpersonal relationships, it is difficult for American people to receive and benefit from Naikan therapy. This illustrates that the transcultural application of certain healing practices is limited if those practices are particularly culturally flavored.

F. ERHARD SEMINARS TRAINING

Founded by Werner Erhard, a layman whose formal education only included high school, est was fashionable among well-educated adults in the United States during the 1970s. It consisted of a structured, two weekend (60-hour) program for self-improvement. The program was organized with certain rules, including a strict 7 hours between bathroom breaks — thus it was nicknamed "no-piss training."

As a program, est is concerned primarily with a philosophy of life and self. The seminar is conducted in such a way as to stimulate enlightenment about life. The participants might be humiliated by the seminar leader by being called "assholes," "machines," and so on, but the key point is to help them recognize that life is only what it is, not the way it used to be, ought to be, or might be. Life does not work. There is nothing one can do to make it work, so stop trying. There is nothing to do in life except to live it. As recognized by the founder, the training has philosophical views similar to Zen's attitude toward life.

Coupled with this philosophical attitude, the purpose of the training is to transform a person's ability to experience — to expand his or her experience of aliveness and full self-expression. It is aimed at intensifying a person's own awareness that an individual runs his own show, whatever he chooses it to be. The ultimate goal is for the participants to develop the sense that: "I had total responsibility for my life — all of it, the happiness and the sorrow."

From a cultural perspective, est appealed to well-educated adults during the 1970s because it provided a philosophy of life that was radically different from the beliefs of the contemporary society. In Torrey's interpretation (1986), est tends to affect the participant through the "superman syndrome," i.e., making a person believe that he has the power to handle his own life.

Est is primarily oriented philosophically and psychologically. Instruction by the therapist for enlightenment toward life is accomplished in a group setting. Reexamination of the self and correction of one's views of life are the mechanisms of therapy, with the goal of psychosocial change of the self.

G. MORITA THERAPY

Morita therapy was originally founded by a Japanese psychiatrist, Shoma Morita (see Fig. 33-1a), in 1919, about the same time that Sigmund Freud developed psychoanalysis in Austria. Morita developed his therapy primarily for the treatment of anthrophobia — a common minor psychiatric disorder recognized in Japan at the time (Iwai & Reynolds, 1970; A. Kondo, 1953; K. Kondo, 1976). Around the turn of the 20th century, industrialization and modernization began to take hold in Japan. It was also the era in which Western psychiatry began to be imported from Europe to Japan. In clinical psychiatry at that time, the major focus was on the treatment and care of patients who were hospitalized with diagnoses of psychoses. However, associated with rapid social change, many neurotic patients with diagnoses of "neurasthenia" appeared in clinics without any relevant therapy. Morita himself had been troubled by the fear of death and neurasthenia since his childhood and had over-

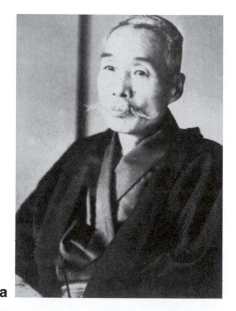

a

FIGURE 33-1 **Morita therapy originated in Japan.** (a) A Japanese psychiatrist, Shoma Morita, founded the experiential therapy, which was later named after him. *(Figure continues)*

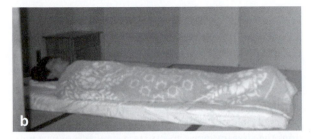

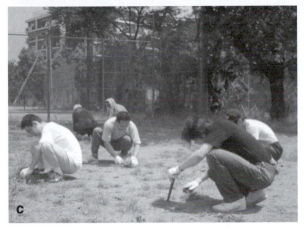

FIGURE 33-1 (continued)   (b) A young male suffering from *taijinkyofusho* resting in bed during the first stage of therapy. (c) A group of male patients doing yard work in the second stage of therapy. (d) A patient's diary with comments by his therapist in red pen as a part of the therapeutic activities. [Courtesy of Kenji Kitanish, M.D.].

come the problem on his own. Based on his personal experience, Morita was very interested in the treatment of patients diagnosed with neurasthenia, *shinkeishitus* (nervous temperament), and *taijinkyofusho* (interpersonal relation phobia). According to Kitanish and Mori (1995), Morita tried to replicate Silas Weir Mitchell's "rest therapy," Otto Binswanger's method of "life normalization," and Dubois' "persuasion method," but did not obtain favorable results. After attempting a variety of treatment methods, he created a new therapy of his own, which he called "experiential therapy."

In experiential therapy, Morita treated patients in his own home, letting them go through different stages of experience, including rest, life renormalization, and life rehabilitation. In the first stage, the patients were asked to take bed rest. On addition to taking three meals or going to the rest room occasionally, patients were confined to bed day and night for 1 or 2 weeks. No talking or reading was allowed through this stage so that sensory and social activity deprivation would occur, often making patients eager to reenter normal life (see Fig. 33-1b). Then patients were permitted to wake up, starting to engage in simple life with light chore work, such as washing dishes, cleaning the yard, or taking a walk, often experiencing appreciation of life around them rather than obsessing about their mental symptoms as they had done before (see Fig. 33-1c). Starting this second stage, the patients were asked to write a diary, which would be commented on by the therapist, with an emphasis on how to establish a new attitude about life, i.e., to accept reality (including symptoms or suffering) as it was (see Fig. 33-1d).

Most important is that through all stages of therapy, patients were discouraged from talking about their problems and complaining about their symptoms. A life atmosphere was set up to encourage the patient to learn to accept his self "as it is" (*arugamama* in Japanese, which literally means thing-as-it-is-ness) and to concentrate on enjoying his own life as it was. Perhaps Japanese patients were not used to talking about their internal emotional lives in face-to-face situations with others, thus, instead of talking to a therapist individually, each patient was asked to write a daily diary in which various therapeutic comments were made by the therapist. *Arugamama* (accepting things as they are), *shizen-fukuziu* (obedience to nature), *kohdo-honyi* (action-orientation), *ichi-nich kore koji* (every day is a good day), and *heijosin kore michi* (to keep an ordinary mind is the way of life) are some examples or comments that were often used by the therapist (Ohara & Ohara, 1993). The latter two comments are direct quotations from Zen teaching. These comments were used as slogans in the patient's daily life, with the intention of changing this basic life attitude.

Morita theorized that the disorder of *shinkeishitus* was a result of the disposition of a hypochondriacal temperament, exposure to internal or external mental stimulation, and psychic interaction with a patient's own reaction. The patient sees the "natural" emotional reaction toward stress as a negative one. Excessive attention is given to his own reaction. As a result, symptoms are formed and fixated from this negative relation between sensation and attention. In order to solve the malicious prepossession *(toraware)* resulting from this negative psychic interaction, the core of the therapy is to help the patient accept himself and ignore the symptoms. The change in attitude is achieved through actual life experience with the therapist.

Although Morita himself denied that he was influenced directly by Zen philosophy, many scholars have pointed out that his therapeutic principles were very much rooted in Oriental philosophical concepts (T.S. Lebra & Lebra, 1974; Miura & Usa, 1970; Reynolds, 1980). To learn things through life experience with a master was a common concept and practice in Japan-

ese traditional life. In general, people in Japan do not feel comfortable communicating personal feelings toward others. Instead, communication through writing a diary was very comfortable and acceptable to ordinary Japanese. In other words, the practice of Morita therapy was strongly shaped by the lifestyle of the Japanese. Thus, through programmed and staged life experiences, coupled with philosophical instruction, the therapy aims to create a new life experience for the patient. Through therapeutic mechanisms such as enlightenment about life, the therapy encouraged the patient to reach the psychological condition of accepting the self as it is.

Of interest is that during the past 75 years there have been many changes in the practice of Morita therapy. The original target population, diagnosed with *shinkeishitus,* has declined, and now more patients with obsession are being treated by the therapy. Needless to say, all therapy takes place in hospitals, not at a therapist's personal residence, as it was originally conducted by Morita. The 2-week complete rest therapy is not strictly observed and is less tolerated by young, contemporary Japanese patients. Drug therapy is frequently combined with work and recreational therapy. In other words, there has been considerable modification of therapy procedures so that it is now called neo-Morita therapy (Ohara & Ohara, 1993). One of Morita's major successors, Kenjiro Ohara, pointed out that the core of the therapy that remained was the emphasis on creating new life experiences. Thus, he preferred to call it "creative experiential therapy."

Another interesting point that deserves attention is that while the practice of Morita therapy is gradually declining in Japan (Kitanish & Mori, 1995), a new, rising Morita therapy movement has been observed recently on mainland China. According to Chinese psychiatrists, Morita therapy has become popular for various reasons: eagerness to develop psychotherapy after the period of vacancy following the Cultural Revolution, availability of funding from the Morita Foundation, and the relative ease of mastering the techniques of Morita therapy. Most important, according to Cui (1997), is that the basic therapeutic attitude and ideology emphasized in Morita therapy, as illustrated by the concept of "acceptance (of symptom or illness) as it is," is related to the teaching of Zen Buddhism, which originated in China. Therefore, the therapeutic ideology is very easy for patients in China to understand and accept. What Cui is referring to is the cultural compatibility of such therapy with the Chinese people.

There have been several attempts to carry out Morita therapy in Western societies. According to Iwai and Reynolds (1970), K. Leonhard has tried the therapy in East Germany and reported in 1965 that "it was almost impossible for the neurotic European patient to undergo the stage of absolute bed rest for therapy; besides, recreational activities rather than work activities were more effective for anxiety reduction in his patients." According to Reynolds and Kiefer (1977), several therapists implemented Morita therapy in West Coast areas of the United States with reasonable success among certain populations of clients. If this is true, it is worth examining the kinds of modifications needed for this imported Japanese-culture related therapy to work for American patients.

H. Existential Psychotherapy

Existential psychotherapy is a general term used to refer to the basic approach concerned with understanding the client as he exists in his world. In a strict sense, it is not a particular type of therapy with a special theory, method, or technique. It is an attitude and approach to human beings. The incorporation of an existential approach into psychotherapy was developed independently in various parts of Europe around the 1960s by a group of trained analysts and scholars, including Binswanger, Boss, Frankle, Marcel, and Sonneman (Patterson, 1966).

Existential psychotherapy is based on existential philosophy, which holds that man is responsible for his own existence. From an operational perspective, the therapy emphasizes confrontation, primarily in the here-and-now interaction, and on feeling experiences. The therapeutic relationship is regarded as an encounter, a new relationship opening up new horizons. The goal of the therapy is to encourage the client to actualize himself and to fulfill his inner potential.

From a cultural point of view, Kelman (1960) pointed out that the orientation of existential psychotherapy is a phenomenon of the West. He explained that the East in characterized by a subjectifying attitude, the West by an objectifying one. Eastern cognition is interested in consciousness itself. Western cognition is interested in the objects of consciousness. According to Kelman, existentialism is the formulated awareness of Westerners' estrangement and alienation from their roots and from all otherness. He regards the emergence of and interest in existentialism as evidence that Western man is aware that his philosophic roots are inadequate.

III. COMMENTS

From a clinical point of view, culturally influenced unique therapies, as a subgroup, share some characteristics. First, the therapies are often invented originally to treat a particular set of clients or patients with a certain pathology so that the treatment is often applicable only to a limited group of subjects, such as Mesmerism for neurotic women in Europe in the late 18th century, rest therapy for patients who seemed exhausted and were thought to have an "anemic" brain (neurasthenia), Naikan therapy for juvenile delinquency (in the beginning stages), rapid integrated therapy for neurasthenic patients who failed to participate fully in the social and economic production expected during the era of "Great Leap Movement," est for relatively well-educated clients who were frustrated by the contemporary beliefs of American society and were looking for self-improvement during the 1970s, or Morita therapy for anthrophobia (taijinkyofusho), a special form of social phobia often observed in Japan. Each therapy has been developed more or less specifically for a particular subpopulation of patients. Therefore, the treatment tends to have limited value when applied to broader psychiatric populations.

Second, each therapy is strongly influenced by cultural factors, and is based on a certain set of beliefs, value systems, and underlying philosophy. It is useful clinically only in a particular sociocultural environment in a given era. Thus, it is unlikely to gain favor in other cultural settings, or during different periods of time in the same society. This is best exemplified by the rapid integrated therapy, invented and popularized in China during the period of "Great Leap Movement," but abandoned in conjunction with the dramatic social changes of the Cultural Revolution. There is no current interest in reviving this method of treatment that was once considered so effective. Another example is the decline in use of Morita therapy in contemporary Japan. Today's younger generation is unlikely to tolerate lying quietly on a bed for a week without listening to loud jazz music or navigating the internet. As a consequence, neo-Morita therapy no longer practices strict bed confinement as the initial stage of treatment and, instead, concentrates on cognitive approaches in order to help patients establish a new life philosophy and attitude, which is now claimed as the core of the therapy.

Third, there is often a tendency for the therapist to emphasize the uniqueness of the invented therapy. This is frequently coupled with a subjective claim that the therapy is very effective, despite the lack of objective scientific data to support it. Nevertheless, such treatment may be favorably received by clients who eagerly try any unique therapy that appears to satisfy their psychological needs and complies with their cultural beliefs. However, from a scientific perspective, these unique therapies are often atheoretical, without comprehensive theories of psychopathology, or consistency in the proposed mechanisms of therapy. Thus, the application of the therapy may rely heavily on the therapist's personal charisma or the contextual social and group dynamics. Thus, from a professional point of view, there tends to be many limitations and shortcomings when considering the unique therapy as a psychotherapy.

In spite of this, from a cultural perspective, a culture-influenced unique psychotherapy provides an opportunity to examine important social and cultural trends. For instance, many therapies are heavily oriented toward social, religious, and political dimensions that are seldom utilized in individual therapy in the mainstream. Examples include the emphasis on religious faith in folk family therapy, ho'oponopono, to set right the problem; the utilization of social and group influences in A.A.; and sociopolitical psychology in rapid integrated therapy. Unique therapies are also often organized around explicit philosophical issues or viewpoints, such as in Naikan therapy, est, Morita therapy, or existential psychotherapy. In any therapy, the therapist's personal philosophy is often important in influencing the style and direction of treatment, yet this is almost ignored, if not denied, in "psychology-oriented," contemporary empirically-based psychotherapies. By studying culture-influenced unique psychotherapies, we may recognize more clearly the therapeutic factors operating in treatment that involve broad social, religious, philosophical dimensions, beyond the individual psychology to which we are more sensitive.

Cultural analysis readily demonstrates the cultural influences in these unique therapies. For instance, folk family therapy of ho'oponopono utilizes the cultural value of harmony without conflict within a family, Nikan therapy makes use of a particular culturally sanctioned filial attitude toward parental figures, and Morita therapy stresses the philosophy that it is desirably to accept things as they are. These therapies thus affirm and make therapeutic use of cultural values. In contrast to this, est proposes the possibility of self assurance and improvement in order to contrast with the cultural emphasis of social confinement; rest therapy provides cultural time out temporary from sociocultural pressure; and ho'oponopono provides temporary permission to express anger or resentment during the healing session. Culture-influenced unique psychotherapies teach us that the cultural implications of psychotherapy in general are many. Among them are the affirmation of central cultural values and reinforcement of culturally sanctioned coping patterns on one hand, and the exploration of alternative cultural approaches to conflict resolution (or permission for cultural "time out") on other hand. Indeed, the practice of any psychotherapy can not operate without cultural implications [cross-reference to Chapter 37: Culture-Relevant Psychotherapy (Section III, B)].

Finally, from an academic point of view, there is a great need to investigate the actual factors that contribute to the therapy, if it is effective. For instance, regarding Morita therapy, there are a number of academic questions waiting to be researched. What is the clinical significance of having a two-week-long bed rest during the initial stage of therapy? Why is it necessary to carry out therapeutic intervention through comments in the client's diary rather than through a face-to-face interview method? Is such a therapy useful only for social anthrophobia, for which it was originally applied, or is it applicable to other kinds of psychopathologies as well? What would the clinical effect be if such a therapy were applied in other cultural settings with different views of the world and life? These are issues that remain to be explored.

REFERENCES

Alexander, F.G., & Selesnick, S.T. (1966). *The history of psychiatry: An evaluation of psychiatric thought and practice from prehistoric times to the present.* New York: Harper & Row.

Beard, G.M. (1880). *A practical treatise on nervous exhaustion (neurasthenia), its symptoms, nature, sequences, treatment.* New York: William Wood.

Cui, Y.H. (1997). Review of the experience of Japanese Morita therapy in China. In W.S. Tseng (Ed.), *Chinese mind and therapy* (pp. 508–525). Beijing: Beijing Medical University Press (in Chinese).

Ito, K.L. (1985). Ho'oponopono, "to make right": Hawaiian conflict resolution nd metaphor in the construction of a family therapy. *Culture, Medicine and Psychiatry, 9*(2), 201–217.

Iwai, H., & Reynolds, D.K. (1970). Morita psychotherapy: The views from the West. *American Journal of Psychiatry, 126*(7), 1031–1036.

Jilek, W.G. (1994). Traditional healing in the prevention and treatment of alcohol and drug abuse. *Transcultural Psychiatric Research Review, 31*(3), 219–258.

Jilek-Aall, L. (1981). Acculturation, alcoholism and Indian-style Alcoholics Anonymous. *Journal of Studies on Alcohol, Supplement, 9,* 143–158.

Kelman, H. (1960). Existentialism: A phenomenon of the West. *International Journal of Social Psychiatry, 5,* 299–302.

Kitanish, K., & Mori, A. (1995). Morita therapy: 1919 to 1995. *Psychiatry and Clinical Neurosciences, 49,* 245–254.

Kondo, A. (1953), Morita therapy — A Japanese therapy for neurosis. *American Journal of Psychoanalysis, 13,* 31–37.

Kondo, K. (1976). The origin of Morita therapy. In W.P. Lebra (Ed.), *Culture-bound syndromes, ethnopsychiatry, and alternate therapies* (pp. 250–258). Honolulu: University Press of Hawaii.

Lebra, T.S., & Lebra, W.P. (Eds.). (1974). *Japanese culture and behavior: Selected readings.* Honolulu: University Press of Hawaii.

Lebra, W.P. (Ed.). (1976). *Culture-bound syndromes, ethnopsychiatry, and alternate therapies.* Honolulu: University Press of Hawaii.

Li, C.P. (1997). Integrative rapid therapy: Sociocultural background and clinical experience. In W.S. Tseng (Ed.), *Chinese mind and therapy.* Beijing: Beijing Medical University Press (in Chinese).

Makela, K. (1993). International comparisons of alcoholics anonymous. *Alcohol Health & Research World, 17*(3), 228–234.

Miura, M.S., & Usa, S.I. (1970). A psychotherapy of neurosis: Morita therapy. *Yonago Acta Medica, 14*(1), 1–17.

Murase, T. (1976). Naikan therapy. In W.P. Lebra (Ed.), *Culture-bound syndromes, ethnopsychiatry, and alternate therapies.* Honolulu: University Press of Hawaii.

Murase, T. (1984). *Sunao:* A central value in Japanese psychotherapy. In A.J. Marsella & G.M. White (Eds.), *Cultural conceptions of mental health and therapy* (pp. 317–329) (pp. 259–269). Dordrecht; The Netherlands Reidel.

Ohara, K., & Ohara, K.I. (1993). *Morita therapy and neo-Morita therapy* (in Japanese). Tokyo: Nihon Bunka Kagakusha.

Patterson, C.H. (1966). *Theories of counseling and psychotherapy.* New York: Harper & Row.

Reynolds, D.K. (1977). Naikan therapy: An experiential view. *International Journal of Social Psychiatry, 23*(4), 252–263.

Reynolds, D.K. (1980). *The quiet therapies: Japanese pathways to personal growth.* Honolulu: University Press of Hawaii.

Reynolds, D.K. (1983). *Naikan psychotherapy: Meditation for self-development* (pp. 137–147). Chicago: University of Chicago Press.

Reynolds, D.K., & Kiefer, C.W. (1977). Cultural adaptability as an attribute of therapies: The case of Morita psychotherapy. *Culture, Medicine and Psychiatry, 1*(4), 395–412.

Schneck, J.M. (1975). United States of America. In J.G. Howells (Ed.), *World history of psychiatry* (pp. 432–475). New York: Brunner/Mazel.

Shook, E.V. (1985). *Ho oponopono: Contemporary use of a Hawaiian problem-solving process.* Honolulu: University of Hawaii Press.

Torrey, E.F. (1986). *Witchdoctors and psychiatrists: The common roots of psychotherapy and its future* (pp. 73–74). New York: Harper & Row.

34

Culture-Related "Common" Psychotherapies

I. WHAT ARE CULTURE-RELATED COMMON PSYCHOTHERAPIES?

As pointed out at the beginning of this section, psychotherapeutic activities, as cultural products of humankind, are connected to and shaped by culture in their theory and practice to some degree. In this section, the terms "culture-embedded," "culture-influenced," and "culture-related" are used to denote various degrees of cultural impact. As described previously, "culture-embedded" implies that a healing practice is heavily bound to a particular cultural context, and that it is almost impossible to transplant it to another cultural setting. The term "culture-influenced" indicates that a therapy is very strongly colored by cultural elements, and may have some limited application to other cultural environments. "Culture-related" indicates that, while a practice is influenced by culture, the impact is less recognized and emphasized.

Based on these general concepts, in Chapters 32 and 33, indigenous healing practices, which are heavily embedded in their cultural contexts, and unique therapies, which are strongly culture-influenced, have been reviewed. In this chapter, modern, contemporary "common" therapies, which are culture-related, will be examined.

In this chapter, "common" psychotherapies refer to the ordinary, mainstream therapies that are recognized by contemporary professionals in European-American societies. This group of psychotherapies is in significant contrast to indigenous, folk, or nonmodern therapies in many ways. It is characterized by a psychological orientation and operates as a professional activity with a scientific nature — allowing for objective evaluation and criticism of its theories and its effectiveness as a therapy. However, it needs to be recognized that the distinction between so-called common or mainstream therapies and unique, alternative or folk therapies is arbitrary and artificially determined, depending on who is viewing the phenomena and defining the terms.

Because common psychotherapies tend to be viewed as "scientific" medical practices, are assumed to be "universally" applicable, and have, in fact, been practiced as major, orthodox therapies in European-American societies, they are seldom studied from cultural perspectives. They are products of ethnocentrism or cultural scotoma. However, if one takes the view that these "common" or "regular" therapies are cultural products, then there is room to evaluate them in their cultural dimensions. This section attempts to review the cultural aspects of these "mainstream" psychotherapies. Because it would be impossible to examine every kind of regular psychotherapy that exists, only those that have appeared in literature on the ways in which therapies are culture-related will be reviewed here.

II. CULTURAL ELEMENTS IN VARIOUS COMMON PSYCHOTHERAPIES

A. INDIVIDUAL PSYCHOTHERAPIES

1. Psychoanalysis

Even though many psychoanalysts take the view that psychoanalysis deals with the basic aspects of the human mind and is universally applicable, some clinicians do not agree. Some scholars have pointed out that the theory and practice of psychoanalysis are very culturally influenced: by the ethnic cultural background of their founder, Sigmund Freud, and the sociocultural environment of Vienna, where they originated.

For example, Meadow and Vetter (1959) indicated how the Judaic cultural value system influenced the Freudian theory of psychotherapy. In contrast to Christianity, Judaism maintains that the ultimate goal of human happiness is attainable in the real world (not in heaven) and that any unhappiness in the real world is evil and needs to be fixed. This is the basic attitude reflected in psychoanalytic theory, and the purpose of therapy. While psychoanalytic therapy views heterosexual relationships as a *sine qua non* for happiness, it is the aim of psychoanalysis to aid the individual in establishing rational control over his sexual drive. This affirmation of rational control is consistent with a major emphasis in the Jewish cultural pattern. To the Talmudic scholar, a word is presumed to possess a special hidden significance in addition to its simple and direct meaning. A similarity is found between Talmudic and psychoanalytic attitudes toward the mean-

ing of words. The Freudian concept of family relations and the development of the Oedipus complex are closely related to the typical family pattern in Jewish culture: the mother–son relationship is more intense and complete than the relationship between husband and wife and the ideal marital relationship is one in which the wife treats her husband as a child. From a cultural point of view, it can be explained that most psychoanalysts have Jewish backgrounds, and most of the patients who seek psychoanalysis are also Jewish. At least this is true in New York, where there is a high percentage of Jewish people.

The Eastern psychiatrist Pande (1968) offered an Eastern interpretation of why psychoanalysis, as a "Western" psychotherapy, fit people in contemporary Western societies. He pointed out that in Eastern, relationship-oriented societies, no agenda as such was necessary for the cultivation of a relationship; however, in Western working- and activity-oriented societies, the absence of an agenda would be disturbing. Although the language of psychoanalysis is of understanding and insight, its metalanguage is of love and human involvement in an activity-oriented society. There is a general tendency in Western societies to rush a person from infancy into adulthood. The rush toward adulthood may be compelling, but it leaves much unfinished business, which at times needs to be dealt with in psychotherapy. The "working through" of childhood experiences in psychotherapy, particularly in psychoanalysis, becomes a meaningful and worthwhile experience for patients in this regard. Thus, the institution of psychotherapy may be viewed as a symbolic and substantive cultural undertaking to meet the deficits in Western societies.

On a different level, Gellner (1985) suggested that one of the reasons for the dramatic rise of psychoanalysis in the Western world is that it filled a gap left by religion, providing a doctrine that allowed post-Darwinian man to accept his place in the natural world. He pointed out that many hours of analysis, which combines confession, authority, and closely applied attention, inevitably develops a strong bond of loyalty between the analyst and the patient, strengthening the belief system.

However, psychoanalytic practices have difficulty taking root in various societies for various reasons. One of the main factors is cultural background. For instance, as pointed out by Doi (1964), even though psychoanalytic thought was introduced in Japan around the 1930s, the practice of psychoanalysis had barely reached beyond a small circle of interested people to the majority of Japanese psychiatrists by the 1970s. According to Doi, Japanese culture and society lacked a certain quality — respect for potential independence and basic freedom — that favors the practice of such therapy. Dividing psychotherapy into the two main categories of analytic-psychological and directive-organic, Redlich (1958) pointed out that the former, exemplified by psychoanalysis, requires a tolerant and permissive culture for its development. It will not grow in a totalitarian or dogmatic culture. This is well illustrated by the situation in Russia during Stalin's time, Germany in the Nazi era, and China in Mao's time.

It is well known that due to political ideology and cultural factors, psychoanalytic theory and practice were opposed in communist societies. In Russia, despite the development of a small psychoanalytic movement, based mainly in Moscow during the early Soviet years, the movement began to die out after the Russian Psychoanalytic Society was disbanded in 1933 (Calloway, 1992–1993). Psychoanalytic theory fell out of favor on ideological grounds. In China, during the Cultural Revolution, psychoanalysis was criticized as the product of (Western) capitalism, which benefits only the individual, ignoring society's collective needs, and is applicable only to a privileged minority.

2. Client-Centered Psychotherapy

This therapy was developed in the 1940s by Carl R. Rogers, a psychologist with a Freudian background. His method of counseling was originally called "nondirective" and, later, "client-centered." In drastic contrast to the orientations of classic psychoanalysis that were most influential at the time in the United States, Rogers developed a unique mode of counseling

with several emphases. The cornerstones of his method were the basic knowableness and trustworthiness of an individual's own inner awareness, and his or her ability to accurately symbolize these inner data and use them to reorganize and make choices (Wexler & Rice, 1974). The fundamental assumption of the therapy was a person's basic motivation toward growth and differentiation. Thus, the therapy focused on the enormous potential of the individual and freeing the client for normal growth and development (Rogers, 1974).

It is interesting to note that Meadow (1964) made cultural comments about client-centered therapy and its relation to the basic American ethos. He pointed out that client-centered therapy is an expression of the fundamental individual "distrust of the expert" theme in American culture. Reflecting the tendency of American culture to deemphasize the past, client-centered therapy places greater stress upon the immediate situation. Most important is that client-centered therapy gives particular attention to the client's need for autonomy or independence. It is closely related to the American ethos: The American not only seeks independence for himself but feels it is his moral duty to make others independent. No wonder such a therapeutic approach is not particularly welcomed by clients in cultural settings where dependence on authority is expected and personal autonomy is less emphasized.

3. Behavior Therapy

Among the different kinds of individual psychotherapy, behavior therapy is oriented most heavily toward the purely psychological aspects of behavioral change and is less colored by culture elements. In Russia, behavior therapy is called "condition-reflex therapy," implying that it is embedded in the biological–behavioral nature of therapy. However, by examining the cultural dimensions of therapy models, one recognizes that behavior therapy is not immune from cultural impact. Contemporary behavior therapists have discovered that the application of the principles of learning theory requires attention to the sociocultural determinants of behavior as part of behavior assessment and treatment planning. The practitioner needs to understand the norms in the patient's sociocultural milieu for presenting problem behaviors. Who are the most significant persons in the patient's life and current environment? How will improvement in the patient affect the patient's relationships in his current environment?

From a technical standpoint, an emphasis on action and presumably concretely identifiable change are the targeted outcomes of behavior therapy, which may be accepted more favorably in some cultures than in others. The distinction between mind and body takes on a phenomenological tone rather than an explanatory or causal one. This might be more understandable or acceptable in some cultural groups than others. The use of relaxation training, some forms of biofeedback, and other techniques can be used within the context of cultural values with little adaptation of interventions. One of the advantages of behavior therapy is the objectivity and systematization of the teaching and practicing of its protocols or techniques. These elements tend to be accepted more easily by people from cultural backgrounds that favor such approaches to life. In other words, there are numerous ways in which culture influences the practice of behavior therapy.

4. Cognitive Therapy

Cognitive therapy has been developed with emphasis to work on therapeutic issues mainly at the level of cognition. It is based on the assumption that if the dysfunctional cognition is corrected, the ill-functioning behavior and affection will be improved accordingly. It is considered easier to apply clinically to a beginner in therapy. However, from a cultural point of view, it is considered more beneficial to people who are oriented toward reviewing and discussing psychological issues at a cognitive rather than an emotional level and who focus on the present rather than their roots in the past.

It is interesting to note that in China recently, associated with the rapid increase in the popularization of psychotherapy — after nearly two decades of the inhibition of individual-focused psychotherapy during the Cultural Revolution for reasons of political ideology — Taoist thought-oriented cognitive therapy has been experimented with and examined (Young, 1997). Taoist thought is characterized by a philosophical attitude that views things beyond realistic and practical needs. It has been claimed to be useful in cognitive therapy for patients who have indulged in and are suffering from the pursuit of achievement and gain in reality. This is culture-modified cognitive therapy.

B. INTERPERSONAL PSYCHOTHERAPY

Interpersonal psychotherapy refers to therapy that is focused primarily on interpersonal issues rather than on the individual. It includes couple or marital therapy, family therapy, and group therapy. The interpersonal issues of communication, interaction patterns, and role playing, as well as attitudes, opinions, views, and value systems relating to interpersonal interaction, receive primary attention. Therefore, the cultural aspects of human behavior are dealt with more explicitly in these therapeutic processes.

1. Marital Therapy

In marital therapy, the therapist usually works on several different areas, including the partners' expectations of and commitment to marriage, the division of roles between husband and wife, ways of rearing children, relationships with families of origin, communication and sharing between partners, and methods of coping when problems arise. Obviously, all of these issues are subject to cultural factors. Thus, there is a great need for cultural consideration in marital therapy.

In practice, the marital therapist needs to pay attention to the culturally defined roles of man and woman, husband and wife, or father and mother. These roles vary greatly in different cultural groups. For instance, even in trivial matters, which partner should be encouraged or allowed to start the conversation or make the complaint is important from the first session. In a culture that places great emphasis on the dominant role of the man, husband, or father, it is very important to follow the cultural pattern and respect the male participant and allow him to open the conversation or lead in the revealing of problems. Otherwise, there may be an unfavorable outcome, including the discontinuation of therapy by the male for not respecting him as the "boss" in man–woman, husband–wife, or father–mother relations.

One of the basic rules in couple therapy is to avoid alienating one partner and neglecting the other. Taking sides with one of the partners can occur for a number of reasons, including gender or age factors. Similarity or dissimilarity of personal, ethnic, or cultural backgrounds are additional factors that may affect the therapist–client relationship and need careful attention.

The acceptable and effective ways of dealing with marital problems vary from culture to culture. For instance, openly acknowledging and facing problems and actively, even aggressively, dealing with problems to resolve them are coping patterns favored in some cultures, whereas passively enduring and concealing problems to maintain harmony may be considered virtues in other cultures. It is the therapist's job to consider and check with the partner–clients to learn the nature and direction of their cultural coping patterns. The goal and outcome of therapy need to be clarified with the clients from the beginning of therapy and throughout the course of treatment.

In general, cultural issues will become more explicit if therapy is undertaken for problems related to intercultural marriage (Tseng, McDermott, & Maretzki, 1997). In therapy for intercultural marriage-related problems, the therapeutic maneuvers should focus on the promotion of awareness and understanding of differences in values between the partners; encouragement of negotiation and compromise in the resolution of differences; allowing time for the gradual change of culture-related emotions; and permitting a cultural holiday for both partners as needed.

2. Family Therapy

A family is the basic social unit in life. The cultural aspects of family therapy have been discussed from several perspectives. Regarding the applicability of family therapy, the question has been raised whether ethnic–cultural groups that give greater importance to the family (such as Italian, Portuguese, or Chinese) are better suited for family therapy. Based on clinical experience, it has been pointed out that an emphasis on close family interrelations does not necessarily favor the family therapy approach. For instance, Moitoza (1982) pointed out that Portuguese families' closed family systems prevents them from actively seeking family therapy; instead, they attempt to solve their problems via their own family resources and support systems. Chinese families are concerned that "internal disgrace not be known by outsiders"; thus, until a family trusts a therapist, it is relatively difficult to work on their family "secrets" (Hsu, 1983, 1995). Also, it usually takes considerable effort to help a family with culturally fixed, preexisting behavior patterns to unlearn its way of dealing with problems (Tseng & Hsu, 1991).

Concerning the therapist–family relationship, it has been pointed out that it is desirable for the therapist to respect and utilize the culturally defined and sanctioned family hierarchy and relations and constantly evaluate the cultural transference that could occur in family therapy. For instance, McGoldrick and Pearce (1981) pointed out that the Irish cultural attitude toward authority figures will often lead members of an Irish family to show extreme loyalty and willingness to follow through on therapeutic suggestions. In Chinese families, Hsu (1983) suggested that, based on the concept of extended family social relationships, members may feel more comfortable if they are allowed to address the therapist with a pseudokin term (e.g., if the therapist is a woman close to the mother's age, she may be referred to as "auntie").

Numerous points are made by various clinicians concerning cultural aspects directly related to therapeutic strategies. In working with Japanese families, it is necessary to deal with family matters according to cultural priorities, i.e., to work on parent–child relations before beginning work on husband–wife issues, according to the Japanese cultural priority of dyad within a family (Suzuki, 1987). Working with Chicano families, several clinicians (Falicov, 1982; Minuchin, Montalvo, Guerney, Rosman, & Schumer, 1967) have proposed that it is better to use a structural family therapy approach to satisfy the cultural emphasis on hierarchies within families. McGoldrick and Pearce (1981) have pointed out that Irish families are apt to be threatened by therapy directed at uncovering hostile or erotic feelings and may respond better to a positive reframing of the strategic therapy model. Regarding Jewish families, Herz and Rosen (1982) have mentioned that, closely related to their cultural tendency to treasure suffering as a shared value, the verbal expression of feelings in family therapy may be emphasized.

In sum, a family therapist needs to be familiar with cultural variations of family systems, structures, and interactional patterns, including role playing, communication, and value systems that are emphasized. The therapist also needs to know how to select culturally suitable intervention techniques so that culturally relevant family therapies can be applied for families with different cultural backgrounds (Tseng & Hsu, 1991). If the therapist is working with ethnic minorities, as stressed by Ho (1987), his role is to serve as a "culture broker" rather than an intruder; to facilitate negotiations between systems; and, usually, to work closely with the more acculturated members to promote change within the whole family, facilitating its adjustment to the host society. A similar view has been raised by Jalali (1988), who pointed out that, in treating ethnic families, the therapist is often confronted with a clash of two cultures, two generations, and problems in acculturation. The therapist, at the time of the conflict, explains and teaches the values and norms of both sides and acts as a cultural mediator, encouraging all to become multicultural, or to have a foot in both cultures. Thus, it is clearly indicated that family therapy is focused on cultural adjustment within the family or among family members.

3. Group Therapy

By definition, group therapy works with a group of members in therapeutic activities. Naturally, it involves group formation, interaction, and many other aspects of group processes and phenomena. In addition to the basic factors relating to group composition, including age, gender, personality, and the psychopathology of the group members, the group transactions will obviously be influenced by the ethnic and cultural backgrounds of the members and the therapist.

A psychiatrist from Nigeria, Asuni (1967), reported that due to the extreme shortage of therapists for standardized individual psychotherapy, an attempt has been made to develop group therapy mainly for hospitalized patients. As for the style of therapy, a nondirective, nonformal procedure was adopted for open group therapy for selected inpatients to fit their local situation and cultural background.

Working with Greek immigrants in group therapy, Dunkas and Nikelly (1975) commented that a Greek was more attuned to group goals than to individual fulfillment. He did what the group approved of and expected, receiving cues through its tacit or obvious approval. Instead of self-actualization and personal happiness, the Greek pursued love, esteem, and admiration from members of his group. The group members tended to maintain an attitude of servility and passivity; they looked up to the therapist and expected him to do the work. Such ethnic-related personality attributes were clearly manifested in transactions of the group during therapy.

Based on his working experience with Orthodox Jewish patients in New York, an Orthodox Jewish therapist, R.Y. Shapiro (1996), raised issues that are pertinent to treating such a population in group therapy. For instance, due to the small and close ethnic population in the community, individual anonymity was almost impossible to maintain. The mixture of gender in the group was quite untraditional and culturally unfamiliar, and resulted in heightened resistance to therapy. Because verbal propriety is a cultural requirement, group members were self-restricting in their language and verbal style and the topics they were willing to discuss.

Leading group therapy for Chicanos in Texas, Martinez (1977) pointed out that there was a Mexican tradition of close-mouthedness and not opening up to others *(no te rajes)*. This worked against communication and expression of feelings in group situations. Also, there was a built-in formality in interpersonal relations among Spanish-speaking people, as reflected in their language usage. This greater formality made it difficult for group members to relate to one another candidly as equals and inhibited the voicing of negative feelings toward the therapist.

Based on group therapy experiences with Chinese clients in Canada, Chen (1995) noted that the Chinese tended to expect the therapist to maintain the image of an authority figure with expertise, to educate the group members, and to provide structure for the group process. It was also better for the therapist to define rules and boundaries for the members to follow.

All of the points just raised indicate that the behavior of group members is influenced greatly by their cultural backgrounds in the areas of communication style, relational patterns, and interaction with the therapist, all of which, in turn, impact the process of group therapy. In contrast to individual psychotherapy, which focuses mainly on the psychopathology of an individual, interpersonal psychotherapy deals primarily with problems related to interpersonal issues; thus, there is more of a need to consider and understand cultural impact on interactional human behavior.

III. INTEGRATION: COMPARISON OF VARIOUS MODES OF THERAPY

The various kinds of psychotherapy broadly defined in the previous two chapters — **culture-embedded** indigenous healing practices and **culture-influenced** unique psychotherapies — and, in this chapter, **culture-related** common psychotherapies are all included for comparison here. Historically, when cultural psychiatrists became interested in indigenous healing practices, their efforts were concentrated on discovering the similarities between folk and modern therapy. They focused on the universal therapeutic mechanisms utilized (Frank, 1961; Torrey, 1986). Here, instead, the aim is to compare the differences

between them. This will be done in several areas, including the orientation of the practices, the operations and mechanisms of therapy, and the goals of therapy (see Table 34-1). The purpose of these comparisons is to provide a panoramic view of the nature of "psychotherapy" from different perspectives.

A. ORIENTATION AND THERAPEUTIC OPERATION

The most distinguishable variables among the indigenous, unique, and regular psychotherapies listed in Table 34-1 are the orientations on which they are based. Most indigenous healing practices, such as spirit mediumship, religious healing ceremonies, and divination, are founded on the basic assumption of the existence of a supernatural power. It is believed that the mediator, a special person such as a shaman, priest, or diviner, has the power to communicate with spirits and to use supernatural powers to solve the client's problems. Based on this premise, the causes of the problems are usually perceived as having to do with loss of soul, sorcery, spirit intrusion, or violation of taboos. By interpreting for the client the idea that a god, a devil, or a soul is the potential source of interference, the healer provides a concrete way to counteract the "identified" cause of the problems. The suggested coping methods are usually magical, such as prayer, the use of a charm, or the performance of a ritual ceremony for extraction or exorcism. Even though these therapies are based on a supernatural orientation, clearly there are psychological implications and effects in their interpretations and suggested remedies. That is, the interpretation of the shaman is symbolic, containing psychological and therapeutic effects. Emotional catharsis, gratification of unfulfilled wishes, or obtaining concrete and decisive "answers" are in operation.

Unlike spirit mediumship, such as shamanism or Zar ceremonies, religious healing does not necessarily involve the therapeutic operation of the healer going into an altered state of consciousness; a trance or possessed state. However, it is still supernaturally ori-

TABLE 34-1 Comparison of Therapeutic Orientations, Operations, Mechanisms, and Goals among Different Indigenous and Modern Therapeutic Modes[*]

Therapeutic mode	Example of therapy	Orientation	Therapeutic operation	Special healing mechanism	Goals of practice (aims of therapy)
Culture embedded **Indigenous healing practices**	Spirit mediumship	Supernatural	Altered state of consciousness	Belief in supernatural power suggestions	Resolving "problems"
	Shamanism Zar Ceremony		Symbolic interpretation Revealing of wishes	Magical counteracting Emotional catharsis Gratification of unfulfilled wishes	Restoring balance in life
	Religious healing ceremony	Supernatural	Healing ceremony Prayer, sacrifice	Assurance, suggestions Generation of conviction	Healing problems
	Divination	Supernatural	Providing an "answer"	Finding a way to adjust "Naming" effects	Complying with divine instruction
	Fortune-telling Astrology/ physiognomy	Natural-supernatural	Providing guidance in making choices Folk interpretation	Helping make decisions Suggestion for counteracting	Complying with rules of nature
	Meditation Yoga/qigong	Somato-natural	Practice of meditation Regulation of vitality	Tranquilizing effects	Harmonizing with nature
Culture influenced **Unique therapy**	Somatotherapy Mesmerism Rest therapy	Somato-psychological	Supplementation Recuperation	Suggestions Legitimizing complaint	Restoring natural conditions
	Ho'oponopono	Socioreligious psychological	Group revealing and elaboration of conflict	Confession and apology	Restoring family–group relationships
	AA group	Sociopsychological	Group confession and testimony	Group support and enforcement	Restoring normal life
	Rapid integrated therapy	Sociopolitical psychological	Instruction and group activities	Sociopolitical sanction Group activation for recovery	Resuming status of normal member of society
	Naikan therapy	Philosophical– psychological	Self-examination	Reappraisal of relationships	Resuming ordinary family relationships
	est	Philosophical– psychological	Instruction and group enlightment	Re-examination of self	Psychosocial change of self
	Morita therapy	Philosophical– psychological	Programmed experience	Creating new life experience	Accepting self as it is
	Existential psychotherapy	Philosophical– psychological	Emphasis on confrontation' feeling experiences	Change attitude and view	Fulfill self potentialities
Culture related **Common therapy**	Psychoanalysis	Psychological	Listening with empathy Analytic interpretation	Transference Insight	Resolving "conflict" Striving for "maturity"
	Client-centered therapy	Psychological	Self-actualization	Sanction of self-independence	Improving self
	Behavior therapy	Psychological	Behavior manipulation	Relearning of behavior	Establishing "functional, adaptive" behavior
	Family therapy	Psychological	Working on family structure and relationships	Restoring family relations	Working toward a functional family
	Group therapy	Psychological	Working on group interaction	Group learning and interaction	Improving social relations

[*] From W.S. Tseng, *Transcultural Psychiatry, 36* (2), 131–179, 1999.

ented. Healing ceremonies, including prayer, sacrifice, and testimony, are often utilized for assurance and suggestions. In divination, the client seeks answers from the supernatural being on ways of dealing with his problems. The naming effect is the primary mechanism for healing.

In some indigenous, folk-healing practices, the basic orientation shifts from the supernatural to the natural. This is true in fortune-telling, physiognomy, and meditation, all of which emphasize that the principles of the universe rule nature, including human life and behavior. The concepts of microcosm and macrocosm are used to explain the corresponding relationships between nature and human phenomena. Problems are considered to result from an imbalance or disharmony with the underlying natural principles that rule the universe. The objectives of these practices are to help the client find out how to live compatibly with nature and to adjust to the environment more harmoniously and with stability. Providing guidance in making choices is the major therapeutic operation. The psychological interaction between the fortune-teller or astrologer and the client is an important variable in the effectiveness of the therapy.

Specific modes of therapy developed by professionals in the past, such as Mesmerism and rest therapy or current homeopathic therapies, are characterized as physiologically based treatments for psychological problems. They are basically oriented toward the somatopsychological system. The causes of problems are interpreted as the results of disequilibrium, insufficiency, or decompensation of the individual's physiological system, particularly the nervous system. Thus, supplementation of deficiencies, recuperation, and compensation are the methods generally employed in this mode of therapy, although suggestion is an important variable in the healing process.

Next is a group of therapeutic modes basically characterized by a philosophical–psychological orientation. These therapies recognize problems as psychological in nature and attempt to resolve them through psychological means. Therefore, they belong to psychotherapy in its stricter definition. However, they are heavily colored by a philosophical tone in their operation. The philosophical ideas of the self, how to behave as a person, and how to live life encompass the whole therapeutic operation. Specific preprogrammed therapeutic procedures are constructed for application — through individual introspection, group discussion, or creation of new life experience. Philosophical enlightenment, new life experience, or group activities are the mechanisms utilized for recovery.

Finally, there is a group of common therapies that are primarily oriented to the psychological level. Problems are seen as the result of psychological reactions to the stress of internal conflict or external maladjustment. The essential core of these therapies is to work on the psychological problems through the mechanisms of obtaining insight, learning new behavior, changing coping patterns, and working on interpersonal relations at the family or group level.

Among these therapies, there is obviously a shift in orientation from the supernatural to the natural, to the physical person, to the philosophical–psychological, and finally to the psychological. The nature of the psychological healing process may have developed historically in this sequence. It is also apparent that psychologically oriented modern psychotherapies may miss other dimensions — the supernatural, the natural, the physical, and the philosophical — that should be addressed in the healing process to meet the needs of the patient from a cultural perspective.

B. MECHANISMS OF HEALING

The healing mechanisms utilized in these different modes of therapy cover a broad spectrum. Among the supernaturally oriented healing practices (such as shamanism or divination), belief in a supernatural power itself is an important healing mechanism. Associated with this, magical counteracting or generation of conviction often works in such healing systems as well. In addition, basic, supportive therapeutic mechanisms, such as emotional catharsis, assurance, suggestion, "naming" effect, or gratification of unfulfilled wishes, are operating.

Among socioreligious or philosophical–psychological therapies, many healing mechanisms of psychological natures are operating. Confession and apology *(ho'oponopono),* group support and enforcement (AA group), reappraisal of interpersonal relationships (Naikan therapy), creating new life experience (Morita therapy), or reexamination of self (est) are some of the examples.

Primarily, psychologically focused therapies focus on and utilize certain specifically conceptualized psychological mechanisms, such as transference or insight (psychoanalysis), relearning of behavior (behavior therapy), and learning and restoring relations (family or group therapy) in their therapeutic work.

C. Goals of Therapy

When the aims of therapy, or the goals of practice, are examined, considerable differences are found among different therapeutic modes. The goals of therapy vary in close relation to its basic orientation. In the supernaturally oriented healing practice, the final goal of healing is to comply with the divine power. Based on this, an attempt is made to find a way to resolve problems and to restore life. There is no intention of changing a person's life radically. The therapy emphasizes finding a supernaturally blessed and correct way to deal with problems within the existing world. It takes the view that an individual is limited in his dealings with the supernatural being.

In a nature-oriented system, the goal of therapy is also to find a way to comply with the rules of nature. The primary effort is to seek a way to harmonize with nature or to restore natural conditions. Although it shifts from a supernatural to a natural orientation, it still takes the basic view that an individual is a small part of the natural universe.

When the orientation shifts to a philosophical and psychological one, the aim of therapy becomes accepting the self (as it is), restoring family or group relations (as they should be, according to sociocultural definition), or resuming the social role of the self (as politically demanded). A person is still seen as an individual member of a family, group, or society. The main purpose of this kind of therapy is to find a proper way to perform externally defined roles and to be accepted as a member of the family, group, or society.

Finally, when the therapy is psychologically oriented, such as contemporary, regular psychotherapy, the emphasis is on "improving" the self, becoming a "mature" person and a "functional" family member or "healthy" group member. Conceptually, it is expected that, through therapy, the patient will become more "mature," "healthy," or "functional." Whether such goals are practical and attainable is not the question here. We are merely pointing out that the aims of therapy become increasingly demanding for patients in philosophically and psychologically oriented therapies. Whether this is the natural evolution of psychotherapy — starting from a passive expectation to an active demand for the patient to make changes — or merely a reflection of Euro-American cultures deserves careful theoretical examination. Otherwise, modern therapists (or rather Euro-American therapists) are conducting psychotherapy with unspoken goals that can never be accomplished in reality. This may be one of the reasons that modern Euro-American psychotherapies are limited, or encounter difficulties, in their application to other cultural settings.

REFERENCES

Asuni, T. (1967). Nigerian experiment in group psychotherapy. *American Journal of Psychotherapy, 12,* 95–104.

Calloway, P. (1992–1993). *Russian/Soviet and Western psychiatry: A contemporary comparative study.* New York: Wiley.

Chen, C.P. (1995). Group counseling in a different cultural context: Several primary issues in dealing with Chinese clients. *Group, 19*(1), 45–55.

Doi, T. (1964). Psychoanalytic therapy and "Western man": A Japanese view [Special edition]. *International Journal of Social Psychiatry, 1,* 13–18.

Dunkas, N., & Nikelly, A.G. (1975). Group psychotherapy with Greek immigrants. *International Journal of Group Psychotherapy, 25,* 402–409.

Falicov, C.J. (1982). Mexican families. In M. McGoldrick, J.K. Pearce, & J. Giordano (Eds.), *Ethnicity and family therapy* (pp. 134–163). New York: Guilford Press.

Frank, J.D. (1961). *Persuasion and healing: A comparative study of psychotherapy.* (p. 62). New York: Schocken Books.

Gellner, E. (1985). *The psychoanalytic movement: The coming of unreason.* London: Paladin.

Herz, F.M., & Rosen, E.J. (1982). Jewish families. In M. McGoldrick, J.K., Pearce, & J., Giordano (Eds.), *Ethnicity and family therapy* (pp. 364–392). New York: Guilford Press.

Ho, M.K. (1987). *Family therapy with ethnic minorities.* Newbury Park, CA: Sage.

Hsu, J. (1983). Asian family interaction patterns and their therapeutic implication. *International Journal of Family Psychiatry, 4,* 307–320.

Hsu, J. (1995). Family therapy for the Chinese: Problems and strategies. In T.Y., Lin, W.S., Tseng, and E.K., Yeh (Eds.), *Chinese societies and mental health* (pp. 295–307). Hong Kong: Oxford University Press.

Jalali, B. (1988). Ethnicity, cultural adjustment, and behavior: Implications for family therapy. In L. Comas-Díaz & E.E.H. Griffith (Eds.), *Clinical guidelines in cross-cultural mental health* (pp. 9–32). New York: Wiley.

Martinez, C. (1977). Group process and the Chicano: Clinical issues. *International Journal of Group Psychotherapy, 27,* 225–231.

McGoldrick, M., & Pearce, J.K. (1981). Family therapy with Irish-Americans. *Family Process, 20,* 223–244.

Meadow, A. (1964). Client-centered therapy and the American ethos. *International Journal of Social Psychiatry, 10*(4), 246–259.

Meadow, A., & Vetter, H.J. (1959). Freudian theory and the Judaic value system. *International Journal of Social Psychiatry, 5*(3), 197–207.

Minuchin, S., Montalvo, B., Guerney, B.G., Rosman, B.L., & Schumer, G.G. (1967). *Families of the slums.* New York: Basic Books.

Moitoza, E. (1982). Portuguese families. In M. McGoldrick, J.K. Pearce, & J. Giordano (Eds.), *Ethnicity and family therapy* (pp. 412–437). New York: Guilford Press.

Pande, S.K. (1968). The mystique of "Western" psychotherapy: An eastern interpretation. *Journal of Nervous and Mental Disease, 146*(6), 425–432.

Redlich, F.C. (1958). Social aspects of psychotherapy. *American Journal of Psychiatry, 114,* 800–804.

Rogers, C.R. (1974). Remarks on the future of client-centered therapy. In D.A. Wexler & L.N. Rice (Eds.), *Innovations in client-centered therapy.* New York: Wiley.

Shapiro, R.Y. (1996, May). *Group psychotherapy with Orthodox Jewish patients.* Presented at the meeting of the American Psychiatric Association Symposium on the Psychiatric Treatment of Orthodox Jews, New York.

Suzuki, K. (1987). Family therapy in Japan. *AFTA Newsletter, 27,* 15–18.

Torrey, E.F. (1986). *Witchdoctors and psychiatrists: The common roots of psychotherapy and its future* (pp. 73–74). New York: Harper & Row.

Tseng, W.S. (1999). Culture and Psychotherapy: Review and practical guidelines. *Transcultural Psychiatry, 36* (2), 131–179.

Tseng, W.S., & Hsu, J. (1991). *Culture and family: Problems and therapy.* New York: Haworth Press.

Tseng, W.S., McDermott, J.F., Jr., & Maretzki, T.W. (Eds.), (1977). *Adjustment in intercultural marriage.* Honolulu: University of Hawaii, Department of Psychiatry, John A. Burns School of Medicine.

Wexler, D.A., & Rice, L.N. (1974). *Innovations in client-centered therapy* (pp. 1–6). New York: Wiley.

Young, D.S. (1997). Chinese mind and unique Chinese psychotherapy. In W.S. Tseng (Ed.), *Chinese mind and therapy* (pp. 22–38). Beijing: Beijing University Press (in Chinese).

35

The Practice of Psychotherapy in Various Cultures

I. INTRODUCTION

Historically, it has been clearly demonstrated that the development of psychotherapy has been influenced not only by medical knowledge and professional theories, but also by social and cultural factors. As mentioned earlier, the acceptance of psychotherapy has been obstructed by political ideology, as in Germany during the Nazi era, Russia during Stalin's time, and China during the Cultural Revolution. The prevalence of psychotherapy has been influenced by socioeconomic–medical systems, as in Scandinavian societies, where medical practice is heavily oriented toward socialism, which emphasizes community-related health programs that are not conducive to individually focused psychotherapy (Kelman, 1964). No doubt the sociocultural environment also contributes to the practice of psychotherapy in a society. For example, psychoanalysis never flourished in Old Vienna, where it originated. Vienna was a conservative society with many other traditional ways of providing mental tranquility for people, and it did not respond enthusiastically to this new method of treatment. However, psychotherapy became popular in the new world of America, where changing society and creating one's own life were valued in the country's pioneer atmosphere (Schick, 1973). How cultural factors affect psychotherapy and the kinds of cultural adjustments that are needed to provide effective therapy are common concerns that deserve attention not only from a scientific point of view, but also from a practical perspective.

Many clinicians have begun to call attention to the considerations and modifications that are needed when psychotherapy is practiced within a particular ethnic–cultural group, especially in their own societies or countries. In this case, the therapist and patient usually belong to the same ethnic–cultural background. Theoretically speaking, there is no severe cultural barrier between them, as there is in intercultural therapy, which will be discussed in Chapter 36. Still, the ethnic–cultural background of the population, the sociocultural environment, in terms of time and place, and the general attitudes, understandings, and beliefs of the people toward psychotherapy all significantly affect the nature and process of therapy and necessitate certain cultural adjustments in the way therapeutic services are offered (see Fig. 35-1).

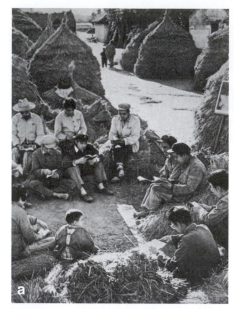
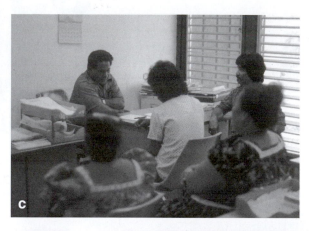
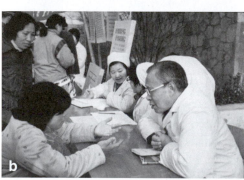
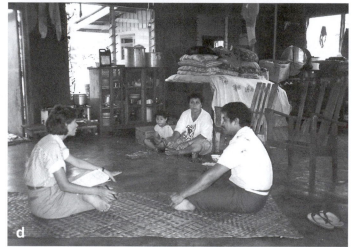

FIGURE 35-1   Pschotherapy in different cultures. (a) A group study of Mao's teachings in China during the Great Forward Movement era, utilizing political ideology for the improvement of life (source unknown). (b) Chinese child psychiatrists counseling parents at the road-side to promote child mental health in Nanjing. Privacy and confidentiality are not concerns in this public situation. [Courtesy of Tao Kuo-Tai, M.D.] (c) Medical officers in Truk, Micronesia, providing counseling to a patient with his family members around — a natural setting for family-involved therapy. (d) A psychiatrist visiting a home in the island society of Samoa to study the mental health of the family members. [Courtesy of Gail Ingram, M.D.].

II. PSYCHOTHERAPEUTIC PRACTICES IN DIFFERENT SOCIETIES

The development and vicissitude of psychotherapy in various societies around the globe will be reviewed to illustrate how sociocultural factors influence the practice and evolution of psychotherapy. Information on this subject is still very limited and lacks systematic evaluation. Based on the literature available, only situations in several selected societies will be reviewed here.

A. IN JAPAN

Let us first look at the situation in Japan. Knowledge of psychoanalysis was introduced into Japan as early as 1912, two different translations of Freud's selected papers were already published in 1929, and a branch of the International Psychoanalytic Association was established in 1934. Still, as pointed out by Kato (1959), the former head of the National Institute of Mental Health in Japan, the psychoanalytic or psychotherapy movement never became popular in Japan. Kato cited Japanese psychiatrists' heavy orientation toward Kraepelinian psychiatry and Japanese patients' requests for somatic treatment as among the main reasons. From a financial standpoint, because Japanese psychiatrists could not charge high fees for psychotherapy, very few were interested in practicing it.

Beyond such practical considerations, many scholars have pointed out psychological and cultural factors that explain why psychotherapy is not prevalent in Japan. For instance, Tatara (1982), a psychoanalyst practicing in Japan, indicated that the typical Japanese psychotherapy patient is action oriented and seeks direct guidance from the therapist rather than oriented toward intrapsychic inspection. Further, based on culturally patterned expectations, Japanese patients tend to assume a "pathological" dependent role and do not appreciate the goal of autonomy or independence emphasized in psychotherapy. One of the leading psychotherapists in Japan, Doi (1962), indicated that "benevolent dependency" *(amae)* — a key concept for understanding Japanese personality structure — is highly valued in interpersonal relationships in Japan. The American cultural psychologist DeVos (1980), based on his long-time observations in Japan, commented that psychoanalysis is emotionally impossible for the Japanese, who live in a culture that is concerned with hierarchy and obligation to society and do not value the concept of individual autonomy.

Based on clinical work in Japan, India, and the United States, Roland (1991) pointed out that modification is needed to understand the ego structure of the Japanese and the Indian. For them, the outer ego boundary is much more permeable and vague than it is for Westerners, with more of a sense of merging with others. However, there is another kind of ego boundary that is observed among the Japanese and Indians. It is an inner boundary that enables them to keep a highly private self, to maintain an inner sanc-

tum of feelings and thoughts, while being partially merged with others in the family or other group. The concept of such a "private self" is not yet formulated in Western psychoanalytic theory, but it is useful in understanding the psychology of the Japanese and Indians.

B. IN CHINA

Let us now focus on China. It should be pointed out first that due to political ideology, psychotherapy was severely suppressed in China during the period of the Cultural Revolution. Individually focused psychotherapy was considered the product of capitalism and was criticized as not suitable to a socialistic country. Since the end of the Cultural Revolution, China has opened itself to Western influence and ideas, including those of psychotherapeutic theory and practice. As pointed out by Li and colleagues (1994), there is a great need for psychotherapy, yet currently there is a lack of psychotherapeutic skills within the Chinese medical profession.

In order to provide culture-relevant psychotherapy for the Chinese, Tseng (1995) has made suggestions in the areas of technical adjustment, theoretical modification, and philosophical reorientation. He has pointed out that in addition to a series of technical adjustments, there is a need to modify certain theories in order to understand the Chinese mind. These include the basic concepts of the self, ego-boundary, and interpersonal relations, among others.

C. IN INDIA

Concerning the practice of psychotherapy in India, Varma (1982), an Indian psychiatrist trained in the West, pointed out that the major factors to consider are the fundamental philosophico-religious beliefs of the culture. Psychotherapy has a limited role for utterly fatalistic people who believe that their present suffering is the result of sins committed in earlier incarnations.

Varma's view is echoed by a psychiatrist from Switzerland, Hoch (1990), who, based on three decades of psychiatric activity in India, revealed that the basic difficulty encountered in psychotherapy there was the traditional Hindu philosophy. A deep-rooted, ancient worldview, represented by the doctrine of "karma" and the concept of reincarnation, shapes the basic Hindu mentality. Hindu life lacks an anthropocentric orientation and discourages egoistic and individualistic striving, leaving very little that can be done with the tools and methods of Western psychotherapy.

Desai (1982) listed several cultural issues that need to be addressed for the practice of psychotherapy in India. The basic unit of Hindu society is the family, rather than the individual. Thus, individual growth is subordinated to family integrity. The matter of collaboration versus individuation needs to be handled carefully. A Hindu family strives to maintain integrity by prohibiting the expression of anger and hostility. Suppression versus expression is another matter that needs delicate management in therapeutic situations.

D. In Africa

As pointed out by the pioneer psychiatrist Lambo (1982), it is impossible to speak of a single African situation, as the continent contains a broad range of cultures. However, the basis of most African value systems is the concept of the "unity" of life and time. African thought draws no sharp distinction between animate and inanimate, natural and supernatural, material and mental. Furthermore, there is continuous communication between the dead and the living. He pointed out that in working with African patients, it is important to understand this worldview.

A psychiatrist from Nigeria, Asuni (1967), correctly pointed out that the situation in sub-Sahara Africa is the result of colonial domination in the past. The continuing colonial influence is manifested in the extreme shortage of trained indigenous personnel in all fields, especially psychiatry. Strongly reflecting the reality of the society, psychiatry in Africa is the psychiatry of psychosis. Limited manpower is available to focus on minor psychiatric disturbances, particularly in the format of psychotherapy.

Based on clinical experiences with Tanzanians over a number of years, Neki, Joinet, Hogan, Hauli, and Kilonzo, (1985) pointed out that the central notion that talk therapy is "good for you" is undoubtedly a product of Western culture. The Western patient, by and large, understands the rules of the game, the roles of the patient and therapist, and the purpose of the therapy. For the African, these rules and roles are essentially foreign, and the therapist's overtures tend to be misinterpreted and mistrusted. The African worldview appears to revolve around a humanized supernatural that influences the lives of men. As mentioned previously, no sharp distinctions are drawn between animate and inanimate, natural and supernatural, and physical and psychic.

A Western-trained Nigerian psychiatrist, Oyewumi (1986), reviewed the difficulties encountered in practicing psychotherapy in his home country. Insight-oriented psychotherapy is difficult to achieve in the absence of the capacity for self-criticism and introspection. The Nigerian always attributes whatever happens to him to someone else. It is always "they," not "me" or "I." The tendency of the Nigerian to externalize, and the apparent lack of introspection, hinders the psychotherapeutic process and its success. Based on their traditional orientation, Nigerian patients expect benevolent authoritarian treatment and are confused by therapeutic endeavors that leave them to decide what to do next.

Uzoka (1983) conducted clinical experiments in Nigeria and found that when the therapist spoke a lot, the patients attended more and made substantially more self-disclosures. Based on such findings, Uzoka concluded that, for African patients, the therapist needed to appear actively involved if therapy was to be credible.

Ilechukwu (1989) pointed out that many generalizations made in the past about psychotherapy in Africa, such as Africans patients are unsophisticated, talk only of symptoms and never of feelings, must be told what to do, and always return to their root beliefs, were misguided. These assumptions need careful assessment or they will discourage attempts at psychotherapy.

E. In Muslim Societies

As pointed out by El-Islam (1982), because the characteristics of Arabs vary so much from one community to another, the validity of generalizations about Arabs as a whole can be doubted. Nevertheless, there are certain widely shared features of general relevance to psychiatry that can be recognized, such as traditional beliefs regarding spirits and the "evil eye," unique family structures and relationships, particularly regarding the status of women, and healing practices. Concerning psychotherapy, El-Islam (1967) pointed out that the Arab patient may not accept "talking" as a treatment that can replace a prescription. Most Arab patients have a dependent attitude toward doctors and are not interested in active participation in their own treatment (such as through behavior therapy).

Regarding the situation in the eastern province of Saudi Arabia, West (1987) explained that the Islamic influence on Arab psychology was revealed in the acceptance of life now and in the future as being in the hands of Allah. Many patients believed that the therapist was *hakeem* (wise man and healer), a professional working through the hands of Allah. Many patients expected the therapist to take an active, authoritarian role, while they took a passive and dependent role. Thus, the therapy had to be directive if it was to be effective. From a psychological point of view, denial of anger was common, as anger was not recognized in the Qu'ran (Koran) and a constricted life was never described as a painful problem. Somatized behavior appeared to be an important adaptive coping mechanism. The therapist had to be familiar with these issues in treating Arab patients.

Several cultural issues need special consideration in the treatment of Arab patients. As pointed out by El-Islam (in press), based on the traditional Arabs concepts of the roles of men and women, the issue of how to assist and support women in the revealing of their desires and opinions has to be handled carefully and delicately in therapy.

F. In Russia

There is considerable academic interest among scholars as to how psychiatry and psychotherapy were practiced in Russia during the communist regime and after *glasnost* (openness). However, there are few articles available in English (Calloway, 1992–1993; Gilbert & Shiryaev, 1992; Lauterbach, 1984).

A German psychologist, W. Lauterbach, published the book, *Soviet Psychotherapy,* in 1984, in which he described how Soviet psychotherapists differed from their Western colleagues in their view of psychological disorders as accompanied by somatic disorders. Therefore, they tended to administer complex treatment by supplementing psychotherapy and conventional psychopharmacological medication with the prescription of energy-boosting medications as well as involvement in sports and cultural activities (pp. 190–191).

An article written jointly by an American psychologist and a Russian psychologist (Gilbert & Shiryaev) in 1992 provided useful and insightful comments about the practice of psychotherapy in Russia. According to the authors, psychoanalysis was considered ideologically unacceptable prior to *glasnost,* but there was now considerable interest among clinicians in its theory and practice. It was also surprising to find out that in the nation where Pavlov discovered the process of classical conditioning, behavior therapy was not very popular. Instead, humanistic-existential approaches were more common. This was consistent with the prominent role that existential thought played in Russian culture as a whole.

In terms of psychotherapeutic formats, group therapy was far more popular and widely practiced in Russia. There were practical reasons for this trend. First, the total number of therapists was very limited. It was estimated that there were approximately 2000 practicing psychotherapists in all of Russia. The majority of these had just begun their clinical work in the several years after *glasnost,* and few had had the opportunity to be trained in individual therapy. Second, group therapy was less expensive than individual treatment. Russia, especially during the years of Soviet domination, was traditionally a group-oriented society. The forces of social influence that were present in group therapy could exert a powerful effect on the behavior and attitudes of Russians.

Regarding individual therapy, it was noted that the therapist–patient relationship was very much shaped by Russian culture. For centuries, Russia had been a highly paternalistic and authoritarian culture. Therefore, it was adaptive for the individual to exhibit an attitude of deference to authority and to hope and expect that this deference would be rewarded by the authority figure taking care of him. As pointed out by Gilbert and Shiryaev, this cultural legacy of authoritarianism had an important influence on the patient's expectations of psychotherapy. Many patients approached the therapist as a figure of authority with the implicit expectation that the therapist would intervene on their behalf or provide them with solutions that did not require a great deal of work on their part. It is interesting to note that, in this context, hypnosis was one of the most desired methods of treatment for Russian patients.

In the book *Russian/Soviet and Western Psychiatry* by Calloway (1992–1993), there is a chapter on psychotherapy. According to the author, the main Soviet criticism of Western psychotherapy, particularly of psychoanalysis, is that it is too concerned with "intrapsychic" and individualistic aspects of man and does not adequately take into account environmental and social factors. Calloway reported that during the early Soviet years, there was a small psychoanalytic movement, based mainly in Moscow. However, the movement began to die out after the Russian Psychoanalytic Society was disbanded in 1933, mainly because it fell out of favor on ideological grounds. Calloway pointed out that psychotherapy in the Soviet Union has traditionally been short term and directive. The therapy also covers a wide range of therapeutic activities, such as exercise, gymnastics, sports, art, games, music, psychodrama, and group discussion based on watching films or reading books.

Russian psychiatrist C. Korolenko, working mainly in eastern Russia, pointed out that due to geographical factors, the practice of psychiatry varies widely in Russia in the present, as it did in Soviet society in the past. This is true of psychotherapy as well. He warned that reports by outsiders, (Westerners), who obtained information mainly from the capital or other large cities, such as Moscow, hardly reflect the situation in Russia in general. In rural areas, or the eastern parts of Russia, far from the capital, situations can vary widely. For instance, folk healing may still be secretly practiced, and formal psychotherapy is unknown to many laypeople.

G. In Italy

Cultural psychiatrist Goffredo Bartocci and his colleague, Nicola Lalli (1992), stated that there was a historical delay in the development of psychotherapy in Italy. They explained that psychiatry was based on the German model, fundamentally biological and constitutional, to the extent that psychiatry was regarded as the poor and neglected sister of neurology. Further, the presence of the church in the almost entirely Catholic society did not permit any type of research into the unconsciousness and irrational aspects of man, as this was already contained in and explained by the generic concept of evil and sin. Actually, psychology as a teaching subject was withdrawn in 1920s from all universities and psychoanalysis was defined either perversely (from the Catholic point of view) or incoherently and inconsistently (from the philosophical point of view).

It was only in the 1950s that psychotherapy appeared on the scene. Nevertheless, the prominent trend was to use public service, with the ever-present Catholic charities as a base, for "looking after" patients. Numerous methodologies and techniques of psychotherapy were imported from America, but, in fact, formal and long-term training was lacking. Most of the private centers offering psychotherapy were based on autogenous training, biofeedback, and hypnosis, which were defined as "psychological learning techniques." Bartocci and Lalli (1992) commented that religious thought was based on cultural and moral values and avoided any critical knowledge offered by scientific methods.

H. In South America

Information about psychiatry, particularly the practice of psychotherapy, in South America is generally scarce. There is only a handful of English publications available on some South American regions. It is especially necessary to recognize that there are vast variations within the numerous countries and societies of South America.

Two interesting themes emerged through a review of the available literature. One was related to Chile, where the society has long been marked by violence, torture, and political repression. Jimenez de la Jara (1991) pointed out how it was possible to practice psychoanalysis and psychotherapy under a military dictatorship. An emphasis on neutrality and the avoidance of political subjects were necessary. Dominguez and Weinstein (1987) suggested that it was important in the therapeutic relationship that the patient knew the therapist believed in human rights. Becker, Castillo, Gomez, and Kovalskys (1989) and Becker, Lira, Castillo, and Gomez (1990) stressed the need for working on the patient's loss, grief, and mourning associated with extreme traumatization, and the importance of societal reparation.

Another theme is how to provide psychotherapy for poor people. This issue was of particular concern in Brazil and Peru. In Brazil, psychotherapy provided by psychiatrists and clinical psychologists was built around middle- and upper-class minority populations. Loreto (1984) suggested that brief forms of supportive psychotherapy, characterized by problem solving and symptom relieving, be provided for the majority of the population, who were underprivileged. In Peru, Rodriguez-Rabanal (1990) stressed the need to provide psychotherapeutic work for slum-dwellers in Lima, paying particular attention to survival strategies.

I. In the Island Society of Micronesia

The island society of Micronesia offers a unique opportunity to examine and discuss a mental health service delivery system from an academic point of view. Micronesia and the island societies of Polynesia and Melanesia are characterized by several factors. First, from a geographic point of view, they are composed of numerous tiny islands, very far apart from each other, located in the middle of the vast Pacific Ocean, with very limited opportunities for and means of communication or contact with the outside world. The islands have small populations: several hundred to several thousand people at most. Besides the geographic isolation and the small size of the communities, there are also unique cultural systems that shape the behavior and lives of the islanders. These include the family systems. The islanders observe matrilineal family systems, which shape their intra- and interfamily relationships. They hold different worldviews, economic systems, and sets of life values. For instance, the female holds a significant position in the society, as the family heritage is traced through the mother–daughter lineal system (rather than the father–son, as in patrilineal family systems). While families have large numbers of children, multiple adoption is also practiced to enforce interfamily dependency and support in these island socieites in which the resources of food and supply can become scarce unexpectedly. There is a unique social etiquette, and various taboos are observed, including gestation and brother–sister taboos. Caste systems are still observed within the communities, subdividing people according to certain hierarchies.

Such unique geographical and cultural backgrounds present a special challenge for mental health service delivery, including the practice of psychotherapy. For instance, there are always a limited number of specialized professionals, including health workers. There are only a few physicians available on each island, who perform multiple specialities as family-practice physicians. Based on the need, a physician may give a vaccination shot to a child in the morning, delivery a baby at noon, perform an operation on an injured person in the afternoon, and an autopsy in the evening. The same physician may function as a priest on the weekend and a political candidate running for the senate at election time. He may be asked to diagnosis a psychotic patient and to offer psychotherapy for those who are in need of it. Thus, it is a luxury to talk about specialization, and impossible to consider the sole practice of psychotherapy. Actually, the need for psychotherapy is low on the list of priorities in these societies. High on the list are the surgical treatment of injuries, treatment of infections, and delivery of babies.

From a technical standpoint, there are some obstacles to overcome. If the therapist is from outside of the island society, there is the problem of how much he or she knows about the island lifestyle and how much he or she is permitted to know about island matters. If the therapist is from the patient's own island, different problems may be encountered. There is particularly the matter of caste hierarchy, who belongs to which caste, and who, patient or therapist, is superior to the other according to the caste system. By the nature of the caste system, the therapist has to belong to a higher caste than the patient because he cannot offer any suggestions or counseling to a person who is above his caste position. These are unique cultural issues that exist in island societies and may seldom be encountered in other kinds of societies — highlighting how culture significantly influences the practice of psychotherapy.

III. GENERAL FINDINGS AND COMMENTS

A. FACTORS THAT AFFECT THE PRACTICE OF PSYCHOTHERAPY IN A SOCIETY

Through the just-discussed review of psychotherapeutic practices in various societies, it is found that numerous factors affect the development and vicissi-

tude of psychotherapy within any society. Some stem from the social reality, some from the medical system, and others from the culture. Let us list those factors.

1. Socioeconomic Reality

It cannot be denied that socioeconomic conditions have a direct impact on the development of psychotherapy in society. Social conditions involve many aspects. For instance, the size of the population in the community will determine the kind of need that exists in the health delivery system. This is well illustrated in the island society of Micronesia, where the population of each island is so small that the specialization of professionals, including psychotherapists, is not practical. The level of economic development is also always a crucial factor. As in many underdeveloped societies where an adequate food supply, housing, and other minimum requirements for living are the highest priorities, mental health and psychological care are at the bottom of list. There is a need to modify psychotherapeutic service toward survival strategies for the economically underpriviliged population, as exemplified in Peru or Brazil.

Closely related to these conditions is the stability of a society. If a society is constantly faced with danger and destruction, such as during wartime, there is no way to nourish the development of psychotherapy. This was the situation in China in the past half-century.

2. Political Ideology and Attitudes

As exemplified by the Nazi era in Germany, the Soviet Union during Stalin's time, and the period of the Cultural Revolution in China, political ideology has a powerful effect on the fate of psychotherapeutic practice. Psychotherapy, which advocates the importance of the individual's mental life, tends to be viewed as an obstacle to an autocratic political system and is strongly suppressed. The practice of psychotherapy becomes extremely difficult under a military dictatorship, as illustrated in Chile. Closely related to this is how the administration views the need for mental health care and what kind of support it offers for the delivery of psychotherapy to people in the community at large.

3. Medical Systems

Due to different medical orientations or historical backgrounds, different societies have different medical systems, which, in turn, influence the development of psychotherapy. For instance, a medical system may be characterized as a public or a private delivery system. A medical system may stress primary or tertiary care. Such different medical systems will affect the nature of the health delivery style, including the ratio of service between physician and the population, as well as priorities of care, e.g., either major or minor disorders. How the payment for care is handled also has a direct impact on the practice of psychotherapy. Generally, in medical systems that emphasize the public and community, as exemplified by Scandinavian countries or the previously existing communist societies of China and the Soviet Union, individually focused psychotherapy tends to be ignored. In contrast, in capitalist societies, where payment for psychotherapy is taken care of by medical insurance systems, the practice of psychotherapy flourishes.

Closely related to the nature of the medical system is the need for a health service within a society. For instance, as pointed out by Asuni (1967), regarding his home country of Nigeria in Africa, the primary psychiatric mission is to take care of major psychiatric disorders, namely acute or chronic psychoses; there is no room to consider the minor psychiatric disorders that are usually dealt with in psychotherapy.

4. Psychiatric Orientation

Within the field of psychiatry, there are different fundamental professional orientations. If the psychiatric orientation is heavily biological, as in the Soviet Union and China in the past, or professional, as is still the case in Japan and Germany, the practice of psychotherapy will not be emphasized strongly. The fate of the psychotherapy movement is closely associated with the orientation of psychiatry held by clinicians at large. Psychotherapy becomes the active style of service if it is primarily oriented toward dynamic psychiatry, as in the United States almost a half-century ago.

5. Laymen's Perception and Understanding

Besides the orientation of professionals, how laymen perceive and understand psychotherapy will greatly affect the practice of therapy. Familiarity with psychotherapy is also an influential factor. As indicated by Neki and colleagues (1985) in Africa, most people do not believe that "psychotherapy is good for you." Thus, people are not keen to seek help through psychotherapy as they do in most Western societies, where people have a positive view of its nature and function.

6. People's Psychological Structure

Culture-shaped personality and psychological structures will determine whether people will utilize a special mode of service, i.e., psychotherapy, to heal their psychological problems. This is illustrated in Japan, where, explained American medical anthropologist DeVos (1980), people are more concerned with interpersonal relations in a social context, rather than indiviudal psychology, and do not favor autonomy-emphasizing psychotherapy. In Nigeria, according to Oyewumi (1986), people tend to attribute whatever happens to them to someone else. This tendency of externalization, rather than introspection into the self, hinders the process and goals of therapy. In contrast, Jewish people, very much influenced by their tradition, value intrapsychic examination of self and analysis of thought and word, and tend to have a high regard for psychotherapy.

7. Philosophical Orientation

The impact of the philosophical view held by the common people on the acceptance of psychotherapy is well demonstrated in many cultures. For instance, in Muslim societies, as pointed out by West (1987), people believe that their lives are in the hands of their god, Allah. Therefore, they lack the psychological motivation to seek solutions or to improve themselves through therapy. A similar situation is noted in India and Africa. As pointed out by Varma (1982), Indians, due to their fatalistic view of life, are seldom interested in improving their individual lives through psychotherapy.

Among the factors listed earlier, some are strictly related to matters of society, such as the political, economic, or medical service systems, whereas others, such as people's perception and understanding of therapy or their philosophical orientation to their life problems and views of the world, are related more to cultural factors.

B. THE NEED FOR CULTURAL MODIFICATIONS IN THE DEVELOPMENT OF PSYCHOTHERAPY

It is apparent that there are numerous reasons for modifying and adjusting psychotherapy in different societies. One reason may be the basic personality or ethnic character of the population concerned (Doi, 1964), commonly shared belief and value systems (Hoch, 1990), basic philosophical attitudes (Rhee, 1990; Varma, 1982), or orientations toward and expectations of psychotherapy (Neki et al., 1985; Ng, 1985; Tseng, Lu & Yin 1995; Tung, 1991).

No matter what the reasons, it is clear that cultural adjustment is needed in the practice of psychotherapy in various societies. The cultural adjustment of psychotherapy can be carried out at different levels, including the technical, theoretical, and philosophical. This will be elaborated in detail later in Chapter 37.

REFERENCES

Asuni, T. (1967). Nigerian experiment in group psychotherapy. *American Journal of Psychotherapy, 12*, 95–104.

Bartocci, G., & Lalli, N. (1992). Psicoterapia e cultura: L'esperineza Italiana (Psychotherapy and culture: The Italian experi-

ence). *Rivista Europea di Psichiatria, 4*(2/3), 12–24 (in both Italian and English).

Becker, D., Castillo, M.I., Gomez, E., & Kovalskys, J. (1989). Subjectivity and politics: The psychotherapy of extreme traumatization in Chile. *International Journal of Mental Health, 18*(2), 80–97.

Becker, D., Lira, E., Castillo, M.I., & Gomez, E. (1990). Therapy with victims of political repression in Chile: The challenge of social reparation. *Journal of Social Issues, 46*(30), 133–149.

Calloway, P. (1992–1993). *Russian/Soviet and Western psychiatry: A contemporary comparative study.* New York: Wiley.

Desai, P.N. (1982). Learning psychotherapy: A cultural perspective. *Journal of Operational Psychiatry, 13*(2), 82–87.

DeVos, G. (1980). Afterword. In D.K. Reynolds (Ed.), *The quiet therapies: Japanese pathways to personal growth* (pp. 113–132). Honolulu: University Press of Hawaii.

Doi, T. (1962). Amae — A key concept for understanding Japanese personality structure. In R.J. Smith & R.K. Beardsley (Eds.), *Japanese culture: Its development and characteristics.* Chicago: Aldine.

Doi, T. (1964). Psychoanalytic therapy and "Western man": A Japanese view [Special edition]. *International Journal of Social Psychiatry, 1,* 13–18.

Dominguez, R., & Weinstein, E. (1987). Aiding victims of political repression in Chile: A psychological and psychotherapeutic approach. *Tidsskrift for Norske Psykolgforening, 24*(2), 75–81.

El-Islam, M.F. (1967). The psychotherapeutic basis of some Arab rituals. *International Journal of Social Psychiatry, 13*(4), 265–268.

El-Islam, M.F. (1982). Arabic cultural psychiatry. *Transcultural Psychiatric Research Review, 19*(1), 5–24.

El-Islam, M.F. (2001). One foot in the past and the other foot in the present. In W.S. Tseng & J. Streltzer (Eds.), *Culture and psychotherapy: A guide to clinical practice* (pp. 27–41). Washington, DC: American Psychiatric Press.

Gilbert, R.K., & Shiryaev, E. (1992). Clinical psychology and psychotherapy in Russia: Current status and future prospects. *Journal of Humanistic Psychology, 32*(3), 28–49.

Hoch, E.M. (1990). Experiences with psychotherapy training in India. *Psychotherapy and Psychosomatics, 53,* 14–20.

Ilechukwu, S.T. (1989). Approaches to psychotherapy in Africans: Do they have to be non-medical? *Culture, Medicine and Psychiatry, 13,* 419–435.

Jimenez de la Jara (1991). Einige uberlegungen zur praxis von psychoanalyse und psychotherapie in Chile under der militardiktatur (Some reflections on the practice of psychoanalysis and psychotherapy in Chile under the military dictatorship). *Psyche Zeitschrift fur Psychoanalyse und ihre Anwendungen, 45*(2), 157–176 (in German).

Kato, M. (1959). Report on psychotherapy in Japan. *International Journal of Social Psychiatry, 5*(1), 56–60.

Kelman, H. (1964). Psychotherapy in Scandinavia — An American viewpoint. *International Journal of Social Psychiatry, 10*(1), 64–72.

Lambo, T.A. (1982). Psychotherapy in Africa. *African Journal of Mental Health, 1*(1), 4–14.

Lauterbach, W. (1984). *Soviety psychotherapy.* Oxford: Pergamon Press.

Li, M.G., Duan, C.M., Ding, B.K., Yue, D.M. et al. (1994). Psychotherapy integration in modern China. *Journal of Psychotherapy Practice and Research, 3*(4), 277–283.

Loreto, G. (1984). Necessidade de uma psicoterapia para os clientes de condicao socio-economica desfavorecida (The need to develop a psychotherapy that will meet the needs of clients from lower socioeconomic class). *Neurobiologia, 47*(1), 21–32 (in Portuguese).

Neki, J.S., Joinet, B., Hogan, M., Hauli, J.G., & Kilonzo, G. (1985). The cultural perspective of therapeutic relationship — A viewpoint from Africa. *Acta Psychiatrica Scandinavica, 71*, 543–550.

Ng, M.L. (1985). Psychoanalysis for the Chinese — Applicable or not applicable? *International Review of Psychoanalysis, 12*(4), 449–460.

Oyewumi, L.K. (1986). Psychotherapy in Nigerian psychiatric practice: An overview. *Psychiatric Journal of the University of Ottawa, 11*(1), 19–22.

Rhee, D.S. (1990). The Tao, psychoanalysis and existential thought. *Psychotherapy and Psychosomatics, 53*, 21–27.

Rodriguez-Rabanal, C. (1990). Psychoanalytishce gesprache mit slum-bewohnern in Lima (Psychoanalytic interviews with slum-dwellers in Lima). *Psyche Zeitschrift fur Psychoanalyse und ihre Anwendungen, 44*(7), 593–611 (in German with an English abstract).

Roland, A. (1991). Psychoanalysis in India and Japan: Toward a comparative psychoanalysis. *American Journal of Psychoanalysis, 51*(1), 1–10.

Schick, A. (1973). Psychotherapy in old Vienna and New York: Cultural comparisons. *The Psychoanalytic Review, 60*(1), 111–126.

Tatara, M. (1982). Psychoanalytic psychotherapy in Japan: The issue of dependency pattern and the resolution of psychopathology. *Journal of the American Academy of Psychoanalysis, 10*, 225–239.

Tseng, W.S. (1995). Psychotherapy for the Chinese: Cultural adjustments. In L.Y.C. Cheng, H. Baxter, & F.M.C. Cheung (Eds.), *Psychotherapy for the Chinese: II Selected papers from the Second International Conference on Psychotherapy for the Chinese* (pp. 1–22). Hong Kong: Chinese University of Hong Kong, Department of Psychiatry.

Tseng, W.S., Lu, Q.Y., & Yin, P.Y. (1995). Psychotherapy for the Chinese: Cultural considerations. In T.Y. Lin, W.S. Tseng, & E.K. Yeh, (Eds.), *Chinese societies and mental health* (pp. 281–294). Hong Kong: Oxford University Press.

Tung, M. (1991). Insight-oriented psychotherapy and the Chinese patient. *American Journal of Orthopsychiatry, 61*(2), 186–194.

Uzoka, A.F. (1983). Active versus passive therapist role in didactic psychotherapy with Nigerian patients. *Social Psychiatry, 18*, 1–6.

Varma, V.K. (1982). Present state of psychotherapy in India. *Indian Journal of Psychiatry, 24*, 209–226. (Reviewed in *Transcultural Psychiatric Research Review, 21*(4), 291–291 [1984]).

West, J. (1987). Psychotherapy in the Eastern Province of Saudi Arabia. *Psychotherapy, 24*, 105–107.

36

Intercultural Psychotherapy

I. WHAT IS "INTERCULTURAL PSYCHOTHERAPY?"

Intercultural psychotherapy is psychotherapy that is delivered to patients with ethnic or cultural backgrounds considerably different from that of the therapist. With significant differences or gaps between the culture of the therapist and that of the patient, the **interaction** of cultural components is, either consciously or unconsciously, heavily involved in and significantly influences the process of psychotherapy. Thus, it is specifically addressed as "intercultural therapy" (Hsu & Tseng, 1972) in contrast to "intracultural therapy," which takes place between a therapist and patient with basically the same cultural backgrounds. As there is a need to transcend cultural barriers between the therapist and the patient, it is also called "transcultural psychotherapy." It is a challenge to clinicians to be aware of the ethnocultural impact in such intercultural therapy processes. In a way, in "culture-reactive" psychotherapy, a term coined by Koss-Chioino and Vargas (1992), it becomes necessary for the therapist to work "actively" on cultural issues and overcome the potential difficulties associated with cultural barriers. From an academic point of view, intercultural psychotherapy offers a splendid opportunity to examine the role and impact of culture at a clinical level, with a microscopic focus on the delivery of therapy.

Associated with clinical experiences working with patients in foreign societies, or with minority groups, literature concerning "cross-cultural" psychotherapy began to appear in the 1960s (Bishop & Winokur, 1956; Bolman, 1968; Carstairs, 1961). Hsu and Tseng (1972) pointed out the influence of cultural factors on the process of intercultural psychotherapy broadly in the areas of communication, assessment, therapist–patient relationship, interpretation, advice-giving, and treatment goals. Kinzie (1972) emphasized that an open system model is important when a therapist is engaged in cross-cultural psychotherapy. Various terms, such as "intercultural" (Hsu & Tseng, 1972) or "cross-cultural" psychotherapy (Bishop & Winokur, 1956; Bolman, 1968; Carstairs, 1961; Cheng & Lo, 1991), psychotherapy "across cultures" (Foulks, Bland, & Shervington, 1995; Pedersen, Draguns, Lonner, & Trimble, 1989; Pedersen, Lonner, & Draguns, 1976), or "transcultural" psychotherapy, have been used by different scholars. The adjective "transcultural" was originally used by Wittkower to indicate clinical work that needed to "trans-across" the barriers of culture, whereas the term "intercultural" highlights the unique nature of the therapy, which involves the bilateral **interaction** of the cultures of the patient and therapist. For the sake of convenience and consistency, and to reflect the core nature of the therapeutic process, in this chapter, the term "intercultural psychotherapy" will be used.

Closely related to the emerging human rights movement in the United States, as well as the increased migration of non-European minority groups into European countries, there was increased concern in the 1970s and 1980s with how to deliver mental health counseling for minorities, migrants, refugees, sojourns, and foreign students. The monograph, *Transcultural Counseling,* by Walz and Benjamin, appeared in 1978, suggesting ways to provide counseling for various minority groups in the United States. The book, *Counseling Across Cultures,* by Pedersen and colleagues (1976), followed by several revisions (1989, 1996), is another example of the work that has been done in this area. Numerous books have appeared recently that focus on intercultural therapy among particular groups, such as immigrants (Samuda & Wolfgang, 1985), refugees (van der Veer, 1992), and minorities (Aponte, Rivers, & Wohl, 1995), indicating increased awareness of and experience in this area.

A search will show that from the early 1980s, many works have appeared that offer specific suggestions on how to provide psychotherapy for patients of particular ethnic/cultural backgrounds (Kinzie, Tran, Breckenridge, & Bloom, 1980; Marcos, 1988; Sanchez & Mohl, 1992; Tseng, McDermott, & Maretzki, 1974; Walz & Benjamin, 1978). Generally, it has been suggested that in addition to concerns about how cultural factors may influence the process of therapy, the therapist should be equipped with certain knowledge about the culture of his patients, and that certain issues require care in treating each particular cultural group. Also, it has been warned that cultural differences may fascinate the therapist to the point that he tries to gain information of a more anthropological nature and becomes distracted from the reality of the patient's core problems (Foulks et al., 1995). This may occur when a clinician encounters a patient with an "exotic" cultural background.

Numerous specific issues have been brought up in the clinical experience of intercultural psychotherapy, such as the need for examining the congruence and incongruence of cultural backgrounds between therapist and patient; how to communicate with patients on verbal as well as nonverbal levels (Wolfgang, 1985); how racism may affect interracial counseling (Burke, 1986; Geller, 1988; Pinderhughes, 1989); the problem of ethnic or cultural identification with the therapist; the management of cultural transference and countertransference; how to deal with a therapist's cultural rigidity or cultural blindness; how to provide appropriate therapy for patients who were refugees (van der Veer, 1992); and how to provide culture-fair, -matched, -sensitive, -relevant, or -reactive therapy. It is certainly stimulating for a clinician to consider the impact of culture on the practice of psychotherapy (Hsu & Tseng, 1972).

II. VARIOUS ISSUES ENCOUNTERED IN INTERCULTURAL THERAPY

A. ORIENTATION TO, FAMILIARITY WITH, AND EXPECTATIONS OF PSYCHOTHERAPY

1. Familiarity and Orientation

The first thing that needs attention in the practice of intercultural psychotherapy is the matter of the patient's familiarity with psychotherapy, and his or her expectations of it. This is particularly true if the patient comes from a place where psychotherapy is not a common professional practice or there are certain biases against it as a healing practice. In many societies, due to tradition and orientation, people value medically oriented service, which includes prescriptions, injections, or operations. They see medical practices as effective and valuable. In contrast, "talking" therapy to them is nothing but talk and is not going to solve their sleeping problems or stomach tension. They may never have seen a movie or read a book describing the psychotherapeutic method of lying on a couch in order to associate freely about "whatever comes to their mind." They may not understand why a father needs to see the therapist when his son has problems relating to his classmates at school or why a husband and wife both need to talk to the therapist when the wife is the one complaining of frequent tension headaches. They may be puzzled as to why the therapist wants the patient to recall and describe his childhood experiences when he is having a nervous attack at work that relates to his boss. The therapist must first explain the nature of therapy, to orient and prepare the client for it, and not assume that he or she is familiar with its procedures. This is particularly crucial in situations of intercultural therapy, where patients are not familiar with psychotherapy.

2. Expectation, Rules, and Agreement

Closely related to the understanding of psychotherapy is the need to find out and clarify what the patient expects of it and what he assumes to be his role as patient. The roles of the patient and therapist, who reflects cultural concepts of authority and healer, can be perceived and defined differently in various cultures.

For professional reasons, based on past clinical experience, contemporary psychotherapists have set up certain rules and agreements with which patients must comply. For instance, in order to carry out successful psychotherapy, modern therapists feel strongly that it is essential for the patient to be on time for his appointments and follow his agreement to see the therapist regularly for a determined period of time. These rules are made partly for clinical reasons, but they also reflect the habits demanded by modern industrialized society. These practices are seldom evaluated carefully for their clinical relevance and cultural implications. For many people, there is no custom of keeping preset appointments. There is no concept of treatment requiring regular visits, even after the initial problems have been resolved or cardinal symptoms have subsided.

Further, if people live in a place where there is no convenient transportation, it is rather difficult to see a therapist regularly. When a person lives in a rural area and has to climb a mountain, cross a river, or walk a long way to reach a clinic, it is not easy to show up on time for a session. When a person rides a bus, there is always the possibility of missing it and having to wait for another, and taking several hours to reach a destination. The demand for regular visits should be evaluated from the standpoint of such practical matters, in addition to culture-patterned habits of being on time. It would be culturally careless and a great mistake to interpret a no-show or delayed appointment simply as "resistance" to therapy.

As part of their agreement, patients are expected to pay the therapist for their visits. However, how and how much to pay are not merely technical issues, but also cultural matters. According to traditional custom, people in nonindustrialized societies seldom make cash payments to healers; only voluntary donations are made, in the form of gifts of appreciation. Being asked to make cash payments according to a preset agreement makes the therapy seem like a "commercial business" rather than the charitable work done by folk healers. Making a payment agreement is a delicate and sensitive matter that needs to be handled carefully in intercultural therapy with patients who are not used to business-like payment systems.

B. COMMUNICATION

Communication between the therapist and the patient is considered by psychotherapists to be a core element of therapy. Determining how to achieve informative, comprehensive, meaningful, and therapeutic communication is necessary for effective results. In intercultural psychotherapy, many issues in the area of communication need attention.

1. Spectrum of Words in Language

Human beings around the world use different languages for communication. Chinese, English, or

Spanish are some of the main languages used by different ethnic groups. The natures of different languages, including their words, grammar, and communication patterns, vary greatly. For instance, differences in gender among subjects are noted in some language, such as English, Russian, French, or Spanish, but not in Japanese or Chinese. This is related to the basic structure of language, but it may also reflect the cognitive style and perceptional and conceptional aspects of the people who use it. For instance, for the hierarchically concerned Japanese, the vocabulary and grammar of their language change depending on who you are speaking to. For example, the word for "self" changes depending on the gender of the speaker and his relationship with the person being spoken to. It is *boku* when a man refers to himself to his friends, *watakushi* when he is talking to his superior, and *watashi* when a woman addresses herself. The word reflects the concern for gender and social status in Japanese culture. It would be a mistake, and cause confusion, if a woman addressed herself as *boku* or if a man addressed himself as *watashi*.

The more differentiated a word, or the richness of variations of certain words, often indicates the level of concern for the subject in the culture. For instance, Eskimo people have many different words for "snow," reflecting the reality of their lives in the snow, while in English there is only one word for it. People living in an island society in the Pacific, out of necessity, have developed numerous words for "cloud" to help them predict and adjust to weather changes in the middle of the ocean. Westerners use different words to describe various kinds of wine or liquor, whereas the Chinese have only one inclusive word, "wine." In contrast, the Chinese use several different terms to address uncles or aunts, distinguishing paternal from maternal relatives, as well as age hierarchy. This illustrates the importance to the Chinese of discriminating among different relatives and ages.

It was the Japanese psychiatrist Takeo Doi (1962) who, through clinical experience, realized that, in the Japanese language, in contrast to English or other languages, numerous words are used to refer to the nature of human relationships, or *amae* (benevolent depend-

ence), such as *amaeru, amayakasu*. Doi proposed that the richness of the Japanese word centering on *amae* reflects that Japanese values allow benevolent dependence in interpersonal relationships — a unique aspect of Japanese behavior.

2. Meaning of Words for Communication

In the process of psychotherapy, it is important to grasp the meaning of words expressed explicitly, subtly, or in a symbolic way. Transculturally, it is difficult to comprehend the subtle or symbolic meaning of words. The meaning needs to be understood through cultural context and with cultural knowledge. For instance, there is no problem understanding what the word "like" means in the English language. However, it would be difficult to comprehend accurately what it really means when an Asian girl says, "I like you." You need to know that conservative Asian men and women never say "I love you" to each other. At most, they may say "I like you." Thus, when a traditional Asian girl uses the word "like," it does not merely indicate a positive feeling toward another (equivalent to "fond of"), but could be equivalent to serious and intense affection toward a person of the opposite sex (equivalent to "love" for Occidentals). This illustrates that the issue is not simply understanding a word, but comprehending the cultural meaning beyond it (Hsu & Tseng, 1972).

From a cultural point of view, there are numerous words, phrases, or idioms commonly used by certain cultural groups to convey specific, but subtle, meanings. For instance, if someone says: "My house is far away," it means that you are not welcome to visit it. If someone asks you whether you already ate or not, it does not mean that he is concerned about you meal or interested in offering you a meal, it is simply a social greeting, like asking, "How are you?"

As an extension of this, it is important to know that, in the field of psychiatry, clinicians and patients use some psychiatric terms in their communication, such as "depression" and "hypochondriacal," which deserve careful elaboration and clarification to understand their actual meaning. Even when a patient reveals a wish to kill himself, it should not be taken literally, but requires a clinical judgment about the patient, his psychopathology, and his possible motivation for such a revelation. In addition, a cultural judgment is necessary to understand the general custom of people in the patient's culture of revealing a wish to end their lives, its common implication, and the possible message that the person wants to communicate. For example, if a Muslim person, whose faith forbids self-killing, says that he wishes he were dead, this suicidal idea must be interpreted and reacted to in a delicate manner.

In the practice of psychoanalysis, primary thinking material is often analyzed through the interpretation of dreams, fantasies, or slips of the tongue. Interpretation of symbolism becomes important in the process of analysis. It is already recognized that things are associated with different symbolic meanings, depending on universal rules and personal factors, as well as social and cultural interpretations. The same subject can be an opposite symbol in different cultures. For instance, a snake is generally considered a symbol for a male (due to its physical similarity with the male sex organ). However, for the Chinese, the snake usually symbolizes a female (due to its seductive physical movements). A dragon is interpreted as a symbol of evil by Westerners due to past legends (such as the fairy tale about a young man killing a dragon). However, for the Chinese, a dragon is a symbol of nobility, power, and benign authority. Thus, it is used to represent an emperor or a rain god, who brings the rain needed by the farmers. Thus, the interpretation of symbolism needs to be carried out subjectively, based on the patient's personal and cultural orientation.

3. Culture-Shaped Communication Patterns

Beyond the words and language used for communication, cultural factors influence how a person communicates with others, which has an impact on the clinical setting. The best example is derived from Micronesia. According to Micronesian tradition, woman are not permitted to talk directly to a stranger, even to a physician. If a stranger wants to talk to her, she is permitted to communicate only through her husband (if she is married) or through her mother (if not yet married). Imagine yourself — as an outside psychiatrist — interviewing a Micronesian couple. Whatever question you ask the wife, she will only reply in her native language to her husband and her husband will translate what she said. This applies even when the wife understands and can speak English. With the conversation going through her husband, it is difficult for you to know to what extent the communication has been screened or distorted by him. This highlights a culture-shaped communication pattern that becomes a challenge in intercultural psychotherapy.

It is also well known that the Japanese tend to respond by saying, *"Hai! Hai!"* when you are talking to them. Although *hai* in Japanese literally means "yes," it does not mean that the person is saying "yes" to you or responding affirmatively to whatever is said. It simply indicates that he is listening to what you are saying (even though he may disagree with you). The therapist needs to be aware of this to avoid any misunderstanding.

4. Nonverbal Communication

Difficulties occur in the area of nonverbal communication as well, including facial expressions, gestures, or behavior. Even though human beings share certain universal nonverbal communication, such as nodding their heads to indicate affirmation, shaking their heads to express denial or disagreement, and using certain facial expressions to demonstrate emotions of pleasure and displeasure, certain nonverbal communication is culture-patterned in specific ways. Without knowing this, a person's message may be missed or misunderstood.

For instance, one Egyptian patient made a sound, "che, che," whenever the therapist said something. This puzzled the therapist until he finally asked the patient what he meant by this. He learned that, in Egypt, such a sound indicates agreement (Hsu & Tseng, 1972). An outside psychiatrist was very much frustrated at his first encounter with a Micronesian patient. No matter what the therapist said to the patient, the latter never made any response, either verbal or nonverbal. After the therapist raised this issue to the patient, almost in an accusing way, the patient protested that he was acknowledging the therapist the whole time in his (cultural) way — raising his eyebrows. Instead of saying "yes," people in Micronesia raise their eyebrows. A Japanese psychiatrist was upset by a Chinese patient who stuck out his tongue in response to certain subjects in the middle of conversation. The therapist was upset because, for the Japanese, sticking out the tongue toward another is an insult. Fortunately, the therapist consulted his Chinese colleagues and learned that, for the Chinese, this is a customary way to indicate astonishment. These examples show that many nonverbal expressions, body gestures, or behavior are specifically culture-patterned, with particular meanings. Once the therapist observes and discovers such expressions, he should inquire into and clarify them to avoid any miscommunication.

5. Styles of Problem Presentation

As a physician, particularly a psychiatrist, and more so as a psychotherapist, it is important to recognize that there are culturally molded styles of problem presentation. A good example is that a patient may make a somatic complaint, not because he actually suffers from a somatic problem, but simply because it is a culture-patterned behavior to present somatic problems (initially) to a physician, or even to a psychiatrist. After proper inquiry or guidance, it will be easy for the patient to reveal any emotional problems that he may have (Tseng, 1975). In contrast, the patient may present a psychologized complaint, such as how much he hates his father, a trauma he encountered in his early childhood, and so on, at his first session with the therapist, as if he were very much psychologically minded and aware of his psychological problems. However, as the therapy goes on, it may shown that the patient learned to present such "psychoanalytical" material from mass media or from his friends, while he actually knew nothing about his own psychological problems.

If you interviewed Japanese patients diagnosed with *taijinkyofusho* (a special form of social phobia) you would be very surprised to learn that they tend to present their complaints at the initial session in a certain style. They will use the Japanese *sekimen-kyofu* (erythrophobia), *shisen-kyofu* (fear of eye contact), or *taishiu-kyofu* (fear of having a bad body smell that bothers others) or other professionalized terms to describe their symptoms, and even mention that they are suffering from *taijinkyofusho:* a medical diagnostic term for interpersonal relationship phobia (equivalent to social phobia). This is because the concept of *taijinkyofusho* has become popular in Japan, and even laymen use the medical term that describes this morbid condition. Used to such a stylized way of symptom presentation, Japanese psychiatrists had no difficulty diagnosing social phobia in Japanese patients. However, Japanese-American patients living in the United States do not use this style of problem presentation. When they were seen by Japanese psychiatrists, the psychiatrists had problems diagnosing their social phobia accurately (Tseng, Asai, Kitanishi, McLaughlin, & Kyomen, 1992).

This illustrates that, without knowing it, patients learn a culturally patterned way of presenting their complaints, particularly in the initial stage of therapy. A therapist needs to know about such culturally stylized problem presentation and know to deal with it. When a young male patient (either from India or China), concerned about the leaking of his semen, asks for a urine examination, or requests a tonic to nourish his kidneys, a therapist should understand that he is presenting his problem according to the folk concept of *daht* syndrome (in the case of an Indian) or *senkui* syndrome (in the case of a Chinese).

6. Disclosure of Private Matters or Taboo Subjects

In general, a therapist would like to have his patient disclose as much personal information about himself as possible so that a proper, in-depth understanding of the patient can be achieved. Based on a comprehensive and dynamic understanding of the patient, proper therapy can be performed. However, to what extent a therapist should encourage a patient to reveal private matters and how much a patient should open his mind and share very personal issues with an outsider are rather delicate clinical matters. This is particularly true when a therapist is dealing with a patient of a different cultural background. From a cultural point of view, there are many customs regarding how much internal information a person should reveal to an outsider, and what issues are taboo.

For instance, in Micronesia, it is taboo to mention the death of an ancestor. Even a physician, as an outsider, should not ask his patient about how his parents or grandparents died, although it is desirable for the physician to know about the medical history of the family. The physician may hint to his patient that it is important to know the family's medical history so that a proper diagnosis can be made of the patient's present illness. Nevertheless, the physician should not blatantly ask: "When did your father die?" or "What was the cause of your grandmother's death?" For the patient to reply to these questions is culturally forbidden, and the physician would be asking him to break his taboos.

For people in many cultures, including Asians, it is taboo to discuss death in the future. Even if a person is suffering from a terminal disease and death is imminent, it is perferred that the possibility of death not be mentioned. In such a circumstance, breaking the social taboo and helping the person to face reality and prepare for the end of his life, including making a living will and making plans for a funeral, for instance, has to be dealt with delicately and subtly, and cannot be discussed openly and liberally. Otherwise, the patient will misinterpret the therapist as wishing him to die soon.

In a less serious way, people from many cultures do not feel comfortable revealing certain family secrets. To reveal that some family member suffered from tuberculosis, indulged in gambling, had an extramarital affair, and so on is considered a shameful thing. "Not to reveal ugly family matters to the outside" is a common saying observed by the Chinese and people of many other cultures. How to take proper personal and family histories and how to deal with "cultural resistence" to information needed for dynamic case formulation become challenging matters in intercultural therapy. They become compound matters beyond the simple concerns and management of "resistence" understood by psychoanalysts.

7. The Matter of Confidentiality

Closely related to revealing private matters is how confidentiality is conceived and practiced in various cultural settings. If, in the patient's social setting, the rights of the individual are more or less emphasized and personal boundaries are relatively well established, confidentiality can be observed and maintained in the clinical situation. However, in a society where the group (or family) is emphasized, and the boundaries between individual members are not so restrictively stressed, the matter of confidentiality needs to be interpreted and observed in a slightly different way. For example, a conversation with an adolescent child is expected to be shared with his parents in a society where parents have a strong position of authority. If a therapist refuses to share information about adolescent children with their parents, under the concept of confidentially as conceived by the therapist according to his professional and cultural background, his behavior may be interpreted by the parents as offending parental authority. A similar situation may occur in a society where a husband's status is superior to his wife's. The husband may become angry if he finds that the therapist is withholding information about his wife. Thus, confidentiality needs to be interpreted and carried out differently according to the patient's cultural background. Otherwise, it may cause unexpected trouble.

8. The Art of Using an Interpreter

For intercultural psychotherapy, language can be a major obstacle, requiring an interpreter in the process of therapy. It is necessary for the clinician to be aware that there are three different ways for interpreters to function in a therapeutic situation, depending on how the interpreter performs his role and what modes of interpretation are undertaken.

a. Simple Translation

This refers to the situation in which the interpreter performs straightforward, semantic translation. The interpreter can be instructed to performed slightly differently, according to the nature of the interview. For instance, if the interview focuses on a very crucial area or a delicate emotional matter, the interpreter should be asked to carry out "word by word" translation so that the therapist will not miss the details of the content or flow of the patient's thoughts. If it is to gather information on a certain subject, such as family history, marital history, or medical history, the interpreter may be instructed to offer a condensed or reintegrated summary of what has been described by the patient on that particular subject. In this way, time can be saved. Interviews conducted through interpreter usually take more time, more than double that of ordinary interviews. Saving time becomes an important matter.

This type of interpretation is required when the therapist has no background of the patient's language. When the interview takes place, the therapist and the patient are encouraged to face each other, as if they were talking to each other. This will help the therapist establish a relationship with the patient (rather than establishing a relationship between the interpreter and the patient). Also, nonverbal responses can be transmitted between the therapist and the patient to increase the level of mutual understanding. This will make up, to some extent, for the disadvantages of conducting the interview through an interpreter.

For this type of interpretation, the interpreter does not necessarily need a scholarly or comprehensive knowledge of the language in question. Any laymen, including family members or friends, can do it, providing that the interviewer can command a flow of conversational small-talk.

b. Cultural Interpretation

This is when, in addition to the function just described, the interpreter is asked to give his or her interpretation of a word, a segment of information, or the whole matter communicated from a culture per-

spective. This may take place bilaterally, in interpretation for the therapist as well as for the patient. Thus, the interpreter serves as a culture broker, so to speak. Needless to say, there is no way to guarantee that the cultural interpretation made will be objective and accurate rather than subjective and biased. The therapist should check into it for its accuracy or offer instruction and suggestions on how to do such interpretation without distortion. This level of work requires the interpretator to have a certain level of knowledge, ability, and skill.

c. Adjunct Therapy

This is another function that some interpreters may perform: that is, as an assistant to the therapist in carrying out his therapeutic work. For this, the interpreter needs certain training and experience. It would be preferable if the interpretator had training in mental health counseling. In this circumstance, the therapist and the interpretator (or adjunct therapist) act as cotherapists. As a team, they need to practice and constantly review their performance to ensure that their approach is congruent and complementary and without conflict.

Among numerous factors needing consideration, one that deserves particular attention is, if there is a choice, whether to use an interpreter from the same ethnic group as the patient (ingroup) or someone outside the patient's ethnic group (outgroup). Clearly, an ingroup interpreter will possess more knowledge of the patient's cultural and greater language efficiency, which will increase the cultural accuracy of the interpretation.

However, clinical experience has pointed out that some potential problems exist in using interpreters from the same ethnic group as the patient. The interpreter will explicity or implicitly identify with a patient of his own ethnic group. He may feel ashamed to reveal the "ugly" information about a person who shares his ethnicity or project his own ethnic views and feelings in the process of interpreting. Furthermore, the patient may hesitate to reveal his or her own personal life to the therapist through his or her ethnic-fellow interpreter, with the concern, or even fear, that his or her secret may become known to his ethnic fellows in the community. This is particularly true when the ethnic fellows congregate in a small community.

It cannot be denied that if there is a language barrier between the therapist and the patient, extra effort is required to work through it. There are always considerable limitations in communication in therapeutic work. However, such circumstances are not entirely negative. Language barriers provide a legitimate excuse for the therapist to ask the patient to clarify an obscure word or concept so that new light is thrown on the subject — a process that is highly valued in dynamic therapy (Carstairs, 1961).

C. Therapist–Patient Relationship

1. Culture-Shaped Therapist–Patient Relationship

The therapist–patient relationship usually plays a significant role in the process of psychotherapy and is therefore often closely examined and regulated by the therapist. As clinicians know, the nature of the therapist–patient relationship is subject to numerous factors, including the personalities of the therapist and patient, their gender and age, the nature of the psychopathology, and process of therapy. Beyond these factors, the therapist should comprehend and manage the aspects of the therapist–patient relationship that are culturally molded. Attitudes toward and relationships with authority vary widely among different cultural groups. Patients who come from a background where authority tends to be autocratic will expect the therapist to be active, instructive, and responsible, while the patient plays a submissive role and hesitates to make any responses that may be considered disobedient. In contrast, patients who are used to relating with authority in a more democratic way will prefer a more equal relationship, and will expect the therapist not to manipulate them.

For instance, Filipino patients, following the traditional concept of the "powerful" physician as an almost "almighty" authority figure, tend to relate to physicians, including psychiatrists and psychotherapists, in a subordinate way, demonstrating obedience and shying away from any disagreement. "Yes, doctor!" is the common response given to physicians and psychotherapists. An interesting case vignette was described by Streltzer (1998) from his liaison–consultation psychiatric experience. A middle-aged Filipino man suffered from hypertension. He came to visit his American internist faithfully for several months, as he was instructed. Medication for hypertension was prescribed and an explanation was given on how to take it. The patient replied "Yes, doctor!" When there was no response to the medication, the dose was increased, but still there was no favorable response. When the physician asked the patient whether he was taking the medication as prescribed, the patient replied, "Yes, doctor." As the increased dose did not have any effect, another kind of medication was prescribed. After taking the patient's blood pressure, the doctor informed him that there was still no response. The patient replied: "I am sorry, doctor!" Finally, the physician checked with the patient's spouse and found that the patient never took any of the medication that was prescibed. When the patient experienced undesirable side effects, he stopped taking the medication right away, believing that medicine that causes side effects is not good. However, he never mentioned his mistrust of the drug prescribed or any disagreement toward the physician, continuing to give his patterned response of, "Yes, doctor!"

The relationship between patient and therapist will be affected by the cultural view of man–woman relations. If there is a strong cultural view about the role and status of men and women, such as the man being superior and the woman inferior, it can become problematic if a male patient is treated by a female therapist. This may be true in Muslim societies or in some Asian societies, where the role and status of man and woman are clearly defined and strikingly differentiated. Such a situation will occur not only in intracultural situations, but in intercultural situations across country boundaries. A clinical situation has been reported by Bishop and Winokur (1956) concerning a Japanese man–patient treated by an American woman–therapist. They described that, influenced by traditional attitudes about gender, the patient had difficulty accepting help from a woman (therapist). He tended to show excessive and impeccable Asian courtesy with minimal emotional coloring, particularly in the early part of the treatment sessions.

2. Ethnic/Cultural Trasference and Countertransference Issues

The ethnic and cultural transference and countertransference that are observed in interethnic or intercultural psychotherapy have attracted attention among therapists for some time (Hsu & Tseng, 1972; Schachter & Butts, 1968). Cultural transference is when a patient develops a certain relationship, feeling, or attitude toward the therapist because of the ethnic/cultural background of the therapist. Cultural countertransference is the reverse phenomenon, when a therapist develops a certain relationship with the patient mainly because of the patient's ethnic/cultural background. Transference and countertransference are based primarily on the previous knowledge, impression, bias, or experience of a therapist or a patient in relation to a particular ethnic group or people of a certain cultural system. Because it is easier to identify and react to ethnicity and race, this phenomenon occurs, in fact, as ethnic/racial transference or countertransference.

In the same way as personal transference or countertransference, ethnic or racial transference or countertransference can be positive or negative, severely influencing the process of therapy, and, therefore, needing prompt attention and management.

Concerning ethnocultural transference, which may be observed in a clinical situation, Comas-Díaz & Jacobsen (1991) indicated that the transference may be manifested as denial of ethnicity and culture; mistrust, suspicion, and hostility; ambivalence toward the therapist; or overcompliance and friendliness. Likewise, countertransference can be shown as denial of ethnocultural differences; being overly curious about the patient's ethnocultural background and developing a clinical anthropological syndrome; or demonstrating

excessive feelings of guilt, anger, or ambivalence toward the patient.

3. Impact of Racism on Intercultural Therapy

The possible negative impact or obstacle of racism on psychotherapy has attracted a great deal of attention (Carter, 1995). This is quite true if negative, or even hostile, relations preexist between the two racial groups concerned. The difficulty of psychotherapy involving racial factors has been demonstrated by extreme circumstances. For example, in South Africa, as pointed out by Lambley and Cooper (1975), individual contact between a white therapist and a black client contained elements of the overall relationship between blacks and whites in apartheid society, and these elements severely affected the therapeutic relationship. The black patient had difficulty trusting the white therapist. The therapist always had difficulty handling the black patient's anger and hatred toward whites in general, which tended to project onto the therapist. Furthermore, if the therapist was genuinely concerned for a black patient and demonstrated too much sympathy for him, the therapist ran the risk of being arrested by the government under the circumstances of apartheid. It was a political reality.

The psychotherapy of an Arab patient by a Jewish therapist in Isreal during the Intifada — an exacerbation of a historical political conflict — as described by Bizi-Nathaniel, Granek, and Golomb (1991), is another example of how political reality may intrude into interracial psychotherapy and interfere with the therapist–patient relationship. Being open with patients at an early stage of therapy about the possible effects of race and ethnic differences on therapy is encouraged (Brantley, 1983), and working on a suitable therapeutic relationship is suggested to minimize the ill effects that are always associated with such negative interracial relations.

4. Matching of Therapist and Patient

Griffith (1977) addressed different issues that are of concern in certain racial matches between therapist and patients. He pointed out, for instance, that the main issue in the white therapist–black client relationship is "trust"; in the black therapist–black client relationship, "identity"; and in the black therapist–white client relationship, "status contradiction." Resolving these special issues in each different racial match becomes a challenge.

Probably influenced by the minority and human rights movements, some groups have stressed the importance of having ethnic/culture-matched therapy. They assume that, in order to obtain effective therapy, every client is better treated by a therapist of the same ethnic–cultural background and by applying certain culture-relevant models of therapy (Sue & Morishima, 1982).

There is no doubt that the congruence of ethnic–cultural background between the therapist and the patient would definitely benefit the therapy process, particularly during the initial stage, making engagement and meaningful communication relatively easier. However, from a clinical point of view, it has been shown that the congruence of ethnic–cultural background alone is not sufficient. In fact, as pointed out by Kareem and Littlewood (1992), ethnic matching of the client and therapist is not the solution to improving intercultural therapy, as it imprisons the professional and the client in their own racial and cultural identities and diminishes the human element.

A unique clinical case in which a client was treated by three therapists (one with a different ethnic background and two with the same ethnic background as the patient) serves as a good example of therapist–patient ethnic matching (Carlton, 2001). A Chinese-American man was initially treated as an inpatient by a Caucasian psychiatrist. The patient developed acute depression and anxiety after he was scolded one day by his boss at work for being unable to function properly. Fearing he might lose his job and be unable to support his family, he panicked and became depressed, with many somatic complaints. Without too much concern that the Asian patient needed less of a dose than a white patient, a high dose of medication was prescribed by the psychiatrist to treat the patient's severe emotional condition. The patient had a fainting episode, which he suspected was

a serious side effect of the "too-strong Western medication," whereas the episode was interpreted by his Caucasian psychiatrist as the manifestation of a "hysterical attack." The fainting episode occurred on the day that the patient was urged to return to work as soon as he could. The patient as well as his spouse were not happy with the situation. They complained that the psychiatrist did not really understand his illness and did not comprehend the difficulties that he was encountering. The patient refused to take the medication again and used language problems as an excuse to request a Mandarin-speaking psychiatrist upon his discharge. The Caucasian psychiatrist, who was already frustrated by this "noncomplying," "not psychologically sophisticated," "too dependent" patient, was glad to make arrangements to transfer him to see a Chinese psychiatrist.

The second psychiatrist spoke Mandarin so there was no longer a language problem. However, the patient was still no satisfied with the second psychiatrist, even though he was Chinese. He felt that he was too busy with his clinical work, did not spend as much time talking to the patient as the patient wished, and only prescribed medication for him. Because the patient was very sensitive to the medication and complained readily about side effects he was having, medication for him become difficult. Several different kinds of medication had been tried, but all in vain. The patient soon became frustrated by the second psychiatrist. In his interpretation, he did not know how to treat him. The Chinese psychiatrist was very much frustrated by the patient, also, because he made too frequent visits to the clinic without appointments and was always presenting many somatic complaints. Very much annoyed by this "noncomplying," "too hypochondriacal," "too doctor-dependent" patient, the patient was referred to a third psychiatrist and the second Chinese psychiatrist.

The third psychiatrist was introduced by the second psychiatrist as "a more senior and more experienced" clinician in the community. The patient was satisfied that this third psychiatrist was an "authoritative" figure. Although this psychiatrist set firm rules with the patient, including complying with the psychiatrist's orders, taking his medication, how often he should come to visit the therapist, and not dropping into the clinic without an appointment, the patient liked that this doctor took time to understand him and that the doctor knew what he was doing. Very soon he followed the doctor's recommendation of taking a gradually increasing dose of medication, trying to tolerate its side effects. It was the same medication that the first and second psychiatrists had tried on him without success. This time he complied and began to show considerable improvement. When he was asked why he took the medication as prescribed this time, he replied that it was because the medication was prescribed by a "doctor" who reminded him of his "father." He felt that the doctor knew what he was doing and he trusted him.

The case did not have a rosy ending. The third psychiatrist treated the patient rather smoothly with moderate improvement for almost a year, but the patient did not recover fully. He still was often preoccupied and complained about his somatic discomfort in a hypochondriacal way, calling the doctor on the phone for trivial matters. He felt that by seeing the doctor only once a month as his medical insurance allowed was not enough for him. He wanted to see the doctor more often to satisfy his needs. His frequent telephone calls began to annoy and disturb the psychiatrist, who worked primarily as a teacher. Even though the psychiatrist reminded the patient that he should continue to take the medication, he stopped taking it after visiting his elder sister in mainland China. His sister advised him that the Western medicine was too strong and it would damage his body. His grade-school-educated sister advised him to take an herb medicine instead.

The patient's personal history revealed that he had lost his father when he was little. His mother worked hard to support the family and was seldom available for the patient when he was a child. As a result, he was raised by his 3-year-older sister. He remembered that, as a little boy, he was very insecure and that it was his sister who comforted him whenever he complained about any discomfort. It was his sister who suggested that he quit taking the medication. He did immedi-

ately, without consulting his doctor. One month later, when he went back to see the psychiatrist, the latter was upset to learn what the patient had done — ruining all the progress that had been made during the past year and making it necessary to start from the very beginning. The Chinese psychiatrist was not able to continue to see the patient due to a change in his daily work schedule, and the patient returned to the first Chinese psychiatrist, who agreed to see the patient only on an intermittent, supportive basis.

This case, which occurred in a natural setting, offers the opportunity to examine how the matching of a therapist–patient might bring about different effects. Clearly the patient demonstrated resistance to being seen by a therapist of a different ethnic background. Besides the language limitation, lack of cultural empathy was the reason given by the patient. Rather severe conditions in the initial stage were other clinical factors with which the first psychiatrist had to deal with. The second psychiatrist did not have the language problem, but, for some reason, the patient failed to develop trust in him, even though he had the same ethnic background. Personal and ethnic transference developed with the second Chinese psychiatrist, who was able to utilize the relationship to manage the medication — a difficult task with a hypochondriacal patient. We see how the three therapists handled the patient with different styles and results. This case illustrates how ethnic background, interacting with other factors (such as professional orientation, clinical experience, and cultural empathy), affects the outcome of treatment for the patient. Clearly, matching ethnicity alone is not the only answer.

Chinese-American psychologists Sue and Zane (1987), based on their clinical work, have pointed out that, in intercultural psychotherapy, it is not enough for the therapist to merely have a cultural sensitivity to and knowledge of the cultural background of the client. Additional factors are needed. Cultural knowledge and culture-consistent strategies need to be linked to two basic processes — credibility and giving — to make the therapy successful.

It is seldom pointed out in literature that there are several negative factors associated with the treatment of minority patients by therapists of the same minority background. The matter of confidentiality becomes a real concern if the minority population is relatively small in the community. Patients of a minority background may prefer to be treated by a therapist from outside of their own group. Negative ethnic transference may also occur. The patient may not trust a therapist of his own kind, with a minority or disadvantaged background, and may prefer to be treated by a therapist from a majority group. Identification with a therapist with an advantaged background may operate in such circumstances. Regarding the situation in Israel, despite the racial problems that exist between people of Arab and Jewish backgrounds, interestingly enough, as pointed out by Bizi-Nathaniel and colleagues (1991), many Arab patients in Israel prefer Jewish rather than Arab therapists. Possible explanations offered by Bizi-Nathaniel are self-hatred, "identification with the aggressor," higher evaluation of therapists' skills, and confidentiality from their own ethnic group.

5. Reverse Matching of Therapist and Patient

Reverse matching of therapist and patient has seldom been elaborated and examined in the past. It refers to the situation in which a patient of a majority background with social privilege is treated by a therapist from a minority background who is socially disadvantaged. Thus, it is a reverse of the common situation in which a minority patient is treated by a majority therapist. What happens in the matter of identification with the therapist? What about ethnic transference and countertransference? Do they tend to become negative? How does the therapist of a minority background affect the process of therapy from the point of view of value systems? These are questions waiting to be answered. In an interesting way, Cheng and Lo (1991) pointed out the advantages of intercultural psychotherapy when it was undertaken with the minority therapist-mainstream patient dyad. They pointed out that in this reversed intercultural therapy situation, the therapist, as an outsider, may provide cultural objectivity and neutrality for the patient in coping with the stresses of life.

D. Assessment, Diagnosis, and Understanding of Problems

As a part of medical practice, psychotherapy follows the medical model and procedure of making a clinical assessment and establishing a diagnosis based on which therapeutic work can proceed. The only difference is that, in psychotherapy, the nature of the assessment or diagnosis is not entirely focused on biological or physical aspects, but predominantly addresses the psychological perspective. It is not descriptive but dynamic. Understanding the nature of the problems and comprehending the causal factors in the occurrence of emotional problems are crucial parts of assessment in psychotherapeutic work. Such assessment is not carried out merely at the initial stage of therapy, but is continued throughout the process of treatment, in an accumulative and progressive way (cross-reference to Chapter 27: Clinical Assessment and Diagnosis).

From a cultural point of view, it is crucial whether the therapist can accurately understand the nature of the patient's behavior, emotional reactions, psychological problems, and coping patterns, which are all subject to cultural influence. The therapist not only needs basic knowledge of the patient's culture, but also "culture empathy," i.e., the ability to comprehend the patient's psychology and behavior at an emotional level in a culturally relevant and accurate way. This is a challenging task for any therapist performing intercultural psychotherapy.

In order to illustrate this point, let us present two clinical examples.

A Vietnamese wife, who migrated to the United States with her husband, went to see an American psychiatrist (Young, 1997). Her initial complaint was a headache and sensation of pressure on her chest. After skillful exploration, it was gradually revealed that the underlying problem was that she was feeling bad about herself. Her history revealed that while she was in Vietnam, her husband and his relatives all lost contact in the middle of the war. When the war ended, the government gave a limited time span for people to reregister their property. Without knowing whether her husband was still alive or not, her mother-in-law suggested she register the family property under her name. However, shortly after this, her husband safely returned home. Discovering that his wife had registered all the property in her name, he became very furious at her. According to Vietnam custom, family property is always registered under a man's name, the grandfather's, the father's, or the son's; it was never registered under a woman's name. The wife was accused of doing something improper, with the intention of stealing the family property. Despite her explanation that it was the only way under the circumstances to protect the property, and done at her mother-in-law's suggestion, her husband still never forgave her. The marital displeasure continued even after they took refuge in the United States, leaving all their property behind. After hearing this story, the American therapist could understand, at a *cognitive* level, the dilemma the patient encountered, but without having the experience of living in Vietnam and not having in-depth cultural knowledge, the therapist still faced limitations, at the *affective* level, in really comprehending the "disgraceful" thing that the wife had done and the kind of "shame" she was facing. Needless to say, this limited cultural empathy interfered with the progress of the therapy.

An old Samoan woman with multiple somatic disorders, including diabetes, hypertension, and kidney problems, was admitted to the hospital under her physician's advice (Streltzer, 1998). Emergency psychiatric consultation was requested as she was found tying the string for the bedside light around her neck, and suicidal intentions were suspected by the medical staff. After a skillful interview by the Caucasian-consulting psychiatrist, who established a rapport first by praising the patient on how she was a successful woman, raising a large family by herself after her husband's death, the patient began to open up and reveal her frustration. She described that she was very reluctant to stay at the hospital to begin with. It was her family doctor who promised that she needed to stay at the hospital only for several days for a workup. But

now, she had been confined to the hospital for more than 2 weeks, and she was not allowed to return home. She became resentful and tied the rope around her neck — not wanting to kill herself — but to show her anger toward her physician for his being untruthful and unable to keep his promise. A sensitive therapist was required, who knew how to engage a patient of a different ethnic background, how to establish a rapport by "talking story" about her family, and how to show cultural empathy so that the patient eventually was willing to share her inner feelings and allow the consultant to work on her problems. Otherwise, the patient might have been simply treated as a person with suicidal tendencies and transferred to a psychiatric ward with a diagnosis of major depression.

E. INTERPRETATION AND GIVING ADVICE

For clinicians, it is a common knowledge that a therapist needs to know how to provide interpretation or advice at the proper time in a suitable way. It is a matter of clinical judgement, depending on the therapeutic process and numerous other factors, including the patient's psychopathological condition, ego strength, readiness for explanation, level of psychological sophistication, and so on. Intercultural psychotherapy needs to consider further how to make interpretations that are culturally suitable, proper, meaningful, and effective. The best language and concepts are those familiar to the patient so that he can receive the explanations with ease and will find them meaningful.

For instance, an American psychiatrist was treating a young male hypochondriacal Korean patient and his parents in a family session in Korea when he was visiting there as a consultant. The therapist observed that the patient, an only son, had been using multiple somatic symptoms as excuses to stay close to his mother, even sleeping in the same bedroom with her, despite being an adolescent. This analytically oriented family therapist, with professional intentions and deliberately chosen strategies, made a direct comment to the young patient in his broken Korean: "You want to kill your father and marry your mother?!" This may have been all right for an (American) patient and his parents if they were familiar with the psychoanalytic concept of the Oedipus wish. Such a direct comment would certainly point out the core of the problem and wake up their conscious awareness of the unresolved parent–child relationship. However, for the Korean patient and his parents, without any preparation, it was a shocking comment that was difficult for them to understand, accept, and react to. Actually, from a cultural point of view, it was extremely inappropriate to make such an interpretative comment to them. Within a conservative, family-oriented society like traditional Korea, it was almost taboo to stir up conflicts within a family. It might be a psychoanalytically correct understanding (from a theoretical, conceptual point of view), but it was a premature dynamic interpretation (from a clinical perspective) and an inappropriate therapeutic attempt (on a cultural level). Even though the therapist conceptualized the patient and the family pathology in such a way, practically he should simply have encouraged the patient to grow up and learn how to become a man like his father. There was no need to sexualize the situation and stimulate conflict within the parent–child triangular relationship, the last thing that was desirable within such a cultural system.

In many societies, there are numerous proverbs hinting at how a person should lead his life. "A rolling stone never gathers moss," "the grass on the other side of the fence is greener," or "it is better not to gather all your eggs in one basket" are some Western examples. "A protruding nail will be hit by a hammer" (do not speak up too loudly or you will invite a punitive reaction), "a leaf will fall and return to the root of the tree" (a person in crisis will seek support from his family or an aged person will seek to return to his home in their later life), "a *samurai* will use a toothpick even if he is hungry" (pretending he just had a meal — not showing his weakness in case of any unexpected fighting) are some Eastern examples. These proverbs reflect the cultural wisdom accumulated from life experiences in the past. It is useful in therapy if the proper sayings or proverbs are selected for particular purposes. They will especially make it easier for the patient to understand and obtain insight. Naturally, it will be desirable for the therapist to know some of the sayings that exist in the patient's culture so that he will be able to utilize them when they are needed.

Contemporary Western psychotherapists are trained not to offer any advice to their patients, particularly relating to major life matters, such as decisions about adoption, separation, divorce, or remarriage. This is based on the belief that patients should be respected for making their own decisions. This reflects a cultural belief in basic human rights, and a professional orientation rooted in the psychoanalytic approach. However, it cannot be denied that no matter how the therapist pretends he is not making any decisions for the patient, the patient is always looking for clues given by the therapist, and the therapist *does* send messages to the patient regarding choices that he should make — with or without knowing that he is doing so through verbal or nonverbal communication.

Many patients suffer from dilemmas that they encounter in their daily lives. Therefore, they need to see psychiatrists for guidance. How to relate to parental authority; the proper role of a wife; whether to decide situations for the sake of the individual self or for the family; is it all right to have premarital sexual relations, an abortion, or extramarital affairs; what is the proper choice to make, separation, divorce, remarriage, or to continue in the present unhappy marriage? Those are common psychological problems encountered by patients and the choices they make are subject to personal as well as cultural considerations. Offering advice on these daily life matters is a challenge for the therapist — one that cannot be avoided in intercultural psychotherapy. A culturally relevant therapist should actively explore with the patient the implications of each choice the patient has and elaborate on the implications of difference decisions that the patient is going to make — from the different levels of the personal self, the family, the group, and social and cultural perspectives.

H. GOALS OF THERAPY

The final issue that needs attention in intercultural psychotherapy is the matter of the goals of therapy. Defining a normal, healthy, or mature person is subject to cultural influence. What route should be taken to resolve problems and which coping mechanisms should be utilized are subject to cultural determination.

The process of psychotherapy can be viewed as a communication and exchange of values between two partners: the therapist and the patient. It has been said that patients who have shown greater clinical improvement have displayed a significantly greater change in moral values in the direction of their therapists' values. This is the situation in intracultural psychotherapy. To what extent this is true in intercultural psychotherapy is waiting for validation. If a therapist is working with a patient with a different value system, he needs to carefully assess his values. Questions such as, "Shall a wife show her resentfulness toward her husband more openly?" or "Shall a woman learn to express her sexual desire more directly in a public setting?" should be examined carefully and constantly in terms of the patient's culture. It is important that the therapist not impose values and goals that, although appropriate in the therapist's culture, may not be suitable for the patient.

At the philosophical level, many things have to be elaborated carefully. Encouraging a patient to accept suffering or advising him to deal with obstacles are philosophical matters that deserve assessment from a cultural perspective. For an ordinary contemporary American, it may be ideal to be self-directed and independent, to emphasize work and socialization, and to have a problem-solving approach to life's conflicts. For many Eastern people, it may be better to be dependent, to learn rational control over emotions and desire, and to be harmonious with others and with nature. Therefore, it is very important for the therapist to consider the patient's prior life, patterns of enculturation, the kind of cultural environment he is going to live in (in his home community or in a new place), and then to elaborate and discover with the patient which direction he should take to improve his life. The

therapist may lend his value system to the patient for the latter's reference, but it is the patient who, under the therapist's guidance, should develop goals for improvement.

In summary, numerous obstacles may be encountered and many challenges need to be resolved when a therapist is treating a patient with a diversely different cultural background. As a result of his work with Malaysians, Kinzie (1972), stressed the importance of openness and flexibility in intercultural therapy.

III. COMPETENT INTERCULTURAL PSYCHOTHERAPY

It is a fact that the practice of psychotherapy is complex. The therapist needs to pay attention to various factors, including the nature of psychopathology and psychological problems from which the patient suffers, the ego strength of the patient, the coping mechanisms customarily utilized by the patient, the patient's motivation for therapy, the therapist–patient relationship, the strategies to be used in therapy, the process and stages of treatment, the defined goals of therapy, and the socioeconomic condition of the patient, including medical insurance to pay for therapy. Beyond such general clinical and social factors, cultural aspects deserve special attention, and an effort is needed to make the therapy culturally relevant and meaningful for the patient.

A. QUALITIES REQUIRED FOR SUCCESSFUL, CULTURALLY COMPETENT THERAPY

It is a fundamental requirement that the therapist needs to be clinically competent. This includes being sensitive, caring, equipped with clinical knowledge and theories of human behavior, and experienced in clinical work. In order to be successful in conducting culturally relevant psychotherapy, many additional qualities are desired. These include cultural sensitivity, knowledge, empathy, and insight, with the ability to offer objective cultural guidance to the patient (Tseng & Streltzer, 2000).

1. Cultural Sensitivity

This refers to the clinical quality of being able to be open and sensitive about the dimensions of culture with regard to human behavior and to appreciate the different views that people of different cultural groups may hold. There is a tendency to be ethnocentric and an effort will be made to understand and accept potential differences that may exist between people of various socioeconomic backgrounds.

2. Cultural Knowledge

In order to perform culturally appropriate therapy, the therapist needs to have a certain knowledge about the patient's cultural background. It does not need to be comprehensive and in-depth, but it should cover the basic and relevant issues so that the therapeutic work can be carried out relevantly. Anthropological reading, medical anthropological consultation, and relying on cultural informants are general ways to approach such needed knowledge. The patient or the patient's family or friends are also good resources from whom knowledge can be acquired.

3. Cultural Empathy

A therapist not only needs to be equipped cognitively with cultural knowledge, but also to be able to affectively understand and empathetically feel the patient's cultural views. Otherwise there will be a wide gap in the therapist's understanding and ability to share the emotions of the patient — an important issue that will determine the quality of the psychotherapy.

4. Cultural Insight

Finally, based on relevant insight into the nature of culture, the therapist should have the ability to view the patient's situation from cultural perspectives, as well as other clinical issues. The therapist should further be able to offer appropriate suggestions or guidance to the patient on how to make cultural changes, adjustments, or resolutions that will lead to more culturally sound, successful solutions for the patient in his or her sociocultural environment.

In summary, beyond this basic clinical competence, additional clinical qualities are needed to perform culturally sensitive and relevant therapy, which will be greatly beneficial to the patient. Such culturally oriented qualities can be obtained through knowledge, training, and adequate experience. They are desirable qualities for every contemporary therapist to have in order to offer relevant and meaningful service to his or her patients.

B. LESSONS FROM INTERCULTURAL PSYCHOTHERAPY

Intercultural psychotherapy — treating patients of very diverse cultural backgrounds — helps clinicians realize and examine the cultural dimensions that are involved in the practice of psychotherapy. Such "extreme" situations make us aware that culture cannot be ignored even in "regular" or "intracultural" psychotherapy, whether the clinician is dealing with a patient of the same cultural background or treating a member of the majority group in a society. How to assess different situations in which cultural matters are involved and how to handle them at the clinical level are issues that deserve particular attention. They will be elaborated in more detail in the following chapter on culturally relevant psychotherapy.

Among several issues involved in intercultural psychotherapy that can also be applied to intracultural (or homocultural) psychotherapy are communication and values. Even if the therapist and patient speak the same language, there is always a need to check whether the communication is carried out properly and accurately, without the influence of preoccupation or misunderstanding; whether or not the verbally communicated material reflects the actual meaning and feeling; and how to understand and empathize relevantly and meaningfully with a patient's mental life and experience. These are always challenges for the clinician, even one who shares the same cultural system as the client, but has a different socioeconomic or geographic background.

How the therapist's own value system is going to explicitly or indirectly affect the content and direction of therapy is another matter that calls for the therapist's attention (Buhler, 1962). This is true even when the therapist and patient have the same sociocultural background. Every person has a certain individual value system, beyond the collective one, that shapes his or her own thinking, affects his or her behavior, and molds the direction of his or her actions. The therapist is no exception, even though he is trained to be "neutral," "professional," and "nonpersonal" in his therapeutic actions. It cannot be denied that the therapist is a human being and that his personality, way of thinking, and attitudes and beliefs will come across in his therapeutic interaction with the patient. As a therapist, he is advised to be aware of his own personal and professional value systems and to examine constantly how they are affecting the process of therapy with the patient, who often has a different set of individual, family, and collective value systems. These are lessons we can learn from the extreme area of intercultural psychotherapy.

REFERENCES

Aponte, J.F., Rivers, R.Y., & Wohl, J. (Eds.). (1995). *Psychological interventions and cultural diversity.* Boston: Allyn & Bacon.

Bishop, M.M., & Winokur, G. (1956). Cross-cultural psychotherapy. *Journal of Nervous and Mental Disease, 123,* 369–375.

Bizi-Nathaniel, S., Granek, M., & Golomb, M. (1991). Psychotherapy of an Arab patient by a Jewish therapist in Israel during the Intifada. *American Journal of Psychotherapy, 45,* 594–603.

Bolman, W.M. (1968). Cross-cultural psychotherapy. *American Journal of Psychiatry, 124*(9), 1237–1244.

Brantley, T. (1983). Racism and its impact on psychotherapy. *American Journal of Psychiatry, 140,* 1605–1608.

Buhler, C. (1962). *Values in psychotherapy* (pp. 172–221). New York: Free Press of Glencoe.

Burke, A.W. (1986). Racism, prejudice and mental illness. In J.L. Cox (Ed.), *Transcultural psychiatry* (pp. 134–157). London: Croom Helm.

Carlton, B. (2001). One patient, three therapists. In W.S. Tseng & J Streltzer (Eds.); *Culture and psychotherapy: A guide for clinical practice* (pp. 67–78). Washington, DC: American Psychiatric Press.

Carstairs, G.M. (1961). Cross-cultural psychiatric interviewing. In B. Kaplan (Ed.), *Studying personality cross-culturally* (pp. 532–548). New York: Harper & Row.

Carter, R.T. (1995). *The influence of race and racial identity in psychotherapy: Toward a racially inclusive model.* New York: Wiley-Interscience.

Cheng, L., & Lo, H. (1991). On the advantages of cross-cultural psychotherapy: The minority therapist/mainstream patient dyad. *Psychiatry, 54,* 386–396.

Comas-Díaz, L., & Jacobsen, F.M. (1991). Ethno cultural transference and countertransference in the therapeutic dyad. *American Journal of Orthopsychiatry, 61,* 392–402.

Doi, T. (1962). Amae — A key concept for understanding Japanese personality structure. In R.J. Smith & R.K. Beardsley (Eds.), *Japanese culture: Its development and characteristics.* Chicago: Aldine.

Foulks, E.F., Bland, I., & Shervington, D. (1995). Psychotherapy across cultures. In J.M. Oldham & M.B. Riba (Eds.), *Review of psychiatry* (Vol. 14; Sect. IV, pp. 511–528). Washington, DC: American Psychiatric Press.

Geller, J.D. (1988). Racial bias in the evaluation of patients for psychotherapy. In L. Comas-Díaz & E.E.H. Griffith (Eds.), *Clinical guidelines in cross-cultural mental health* (pp. 112–134). New York: Wiley.

Griffith, M.S. (1977). The influences of race on the psychotherapeutic relationship. *Psychiatry, 40,* 27–40.

Hsu, J., & Tseng, W.S. (1972). Intercultural psychotherapy. *Archives of General Psychiatry, 27,* 700–705.

Kareem, J., & Littewood, R. (Eds.). (1992). *Intercultural therapy: Themes, interpretations and practice.* Oxford: Blackwell.

Kinzie, J.D. (1972). Cross-cultural psychotherapy: The Malaysian experience. *American Journal of Psychotherapy, 26,* 220–231.

Kinzie, J.D., Tran, K.A., Breckenridge, A., & Bloom, J.D. (1980). An Indochinese refugee psychiatric clinic: Culturally accepted treatment approaches. *American Journal of Psychiatry, 137,* 1429–1432.

Koss-Chioino, J.D., & Vargas, L.A. (1992). Through the culture looking glass: A model for understanding culturally responsive psychotherapies. In A. Vargas & J.D. Koss-Chioino (Eds.), *Working with culture: psychotherapeutic interventions with ethnic minority children and adolescents.* San Francisco: Jossey-Bass.

Lambley, P., & Cooper, P. (1975). Psychotherapy and race: Interracial therapy under apartheid. *American Journal of Psychotherapy, 29,* 179–184.

Marcos, L. (1988). Understanding ethnicity in psychotherapy with Hispanic patients. *American Journal of Psychoanalysis, 48,* 25–42.

Pedersen, P.B., Draguns, J.G., Lonner, W.J., & Trimble, J.E. (Eds.). (1989). *Counseling across Cultures* (3rd ed.). Honolulu: University of Hawaii Press.

Pedersen, P.B., Draguns, J.G., Lonner, W.J., & Trimble, J.E. (Eds.). (1996). *Counseling across cultures* (4th ed.). Thousand Oaks, CA: Sage.

Pedersen, P.B., Lonner, W.J., & Draguns, J.G. (Eds.). (1976). *Counseling across cultures.* Honolulu: University Press of Hawaii.

Pinderhughes, E. (1989). *Understanding race, ethnicity, and power: The key to efficacy in clinical practice.* New York: Free Press.

Samuda, R.J., & Wolfgang, A. (1985). *Intercultural counseling and assessment: Global perspectives.* Lewiston, NY: C.J. Hogrefe.

Sanchez, E., & Mohl, P. (1992). Psychotherapy with Mexican American patients. *American Journal of Psychiatry, 149,* 626–630.

Schachter, J.S., & Butts, H.F. (1968). Transference and contertransference in interracial analysis. *Journal of the American Psychoanalytic Association, 16,* 792–808.

Streltzer, J. (1998). Cultural impact on consultation-interaction liaison psychiatric services. Presented at the American Psychiatric Association annual meeting workshorp on Cultural Issues in Consultation-Liaison Psychiatry, at Toronto, Canada.

Sue, S., & Morishima, J.K. (Eds.). (1982). *The mental health of Asian Americans.* San Francisco: Jossey-Bass.

Sue, S., & Zane, N. (1987). The role of culture and cultural techniques in psychotherapy: A critique and reformulation. *American Psychologist, 42,* 37–45.

Tseng, W.S. (1975). The nature of somatic complaints among psychiatric patients: The Chinese case. *Comprehensive Psychiatry, 16,* 237–245.

Tseng, W.S., Asai, M.H., Kitanishi, K.J., McLaughlin, D., & Kyomen, H. (1992). Diagnostic pattern of social phobia: Comparison in Tokyo and Hawaii. *Journal of Nervous and Mental Disease, 180,* 380–385.

Tseng, W.S., McDermott, J.F., Jr., & Maretzki, T.W. (Eds.). (1974). *People and cultures in Hawaii: An introduction for mental health workers.* Honolulu: University of Hawaii School of Medicine, Department of Psychiatry, Transcultural Psychiatry Committee.

Tseng, W.S., & Streltzer, J. (2000). *Culture and psychotherapy: A guide for clinical practice.* Washington, DC: American Psychiatric Press.

van der Veer, G. (1992). *Counseling and therapy with refugees: Psychological problems of victims of war, torture and repression.* Chichester: Wiley.

Walz, C.R., & Benjamin, L. (Eds.). (1978). *Transcultural counseling: Needs, programs, and techniques.* New York: Human Sciences Press.

Wolfgang, A. (1985). Intercultural counselling and nonverbal behavior: An overview. In R.J., Samuda & A. Wolfgang (Eds.), *Intercultural counseling and assessment.* Lewiston, NY: C.J. Hogrefe.

Young, D. (1997). *Psychotherapy for a Vietnam woman.* Presented at the Culture and Psychotherapy Symposium, University of Hawaii School of Medicine, Department of Psychiatry, Honolulu.

37

Culture-Relevant Psychotherapy

I. INTRODUCTION

In this section, in Chapters 32 through 36, the subject of "culture and psychotherapy" has been elaborated broadly from various perspectives. It started with a review of indigenous healing practices that exist in various societies (Chapter 32); was followed by an examination of culture-influenced unique psychotherapies invented by laymen or professionals (Chapter 33); and ended with an analysis of common psychotherapies applied by contemporary professionals (Chapter 34). Thus, various modes of psychotherapy, including folk and professional, are reviewed comprehensively in order to understand the common elements as well as the differences among them. Furthermore, the practice of psychotherapy in selected societies around the world was examined (Chapter 35), and a particular psychotherapeutic situation, namely intercultural psychotherapy, was analyzed in detail for clinical application (Chapter 36). These extensive reviews assist us in realizing that the practice of psychotherapy, as one kind of healing practice, is indeed influenced heavily by cultural factors.

These elaborations affirm our view that the definition of psychotherapy needs to be broadened to embrace different practices, whether indigenous or universal, folk or professional, that are utilized to treat disorders and promote health (Prince, 1980). It also confirms our opinion that the orientations of psychotherapy are broad and need to be expanded from the medical and psychological to embrace the supernatural, natural, and philosophical.

It is apparent that the practice of psychotherapy should always be carried out in a way that is relevant to the patient and to the social setting where the practice takes place, including political background, social class, economical situation, ethnic and racial factors, and cultural diversity. Cultural influence on the practice of psychotherapy should be examined and dealt with actively by the therapist (Tseng & Streltzer, 2001). Culture-adjusted psychotherapy is needed at the microscopic level for individual patients and at the macroscopic level for societies. How to perform culture-relevant or culture-responsive psychotherapy for clients of cultural diversity, patients of different socioeconomic backgrounds, and minorities is a challenge for modern mental health workers (Abel & Metraux, 1974; Acosta, Yamamoto, & Evans, 1982; Koss-Chioino & Vargas, 1992). This is the focus of the final chapter in this section.

II. ADJUSTMENTS NEEDED FOR PSYCHOTHERAPY IN DIFFERENT CULTURES

In order to carry out culture-relevant psychotherapy, there is a need to make adjustments at the technical, theoretical, and philosophical levels (Tseng, 1995, 2001).

A. TECHNICAL ADJUSTMENTS

Clinically, technical adjustments in psychotherapy refer to the need for the therapist to make proper choices of skills or techniques in therapy to fit the background of the patient. It is commonly known by clinicians that the practice of therapy needs to be adjusted in accordance with various factors, including the patient's age, gender, personality, level of cognitive sophistication, style of psychological orientation, and the nature and severity of the psychopathology. Such technical adjustments are needed, furthermore, to fit the cultural background of the patient.

Generally speaking, from a cultural point of view, numerous areas need technical adjustment. Following are some of the areas that deserve consideration.

1. Preparation for Starting Therapy

Based on the patient's orientation toward and understanding of psychotherapy, suitable preparation is needed in the way therapy is started. It includes to what extent an explanation regarding psychotherapy is needed and what kind of contract needs to be established, including the rules to be observed and the payment that is expected.

2. Adjustment of the Therapist–Patient Relationship

The relationship between the therapist and patient, in addition to following professional considerations, also needs proper modification to conform to a cultur-

ally sanctioned therapist–patient relationship; in particular, what kind of role a therapist needs to undertake: authoritative or egalitarian.

3. Management of Cultural Transference and Countertransference

In addition to the general phenomena of transference and countertransference that may be observed in therapy, ethnic/culture transference and countertransference may occur when there is a difference in the ethnic or cultural backgrounds of the therapist and patient, and a strong feeling or bias toward the ethnicity or culture of either one. Such phenomena will significantly influence the relationship between the therapist and patient, and have tremendous impact on the process of therapy, requiring suitable management from the beginning of therapy.

4. Performing Culturally Suitable Communication and Interpretation

The style and content of communication need cultural adjustment. This includes the concept of illness and an explanation of the cause of the problems, the use of cultural idioms, and the level of sophistication of interpretation.

5. Selection of Modes of Therapy

There are numerous modes of therapy to be selected for treatment of a targeted patient(s). How to select proper modes of therapy to maximize therapeutic effects is a matter of clinical consideration. In addition, cultural factors should be included in the consideration of therapeutic modes.

6. Choice of the Goal of Therapy

The goals of therapy need to be determined according to the patient's psychological strength, the nature of the pathology, the expectations of therapy, and other practical factors. Cultural factors are certainly considerations in the proper determination of the goals of therapy if the cultural expectations of therapy are to be met.

Descriptions of the these technical adjustments were presented in detail in Chapter 36.

B. THEORETICAL MODIFICATIONS

Beyond technical adjustments, it is also necessary to make conceptual or theoretical modifications relating to therapy to fit the patient's cultural background. At present, several theories, particularly psychoanalytic ones, are utilized by therapists to understand the patient's personality and behavior. However, these theories are subject to cross-cultural modifications if they are to be used for people living in different sociocultural settings. Ethnicity and culture are to be recognized as significant parameters in understanding psychological processes (American Psychological Association, 1993).

1. Concepts of Self and Ego Boundaries

How to view the "self," how to hold an image of the "self," and how to maintain boundaries between the self and others and relationships with others are psychological issues that are often of concern and dealt with in the process of therapy. The concept of the "self" and its boundaries (ego boundaries) have been elaborated cross-culturally by several scholars (Kirmayer, 1989; Marsella, DeVos, & Hsu, 1985; Roland, 1991). Cultural anthropologist F.L.K. Hsu (1985) has pointed out that, in contrast to Americans, the Chinese tend to view the self as a member–partner who is embedded in the group surrounding him rather than a clearly defined, independent, individual entity. This does not imply that the ego boundary for the Chinese is "blurred," but indicates that the Chinese person is relatively more heavily bound to immediate family members, relatives, or friends who are living around him. This is the natural result of living in a society that is characterized by situation orientation rather than individual orientation. Thus, although human beings share a fundamental psychological structure, the psy-

chology of the "self" varies according to the sociocultural background of the person concerned (see Fig. 49-1). Such variations in concepts of the self and ego boundaries need to be recognized in dealing with patients from different cultural backgrounds.

2. Interpersonal Relations

How to maintain suitable and functional social relations is often of great concern in therapy. However, suitable and functional social relations need to be maintained in the various groups, including family, friends, colleagues, social groups, that are subject to sociocultural definitions and sanctions.

In terms of culturally patterned interpersonal relations, Japanese psychiatrist Doi (1962) raised the issue of *amae* (benevolent dependence) in understanding Japanese behavior. A rather positive value is given to mutual dependence in interpersonal relations among Japanese. This is quite a contrast to the West, where "dependency" on others is consciously devalued, while independence is emphasized. Thus, defining proper and healthy interpersonal relations from a cultural perspective is certainly a subject that needs further theoretical elaboration.

3. Theories of Personality Development

Several theories have been proposed by scholars for understanding and interpreting psychological development. These include Freud's psychosexual theory, Erikson's psychosocial theory, and Piaget's cognitive theory. The first two are focused more on personality development and are subject to cultural influences and deserve more theoretical clarification for cross-cultural application.

The psychosexual developmental theory proposed by Sigmund Freud is focused on the biological-drive aspect of individual development and is regarded, in principle, as universal. However, Freud himself speculated that due to the individual's unique developmental course, the drive that emerges in each developmental stage may be subject to variations. This is particularly true regarding the parent–child relationship conflict that occurs at the phallic stage or the so-called Oedipal complex: the core of psychoanalytic theory. It has been pointed out that the intensity of this triangular complex, which a child needs to overcome, depends on the sexual attitude that exists in the environment. It is subject to variations based on the family system and structure that exist with the society [cross-reference to Chapter 4: Child Development and Enculturation (Section III,A)].

The psychosocial theory proposed by Erikson (1963) is concerned with the psychosocial theme emphasized at each stage of development. Erikson has indicated that the psychosocial view of personality development needs cultural adjustment in terms of the pace of the stages that an individual may go through and the major tasks that need to be mastered in each stage. Following his notion, the cultural modification of psychosocial development can be elaborated in terms of variations of the themes in each developmental stages as well as the pace of development between stages [cross-reference to Chapter 49: Culture and Psychiatric Theories (Section IV,B)].

4. Theories of Defense Mechanisms

The theories of defense mechanisms were considered by analysts to be universally applicable for understanding human nature. Defense mechanisms are systematically subgrouped into a theoretical hierarchy of narcissistic, immature, neurotic, and mature defense mechanisms according to a person's level of pathology and maturity (Vaillant, 1971).

Although empirical studies of ego mechanisms have begun to emerge (Vaillant, 1986), the theories have not been tested thoroughly from a cross-cultural perspective. Transcultural clinical experience has shown that there is still room for cross-cultural modification of the theoretical structure of defense mechanisms. For example, elaboration is needed on which defense mechanisms are utilized more in one cultural group than in another, particularly concerning neurotic or mature mechanisms. There is a possibility that there are defense mechanisms utilized in some cultures that have not been included in existing theories.

A unique culturally rooted defense mechanism, referred to as "Ah-Q's way," often used by the Chinese in dealing with problems, is one such example [cross-reference to Chapter 49: Culture and Psychiatric Theories (Section IV,C)].

5. Therapeutic Mechanisms: Expression or Suppression

Deeply influenced by early psychoanalytic concepts, it has been theorized by analysts that the major therapeutic mechanism for healing neurotic patients is helping them learn how to express their inhibited desires and demonstrate their hidden emotions. Fulfillment of desire and expression of emotion is considered to be a healthy way to overcome neurotic problems. Although such id-centered psychoanalysis has been more or less replaced by the ego-focused psychotherapy of the present, such therapeutic views need reconsideration from a cross-cultural perspective. Instead of expression, suppression can be considered a more functional and healthy way to cope with problems in certain cultures, particularly interpersonally oriented societies (such as many Asian or Arabic societies), and should be utilized as a healthy therapeutic mechanism in therapy. In some societies, superego-emphasized therapy is more culturally appropriate.

This point is elaborated well by Dwairy (1997, p. 1) concerning Arabic clients. He explained that, compared to Western families, the traditional Arabic family plays a relatively greater role in providing support for adult progeny. This conditions adult offspring to continue to comply with the will and values of the family. From the aspect of ego psychology, Arabic individuals learn to repress authentic needs and emotions, and within that process they relinquish the need for self-actualization. The important point is that if Western psychotherapy is applied to Arabic patients, with its emphasis on reliving and activating repressed needs and emotions and ultimately promote self-actualization, it will transform intrapsychic conflicts into interpersonal and social ones. As a result, the therapy will often lead the Arabic client to become more helpless, as such wishes of self-actualization will rarely be socially sanctioned or satisfactorily fulfilled.

In summary, based on limited resources of knowledge and information, only a handful of examples from some cultures are used here to elaborate the subject and support the views concerned. However, it is believed that the concepts or theories about human nature or behavior need to be reexamined and modified for all cultural groups, whether Japanese, Indian, Hispanic, Italian, Russian, Arabic, or others. The concepts or theories discussed earlier are primarily used to understand the nature of human behavior. Clearly, there is a need to elaborate on theories that deal with the formation of psychopathology and the therapy itself. This is an area that has not yet been studied sufficiently, but deserves further attention in the future.

C. Philosophical Considerations

It is becoming clear to cultural psychiatrists that in the practice of psychotherapy, the therapist needs to take into consideration the patient's (as well as the therapist's) philosophical orientation. A patient's basic view of and attitude toward human beings, society, and life, closely related to concepts of normality, maturity, and health, will have an obvious impact on the patient in his search for improvement. The therapist's own values system and philosophical attitude toward life and problems will explicitly or implicitly guide the direction of therapy, particularly regarding how to encourage the patient to resolve the problems.

For instance, Indian psychiatrist V.K. Varma (1982) pointed out that in India, where people have a fatalistic view of life, believing their present suffering is the result of sins committed in an earlier incarnations, psychological therapy, aimed at resolution in life, has a relatively difficult time flourishing. It is not easily accepted by patients, or even by therapists in training (Hoch, 1990). Therefore, attention to philosophical reorientation is necessary in providing therapy for patients of any ethnic–cultural group.

In a similar way, Muslims, based on their faith, tend to believe that their lives are in the hands of their almighty god, Allah. Thus, devotion to Alah is considered the most important and best way to solve their problems rather than seeking help from a healer of mental problems. Within such a belief system, the practice of psychotherapy also has a difficult time flourishing.

In contrast to this, within contemporary European-American societies, people tend to hold the philosophical view that any problem can be solved by humans, as long as they are willing to solve it. Based on such a philosophical premise, people are encouraged to seek solutions through therapy when they encounter emotional problems. However, this also adds a psychological burden on the patients, as it becomes their individual responsibility to cope their problems, which could exceed the actual limits of reality. This is an issue deserving attention from a culture perspective: how to relevantly set up the ultimate goals of therapy.

III. CULTURALLY RELEVANT PSYCHOTHERAPY: INTEGRATION

A. Practical Guidance for Culturally Relevant Psychotherapy

The areas of impact of culture on psychotherapy are broad. In order to carry out culturally relevant, compatible, sensitive, or responsive therapy, attention must be paid to various aspects (Tseng & Streltzer, 2001).

1. Thoughtful Consideration of the Sociocultural Setting within Which the Therapy Takes Place

This refers to how the society at large recognizes and understands the practice of psychotherapy. Specifically, political ideology, economic conditions, the medical system itself, the history of medicine and psychiatry, and the population's general understanding of and attitude toward mental illness, as well as psychotherapy, are all factors that influence the practice of psychotherapy in practical ways. The factors may resist or even present obstacles to the practice of psychotherapy, may discourage such a treatment method, or may greatly favor it.

Attention must also be paid to the basic philosophical orientation held by the society and the individual toward the nature, purpose, and meaning of life. This fundamental philosophical orientation may affect the nature, process, and goal of the therapy as a whole.

2. Full Attention to the Patient's Cultural Orientation Toward and Expectation of Psychotherapy

At a clinical level, the issues of concern are the patient's familiarity with and orientation and attitude toward psychotherapy. These may vary from society to society, as well as from individual to individual, based on the general attitude toward mental illness or emotional problems, medical knowledge, and understanding of and orientation toward psychotherapy. A therapist needs to pay attention to these factors and make necessary preparations for psychotherapy, particularly in the initial stages of treatment. This is particularly true when a therapist is working with a patient from a society in which people have little knowledge of or hold biased impressions about psychotherapy.

As professionals, psychotherapists establish certain rules for patients to follow and agreements for them to observe in order to facilitate the process of therapy. However, many patients are unfamiliar with such rules or unable to comprehend such agreements, in which case they need to be explained and discussed. This is especially true when a therapist is treating a patient without too much knowledge of or experience with psychotherapy. This is often the case when the patient comes from another cultural background.

Psychotherapists have developed and utilized various specific therapeutic techniques in their practices, e.g., dream analysis, free association, or interpretation of unconscious dynamics in psychoanalysis; reframing or paradox suggestions in family therapy; or positive enforcement or punishment in behavior therapy. Careful explanation of the purpose of such maneuvers

and guidance on how to follow them are always needed if such specific therapeutic manipulations or techniques are utilized.

3. Careful Adjustment of Culturally Suitable Therapist–Patient Relations

How to develop and maintain a certain relationship between therapist and patient is a crucial issue in psychotherapy. The desirable "therapeutic" relationship is defined differently in different therapeutic modes. However, there are three factors that generally need to be considered: to fit the individual patient's condition and need; to be "therapeutic", and to be culturally relevant. From a cultural point of view, the relationship should be culturally relevant and therapeutic. This requires consideration of how the patient views and relates to authority in his society and the role the "therapist" is expected to take according to his cultural perspectives. Some patients expect the therapist to take an authoritative, active, and giving role in relating to them, whereas others expect him to relate on an equal basis, without interfering with their autonomy and independence.

Clinically, it is understood that in therapy, in addition to an ordinary and realistic therapist–patient relationship, personal transference and countertransference usually occur between them. From an ethnic and cultural point of view, it is necessary to note that there is additional ethnic/cultural transference and countertransference. This is particularly true if the therapist and patient belong to different ethnic or cultural backgrounds. Such ethnic/cultural transference and countertransference, as with personal transference and countertransference, can be manifested in various ways, provide different impacts on the process of therapy, and are in need of proper management, even from the very beginning of therapy.

4. Relevant Modification of Communication Styles to Fit the Culture of the Patient

Special attention and consideration need to be given to the nature of communication that takes place between the therapist and the patient. This includes the content, level of sophistication, and focus of communication. This is particularly true when a therapist is going to provide explanations and interpretations as well as suggestions for the patient or his family. It is desirable that such communication be culturally geared and suitable.

The chief problem presented by the patient usually leads the direction of therapy, at least in the initial stage. As a part of the illness behavior, the patient's style of problem presentation or complaining of suffering will be shaped by cultural factors. How a person chooses a topic or focuses in presenting clinical problems is subject to individual need and understanding of the health system, but is also very much influenced by the culturally patterned style of problem presentation. The patient's orientation and explanation of problems may cover a broad spectrum of the supernatural, natural, biophysical, medical, and psychological. The nature of the problems may be presented as "somatic" or "psychological" or a mixture of the two. By its very nature, psychotherapy welcomes psychological presentation. However, this does not mean that a patient with a psychological presentation is easier to treat than a patient with a somatic presentation. Sometimes the situation is reversed, i.e., it is easier to treat a patient who does not overpsychologize his problems, merely presenting somatic problems in his initial contact with the therapist. The patient's problem presentation needs to be understood dynamically within the context of the patient's cultural background. It is part of the art of psychotherapy for the therapist and patient to collaborate together regarding which direction the therapy needs to take.

5. Appropriate Understanding of the Patient's Behavior and Pathology with Culturally Adjusted Theories

In order to have an in-depth understanding of the patient's behavior, personality, and coping patterns, a clinician makes use of available theories regarding the basic nature of the human mind, personality development, coping mechanisms, and so on. However, from a cultural point of view, these "basic" theories need cultural adjustment or modification so that they can be applied relevantly and meaningfully to people from different cultural backgrounds. They include theories about the self, personality structure, character formation, personality development, defense mechanisms, and so on.

It is a salient fact that, clinically, there are always variations in the manifestation of psychopathology. This is particularly true in situations relating to minor psychiatric disorders or primary emotional problems. The psychopathology manifested by the patient needs to be interpreted and understood carefully at individual, family, social, and cultural levels. This is especially true if the psychopathology is culture-related psychological problems. A clinician needs to understand the dynamic meaning of the problems presented. Based on this understanding, appropriate therapeutic strategies can be planned.

6. Suitable Selection of Therapeutic Models That Match the Patient's Cultural Style

Clinicians are still at the stage of debating which therapeutic models are best suited for patients with certain psychopathologies or personality backgrounds. As an extension of this, there is room for clinicians to consider which therapeutic models are best suited for patients of which ethnic or cultural backgrounds. For instance, issues needing further investigation include whether directive or nondirective therapy is better suited to people who culturally tend to view the therapist as an authoritative figure in a position of offering suggestions and making decisions for the patient; whether individually focused therapy or family-oriented therapy is better suited for people who are strongly influenced by close family relations and emphasize the family as a whole in their behavior; or whether it makes any difference if analytic therapy or behavior therapy is used, depending on culturally patterned preferences for introspection or an action-oriented approach to solving problems,

7. Maximal Utilization of Universal Therapeutic Mechanisms as Well as Culture-Specific Coping Patterns

Professional therapists are fully aware that the effects of psychotherapy can be attributed to nonspecific universal therapeutic factors in addition to specific therapeutic mechanisms. Through the study of various forms of psychotherapy, particularly indigenous healing practices, it is known that the exercise of a powerful, authoritative figure, establishment of an influential setting, involvement and mobilization of resource persons in the family or community, arising need emotions, making suggestions, allowing emotional ventilation, channeling inhibited expressions or desires, provision of cultural time out, and cultivation of hope are some of the basic therapeutic mechanisms that work on the patient. Modern, professional psychotherapists tend to be concerned with specific therapeutic mechanisms and need to pay attention to and make good use of them in treating the patient.

Various coping patterns are enhanced in therapy. For example, for an internal emotional complex, the patient might be assisted by the therapist in "uncovering" so that the emotional complex may be worked out consciously or, on the contrary, the patient might be encouraged to suppress the complex to maintain the stability of his mind. This is a matter of clinical judgment that requires the consideration of many factors, including the nature of the complex, the patient's ego strength, and the patient's preference. In addition, cultural consideration is necessary, depending on the kinds of coping mechanisms that are sanctioned by and function better within the patient's cultural setting. Seeking harmony with others or resolving conflicts are other examples of coping patterns that may be thought of differently in different sociocultural settings, depending on the extent to which social harmony is emphasized and active solutions of identified problems are favored. Cultural consideration is needed in selecting the style of coping.

8. Careful Evaluation of the Goals of Therapy in Relation to the Needs of the Individual, Family, and Culture

Finally, it is important to recognize that the goal of psychotherapy needs to be evaluated from a cultural as well as a clinical point of view. We all know that the concept of "normality" may be approached by defini-

tion by a professional expert, by evaluation from a mathematical standpoint, by judgment from a functional perspective, or by definition from a sociocultural point of view (Offer & Sabshin, 1975). Clearly the definition of a healthy, mature, adaptive person is very different depending on the value system held by a group of people in a particular cultural setting. The philosophical aspects of life need to be taken into consideration in order to set up the ultimate goals of psychotherapy.

In summary, it needs to be pointed out that in addition to a therapist's medical knowledge, psychotherapeutic orientation, personal view, and clinical experience, his value system will have a direct or indirect impact on the practice of psychotherapy. A clinician needs to be aware of this and constantly assess and regulate the therapy to maintain its relevance to the patient from a cultural point of view.

B. Cultural Implications of Psychotherapy

Various modes of psychotherapy — from indigenous, folk healing practices to modern, professional therapy — have been reviewed in this section. It is realized that, despite the differences in major orientations, therapeutic operations, and healing mechanisms among various forms of psychotherapy, there are common cultural implications of therapeutic activities (Tseng & Hsu, 1979). These implications are summarized as follows.

1. Provision of Culturally Permitted Channels for Fulfilling Wishes or Desires

In many societies, it is difficult for some of the members, particularly those who are in underprivileged or culturally suppressed subgroups, to express their unsatisfied needs or desires. Healing ceremonies or therapies become channels for them to reveal their unexpressed wishes. The practice of the Zar ceremony illustrates this point. Through institutionalization, clients were given the opportunity and means to express the inhibited wishes and unsatisfied desires that they were not permitted to express in ordinary life. Because their revelations were made through possessing spirits, the clients were not held responsible. At the same time, they were able to fulfill their wishes, either symbolically or in actuality [cross-reference to Chapter 32: Culture-Embedded Indigenous Healing Practices (Section II,A,2)]. The practice of free association in psychoanalysis is another example in which clients are given the opportunity to express their inner thoughts or desires without social inhibition.

2. Reinforcement of Culturally Sanctioned Coping Patterns

One of the functions of psychotherapy is to serve as a process of reinforcing culturally sanctioned coping patterns. This is exemplified by the Chinese *chien* divination practice in which the traditional Chinese way of remaining "patient," "nonaggressive," and "accepting" of the situation is emphasized for coping with problems encountered in daily life (J. Hsu, 1976). In contrast to this, Alcoholics Anonymous (AA), which originated in the United States, encourages members to reveal and face their problems, to work them out according to a "program" and through concretely defined "steps" — a reflection of coping patterns sanctioned in a society that emphasizes openness, action, and dealing with things through a "program." AA is based on the acceptance of a "higher power" and His help in achieving a cure.

3. Affirmation of Central Cultural Values

Psychotherapy becomes an institution through which the basic philosophy or value system emphasized by a culture is stressed and implanted into the clients. The emphasis on the *argamama* (as it is) attitude toward life and illness in Morita therapy, the stress of becoming *sunao* in Naikan therapy in Japan, and the regaining of self-confidence and becoming socially productive members to comply with the politics of the Great Leap Movement in integrated rapid therapy in China all illustrate this point. Western

client-centered therapy emphasizes a nondirective counseling approach to reinforce a coping pattern and to solve problems by oneself. This is a style of dealing with problems that is valued in American culture (Meadow, 1964).

4. Permission for Cultural "Time Out"

In an unusual way, therapy may offer a cultural "time out" to clients during the therapeutic process. For example, in the Hawaiian folk healing practice ho'oponopono, the family members who have concerns are permitted to express their anger or resentment during the healing meeting. In this therapeutically protected situation, the clients are allowed to temporarily ignore the ordinary cultural emphases on harmony and not expressing negative feelings in public. After revealing the source of the conflict, an apology is required from the person responsible for causing the problem. Once the therapy session is over, it is required that the patient forget the uncomfortable issues explored and return to a normal life.

5. Exploration of Alternative Cultural Approaches to Resolution

Instead of enforcing culturally sanctioned, traditional coping mechanisms, therapy may urge the clients to explore alternative approaches for solving problems. Encouraging a culturally sanctioned, "submissive" wife to become "assertive" and stand up for her rights in her relationship with her husband is an example of searching for an alternative resolution. Guiding a man to become relaxed and not overly concerned with his success in an achievement-oriented society is another example of finding a balance and resolution that goes against the mainstream cultural trend.

6. Elaboration and Incorporation of "New" Cultural Systems

The nature of psychotherapy can be perceived as the interaction of two value systems: the client's and the therapist's. Through the process of therapy, a client is exposed to the therapist's way of viewing things, which is supposedly more healthy and functional than the client's. After the process of exchange and incorporation, the client gradually absorbs the "healthier" value system. Therefore, in a microscopic way, a leveling of the acculturation process takes place.

IV. SITUATIONS IN WHICH THE FOCUS NEEDS TO BE ON CULTURE

Although the impact of culture on the practice of psychotherapy has been examined intensively through intercultural psychotherapy in the previous chapter, it is important for clinicians to realize the attention to culture is needed in various ways in different situations and for different reasons. The culture is not to be focused on *simply* because the patient has a different ethnic or cultural background than that of the therapist or *merely* because the patient belongs to a minority group or is a foreigner. The impact of culture on an individual or a family varies in different ways according to various circumstances. Therefore, an appropriate "cultural differential diagnosis of a case" is necessary in clinical application (Kinzie, 1977; Tseng & McDermott, 1981). Appropriately distinguishing and understanding is needed case by case. The different roles cultural issues play in clinical cases are analyzed and distinguished as follows.

A. VARIOUS SITUATIONS IN WHICH CULTURE PLAYS A ROLE IN CLINICAL CASES

1. Psychiatric Cases Directly Imbedded in Cultural Matters

These are cases in which the clinically presented problems are closely related to culture-induced stress or problems. Thus, how to solve the culture-related conflict or dilemma is the primary focus of the case. Several case vignettes will be given here to illustrate such situations.

A young physician was considering double suicide with his girlfriend in a traditional, conservative Japanese society because their love relationship was not accepted or approved by either their parents or their society. His girlfriend was a nurse, but unfortunately she was a widow with a young son. Her husband had died in an accident. In their society, it was unthinkable for a socially respectable man to marry a woman who was married before, particularly with children from the previous marriage. The situation became worse, as this young physician was expected to succeed his father as superintendent of the hospital. It was considered absolutely impossible for him to marry such a "disgraceful" woman and a nurse in the hospital. In traditional Japan, where hierarchy was emphasized, a nurse was considered subordinate to a physician and not a suitable candidate for the wife of the hospital's superintendent-to-be. There was no way out of this culturally entangled problem.

2. Psychiatric Cases Related Only Indirectly to Cultural Issues

In some cases, the problem is indirectly related to cultural matters, or cultural factors play only a secondary role in the total problem. For instance, marital therapy was arranged for a Filipino-American wife after she attempted suicide. She had migrated from the Philippines to the United States several years before and married a Caucasian man. After she became pregnant, her husband was so happy that he invited his parents to visit them at their new house. His mother had suffered a minor stroke and was not able to attend their wedding. He thought that it was a good time for his parents to meet his wife and become close as a family. However, things went the opposite way. The wife suffered from severe morning sickness and was very much annoyed that her husband spent more time with his parents than with her when she was in need of attention. Despite her warnings, he continued to spend considerable time showing his parents around, hoping that they would have a good time. With his mother physically disabled now, he thought that it might be his only chance to be close to her and be nice to her.

However, his wife, not having her own parents nearby (they were far away in the Philippines), felt terribly lonely, and that she was not being treated tenderly enough by her husband at a time when she needed his support. She became emotionally hysterical, overdosed, and ended up being sent to a hospital emergency room.

Her history revealed that this was not the first time the wife had suffered emotional turmoil. Shortly after their marriage, the husband's sister had come to visit them. The wife had a serious quarrel with her husband when he prepared the bed for his sister rather than let his wife, as hostess, do it. Furthermore, it upset her very much when the three of them went out in the car. The husband drove the car as usual, but asked his sister to sit next to him, letting his wife sit in the back seat. He explained that because it was the first time his sister had come to this new place, letting her sit on the front seat would allow her to sightsee better. However, the wife became very upset, feeling that her husband cared more for his sister than he did for his own wife. She cried, caused a scene at home, and her sister-in-law left the uncomfortable situation.

In this case, multiple factors contributed to the problems. The interracial marriage might have contributed indirectly, in matters such as the roles of husband, brother, and son in different circumstances as perceived in different cultures. A certain attitude and reaction may be expected from a husband when his wife is pregnant and experiencing morning sickness. There is a need to explore those issues from a Filipino as well as an American point of view. However, personality and interpersonal relationship patterns certainly played a part for the husband and the wife, at both the individual and marital levels, which are outside of cultural issues. Thus, a comprehensive understanding is needed.

3. Psychiatric Cases in Which Culture is a Disguise for Psychiatric Problems

An Irish-American woman in her 40s was referred by her family doctor for psychiatric treatment because she suffered from asthma that was difficult to control by medication. Besides, the doctor suspected that she had some kind of marital displeasure that needed psychiatric attention. This woman had married an African-American man several years before. After the marriage, she discovered that her husband tended to ignore her at home. For instance, in the morning, while both of them were having breakfast, her husband would concentrate on reading the newspaper, hiding his face from her. Unable to tolerate being ignored, she would push the newspaper away from her husband's face and try to talk, but their conversation would only last for a couple of minutes. Then he would sink into the newspaper again. Finally, she would start to cry, provoking an asthma attack, which would finally get his attention, and he would take her to see the doctor. Thus, their marital problems contributed indirectly to her repeated asthma attacks. She blamed her mistake in getting into a mixed marriage as the cause of her problems.

History revealed that she had feelings of inferiority since she was young. She had always felt that she was not good enough as a woman and had difficultly maintaining a meaningful relationship with a man. In order to cope with this chronic feeling of inferiority, she decided to marry a black man because she viewed African-Americans as an "inferior" group. She thought that marrying such an inferior man might balance her psychological problems. Her husband married her for the opposite reason. He used to despise white people for their superiority. He thought that marrying a white woman would give him satisfaction by counteracting his fear of being inferior to white people. Thus, subconsciously, he despised his white wife and used her for his own psychological gratification, until she became sick, then he would take care of her out of pity. Because of their racially mixed marriage, they had difficulty establishing and maintaining a social network with either whites or blacks, as they were not accepted by either. Based on this social isolation, the wife felt a greater need to rely on her husband for emotional support. However, in return, what she received was intentional ignoring and despising that aggravated her feelings of rejection.

In this case, intermarriage associated with racial issues seemed to be the core problem. However, a case analysis revealed that race was merely used as an excuse to solve their individual, preexisting, internal psychological problems. Race was merely disguised as the major problem.

4. Psychiatric Cases in Which Culture Is Not a Clinical Issue

Psychiatric problems may not be related to cultural matters at all in many cases, even though the patient may belong to a minority, foreign ethnic group, or be part of an interethnic married couple. The psychiatric problems may be primarily of a biological nature, such as dementia, mental subnormality, autism, or organic mental disorder induced by trauma, intoxication, infection, or metabolic or vascular disturbance. Even with major psychoses, such as schizophrenia and bipolar disorders, there is little room for cultural influence except in a secondary way. Race, ethnicity, or culture should not be easily considered the direct or primary cause for this group of psychiatric disorders.

For instance, a young woman of Laotian origin was brought by police to a psychiatric hospital after she entered a woman's house and physically assaulted her, trying to take away the woman's daughter. She claimed that the daughter was her own. Even though the police were called in and it was explained to her that the girl was the other woman's daughter, the Laotian woman did not want to listen. After being admitted to the hospital, it was revealed that she and her husband had come to the United States as war refugees from her home country. Her husband had been killed in a traffic accident the year before. In reaction to this tragic loss, she developed the idea that the communists in Laos were still trying to persecute them. She interpreted her husband's death not as accidental, but as an assassination because he was anticommunist. After this incident, she began to suspect that someone was following her when she was walking on the street and watching her from outside of her house when she returned home. When she began to deteriorate in her daily life, becoming unable to take care of her young daughter, a social worker had to remove the daughter from her house and place her in a foster home not known to the patient. She missed her daughter very much and wandered the street day and night, looking for her, until she found a girl who looked like her and insisted on bringing back "her own daughter!"

In this case, it is quite a temptation to interpret the woman as a victim of war in her home country who became vulnerable in the host society, especially after her husband's tragic death. The role of ethnicity and culture may be entertained and hysterical psychosis rather than paranoid psychosis considered as a clinical diagnosis. Actually, in this case, when the patient was treated by a dynamically oriented psychiatrist, intensive psychotherapy was given for a month without any improvement. After consultation with a cultural psychiatrist, the attending psychiatrist reluctantly revised his diagnosis, accepting the suggestion of prescribing antipsychotics for the patient, which later improved her psychotic condition considerably.

Sometimes, clinicians will overemphasize ethnic or cultural factors in case formulations and overinterpret culture as the cause of the problems. This is illustrated in the psychotic case just given. Even in the case of minor psychiatric disorders, and common psychological problems, unless there is sufficient solid evidence that culture played a significant role in the cause and formation of the disorders, a clinician should not loosely entertain cultural considerations as psychogenetic factors. A proper clinical differential diagnosis, including cultural dimensions, is necessary for proper management and treatment.

Finally, it needs to be said that a clinician should pay attention to social factors, particularly economic condition and social class, different educational levels, style of communication and expression of emotion, and familiarity and suitability of "regular" psychotherapy. Such "social" factors, paralleling "culture" factors (manifested mostly in the area of attitude and belief), are going to affect the process, style, and effectiveness of psychotherapy and deserve more exploration and understanding (Acosta et al., 1982; Prince, 1987).

B. Various Circumstances That Warrant Attention to Cultural Matters

Although conceptually culture is an important issue that needs to be addressed, strictly speaking, it is not necessary to focus primarily on cultural factors all the time in all clinical situations. Attention to culture is needed for different reasons under different circumstances, and perhaps with different kinds of attention and clinical management. For the sake of simplicity, several circumstances will be listed and elaborated here.

1. Working on Culture-Related Particular Issues in Therapy

In clinical settings, the primary focus of therapy needs to be on different areas or dimensions, depending on the nature of the problems presented by the patient or perceived by the therapist. If the problems are closely culture related, then there is a great need to address such culture-related problems in therapy.

For instance, when a patient's clinical problems are associated with adjustment problems due to transcultural migration, related to the matter of ethnic or cultural identity confusion, or connected to intercultural marital problems, all will be considered as primarily related to cultural issues. There is a need for specific therapeutic considerations and strategies to work on such issues.

For example, for problems encountered by minority groups with ethnic identity confusion, Chin, De La Cancela, and Jenkins (1993) suggested that ethnic identity needs to be viewed as bicultural rather than moving along a linear continuum of acculturation. Many factors have been identified that will contribute to the success or failure of transcultural adjustment after migration to a foreign society. The personality of the migrant, the motivation for migration, the attitude toward the hosting society, and acceptance by the hosting society are all issues that need to be considered for therapy. In general, based on recently accumulated professional knowledge and experience, clinicians are gaining more insight into culture-related psychological problems and how to work on them — opening new clinical areas for exploration in culture and psychotherapy.

2. Working in Situations of "Intercultural Psychotherapy"

Cultural impact on psychotherapy needs special and active attention in situations of interethnic and/or intercultural psychotherapy, even though the primary clinical problems are not related directly to cultural issues. It is because cultural factors have a direct impact on every aspect of the therapeutic process, including communication, therapist–patient relations, and so on, as elaborated in the previous chapter, that there is a need for special attention and management by the therapist. This is always more important if the cultural gap is more diverse, a language barrier exists, and the therapist is relatively unfamiliar with the patient's cultural background.

3. Working with "Special" or "Minority" Populations Needing Cultural Consideration

When a therapist is working with a patient from a special population, such as a different gender (particularly women), different sexual orientation, different physical condition (handicapped or disabled), different age (children or aged persons), or a different social class (underprivileged lower class), the therapist needs to make an extra effort to consider cultural perspectives, even if the patient belongs to the same ethnic group as the therapist. This is because these special populations have grown up with different personal experiences than those of the therapist, have different views of the world and life, and different value systems. They usually have different kinds of psychological issues and problems that require special understanding and approaches in treating them.

The differences among these special groups will be compounded if they are of different ethnic, racial, or sociopolitical backgrounds. Thus, they provide new areas for clinical exploration beyond the experience and knowledge of working with the ordinary, mainstream adult population. These issues, which are getting more recognition among clinicians and are addressed more in writings (Pedersen, Draguns, Lonner, & Trimble, 1996; Pedersen, Lonner, & Draguns, 1976 Sue & Sue, 1999), include how to work with children of minority groups (Powell, 1983; Vargas & Koss-Chioino, 1992), ethnic elders (Baker & Lightfoot, 1993), and gay men and lesbians (Krajeski, 1993).

4. Working with "Common" or "Majority" Populations in Therapy

Finally, from a cultural perspective, the impact of culture on the process of psychotherapy cannot be ignored, even if the therapist is treating a patient of the same cultural background as the general population. There is always a communication problem to overcome, even if the therapist and the patient speak the same language. A metaphor might be different from one person to another. There is always some degree of value differences at the individual level — there are broad differences in attitudes toward birth control, abortion, or divorce, for example, even among Christian groups. There are always different personal views, to some extent, between two individuals that need to be faced, adjusted, or resolved in ordinary daily life as well as in therapeutic situations. This is the dilemma that the psychotherapist has to manage with any kind of patient.

Thus, as pointed out by Wohl (1989), all psychotherapy is "intercultural" in that no two people have internalized identical constructions of their cultural worlds. Cultural issues tend to be noticed only when cultural differences among the patient and therapist are clearly evident. There is no sharp difference between intracultural and intercultural psychotherapy. They are merely different situations on a continuum.

V. SUGGESTIONS FOR THE FUTURE

In order to stimulate further improvement in the field of culture and psychotherapy, several areas need to be worked out in the immediate future.

A. IMPROVEMENT IN TRAINING FOR CULTURE-RELEVANT PSYCHOTHERAPY

1. Promotion of Awareness and Training on the Subject of Culture and Psychotherapy

Because culture has a direct or indirect impact on the therapy of any patient — whether he is from a majority or a minority population or from a different cultural background — it is important that culture and psychotherapy be a part of the regular training program for psychiatrists, clinical psychologists, and allied mental health workers who plan to be involved in psychotherapeutic work. The training should involve not only basic knowledge, but also actual clinical experience working with patients of various cultural backgrounds [cross-reference to Chapter 50: Cultural Psychiatry Training (Section III,A–C)].

2. Development of Special Training Programs for Improving Intercultural Psychotherapy

Dealing with patients of different ethnic and cultural backgrounds is becoming a part of daily psychiatric practice for clinicians. Associated with an increase in international travel and moving, mass transcultural migration, and multiethnic societies, increased attention is given to culturally relevant mental health care for minorities. In order to deal with this reality, there is a need to develop training programs for psychiatrists on how to provide proper intercultural psychotherapy for patients of diverse cultural backgrounds.

3. Attention to Transcultural Supervision in Psychotherapy

One area that tends to be neglected or ignored is that of transcultural (or cross-cultural) supervision in psychotherapy. In order to master the knowledge and skill of psychotherapy, trainees are required to receive individual guidance from supervisors on how to carry out psychotherapy. There is always the possibility that the patient, the supervisee, and the supervisor will not share the same ethnic or cultural background. Therefore, the need for transcultural supervision in therapy will occur. For instance, a Caucasian supervisor may supervise an Asian supervisee in treating an African-American or Hispanic patient. In this situation, there arises the matter of the ethnic or cultural differences among the three partners in therapy: the supervisor, the supervisee, and the patient. In addition to the ordinary clinical concern with how to provide supervision relating to common clinical issues, including making an assessment, formulating the nature of the problem, selecting the choice of therapeutic strategies, and so on, there is the matter of how to deal with or overcome the incongruence of ethnic or cultural factors among the three partners involved. This is a challenging issue that has seldom been examined in the past. If it is colored by racism, then how to deal with privilege, power, trust, and communication among partners of different racial backgrounds, as well as ethnic/racial transference and countertransference, all become essential issues that need to be carefully worked out (Fong & Lease, 1997; Katsnelson, 1998).

The supervisor's ability and competence relating to cultural sensitivity, cultural knowledge, cultural empathy, and cultural guidance all become critical matters. Certainly there is an urgent need to explore this subject in order to improve culturally relevant supervision.

B. Accumulation of More Clinical Knowledge and Experience

Although the awareness of the need for culturally relevant therapy is becoming more prevalent among clinicians, the next step is to accumulate more comprehensive clinical experience and knowledge on how to provide psychotherapy for patients with diverse cultural backgrounds. This includes trying modified or radically alternative therapy models for patients of different ethnic–cultural backgrounds, coupled with comprehensive evaluation and assessment of these various therapeutic approaches. Based on such systematic clinical exploration, we can obtain better insight into the subject of culture and psychotherapy.

C. More Theoretical Exploration and Comprehensive Research

Up until now, most of the concern with the subject of culture and psychotherapy has focused on how to modify the "technical" aspects of psychotherapy to fit cultural factors. Few scholars pay attention to theoretical issues. Theories for understanding human behavior at cross-cultural levels, theories for explaining how certain therapies work better for patients from particular cultural contexts, and theories concerning cultural aspects of therapeutic mechanisms all need further exploration.

One cannot deny that only a handful of investigations have been done on the subject of culture and psychotherapy, particularly concerning the outcome of therapy with relation to cultural factors. We need more solid and empirical investigation to push our knowledge beyond clinical impressions and speculation regarding the impact of cultural factors on the practice of psychotherapy.

REFERENCES

Abel, T.M., & Metraux, R. (1974). *Culture and psychotherapy.* New Haven, CT: College & University Press.

Acosta, F.X., Yamamoto, J., & Evans, L.A. (1982). *Effective psychotherapy for low income and minority patients.* New York: Plenum Press.

American Psychological Association. (1993). Guidelines for providers of psychological services to ethnic, linguistic, and culturally diverse populations. *American Psychologist, 48*(1), 45–48.

Baker, F.M., & Lightfoot, O.B. (1993). Psychiatric care of ethnic elders. In A.C. Gaw (Ed.), *Culture, ethnicity, and mental illness* (pp. 517–552). Washington, DC: American Psychiatric Press.

Chin, J.L., De La Cancela, V., & Jenkins, Y.M. (1993). *The politics of race, ethnicity, and gender.* Westport, CT: Praeger.

Doi, T. (1962). *Amae* — A key concept for understanding Japanese personality structure. In R.J., Smith & R.K., Beardsley (Eds.), *Japanese culture: Its development and characteristics.* Chicago: Aldine.

Dwairy, M. (1997). Addressing the repressed needs of the Arabic cllient. *Cultural Diversity and Mental Health, 3*(1), 1–12.

Erikson, E.H. (1963). *Childhood and society* (2nd ed.). New York: W.W. Norton.

Fong, M.L., & Lease, S.H. (1997). Crosscultural supervision: Issues for the White supervisor. In D.B., Pope-Davis & H.L.K., Coleman (Eds.), *Multicultural counseling competencies: Assessment, education and training, and supervision.* Thousand Oaks, CA: Sage.

Hoch, E.M. (1990). Experiences with psychotherapy training in India. *Psychotherapy and Psychosomatics, 53,* 14–20.

Hsu, F.L.K. (1985). The self in cross-cultural perspective. In A. Marsella, G. DeVos, & F.L.K. Hsu (Eds.), *Culture and self.* New York: Tavistock.

Hsu, J. (1976). Counseling in the Chinese Temple: A psychological study of divination by Chien drawing. In W.P. Lebra (Ed.), *Culture-bound syndromes, ethnopsychiatry, and alternate therapies* (pp. 210–221). Honolulu: University Press of Hawaii.

Katsnelson, N. (1998). *Transferance and countertransference in cross-cultural supervision.* Presented at the annual meeting of the Society for the Study of Psychiatry and Culture, Portland, OR.

Kinzie, J.D. (1977). Intercultural marriages: Problems and challenges for psychiatric treatment. In W.S. Tseng, J.F. McDermott, Jr., & T.W. Maretzki (Eds.), *Adjustment in intercultural marriage* (pp. 104–112). Honolulu: University of Hawaii, Department of Psychiatry, School of Medicine.

Kirmayer, L.J. (1989). Psychotherapy and the culture concept of the person. *Sante, Culture, Health, 6*(3), 241–270.

Koss-Chioino, J.D., & Vargas, L.A. (1992). Through the culture looking glass: A model for understanding culturally responsive psychotherapies. In A. Vargas & J.D. Koss-Chioino (Eds.), *Working with culture: psychotherapeutic interventions with ethnic minority children and adolescents.* San Francisco: Jossey-Bass.

Krajeski, J.P. (1993). Cultural considerations in the psychiatric care of gay men and lesbians. In A.C., Gaw (Ed.), *Culture, ethnicity, and mental illness* (pp. 553–572). Washington, DC: American Psychiatric Press.

Marsella, A., DeVos, G., & Hsu, F.L.K. (Eds.). (1985). *Culture and self.* New York: Tavistock.

Meadow, A. (1964). Client-centered therapy and the American ethos. *International Journal of Social Psychiatry, 10*(4), 246–259.

Offer, D., & Sabshin, M. (1975). Normality. In A.M. Freedman, H.I. Kaplan, & B.J. Sadock (Eds.), *Comprehensive textbook of psychiatry* (2nd ed., Vol. 1). Baltimore: Williams & Wilkins Co.

Pedersen, P.B., Draguns, J.G., Lonner, W.J., & Trimble, J.E. (Eds.). (1996). *Counseling across cultures* (4th ed.). Thousand Oaks; CA: Sage.

Pedersen, P.B., Lonner, W.J., & Draguns, J.G. (Eds.). (1976). *Counseling across cultures.* Honolulu: University Press of Hawaii.

Powell, G.J. (Ed.). (1983). *The psychosocial development of minority group children.* New York: Brunner/Mazel.

Prince, R. (1980). Variations in psychotherapy procedures. In H.C. Triandis & J.G. Draguns (Eds.), *Handbook of cross-cultural psychology: Psychopathology* (Vol. 6). Boston: Allyn & Bacon.

Prince, R. (1987). Alexithymia and verbal psychotherapies in cultural context. *Transcultural Psychiatric Research Review, 24*(2), 107–118.

Roland, A. (1991). Psychoanalysis in India and Japan: Toward a comparative psychoanalysis. *American Journal of Psychoanalysis, 51*(1), 1–10.

Sue, D.W., & Sue, D. (1999). *Counseling the culturally different: Theory and practice* (3rd ed.). New York: Wiley.

Tseng, W.S. (1995). Psychotherapy for the Chinese: Cultural considerations. In T.Y. Lin, W.S. Tseng, and E.K. Yeh (Eds.), *Chinese societies and mental health.* Hong Kong: Oxford University Press.

Tseng, W.S. (2001). Culture and psychotherapy: Overview. In W.S. Tseng & J Streltzer (Eds.), *Culture and psychotherapy: A guide to clinical practice* (pp. 3–12). Washington, DC: American Psychiatric Press.

Tseng, W.S., & Hsu, J. (1979). Culture and psychotherapy. In A.J. Marsella, R.G. Tharp, & T.J. Ciborowski (Eds.), *Perspectives on cross-cultural psychology.* New York: Academic Press.

Tseng, W.S., & McDermott, J.F., Jr. (1981). *Culture, mind and therapy: An introduction to cultural psychiatry.* New York: Brunner/Mazel.

Tseng, W.S., & Streltzer, J. (Eds.). (2001). *Culture and psychotherapy: A guide to clinical practice.* Washington, DC: American Psychiatric Press.

Vaillant, G.E. (1971). Theoretical hierarchy of adaptive ego mechanisms. *Archives of General Psychiatry, 24,* 107–118.

Vaillant, G.E. (1986). *Empirical studies of ego mechanism of defense.* Washington, DC: American Psychiatric Press.

Vargas, L.A., & Koss-Chioino, J.D. (1992). *Working with culture: psychotherapeutic interventions with ethnic minority children and adolescents.* San Francisco: Jossey-Bass.

Varma, V.K. (1982). Present state of psychotherapy in India. *Indian Journal of Psychiatry, 24,* 209–226. (Reviewed in *Transcultural Psychiatric Research Review, 21*(4), 291–291 [1984])

Wohl, J. (1989). Integration of cultural awareness into psychotherapy. *American Journal of Psychotherapy, 43,* 343–355.

Section G

Culture and Therapy with Special Subpopulations

Following the systematic review of cultural influence on psychological therapy in the previous section, this section is devoted to further elaboration on working psychotherapeutically with special subpopulations. Following the developmental stages of life, the subpopulations of children and adolescents, couples and spouses, families, and aged persons are addressed. In each chapter, common culture-related psychological problems are reviewed briefly with regard to the subpopulation concerned. Then, basic considerations and specific skills involved in psychotherapeutic work with these subpopulations are discussed in detail from cultural perspectives.

The role of culture becomes prominent when clinical practice is focused on psychotherapy. The impact of culture on psychological problems and ways of treating these problems through therapist–patient interpersonal interaction are highlighted. Thus, culture and therapy are reelaborated in this section from different perspectives, by focusing on the whole life span. Clinical cases are utilized to illustrate the practical perspective of cultural influence on problems and therapies.

At the end of the section, medically ill patients as a special subpopulation are addressed. Psychiatrists often need to deal with medically ill persons in their clinical practice, particularly in consultation–liaison service. The ethnic–cultural impact on medically ill patients cannot be ignored. An examination of cultural influence on illness behavior and medical care will assist psychiatrists in providing culturally geared consultation–liaison in medical settings.

38

Working with Children and Adolescents

I. INTRODUCTION: COMMON GROUND

Children and adolescents are persons who have not yet grown to adulthood. They are still in the early stages of the life cycle. Due to their level of mental development, as a special subpopulation, they need certain specific attention in therapy. Strictly speaking, children are younger than adolescents. They are artificially subdivided by the developmental landmark of puberty. However, they share the common element of being psychologically growing and developing individuals. From cultural and psychotherapeutic perspectives, several common considerations are needed.

A. DEVELOPMENTAL ASPECTS OF CHILDREN AND ADOLESCENTS

1. Adjustment of Developmental Stages and Scales

Both children and adolescents are in the process of psychological development and maturity. However, the developmental stages and scales of growth pro-

posed by scholars, although they are claimed to be universally applicable, need cultural adjustment for clinical application (Powell, 1983). As has been elaborated previously [cross-reference to Chapter 4: Child Development and Enculturation (Section III,A–E)], for instance, the stage of adolescense is relatively short in some societies (particularly agricultural), and children are pushed into young adult life rather abruptly — encouraged to marry shortly after reaching puberty and engage in adult, productive work; whereas in others (particularly industrialized societies), the adolescent period is prolonged, and entry into adult life delayed — with many years of formal education and late marriage, sometimes after the age of 30.

Furthermore, the transition between stages can take place rather smoothly in certain cultures, while it can be abrupt in others. For instance, in the Amazon, it was reported that although infants are generally well taken care of by their mothers (during the oral stage), once the young children are able to walk around (reaching the anal stage), they tend to be abruptly left alone or even neglected by their mothers. In contrast, in other cultures, such as China or Japan, infants are indulged by their mothers or other caretakers (such as grandmothers) from the very beginning (oral) stage, through the toddler (anal) and preschool (phallic) stages. Then, when they enter school (early latency stage), they are expected to grow up suddenly and meet the social expectations of studying diligently and behaving correctly in school. Thus, the pace and transition between stages in their early life cycle are different depending on their cultural backgrounds.

2. Variation of Themes Emphasized at Different Stages of Development

Closely related with variations in the pace of development, there is also the modification of themes stressed at different stages of growth in different cultural settings. Self-control and regulation may be emphasized as soon as a child learns how to move around — the so-called anal stage, in societies in which discipline is stressed, whereas indulgence and flexibility may be allowed among children of the same age or in societies in which irregularity is tolerated. Similarly, in the latency stage, as described by Erick Erikson, industry is generally emphasized; however, in addition, in many societies, particularly in agricultural or so-called underdeveloped societies, responsibility is stressed. It is not so important to study and to join the adults to work diligently in the field, but often to take full responsibility, almost as adult substitutes, in performing many important tasks, such as caring for younger siblings, or even learning to cook for the family. In other words, youngsters are expected to learn to take responsibility in association with the rapid entry into adult life and to take part in production [cross-reference to Chapter 49: Culture and Psychiatric Theories (Section IV,B)].

B. Family Impact on Psychological Growth

1. Importance of the Family in Actual Daily Life

Generally speaking, the importance of the family in the lives of children and adolescents cannot be denied.

However, the importance of the family is more so in societies that emphasize close family ties in daily life, for both children and adults. The relationship between children and their parents, adolescents and adults, is much more tightly interwoven so that they are almost inseparable. This cannot be ignored when clinicians are working with children.

2. Consideration of Cultural Variations of Family Systems and Structures

Associated with this, it is necessary to recognize that there are anthropological variations of family systems around the world (Tseng & Hsu, 1991), and even among different ethnic subgroups within the same multiethnic society (McGoldrick, Giordano, & Pearce, 1996; McGoldrick, Pearce, & Giordano, 1982). This is reflected in the family system: patrilineal or matralineal; monogamous or polygamous; offering postmarital residential choice or not; family structure (nuclear, stem, extended, or single-parent); and so on. The impact of variations in family systems and structures on the lives of children needs careful consideration and understanding.

C. Socioenvironmental Influence on Socialization

1. Direct Impact from the Environment

Beyond the family, children's lives are influenced directly or indirectly by the actual environment in which they are living. If society's conditions are undesirable in terms of health and economics, the children's lives will be subject to greater risk. For instance, the mortality of children in some underdeveloped countries is so high that nearly half of them do not survive beyond childhood — a terrifying contrast to the situation in developed societies, in which the majority of babies live beyond childhood. Malnutrition, sickness, and neglect are the major issues for children living in undesirable social conditions.

It is assumed in developed societies that every child will go to school to receive a formal education and experience socialization, but this is not necessarily true in underdeveloped societies. It is common in some of these countries for children to help their parents with chores, take care of younger siblings, and even join their parents in working for a living rather than reading books, taking physical exercise classes, playing various sports, and indulging in TV games. Thus, children's lives and patterns of growth are widely diversified.

2. Rapidly Changing Society

When a society is going through rapid social change, the impact is great on the lives of the people in it. This is true for children as well as adults. Depending on the nature of the change, the lives of children will be modified greatly also. For instance, associated with improvements in economic conditions, the basic needs of children, in terms of health, food, and care, will be much improved. Improvements in transportation (going to school by bus rather than walking) and the availability of television (watching it at home rather than playing games outside) will decrease greatly the amount of daily exercise the children receive. Coupled with improvements in food, overweight could become a new problem that was not encountered before [cross-reference to Chapter 25: Childhood-Related Disorders (Section III,G)].

Following changes in value systems, physical discipline is prohibited in modern life, changing ways of child-rearing from the past, when spanking children was the norm for disciplining them. Following family planning concepts and practices, the number of children within a household has declined greatly during the past half-century. This is often coupled with another phenomenon, the greater prevalence of nuclear families, particularly in urban settings, where traditional extended family ties are becoming history. Also, associated with increased divorce, children raised by single parents (mostly mothers) have increased remarkably in some developed societies in which divorce is rather common. Changes in family structure associated with cultural changes impact the lives of children greatly.

How sociocultural change can revise child-rearing patterns and the mental health of youngsters is well exemplified by the situation in Micronesia. As described by Untalan and Camacho (1997), prior to World War II (when Micronesia was occupied by the Japanese), family structure was characterized by the extended family, rules and responsibilities were clearly defined for children, and discipline was strict. As a result, teen pregnancy was rare, alcohol and substance abuse were unknown, and suicide among youngsters was hardly ever observed. However, after World War II, when Micronesia become a territory of the United States, there was significant and rapid sociocultural change. Associated with changes in the political system, there were improvements in the educational and health systems. However, the traditional economy and ways of living by fishing and farming changed, and many people relied on salaries from government employment. The past restrictions on alcohol for indigenous people were removed and much beer and liquor were imported. Large towns were formed for commercial and administrative purposes, and nuclear families began to appear due to internal migration to these towns. Associated with changes in the value system, with a new emphasis on democracy, freedom, and equality, many parents began to lose their authority, and patterns of child-rearing began to change accordingly. Discipline became lax, and rules and roles for children (as well as parents) became confusing. Drug and substance abuse among youngsters increased, as did juvenile delinquency, suicide, and homicide.

In other words, the lives of children can change, even in the space of one generation in the same society, associated with rapid changes in the society, including quality of life, family structure, attitudes, and ways of child-rearing.

3. Effects of Transcultural Migration

Similarly to the social change that takes place in one's own society, cultural change is experienced when people migrate to a host society with a different cultural background. The sociocultural change associated with transcultural migration often has superimposed on it a minority status in the hosting society. These factors all affect the lives of youngsters, significantly, starting from childhood, but more so those in the stage of adolescence. One commonly observed phenomenon is the change in or challenge to the status and role of parents in the hosting society. Associated with confusion in value systems, parents lose their ideas of disciplining their children. When the immigrants are from a society with a different language than that of the hosting society, very often, due to the language barrier, the youngsters have more knowledge about their new environment and their parents have to rely on them. This creates an unusual family phenomenon, namely a reversal of the parent–child relationship. This often occurs when east or south Asian families migrate to North America, such as Hmong people to the United States (Westermeyer, Bouafuely-Kersey, & Her, 1997) or west Asian families to Europa [cross-reference to Chapter 44: Migration, Refuge, and Adjustment (Section V,B,2 and C)].

D. Enculturaltion and Ethnic/Racial Identification

1. Enculturation as One of the Key Dimensions in Growth

A child encounters numerous tasks in the process of development. Generally speaking, these include physical growth, psychological development, and the experience of socialization. From a cultural perspective, development also involves the process of enculturation. Enculturation refers to the process through which an individual, starting from early childhood, acquires a cultural system from his environment, particularly from his parents, family, neighbors, school, and society at large. Apparently, the content of enculturation will vary according to the cultural environment to which the child was exposed and issues emphasized by the child's parents, neighbors, school, and society. For instance, whether a person should live life harmoniously or competitively with others,

whether a person should respect authority or relate as an equal even with authority figures, or whether a person should strive for individual independence or value mutual dependence are some of the issues that are shaped through the process of enculturation throughout childhood until adulthood [cross-reference to Chapter 4: Child Development and Enculturation (Section IV)].

2. Ethnic/Racial Identification Starts Early

Identification is a part of personal psychology. It involves multiple levels, such as self-identification, gender identification, family identification, group identification (such as school, neighborhood, or working group), and ethnic/racial identification. The development of identification is associated with cognitive development. For instance, without cognitive awareness of gender differences, there can be no gender identification issues. It is also subject to emotional relations and experiences. Without strong ties with members of a group, such as classmates, no intense sense of group identification will be developed. Identification also relies on situations of contrast or competition with others, enhancing the sense of identity. This is particularly true for collective identity. Games between schools provoke a sense of school identity. Wars against other countries stimulate national identity. When there is an issue regarding ethnicity or race, it cultivates ethnic or racial identity. Certainly, a certain level of cognitive development is required to comprehend the differences between different ethnic groups (if different languages or customs are demonstrated explicitly) or racial groups (as characterized by different external features), opportunities to be exposed to and stimulated by such differences, and how parents and other people stimulate such identity issues. Immigrants to different ethnic societies, members of an ethnic minority group, and members of multiethnic societies all tend to induce a sense of ethnic or racial identity earlier and more firmly. Even a 2- or 3-year-old child can recognize that he or she is black or white, Japanese or Italian, if the surroundings stimulate a sense of those differences. In other words, ethnic or racial identity starts early, in childhood, it does not wait for adolescence or young adulthood [cross-reference to Chapter 6: Psychology, Customary Behavior, and Ethnic Identity (Section, IV,A, and B)].

II. WORKING WITH CHILDREN

A. BASIC STRATEGIES FOR WORKING WITH CHILDREN

1. Work on the Family as a Unit, Including Grandparents

It is a general rule that the family, particularly the parents, needs to be involved in the care of the children. The family is defined broadly to include any person who has an impact on the lives of the children, whether living in the same household or not. In many cultures, grandparents play a significant role in child-rearing, so they need to be involved, too. Based on different family systems, structures, and functions, the ways of working with families need careful adjustment (Canino & Spurlock, 1994; Hsu, 1983, pp. 138–139). For instance, in cultures where parental figures are highly respected, caution is needed to respect them (particularly the father, as the master of the household) in family sessions. Any comments toward parents are better not made in the presence of the children so that the parents do not feel offended. When a culture does not encourage open expression of opinions and demonstrating emotion, it is wise not to provoke family members (particularly of the younger generation) to speak out against the older generation. For people who are used to identifying an individual (particularly an identified youngster) as the person having problems, parents often take the view that the therapist should fix the problems of the identified child for them. The suggestion of family therapy to work on family problems would sound awkward to these parents. When families have such an orientation, it is suggested that the parents be invited to come to the session "to help the therapist decide how to treat the youngster–patient," not to treat (or even work on) family problems.

2. Working Closely with Parents, Particularly Mothers

It has to be determined and understood quickly who is more in charge of the rearing and discipline of the children in actual family life so that proper attention may be focused on that person or persons. In many Asian societies, taking care of the children is left entirely in the mother's hands. The father is often busy at his work outside the home and has no time to be involved in raising and disciplining the children. Actually, the contact between the father and the children might be very minimal, as in Japan. This is not merely a fact, but also a cultural assumption and expectation. Thus, this needs to be kept in mind when the therapist works with the parents — focusing on the mother, primarily. In some cultures, it is the older siblings' job to take care of the younger siblings if the mother is working outside in the fields or in a store or perhaps it is the grandparents who take care of the youngsters rather than the parents. In therapy, involving the actual primary caretakers (older siblings, grandmother, or other) is essential.

B. CULTURAL ISSUES NEEDING SPECIAL CONSIDERATION

1. Attachment and Dependency within a Cultural Context

Among variables that are encountered in child development, the issue of independence versus dependence is one that is viewed very differently by different cultures, particularly between the East and the West. Take the concrete example of when it is the appropriate time for a child to sleep separately from his parents — as a sign of independence. Most contemporary European or American parents will arrange for their newborn baby to sleep in a cradle in a separate room as soon as they feel ready to do so — perhaps several days or weeks, at most, after the baby is born. Most Asian parents, however, will let their baby sleep with them in the same bed or, at least, in the same room in the baby's own small bed for many years. It is not unusual to let young children sleep in their parents' room until the children reach school age, or even after that. Besides the reality that there is a shortage of rooms in the household, there is no concept of "separating" the children from the parents as soon as possible.

Besides sleeping arrangements, physical contact between parents and young children varies greatly among different cultures as well. In contemporary times, many Western parents use baby carriers to hold their babies, whereas Eastern mothers carry their babies on their backs or hold them in their arms. When the children reach the age when they can walk, their parents still hold them when walking in the street, or at least hold the child's hand when they are walking together. For Eastern parents to see Western parents walking their children on leashes, as if they were walking their dogs, is surprising.

These examples of child-rearing practices merely reflect how autonomy and independence are encouraged in one culture and attachment and dependence are allowed in another. When clinicians are working with children, this is just one area that needs careful evaluation in making clinical judgements and offering therapy.

2. Physical Discipline versus Child Abuse

Another area that is easily confused and even mistaken by clinicians is the matter of physical discipline versus physical abuse practiced by parents on children. In many cultures, it is a fact that parents use physical punishment to discipline their children. Even schoolteachers in the past were sometimes allowed to physically discipline students who did not behave well in school, although this is strictly prohibited now in most cultures. Clinically it becomes a challenge to distinguish between corporal discipline and physical abuse inflicted by parents. It is a gray area, but certain rules apply. If the physical punishment is given with the clear intention of disciplining a child's wrong behavior, it is given by parents in a relatively calm way, without emotional upset, and the degree of severity is relatively mild and the body location chosen for punishment is well selected to avoid causing severe damage, then such behavior may be considered "discipline." In contrast, if the physical attack occurs as the result of a parent's emotional upset, an instrument (such as a stick or a club) is used rather than the hand, or the discipline is carried out in an "unusual" way, such as pouring hot water on the child or burning him with a heated iron bar, the damage is obviously severe, causing physical injury, and the action occurs repeatedly, then it is definitely abusive in nature. Detail information and careful assessment will help clinicians to make a judgement.

In various cultures, people in the community distinguish between discipline and abuse according to their social judgements and cultural criteria. For instance, Pacific Islanders consider the head to be where the soul resides. If anybody, including his own parents, hits a child's head, it is considered abuse. It is a cultural custom to hit the child's buttocks, legs, or arms, but not the head, for discipline.

3. Transracial Adoption of Children

There is an increasing trend among many Caucasian people in Western societies to adopt children of different racial backgrounds: either African, Asian, or other. This is mainly because the parents cannot bear children of their own and there are not enough Caucasian children for adoption. It has become a choice to adopt African-American or Asian children. Sometimes parents, even though they already have their own children, still want to adopt children of other races for different reasons. Helping deserted orphans is one, wanting "different" kinds of children is another.

Transracial adoption, particularly the adoption of black children by white parents, has attracted attention and debate regarding its social and legal merits. However, as pointed out by African-American psychiatrist Ezra E.H. Griffith (1995b), little attention has been made from a forensic psychiatric point of view. Major concern is related to several matters, namely the community's reaction to black–white transractial adoption (based on feelings associated with the preexisting relations between the majority and the minority), the parents' motivation in adopting a child of a different racial background (particularly children distinctly identified with minority racial backgrounds), and the psychological and cultural impact on the process of enculturation (Griffith, 1995a). General claims made by some professionals as well as laypersons (with African-American backgrounds) are that "only Black families can teach Black culture to their children" and "African-American parents have a unique ability to pass along to their children the coping skills needed for a minority person to manage in American society."

As reviewed by Griffith and Silverman (1995), a handful of empirical studies have been carried out regarding the outcome of transracial adoption of African-American children by Caucasian-American parents. Regarding their overall adjustment, Silverman (1993) summarized that these studies indicated that a majority (75%) of the adopted preadolescent and younger children adjusted well in their adoptive homes — a similar success rate for white–white inracial infant adoptions.

Concerning self-esteem and identity issues, McRoy, Zurcher, Lauderdale, and Anderson (1982) compared a group of white families that had transracially adopted black children to a group of black families that had inracially adopted black children. They reported that there were no significant differences in the self-esteem scores of the black children who were adopted transracially or interracially. As for racial identity, the issues were more complex. The transracially adopted black children were often influenced by their white parents' views. The white parents who viewed their black child as being mixed or part-white tended to have the black child voice the same view of his or her own racial identity. Some of the transracially adopted black children who had little contact with blacks tended to devalue their black heritage.

A burning question that always arises is what will happen to the transracially adopted children when they reach adolescence or adulthood? Based on a 20-year longitudinal follow-up study of transracially adopted children who were now adults, Simon (1993) reported that, as adults, the transracial adoptees were aware of and comfortable with their racial identity. It seems that strong opposition expressed (by people of African-American backgrounds) in the past regarding the potential ill-effects of black–white transracial adoption was not supported by empirical studies.

Asian-Caucasian transracial adoptions have not received as serious objections as African-Caucasian adoptions. There have not been many studies regarding Asian-Caucasian adoptions, and we are awaiting more investigation into this area.

Regarding transethnic adoption, one unique study was reported by Tseng, Ebata, Miguchi, Egawa, and McLaughlin (1990). It related to the Japanese war orphans left in China at the end of World War II who were adopted by Chinese foster parents. Almost four decades later, the adult war orphans were interviewed (when they were about middle-aged) and it was found that they still retained some (Japanese) personality traits, such as a fondness for sweets, keeping things clean, taking frequent baths, being hardworking, and being polite, even though they had become war orphans at about the age of 5 or 6.

III. WORKING WITH ADOLESCENTS

A. Fundamental Considerations in Working with Adolescents

After puberty, children enter the stage of adolescence. From childhood to adolescence, the youngsters continue the process of growing physically and psychologically. Thus, most of the issues raised earlier, regarding children, also apply to adolescents. However, as the ego reaches a certain level of maturity, there are issues that need more attention in the stage of adolescence. These are as follows.

1. Continuous Attention to the Stages of Development

As a part of the growing process, adolescents continue through different stages of development. Within the period of adolescence, three substages of development are recognized by scholars: early, mid-, and late adolescence. As stated by child psychiatrist Danilo Ponce (in press), in early adolescence, issues are primarily organized around puberty and hormonal changes, and the corresponding impact of these changes on the youngsters. In contrast, the midadolescent is poised to move from same-sex issues to exploring opposite-sex issues. Tasks and activities are more or less bisexual, wanting to be with one's same-sex friends, while being interested in opposite-sex friends. The late adolescent, emerging from the struggles of the previous substage, is more focused on gearing up for formal initiation into the world of grownups. Culture impacts these three adolescent substages by shaping acceptable responses to or ways of dealing with substage issues.

2. Privacy and Confidentiality in Therapy

One of the characteristics of the psychology of adolescence is the need for keeping personal matters secret from parents. Thus, it brings up the issue of how to respect the adolescent's privacy in therapy and observe confidentiality between the adolescent and his parents, as there are different views and practices in different cultures regarding privacy among family members. This is particularly true regarding how much the parents have the right to know about their youngsters. In cultures that stress parental authority, it is a basic assumption made by parents that they have the right to know everything about their offspring. To propose confidentiality between parents and children would be unthinkable, and would certainly offend the parents. In contrast, in cultures where individuality is the ethos, it is considered that after children reach a certain age, they have the right to keep their personal matters confidential from their parents.

This creates a dilemma for therapists regarding the extent to which they should keep information about their adolescent patients confidential from their parents. There is a need for clarification from the very beginning, and adjustment should be made in each case according to cultural considerations.

3. The Mode of Therapy: Individual, Family, or Group?

It is the judgment call of the therapist which mode of therapy to adopt — whether to work primarily with the adolescent patient or the whole family together, or to try peer-group therapy. Depending on the extent to which individuality, mutuality, and collectiveness are emphasized in daily life, the therapist could decide to match such cultural norms in the therapeutic process. For instance, if an individual is not used to expressing his or her personal opinions or feelings in his culture-shaped daily life, peer-group therapy sessions may be more comfortable for the youngster than one-to-one sessions. If the parents are closely related to their children and are eager to know everything about them, it may be a good idea to have individual sessions with the adolescent, family sessions, and sessions with the parents alternated in the course of therapy to enhance the adolescent patient's individualization and, at the same time, gratifying the parents' wishes and needs and involving them properly in the therapeutic work.

4. The Matching of Therapist and the Adolescent Patient: Gender, Age, and Ethnicity

Associated with cognitive development, recognizing ethnic or racial differences more explicitly in adolescence, the matching of the therapist and the adolescent patient becomes more of an issue where ethnicity or racial background is concerned, in addition to gender and age factors. The general rule is that if the adolescent patient is matched with a therapist of the same ethnic or racial background, it will be easier to start a relationship, avoiding potential negative ethnic or racial transference that could be observed from the very beginning. During the course of treatment, it helps the patient to identify with the therapist, not only on a personal level, but also at ethnic or racial levels — an important treatment mechanism for an adolescent patient in therapy.

If the therapist happens to be different from the adolescent patient in ethnic or racial background, these issues should be brought up from the very beginning and dealt with continuously throughout the course of treatment. Cultural knowledge should be obtained and cultural empathy exercised to make up for the differences that exist in such transcultural interethnic or interracial therapy [cross-reference to Chapter 36: Intercultural Psychotherapy (Section II,C,4)].

B. Common Themes to Be Addressed in Therapy

1. Autonomy and Independence

As in the treatment of young children, the issue of independence versus dependence needs careful attention, but more so in the stage of adolescence, as autonomy and independence are more emphasized in this stage of development. The extent to which autonomy is desirable and independence is acceptable is subject to cultural definition. In addition to professional judgement, cultural consideration is necessary in this matter.

It is a common desire for the adolescent to be separated from his parents as he is searching for individuality. This is often manifested by the need for privacy, setting personal boundaries from the parents, and being sensitive about intrusion of the parents. However, this developmental need is often reacted to differently by parents of different cultural backgrounds. Parents who strongly believe that their children are their possessions and that children should be filial to their parents and obey them often consider it their parental right to oversee their children's personal lives and inspect their personal belongings, such as reading their letters and diaries and inquiring into their

private matters, for example, what happens on dates. There is less of a sense that the adolescent needs to be respected as a growing-up individual and that his privacy and desire for individuality should be considered. In such cases, there is a need to help the parents redefine their roles and adjust the extent to which they should respect their children's personal lives. This is not so much a problem for parents who, according to cultural influence, recognize that every person should be treated as an individual, even

2. Cultural Gap with Their Parents

The generational gap between parents and youngsters is often one of the issues that needs to be focused on in therapy. The cultural gap between generations is often widened when there is rapid cultural change or when the family immigrates to a foreign country. It becomes the therapist's job to deal with the generational gap by helping the parents and youngsters communicate, exchange views, and make compromises between them, if possible. It is important to stress to both parents and children that there is no "wrong or right," but that things are viewed "differently" according to different life experiences and cultural beliefs in different times and circumstances. How to work out difference between generations is the main issue. In addition to clinical skill, the therapist needs to have a comprehensive and proper understanding of the cultural aspects of the lives of both the parents and the youngsters so that proper advice and suggestions can be made to narrow the gap between them, making compromises, or at least understanding and feeling comfortable with the existence of differences between the generations.

3. Psychosexual Development within the Context of Society

Among the cultural variables that need special consideration in adolescent therapy are psychosexual issues. Because views and attitudes toward sexual matters vary greatly among different cultures, so also do the problems experienced by adolescents in this area. In conservative societies, the issues faced by adolescents are often related to inhibiting their sexual interests, avoiding masturbation (as it is considered undesirable by folk belief), or controlling their sexual desires; whereas in sexually liberated societies, the matters concerning adolescents are how they appear to friends of the opposite sex, how to date boy- or girl-friends, how to be popular among their peers of the opposite sex, and so on. What is normal psychosexual development as measured by their sexual interest, knowledge, and experience needs careful consideration from cultural perspectives. How to adjust their sexual development within their cultural context is a challenging matter.

4. Ethnic or Racial Identity Issues

Adolescence is the stage in which ethnic or racial identity becomes a major issue in psychological development. The sense of self-identity is heightened at this stage of development, as does ethnic or racial identity. In addition to asking, What kind of person am I? Do others like me or not? and Which group do I belong to? there are similar questions about what kind of ethnic or racial group I belong to, how others see me as part of a particular ethnic or racial group, and with which ethnic or racial group I should identify. Thus, the issues of identity become more complicated.

If the youngsters are surrounded by people of the same ethnic or racial group, such as in homogeneous societies, ethnic or racial identity issues seldom become apparent unless they go abroad and interact with people of distinctly different ethnic or racial groups. However, if the youngsters are surrounded by people of different ethnic or racial groups in their living environment, their ethnic or racial identity will be stimulated early in their development and can become an issue when they reach the adolescent stage. This is particularly so if they belong to an ethnic minority and experience ethnic or racial discrimination. Depending on their actual experiences in life, the ethnic- or race-related identity can be either a positive or a negative one, affecting their psychology differently. Some-

times, they are unclear or confused about their ethnic or racial identity, which can influence their mental health, and require professional help.

C. Special Issues to Be Concerned in Treatment

1. Socioculturally Deprived Minority Youth

Sociocultural deprivation refers to a person experiencing less than desirable conditions from social and cultural perspectives. In a concrete sense, the person suffers from poor economic conditions, less opportunity for education or employment, is exposed to confused values systems (as traditional cultural systems are uprooted), experiences unfair treatment from others, and lacks a positive group or ethnic/racial identification. This is often observed among indigenous minority people whose sociocultural system is destroyed by (invading) outsiders or due to exposure to rapid social and culture change associated with "modernization."

The youngsters of such backgrounds often experience undesirable mental health conditions manifested by a prevalence of drinking problems, substance abuse, behavior problems, including juvenile delinquency, and self-destructive behavior, such as suicide. These are rather universally observed phenomena among young people who are members of a minority growing up in a socioculturally deprived environment. They are reactions to and the products of such circumstances.

Clinical experience has suggested that ethnic and cultural issues need to be dealt with actively in therapeutic intervention (Vargas & Koss-Chioino, 1992). Furthermore, for youngsters with these kinds of mental health problems, group and social-activity approaches are more meaningful and useful than traditional, individual therapy. In other words, the whole community needs to be focused and worked on rather than merely the single person. It is quite a challenge for the clinician, as it takes a lot of energy, effort, and time.

2. The Immigrated Youngster

When people migrate from one society to another, it often disrupts the growing process of the youngsters in terms of language, ways of behavior, education, and socialization. The youngsters have to adjust to changes in their personal lives, family situations, and society at large. If the youngsters have difficulty going through this migration-related adjustment, many mental health problems may occur, the same as those for socioculturally deprived minority groups. However, if they learn the new language and new ways of life, make good use of the educational system, and are successful in adjusting their family life and socialization with others, they can adjust well and become successful in their later lives. While they are vulnerable because of migration, there is a chance for their adjustment and improvement (Nguyen & Williams, 1989).

In therapy, they need to be encouraged to improve in their new language, to learn about the ways of behaving and doing things in the host society, and to activate their socialization. If the youngsters receive sufficient attention from their teachers at school, proper care at home, and are welcomed by their peers, there is always a good chance for their successful adjustment to the hosting society. The role of the therapist is to facilitate these issues in all dimensions.

3. Traumatized Refugee Children

Refugee children are generally considered to be at high risk for mental health problems because of the extreme stressors they experienced in the past. From a therapeutic standpoint, a debate often occurs over the question of whether to break the silence surrounding the war and repression that have become part of family and social relationships. According to Rousseau (1995), who reviewed the available literature, most Latin American authors considered social silence to be a consequence desired by oppressive political regimes. Given this situation, some clinicians, such as Becker, Lira, Castillo, Gomez, and Kovalskys (1990), suggest that group therapy creates a space to hold past experiences and all their associated emotions, allowing symbolization to begin. Giving testimony is in itself therapeutic, providing an instrument of struggle and protest against the aggressor and an act of recognition of the emotional hurt. Otherwise, children may become "unintentional transmitters of undiscussable traumatic life events" (Bar-On, 1993). For some clinicians, intervention in the form of community or school programs has been applied. In general, it is considered that mental health intervention for refugee children cannot be confined to a psychiatric approach centered on psychopatholpogy. Cultural, social, political, and even historical dimensions must be incorporated.

4. The Mixed-Race Child

Associated with the increase in interracial or interethnic marriage, there is an increase in the number of mixed-race or -ethnic children. The common concerns related to mixed-race adolescents are the matters of social marginality, sexual identity, and racial identity (Gibbs, 1987). When parents are joined together in interethnic or -racial marriages, they often encounter certain issues in their marital lives. One issue is how to raise their children, who are the products of their intermarriage [cross-reference to Chapter 46: Intercultural Marriage (Section III,D)].

If parents know how to care for their mixed children with affection, basically there will be no problems for the youngsters. However, if there are problems between the parents, that the youngsters are mixed could aggravate triangular relationship problems with the parents. For instance, in a black (husband)–white (wife) interracial marriage, if the son happens to have more white features, the black father may see him as the wife's son rather than theirs (unconsciously or consciously) and treat him with certain negative feelings, or hate and resent him, in the worst case. It could obstruct the father–son identification and intensify the triangular conflict if the white mother tended to take a sympathetic and protective attitude toward the son. It needs to be clarified that it is not the racial appearance of the youngster alone that creates such conflict and problems, but the preexisting problems between the husband and wife that are provoked or aggravated by the racial appearance of the child. The same situation could occur with a daughter depending on her racial appearance. Because each child would be different, different situations could occur for him or her.

It is not only racial appearance that can provoke conflict between the parents and induce family problems, but also the different value systems held by the parents, widened by the intercultural marriage situation. Again, if the marital adjustment is successful, the problems of mixed-racial or -ethnic youngsters will not occur, or will be minor issues.

In Hawaii, Danko and colleagues (1997) examined adolescents who were offspring of interracial or -ethnic married parents versus homoracial or -ethnic married parents. They reported that there was no difference among the groups compared in terms of reported psychiatric symptoms. Because Hawaii is a multiethnic society in which many people are intermarried, living in a relatively harmonious setting in terms of inter-racial or -ethnic relations, it may explained that such a social environment minimizes any differences due to interracial or -ethnic marriage.

IV. CLOSING REMARKS

It has been pointed out that the psychological lives of children and adolescents need to be comprehended from cultural perspectives in addition to those of development, family, and social environment. Understanding through multiple dimensions is necessary (Ponce, 2001). Despite this recognition, there is not yet any sufficient and systematic knowledge for clinicians to grasp in terms of how children's and adolescents' lives are actually shaped by culture and the kinds of practical cultural considerations that are needed in their care. This is because there is a shortage of child psychiatrists around the world to accumulate such transcultural knowledge in diverse cultural settings. However, there is a rising awareness among clinicians that cultural concern is necessary in working with youngsters of different ethnic, racial, and cultural backgrounds. It is hoped that more systematic and rich information will be available in the future that will give us a better understanding of this subject for culture-relevant clinical application.

REFERENCES

Bar-On, D. (1993). *Children as unintentional transmitters of undiscussable traumatic life events.* Presented at the Congress on Children — War and Persecution, Hamburg, Germany.

Becker, D., Lira, E., Castillo, M.I., Gomez, E., & Kovalskys, J. (1990). Therapy with victims of pollitical repression in Chile: The challenge of social reparation. *Journal of Social Issues, 46*(3), 133–149.

Canino, I., & Spurlock, J. (1994). *Culturally diverse children and adolescents: Assessment, diagnosis, and treatment.* New York: Guilford Press.

Danko, G.P., Miyamoto, R.H., Poster, J.E., Johnson, R.C., Andrade, N.N., Yates, A., & Edman, J.L. (1997). Psychiatric symptoms in offspring of within vs. Across racial/ethnic marriages. *Cultural Diversity and Mental Health, 3*(4), 273–277.

Gibbs, J.T. (1987). Identity and marginality: Issues in the treatment of biracial adolescents. *American Journal of Orthopsychiatry, 57*(2), 265–278.

Griffith, E.E.H. (1995a). Culture and the debate on adoption of Black children by White families. In J.M., Oldham & M.B., Riba (Eds.), *American Psychiatric Press review of psychiatry* (Vol. 14) (pp. 543–564). Washington, DC: American Psychiatric Press.

Griffith, E.E.H. (1995b). Forensic and policy implications of the transracial adoption debate. *Bulletin of the American Academic Psychiatry and Law, 23*(4), 501–512.

Griffith, E.E.H., & Silverman, I.L. (1995). Transracial adoptions and the continuing debate on the racial identity of families. In H.W., Harris, H.C., Blue, & E.E.H., Griffith (Eds.), *Racial and ethnic identity: Psychological development and creative expression.* New York: Routledge.

Hsu, J. (1983). Asian family interaction patterns and their therapeutic implications. *International Journal of Family Psychiatry, 4*(4), 307–320.

McGoldrick, M., Giordano, J., & Pearce, J.K. (1996). *Ethnicity and family therapy,* (2nd ed.). New York: Guilford Press.

McGoldrick, M., Pearce, J.K., & Giordano, J. (1982). *Ethnicity and family therapy.* New York: Guilford Press.

McRoy, R.G., Zurcher, L.A., Lauderdale, M.L., & Anderson, R.N. (1982). Self-esteem and racial identity in transracial and inracial adoptees. *Social Work, 27,* 522–526.

Nguyen, N., & Willams, H. (1989). Transition from East to West: Vietnamese adolescents and their parents. *Journal of the American Academy of Child and Adolescent Psychiatry, 28,* 505–515.

Ponce, D.E. (2001). The adolescent. In W.S. Tseng & J. Streltzer (Eds.), *Culture and psychotherapy: A guide for clinical practice* (pp. 193–208). Washington, DC: American Psychiatric Press.

Powell, G.J. (Ed.). (1983). *The psychosocial development of minority group children.* New York: Brunner/Mazel.

Rousseau, C. (1995). The mental health of refugee children. *Transcultural Psychiatric Research Review, 32*(3), 299–331.

Silverman, A.R. (1993). Outcomes of transracial adoption. *The Future of Children, 3*(1), 104–118.

Simon, R. (1993). Transracial adoption: Highlights of a twenty-year study. *Reconstruction, 2*(2), 130–131.

Tseng, W.S., Ebata, K., Miguchi, M., Egawa, M., & McLaughlin, D.G. (1990). Transethnic adoption and personality traits: A lesson from Japanese orphans returned from China. *American Journal of Psychiatry, 147,* 330–335.

Tseng, W.S., & Hsu, J. (1991). *Culture and family: Problems and therapy.* New York: Haworth Press.

Untalan, F.F., & Camacho, J.M. (1997). Children of Micronesia. In G. Johnson-Powell, J. Yamamoto, G.E. Wyatt, & W. Arroyo (Eds.), *Transcultural child development: Psychological assessment and treatment* (pp. 304–327). New York: Wiley.

Vargas, L.A., & Koss-Chioino, J.D. (1992). *Working with culture: Psychotherapeutic interventions with ethnic minority children and adolescents.* San Francisco: Jossey-Bass.

Westermeyer, J., Bouafuely-Kersey, M., & Her, C. (1997). Hmong children. In G. Johnson-Powell, J. Yamamoto, G.E. Wyatt, & W. Arroyo (Eds.), *Transcultural child development: Psychological assessment and treatment* (pp. 162–182). New York: Wiley.

39

Working with Couples and Spouses

I. INTRODUCTION

From a psychological point of view, men and women are different in some perspectives even when they grow up within the same village or community. When they marry partners of the same cultural background, a so-called "homocultural" marriage, they still have to learn to adjust to the differences that exist between them. One of the main purposes of couple therapy is helping a couple resolve their differences in terms of the way they view or feel about things. If the couple is from different social or cultural backgrounds, then their marriage is "intercultural" (or "heterocultural"), and the differences that may exist between them are potentially greater and their marital problems more complicated.

Based on the similarity or differences in the cultural backgrounds of the therapist and the couple–partners, three situations can occur (see Fig. 39-1). In **intercultural-marriage therapy** (or marital therapy for interculturally married couple), even though the therapist shares the same cultural background with one of the couple, dealing with the cultural differences that exist between the partners is often the main thrust of the therapy. Another situation

that requires cultural concern is **intercultural couple-therapy** (or **transcultural marital-therapy** for homoculturally married couple). This refers to the situation in which the couple in therapy is homocultural (of the same cultural background), but the therapist's cultural background is different. Therefore, the therapist needs to determine how best to offer the couple therapy by transcending the cultural barriers that exist between the therapist and the couple. Another more complicated situation is **triad-intercultural couple-therapy.** This is when the three parties involved, the therapist and the intercultural married couple, all have different cultural backgrounds so that a triad transcultural interaction may take place in the therapeutic situation. For instance, an Italian couple therapist treats a Japanese husband married to a Hispanic wife. Thus, culture becomes a crucial issue in couple therapy, depending on the cultural background of the therapist and the partners undergoing therapy.

Conventional couple therapy ordinarily refers to therapy for heterosexual partners or spouses, but it may include therapy for homosexual partners as well. Homosexually bound partners have different relationship issues in terms of commitment, role division, function, and goals of the relationship than heterosex-

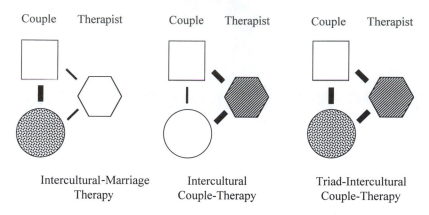

FIGURE 39-1 **Different therapist–couple combinations associated with cultural background.**

ual partners, so that such **homosexual partner couple therapy** will require a different focus, skill, and approach. Traditional marital therapy involves a married couple, i.e., a husband and wife, that is different than a couple that is not formally married. Because many couples nowadays live together in long-term relationships without marriage, the difference between them and married spouses is becoming less, particularly if the married spouses do not bear offspring, forming a family. Thus, for the sake of convenience, in this chapter therapy for these both types of couples will be addressed interchangeably either as "couple therapy" or "marital therapy," without making a distinction between them.

Issues relating to intercultural psychotherapy, in which the therapist and the patient have divergent cultural backgrounds, have been discussed previously (Chapter 36: Intercultural Psychotherapy). The basic principles and considerations of intercultural therapy (for an individual patient) also apply to intercultural couple therapy (for partners in a couple). The nature of the problems and adjustments found in interculturally married couples, as well as some therapeutic considerations for treating them, will be elaborated in detail later (Chapter 46: Intercultural Marriage: Problems and Therapy). Thus, the primary focus of this chapter will be on how to provide culturally relevant marital therapy for (homoculturally married) couples

from various ethnic–cultures. This is based on the assumption that couples from different ethnic–cultures, such as couples from Euro-America, the Mideast, Asia, India, and Micronesia, have culture-related special issues that need to be worked out in therapy. It also suggests that certain skills and approaches need to be considered in dealing with couples from different ethnic–cultures.

In order to carry out culturally geared marital therapy, it is very important for the therapist to have a basic knowledge of the cultural aspects of marriage, including how cultural factors influence the martial system and marital relations. Furthermore, the therapist should be aware of how cultural factors, in addition to many other factors, contribute to marital problems. Based on this basic knowledge, issues can then be discussed to determine how to conduct marital therapy in a culturally relevant way. This chapter is devoted to these subjects in this order.

II. CULTURE AND MARRIAGE

As elaborated previously, the system of marriage is subject to culture [cross-reference to Chapter 3: Marriage and the Family (Section II, A–C)]. This is exemplified by how culture determines the number of spouses who may be joined in marriage, as either a monogamous or polygamous marriage (the latter could be either polyandry or polygamy). Culture also encourages a certain choice of mates, such as someone from the same background (endogamy, within the same cultural group) or a different background (exogamy, across culture boundaries). Culture also favors certain methods of selecting a mate, such as arranged marriage or self-selection. Culture also has a strong impact on the choice of residence after marriage, either patrilocal, matrilocal, or neolocal residence, which in turn shapes the relationship with the family of origin.

Besides the direct impact on the form and structure of marriage, culture also strongly influences the nature of marriage. This is demonstrated by how marriage is considered — whether it is a firm, lifelong commitment that does not allow for the possibility of separation or divorce under any circumstances, or a rather flexible joining that can be terminated easily if there is not enough affection to bind the spouse–partners. From a functional point of view, culture will shape the role divisions between husband and wife, determine the responsibilities to be shared between marriage partners, and mold the way they bear and raise their offspring.

In summary, marriage form, structure, and function are significantly subject to cultural factors. The impact is either direct or indirect, but the influence cannot be ignored. This is the basic orientation that is needed to discuss the cultural aspects of marital therapy.

III. CULTURE AND MARITAL PROBLEMS

The psychological problems encountered by a married couple can be caused by many factors. Some problems are social, such as financial problems or the separation of the husband and wife due to social demands or war, whereas others are psychological, such as the incompatibility of the personalities of the spouses or an unhealthy motive for marriage. However, at another level, there are numerous ways in which martial problems are related to cultural factors. These are elaborated as follows.

A. MARITAL PROBLEMS ASSOCIATED WITH THE SYSTEM OF MARRIAGE ITSELF

1. Arranged Marriage versus Love Marriage

Even though the self-selection of marital partners is the most common and favored way to marry in most European-American societies, in many parts of the world, arranged marriages are still practiced. In many Asian societies, gradually shifting from the traditional arranged marriage system toward free marriage, parents still play a significant role in guiding their children in the selection of a mate — at least, the young people still need their parents' agreement or sanction to get married.

There are certain advantages and disadvantages to both arranged marriages and love marriages, or structured versus unstructured marriages, as defined and elaborated by Japanese-American sociologist T.S. Lebra (1978). Marriage according to free love sounds romantic, but if a person is not socially sophisticated and experienced in heterosexual interactions, he or she may be at a disadvantage, not knowing how to objectively select a proper and suitable mate. In some societies, where love marriage is a newly adopted phenomenon, it has been observed that separation and divorce are relatively frequent among those who wed for love, as opposed to those who marry through parental arrangement. In arranged marriages, the parents assist the young couple in selecting a partner with consideration of objective factors, including the realistic aspects of life, such as level of education, occupational skill, the background of the family of origin, and past history of behavior and performance. Besides, theoretically, the relations between in-laws tend to be better from the beginning if the wedded partner has been selected or screened by the prospective in-laws.

However, arranged marriages tend to have inherent problems that may emerge after the marriage. The partners selected by the parents may not like each other, and intimate affection may not develop or may be delayed. Unsatisfied with his arranged wife, the husband may seek romance outside of the marriage.

2. Other Culture-Based Unique Marriage Customs

Besides the way in which partners are married, there are certain unique culture-related marriage customs in many societies that deserve attention. For instance, the custom of an "adopted husband" (or "adopted son-in-law" from the parents' perspective) is still observed in some societies in Asia, such as Japan and China (Tseng & Hsu, 1991, p. 12). This is rooted in a cultural system that views it as very important for a son to carry on the family name. If parents do not bear a son, their daughter may be expected to marry a man who will be willing to give up his own family name and adopt his wife's surname so that his parents-in-law's family lineage can be maintained. This is usually a man who is not an elder son and has no obligation to succeed his own family. It is considered culturally unfavorable behavior for a man to give up his surname of origin, even if he does so to comply with a culture-based family requirement. Usually the wife's family is rather affluent and the man who is adopted as a son-in-law and becomes a "husband" tends to do so for financial gain. Such an "adopted husband" is in a weak position in his relationship with his wife. He also has to fulfill his responsibility to the family that has adopted him as a son-in-law. This complicated situation tends to stir up marital problems for the couple involved.

Another unique marital custom is "spouse substituted by a sibling." This refers to the situation in which a spouse dies young, and his or her unmarried sibling has an obligation to marry the widow or widower. In Micronesia, for instance, when a husband dies young, his single brother or cousin is expected to marry his widow. In Japan, if a wife dies young, the wife's sister, if she is still single, is culturally expected to marry her brother-in-law, the widower. This custom is based on the cultural consideration that such a spouse substitute will maintain the relations of the families on both sides and is a favorable substitute for the lost spouse if the couple has young children. It is believed that the orphans will be well taken care of by their new parent, who is an uncle or aunt by blood.

However, this spouse substitute custom has certain inherent problems. The person who is expected to substitute for the deceased spouse has no choice of his or her own mate and is expected to accept the fate of marrying his or her sibling-in-law and to serve as a stepparent for his brother or sister's children. Sometimes, jealousy may occur when comparisons are made between the deceased spouse and the sibling substitute. For instance, a Micronesian man who married his elder brother's wife after his elder brother passed away was troubled because he was sometimes less competent as a "husband" than his elder brother. Actually, he visited a psychiatrist with the complaint that his penis was smaller than his brother's, and he failed to satisfy his wife. Apparently, his inferior feelings of himself in relation to his elder brother were heightened by this marriage custom.

B. PROBLEMS ASSOCIATED WITH CULTURALLY EXPECTED RELATIONS WITH THE FAMILIES OF ORIGIN

In an individual-emphasizing society, marriage is considered the binding of two persons. The neolocal residence system, namely living in a new place of their own parting from the parents on both sides, is practiced. The families of origin or marriage-related families are kept at a certain distance from the new couple, according to the nuclear family structure. The relations are characterized by periodic telephone contact supplemented by occasional visits. This is common practice for people living in urban settings who move frequently. However, this is not true in other societies in which either paterlocal or materlocal residence systems are observed and the families of origin or marriage-related family live close together. Even though the families do not live together physically, the nature of a stem or extended family is maintained. Under such circumstances, relations with parent-in-laws, sibling-in-laws, and other members of the family or clan are close, influencing marital relations intensely and significantly. It is almost impossible to ignore the existence and impact of families of origin or families by marriage. No doubt these close, extended ties with families have their advantages. Often support is available when it is needed. However, there are always certain restraints for married couples as they have to take into consideration the impact of their marital life on their families. This creates certain conflicts, even though harmony may be ideally emphasized in such extended and complicated family ties.

A Hawaiian couple came to see a marital therapist for tensions they were experiencing after the birth of their first child. The conflict derived from an argument they had about what middle names to give their newborn child. It is Hawaiian custom, in addition to the first and last names, for a person to have several middle names, which are given after the first names of respected uncles or aunties from both the paternal and the maternal sides of the family. In order to show respect, the young couple argued about how many names should be given, from which side of the family, in which order. This involved matters of ties, obligations, and favoritism on both sides of the family. Obviously, this kind of conflict will arise only in a culture in which ties with the families of origin are strongly emphasized. A newborn child is considered the product of the (extended) "family" or clan rather than of the couple themselves.

C. Conflict Originating from Culturally Prescribed Role Divisions between Spouses

The roles to be performed by a husband and wife are individual and private matters. However, beyond the personal level, they are often influenced by culture in either explicit or subtle ways. While the culturally prescribed role divisions between spouses tend to guide and stabilize their relations and interactions, they may also induce certain conflicts. Following are some examples.

In Korea, it is not considered a virtue for a woman to work outside the home after becoming a wife. A wife is expected to stay at home and devote herself primarily to domestic matters, including serving her husband and raising the children. It would be viewed as "disgraceful" for a wife to work outside of the house. Therefore, it is almost a rule that women quit their jobs and become housewives when they are married. It does not matter if the woman is a highly educated professional woman. Less than 20% of women still work as professionals after marriage, even in contemporary Korea. Due to this custom, many young women, as housewives, have to confine themselves to their houses for the rest of their lives. In the past, housewives were kept busy doing many household chores and raising their children. However, in present-day Korea, housewives give birth to only a couple of children. The modern household is equipped with appliances such as refrigerators, ovens, microovens, dishwashing machines, and laundry machines, making it relatively easy for housewives to take care of their domestic work. Thus, modern Korean wives are not as busy as they were in the past. After their children enter school, they find life at home becomes boring. Many Korean wives develop emotional problems in these circumstances, complaining of feelings of loneliness, emptiness, and boredom. This phenomenon is referred to by Korean psychiatrists as the "housewife syndrome" (Chang & Kim, 1988).

In many parts of the Mideast, Muslim wives are also expected to be subordinate to their husbands, to keep busy with household work, and to not raise their voices to express their opinions, complain, or make demands of their husbands. Some wives suffer as a result of this underprivileged life. They express their unhappiness and satisfy their demands through folk ways, such as participation in the Zar cult. During the religious ceremony, in a dissociated state, through the voice of the spirit of Zar, they make demands on their husbands for their unfulfilled desires. This folk healing practice functions as a way of solving marital problems in a culture that tends to suppress wives [cross-reference to Chapter 32: Culture-Embedded Indigenous Healing Practices (Section II, A,2)].

A Vietnam wife suffered from chronic depression associated with guilt feelings because she was not able to obtain her husband's pardon for the "awful" thing that she did during the war. During the Vietnam war, her husband was drafted as a soldier and lost contact with his family. At the end of the war, the new government asked people to reregister their houses and lands. Without knowing the fate of her husband — whether he was deceased or not — she followed her mother-in-law's suggestion and registered the land under her own name, as it was the only way to keep the property. Shortly after this, her husband returned alive from the war. He had been wounded and delayed in coming home. When he discovered that his wife had registered the property in her name, he became very angry. As this was an unusual thing for a woman to do in a male-dominant society, he interpreted it as her trying to take over the household. He described her, in a folk way, as "a hen trying to crow in the morning." He was very upset by her "disgraceful" behavior and never excused her for it, even after many years had passed (Young, 1998).

D. PROBLEMS STEMMING FROM CULTURE-SHAPED COMMUNICATION PATTERNS BETWEEN SPOUSES

In contemporary American society, it is common for a husband and wife to communicate openly with each other about how they think and feel. Sharing between spouses is one of the most important elements in maintaining their affection for each other and preserving their relationship. It is also a cultural habit for partners to praise each other as often as possible and to express appreciation whenever it is appropriate. This is a means of offering assurance and making the relationship work.

However, it is important for a marital therapist to know that this concept and habit of open communication to maintain closeness is not necessarily shared by couples in other cultures. In some cultures, it is considered "awkward" for intimate persons, such as a

husband and wife, to praise each other verbally and to express gratitude. It is considered necessary to say thank you only to "outsiders," but not to intimate "insiders," particularly spouses. Physical intimacy, such as touching, holding, and hugging, between husband and wife in a public setting is considered impolite or improper behavior. Kissing each other in front of others is considered "disgusting," uncivilized, "animal" behavior. These differences in cultural views and attitudes regarding communication and expression of affection between husband and wife need to be taken into consideration when the therapist assesses the relations between couples from other cultures. Otherwise, a great misunderstanding may take place. Needless to say, there are subtle ways that couples from such cultural backgrounds express their opinions and feelings. These usually involve nonverbal expressions, which can be perceived if the therapist is knowledgeable about and sensitive to them.

When subtle ways of communicating are applied, sometimes even the husband and wife themselves fail to perceive the message, confusing or misunderstanding it, and feeling frustrated. Such culture-shaped communication patterns can be the source of potential problems.

E. DIFFICULTIES RELATED TO CULTURE-SHAPED CHILD-REARING PATTERNS

Another source of problems and disagreement may be child-rearing patterns. The husband and wife may not necessarily share the same views on how to raise and discipline their children. This is particularly so if the society is experiencing sociocultural change and many parents have lost their values and beliefs on how to raise their children.

In many societies, the care and discipline of the children are assigned solely to the wife, while the husband concentrates only on business matters outside of the household. As a result, potential problems may occur. The wife may be overinvolved with the children and neglect her husband, or she may feel overwhelmed by the responsibility of taking care of the children by herself without any help from her husband.

F. Culture Sanctioned Violence against Wives by Husbands

The physical abuse of wives by their husbands has been documented in almost every culture in the world (Levinson, 1989). Krane (1996) pointed out that research findings from developed and developing societies suggest that from 20 to 67% of women have experienced violence in intimate heterosexual relationships. Such information reveals that women, in their capacities as wives or partners, are not safe. Battered wives often internalize deep feelings of self-blame and shame. Suicide may be one of the ways they react to abuse. Abuse of women in marital relationships has been identified as possibly the most important precipitant of female suicides cross-culturally (Counts, 1987). In Papua New Guinea, suicide is considered a "reasonable and culturally valid response to abuse" of women by men (Counts, 1987, p. 198). Marital violence is cited as a significant factor in suicide among Fijian Indian families (Lateef, 1992). Similarly, in Egypt, family quarrel was the leading cause of all suicides reported, particularly among young women (Heise, Raikes, Watts, & Zwi, 1994). Another consequence associated with physical abuse is homicide. Studies from India, Bangladesh, Kenya, and Thailand verify that murder frequently takes place within the family and most often the victim is a woman (United Nations, 1989). A review of research across the globe found many of the same risk factors. The young wife, in the early years of her marriage, was at great risk (United Nations, 1989). Unfounded sexual jealousy or protest against the woman's threat to terminate the relationship were some other risk factors. It was the real or perceived challenges to the man's possession, authority, and control of his wife that most often resulted in the use of violence. Despite these similar-

ities, there was good reason to speculate that there were sociocultural factors that contributed to the low or high frequency of violence against wives.

G. Problems Rooted in Cultural Views and the Commitment to Marriage

Finally, there may be problems related to the way the couple viewed their commitment to their marriage. Most Western societies believe that marriage should be monogamous. Also, it is basically considered that marriage is a life-long commitment. Therefore, during a religious ceremony, the couple is often officially asked to swear that they will be bonded and take care of each other for the rest of their lives. However, in reality, for couples whose marriages are not working, divorce is a common contemporary solution that is easily entertained and practiced. In contrast, in many other cultures, it is still believed that marriage is a life-long commitment. Even though there are problems, termination of the marriage is seldom considered. When a couple has such a cultural background, separation or divorce as a solution to problems should not be proposed by the therapist. Such a suggestion would be misinterpreted as an attempt to "break up" the marriage, when the couple came to see the therapist with the intention of saving it.

In most monogamous societies, in theory, extramarital affairs are not accepted. However, in some, a husband having affairs outside of the marriage is tolerated. Multiple wives are permitted in some cultures (such as in China in the past and in Muslim societies even in the present) if the husband is affluent enough to support them. The rivalry and conflict between wives may be minimized by certain cultural rules and practices. For instance, the first wife is always respected as the primary spouse, with a certain prestige and power, even though the husband may accumulate other wives or concubines. Still, there is potential competition and conflict in such polygamous situations.

IV. CULTURAL CONSIDERATIONS IN WORKING WITH COUPLES

In addition to using the fundamental therapeutic strategies and basic techniques utilized in "regular" marital therapy, the following issues need attention when working with couples whose cultural backgrounds are different from the therapist's or when the partners are having culture-related marital problems.

A. CAREFUL ESTABLISHMENT OF THE THERAPIST'S RELATIONSHIP WITH SPOUSE–PARTNERS

It is generally the rule for the marital therapist to be careful to maintain a well-balanced relationship between the husband and the wife in treatment, avoiding any possibility of taking sides. The similarities or dissimilarities of personal backgrounds, personalities, and gender are some common factors that may lead to complications in therapy. In terms of gender, the therapist may be seen by the couple in treatment as taking the side of the partner of the same or different gender. As an extension of this, the ethnic or racial background of the therapist and the couple can provoke the "joining" of problems between the husband and wife associated with the tendency of "identification" of the therapist with one of the partners.

In individual therapy, the ethnic or racial background of the therapist could have a significant impact on the therapist–patient relationship, either in a positive or in a negative way [cross-reference to Chapter 36: Intercultural Psychotherapy (Section II,C)]. In marital therapy, in addition to the impact on the dyad, there may be a forceful influence on the triad relations among the therapist and the two partners that deserves careful management.

B. RELEVANT RESPECT OF CULTURALLY DEFINED ROLES AND COMMUNICATION PATTERNS

Based on their cultural background, the roles of a husband and wife are defined in terms of how they behave, interact, and relate to other people. As a therapist, it is important to recognize the preexistence of such culturally defined roles of the husband and wife and, based on this knowledge, to decide how to relate to the couple.

The best example to illustrate this point is that of a therapist treating a Micronesian couple. According to their traditional culture, the wife was not supposed to speak directly to a man other than her own husband, particularly on very private matters. The Micronesian husband was referred by his family physician to a psychiatrist, with the complaint that his penis was too small and he was not able to satisfy his wife sexually. Thinking that this was related to a matter between the man and his wife, the therapist advised the patient's wife to come with him so that a more comprehensive interview could be conducted in a joint session. However, the therapist soon discovered that no matter how he addressed his questions to the wife, even though she could speak reasonably good English, she would turn around to speak to her husband in their native language and her husband, acting as a mediator and translator, would then give her answer in English to the therapist. Clearly the wife was following their custom of not talking directly to a male stranger (the therapist). The therapist questioned whether the husband was translating his wife's replies accurately. However, he was left with no other choice but to respect and follow the couple's culture. Otherwise, there would have been no way to continue the session.

In many cultures, particularly those with Asian or Muslim backgrounds, there is a cultural expectation that the wife should behave submissively toward her husband. If the therapist ignores this cultural expectation and asks the wife to openly and directly give her opinions — without asking permission from her husband — there is a potential risk of ignoring the culture-defined roles of husband and wife. This goes beyond the matter of communication patterns and is related to respecting the cultural roles expected of the husband and wife in their own cultural system, even if it is desirable from a therapeutic point of view that the two express their own opinions and communicate freely.

C. Dynamic Understanding of Problems with Cultural Insight

When the therapist does not share the same ethnic–culture with the couple–partners, in such interculture marital therapy, as in intercultural psychotherapy in general, he needs to make an effort to understand the nature of the problems presented by the couple with cultural knowledge and insight (Hsu, 2001). After relevant and meaningful understanding of the problems, culture-relevant coping and solutions can be suggested or prescribed. This is illustrated in the following case vignette.

A Chinese husband became depressed after his wife deserted him, returning to her family of origin. She complained that her husband was "a mother's son, but not her husband!" The family history revealed that the husband was the only and youngest son, with three elder sisters. As his father was deceased shortly after he was born, he was raised by his widowed mother alone. The mother took extra precautions in raising him and indulged him a lot because he was the only boy in the family. She would not spend any money on herself, but would not hesitate to buy good food and clothes for him. In return, he became a filial son — thoughtful and obedient and almost dependent on her. This situation become more so after his three elder sisters married and moved out, leaving the mother and son living together. He married late. Through a matchmaker, he married a woman a couple of years older than he. His wife married him thinking that if he was obedient and filial to his mother, he would be a good husband who would be nice to his wife.

Things did not turn out the way the wife wished. Very soon, she found out that the tie between the mother and son was so strong that it interfered with their martial relations. For instance, even though her son was now married, the mother still kept her old habit of coming into his bedroom at night to make sure that he was properly covered with a quilt and not catching cold. The mother-in-law's behavior became intolerable to the wife and upset her more when she discovered that her husband did not have the guts to complain to his mother and stop her intrusion on their privacy.

When the couple and the mother had meals together, the husband, out of respect, would pick out some food to offer to his mother. However, he did not pick out any food for his wife. The turning point came one day when the wife bought a new bicycle. At the time of this story, it was considered an expensive item, and it took a lot of saving to purchase it. She wanted to keep her new bike inside the house when it rained. As the house was rather small, the mother-in-law complained that the bike, which was in the corridor, interfered with her walking. Her husband did not speak up on his wife's behalf. Instead, he advised her to move her new bike outside. She realized that her husband was his mother's son, and not her husband. She packed her belongings and returned to her own family.

From a clinical point of view, it can be said that the husband had not mastered his own individualization and was not functioning in his role as a husband. However, from a cultural point of view, the case should not be formulated so quickly. It needs to be considered that filial behavior is considered a virtue in Chinese culture. Close mother–son relationships are not only permitted, but have traditionally been glorified under the concept of filial piety. Even now, it is "morally" and "legally" expected for a child to support his aged parents, particularly a widowed mother who devoted her life to raising her son. It would be hasty for the therapist to suggest that the husband "grow up," "become autonomous," "be a man," and "join his wife as a husband!" His personal background and culture situation need to be understood from his perspective. Obviously he needs to restructure his intrapsychic feelings toward his mother and develop his new relationship with his wife as a husband, but this needs to be done gradually and steadily, not abruptly. To suggest a "mother-sectomy" — cutting his bonds with his mother — would be fatal and would only increase his guilt feelings and aggravate his depression. This case illustrates that cultural knowledge is not necessarily an excuse to ignore a psychopathology, but it gives the therapist a more relevant perspective for understanding, reacting to, and dealing with the therapeutic situation.

D. Delicate Adjustment of Therapeutic Changes between Spouses

It is clear from the case vignette just described that the therapeutic process needs to be performed at a certain pace, with tenderness and in a correct direction. This is quite true in marital therapy in general. The balance between interpersonal relations and individual intrapsychic homostatis always needs consideration. This is particularly so from a culture perspective, as emotionally embedded cultural beliefs and attitudes take time to revise. Balancing changes between husband and wife in the therapeutic process needs to be managed delicately. The following case vignette illustrates this.

The case concerns a Muslim wife in Cairo who sought psychiatric therapy with multiple somatic complaints (El-Islam, 2001). In therapy, it was soon realized that her problems were centered around her relations with her husband. She felt that, as usual in a Muslim family, she did not have the status to express her opinions and desires and to protect her needs — she could only be submissive.

Based on understanding and formulation of the problem, therapy was aimed to improve the wife's status and help her protect her rights and benefits. However, this would certainly encounter a vigorous reaction and resistance from her husband, as it would challenge his traditional status as a husband and take away his culture-given privileges as a man. Even though the goal of therapy would be good for the suppressed wife, it would not be beneficial for the privileged husband. He was going to reactive negatively toward the direction of the therapy, and even pull out of the therapy if he sensed that he would be asked to change his role, status, and behavior as a husband in such a way that he would look like a "fool" in his men-friends' eyes. Therapy needs to be undertaken in such a way that the change between husband and wife will occur gradually in a dedicated and balanced way.

E. Relevant Application of Special Marital Therapeutic Maneuvers

Based on clinical experiences (Western), marital therapists have developed some special marital therapeutic maneuvers, such as "role playing" and "family sculpturing," during therapeutic sessions or the application of "paradox" approaches to deal with therapy-resistant couples of Euro-American backgrounds. However, such special therapeutic maneuvers need careful consideration for application to couples from other cultures. This is not merely because couples from other cultures are often not familiar with such therapeutic maneuvers and need more explanation and preparation before application, but because the cultural background of the couple in therapy may make the application of such special maneuvers difficult or even contraindicated.

For a family hierarchy-oriented culture, "family sculpturing" will encounter less difficulty. Actually, it can become an objective way to illustrate the dysfunctional family structure and hierarchy that has been established by the couple and their children. However, "role playing" is difficult for those couples who are not used to playing (or to performing certain roles) in front of others (the therapist). This is particularly true when they are asked to reverse role play, i.e., for the wife to play the role of the husband, and vice versa. Imagine how the husband and wife would feel if they came from a society that strongly emphasized dominant men and subordinate women, such as many Asian and Muslim cultures. The husband would certainly feel very insulted when asked by the therapist to play a woman's role, and the wife would feel very hesitant to play a man's role — it would be almost taboo to ask the couple to go through such a "therapeutic maneuver." In theory, it could be a useful maneuver to increase the understanding, empathy, and insight between the husband and wife, but, in practice, it could be a disaster when applied to couples from other cultures.

The "paradox approach" has been developed by marital therapists for couples who are resistant to therapeutic work. Instead of working toward improvement, the therapist might work the other way (paradoxically), e.g., commenting that the couple is untreatable and suggesting that they end their troubled relationship. The intention is to provoke the couple to work together against the therapist for a therapeutic effect: to combat the couple that tends to react negatively to each other and resist therapy. However, this paradoxical approach has inherent risks. To make paradoxical comments, such as "You, as a couple, fight against each other all the time and negatively criticize each other all the time. I do not think there is a chance to improve your relationship. Separation or divorce may be the only chance to solve the problem," can bring unexpected results even for Western couples, who may be confused and misunderstand the therapist's (therapeutic) intention. If this technique is applied to a couple from a traditional culture, they may faint or become very angry at the therapist's (paradoxical) negative suggestion.

F. Proper Utilization of Culture-Rooted Coping in Therapy

From a cultural perspective, it is desirable to utilize any existing culture-rooted coping concepts or mechanisms available. They are not merely more familiar to the patients, but have also been proven to work in the cultural environment. For instance, in Chinese societies, many proverbs or daily-life sayings have been accumulated from history. Some of them are related to marital relations, such as "Fruit forcefully picked is not sweet; a wedding forcefully arranged is not wise" — stressing that affection between partners is still important, even though arranged marriage is practiced; "Even though he looks ugly, a spouse bounded is still better; even though of rough material, stout cloth can be worn long" — describing the practical aspects of marital relations; "If a hen starts to crow in the morning, the day will end with disaster" —

emphasizing that proper roles should be observed by the spouses; and "Man busy in farming, woman devoted to weaving, enough food and cloth" — explaining that if both husband and wife work hard and complementarily, their lives will be sufficient and happy.

When such common folk sayings are used, it is easier for the couple to grasp their meaning and to apprehend concretely the essense behind them. If the therapist is not familiar with such marriage-related cultural views and coping mechanisms, or there is no knowledge or wisdom reflected in folk sayings, the therapist may ask the couple to explore and elaborate on folk coping concepts that are commonly acknowledged and utlized in their culture. This is not only to identify such traditional concepts and folk suggestions, but provides an opportunity to elaborate with the couple on finding solutions to their problems that are culturally relevant and workable.

G. Relevant Concepts and Definitions of "Healthy" Couples

For therapy with an individual patient, the therapist needs to constantly check the definition of normality and health for an individual within his cultural context. In the same way, in marital therapy, the therapist is advised to examine what constitutes a functional, healthy couple within their own culture framework. Otherwise, the therapy may be misdirected.

For most couples in contemporary Euro-American cultures, it is considered desirable to communicate openly, to share their feelings, to maintain affection, and to exercise mutual respect. For couples in other cultures, such as most Eastern societies, it is considered more important to be faithful to each other, to perform complementary roles, and to maintain clear roles with divided functions. Thus, the concept of desirable couples or the definition of a healthy couple varies in different cultural settings. This needs to be examined in therapy with each couple.

H. Thoughtful Balancing between Cultural Requirements and Professional Theory

Finally, it needs to be mentioned that there should always be a proper balance between what is expected by culture and the theoretic goals suggested by professional therapy.

Marital therapy can be viewed as working with a couple suffering from differences existing between them — they can be differences in their ways of viewing things, their belief systems, or their feelings. In a way, the therapist works as a broker between the troubled couple–partners to improve mutual understanding and empathy to promote better and "healthier" relations. This is the general goal of marital therapy, based on the knowledge, experience, and theories accumulated by marital therapists. However, these professional theories are mainly derived from clinical experiences with Euro-American populations and are embedded in Western culture. It is very important for marital therapists to adjust such (Western) marital therapy theories for application to couples from non-Western backgrounds. The cultural adjustment of therapeutic techniques, approaches, and goals of therapy is essential.

Furthermore, it is necessary to consider the sociocultural environment within which the couple is going to live and function. Compliance and adjustment to the living environment are important parts of life. Depending on whether a Muslim couple is living in the Mideast, in the midst of Muslim culture, or has immigrated to a Euro-American society, the emphasis on adjustment of marital relations can be very different. Cultural compatibility with the living environment needs to be considered and emphasized so that meaningful, culturally relevant marital therapy can be implemented.

REFERENCES

Chang, H.I., & Kim, H.W. (1988). The study of the "house-wife syndrome" in Korea — with special concern with neurotic symptoms and family strains. *Asian Family Mental Health Conference Proceedings.* Tokyo: Psychiatric Research Institute of Tokyo.

Counts, D.A. (1987). Female suicide and wife abuse: A cross-cultural perspective. *Suicide and Life-Threatening Behavior, 17*(3), 194–204.

El-Islam, F.M. (2001). The woman with one foot in the past. In W.S. Tseng & J. Streltzer (Eds.), *Culture and psychotherapy: A guide to clinical practice* (pp. 27–41). Washington, DC: American Psychiatric Press.

Heise, L., Raikes, A., Watts, C., & Zwi, A. (1994). Violence against women: A neglected public health issues in less developed countries. *Social Science Medicine, 39*(9), 1165–1179.

Hsu, J. (2001). Marital therapy for intermarried couples. In W.S. Tseng & J. Streltzer (Eds.), *Culture and psychotherapy: A guide to clinical practice* (pp. 225–242). Washington, DC: American Psychiatric Press.

Krane, J.E. (1996). Violence against women in intimate relations: Insight from cross-cultural analysis. *Transcultural Psychiatric Research Review, 33*(4), 435–465.

Lateef, S. (1992). Wife abuse among Indo-Fijians. In D.A. Counts, J. Brown, & J. Campbell (Eds.), *Sanctions and sanctuary: Cultural perspectives on the beating of wives.* Boulder, CO: Westview Press.

Lebra, T.S. (1978). Japanese women and marital strain. *Ethos, 6,* 22–41.

Levinson, D. (1989). *Family violence in cross-cultural perspective.* Newbury Park, CA: Sage.

Tseng, W.S., & Hsu, J. (1991). *Culture and family: Problems and therapy.* New York: Haworth Press.

United Nations. (1989). *Violence against women in the family.* New York: United Nations Publication.

Young, D. (1998). A *Vietnam woman who was never forgiven by her husband.* Presented at the Culture and Psychotherapy Semina, organized by the University of Hawaii School of Medicine, Department of Psychiatry, Honolulu.

40

Working with Families

I. INTRODUCTION

As elaborated previously (cross-reference to Chapter 3: Marriage and the Family), the family is a special kind of small group that consists of members of different genders (bound by marriage) and generations (related by blood or by adoption), who maintain intense relations for a prolonged period of time. The family is the basic social unit through which culture is transmitted. From a clinical point of view, the family may manifest unique psychological problems or psychopathologies that are different from an individual perspective and need a special approach in treatment.

A clinician must have special knowledge and skills to work with a family that is having problems. Additionally, cultural considerations are essential in family therapy, as the family life and behavior of family members are heavily subject to cultural impact (Ariel, 1999; DiNicola, 1985; Falicov, 1983; Mindel & Habenstein, 1981). If the clinician is working with a family of a different cultural background, it is called **intercultural** or **transcultural family therapy,** and the therapist will need a certain cultural orientation and knowledge in order to understand the family transculturally and to deal with its problems in a culturally

appropriate way (McGoldrick, Giordano, & Pearce, 1996; Sue & Sue, 1990).

The focus of this chapter is understanding culture-related family psychopathology, elaborating on how to perform culturally relevant family assessment, and, finally, suggesting ways to conduct culturally appropriate family therapy.

II. FAMILY PSYCHOPATHOLOGY

A. FORMULATIONS OF FAMILY AND PSYCHOPATHOLOGY

In order to elaborate on family pathology, it is useful to first clarify from a conceptual point of view the potential relations that may exist between individual and family pathology. The various ways to formulate family psychopathology are as follows.

1. The Family as a System of Pathology

According to family scholars, one way to understand the relations between individual pathology and family pathology is to consider the possibility that the manifested individual abnormality is a part of the display of the total family psychopathology. Although individual psychopathology may initially receive clinical attention, individual psychopathology is merely an expression of the pathological function of the whole family. Closer examination generally reveals a particular set of dysfunctional family relationships that deserve therapeutic intervention. For example, a person with a psychosomatic disorder is often associated with a family characterized by enmeshed subsystem boundaries, requiring therapy for the family as a whole rather than focusing on the individual patient (Minuchin, Rosman, & Baker, 1978).

2. The Family as the Cradle of Pathology

The next formulation is that family dynamics and environment are the sources of the development of certain individual vulnerabilities, particularly throughout his or her early life. Based on these developmental predispositions rooted in the family, the pathology of an individual will be manifested when he or she reaches a certain age, particularly when he or she is exposed to certain stressful situations. For instance, a child repeatedly abandoned by his or her parents may become an insecure person who fails to develop basic trust toward others. In another example, an only male grandchild may be overindulged by his grandparents to such an extent that even his own parents are not allowed by the grandparents to provide any discipline. With these three-generation boundary problems, this family is very likely to raise a child who will have conduct problems.

3. Family Pathology as a Concomitant Manifestation of Individual Pathology

This formulation takes the position that the expressions of certain observed family behavior patterns are the manifestations of subclinical pathologies of parents or family members who have the same spectrum of genetic predispositions as an individual's identified disorder. Therefore, the pathologies manifested among family members are concomitant in nature, even though they may appear superficially to be different. Thus, the irrational thoughts and pseudomutual communication patterns manifested among the members of a schizophrenic family (Wyne, Ryckoff, Day, & Hirsch, 1958) may be viewed as the concomitant, but subclinical, individual manifestations of the same schizophrenic disorder (Wender, Rosenthal, Kety, Schulsinger, & Welner, 1974).

4. The Family as the Catalyst of Pathology

Pathology or disorders are primarily related to an individual predisposition, yet the unique environment and dynamic of the family provoke, maintain, or aggravate the individual psychopathology. This position is supported by experiments conducted by Purcel and associates (1969) on children with asthma. Although a child may suffer from asthma caused by an allergenic situation that exists in the house, children with a history of emotionally precipitated asthma attacks had fewer attacks when family members were (experimentally) removed from the house and were replaced by substitute parents. This illustrates indirectly that the original family member, through certain interactions, provided a catalytic effect for the occurrence of the child's asthma attack. Once the provoking factor was minimized the pathology subsided considerably.

5. Family Reactions to Individual Pathology

Situations may occur when family problems or dysfunctions are manifested as secondary reactions to the presence of the disorder or malfunction of an individual family member. An illustration is a situation in which there is an extremely hyperactive and destructive child in the house who upsets everybody and induces chaotic conditions for the whole family. Although the occurrence of attention deficit disorder in children is considered organic in nature, the family's reaction to such a behavior disorder is psychological and secondary.

6. Comorbid Existence of Individual and Family Pathology

This is a situation in which there is both an individual pathology and a family pathology that have little interactional relation and occur coincidently. An example is the presence of an epileptic child in a substance-abusing family.

B. CLASSIFICATION OF FAMILY PATHOLOGY

Since the 1960s, there have been several attempts by family psychiatrists to classify all possible existing family pathologies, as clinical psychiatrists do for individual pathologies. For instance, two pioneer family therapists, Ackerman and Behrens (1956), identified seven deviant family groups, focusing primarily on how a family, as a unique social unit, integrates with its community. Titchener and Emerson (1958) devised six experimental typologies of families based on the cohesiveness of a family in reacting to emotional conflict. Other family researchers have described certain types of family pathology associated with specific individual psychopathologies, such as the pseudomutuality in families of schizophrenics described by Wynne and colleagues (1958) and the schism and skew in families of schizophrenics illustrated by Lidz, Cornelison, Fleck, and Terry (1957).

Based on the perspectives of family development and family interaction patterns, and focusing on the members of the family involved in the manifestation of the pathology, Tseng, Arensdorf, McDermott, Hansen, and Fukunaga (1976) identified six major categories of family pathology: the child-reactive family, the parent-reactive family, the marital-reactive family, the unresolved triangular family, the special-theme family, and the panpathological family.

Clearly the nature of family psychopathology is very different from that of individual psychopathology (N.J. Kaslow, Celano, & Dreelin, 1995). It is not easy to find a satisfactory method and framework in which to develop a comprehensive classification of family psychopathologies for clinical and research use.

C. EXAMPLES OF CULTURE-RELATED FAMILY PROBLEMS

From a family psychiatric point of view, there are various recognized family pathologies that are difficult to describe exhaustively. For the purpose of this chapter, some examples will be listed here regarding family problems that are closely related to cultural factors.

1. Wide Cultural Differences between Generations

It is common for certain differences in viewpoint and opinion between parents and children to be brought about by age, developmental factors, and the different environments in which each generation has grown up. However, when a family faces a rapidly changing cultural environment in its own society or encounters a different sociocultural environment after migrating to an alien culture, the differences between parents and children can become great and create a large schism between generations, resulting in serious family problems. In general, the parents still stick to the traditional ways of viewing and doing things, finding it difficult to adjust to the new changes, whereas the young generation adopts the new ways of life and value systems rather quickly, tending to ignore or even despise the old views and style of life, creating a wide difference between the parents and the children. In association with this, there are confusion and conflict about how to raise and discipline children, which threatens the function and role of the parents.

This phenomenon is often observed among immigrant families. If the transculturally migrated family needs to learn a new language in the hosting society, often the parents have more difficulty in language adjustment. Consequently, the younger generation has more access to knowledge about the hosting society than the parents. The children become the sources of information, reversing the role of parents and children, which often aggravates the confusion in the family and threatens the authority of the parents.

2. Culturally Uprooted Families among Deprived Minorities

When the sociocultural system of a group of people has been rapidly destroyed, families within that system will suffer from a loss of their cultural roots, resulting in deterioration of the family as a whole. This is usually manifested by parents losing their cultural methods of organizing the family and subsequently experiencing confusion about how to properly perform their parental functions. The children, meanwhile, often dissociate themselves from their parents both cognitively and emotionally and are unsure of their identities and directions in life. Such families have not only lost their own identity, but have also lost their cultural guidelines for functioning. This culture-uprooted phenomenon is observed frequently among families of many ethnic minority groups in the United States, including Native Americans, African-Americans, and south Asian refugees, as well as many other ethnic groups around the world who are facing the situation of rapidly losing their traditional culture without establishing a new one.

3. Some Special Family Problems Observed

a. Daughter-in-Law Abused in Hindu Family

The traditional Hindu family is characterized as a mother–son dyad. Based on this household structure, the daughter-in-law holds an inferior position in the family, not only to her mother-in-law but also to her brother-in-law. This creates a potential situation for the daughter-in-law to be physically and/or mentally abused by members of the extended family. These culture-shaped family problems are exemplified in the following case.

A daughter-in-law of Hindu background was brought to the emergency room after she was found attempting to hang herself. Physical examination revealed that not only was there a fresh mark around her neck, indicating that she had tried to end her life by hanging, it was also found that there were numerous scars over her body. Suspecting that she was beaten by others, an inquiry was made by the physi-

cian. However, the patient kept her mouth shut, refusing to admit any intention of self-killing and denying any abuse she received. It took a while for the clinician to finally obtain information through other family members. The patient had just given birth several weeks before. As was the custom, her mother-in-law came to visit her and to see the newborn baby. The mother-in-law decided to stay with them for a couple of days. As the new mother felt weak, she asked her mother-in-law to do the laundry for her. When this was discovered by her brother-in-law, he became upset. According to custom, it was not polite for the daughter-in-law to ask the mother-in-law to do household work, even if she had just given birth and was physically weak. The brother-in-law beat the patient (his sister-in-law) severely as punishment for her impolite behavior toward his mother. When her husband found out about this, he felt that his wife had brought disgrace to the family and beat her again. After facing such harsh treatment not only from her brother-in-law but also from her own husband, she was so frustrated that she tried to end her life.

This case shows that culturally, a certain relationship is described between a mother-in-law and a daughter-in-law, and breaking the rules of such a relationship is not tolerated. Also, according to the Hindu family system, even a brother-in-law has the authority to "discipline" his sister-in-law if the latter does not properly follow the etiquette and rules required by the culture between a mother-in-law and a daughter-in-law.

b. "Parental Abuse Syndrome" Described in Japan

Traditionally, Japanese culture emphasizes the virtue of respecting parents and authority. Therefore, it is almost unbelievable that grown-up children physically abuse their parents nowadays, but the fact is that this is happening, according to Japanese psychiatrists.

After World War II, the number of children in families declined remarkably in Japan. There were usually only two or three at most. There was a high probability that there was only one boy in the household. As a result, the boy was very indulged by his parents, not to mention his grandparents. The situation was complicated by the fact that the Japanese father was usually busy with his work, leaving early and returning home late, seldom having the opportunity to interact with his children. From a cultural point of view, it was considered the mother's job to raise the children. Thus, boys were raised and disciplined mostly by their mothers. According to Yoshimatsu (1984), even when the fathers were at home, the authority of the father was generally questioned and weakened; after the war, the generation of middle-age fathers lost its confidence in providing discipline for its teenage sons. The mother, who seldom had the opportunity to be with her husband, usually devoted her attention and emotion to her children, especially her son. Thus, there was close contact between mother and son (even though from an anthropological point of view, the Japanese family had been described theoretically as a father–son dyad family). As a result, some boys were raised exclusively by their mothers and indulged without a prominent father figure in the household. When these boys reached adolescence, they psychologically felt the need to develop a distance from their parent of the opposite sex (namely, their mothers), tended to react violently when approached by their mothers, reacting to them with repelling action and aggression, resulting in the so-called "parent-abuse" phenomenon.

This culture-related, unique family pathology was observed not only in Japan, but was also becoming rather frequent in China, due primarily to the fact that, under the one-child-per-couple official policy, many boys were spoiled by their parents and grandparents when they are small and became violent toward their parents when they became teenagers and their demands at home were not satisfied.

c. Collective Family Mental Disorder

Psychiatric literatures have shown that occasionally more than one member of a family may become mentally ill through a process of contagion — forming so-called "double insanity" or "family insanity" (*folie à deu* or *folie à familie,* in French). This psychiatric condition may take the form of dissociation, conversion, delusion, or abnormal behaviors. Although the phenomenon of *folie á familie* is considered rare, sporadic occurrences have been reported from Malaysia (Woon, 1976), Taiwan (Tseng, 1969) [cross-reference to to Chapter 14: Epidemic Mental Disorders (Sections III,B,4 and D,1, respectively], or the Philippines (Goduco-Angular & Wintrob, 1964).

A review of such contagious collective family mental disorders made it apparent that in addition to the existing premorbid personality of the family members, a strong emotional bond between family members facilitated the occurrence of a collective psychiatric condition in the family, particularly when it faced a stressful situation together. To share and be involved in a similar psychiatric condition appeared to be an alternative way for family members to deal with the common crisis they encountered. It was speculated that such an unusual contagious family reaction tended to be observed in societies where family ties were stressed.

d. Family Suicide Observed in Japan

Another unique family pathology is family suicide (or *ikkasinjiu*) in Japan (Ohara, 1963). Family suicide refers to situations in which suicidal behavior involves multiple members of a family. In a strict sense, this phenomenon occurs as the double suicide of the parents coupled with the murders of their children. Family suicide is frequently observed in Japan. It usually occurs when one of the parents encounters a culturally unbearable situation, such as severe debt or an incurable disease, or becomes involved in socially disgraceful events and decides to solve the problem by ending his or her life. The spouse, upon learning of the contemplated suicide, consents to die with his or her mate. Eventually the parents kill their young children and finally kill themselves, i.e., homicide and suicide are combined, or they make plans for the whole family to die together, perhaps by taking poison. Recently, a more modernized method of family suicide has been through drowning after driving their automobile into the sea (see Fig. 13-13).

As elaborated earlier [cross-reference to Chapter 22: Suicidal Behavior (Section III,A,2)], there are several motives behind family suicide. One is the cultural belief that death is one way to resolve problems in life. The other is the cultural assumption that no one will care for the orphaned children, and that they are best cared for by their parents. Family suicide occurs in a society that greatly values the ties between parent and child; it is believed that it is better to die together as a family than to leave behind a member of a broken family. Although it has long been forbidden legally in Japan for parents to carry out family suicide, this phenomenon is still observed. The reaction of society is usually sympathetic rather than critical.

III. CULTURE AND FAMILY ASSESSMENT

A. Cultural Considerations in Family Assessment

1. Expansion of the Understanding of Family Dimensions

If we are clinically working with families of different ethnic/cultural groups, we must extend our orientation and understanding of the dimensions of the family. In addition to the conventional dimensions with which family researchers and therapists are concerned (i.e., family development, family subsystems, and family groups), it is necessary to expand our knowledge and understanding of the cultural aspects of family systems focused on by cultural anthropologists. These include anthropological aspects of marriage forms, marital residential choice, kinship relations, and family values as observed by the family under consideration.

2. Clarification of the Concepts of Normality and Dysfunction

When an evaluator is assessing a person with a cultural background different from his/her own, the concepts and definitions of normality and pathology must be considered cautiously (Westermeyer, 1985). Such caution should also be applied and exercised when examining a family. The definitions of "functional" versus "dysfunctional," or "healthy" versus "pathological" vary among families of different cultural backgrounds.

Various definitions of normality have been applied when dealing with individuals, namely normality construed as "healthy," "utopian," "average," "processing," or "coping and adaptation" (Offer & Sabshin, 1974). In a similar way, family functioning may be approached in different ways, such as "asymptomatic," "optional," "average," "transactional," or "adaptive" family functioning (Walsh, 1982).

B. Process of Culture-Adjusted Family Evaluation

1. Cultural Engagement

In a family session it is essential that the evaluator or therapist be able to engage the family in accordance with the background of the family members, which includes their personal style, educational level, and social class. Along the same lines, it is desirable for the family therapist to engage culturally with the family (Faulkner & Kich, 1983). By simply learning how to extend social greetings or demonstrate etiquette in accordance with the family's ethnic or cultural background, the therapist will show respect and understanding of the ethnic or cultural background of the family. Such actions will assist the therapist in establishing a rapport with the family more rapidly.

2. Gearing to an Existing Authority Hierarchy

Families of different cultural backgrounds may observe and practice different hierarchial patterns of authority. It is very important to recognize such hierarchical patterns early in the therapy sessions and to try to comply with and utilize these systems, even though they may be subtle or almost invisible.

For instance, in dealing with Asian families, which traditionally show great respect for the father's authority, it is important to begin by paying respects to the father and addressing questions to him, inviting him to start the conversation or asking his permission to begin dialogue with the other family members. In many Pacific families, which are traditionally characterized by a maternal hierarchy, the therapist should show respect to the grandmother of the family, no matter how quiet she may appear and even if she does not exercise her culturally inherited authority in front of the other family members. After all, she is the person behind the scenes who ultimately makes the final decisions regarding the family. If the therapist does not handle her correctly, the cooperation of the entire family could be lost.

3. Culture-Relevant Exposure of Private Matters

The subjects that can be revealed to outsiders and the way disclosures are made are closely related to cultural practices. In the process of exploring family life, certain rules need to be observed in dealing with some private matters. For instance, when examining family history in Micronesian families, direct inquiries about the death of parents or grandparents must never be made, as it is taboo for them to mention the death of an ancestor. Micronesians have indirect and subtle ways of mentioning the demise of their ancestors; one must learn subtle ways of inquiring about such matters. In dealing with a family that customarily respects parental authority, it is very important not to let the parents disclose their shortcomings or faults in front of their children, as these disclosures could hurt their images as authoritative parents.

C. The Scope of Culture-Oriented Family Assessment

In order to conduct comprehensive family assessments, a certain format for evaluating various aspects of the family has been proposed by family therapists. The format is expanded and revised for cross-cultural application with more elaboration on the cultural aspects of family function (Tseng & Hsu, 1991) as follows.

1. Basic Information

Genogram: Description of the relations among three generations.
Background of each family member, including age, sex, education, occupation, and religion.
Medical/psychiatric/legal history of family members.

2. Presenting Problems

Identification of current problems that primarily concern the family.
Any precipitating factors or circumstances for the development of problems.
The understanding of the nature of the problem by the family.
The family's goals and expectations for treatment.

3. Ethnic/Cultural Background of the Family

Marriage form: Refers to the number of spouses in a marriage, such as monogamy, polygamy (polygyny, or polyandry), and other forms of marriage (such as group marriage).
Descent system: Rule that defines how descent is affiliated with sets of kin, such as patrilineal (through men's kin), matrilineal (through women's kin), bilineal (through both men's and women's kin), and ambilateral (through either men's or women's kin).
Rule of marital choice: Exogamous (partner to be chosen from outside the group) or endogamous (partner to be chosen from inside the group. Arranged by family or clan or by self-choice by the partners themselves.
Postmarital residence: Matrilocal (with or near the wife's parents' place of residence), patrilocal (with or near the husband's parents' place), bilocal (with either the wife's or the husband's

parents' place), or neolocal (at a new place of their own).

Households: Nuclear (only the couple and their unmarried children), stem (the couple, their parents, and the couple's unmarried children), joint (the couple and their children, their parents, and the couple's unmarried siblings), or extended (the couple, their children, their parents, and the couple's married siblings and their children).

Authority and power distribution: Patriarchal (father or grandfather), matriarchal (mother or grandmother), egalitarian (both father and mother), or democratic (all members of the household).

Primary axis (dyad): Conjugal (horizontal between husband and wife), consanguineal (vertical between parent and child of one gender), or sibling (such as between brother and sister).

Family values/beliefs/attitudes: A particular set of value systems or beliefs jointly shared and firmly held by a family. It may cover many areas, including concept of marriage and family, role expectations for family members, child-rearing practices and child discipline, moral issues, life philosophy, religion, sexual attitudes, family planning, generational relationship and gap, and attitude toward aging and death.

4. Family Developmental History

A longitudinal and chronological review of family development through the stage of marital formation, childbearing, child rearing, family maturing, family contraction, and any developmental variations, including separation, divorce, single parent family, and remarriage.

5. Family–Group Interactional Patterns

Assessment through parameters of boundaries, alignment, cohesion, power/control, communication, affection, hierarchial formation, and role divisions.

6. Family Stress/Problems

The life events, changes, or situations that cause significant psychological distress in a family. The problems may rise due to the situations for which the family has had little preparation, any decisive changes for which old patterns of adjustment are not adequate, or any emotional tensions, anxiety, or dysphoria related to intrafamily matter.

7. Family Coping Patterns

Some examples of coping that can be utilized to solve family problems are negotiation, compromise, active problem-solving, reframing, passive appraisal, conflict avoidance, scapegoating, or paralysis by ambivalence.

IV. CULTURE AND FAMILY THERAPY

A. CULTURAL CONSIDERATIONS OF FAMILY THERAPY

1. Applicability of Family Therapy

Family therapy should be considered and applied whenever it is indicated and necessary, as long as the problems are dynamic or closely related to family relations or there is a need to mobilize family resources and make good use of the input of family members to cope with and adjust to problems.

It has been suggested that family therapy is particularly appropriate and indicated for ethnic–cultural groups that emphasize family structure in their life patterns, such as the Italians, Portuguese, or Chinese. Clinical experience, however, has shown that an emphasis on family and close family interrelations does not directly favor the family therapy approach. As pointed out by Moitoza (1982), Portuguese families' closed family system prevents them from actively seeking family therapy; instead, they attempt to solve their problems via their own family resources and support systems. When a close family seeks therapy, the family's values and tight intermember relations can be utilized; it will usually take considerable effort, however, for a therapist to work on the intense and complicated family dynamics.

Alternatively, it cannot be assumed that family-oriented therapy is unsuitable for families of cultural groups that deemphasize the family system and place more relative value on an individual system. Family therapy may actually prove to be particularly useful to such unlikely candidates by providing an opportunity for self-examination of the relatively neglected aspects of their lives (i.e., the family system) as well as by encouraging them to place more value on the function of the family.

2. Members to be Included for Therapy

Family therapy traditionally emphasized the importance of including all family members living under the same roof in the treatment sessions. This was based on the view that family members, no matter how old or young, interacted with each other as a system. Any meaningful therapeutic improvements needed to involve all the members who were related in their actual daily lives. Contemporary family therapy has revised this treatment approach, regarding it as not absolutely necessary to have all family members present together in the therapeutic session. As long as the therapy is oriented conceptually toward the "family," it is considered family therapy.

No matter which approach is undertaken, it is very important to conceive the unit of family broadly depending on who is living together and who has a significant impact on daily family life. This is particularly true from a cultural point of view. As pointed out by Wilson, Phillip, Kohn, and Curry-El (1995), if the identified family is composed of an extended family, then the therapy needs to accommodate the characteristics of the extended family structure. Within this structure there exist reciprocal obligations and mutual influence on decision-making and membership roles. The presence of grandparents as well as other extended family members in many minorities families speaks to the necessary inclusion of these members in therapy.

3. Therapist–Family Relationship

When the family to be treated has a different cultural background than the therapist, cultural effects on the therapist–family relationship need to be closely examined from the very beginning of contact. Three areas need special attention. First, ethnic/racial/cultural transference in the therapist–client relationship needs to be evaluated and addressed. The same principle and management applied in individual therapy may be extended to family therapy (cross-reference to Chapter 36: Intercultural Psychotherapy).

Second, there is a need to respect and utilize the culturally defined and sanctioned family hierarchy and relations already existing within the family. Who is the ultimate authority in the household (father, mother, or the grandmother)? Who needs to be respected and needs to utilize his or her power to control the family behavior? Does any hierarchical relation exist between the husband and the wife or do they relate and function equally? These things need to be found out and caution taken not to ignore them. Even among children, does any hierarchy exist due to gender or birth order? It would be a mistake to allow a younger sister to make comments that indicated a lack of respect toward older brothers if a gender/age hierarchy is valued among the siblings (cross-reference to Chapter 3: Marriage and Family).

Finally, there is a need to be aware of and carefully manage the effect of the therapist's own cultural background and value system on the process and direction of treatment, particularly if the therapist and the family have ethnic/cultural differences. These include basic family issues, such as how a family should relate to each other, how to make decisions, who has the final authority, what kind of coping is considered functional, and so on — all aspects subject to cultural impact and bias beyond therapeutic choice.

4. Matching of Treatment Methods

Many different schools or modalities of therapy have been described and emphasized by various groups of therapists (Crespi, 1988; F.W. Kaslow,

1982). There has been a recent tendency to integrate these diverse modalities into a set of unified and comprehensive systematic models. Is there any particular fitness between the family types and the choice of treatment? Unfortunately, this issue has not yet been examined thoroughly, particularly from a cross-cultural perspective. However, there are some suggestions derived from clinical experience. For example, Falicov (1982), investigating Mexican families, and Minuchin, Montalvo, Guerney, Rosman, and Schumer (1967), working with Chicano families, have proposed that the cultural emphasis on hierarchies within these families lends itself to a structural family therapy approach. In contrast, Herz and Rosen (1982) mentioned that the Jewish family closely relates to a cultural tendency of treasuring suffering as a shared value. By emphasizing the verbal expression of feelings in family therapy, the focus of therapy on this process and interaction can motivate Jewish families to see talking and insight as relevant solutions. Zuk (1978) has pointed out that Jews generally do well in family therapy. The favorable response of Jewish families stems from their cultural emphasis on high familism, high egalitarianism, maternal intrusiveness, verbal rather than physical aggressiveness, an assertive stance toward problem-solving, and the maintenance of a scapegoat theme. It has been suggested by Zuk that in treating Jewish families, it is important to keep this entire set of values in mind rather than any one particular value.

5. Application of Certain Family Therapy Techniques

In addition to basic family therapy techniques, certain special therapy techniques may be used in family therapy. From a cultural point of view, caution is needed when certain therapy techniques are applied. For instance, special caution must be exercised with families of cultural groups that are not accustomed to direct confrontation. As elaborated by Costello (1977), young children in an Anglo setting might actively voice their opinions on therapeutic intervention. Children in Chicano families, however, are

unlikely to be allowed to participate in their parent's business. If a child were to disagree openly with his or her father, particularly in front of others (including the therapist), the father's shame would be translated into physical discipline of the child as soon as they got home. Thus, the therapist should take pains *not* to allow the child to actively confront his or her father in the family session.

Role playing is one therapeutic technique that can be utilized to induce practical and concrete change in behavior among family members. However, it is necessary to consider how family members will interpret and react to this therapeutic procedure. With a family from a culture that emphasizes hierarchy and formality, it would be rather difficult for the parents and children to act out "informal" and "strange" behavior roles that do not respect hierarchy. Likewise, the technique of "reframing" or "paradox interpretation" should be applied carefully so as not to provoke cultural resistance or misunderstanding.

6. Utilization of Culturally Sanctioned Family Coping Patterns

The strengths and coping mechanisms that already exist in the functioning of a family can often be utilized successfully in family therapy. Within a Chinese family, for example, family life is geared toward the children, and it is considered virtuous for the parents to act benevolently to give their children a better life. With this cultural orientation, if there is a need to mobilize the parents in the course of treatment, to change their behavior or improve their interaction with their children, the therapist can appeal to parental benevolence, reinforcing the parents' intentions "to do the best for the sake of (their) children," as pointed out by Hsu (1983).

After working with American Indian families, Attneave (1982) suggested that the therapist should not hesitate to share the interest that families usually have in keeping alive their own native language, folkways, crafts, and values associated with their tribal identities. Restoration of a sense of innate worth and goodness, of feelings of adequacy, and of the integration of person, place, and family is essential to American Indian families who must constantly work to rebuild their cultural identity.

A unique form of therapy was traditionally practiced in Hawaii in the past, called *ho'oponoppono* (to set things right) [cross-reference to Chapter 33: Culture-Influenced Unique Psychotherapy (Section II,B)]. When there was conflict within a family, or an extended family, this practice was used to heal the conflict between family members. Recognition of wrongness, apology, and acceptance of the apology were encouraged through the session, which was participated in by the family members involved. It is an indigenous family therapy that utilizes culturally sanctioned coping mechanisms to resolve family problems (Ito, 1985).

B. CULTURAL IMPLICATIONS OF FAMILY THERAPY

There are numerous ways to conceptualize the nature of therapy. For instance, from the point of view of nonspecific healing, cultivation of hope for the client is interpreted as the major function of therapy; from an analytic point of view, it is working on resistance; and from an existential perspective, it is working on changing life attitudes. From a culture point of view, there are several implications of family therapy, as follows.

1. To Restore the Cultural Norm of Family Functioning

In each society, there is a setting-dependent, culturally sanctioned way for a family to function, interact, and adapt. If for some reason a family is unable to perform in this way, the purpose of therapy is to help the family restore culturally appropriate functioning.

For instance, within polygamous societies, harmony among the wives of the same husband needs to be maintained if the functioning of the household is to be maintained. The primary goal of family therapy under these circumstances is to help the wives avoid open conflict and rivalry among themselves. However, in a primarily monogamous society, the emphasis of marital therapy is on helping the couple nurture a one-to-one relationship without seeking involvement with others beyond the monogamous system.

2. To Establish a Cultural System in a Family

It is necessary to have certain common rules and principles observed within a family; these are essential to the value system and in some ways can be referred to as the "culture" of the family. If for any reason this family culture is lacking or only vaguely present, family members may not be sure how to behave. The object of therapy should be to help the family establish commonly shared values (Trotzer, 1981), ideologies, beliefs, customs, and rituals (Palazzoli, Boscolo, Cecchin, & Prata, 1977) so that each family member may know and observe them. It would also be useful to help family members strengthen their ethnic identity (McGoldrick & Giordano, 1996). Disorganized and culturally uprooted families are examples of families that need this kind of focus in therapy.

3. To Promote Cultural Exchange within a Family

When there is a great gap in opinions, beliefs, and attitudes among different family members (either between parents and children or between spouses), the goal of family therapy is to promote the exchange of different points of view and to enhance cultural empathy and cultural translation (DiNicola, 1986). This is particularly true for a family that, by culture influence, is not used to open communication and the exchange of ideas among family members, between parents and children, even between spouses. It becomes the therapist's role to enhance the communication among family members, as well as to perform as a "cultural broker" or a "bridge person" for them, offering interpretation and reframing cultural perspectives.

4. To Permit a Cultural Time-Out for a Family

For some families, the nature of stress and subsequent problems are directly related to at least some family members experiencing exhaustion from constant and long-term compliance to a particular set of rules and way of life that are too restrictive or alien. In such cases, the goal of therapy is to provide periodic cultural time-outs or "cultural islands" to which they retreat and take a vacation. This is particularly true for intermarried couples, or transculturally migrated families. To spend some time on certain occasions to resume their original cultural styles of life will help them cope with the new challenges. Every person needs a vacation once in awhile. A family needs a cultural time-out periodically as well.

5. To Supply a Counterculture System for a Family

Family life is sometimes restricted greatly by rules, concepts, and patterns of life that allow only limited ways of coping with situations. Under these circumstances, it is therapeutic to help family members recognize the existence of alternatives and broaden their access to other resources. Occasionally, we can be so trapped in our own tunnel vision of life and value systems that we are unable to receive or consider different attitudes or views. In this situation, bringing in opposite but functional views for consideration will not only neutralize the family's extreme position and attitudes, but will provide an opportunity for family members to reexamine their orientations and belief systems (Hare-Mustin, 1978). This could be a major cultural implication of family therapy.

In summary, the purpose of family therapy can be described from a cultural perspective as working on the cultural system of the family in various ways with the aim of promoting the function of the family. In the treatment of an individual, it is necessary to define what is considered a "healthy" or "functional" persona as a standard to guide the course of therapy. Analogously, in family therapy it is necessary to visualize a well-functioning, normal family as the final goal toward which treatment is directed. The concept of a "functional" or "healthy" family needs to be defined carefully and elaborated further in therapy for families of different cultural groups so that it is consistent with the relevant cultural background.

REFERENCES

Ackerman, N.W., & Behrens, M.L. (1956). A study of family diagnosis. *American Journal of Orthopsychiatry, 26,* 66–78.

Ariel, S. (1999). *Culturally competent family therapy: A general model.* Westport, CT: Greenwood.

Attneave, C. (1982). American Indians and Alaska native families: Emigrants in their own homeland. In M. McGoldrick, J.K. Pearce, & J. Giordano (Eds.), *Ethnicity and family therapy* (pp. 55–83). New York: Guilford Press.

Costello, R.M. (1977). "Chicano liberation" and the Mexican-American marriage. *Psychiatric Annals, 7,* 64–73.

Crespi, T.D. (1988). Specifications and guidelines for specialization in family therapy: Implications for practicum supervisors. *International Journal of Family Psychiatry, 9,* 181–191.

DiNicola, V.F. (1985). Family therapy and transcultural psychiatry: An emerging synthesis. Part II: Portability and cultural change. *Transcultural Psychiatric Research Review, 22,* 151–180.

DiNicola, V.F. (1986). Beyond Babel: Family therapy as cultural translation. *International Journal of Family Psychiatry, 7,* 179–191.

Falicov, C.J. (1982). Mexican families. In M. McGoldrick, J.K. Pearce, & J. Giordano (Eds.), *Ethnicity and family therapy* (pp. 134–163). New York: Guilford Press.

Falicov, C.J. (Vol. Ed.). (1983). *Cultural perspectives in family therapy.* Rockvill, MD: Aspen.

Faulkner, J., & Kich, G.K. (1983). Assessment and engagement stages in therapy with the interracial family. In C.J. Falicov (Vol. Ed.), *Cultural perspectives in family therapy.* Rockvill, MD: Aspen.

Goduco-Angular, C., & Wintrob, R. (1964). *Folie à famille* in the Philippines. *Psychiatric Quarterly, 38,* 278–291.

Hare-Mustin, R.T. (1978). A feminist approach to family therapy. *Family Process, 17,* 181–194.

Herz, F.M., & Rosen, E.J. (1982). Jewish families. In M. McGoldrick, J.K. Pearce, & J. Giordano (Eds.), *Ethnicity and family therapy* (pp. 364–392). New York: Guilford Press.

Hsu, J. (1983). Asian family interaction patterns and their therapeutic implications. *International Journal of Family Psychiatry, 4*(4), 307–320.

Ito, K.L. (1985). Ho'oponopono, "to make right": Hawaiian conflict resolution and metaphor in the construction of a family therapy. *Culture, Medicine and Psychiatry, 9*(2), 201–217.

Kaslow, F.W. (Ed.). (1982). *The international book of family therapy*. New York: Brunner/Mazel.

Kaslow, N.J., Celano, M., & Dreelin, E.D. (1995). A cultural perspective on family theory and therapy. *Psychiatric Clinics of North America, 18*(3), 621–633.

Lidz, T., Cornelison, A.R., Fleck, S., & Terry, D. (1957). The intrafamilial environment of schizophrenic patients. *American Journal of Psychiatry, 114,* 241–248.

McGoldrick, M., & Giordano, J. (1996). Overview: Ethnicity and family therapy. In M. McGoldrick, J. Giordano, & J.K. Pearce (Eds.), *Ethnicity and family therapy* (2nd ed.). New York: Guilford Press.

McGoldrick, M., Giordano, J., & Pearce, J.K. (Eds.). (1996). *Ethnicity and family therapy* (2nd ed.). New York: Guilford Press.

Mindel, C.H., & Habenstein, R.W. (Eds.). (1981). *Ethnic families in America: Patterns and variations* (2nd ed.). New York: Elsevier.

Minuchin, S., Montalvo, B., Guerney, B.G., Rosman, B.L., & Schumer, B.G. (1967). *Families of the slums*. New York: Basic Books.

Minuchin, S., Rosman, B.L., & Baker, L. (1978). *Psychosomatic families: Anorexia nervosa in context*. Cambridge, MA: Harvard University Press.

Moitoza, E. (1982). Portuguese families. In M. McGoldrick, J.K. Pearce, & J. Giordano (Eds.), *Ethnicity and family therapy* (pp. 412–437). New York: Guilford Press.

Offer, D., & Sabshin, M. (1974). *Normality: Theoretical and clinical concepts of mental health* (2nd ed.). New York: Basic Books.

Ohara, K. (1963). Characteristics of suicides in Japan, especially of parent-child double suicide. *American Journal of Psychiatry, 120*(4), 382–385.

Palazzoli, M.S., Boscolo, L., Cecchin, G.F., & Prata, G. (1977). Family rituals: A powerful tool in family therapy. *Family Process, 16,* 445–453.

Purcel, K., Brady, K., Chai, H., Muser, J., Molk, L., Gordon, N., & Means, J. (1969). The effect of asthma in children on experimental separation from the family. *Psychosomatic Medicine, 31,* 144–164.

Sue, D.W., & Sue, D. (1990). Cross-cultural family conseling. In D.W. Sue & D. Sue *Counseling the culturally different: Theory and practice*. New York: Wiley.

Titchener, J., & Emerson, R. (1958). Some methods for the study of family interaction in personality development. *Psychiatric Research Reports, 10,* 72–100.

Trotzer, J.P. (1981). The certrality of values in families and family therapy. *International Journal of Family Therapy, 3,* 42–55.

Tseng, W.S. (1969). A paranoid family in Taiwan: A dynamic study of *folie à famille*. *Archives of General Psychiatry, 21,* 55–63.

Tseng, W.S., Arensdorf, A.M., McDermott, J.F., Jr., Hansen, M.J., & Fukunaga, C. (1976). Family diagnosis and classification. *Journal of the American Academy of Child Psychiatry, 15,* 15–35.

Tseng, W.S., & Hsu, J. (1991). *Culture and family: Problems and therapy*. New York: Haworth Press.

Walsh, F. (1982). Conceptualization of normal family function. In F. Walsh (Ed.), *Normal family process*. New York: Guilford.

Wender, P.H., Rosenthal, D., Kety, S.S., Schulsinger, F., & Welner, J. (1974). Crossfostering: A research strategy for clarifying the role of genetic and experiential factors in the etiology of schizophrenia. *Archives of General Psychiatry, 30,* 121–128.

Westermeyer, J. (1985). Psychiatric diagnosis across cultural boundaries. *American Journal of Psychiatry, 142,* 798–805.

Wilson, M.N., Phillip, D.G., Kohn, L.P., & Curry-El, J.A. (1995). Cultural relativistic approach toward ethnic minorities in family therapy. In J.F. Aponte, R.Y. Rivers, & J. Wohl (Eds.), *Psychological interventions and cultural diversity*. Boston: Allyn & Bacon.

Woon, T.H. (1976). Epidemic hysteria in a Malaysian Chinese extended family. *Medical Journal of Malaysia, 31,* 108–112.

Wyne, L.C., Ryckoff, I.M., Day, J., & Hirsch, S.I. (1958). Pseudomutuality in the family relations of schizophrenia. *Psychiatry, 21,* 205–220.

Yoshimatsu, K. (1984). *Parent abuse in Japanese culture*. Presented at the Japanese Culture and Mental Health Conference, East-West Center, Honolulu.

Zuk, G.H. (1978). A therapist's perspective on Jewish family values. *Journal of marriage and family counseling, 4,* 103–110.

41

Working with Aged Persons

I. UNDERSTANDING PSYCHOLOGICAL PROBLEMS ENCOUNTERED

Aged persons are vulnerable to certain psychiatric disorders. Some of them, such as dementia, are predominantly related to biological or organic factors, whereas others, such as prolonged grief reaction after the loss of a spouse, feelings of insecurity due to aging, and frustrations associated with deteriorating physical conditions, are mainly attributed to psychological factors. The problems that are psychological in nature are usually colored by cultural elements. This chapter discusses the cultural aspects of psychological problems that may be encountered by the elderly of diverse cultural backgrounds. Some of the problems are of an intrapsychic nature, such as views and attitudes toward aging and death; many concern interpersonal matters, such as adjusting to living with their adult children; whereas others are social, such as the availability and utilization of social support systems for the elderly.

A. NEGATIVE VIEWS AND ATTITUDES ABOUT AGING

Negative views and attitudes about aging are fundamental issues related to the psychological problems of aged persons. As elaborated previously, an individual's views and attitudes toward aging will be shaped by cultural attitudes and values toward aged persons [cross-reference to Chapter 7: Late Adult Life: Aging and Death (Sections II,A and B)]. If aging is viewed as negative, aging will become an undesirable stage of life. If getting older is seen as a positive experience, then approaching the later stages of life can be enjoyable and met with optimistism.

In many societies, particularly traditional agricultural societies, the wisdom of past experience is often valued for the improvement of production as well as the regulation of social interaction. Becoming old is equivalent to being experienced in life. In order to maintain social order, the status of the elderly is emphasized. Thus, the elderly are associated with respect and authority. They are often given certain roles in daily life and contribute to the functioning of the family as a whole. Therefore, there is a basic security and dignity associated with the process of aging. It is relatively free from the fear of being alone, neglected, and abandoned.

In contrast, modern, industrial, urban societies, such as those in contemporary Europe and America, are as a whole characterized by an emphasis on youth. When you are young, you can enjoy the opportunities, prospects, beauty, and attractions in life. However, when wrinkles appear on your face and your hair turns gray, this is perceived as the end of the glorious stage of life. Becoming old is considered the beginning of despair and hopelessness. An effort is made to hide age, to pretend that you are still young, and there is an unspoken fear of being alone, ignored, and disabled. This general attitude toward aging in a society will negatively color the life of the elderly.

B. BEING PSYCHOLOGICALLY UNPREPARED FOR THE LATE STAGE OF LIFE

Associated with improvements in social and health conditions, the human life span has increased tremendously during the past several decades. Instead of dying at the age of 40 or 50 at the most, as was the case a mere half-century ago, it is now common to live on average until 70 or 80 in most developed societies. However, as this is still a new experience for human beings, many people are not well prepared to live in such a late stage in life, many decades after their retirement from work.

For instance, in China, the age for retirement from work is officially set at 55 for men and 50 for women. This is intended to give more opportunities for young people to work and for the elderly to enjoy life with their public retirement allowance. Traditionally, Chinese have considered old age a time "to be cared for" by their (adult) children and "to enjoy life" with their young grandchildren. This may still be true in rural agricultural settings, but, associated with rapid social and economic improvements, this style of life for the aged cannot be expected anymore in urban areas. However, the generations that are approaching the ages of 60 or 70 were not raised with the concept of living "independently." Their life expectancy (at birth) suddenly jumped from about 55 to almost 75 within a period of a few decades. They are not psychologically prepared to live "actively" and "enjoyably" for two decades after their official "early" retirement at 50. Many of them feel lost psychologically.

This phenomenon is quite true in many societies, such as Japan, Korean, and Singapore in Asia, and in other areas around the world, where there have been rapid and remarkable social, economic, and health improvements, and the life expectancy has suddenly increased by 20 or so years.

C. LOSS OF MARITAL PARTNER

Associated with the process of getting old, sooner or later, one spouse in a married couple is going to lose his or her marital partner and become a widow or widower. Even though this is an unavoidable and often very sad event in a person's life, the experience of losing a spouse varies among individuals in different societies. From a cultural perspective, the experience varies according to many factors. Most importantly, it depends on how much the marital relationship means to an individual person. In a society in which the spouse is the primary axis in family life — if, in contrast to parent–child or sibling relationships, or other family dyads, the husband–wife dyad has more weight in their lives, and has been the sole resource of emotional support — the loss of the primary partner will have a significant impact on the life of the widow or widower. In contrast, if the spousal relation is embedded in other dyads of the family system, the loss of the spouse will not make as desperate a difference in the life of the person, who will still be surrounded by other family members.

In addition, the fate of the widow or widower will be shaped by cultural expectations and regulations. For instance, as described previously [cross-reference Chapter 7: Late Adult Life: Aging and Death (Section V,B,2)], traditionally, a widow in India has to comply with the restricted social life demanded by her culture. She is not permitted to attend social activities or to meet any men socially besides her father-in-law and brothers-in-law. Based on such a cultural view and practices, widows become vulnerable to depression. In contrast, widows in other cultures are encouraged to observe relatively short, formal mourning periods and then are permitted to engaged in ordinary social activities again, and even to become involved in relationships with men if they wish. This certainly will influence the quality of life of the widows after the loss of their spouses.

Depending on the culture-defined role divisions between husband and wife, the life of a widower will vary greatly after the loss of his wife. For instance, husbands in Japan or Korea are seldom involved in domestic chores. For a man to enter the kitchen is culturally almost taboo. Most men never learned how to cook rice or make tea, not to mention how to cook daily meals or do the laundry. If a man's wife dies and he is living by himself, without children — a common phenomenon occurring more often in urban settings — he is sure to encounter practical problems of daily survival. This is not necessarily true for Chinese men, who do not have such cultural rules and most of whom know how to work in the kitchen if they have to. Thus, the nature and severity of the same experience of losing their spouses are shaped by varying cultural factors.

D. Relationship Problems with Adult Children

When a person becomes old, the nature of the relationship with his or her adult children will change. This is a part of the change associated with an individual's life cycle as well as that of the family. The new generation of adult children begin to have their own life experiences, attitudes toward things, and philosophical views, which may be considerably different from those of their aged parents. This is particularly true if relatively rapid sociocultural change has occurred in the society. Within a family, the locus of power will shift gradually from the aged parents to the adult children. Thus, psychologically, there may be a struggle associated with the reversed parent–child relationship.

This reversed parent–child relationship becomes more severe for immigrants who have migrated to culturally different host societies. In contrast to their young adult children, the aged parents, often become vulnerable. They become underprivileged in terms of

learning the new language, knowledge, and experiences necessary for adjustment to the host society. Their wisdom and experience from their society of origin become useless or even obstacles to their adapting to their new lives. If the host society's language is foreign to them, their problems in communication and catching up on knowledge will become severe. They will have to depend heavily on their adult children for social life outside of the household. If they have grandchildren, they often speak the new language of the host society, but not the native language of the grandparents, while the grandparents speak very little of the new language; thus, severe communications obstacles will exist between them.

If the migration is to a society that puts less emphasis and respect on aged persons, the loss for the migrated aged person is doubled if he or she came originally from a society in which aged persons have a certain status and value. It is difficult for aged persons to follow the family and migrate transculturally — often to a more advanced and developed society. It is often too late for them to learn to drive a car or to learn a new language, and they are shut off from the opportunities of gaining new knowledge and adapting to the new lifestyle. They also have to become humble in their relations with their culturally more privileged adult children, as well as their grandchildren.

E. Loss of Friends and Social Network

It is common for aged persons to gradually lose some of their old friends as time passes. Unless they are socially active and make new friends, their social network is likely to decrease. This is not a very great problem if the society is structured in such a way that every person is closely connected with others. For instance, in a small village, almost everyone knows everyone and is related to them in certain ways in daily life. A person does not have to work hard to make friends; friends and relatives are always around. When a person gets old, he may lose his closer personal friends, but the loss of his social network is relatively minimal. In contrast, in a metropolitan urban setting, where people are secluded in their private apartments, rarely knowing who lives next door, then a person's social network will certainly deteriorate as he ages, unless he keeps active and involved in a social network beyond the family. Thus, the social and cultural systems will affect the nature and severity of the loss of an older person's social relations — a crucial factor that shapes the lives of the aging (Baker, 1996).

F. Availability and Utilization of Social Support Systems

In general, in addition to family life and domestic systems, there are public life and societal systems for networking and support. According to their cultures, some societies concentrate more heavily on the former and less on the latter, whereas others emphasis both. In culturally conservative societies, when a person becomes old, sick, or disabled, he may still prefer living with his own family in a personal setting rather than in a public institution, such as a nursing home. The resistance to living in a nursing home is rather strong in many societies, including Asian. It is considered a "disgrace" to be separated from your family and "dumped" with strangers in a nursing home. It is not only the aged themselves who do not like it, but often their adult children as well. They feel that they will be criticized by their friends or relatives for allowing their aged parents to live in such a "miserable" place. This is rather in great contrast to other societies, which consider it a natural alternative to live in an institutional setting if it becomes difficult to live in a family environment. Views on being placed in a nursing home are only minimally negative.

G. Suffering from Somatic Conditions

One of the common issues encountered in old age is the gradual loss of physical health and increased somatic dysfunction. This includes the functions of vision, hearing, and motor activity. Feelings of inadequacy and frustration result and become common emotional issues that need to be dealt with in working with aged persons. However, the suffering and frustration caused by somatic dysfunction are influenced by an individual's personality, attitudes toward aging, and the nature of the physical problems, as well as the cultural environment that shapes a person's life.

If a person is living in an environment that greatly values youth and physical activity, any somatic dysfunction will be more frustrating. If there is a lack of adequate support from family, friends, and the surrounding environment, the physical problems will be perceived as more or less intolerable. We all know that the problems of the body are not purely physical matters, but are related to how the physical condition is perceived and reacted to psychologically. This applies particularly to the physical problems of aged persons.

H. Feelings of Insecurity

One psychological problem often encountered by the elderly is the feeling of insecurity. This is related to the elderly person having fewer resources and a lessened ability to deal with crises or dangerous situations. The lack of the ability to cope with crises or danger is transferred into a feeling of insecurity. The feeling of insecurity will increase if there are more crises or danger in daily life and less support from external resources, including family, friends, or the community. Needless to say, deterioration of the physical condition will add to feelings of insecurity as well.

There are numerous ways to manifest feelings of insecurity, including fear of crime in the living environment. Although crime occurring in the community is a social phenomenon, the elderly are sensitive about the risks it presents and may react with different degrees of sensitivity. A good cross-societal example has been offered by Ginsberg (1984–1985). He investigated the impact of the fear of crime on the daily behavior of elderly Jews in two racially mixed, deteriorating neighborhoods, one in Boston and the other in

London. He found that the Boston elderly retreated behind locked doors, whereas the London elderly continued their daily routines almost uninterrupted. In Ginsberg's interpretation, the basic difference between these two groups was that the London Jews still felt themselves to be a part of their community, whereas the Boston Jews felt alienated from it, resulting in different coping behavior for their anxiety.

II. PSYCHOTHERAPY FOR THE ELDERLY: TECHNICAL ISSUES

A. Basic Exercise of Practically Oriented, Brief Psychotherapy

It is a general rule among geriatric psychiatrists that it is better to focus on practical aspects of life and realistic problems in therapy for elderly persons. This is particularly true when the therapist is dealing with elderly patients who are unfamiliar with the nature and procedures of psychotherapy. For many, especially those from societies where psychiatry is still not a popular medical specialty, psychological therapy is not commonly practiced, and the concept of analytic psychotherapy is unheard of among most laymen, it is confusing when they are asked to review their psychological lives, to reveal their intrapsychic material, or even to discuss emotional matters (Baker & Takeshita, 2001).

The therapy should focus on how to help the elderly deal with their problems as defined by them and how to eliminate the difficulties they encounter as they see them. How to encourage their adult children to call them more often to offer support, how to deal with sleep problems, and how to minimize their concerns over somatic discomforts are some of the practical issues that need more immediate, primary attention in therapy (Niederehe, 1994).

Regarding ethnic minority elderly, Grant (1995) pointed out that therapists must recognize the diversity within ethnic groups and often must be broad based, multilevel, and direct therapy at the multiple

conditions contributing to the presenting problems. He supported the view that although ethnic minority elderly tend to be unfamiliar with the practice of psychotherapy, it still can be very effective, especially when dealing with depression and anxiety associated with psychological problems.

B. Relevant Attention to Therapist–Patient Relations and Countertransference

It is a common rule that therapist–patient relations should be geared toward the ethnic–cultural background of the patient so that the relations can be more relevant, meaningful, and effective in therapy. This is especially true when dealing with elderly persons. Based on their cultural backgrounds, they have certain views and expectations regarding authority–subordinate relations in various interpersonal situations, including how the elderly should be treated by younger persons. Generally, therapists for elderly patients are younger than their patients. Even though the therapists may be respected by the patients as "physicians" or "healers," at the same time, they are considered "younger" and of a "lower" social status compared to the aged patients. How to show culturally expected respect toward the aged persons and their life-experience authority is one of the issues that needs careful attention. This may not be so important in a society where people are educated to treat each other "equally," disregarding age differences, but it can be a crucial matter for people who come from societies where, culturally, aged persons are expected to be respected.

In many societies, certain views and attitudes are associated with gender. Such views cannot be ignored in the process of interaction between persons of different genders. This is also true when the therapist is treating an elderly patient of a different gender. For instance, when a female therapist treats an elderly male patient, special caution is needed to consider the patient's cultural norms and expectations regarding females and males, especially if the man is from a culture that emphasizes the importance of maintaining male machismo. How to offer advice or suggestions without hurting the elder man's pride becomes a delicate clinical matter. The reverse is true for treating elder women from certain cultures. For instance, in Micronesia, a matrilineal system is practiced and women have a certain social status and weight as those who mainain the lines of inheritance. In such societies, the "grandmother" is regarded as the unspoken head of a household (not the grandfather). Such an elderly grandmother needs to be treated with proper dignity and respect by a young male therapist.

Closely associated with this, it is important to examine and handle the countertransference that the therapist might have toward the elderly person. This is particularly true when the therapist is dealing with a patient from another culture that has different views and attitudes toward the aging process. The therapist's negative attitudes toward aging may reflect on the way the aged patient is handled and the way therapy is directed.

C. Suitable Application of Cultural Knowledge and Empathy

In any situation involving transcultural therapy, it is necessary for the therapist to have a basic knowledge of the cultural background of the patient under care so that proper cultural empathy can occur in the therapeutic purpose. This is particularly true when the patient has a cultural background that is different from that of the therapist. When a therapist is working with an elderly patient from another socioculture background, there is often not only a potential "cultural gap" between them, but a wide "time (or era) gap" as well.

For example, when a patient talks about his World War II experiences in the Pacific, it will sound almost like a historical story to a younger therapist who was born after the war. For a woman patient to share her experiences of traditional life characterized by strict rules about marriage and sexual life (e.g., premarital

sex and adultery viewed as social sins), without the availability of birth control (in a time when it was common for married women to bear more than half-a-dozen children), and the possibility of losing many children in infancy due to health conditions, and so on, might sound unthinkable to a young, contemporary therapist. Transcending the double gap of "culture" and "era" for needed empathy is a technical challenge that therapists have to deal with when they are treating much older patients from other cultures.

D. Reasonable Encouragment to "Talk Story"

As part of the process of aging, the time orientation for a person will shift from the future in youth, the present in adults, and the past in the aged. There are changes observed in psychological orientations to time throughout a person's life span. Seeing less opportunities in the future, perhaps, elderly persons shift their focus to recollections of the past. By utilizing this psychological characteristic, the skillful psychotherapist will encourage elderly patients to talk about their personal lives in the past as a way of stimulating their interest in interaction with the therapist. "Talking story" about their past, without saying it, will indirectly help them to examine the present and to prepare for the future. This is not a waste of time in therapy; rather it may serve as the main part of the therapeutic interaction if it is handled skillfully and utilized properly.

To let the patient "talk story" in therapy sessions is particularly pertinent for elderly patients who have different cultural backgrounds from the therapist. Besides encouraging the patient to interact actively with the therapist, it offers a splendid opportunity to help the therapist learn about not only the patient's personal past history, but also his cultural background, significantly promoting cultural empathy. Talking story is a format that makes elderly patients feel comfortable about engaging with the therapist in therapy sessions, as it is a more "natural" way for them to examine and reveal their lives than a formal psychiatric examination or analytic process.

E. SENSITIVE AVOIDANCE OF MENTAL ILLNESS STIGMA

Based on the background and history of development of psychiatry within their societies, many people around the world still hold rather negative views about psychiatric disorders and are very sensitive about being labeled mentally ill. This is particularly true for elderly persons who were brought up in an era in which there was no optimistic way of treating the mentally ill and many severely disordered mental patients had to be confined to institutional care. This is more so if the elderly are from home countries where the practice of psychiatry is still rather backward.

With this in mind, in therapy, the therapist is advised to avoid labeling the patient as "mentally ill" as much as possible. Mental problems can always be reframed as medical problems that need medical attention by examinations, checkups, and medications. The medicalization rather than psychologicalization of problems is more suitable and acceptable to elder patients. Mental illness is often associated with being "crazy" and having emotional problems is viewed as a personality weakness or failure to "tough it out."

Psychotherapy, or so-called talk therapy, is better conducted as part of a "medical" treatment than as (pure) "psychological" therapy. Taking the patient's blood pressure and using a stethoscope — familiar physicians' medical maneuvers — without hesitation as a part of the session activities, in addition to talking to the patient, or letting the patient talk, will make put the patient more at ease with the therapist.

In other words, from a practical perspective, the dichotomy of medicalization and psychologicalzation should be minimized. Conceptually the distinction between somatic and psychology needs to be reduced as well. The wholistic approach is much more relevant and appreciated in working with elderly persons, who

tend to view the body and mind together without distinction or dichotomatization.

F. PROPER INVOLVEMENT OF FAMILY AND SOCIAL NETWORKS IN THERAPY

When children's therapists are working with child patients, it is important to involve the family, particularly the parents. This is equally true for geriatric therapists when they are working with aged patients. It is desirable to involve the family, namely the spouse (if the patient still has one) and adult children (whether or not they are living together with the patient). The reason is obvious. The lives of elderly persons are very much related to the support and influence of family members, whether they are physically living together or not. Besides, there often exist psychological conflicts, disputes, or crises that are related to family members that need active attention and management. Conceptually, psychotherapy with the elderly needs to be performed almost in the form of family therapy (Richman, 1996).

G. BALANCED ACCEPTANCE OF FOLK HEALING

It is not surprising that many modern people utilize folk or alternative healing services besides modern professional therapies. This is especially true for elderly persons who feel more at home seeking folk ways of healing and using traditionally remedies. This is simply a refection of their time of life, views, and experiences. Based on this understanding, the modern therapist is advised to maintain a rather wholistic view of treatment, a balanced attitude toward alternative therapies, and even take an active interest with patients in nonorthodox approaches. This will help the therapist develop closer therapeutic relations with the patient. Through such a joining (with the patient), the therapist will be be in a better position to make more meaningful and powerful therapeutic suggestions.

H. Adequate Utilization of Culture-Prescribed Coping Patterns

Finally, in terms of technical aspects, another issue that deserves consideration is how to make good use of coping methods that have been prescribed by a patient's culture of origin. This is based on the assumption that culture-prescribed coping mechanisms have more meaning for the patient. In order to encourage utilizing culture-rooted coping patterns, it is necessary for the therapist to have a macroscopic understanding of the patient's personal history as well as his cultural background. Exploring together will help the therapist and the patient reveal traditional ways of coping with the patient's problems. It will certainly facilitate the examination of choices and the utilization of certain coping patterns that are prescribed within the patient's cultural system.

For instance, a Chinese woman in her 60s suffered from a prolonged grief reaction after her husband's sudden death from a heart attack. Besides the emotional injury of losing her beloved husband, she also suffered from the pain of guilt and regret. She regretted badly that she, as a wife, was not able to help her husband seek proper medical treatment to save his life. In order to help this widow, the therapist examined with her the kinds of things that she could do to make up for her regret. After mutual exploration, the patient come up with one idea. She informed the therapist that her deceased husband had a wish for many years to return to his home village to repair the tomb of his ancestors. For practical reasons, he had not been able to carry out his wish while he was still alive. The wife thought that carrying out his uncompleted wish might repair her guilt feelings. According to traditional Chinese culture, it is a virtue to have reasonably decorated the tomb of deceased ancestors to show proper respect for them. Knowing this, the therapist encouraged the patient to do so. The patient returned to her husband's village and used some of her savings to repair his ancestors' tomb. Feeling that she had done what was usually expected of a filial daughter-in-law and a dutiful wife, she was much relieved from her guilt and gradually recovered from her prolonged grief.

In many cultures there are common sayings or proverbs that reflect the wisdom accumulated in the past. Among them, many can be properly chosen and used in therapy to help a patient change his views about things or become more enlightened about life. Some are particularly relevant for elderly persons. For instance, the Chinese have a common saying that, "Older ginger is spicier." This can be used to reinforce the value of being "old." There is another proverb that says, "To ask for help from one's self is much more reliable than from others." This can be used to encourage self-reliance. Because these folk sayings or proverbs are used commonly in society, they are relatively familiar to elderly persons. They can grasp their meanings more easily and use their culture-rooted wisdom for enlightenment. Making use of such cultural insights can be quite a useful education for the elderly person.

III. PSYCHOTHERAPY FOR THE ELDERLY: CONTENT ISSUES

A. Working on Views and Attitudes about Aging

Numerous issues need to be worked on when therapists are caring for aged patients. Among them, the patient's own negative views about aging are fundamental. As pointed out by gerontologist and psychiatrist R.N. Butler (1974), negative views of old age with their outworn stereotypes (particularly "senility") must be changed if the elderly are to have more opportunities for successful aging.

If the therapist is working with elderly patients of culturally deprived ethnic minority groups, there is a great need to help them restore their own images about self as they suffer from the double-negative images of age and ethnicity. Listening to their stories about their ethnicity and appreciating their cultural views is one way to help them restore positive views about their ethnic–cultural backgrounds.

B. Working on Daily Life Adjustment

Technically, psychotherapy with elderly patients, like that with children or adolescents, may take the format of "psycho-education," with a primary focus on how to deal with actual daily life. This may include how to overcome the emotional issue of going out shopping, taking care of family chores, or relating to neighbors. Of course, if the elderly persons have their families, they can be helped by family members in those trivial, practical matters. However, sometimes, emotional issues are involved that cause the elderly person to refuse the suggestions of their adult children. It may take the therapist, as a third person as well as a professional healer, to guide the elderly person in resolving a simple matter — through objective and common-sense suggestions.

For instance, an elderly Korean widow suffered from an anxiety attack after she experienced vertigo episodes. Her condition was aggravated by the thought of what would happen if she fainted and died suddenly. According to her cultural beliefs, it would be a terrible thing for a person to die without being cared for by immediate family members. She had been living alone in her apartment since her husband died several years earlier. Her grown-up daughter, married to an Occidental husband, with three children, was living only one block away from the patient. The patient demanded that her daughter call her by phone at least twice a day to make sure that she was alive and all right. She thought that, according to her culture, it was a simple task for a filial daughter to perform for her widowed mother. However, this arrangement did not last long. The daughter was working outside the home and it was difficult to call her mother during working hours. After work, she was concerned with her husband's feelings, also. She was afraid that the would not understand and appreciate her "overconcerned" behavior and being "overbonded" to her mother, even

after marriage. After a family session, the therapist explained to the patient that there was no danger to her life, and that for her daughter to call her once a day, in the evening, should be enough. Also, it was suggested that the teenage granddaughters could help their mother by taking turns calling their grandmother so that it was not too great a burden on their mother. These were simple, practical suggestions, but they worked for the elderly patient and her family. This is often what is involved in working with elderly patients — helping them deal with daily life problems.

C. Working on Family Relationships with Adult Children

As illustrated by the example just given, working with elderly patients cannot exclude working with their families. This is particularly true when there is conflict between the elderly patients and their adult children, or between or among adult children with regard to their elderly parents. This is particularly so in a society where, culturally, close ties between parents and children are stressed in daily life. When parents become old, preexisting conflicts among children that are rooted in their early childhoods might surface and disturb them again, even though they have become adults.

A Japanese family was referred for family therapy because they were having a serious conflict over who should take care of their elderly widowed mother, who had recently suffered from a minor stroke. After the hospitalization, she recovered considerably, but she still could not walk by herself, could not talk too much, and had some difficulty swallowing. The mother had five married children: four daughters and one son, the youngest. The son, even though he was the youngest, according to his culture, took it as his responsibility to take care of his aged parent. Although all of his four elder sisters had suggested taking turns caring for their disabled mother, he flatly opposed this. He felt that it was time for him to be filial toward his mother. Even though the mother had just been discharged from the hospital, and still needed to sit in a

wheelchair, he took her with him to the football sta-
dium to watch a game. He fed her a hotdog — the only
fast food available there. The mother choked and
almost died from asphyxia. An ambulance was called
and fortunately the mother was resuscitated in time.
However, after this incident, how to take care of their
elderly and disabled mother became an open battle
between the son and his four elder sisters. The problem was not the elderly mother's; it had become the
rearisen conflict among the adult son and his elderly
sisters about who was the mother's favorite child and
who had the right to take care of her to show filial
piety.

Sometimes it is necessary to arrange for elderly
parents to live in institutional settings, such as nursing
homes, if the parents become disabled, either mentally
or physically. Many aged persons could easily be
"dumped" into such public institutions by their careless children, but this is not always the case. The situation can also be the opposite. This could potentially
cause psychological problems for the adult children,
who were raised with the belief that children should
be filial to their parents and take good care of them
when they become old. Making arrangements for their
parents to live in a nursing home could provoke strong
guilt feelings.

At the wife's persuasion, a young couple visited a
clinic for couples counseling. As husband and wife,
they were happy and had good relations, except
regarding the husband's father. The father, who had
been living with them, suffered from severe Parkin-
son's disease, needing medication regularly and frequently around the clock. As a filial son and daughter-
in-law, they had been taking care of the father in their
home for almost 5 years after their marriage. Although
both husband and wife were working outside the
home, during working hours they managed to take
turns coming back home to help the father take his
needed medications. If the father skipped his medications for any reason, he would become unable to move
around by himself and would urinate on the floor.
Because of this situation, the couple had not taken a
vacation together in many years. Even though they
wanted to have children, the wife felt that the condi-

tions at home would not be good for bearing and raising a child. As the father's physical condition deteriorated considerably and progressively, the wife urged
her husband to consider the possibility of arranging
for institutional care for the father, which her husband
strongly resisted, believing that it was the children's
responsibility to care for their parents at home, even
though it was a hardship.

After several therapy sessions, the husband finally
agreed to allow his father to stay in a nursing home on
a trial basis — only temporarily, for several days. It
turned out that the father liked the nursing home, as he
enjoyed being with many other elderly people, and
being cared for by kind attendants who helped him
take his medication on time. The husband's guilt feelings were removed and the wife was happy that they
could have their own life as a couple from then on.
This situation needed the therapist as an objective
third person and as a culture broker to work on the culture-related psychological conflicts encountered by
the family members.

D. WORKING ON THE UTILIZATION OF INFORMAL AND FORMAL SUPPORT SYSTEMS

The case just described illustrates that it is not only
the elderly person but his or her family members who
need to work on issues regarding the support or service systems available in a society. Many cultures hold
the view that aged persons should be cared for by their
own family members in a private setting. It is quite
true that family resources should be fully utilized first
for the elderly person. It is most desirable for the aged
person to live in a familiar setting and to be surrounded and cared for by family members. However,
if this becomes impossible, formal social services and
public systems need to be utilized. This is the trend in
modern urban and industrialized societies. Immediate
family members alone cannot solve all of the elderly
person's problems. Public support systems and institutional services should be maximally utilized if they
are needed. This is an issue that needs to be worked

out for many elderly persons, who tend to hold traditional views and hesitate to make use of the public services available in contemporary society.

Assisting them in learning to attend social clubs for the elderly and make friends there, to participate in social programs available in the community and get involved in activities, and to make good use of public support systems is a common agenda for working with elderly people, who tend to avoid such activities. This avoidance is often rooted in their beliefs and attitudes toward public systems and organizations versus personal family systems. They need a lot of education, persuasion, and encouragement in therapy for proper, balanced, and maximal utilization use of both informal and formal support systems for the elderly.

E. Working on Adjustment to Present Life and Culture

Whatever the traditional cultural background of the patient, he or she has to learn to adjust to contemporary culture. As long as he or she lives in the modern world, the patient has to learn how to live in the modern way. In order to live in a host society, elderly persons have to learn to adapt to it. It is true that it is not easy to learn a new language, a new way of thinking, and different behavior patterns after a certain age. Although it may take a lot encouragement, elderly persons need to be advised and guided in order to make the cultural adjustment to their present lives in the new culture. Making the adjustment will hopefully assist them in developing a sense of having new roots in the new culture, as well as a better way of living for many years to come.

F. Working on Grief and Widowhood

Many married elderly persons will lose their spouses sooner or later and, as this is usually a difficult event, they often need professional help to deal with the loss of this significant person in their lives. As described previously, there is a certain formal process of grief prescribed by culture. There are also certain attitudes and expectations defined by culture for the person who loses a spouse. Beyond this, there are individual and family differences for coping with such loss experiences. The therapist needs to take into consideration all of these factors, to adjust the ways in which he assists the patients through the necessary grieving process and helps them recover from the loss as soon as possible. A balance needs to be created between the psychological conditions, needs, and strengths of the individual and the expectations of the society. The culturally rooted coping process as well as the socially available support systems should be maximally utilized, if possible, in dealing with the psychological trauma.

G. Preparations for the Future

Although the ending of life by death is a natural phenomenon, the subject of death is not faced readily or discussed easily in daily life in many societies. In some cultures, it is even considered taboo to mention death. It is not permitted to discuss openly the possibility of death and how to prepare for it. In such a cultural milieu, the death of elderly persons is a subject that is avoided by immediate family members and ignored by the elderly persons themselves. In such circumstances, it can become the therapist's role to include the subject in the process of therapy with the patient as well as with family members, if necessary.

The concept of life after death varies among different cultures. In some, there is a clear vision based on religious thought. For instance, Christians assume that there is an eternal life after death, and there are two ways to go, either to heaven or to hell. For Buddhists, life is conceptualized as a part of a continuous cycle. You may live an animal life in the next cycle after your human life. Others hold the simple view that life comes from the Earth, and returns to the Earth after death. Still others consider life after death an uncertain issue that is never clearly defined. These different concepts of life after death will impact how people view and prepare for death. It is important to realize that preparation for death is not only for the person who will die, but also for the survivors: their beloved spouses, children, and grandchildren.

How to prepare a will and make arrangements for the surviving family members are issues that need to be faced and discussed openly among family members and with an attorney, if necessary, so that proper preparations can be made not only legally but psychologically. This would be a great help to the elderly and their adult children from a practical perspective. However, different people and cultures have different attitudes about preparing for the end of life. Clinicians need to explore the cultural views on these sensitive subjects, even though it may be very useful to discuss and prepare for them, and eliminate any anxieties that the elderly might have in relation to the end of their lives.

In summary, elderly persons usually encounter certain psychological problems in their lives that might be considerably different from those of other adults. There is a need to modify the "regular" therapeutic techniques and focus of therapy to meet the individual needs of the elderly in their family situations, taking into account the process of aging and their cultural backgrounds in the past and the present.

REFERENCES

Baker, F.M. (1996). Suicide among ethnic elders. In G.J. Kennedy (Ed.), *Suicide and depression in late life: Critical issues in treatment, research, and public policy.* New York: Wiley.

Baker, F.M., & Takeshita, J. (2001). The elderly. In W.S. Tseng, & J. Streltzer (Eds.), *Culture and psychotherapy: A guide for clinical practice* (pp. 209–222). Washington, DC: American Psychiatric Press.

Butler, R.N. (1974). Successful aging and the role of the life review. *Journal of the American Geriatrics Society, 22*(12), 529–535.

Ginsberg, Y. (1984–1985). Fear of crime among elderly Jews in Boston and London. *International Journal of Aging and Human Development, 20*(4), 257–268.

Grant, R.W. (1995). Interventions with ethnic minority elderly. In J.F. Aponte, R.Y. Rivers, & J. Wohl (Eds.), *Psychological interventions and cultural diversity.* Boston: Allyn & Bacon.

Niederehe, G.T. (1994). Psychosocial therapies with depressed older adults. In L.S. Schneider, C.F. Reynolds, III, B.D. Lebowitz & A.J. Friedhoff (Eds.), *Diagnosis and treatment of depression in late life.* Washington, DC: American Psychiatric Press.

Richman, J. (1996). Psychotherapeutic approaches to the depressed and suicidal older person and family. In G.J. Kennedy (Ed.), *Suicide and depression in late life: Critical issues in treatment, research, and public policy.* New York: Wiley.

42

Working with Medically Ill Patients

I. INTRODUCTION

Working with medically ill patients of various ethnic or cultural backgrounds is a challenge in medical practice. It is common enough for general practitioners to encounter medical patients with diverse ethnic or cultural backgrounds so that cultural aspects of medical practice cannot be ignored. Because psychiatrists work in the subfield of consultation–liaison service, it is necessary for them to have the knowledge and experience to provide psychiatric consultation on how to work with patients of different ethnic, racial, and cultural backgrounds.

In the medical setting, three types of culture are present: the culture of the patient, the culture of the physician, and a specific medical culture. The *culture of the patient* will contribute to the patient's way of understanding illness, perception and presentation of symptoms and problems, and adjustment to illness. The patient's expectations of the physician, motivation for treatment, and compliance are also influenced by the culture of the patient. The *culture of the physician,* superimposed on individual style, personal belief, and professional knowledge, will shape the pattern of interaction and communication with the

patient. For example, a physician may have cultural prejudices or biases toward a particular gender (male/female differences), sexual orientation (gay or lesbian), race or ethnicity, specific disease (AIDS, alcohol abuse), or a certain procedure (such as abortion). The *medical culture* refers to traditions and regulations that have developed within the medical service setting beyond medical knowledge and theory. Whether the physician and nurse work together as egalitarian team members or in a distinct hierarchial order depends on the medical culture, as does society's choice of a socialized or privatized medical system. On a clinical level, a patient can be informed about a fatal illness or the actual diagnosis can be concealed from him with the idea of protecting a "vulnerable" patient. Examining medicine practiced in America, anthropologist H. F. Stein (1993) pointed out that for the American doctor, being in control is very important. The physician's dominant values are individualism (the doctor can do it himself), mastery over nature (he can cure the disease), and future orientation (focused on the patient's eventural cure). Actively intervening, aggressively treating, controlling, and fixing the patient are acceptable attitudes and morale for the clinician, strongly reflecting American value systems, which may not necessarily be shared in other cultures.

In order to provide culturally appropriate care, it is essential to first recognize how cultural factors may influence the patient, physician, medical staff, and medical setting. Based on such knowledge, we can then elaborate on the practical aspects of treatment.

II. CULTURAL IMPACT ON MEDICAL PRACTICES

A. PHYSICIAN–PATIENT INTERACTION

1. Basic Physician–Patient Relationship

The physician and patient establish a relationship in which the physician functions as a healer in an authoratative role, taking responsibility over the treatment plan. The patient, in the role of the one being healed, takes a position of dependence on the physician and is a passive participant in the healing process. This is exemplified by an extreme situation, such as a major operation performed under general anesthesia. Once the patient agrees to accept such a healing procedure, he becomes entirely passive under general anesthesia. The surgeon takes an active role in performing the surgical procedure, thus becoming responsible for all activity regarding the patient.

Beyond this basic physician–patient relationship, the healer–client relationship is subject to cultural variations. For example, the extent to which the physician can act in an authoritative role rather than a more egalitarian one is influenced by the cultural system and how authority is assigned to the healing profession.

The general tendency is that if a society is autocratic and the authority figures, such as the head villager, police, or governmental administrator, are authoritative, then the physician can also exercise more power in relating to the patient. In contrast, if the society is democratic, the physician tends to show more respect for the rights of the patient and to relate to the patient in a more egalitarian way.

2. Patient's Relation with the Medical Team

In the medical system, there are personnel with various training, including doctors, nurses, medical technicians, bedside nursing aides, and social workers. Members of the medical team relate to each other, and the team hierarchy is maintained in a manner based not only on treatment needs but also on a medical culture reflecting the general culture in the society. For instance, in Japan, physicians are typically male and nurses are female. The nurses are expected to bow to the physicians and to treat them as masters, thus reflecting the traditional hierarchy in Japanese society where men occupy a superior position to women. In contrast, although American nurses are required to carry out the physicians' medical orders, they are usually given a certain amount of power in carrying out their functions. As the major figures in charge of the wards, nurses can make suggestions to physicians on the management of patient care. Consciously or subconsciously, physicals have to relate to nurses in the same way that men relate to women in American society, with respect and on an equal basis.

Dealing with medical teams with different power structures, patients will learn and adjust to each team. For example, Japanese patients will hesitate to ask questions or make requests directly to the authoritative physician, and instead will try to go through the nurses, with whom they feel more comfortable sharing any problems. In contrast, American patients do not feel the need for such an indirect approach. They will usually communicate directly with the physician concerning their diagnosis or treatment plan, and with nurses on other issues such as what medication the doctor has prescribed. They recognize the different roles performed by various members of the medical team and will interact with them accordingly. However, if a Japanese patient were to be hospitalized in an American hospital, he or she may be confused as to how to relate "appropriately" to the medical team and come across as a "passive" or "uncomplaining" patient. If an American patient were to be admitted to a Japanese hospital, the patient — without knowing it — may behave in a way that would be interpreted as too "direct" and "aggressive" in relating to the physician.

Not all societies have primarily male physicians and female nurses. In Russia, the majority of physicians are women, and in the United States, many men work as nurses. The gender distribution of physicians has also changed with time. An example is in the United States, where obstetricians and gynecologists were predominately male doctors but are now primarily female. How the gender of the physician and nurse influences the medical situation is a challenging question. For instance, how female physicians relate to female nurses or how male physicians relate to male nurses will form a new medical culture that will affect patients as well as medical personnel.

3. Patient's Commitment to a Physician

In the United States and many other Western societies, the medical systems and cultural values expect that a person have an established family physician who they see for care. If there is a need for a specialist for a second opinion, the family physician will usually recommend one and the patient usually follows the recommendation. The general rule is that the patient sticks to one family physician with a commitment to a long-term relationship and seldom changes physicians unless there is a special reason for doing so.

In other societies, such as in many Asian countries, a patient will shop around for physicians without feeling a commitment to remain with any particular family physician. The patient may rely on a friend or relative's recommendation to see a particular physician — usually one with a good reputation in the patient's or his family's point of view. However, there is no long-term commitment, and very often a patient may see several physicians simultaneously or change to another physician. It is not uncommon for a patient to see a modern and a traditional physician at the same time. Therefore, a modern physician should not get too upset upon finding out that the patient is seeing another physician as well. It is mainly a matter of the patient's concept of commitment and does not reflect on the patient's respect of the physician.

4. Patient's Satisfaction with Physician

A patient's satisfaction with the physician is determined by many factors, including how the physician relates to the patient, to what extent explanations are given, and the kind of support given to the patient. Therefore, a patient's satisfaction with the physician may not correlate with the actual success of the medical treatment.

Baider, Ever-Hadani, and De Nour (1995) in Israel carried out a cross-ethnic comparative study of cancer patients' satisfaction with their physicians. The study compared Israel veterans and Russian patients who had immigrated to Israel within the past 4 years. Patients were asked to describe the "actual" physicians they had encountered and their "ideal" physician with the index for satisfaction based on the similarities between the two descriptions. The Russian patients had significantly higher satisfaction scores compared to their Israel counterparts. As there was no reason to suspect that the Russian patients had greater success with their medical treatments than the Israelis, how the patients' satisfaction was affected by their ethnic backgrounds, past medical experiences, or current medical expectations deserves further study.

B. Patient's Illness and Health Behavior

Illness behavior refers to how patients think, react, and cope when they suffer from illness. Health behavior refers to how ordinary people or patients behave in order to maintain their health. This may include how people follow guidance on food intake, exercise, hygiene, preventive exams, and so on. A patient's illness or health behavior is subject to cultural factors in many ways and elaboration is needed from a cultural perspective.

1. Concept of "Disease" and "Illness"

Cultural anthropologists and cultural psychiatrists propose using the term "disease" and "illness" to denote different semantic concepts. Disease refers to the medical definition of sickness and is explained from the perspective of biological and physiological etiology, manifestation, course, and outcome. Disease is considered objective and universal in nature. Illness implies a patient's psychological construct of the perception, experience, and understanding of suffering. Illness is subjective and open to cultural impact [cross-reference to Chapter 9: Mental Illness: Folk Categories and Explanation (Section V,A)].

For instance, a man suffers from seizures. A physician conceptualizes it as a medical "disease" occurring as a result of focal electrical discharges in the brain causing central nervous system dysfunction. Medication is needed to control such a disease, otherwise it will recur and may cause serious injury to the patient. From the patient's point of view, the seizure is an "illness" that may occur suddenly and interfere with daily behavior. It might be interpreted as the result of a force imbalance in his body, being temporarily possessed by an evil spirit, or the consequence of an ancestor's immoral behavior. The illness is a disgraceful condition that needs to be hidden from others, otherwise it may affect the patient's future life in areas such as work or marriage.

The example just given illustrates that the "disease" is the concept utilized by modern medical personnel, whereas "illness" is the concept used by the common people. These two concepts may overlap in certain ways, but in many ways they are different. From a cultural point of view, a physician needs to know and comprehend the whole situation, not only the medically oriented concept of the disease, but also the patient's and his family's perception of the illness.

How different kinds of physical dysfunctions are perceived and managed differently by various ethnic groups is shown by the study carried out by Zuckerman, Guerra, Drossman, Foland, and Gregory (1996). They conducted a survey of a nonpatient population in Texas to examine ethnic differences of health-care-seeking behaviors related to bowel dysfunction. They reported that Hispanic-Americans, probably tending to see bowel dysfunction as a daily problem, were less likely than non-Hispanic (Caucasian) Americans to seek health care for it. Further, they were more likely to self-medicate with folk remedies to maintain good bowel function. Zuckerman and colleagues pointed out that the perception of health and bowel function is in part determined by ethnic differences.

2. Folk and Traditional Medical Concepts

People usually hold certain common knowledge and beliefs about illness. These can be "folk" or "old housewife" cures based on accumulated past experience or well-established traditional medical practices that have deep roots in the society. Traditional Chinese medicine, Ayurvedic medicine in India, and the Galenic-Islamic medicine observed by the Arabian people are examples [cross-reference to Chapter 9: Mental Illness: Folk Categories and Explanation (Sections III, A–C)]. Such beliefs are deep in the patient's and family's mind and it is very important for the modern physician to learn about and deal with them, as they are utilized by the patient and have a significant impact on the patient's illness behavior.

For example, the yin and yang theory is the backbone of traditional Chinese medicine and is often part of the traditional medical beliefs held by patients of Asian backgrounds, such as Japanese, Korean, and Thai. According to the yin and yang theory, patients may inquire whether it is all right to eat certain fruits after childbirth or surgery. Some families may scratch a child's body with a coin to create a "fire-elevated" condition, and physicians not familiar with this folk treatment may wrongly interpret ecchymotic skin injuries as a sign of child abuse. A physician may be puzzled by the burn scars on the back or the belly of a patient if he did not know it was the result of *oqiu* treatment (moxibustion), which some cultures use to treat stomach disorders, back pain, or cancer.

3. Culture-Patterned Problem Presentation

In a subtle way, a patient's style of presenting a chief complaint is influenced by cultural factors. How the major problem and its symptoms are described are subject to the patient's educational level, medical knowledge, and motivation for treatment, as well as culturally patterned modes of problem presentation.

"I feel my heart is empty," "there is a fire elevation within my chest," and "I am concerned that my semen is leaking from my urine" are some examples of culturally flavored problem presentations that may be observed among various ethnic groups in Asia or south Asia. Clearly semantics are involved, but these presentations also reflect folk concepts of illness. For instance, Chinese people may use "empty heart" to describe a depressed mood without any relation to cardiac symptoms. A Korean person may complain of a "fire elevation" (within the trunk) to indicate excessive fire elements, referring to emotionally upsetting conditions. When an Indian man is concerned that his semen might be leaking from his urine, he is using a culture-patterned expression regarding *dhat* illness (known by cultural psychiatrists as "spermatorrhea" to indicate that he has anxieties about some issue [cross-reference to Chapter 13: Culture-Related Specific Syndromes (Section II,A,2)]. A culturally sensitive physician will try to understand the symbolic meaning behind what is said rather than taking the complaint literally.

4. Observation of Recommended Health Examinations

In order to promote or maintain health, many guidelines have been proposed by medical personnel and various health examinations have been suggested. However, people of various backgrounds may not follow such health guidelines faithfully and will not take suggested disease-preventive measures regularly. Ethnic, minority, and cultural factors need to be considered, among others (such as socioeconomic factors) (Luke, 1996).

For instance, concerning ethnic differences in breast cancer-screening behaviors, Friedman and colleagues (1995) examined asymptomatic women, 50 years or older, who participated in a no-cost worksite breast cancer-screening program. Results indicated that African-Americans and Hispanic-Americans were more likely to practice monthly breast self-examination than Caucasian-Americans. African-Americans were more likely to report cancer-related fears and worries as barriers to having mammography examinations, whereas Caucasian-Americans were more likely to report being too busy, inconvenience, and procrastination as barriers.

5. Patients' Medical Knowledge and Attitudes

The following are additional examples of how ethnic or cultural factors may affect medical knowledge or attitudes toward certain medical conditions. These, in turn, have a significant impact on the process and results of medical treatment, such as whether a patient seeks care or is compliant with the treatment plan.

Matsumoto and colleagues (1995) compared first- and second-generation Japanese-American women in San Francisco concerning their attitudes and beliefs about osteoporosis. First-generation Japanese-American women attributed osteoporosis to fate or luck. Second-generation women were much more aware of diet and other risk factors and therefore were potentially more amenable to behavior modification to reduce osteoporosis.

Carpenter and Colwell (1995) pointed out that Latino women are at significantly greater risk of death from cancer than Anglo women in the United States due to a lack of knowledge regarding cancer, lack of access to cancer-screening services, and feelings of fatalism. From their survey of Mexican-American women living in Texas, they reported that increased knowledge is associated with increased self-efficacy for cancer screening.

As a part of a cancer-prevention program aimed at minority and disadvantaged urban women, the cancer beliefs, knowledge, and behaviors were assessed by Morgan, Park and Cortez (1995) among home-health attendants in the Bronx, New York. They found out that nearly 60% of Hispanic women surveyed there did not know what cervical cancer was and that nearly 60% of them believed that surgery causes cancer to spread.

Dancy (1996) surveyed African-American women of different ages and educational levels in Chicago to compare their knowledge and attitudes on AIDS. It was found that the educational level influenced knowledge about AIDS, whereas age influenced not knowledge about AIDS but attitudes and sexual behavior. This illustrated that African-Americans are not a homogeneous group in terms of their knowledge about a specific medical disorder. Age and educational levels are among the variables attributed to differences within the same ethnic group.

Hodes and Teferedegne (1996) interviewed Ethiopian Jews (Falashas) in Ethiopia about the cause of certain medical conditions. They found that interviewees thought epilepsy was caused by spirits and recommended smelling smoke as a treatment. Prolonged labor was due to the evil spirit and miscarriages were due to exposure to sun or cold. Less than 20% of interviewees were able to link malaria to mosquito bite transmission.

C. PHYSICIAN'S SPECIAL PERFORMANCE

1. Physical Examination

It is a basic practice of modern physicians to complete a thorough physical examination of the patient as part of the diagnostic exercise. However, this is not so in some traditional medical practices. In traditional Chinese medicine, in addition to the oral history, holding the patient's wrist to examine the pulse is sometimes the only physical contact needed to be made by the physician. In Chinese history, not even such minimal contact was allowed by (male) physicians in examining the emperor's wife, so a string was tied to the emperor's wife's wrist and the physician held the string through a screen to examine the pulse.

In a modern physical exam, a patient is required to dress in a special gown and be prepared to expose his or her whole body. A manual examination is carried out of the patient's body; however, modern physicians are seldom trained to be aware of cultural differences in the matter of exhibiting the body. For instance, private or erotic zones may differ for cultural groups and

require additional sensitivity and respect to preserve the dignity and comfort of the patient and his or her family. For traditional Japanese women, the back of the neck is considered erotic and not ordinarily exposed, whereas traditional Muslim women may consider it important to cover their hair and face with a veil.

How male physicians should carry out physical examinations of female patients is of special concern in modern medical practice. Professional custom often dictates that a female nurse be present for both the patient's ease as well as for prevention of malpractice suits for inappropriate physician behavior. In some cultures, it is also expected that the husband be present when his wife is examined by a male physician. The professional expectations of a female physician examining a male patient need to be considered from a cultural perspective as well.

2. Informing of Diagnosis and Explanation of Disease

An important part of medical practice is the physician's explanation of the disease to the patient so that he or she may understand and learn how to deal with it. Krauss-Mars and Lachman (1994) studied the ethnic differences in South African parents' reactions to unfavorable news about their children. The parents of white and black preschool children with disabling medical diseases were asked about the explanations provided to them about the illnesses of their children. Despite reporting that explanations were given by physicians, white parents, tended to deny the diagnosis of a mental illness more than other groups. Few black parents reported being asked about their understanding of the diagnosis. The investigators pointed out that the use of a language other than the patient's native tongue had a negative influence on communication between physician and parents. However, because the majority of the physicians are white, racial attitudes held by physicians as well as patients' cultural attitudes toward unfavorable sicknesses may all have contributed to the process of the explanation of disease between physicians and patients.

3. Suggestion for "Psychiatric" Consultation or Referral

Medical or surgical doctors may often encounter patients who they want to refer for a psychiatric consultation. In such cases, the physician needs to know how the patient and his family perceive the meaning of having a "psychiatric" problem and how they understand the function of a psychiatrist. Many people, disregarding their ethnic or cultural background, still hold negative views about mental illness and want to shy away from a "head shrinker," or psychiatrist. At times, it may not be the patient but the physician who is still uncomfortable about referring patients for a psychiatric consultation because of his beliefs about the stigma of mental illness.

Generally speaking, it takes skill and experience for physicians to deal with their patients about a psychiatric referral. It is not a good idea to lie about the situation or disguise the role of psychiatrists. It is better to keep things open and truthful, using terms and explanations that are supportive and proper. For instance, if possible, assurance can be given that the patient is not being referred because he or she is "crazy." The doctor can explain that there is merely concern about how the patient's emotions are affecting his or her physical well-being, and a specialist in the mind and emotions is needed for an expert opinion.

4. Disclosure of "Bad News" about Terminal Illness

Contemporary American health care professionals uphold a model of honest communication and information sharing with dying patients. Physicians are encouraged to inform the patient of the actual diagnosis, even if the disease is a terminal one. This is based on the belief that it is desirable for the individual (the patient) to have the opportunity to take responsibility for medical decisions relating to his or her life. It is tempting to interpret this medical practice as a reflection of an American value. However, it needs to be pointed out that this was not common practice prior to the 1960s, but only began between the 1960s and 1980s, during an atmosphere of antiauthoritarianism and distrust of authority in the United States because of the Vietnam War. Currently, disclosure of medical information to patients is necessary because of the physician's concerns about malpractice suits and the legal need to obtain the patient's consent to treatment.

In many cultures, there is substantial reluctance on the part of physicians and families to share correct diagnoses with the patient. Beyene (1992) points out that for Ethiopians, "bad news" should be told to a close family member or friend of the patient who will divulge the information in a culturally approved time and manner. In the Arabic East, direct mention of death is avoided, and in facing a fatal illness, patients, families, and physicians resort to elaborate forms of denial (Racy, 1969). In modern Japan, the custom of keeping bad news from the patient is based on concerns that it may provoke suicidal ideas. The physician follows the family's wishes and tells the patient he has a less serious illness. If the physician were to inform the patient frankly about his terminal illness, the family may be upset at the "inconsiderateness" of the physician. Clearly, there exist widely different cultural views as to whether the physician should truthfully inform the patient about the diagnosis of a fatal disease.

D. Special Medical Issues

1. Prescribing and Receiving Medication

Western medicine is based on a pharmacotechnology that prepares a drug in a pure abstract form that performs specific pharmacological functions. Modern physicians usually prescribe a single medication for a specific purpose, and for multiple problems they may prescribe multiple medications. Usually fewer medications are prescribed, if possible, to avoid drug interactions. In contrast, herbal medicine used in traditional medical practice is thought to work by combining multiple remedies in their raw form. Multiple herbs are always prescribed, as there is not too much concern over the use of compound medications. In general, in societies where traditional medicine is still used, Western medicine is considered "strong" and useful for combating the specific etiology of a disorder, but there are usually unwelcome side effects. Traditional herbal medicine is viewed as "harmonious," with fewer side effects, and will "strengthen" the body so that it can overcome the disorder.

Another interesting belief that may be held by laypeople from non-Western societies is that medication by injection is much more powerful than oral medication. An injection, even a shot of vitamins, is perceived as a "powerful" remedy. An intravenous medication is considered even more effective than an intramuscular injection. Thus, physicians may give intravenous injections of normal saline or glucose plus vitamins to induce a placebo effect or simply to satisfy a patient's request.

Modern Western physicians make no secret about the name and nature of prescriptions, and often make it a goal to explain to the patient the drug mechanism as well as potential side effects. Traditional physicians, however, sometimes keep prescriptions "secret" and, in some Asian countries, such as Japan, China, and Korea, the patient may not expect the physician to give a full explanation [cross-reference to Chapter 31: Culture, Ethnicity, and Drug Therapy (Section III,A–C)].

Associated with this is the tendency of patients to feel that there is no need to follow the physician's order in taking the medication. If the medicine works immediately (within a day or so), the patient will take it. If the symptoms subside, the patient may decide to discontinue the medication even against the physician's directions. Kandakai, Price, Telljohann, and Holiday-Goodman (1996) examined the use of antibiotics among African-Americans based on gender. Women were more likely to report completing the prescribed trial of antibiotics, whereas older men were more likely to use antibiotics only until the problem stopped. A significant percentage of men (23%) and women (18%) reported sharing their antibiotics with another person.

2. Laboratory Testing

For modern medical practice, it is common to perform various kinds of laboratory testing to assist in making a diagnosis. Various specimens may be needed for such testing. However, due to cultural beliefs regarding the body, certain reactions and preferences may be encountered. People who believe that blood is one of the major fluids in the body, essential for "vitality," may show reluctance to have blood drawn for testing. They will be extremely concerned with how many ccs have been taken. The same situation applies to spinal tapping when spinal fluid — the essence of the "spirit" — is drawn for testing. In contrast, providing urine, feces, or sputum for testing is not a problem, as they are considered "waste."

3. Management of Medical Pain

An examination of a pain disorder, particularly psychologically based pain, has been elaborated in a previous chapter [cross-reference to Chapter 16: Somatoform Disorders, Including Neurasthenia (Section III,E)]. In addition to pain relating to somatoform disorders, there can also be medical pain associated with childbirth, cancer, or surgery. Naturally, there is also room for cultural impact on various factors, such as the patient's perception of pain, interaction between the patient and the caregiver, and general expectations and attitudes about pain-killing medicines.

4. Issues Relating to Surgical Operations

Most people now appreciate that surgery can be effective in treating certain medical conditions, such as appendicitis, and may even be needed to save one's life. However, based on unique cultural beliefs, some patients may have special psychological reactions to certain surgeries, such as those that result in the loss of a part of the body. To lose a part of one's own body may be interpreted as a loss of one's integrity. Influenced by such a belief, a diabetic patient may refuse amputation of a leg necrotic from ulcers, or a woman with breast cancer may choose chemotherapy rather than surgical removal of her breast, even though it may result in a lower rate of cure.

Blood transfusions are also sometimes a necessary part of surgery. While it is common for people to be concerned about how much blood will be lost during an operation, in some cultures, blood is considered a vital body fluid and there might be a strong wish to conserve it as much as possible. In such a case, there might be less opposition toward receiving blood transfusions to gain the needed vital body fluid. In contrast, certain religious beliefs, such as those of Jehovah's Witnesses, might lead to its members to refuse to accept a blood transfusion even as a life-saving treatment.

5. Legal Definition of Death

The professional medical and legal definition of "death" is not uniform around the world. In the United States, "brain death" as verified by an electronic encephalography is sufficient to determine death legally. In contrast, Japan is more conservative, defining "death" as the complete stopping of the heartbeat. These different ways of defining "legal" death have a direct impact on organ donation. For instance, only one heart transplant has ever been performed in Japan, and that was 30 years ago. In 1997, *The Honolulu Advertiser* reported a story by E. Talmadge about an 8-year-old Japanese girl who received $600,000 in donations in Japan for a badly needed heart transplant, but had to come to the United States for the operation. It was 2 years later, after many years' struggle between the professional and legal systems, that Japan finally passed a rule that brain death would be accepted as the criterion for death to facilitate organ donation.

6. Organ Donation and Transplantation

Despite the remarkable medical technology that now exists for organ transplantations, not many people are interested in donating their organs after death. Often even physicians who understand the life-saving benefits of organ donation have great difficulty in suggesting such a concept to the patient or his family.

It has been noticed that donor authorizations tend to be especially low among African-Americans and other minority and ethnic groups in the United States. Rubens (1996) carried out a questionnaire survey of the beliefs and attitudes toward organ transplantation and rates of participation regarding organ donation among a sampling of racially and ethnically mixed university students at a state-assisted university in the Midwest. He reported that African-American students differed significantly from Caucasian students in their attitudes and beliefs toward organ donation. However, a greater percentage of African-American students granted permission for organ donation than African-Americans in the general population.

Among the various reasons that people are reluctant about organ donation is the cultural view that it is very important to keep the body intact, even for burial or cremation. Ross (1981) pointed out that in the Islamic religion, a Muslim does not own his or her body but holds it in a "trust from God." Consequently, a Muslim cannot donate or receive organ transplants, and blood transfusions are permissible only if recommended by a physician who is Muslim for the purpose of saving that person from death. Similarly, traditionally American Indians view the dead body as a seed that is placed in the ground. As a seed is planted whole, so the body should be buried intact. An amputated limb or excised organ may be cliamed for storage in a freezer and retrieved for burial with the body at the time of death.

7. Autopsy

In accordance with the belief of keeping the body intact after death, it is relatively difficult to suggest that the surviving family members agree to an autopsy of the deceased. In many cultures, it is almost impossible to obtain permission for an autopsy unless it is legally required, such as for forensic purposes. The autopsy rate in Arab countries is extremely low, and cadavers are not permitted for use in teaching or research purposes. This is also true in many Asian countries, where the family is not keen about the idea of an autopsy, and cadavers for medical teaching often come only from homeless people who die without family.

8. Death, Grief, and Mourning

Although it is a universal desire for a person to live as long as possible and to find ways to prolong life, attitudes toward death are subject to cultural influences. Prolonging life through intensive care or by mechanical means may not be appreciated in many cultures. In some, it is considered a natural phenomenon to die after a certain age, and death may be treated as a happy occasion rather than a sad one.

In many cultures, it is considered desirable for people to die in their own homes surrounded by their immediate family members. When this is the custom, the family will ask the physician about the prognosis of the patient's medical condition. If the patient is considered to have no hope for recovery, it becomes the physician's responsibility to inform the family of the appropriate time for the patient to be discharged from the hospital so that his last days may be spent at home.

E. CULTURALLY STIGMATIZED MEDICAL DISEASES

Because of their poor prognosis and historically limited effectiveness of treatment, the diagnosis of certain medical diseases still carries a substantial stigma despite an improvement in medical management. The following are some examples of diseases that are still associated with strong negative views as a result of cultural beliefs, and that intensely influence patients' emotional lives as well as their illness behavior.

1. Leprosy

Due to the visible malformation of the face or hands, plus its long history without effective treatment, in many societies leprosy is seen as a terrible disease, and patients are usually isolated from other people.

2. Pulmonary Tuberculosis

Before the appearance of effective antibiotics for treatment, pulmonary tuberculosis ran a chronic and fatal course. People were afraid of this contagious disease and patients tended to keep it secret from others. In China, it was called the "life disease," meaning that once it was contracted, one was going to suffer for a lifetime because there was no cure.

3. Epilepsy

Without knowing the actual cause of epilepsy, many speculations have been made by folk people, such as the patient being possessed by evil spirits or the illness being the result of an ancestor's immoral behavior, and so on.

4. Psychoses

Because of the difficulty in treating this disorder in the past, plus the fact that some psychotic patients manifest strange or violent behavior, in many societies psychotic patients are not welcomed by the people in the community.

5. Venereal Diseases

Because these diseases are usually associated with socially unsanctioned sexual behavior, such as prostitution, promiscuity, premarital intercourse, and extramarital affairs, venereal diseases are considered shameful in many societies, and patients try to conceal them from others, even from their own family members. Patients are hesitant to see physicians, so clinics may be set up in private places where visits will not be easily noticed by others.

6. AIDS

Because of its undesirable outcome, the association with drug abuse or homosexual behavior, and the possibility of contagion — either homosexually (in most Euro-American societies) or heterosexually (in Africa or Asian societies) — AIDS is viewed as an awful disease. Even physicians and dentists have been reluctant to come in contact with and provide care for patients with this disorder. Following a survey of Asian versus

Caucasian dentists practicing in New York City, Raphael, Kunzel, and Sadowsky (1996) reported that Asian dentists expressed significantly more negative attitudes toward and unwillingness to treat HIV-positive patients than Caucasian dentists.

7. Cancer

As a potentially fatal disease, cancer is viewed and reacted to differently by patients of varying backgrounds. Individual personality, family background, age, and gender are some of the factors that influence a patient's reaction to cancer. Ethnic and cultural factors also contribute greatly to different reactions.

For instance, to study cross-ethnic differences among cancer patients' attitudes toward their disease, Ali, Khalil, and Yousef (1993) conducted a structured interview of American patients in a Midwestern hospital and of Egyptian patients at a hospital in Cairo, Egypt. Analysis of the responses found five categories of attitudes among the American patients, including, in order: fighting spirit and adaptation; fear/anxiety/disbelief; hope; passivity in planning; and faith. Among Egyptian patients, seven categories emerged in the order of stoicism and fatalism; dependency; compliance with the medical regimen; anxiety/fear/insecurity; powerlessness; hope and optimism; and family support. This study illustrated how patients of different ethnic backgrounds from different societies (possibly of different medical realities) reacted to the fatal disease of cancer. American patients, based on their cultural attitudes, mostly held views of adaptation and hope. Egyptian patients, based on their philosophical orientation, maintained more fatalistic and powerless views.

F. SEX-RELATED MEDICAL CONDITIONS OR ISSUES

1. Breast Cancer

The varying degrees to which female breasts have a sexual role in different cultures may influence the patient's understanding of the causes of breast cancer. Chavez, Hubbell, McMullin Martinez, and Mishra (1995) interviewed Salvadoran immigrants, Mexican immigrants, Chicanas, and Anglo-Americans in California concerning attitudes toward risk factors for breast cancer. They found two broad cultural models. The Anglo-American model emphasized family history and age as risk factors. The Latin model associated breast trauma and "bad" behaviors (such as alcohol and illegal drug use) as risk factors for breast cancer. A subsequent investigation by Hubbell, Chavez, Mishra, and Valdez (1996) in California found that Latinas were more likely than Anglo-American women to believe that factors such as breast trauma (71% vs. 39%) and breast fondling (27% vs. 6%) increased the risk of breast cancer. The investigators concluded that Latinas' beliefs about breast cancer may reflect the moral framework within which they interpret diseases.

2. Pregnancy, Pre- and Postnatal Care, and Childbirth

Pregnancy and giving birth are major events not only in the parents' lives but also have substantial cultural significance and are impacted by cultural beliefs. Woollet et al. (1995) compared the ideas and experiences of pregnancy and childbirth of Asian and non-Asian women in east London. Although Asian women demonstrated a strong commitment to Western maternity care, they continued to follow traditional cultural practices, such as observing a special diet in pregnancy and following restrictions on certain activities in the postpartum period. Asian women tended to want their partners present at delivery and to express a greater concern with the gender of the child.

In some ethnic groups, great attention is paid to postpartum care. In traditional Chinese belief, a woman is expected to observe 1 month of confinement after giving birth. She is not allowed to go outside of her house, to take "cold" foods (such as fruits), or to bath or even wash her hair. A woman is supposed to eat a lot of "hot" foods (such as chicken cooked with sesame oil and ginger). These were old customs observed in the past — perhaps to prevent postpartum infection — that are still faithfully observed by some traditional women. In Micronesia, a traditional "pregnancy taboo" requires the wife to return to her family of origin once she discovers she is pregnant. She does not return to husband's place until her child is old enough to hold his breath under water or to jump across a ditch, activities that ensure the greater likelihood of his or her survival.

Breast-feeding is a very natural way to feed a newborn baby. However, despite the widely acknowledged evidence supporting the benefits of breast-feeding (fewer childhood infections and allergies), the prevalence of breast-feeding in Western countries remains low. This may be due to the development of baby formula or time demands on a working mom. However, Rodriguez-Garcia and Frazier (1995) pointed out that the cultural notion of the female breast as a primarily sexual object places the act of breast-feeding in a controversial light and can be one of the most influential factors in a woman's decision not to breast-feed.

3. Hysterectomy

In many cultures, reproduction is considered one of the major functions of women, and losing the uterus is considered to be losing the power of being a woman. Many women fear a change in sexual desire after a hysterectomy and that their husbands will not want them because they are "incomplete" woman. As a result, they might refuse to have their uterus removed, or develop anxiety and depression after a hysterectomy.

4. Menopause

Although menopause is a biological phenomenon, the intensity of menopausal symptoms varies among ethnic or racial groups. This may be due partially to diet, with a recent study revealing that Asian women may experience fewer hot flashes because of estrogen derived from soybean products in their meals. To what extent sexual attitudes contribute to emotional adjust-

ment or attitudes toward menopause is a subject that requires future investigation.

G. Culturally and Ethically Controversial Medical Practices

1. Abortion

Abortion is the subject of an intense emotional, political, and ethical debate in many countries. In the United States, there is no foreseeable resolution to the conflict, which has involved radical acts such as the bombing of abortion clinics and the shooting of physicians who perform abortions. However, in many countries, abortion is an accepted part of family planning. This is particularly true in societies where there is societal acceptance of the concept of population control. Thus, abortion is not merely a medical choice, but also a social, cultural, and political matter.

2. Sterilization

From a medical point of view, sterilization is a simple surgical operation and a way of family planning. However, there may be a significant psychological impact depending on how such a procedure is seen by the patient's culture. In some cultures, particularly those that strongly emphasize the need for many children, sterilization can be seen as a very unwelcome procedure. In such cases, sterilization for men may be considered almost equal to castration even though medically it is not.

3. Euthanasia

Whether physicians are allowed to offer active assistance for patients to end their lives is a controversial subject in many societies. In Holland, euthanasia is actively practiced by physicians (Battin, 1991). In Germany, assisted suicide is a legal option, but is usually practiced outside of the medical setting. In the United States, withdrawing or refusing treatment is the only means currently permitted by law, and then only with legal documentation from the patient or family.

H. Systems of Medical Practice in Various Cultures

1. Practices of Indigenous and/or Traditional Healers

Traditional healing refers to healing practices carried over from the past. It comes from another kind of medical system that originated in the past and has a traditional root [cross-reference to Chapter 9: Mental Illness: Folk Categories and Explanation (Section III, A–C)]. Although traditional medicine may be referred to as "nonscientific," in many societies it is accepted as a well-established "medical" system with organized medical knowledge and clinical experiences accumulated over many centuries. Included in this category is Chinese medicine, Ayurvedic medicine in India, and Galenic-Islamic medicine in Arabic countries.

In contrast to traditional medicine, the practice of folk healing through spirit mediumship (such as shamanism) or religious healing is characterized by supernatural orientation [cross-reference to Chapter 32: Culture-Embedded Indigenous Healing Practices (Section II, A)]. Even within the same society there may be different attitudes toward folk healing than toward traditional medicine. For instance, in China, shamanism is strictly forbidden, but the practice of traditional medicine is officially sanctioned. In contrast, in Korea, shamanism is still observed, while traditional medicine is not encouraged officially.

It is important for clinicians to be aware that indigenous healing practices are not only found in developing societies, but may be commonly practiced in developed modern societies. In America, religious healing can be found on daily television programs. It is estimated that over half the people use herbal medicines, and many psychiatric patients have consulted with or are seeing folk healers simultaneously with conventional psychiatrists.

2. Medical Insurance Systems for Payment

Medical insurance differs greatly from one country to another. In many countries, such as Scandinavia, Germany, Canada, and Japan, medical payment is taken care of by a national insurance system. In other countries, such as America, payment is handled primarily by a private insurance system and supplemented by a public social welfare system. In some developing countries, medical expenses are solely the patient's responsibility.

The type of payment system may affect the pattern of medical practice. In Italy, a person relying on the public insurance system may wait a year for a hip joint operation, or only a few weeks if treatment by a private physicians is sought. In contemporary China, a patient can choose a physician if a registration fee is paid according to the rank of the physician. This is very different from when China strongly emphasized communist ideology, and everybody was expected to pay the same minimal fee and receive the same type of treatment. In contrast, in Taiwan in the past, the patient was expected to give a cash gift to the doctors working in a public hospital to ensure that "proper" care was received. This was especially true in the case of surgery. Although it is now officially discouraged, patients and their families still follow this traditional custom.

3. The Matter of Giving Gifts

Gift giving to physicians is a custom that needs careful cultural interpretation. It may be considered against the principles of psychotherapy by classic psychoanalysts or interpreted as unethical bribing to physicians in some societies. However, in others, a gift is considered a sign of appreciation to the physician for the services rendered. This may be especially true where medical practice is considered charity work, so that physicians never ask for payment from patients. Even now, a shaman or herb doctor may not request reimbursement for services, and it is the patient who decides how much cash or what kind of gift should be given in appreciation. Understanding such customs leads to a better understanding of why patients want to give gifts to their physicians.

The many implications of gift giving to physicians need psychological interpretation and caution. Accepting a gift may be interpreted by the patient as assurance that the physician is willing to treat him and that there is a hopeful prognosis. Refusal of a gift may be seen as a sign that the prognosis is bad and that the doctor therefore has no interest or hope in treating the patient. There may also be therapeutic implications, such as making a depressed patient feel appreciated or an insecure patient feel encouraged, and so on. Certain issues, such as whether a gift is too expensive, has any sexual implication, or has the hidden intention of seeking special privileges, must all be considered. However, beyond these factors, the baseline is to find out the cultural meaning and to be aware of the social, ethical, and legal implications of gift giving. In other words, a comprehensive understanding and approach is needed in the matter of gift giving in medical practice, rather than dealing with gifts simply as "gifts," with no further significance.

4. Hospital Service for Minority and Different Ethnic Groups

In addition to the quality of service provided to the patient, as judged from a general medical–social point of view, there are other levels of concern if the patient and his family are members of a minority or different ethnic group. Among these are whether there are adequate interpreting services, whether written information is in the patient's first language, and whether the food is suitable for the patient's ethnic background (Madhok, Bhopal, & Ramaiah, 1992). Associated with the human rights movement, it is becoming a common practice in most health facilities in the United States to offer written instructions or documents in multiple languages. A group of interpreters for different languages is also available for service.

In order to suit the cultural background of the patient and family, many efforts have been made in different societies. For instance, in Bali, Indonesia (Castillo, in press), the hospital is built in the traditional village style with the heads of all the beds facing north (mountain side) to fit the local customs. In Taiwan, the pediatric ward is set up with an additional adult bed so that parents can stay with their sick youngsters day and night. In term of food preparation, in Kashi and Urumuch in Xingjiang, China, there are always two kitchens in each hospital so that different kinds of food can be prepared without "contamination" for patients of different faith: for the Muslim Uygur nationals and the Han Chinese who inhibit the same region. In Hawaii, out of consideration to multiple ethnic groups, different foods are always offered to satisfy patients of different ethnicities.

III. SUGGESTIONS FOR CULTURE-SENSITIVE MEDICAL PRACTICES

Modern medicine emphasizes biopsychosocial approaches in dealing with patients. It stresses the importance of viewing the patient as a whole person with medical problems rather than concentrating on the disease from which the patient suffering. In this approach, the personal background and psychology of the person and his family all need to be taken into consideration. As an extension of this concept, the cultural background of the patient should be included so that a biopsycho-socio-cultural approach can be exercised for maximum benefit (Qureshi, 1994). In order to carry out a culturally oriented psychosomatic medical practice, the following issues are recommended for attention by the physician in dealing with medically ill patients.

A. MAINTAIN BASIC CULTURAL SENSITIVITY

A physician should maintain cultural sensitivity in relating to the patient and his family and in handling the medical care of the patient. He should keep in mind that human life is full of variations that are very much shaped by the patient's cultural background. As a healer, he should keep his mind and his views open and avoid cultural rigidity or cultural blindness.

B. Gain Needed Cultural Knowledge

Because it is practically impossible for a physician to know all the various cultural systems that exist in the world, it is suggested that he make it a habit to gain medically related cultural knowledge about each of his patients.

It is desirable for the physician to keep his mind open and flexible in order to learn from the patient and his family, as they are the most appropriate sources of knowledge for clinical application. It is suggested that overgeneralization and stereotyping be avoided and that the physician try to learn from each person and his family any individual variations of cultural beliefs.

If there are any questions or doubts about cultural issues directly related to medical care, it is recommended that the physician seek cultural expertise for relevant interpretation.

C. Be Aware of Cultural Impact on Various Dimensions of Medical Practice

In addition to paying attention to the basic requirements of medical practice, the physician needs to know in what ways cultural factors have an impact on medical practice, including patient–physician relations, interaction, and communication. Culture also impacts how patients may interpret and react to medical diseases and the ways they respond to the treatments prescribed for them. There also needs to be an awareness of how the medical system and practice are directly or indirectly influenced by the "medical culture" so that changes may be made if necessary.

D. Balancing and Integrating Gaps between Culture and Profession

Quite often, folk attitudes or cultural beliefs may not fit with modern medical approaches. In many cases, they conflict with professional concepts. Balancing and integrating polarized situations is an art form. If it is decided that medical considerations take precedence over cultural beliefs, an effort should be made to carefully explain to the patient and family the medical reasons for this. Finally, a health care delivery person must examine the basis of the decisions made and actions taken in professional behavior: is it due to medical reasons, personal psychology, or cultural impact? Through such an inspection of one's cultural beliefs and attitudes, more culturally appropriate care can be given.

REFERENCES

Ali, N.S., Khalil, H.Z., & Yousef, W. (1993). A comparison of American and Egyptian cancer patients' attitudes and unmet needs. *Cancer Nursing, 16*(3), 193–203.

Baider, L., Ever-Hadani, P., & De Nour, A.K. (1995). The impact of culture on perceptions of patient-physician satisfaction. *Israel Journal of Medical Sciences, 31*(2–3), 179–185.

Battin, M.P. (1991). Euthanasia: The way we do it, the way they do it. In Special Issues: Medical ethics: Physician-assisted suicide and euthanasia. *Journal of Pain & Symptom Management, 6*(5), 298–305.

Beyene, Y. (1992). Medical disclosure and refugees. Telling bad news to Ethiopian patients. *Western Journal of Medicine, 157*(3), 328–332.

Carpenter, V., & Colwell, B. (1995). Cancer knowledge, self-efficacy, and cancer screening behaviors among Mexican-American women. *Journal of Cancer Education, 10*(4), 217–222.

Castillo, R. (2001). Lessons from folk healing practices. In W.S. Tseng & J. Streltzer (Eds.), *Culture and psychotherapy: A guide for clinical practice* (pp. 81–101). Washington, DC: American Psychiatric Press.

Chavez, L.R., Hubbell, F.A., McMullin, J.M., Martinez, R.G., & Mishra, S.I. (1995). Understanding knowledge and attitudes about breast cancer. A cultural analysis. *Archives of Family Medicine, 4*(2), 145–152.

Dancy, B. (1996). What African-American women know, do, and feel about AIDS: A function of age and education. *AIDS Education and Prevention, 8*(1), 26–36.

Friedman, L.C., Webb, J.A., Weinberg, A.D., Lane, M., Cooper, H.P., & Woodruff, A. (1995). *Journal of Cancer Education, 10*(4), 213–216.

Hodes, R.M., & Teferedegne, B. (1996). Traditional beliefs and disease practices of Ethiopian Jews. *Israel Journal of Medical Sciences, 32*(7), 561–567.

Hubbell, F.A., Chavez, L.R., Mishra, S.I., & Valdez, R.B. (1996). Differing beliefs about breast cancer among Latinas and Anglo women. *Western Journal of Medicine, 164*(5), 405–409.

Kandakai, T.L., Price, J.H., Telljohann, S.K., & Holiday-Goodman, M. (1996). Knowledge, beliefs, and use of prescribed antibiotic medications among low-socioeconomic African Americans. *Journal of the National Medical Association, 88*(5), 289–294.

Krauss-Mars, A.H., & Lachman, P. (1994). Breaking bad news to parents with disabled children — a cross-cultural study. *Child: Care, Health and Development, 20*(2), 101–113.

Luke, K. (1996). Cervical cancer screening: Meeting the needs of minority ethnic women. *British Journal of Cancer, 129* (Suppl. 74), S47–S50.

Madhok, R., Bhopal, R.S., & Ramaiah, R.S. (1992). Quality of hospital service: A study comparing Asian and non-Asian patients in Middlesbrough. *Journal of Public Health and Medicine, 14*(3), 271–279.

Matsumoto, D., Pun, K.K., Nakatani, M., Kadowaki, D., Weissman, M., McCarter, L., Fletcher, D., & Takeuchi, S. (1995). Cultural differences in attitudes, values and beliefs about osteoporosis in first and second generation Japanese-American women. *Women Health, 23*(4), 39–56.

Morgan, C., Park, E., & Cortez, D.E. (1995). Beliefs, knowledge, and behavior about cancer among urban Hispanic women. *Journal of the National Cancer Institute, Monographs, 18,* 57–63.

Qureshi, B. (1994). *Transcultural medicine: Dealing with patients from different cultures.* (2nd ed.,). Dordrecht, The Netherlands: Kluwer Academic Publishers.

Racy, J. (1969). Death in an Arab culture. *Annals of the New York Academy of Sciences, 164*(3), 871–880.

Raphael, K.G., Kunzel, C., & Sadowsky, D. (1996). Differences between Asian-American and white American dentists in attitudes toward treatment of HIV-positive patients. *AIDS Education and Prevention, 8*(2), 155–164.

Rodriguez-Garcia, R., & Frazier, L. (1995). Cultural paradoxes relating to sexuality and breast-feeding. *Journal of Human Lactation, 11*(2), 71–74.

Ross, H.M. (1981). Social/cultural views regarding death and dying. *Topics in Clinical Nursing, 3,* 1–16.

Rubens, A.J. (1996). Racial and ethnic differences in students' attitudes and behavior toward organ donation. *Journal of the National Medical Association, 88*(7), 417–421.

Stein, H.F. (1993). *American medicine as culture.* Boulder, CO: Westview Press.

Talmadge, E. (1997, March 27). Girl's need for transplant hindered by Japanese laws. *The Honolulu Advertiser,* Honolulu, p. A3.

Woollet, A., Dosanjh, N., Nicolson, P., Marshall, H., Djhanbakhch, O., & Hadlow, J. (1995). The ideas and experiences of pregnancy and childbirth of Asian and non-Asian women in east London. *British Journal of Medical Psychology, 68*(1), 65–84.

Zuckerman, M.J., Guerra, L.G., Drossman, D.A., Foland, J.A., & Gregory, G.G. (1996). Health-care-seeking behaviors related to bowel complaints. Hispanics versus non-Hispanic whites. *Digestive Diseases and Sciences, 41*(1), 77–82.

Section H

Social Phenomena and Therapeutic Considerations

Clinical practice cannot occur in a vacuum. It has to deal with the social and cultural environment within which the practice takes place. This is particularly true for cultural psychiatry. Many clinical issues go beyond the individual patient or his family. A broader view is needed to understand the social environment and phenomena that take place in the real world around them.

In this section, several social phenomena that are relevant to the lives and mental health of the patients are reviewed and examined from social and cultural perspectives. These include cultural change (Chapter 43); migration and refuge (Chapter 44); minority issues derived from ethnicity, race, and other factors (Chapter 45); intercultural marriage (Chapter 46); and religion (Chapter 47).

There is an almost endless list of topics that we could address in the area of social phenomena. Rather than exhausting the list, only some subjects are selected for discussion here, based on whether material is available from a cross-cultural perspective and whether the subject is relevant to clinical care. This section is intended to assist clinicians in keeping their vision at broader social and cultural levels. It is hoped that a more comprehensive understanding of patients will result and more meaningful care provided.

43

Cultural Change and Coping

I. CULTURAL CHANGE: BASIC CONCEPTS AND ISSUES

Although a society normally undergoes a certain degree of change in any given time frame, occasionally sociocultural change of a remarkable magnitude may occur within a relatively short period of time, significantly impacting the lives of people. Therefore, sociocultural change has been a popular subject of study in the social sciences, including sociology, economics, political science, and anthropology (Berry, 1980).

In this century, in contrast to earlier times, large-scale sociocultural change has been taking place rapidly around the globe. This has been due to the remarkable improvement of communication systems, such as the postal service, newspapers, radio, television, and, now, the internet; as well as the incredible improvement of transportation and the subsequent ease of traveling and migration. These developments have increased transcultural encounters much faster and to a far greater extent than in the past. As pointed out by Zwingle (1999), "Goods move. People move. Ideas move. And cultures change." It is a worldwide phenomenon. As Davis (1999) indicates, "roughly five percent of the global population (about 300 million people) still retain a strong identity as members of an indigenous culture, rooted in history and language and attached by myth and memory to a particular place. Yet, increasingly, their unique visions of life are being lost in a whirlwind of change." As Davis states, there is no better measure of this worldwide crisis of change than the loss of languages. He notes that throughout all of history, something on the order of 10,000 spoken languages have existed on Earth. But "today, of the roughly 6000 languages still spoken, many are not being taught to children — effectively they are already dead — and only 300 are spoken by more than a million people." He predicted that, in another century, fully half of the languages spoken around the world today may be lost. As language disappears, culture dies. This is merely one illustration of the formation of a "global culture." However, paralleling this trend toward globalization, in reaction to cultural universalization, many people are working hard to preserve the uniqueness of their cultures. Thus, it is unlikely that all human beings on Earth will share only one language and one culture — at least not for many centuries to come.

Cultural psychiatrists are interested in this special social phenomenon for theoretical and practical reasons. It is a phenomenon that allows clinicians and scholars to examine the explicit effects of culture on human behavior and psychology. Besides, rapid and great sociocultural change always strongly impacts human life and has a significant influence on the mental health of those who experience it (Murphy, 1961). There is certainly a clinical need to pay attention to such a phenomenon.

A. CLARIFYING SOME TERMS

1. Social and Cultural Change

Any change occurring in a society can be comprehended from a "social" and/or a "cultural" perspective. Sociologists tend to grasp the phenomenon of change in terms of social structures and systems, including economic, demographic, and political. In contrast, cultural anthropologists and psychologists often approach the phenomenon from the perspective of change in habits, customs, attitudes, ways of thinking, beliefs, and value systems. These are merely different angles from which to view change, as if viewing two sides of the same coin. In a sense, any social change usually accompanies cultural change, in terms of lifestyle and belief systems; cultural change also often involves social change to some extent — thus, it is hard to discuss them separately. Therefore, the term **sociocultural change** is often used to indicate the compound nature of the phenomenon.

2. Acculturation

This is a special term originally used by Redfield, Linton, and Herskovits (1936) to indicate cultural change occurring as a group-level phenomenon. As the word itself implies (i.e., ac-culturation), it refers to the acquiring of a new cultural system. It is now used widely for individual-level phenomena as well, stressing the psychological aspects of acculturation. According to the Social Science Research Seminar on Acculturation held by anthropologists in 1954, "accul-

turation" is cultural change that is initiated by the conjunction of two or more autonomous cultural systems. It emphasizes that phenomena occur as the result of direct cultural transmission.

It should be mentioned that the process of **enculturation** is the way an individual, during his lifetime, absorbs and incorporates (or introjects, in analytic terms) the traditions of his family (mostly parents) and immediately surrounding group (neighbors and relatives). As pointed out by Herskovits (1964, p. 151), the process of enculturaltion has two stages: the early life and the adult life of the individual. During early life, a person is conditioned to the basic patterns of his culture. No self-selection is involved. As an adult, he has a certain degree of choice in the process of learning and absorbing new cultures. Thus, enculturation during adult life involves reconditioning rather than conditioning. Based on this concept, **acculturation** can be seen as a special kind of enculturation occurring in adult life that involves great change and the incorporation of new value systems and lifestyles, particularly after encountering new cultural systems from outside.

There are three potential outcomes of the process of interacting with a new culture (Berry, 1980). One is the absorbtion of the new, foreign, or dominant culture in balance with the old, native, or traditional culture and the formation of a new culture. This is called **integration.** Another outcome is giving up one's original or traditional culture almost entirely and making an effort to absorb the new or dominant culture as one's own. This is called **assimilation.** Assimilation may occur voluntarily or as a result of sociopolitical pressure. The last outcome is the conscious refusal to accept the new, foreign, or dominant culture and rigidly adhere to the original or traditional culture. This is defined as active **rejection** with conservatism.

3. Modernization

Modernization refers to one kind of sociocultural change in which social conditions become more "modernized" than in the traditional society. It usually means society becomes more advanced in technology, and things are mechanized in production, transportation, and other social systems. It is often associated with industralization and involves changes in residential patterns: urbanization. It may also involve the adoption of a "new" system of attitudes, views, beliefs, or ways of doing things. It needs to be cautioned that "modernization" does not necessarily mean "improvement" of lifestyle or "progress" of civilization. Modernization itself may bring about a deterioration in the quality of life and have a negative impact on mental health. Also, trying to achieve modernization faster than people can follow and adjust to it often results in some degree of social complication and psychological disturbance.

4. Industrialization

Although this term is often used in conjuction with modernization, in a strict sense, industrialization refers simply to a change in the system of production to mass mechanization. This is in contrast to production in an agricultural, hunting, or food-gathering system. When industrialization occurs, it is often accompanied by social and cultural change.

5. Urbanization

This refers to changes in social structure accompanying the formation of large cities within a society. In modern history, it has usually occurred as the result of industrialization. The urban setting is used primarily for the administration and commercial businesses associated with a high density of population and intense transportation systems. This is the opposite of a rural setting, where the primary function is agricultural and residence is less concentrated. In an urban environment, there is a shift to a wage-earning economic system based on the nuclear family (rather than the collective-labor system and extended families often found in rural, agricultural societies).

Living in urban settings is not considered beneficial by some scholars because of the high population density, heterogeneity of population, and transitory social relations (Milgram, 1970), resulting in a defi-

ciency in meaningful and lasting social bonds (Henderson, Duncan-Jones, Byrne, Adcock, & Scott, 1979). It has been believed that there were more mental health problems among people living in urban settings. However, Krupinski (1979) pointed out that the findings of a study carried out in Victoria, Australia, do not necessarily support the notion that the levels of psychiatric or psychosocial disorders are related to urban living there.

6. Westernization

This term commonly refers to the process by which non-Western (mostly developing) societies, through direct or indirect contact with the West (Europe or North America), absorb some Western culture, resulting in a shift toward a Western lifestyle. The emphasis on a democratic political system, individual autonomy, human rights, freedom, and active change to deal with reality are some characteristic elements of value systems stressed in Western societies. Because modern machine technology originated in the West, the industrialization of a society may be regarded broadly as a form of Westernization. However, strictly speaking, modernization does not necessarily mean Westernization. For instance, in Japan, society is modernized and industrialized, but not entirely Westernized. The Japanese maintain their traditions along with modernization. Thus, even though modernization, in a narrow sense, originated in Western societies during the Renaissance and industrialization, in a broad sense, it should not be equated with Westernization.

In summary, it should be pointed out that, as shown earlier, many terms relating to social and cultural change have been used loosely and interchangeably by laymen as well as professionals that need to be carefully distinguished in academic discussion. It is also important to understand that cultural change can be analyzed from different levels: sociocultural, institutional, and individual. Although clinicians are interested in change primarily at the individual level due to the nature of the phenomenon, attention needs to be given to the social and institutional levels as well in order to comprehend the change as a whole.

B. Sources of Cultural Change

Theoretically, sociocultural change can occur in various circumstances. These include the following.

1. Internally Arising Change

Gradual or abrupt change may occur within a society as a reactive adaptation of its own traditional modes of life, or due to significant changes in its political or economic systems. It may take the form of cultural reformation or political revolution. While the change might be influenced to some extent, indirectly, by the outside, it arises primarily from within the society, initiated and enforced by its own members. The occurrence of democratic movements and industrialization in European societies in the 19th century and the well-known Cultural Revolution that occurred in the 1970s in China are explicit examples of internal change.

2. Externally Influenced Change

This is cultural change within a society that is obviously influenced, or even pressured into happening, by an outside culture. It may occur as the result of direct contact with foreigners, traders, or missionaries or through indirect contact, such as through mass media. This phenomenon may be described as a "cultural invasion by impinging culture."

In the contemporary era, mass media, such as movies and television, are becoming a powerful means of influence by outside cultures. Associated with the convenience of international travel and an increased tendency to go aborad, every society is exposed to outside cultures to some extent and frequently experiences a certain degree of change. However, the social change may occur on a remarkable scale during a rather short period of time. The sociopolitical–economic change that occurred during the Meiji period in Japan was clearly influenced by the West after Japan was forced to open its doors to Westerners.

3. Impact of the Majority

A minority group within a society may be forced to make cultural changes by the majority group through contact or political pressure. Native American people in the United States lost not only their land but also their culture after the European people came to North America. In South America, a similar situation occurred when the Spanish forced the Native Americans there to destroy their own culture. Traditional temples were destroyed and Christian churches were built on the same spots, forcing religious conversion and cultural assimilation on the Native Americans. Similar events occurred in other places, including Asia, Australia, and Africa, where native inhabitants lost their native cultures to the powerful impact of invaders.

4. Results of Transcultral Migration

Cultural change takes place when an individual or a group of people migrates to another place with a considerably different cultural system. In order to survive in the host society, it is usually necessary to make cultural adjustments to its cultural system, with or without political pressure to do so. This is a common phenomenon observed everywhere when a group or individual moves to a society with a different culture, as a voluntary migrant, political exile, war refugee, or transient traveler for education or business purposes.

II. VARIABLES THAT AFFECT THE PROCESS OF ACCULTURATION

As defined previously, acculturation refers to the process of cultural change that takes place in adult life. This process is subject to influence from various factors on individual and social levels, as well as on the level of the cultural system itself.

A. Personal Factors

It is commonly noticed that, at the individual level, age has a certain impact on the process of cultural change. In general, young people adjust to change more easily, whereas for aged persons, change is relatively difficult. Personality often contributes to the process of acculturation. Persons with rigid or obsessive traits do not make drastic adjustments to their lifestyles easily, whereas those who are flexible are more comfortable with changes. Closely related to personality factors are gender differences. It is generally observed that men are relatively slow (or resistant) to lifestyle changes, while women are more flexible.

There are many other personal factors that may contribute to the process of cultural change. These include individual motivation for change. Among immigrants, educational levels and previous occupations affect the outcome of their occupational adjustment in a foreign country. In general, highly skilled (or well-educated) persons and unskilled (or uneducated) persons have a relatively difficult time finding a suitable job in a new place, whereas those in between have a better chance of finding work after settling.

B. Social Factors

At the social level, many factors will shape the outcome of sociocultural adjustment. Needless to say, economic conditions are among the most crucial factors. If a society is affluent, there is relative ease in adjusting to sociocultural change. If it is not, more hardships are encountered. Clearly, the political system and policies and the social atmosphere all have a direct impact on the process of acculturation.

C. Cultural Factors

1. The Nature of the Cultural System Itself

It is not the personal variables or social circumstances but the cultural systems themselves (the old culture versus the new, the original culture versus the foreign, the home culture versus the hosting, etc.) that have the most significant effect on the outcome of acculturation. As pointed out by Fabrega (1969), several features of a culture as a system influence the behavioral responses to acculturation.

a. Boundaries

Certain cultures maintain clear-cut boundaries, whereas others do not. Acculturation will certainly be influenced by the extent to which a culture defends itself from outside cultures. The recognition and function of the boundaries (of a culture) are often closely related to whether the culture is ethnic–centric (or culture–centric).

b. Flexibility

Certain cultures are flexible and open to change, whereas others are rigid. This is analogous to the individual personality, which may be rigid and persistent, or flexible and easily accepting of change. For instance, Hawaiian culture, in contrast to others, such as Japanese culture, is more flexible and open to incorporating outside cultures.

2. The Nature of Cultural Encounters

a. Friendly Encounter or Hostile Invasion

Based on historical background and social circumstance, cultures may have different kinds of contact and relationships between them. As mentioned before, when indigenous cultures in South America encountered Spanish culture, it was in the form of forceful invasion and resulted in hidden hostile relations. When Hawaiian culture encountered European cultures, at least in the beginning, it was with a friendly welcome.

b. Dominant-Subordinate or Equal Encounters

In a similar way, the relationship between two cultures, whether dominant-subordinate or equal, will affect the process of cultural exchange between them.

3. The Relativeness of the Interacting Cultures

a. Compatibility

There may be incompatible or congruent interaction between cultures depending on their natures or characteristics, which in turn depend on the features that are emphasized in each cultural system. For instance, when Jewish people migrated to the United States, they generally had a smoother and higher level of acculturation, simply because of the congruence of their values with those of American culture, specifically in the area of achievement. In contrast, the relationship between Jewish culture and Muslim culture is problematical. This is not merely due to their historical paths, but also to the many incompatible factors within the two cultures, including their religions, systems of marriage, daily life customs, and etiquette, such as patterns of food intake, even at the individual level, making interethnic or interfaith marriages very difficult.

b. Power of Function

Certain elements of life are so forceful in their functions that they will affect other cultures whether they are preferred or not. Mechanization and industrialization are two examples. The impact of computers on information systems and communication is so powerful that most cultures (or societies) will try to adopt them without too much emotional resistance. However, the importation of movies into some cultures, due to the incompatibility of their values and attitudes with those of the culture, could encounter strong resistance from or be prohibited in some cultures.

After reviewing the literature on cultural change and mental health, Favazza (1980) pointed out that the simpler the cultural contexts, the more accurate our predictions about individual mental health and the process of cultural change. In large, complex societies, we are hampered by the limitations of our science in our ability to make meaningful predictions in most areas.

III. DIFFERENT PATTERNS OF REACTION TO CULTURAL CHANGE

When cultures of considerable differences encounter each other, cultural change will occur either

directly or indirectly. Theoretically, the change is bilateral, with a two-way influence, based on interaction between the two cultures. However, in reality, due to differences in their powers of influence or the size of their populations, the direction of change might be predominant in one direction, becoming almost unilateral. This is more so when a minority or inferior culture encounters a majority or superior culture. The former will be forced to change toward the latter. There are different patterns of reaction toward such a powerful influence for change.

A. REJECTION OF THE OTHER (OR NEW) CULTURE

This reaction is characterized by the active rejection of the other culture. The person or group of people sees the other culture as foreign, "harmful," or "evil" and refuses to be influenced. Cultural barriers may be established to protect against the foreign culture. On an individual level, a person may refuse to learn the new language, to adopt to the new custom, or to accept its views or value systems. As a group, people may develop an antimovement against the new cultural system. The establishment of the "iron curtain" in the former Soviet Union during Stalin's era or the "bamboo curtain" in China during Mao's time are concrete and extreme examples at the level of the country as a whole, even though these phenomena were not entirely cultural, but attributed to political and military reasons as well.

B. PRESERVATION OF TRADITIONAL (OR NATIVE) CULTURES

This refers to the situation in which a person or a group of people actively preserve his or her own traditional culture as a way of coping with the influence of a foreign culture. Sometimes, "cultural regression" (returning to or remaining fixated in the original culture) may occur temporarily as a result of stress when the demand for acculturation is too quick or radical and threatens a person's psychological integrity. Occasionally, a person or a group of people may invent or magnify traditional ways of dealing with things when they encounter an invasive culture. It is well known that, in China, during the 19th century, when massive invasion by foreign (Western) powers threatened the integrity of the country and its traditional culture, the *Yi-Ho Tuan* movement occurred (also known as the boxing cult). The leader of the group claimed that by practicing traditional boxing the people could defend themselves against the foreign weapon (gun). This is an extreme but good example of a "preservation" reaction pattern.

C. Integration of Native and Foreign Cultures

When one culture encounters another, it does not simply reject or preserve the culture in a black and white way. Instead, a process of adoption, conversion, and reintegration takes place. Certain elements of the new or foreign culture are partially absorbed, converted, and incorporated into the traditional or native cuture, resulting in a partial reformation of the existing cultural system. For instance, when the American business McDonald's was introduced into India — a society in which people strictly observe the taboo of not consuming cows and many people are vegeterians — it served mutton instead of beef and offered a vegetarian menu acceptable to even the most orthodox Hindu. When the American television show *Sesame Street* was introduced into China, the program was redesigned by Chinese educators to teach children Chinese values and traditions through Big Bird: borrowing the American "box" and putting Chinese content into it (Zwingle, 1999).

Often, only minimal disturbance is experienced in the process of culture conversion. As a result, a new cultural system emerges. This is known as integration and is generally considered a healthy adaptation from a mental health perspective.

D. Assimilation into the Other (More Powerful) Culture

As described at the beginning of this chapter, this is a situation in which a person or a group of people, either voluntarily or involuntarily (under social or political pressure), gives up his or her own culture almost entirely and incorporates the other culture as his or her own. This is referred to as assimilation, from a social perspective.

The degree of assimilation may vary from occasion to occasion. For example, when a person wants to be naturalized as an American citizen, it is normal to expect him to speak minimal English, for reasonable social communication. He is also expected to know a little bit of American history (such as the name of the president of the United States or the governor of the state he lives in) and is willing to vow that he will be loyal to the United States and faithfully pay taxes. These are minimal requirements for political assimilation. The person is not required to change his name to an American one. For example, a person can maintain the native name of Fu-Yong Pak, or only change the first name into an American one, such as Peter Pak, to make it easy for his American friends. In Japan, however, a person is not considered Japanese until, in addition to the basic requirements described earlier for Americans, he changes his native name, for example, Fu-Yong Pak, to a Japanese name, such as Kenjiro Watanabe, which has no trace of the original. Further, the person is expected to learn Japanese daily life etiquette: how to make deep bows in greeting and how to behave properly when bathing in a public bath, for instance. Otherwise, socially, the person will still be treated as a *gaijin* (foreigner).

E. Destruction of the Traditional Culture

At a political level, a "revolution" may take place to affect the radical change of a political system and social structure. In a similar way, at a cultural level, a cultural revolution may occur to achieve the total destruction of the traditional culture and the establishment of a new cultural system. This is exemplified historically by the Chinese Cultural Revolution, which focused on the radical destruction of the traditional culture, including the religious system, authority figures, and any preexisting scholarly thoughts that did not comply with the "revolutionary" ideology. Such a revolution is rare, but can happen, with political intent.

F. Uprooting

In this situation, the original culture is destroyed to such an extent that it is almost like a tree losing its roots. Many indigenous or so-called "primitive" people, encountering powerful ("advanced") cultures from the outside, go through a period of social invasion and destruction, often ending in cultural uprooting. Needless to say, this condition is not healthy and is often associated with grave mental health problems.

The various patterns of reaction just described can occur at the individual, family, small group, or institutional level. The pattern of reaction is not static and often occurs in a dynamic way. It may start with the initial rejection of the other culture, go through a period of preservation of the traditional culture, and end with integration, assimilation, or the uprooting of the original culture.

IV. PSYCHOLOGICAL CONSEQUENCES OF CHANGE

A. Individual Level

While the impact of rapid and drastic sociocultural change on the psychology of an individual is an interesting subject with significant relevance to mental health and clinical work, it has not been investigated throughly. Based on clinical experiences, several issues have been raised.

It is generally considered that the cultural system introjected (through the process of enculturation) in early life tends to remain unchanged, even when new cultural subsystems are acquired in adulthood (through acculturation). In other words, the emotions, views, and attitudes associated with certain value systems that are absorbed in the early stages of development often remain the core part of the individual's psychology. However, the added views, feelings, and attitudes related to new value subsystems are included as added layers, becoming a part of the psychology of the whole self. Throughout life, many new things will be incorporated and endless layers of cultural subsystems will be added so that, analogically, the personality will become like an onion with multiple layers. In general, the various components of the self (the different layers of the "onion") do not differ greatly, allowing interaction among them. They become integrated parts of the total personality manifested as unique patterns of reaction and behavior.

However, if the different cultural subsystems that are absorbed differ widely, or are even oppositional, it is possible for ambivalence, conflict, or confusion to develop within a person's mind. This is often the case with individuals who experience drastic changes in their cultural systems in a short period of time. Shifting from very restrictive views about man–woman relations to very liberal ones, converting from very rigid moral views to very permissive ones, and changing from a loose life orientation to a goal- and achievement-oriented life are some examples of cultural change that can have a serious impact on the psychology of an individual. In the extreme, a person will suffer from cultural confusion and loss of cultural identification. This often results in the formation of various mental health problems.

B. Family Level

Rapid sociocultural change in a society will cause certain psychological disturbances to the family unit. Due to differences in pace and reaction to the new value systems and ways of viewing things, the generation gap between parents and children will be wider than usual. Added to differences between spouses, fragmentation and confusion could occur in the family as a whole. For instance, when a conservative Muslim family is exposed to outside (Euro-American) cultures through the media, whether or not the youngsters should be allowed to watch Western movies can become a serious family issue. The father may not permit any of the children to watch; the mother may secretly allow the sons to watch but not the daughters, creating a split in the family (El-Islam, 2001).

In a stem or extended family, with the presence of a grandparent(s), the gaps among three generations complicate family functioning even further. For example, a three-generation Asian family migrated to the United States. The grandmother stayed at home most of the time, devoting herself to prayer and the worship of Buddhism, and ate only vegetarian food; the adult children, who worked outside the home for a living, went to church on the weekends, where they simply wanted to meet and spend time with their Asian friends; the grandchildren watched TV and played computer games after school, making noise while the grandmother was meditating. There was hardly any conversation between the grandmother and grandchildren because the grandmother hardly spoke English and the grandchildren did not speak their native language. The adult children had difficulty comprehending the kind of education their children were receiving at school and were often upset by their children, who developed the habit of talking back to them. Cultural disconnection and confusion were illustrated in this transculturally migrated stem family.

C. GROUP OR INSTITUTIONAL LEVEL

When sociocultural change takes place in a society, if often occurs in different directions and at different paces among various subgroups. Unless there is a clear goal and direction, and a powerful administrative organization, the change may result in social confusion, imbalance, and disintegration.

At the social level, when people have difficulty following and adjusting to changes, such as modernization, revolution, or reformation, certain social phenomena may be observed. For instance, youth movements may arise that stress antimodernization, antidevelopment, or antiauthority (as examplified by the Hippie movement in the 1960s in the United States, triggered by reactions to the Vietnam War).

Sociologists have noticed the frequent emergence of new cults or peculiar religious groups, or the revitalization of indigenous practices, in reaction to sociocultural change that calls for modernization or mechanization. These special groups or social movements may indicate that the sociocultural change is occurring too fast for many people and needs to be slowed down.

V. RESEARCH RELATED TO SOCIOCULTURAL CHANGE

A. GENERAL CONSIDERATIONS

From the standpoint of research, it is relatively easier to study "social change" by utilizing concrete social indexes, such as the size and density of population, the method and amount of production, financial income, or other social variables. This is not true for the study of "cultural change" — a phenomenon that is based on attitudes, beliefs, value systems, and other abstract variables that are difficult to measure.

One of the most common ways to investigate sociocultural change is to examine longitudinally any changes that might have occurred in a selected society that had undergone rapid and extensive change. This can be done through retrospective or prospective investigations and relies mainly on social demographic data. For example, comparisons might be made of prewar and postwar situations in a target society. In other words, a study is made of the society in different periods of time. An alternative method is to compare two or three different societies that are in different stages of sociocultural change. For instance, comparisons might be made of a society that is already highly industrialized, one that has just begun the process of industrialization, and one that is still at the agricultural level. Cross-sectional comparisons of societies in different stages of change, coupled with the mental health situation in each, can illustrate the possible relation between change and mental health conditions. A comparison of Samoan people living in (traditional) western Samoa, (slightly Westernized) American Samoa, and (very Americanized) Hawaii is a good example of such a cross-comparison conducted at a given time to examine the process of change.

The prevalence of emotional disorders, juvenile behavior problems, drinking problems, substance abuse, and suicidal behavior are some of the variables that are often used as indexes for the total mental health condition of a society (Tseng et al., in press).

It should be mentioned that the prevalence of psychoses, or psychiatric hospital admission rates, is not a suitable index to illustrate the mental health condition of a society. In the past, many scholars, for the sake of convenience, used it as an index for measurement and failed to find any correlation with sociocultural change.

B. Many Social Studies and Reports

Numerous studies of sociocultural change have been carried out in the past, mostly by behavioral or social scientists, and some by psychiatrists. Most of the pioneer studies focused on Native Americans in North America or Aboriginal peoples in Australia. For instance, the studies by Chance (1960, 1968) and Foulks (1980) were concerned with the Alaskan Eskimos' psychological adjustment problems during acculturation. The investigation carried out by Beiser (1980) was related to adaptation to social change in Senegal in west Africa. The publications by Cawte (1974) and Burton-Bradley (1975) were concerned with the Aboriginal peoples' adjustment to modern conditions in Australia. Later studies expanded to include many areas around the globe, indicating that

sociocultural change was a worldwide phenomenon of widespread concern.

C. Some Psychiatric Research Findings

Some investigations have focused primarily on mental health conditions associated with sociocultural change that occured over a period of time. Several will be mentioned here briefly.

1. Psychiatric Problems among Maoris and Pakehas in New Zealand

While they were not formal community epidemiological investigations, several reports were made from New Zealand concerning the time-related differences in psychiatric disorders observed among the indigenous Maoris versus Pakehas, New Zealanders of European origin, before and after World War II, associated with sociocultural change observed there. Concerning mental hospital admission rates, Beaglehole (1939) reported that Maoris had a lower incidence of psychoses than Pakehas. Also, it was noted that, in World War II, Maoris had a lower rate of psychopathological combat reactions than Pakehas. However, three decades later, when Kelly (1973) again studied the mental hospital admission rates, it was found that there were substantial increases in the rates of neuroses and character disorders, but little change in the rate of psychotic disorders among Maori people. It was said that in the 1930s, when Beaglehole conducted his survey, less than 10% of the Maoris lived in urban areas, but in the 1960s, slightly more than 50% of them lived in urabn settings, indicating a significant change in lifestyle associated with internal migration and cultural change during that period of time.

2. Fifteen-Year Follow-Up Study of Mental Disorders in Taiwan

A community psychiatric epidemiological study was originally carried out in three communities in

Taiwan in 1946–1948, shortly after World War II ended (Lin, 1953). Fifteen years later, from 1961 to 1963, a follow-up study was conducted in the same communities by the same research team (Lin, Rin, Yeh, Hsu, & Chu, 1969). During this 15-year period, the community had experienced rapid sociocultural change, as had the whole of Taiwan. The national government retreated to Taiwan when the communists took over the mainland. There was a massive influx of Chinese mainlanders, both civilians and soldiers, and there was military tension across the strait. In addition to the political situation, there were shifts in the common language and the educational system. These were followed by rapid industrialization and urbanization. Thus, during this period, people experienced social upheaval and subcultural changes.

The survey was one of very few follow-up investigations ever conducted of mental health conditions associated with rapid sociocultural changes in the same community. The follow-up study revealed that there was no increase in the observed prevalence of psychotic disorders over the 15-year period. However, in striking contrast, there was a significant increase in nonpsychotic disorders, especially psychoneuroses. The prevalence rate of neuroses increased almost sevenfold, from 1.2 to 7.8 per 1000 population. The interpretation was that psychotic disorders were less affected by environmental (or sociocultural) changes than minor psychiatric disorders (Lin et al., 1969) [cross-reference to Chapter 12: Culture and Psychiatric Epidemiology (Section II, B, 1)].

3. Viscidity of Suicidal Rates before and after World War II in Japan

Japan is one of the few countries in the world in which official household records are well kept and records of suicides are available for nearly a century. It therefore offers information on how the rate of suicide may fluctuate over a period of time when society has gone through drastic changes, including war, postwar social construction, and cultural changes.

As elaborated previously [cross-reference to Chapter 22: Suicidal Behavior (Section II, A, 4)], it was reported that the total suicide rate for the Japanese was rather consistent from 1890 to 1935 — mostly in the range of 15 to 20 per 100,000 population. However, when Japan went through a series of wars in succession, starting with the invasion of China in 1935, and later the attack on Pearl Harbor in 1941, leading to the Pacific War with America and its allies, the suicide rate declined considerably, reaching a bottom of 12 per 100,000 population in 1943, shortly before World War II ended. After the war, the suicide rate increased gradually, reaching a peak of 25 around 1958 — about a decade and a half after the war, when postwar reconstruction was completed and people started to enjoy affluent lives again. After the war, there was considerable subcultural change in daily life with the influence of the West — women and the younger generation were more liberated; the older generation felt a loss of tradition. The increase in the suicide rate between 1955 and 1960 was attributed to the increase in suicide among the elderly (Yoshimatsu, 1992). Although suicide should be regarded as merely one kind of mental health index for a society, the longitudinal study of the viscidity of the suicide rate in a society over many decades certainly provides unique information on how such self-destructive behavior may fluctuate through time and in association with sociocultural changes.

VI. SUMMARY REMARKS

Sociocultural change is a part of our daily lives. It has occurred in every society in the past, is occurring in the present, and will occur in the future. Most people, as members of a society, adjust to change reasonably well. However, it is the general consensus among scholars that, if sociocultural change occurs with great magnitude and within a relatively short period of time, it tends to become stressful, confusing, and disturbing to a society, and some people will find it difficult to adjust, resulting in certain mental health problems. The problems manifested are multiple. They could occur as social problems in daily life, such as family disintegration, with an increase in divorce, the emergence of new religious cults, the revitalization of folk beliefs and indigenous healing practices, and the rise of various youth movements; or as minor psychiatric disorders, such as psychosomatic disorders, neuroses, drinking problems, substance abuse, violent behavior, juvenile delinquency, or suicidal behavior.

It is rather difficult for an individual to directly combat sociocultural changes that occur at a societal level, yet, at the clinical level, it is necessary for the mental health worker to pay attention to the mental health problems that derive indirectly from the macroscopic changes in a society. In other words, there needs to be more mental health care when a society is experiencing gross social and cultural changes with which the ordinary person is unable to deal with.

As mentioned at the beginning of this chapter, sociocultural change may take place from within a society, may occur in association with the special social phenomena of migration or refugees, or may be related to the intense and close interaction between minority and majority groups in a society. These subjects will be elaborated further in Chapter 44 and Chapter 45.

REFERENCES

Beaglehole, E. (1939). Culture and psychosis in New Zealand. *Journal of Polynesian Societies, 48,* 144–155.

Beiser, M. (1980). Coping with past and future: A study of adaptation to social change in West Africa. *Journal of Operational Psychiatry, 11*(2), 140–155.

Berry, J.W. (1980). Social and cultural change. In H.C. Triandis & R.W. Brislin (Eds.), *Handbook of cross-cultural psychology: Vol. 5. Social psychology* (pp. 211–279). Boston: Allyn & Bacon.

Burton-Bradley, B.G. (1975). *Stone age crisis: A psychiatric appraisal.* Nashville, TN: Vanderbilt University Press.

Cawte, J. (1974). *Medicine is the law: Studies in psychiatric anthropology of Australian tribal societies.* Honolulu: University Press of Hawaii.

Chance, N.A. (1960). Culture change and integration: An Eskimo example. *American Anthropologist, 62,* 1028–1044.

Chance, N.A. (Ed.). (1968). *Conflict in culture: Problems of developmental change among the Cree.* Ottawa: Canadian Research Centre for Anthropology.

Davis, W. (1999, August). Vanishing cultures. *National Geographic, 196*(2), 62–89.

El-Islam, M.F. (2001). A women with one foot in the past. In W.S. Tseng & J. Streltzer (Eds.), *Culture and psychotherapy: A guide to clinical practice* (pp. 27–41). Washington, DC: American Psychiatric Press.

Fabrega, H., Jr. (1969). Social psychiatric aspects of acculturation and migration: A general statement. *Comprehensive Psychiatry, 10,* 314–326.

Favazza, A.R. (1980). Culture change and mental health. *Journal of Operational Psychiatry, 11*(2), 101–119.

Foulks, E.F. (1980). Psychological continuities: From dissociative states to alcohol use and suicide in Arctic populations. *Journal of Operational Psychiatry, 11*(2), 157–161.

Henderson, S., Duncan-Jones, P., Byrne, D.G., Adcock, S., & Scott, R. (1979). Neurosis and social bonds in an urban population. *Australian and New Zealand Journal of Psychiatry, 13,* 121–125.

Herskovits, M.J. (1964). *Cultural dynamics.* New York: Alfred A. Knopf.

Kelly, R. (1973). Mental illness in the Maori population of New Zealand. *Acta Psychiatrica Scandinavica, 49,* 722–734.

Krupinski, J. (1979). Urbanization and mental health: Psychiatric morbidity, suicide and violence in the state of Victoria. *Australian and New Zealand Journal of Psychiatry, 13,* 139–145.

Lin, T.Y. (1953). An epidemiological study of the incidence of mental disorder in Chinese and other cultures. *Psychiatry, 16,* 313–336.

Lin, T.Y., Rin, H., Yeh, E.K., Hsu, C.C., & Chu, H.M. (1969). Mental disorders in Taiwan, fifteen years later: A preliminary report. In W. Caudil & T.Y. Lin (Eds.), *Mental health research in Asia and the Pacific* (pp. 66–91). Honolulu: East-West Center Press.

Milgram, S. (1970). The experience of living in cities. *Science, 167,* 1461–1468.

Murphy, H.B.M. (1961). Social change and mental health. *Milbank Memorial Fund Quarterly, 39*(3), 385–445.

Redfield, R., Linton, R., & Herskovits, M.J. (1936). Memorandum on the study of acculturation. *American Anthropologist, 38,* 149–152.

Tseng, W.S., Ebata, K., Kim, K.I., Krahl, W., Kua, E.K., Lu, Q.Y., Shen, Y.C., Tan, E.S., & Yang, M.J. (in press). Asia mental health: Improvement and challenge. *International Journal of Social Psychiatry.*

Yoshimatsu, K. (1992). Suicidal behaviour in Japan. In L.P. Kok & W.S. Tseng (Eds.), *Suicidal behavior in the Asia-Pacific region* (pp. 15–40). Singapore: Singapore University.

Zwingle, E. (1999, August). A world together. *National Geographic, 196* (2), 6–33.

44

Migration, Refuge, and Adjustment

I. INTRODUCTION: MIGRATION AND MENTAL HEALTH

Migration occurs when a person or a group of people move from one place to another, with the intention of staying in the new place for a considerable period of time. Moving to a new place usually causes considerable disruption in life, including changes in work, social relations, community networks, and lifestyle, and requires extra effort for successful adjustment to take place. A person may change residences several times during his or her life, within his or her own society, for education, work, marriage, or other reasons, for example, moving from a rural to an urban area, from the south to the north, or vice versa. Even though such internal or intracultural migrations may involve considerable social changes, such as economics, living environment, or separation from family or friends, in general, adjustment is relatively easy. However, if the migration is transcultural, i.e., to a foreign country or diversely different sociocultural environment, with remarkable differences in language, life patterns, value systems, or social customs, it usually involves considerable cultural change, and calls for special cultural adjustments.

As defined previously, culture refers to a unique lifestyle that is shared by a group of people. It is learned and accumulated experiences, including knowledge, beliefs, value systems, customs, or habits, that are shared and transmitted by the members of a particular society. Cultural change may be the result of different circumstances, most often political change, social or economic revolution, or migration into a different cultural setting [cross-reference to Chapter 43: Cultural Change and Coping (Sections I, A and B)].

The cultural change and adjustment associated with migration often cause psychological stress, emotional strain, and even mental complications while the migrant is adjusting to the new situation. A certain process is involved in coping — at an intrapsychic, interpersonal, or social level. Migration not only impacts a person, but also a family, a community, and a society. Thus, the subject of migration and mental health is an interesting one for examination not only by sociologists and psychologists, but also psychiatrists, particularly cultural psychiatrists. It provides a suitable example of how the sociocultural environment has an impact on our lives, how to anticipate the stress associated with sociocultural change, and how to deal with it. It also challenges clinicians how to provide suitable care for people experiencing mental health problems associated with transcultural migration (Westermeyer, 1989).

II. THE IMPACT OF MIGRATION ON MENTAL DISORDERS

A. FREQUENCY OF MENTAL DISORDERS

The subject of migration and mental health has been studied by cultural psychiatrists for several decades (Al-Issa & Tousignant, 1997). Originally, attention was focused on the prevalence of mental illness among immigrants. This was stimulated by the clinical impression that there were more admissions to mental hospitals among immigrants of certain ethnic groups. In the middle of the 19th century, many European immigrants migrated to North America. The superintendents of many mental hospitals developed the impression that there were more Irish and German peasants than British people admitted to psychiatric hospitals (Wittkower & Prince, 1974). According to Schwab and Schwab (1978, p. 178), Javis, in 1855, noted that, in Massachusetts, the ratio of the mentally ill was higher in the foreign population than in the native population, whereas mental deficiency was much lower among the former than the latter.

B. Malzberg carried out a formal epidemiological investigation of psychiatric patients admitted to mental hospitals in New York. As a result, Malzberg (1935) reported that rates of admission to New York mental institutions were higher among immigrants than among the native-born.

In 1932, Örnulv Ödegaard, a psychiatrist from Oslo, Norway, conducted an epidemiological study at Rochester State Hospital in Minnesota. Based on the patients admitted to the psychiatric hospital during the four decades between 1889 and 1929, he compared the incidence rate between the Norwegian-born and the native-born of Minnesota. He found that the ratio of admissions to the state hospital was higher for the Norwegian-born than for the native-

born. From 1889 to 1899, the rate of admission for the former was 495.8 per 100,000 population, whereas for the latter, it was 338.1 per 100,000 population, with significant differences (more than three times the standard error), indicating a higher incidence of insanity in the former group (namely, the immigrant population). The pattern was the same throughout the four decades investigated.

Ödegaard also compared data with that of the population in his home country of Norway. Although the hospital systems in the United States and Norway are different in terms of how patients are admitted and how the state hospitals are utilized, Ödegaard reported that there was more insanity among the Norwegian immigrants in Minnesota than in their native country. In his interpretation, the difference in rate was too large to be explained by discrepancies in hospital facilities or modes of commitment. Ödegaard concluded that "the higher ratio among the Norwegian-born (immigrants) cannot be due to differences in race or ethnic stock — it must be traced back to the fact that they are immigrants rather than to their being Norwegians" (1932, p. 80).

Two hypotheses have been proposed to explain the relatively higher occurrence of mental disorders among new immigrants. It has been speculated that migration across cultures might bring about mental stress and cause mental disorders. An alternative hypothesis is that those who are mentally vulnerable might have difficulty staying in their own societies and tend to wander and migrate to foreign places.

Later, careful epidemiological studies in other societies revealed that the relationship between migration and frequency of mental disorders was not necessarily a single correlation — immigrants did not necessarily have a higher rate of mental disorders, as illustrated by the immigrants to the United States. For example, Astrup and Ödegaard (1960) found that Swedes and Danes moving into rural areas in Norway had lower first-admission hospital rates than Norwegian nonmigrants in the same areas. In Israel, when its doors were opened to all Jews when it became a nation after World War II, Murphy (1965) reviewed these (Jewish) immigrants from various places. Murphy indicated that immigrants from Asia and Africa (whose socio-cultural experiences were rather dissimilar to those of the hosting society) had higher mental hospitalization rates than the local-born Jewish population. However, those from Europe (whose social status was generally similar to that of the local population) did not have higher rates than the native Jews. In Canada, Murphy (1973) reported that, according to data obtained from the census years 1958 and 1961, immigrants had lower rates of mental hospitalization than native-born Canadians.

The many conflicting results obtained from various investigations prompted scholars to realize that migration is not a singular phenomenon. The person who migrates, the motives for and circumstances of migration, the relationship between the hosting and the original society, and the ways the immigrant is received by the new society are all factors that significantly effect the immigrant's adjustment after migration (Mezey, 1960; Murphy, 1965). Furthermore, it is understood that the process of migration, which is psychologically stressful, might be one of the precipitating factors in the development of certain minor psychiatric disorders, such as anxiety or psychosomatic disorders, but it is not the main reason for the development of major psychiatric disorders (i.e., psychoses), such as schizophrenia.

Originally, for convenience in obtaining data, most investigations focused on the hospital admissions rates of psychoses, particularly chronic psychoses. However, it was realized that hospital admissions rates did not necessarily reflect the occurrence of all mental disorders. They reflected mostly severe psychiatric disorders, and only rarely minor psychiatric disorders or other psychological problems. It is the general view of scholars that the etiology of psychoses is predominantly biological factors and is not a desirable indicator to be used to examine the psychological and sociocultural effects of migration. Many other kinds of mental disorders, which are known to be more susceptible to social factors, such as drinking problems, substance abuse, behavior disorders, depression, or suicidal behavior, can serve as better indicators for examination. The results of such investigations have indicated that those psychologically related mental problems tended to arise when there was sociocultural disruption that may have been caused by migration or some other social phenomenon, such as rapid sociocultural change, socioeconomic deterioration, or sociopolitical instability.

B. TIME SPAN IN THE ONSET OF MENTAL DISORDERS

Several clinicians and scholars have focused on the time span involved in the development of certain mental disorders after migration. This is another way to examine the possible effects of migration on the occurrence of mental disorders.

Ebata, Yoshimatsu, Miguchi, and Ozaki (1983) conducted an investigation of homocultural, or internal migration, specifically, the migration to metropolitan Tokyo from other regions of Japan. They reviewed the medical records of 4899 patients who, during the period of 1968 to 1974, visited a psychiatric outpatient clinic offering services for densely populated downtown Tokyo. Among all the patients, only 508, who were immigrants to Tokyo and had no previous psychiatric histories, were included as subjects. The cases were analyzed by subgroups of psychiatric diagnoses, namely schizophrenia, affective disorders, and neurotic disorders. It was found that the onset of mental disorders in relation to duration of (postmigration) residence in Tokyo could be divided into three periods: the initial highest occurrence period (zero to 1 year); the lowest occurrence period (1 to 4 years); and the later high-occurrence period. The occurrence of mental disorders in the last period varied according to the category of the mental disorder and the gender of the immigrant. For females, there was no difference among the three disorders examined, and the peak rose after 7 to 9 postmigration years. In contrast, among males with schizophrenia, the peak occurred earlier, around 4 to 6 postmigration years, whereas affective disorders occurred later, after 8 to 10 postmigration years. It can be summarized that, within a 1-year period after migration, there is a high risk for the occurrence of mental disorders, regardless of their nature. The risk declined after that, but rose again after several years, with the number of years depending on the gender of the migrant and the nature of the mental disorder. It needs to be pointed out that Ebata's study related specifically to immigration.

In their study of transcultural, international migration, Mavreas and Bebbington (1989) reviewed the hospital records of randomly selected Greek Cypriot immigrants living in London and their history of psychiatric breakdown. They reported that there was no evidence that the risk of mental breakdown was increased in the immediate aftermath of immigration. Among 291 subjects investigated, the 34 who experienced their first mental illness after migration showed a mean interval of 15 years, which was considerably long. Only 9% of them had breakdowns within 2 years after migration.

The studies just described suggest that although migration may contribute to the occurrence of certain mental disorders soon after migration, there is no close correlation to the development of mental disorders in terms of time.

III. MIGRATION AND PSYCHOLOGICAL ADJUSTMENT

In order to comprehend the impact of migration on mental health adjustment, attention is more appropriately focused on the kinds of mental stress that are encountered, the psychological coping mechanisms that are adopted, the resources and supports that are utilized, and the outcomes of mental health based on individual processes of adjustment rather than on time factors. The variables examined may include ethnic–cultural identification, psychological equilibrium, and the mental integration associated with the process of acculturation. Various factors are used by clinicians and investigators to assess conditions of mental health. Psychiatric symptoms are among the indicators that are often used. A person's subjective assessment of adjustment and social adaptation, including educational or occupational achievement, are among

other variables that may be used to evaluate the degree of mental health adjustment associated with migration.

A. Personal Variables that Affect the Process of Adjustment to Migration

It is clear that personal factors will affect the process of cultural adjustment. These may include individual background, age, and gender.

1. Age and Gender

In terms of age, young adults usually have the flexibility to adjust to a new environment much more easily and faster than older people, who tend to be more rigid and fixed in their behavior. However, youth who have not yet established a firm personal and cultural identity may be affected greatly by the cultural confusion associated with migration and become vulnerable in their psychological development.

In terms of gender difference, males, in general, who need to search for new roles in the new social setting, encounter more obstacles, whereas females, whose readjustment is primarily in a domestic setting, have relatively easier outcomes. However, if women are isolated in their home settings, with limited opportunities for socialization, they might suffer from emotional isolation. If job opportunities are more available for women than for men, then men tend to suffer from frustration. In other words, coupled with the issues of male and female roles, working opportunities, and job conditions, males and females will encounter different kinds of outcomes in adjusting to the host society.

From the perspective of mental disorders, Ödegaard (1932), in his study of Norwegian-born immigrants to Minnesota, found that the incidence of mental disorders was higher in females than in males. He explained that in addition to females being more socially isolated, they had more biological burdens, such as pregnancy and childbirth, that made them more vulnerable to mental disorders. Murphy (1977) added later that males are usually the ones who decide to immigrate to the host country, while females simply follow them.

How much these personal factors, namely age, gender, and interacting with the sociocultural environment, might affect the outcome of transcultural adjustment is a challenging question that needs to be investigated.

2. Language

It is a general rule that fluency in the language of the host society will facilitate the process of cultural adjustment. If there is a handicap in learning the new language, there will certainly be difficulties in acculturation. Examining English-speaking Westerners who were temporary residents in Japan, Akiyama (1996) revealed that a higher proficiency in the language of the host society (Japanese, in this case) and being married were related to a lower vulnerability to mental problems, whereas a past history of psychiatric disorders was linked to a higher vulnerability.

3. Personal Background

Israel has an open-door policy for immigrants and provides an opportunity to examine the issues of migration and psychological distress. Zilber and Lerner (1996) carried out a nationwide sample of 600 immigrants who had arrived during the preceding year from various home societies. They reported that the factors that correlated with the immigrants' levels of distress were mostly individual characteristics, such as their professions, religiousness, former residences, and past histories of psychological problems, stressing that personal factors influence the level of adjustment after migration.

4. Occupation and Employment

Educational level and occupational background will obviously influence postmigration adjustment. It is usually the midrange group, with ordinary occupational experience, that has an easier time finding a job in the new society and settling down in the new envi-

ronment. The extremes, either highly educated with a special occupational background or poorly educated with unskilled job experience, have a harder time in obtaining appropriate and satisfactory occupations.

5. Family and Household

Family is the nest for individual life and provides needed emotional support; at the same time, family can become a source for burden and conflict. Depending on the nature of the family system, the household structure, and whether any occurrence of separation of family members is associated with migration, the outcomes of adjustment will differ.

For instance, young Asian people from a developing society coming to the United States to study or work may face separation from their spouses or children. Over the years, they will suffer from nostalgia and encounter strain in their marital relationships due to the long-term separation. At the same time, there is additional psychological pressure for them to achieve and be successful in the host society. People from the Pacific Islands are traditionally bonded with their families. They will receive direct emotional support from immediate family members and other relatives when they are in need of it. However, they also have a responsibility to reciprocate to their families on their home islands by sending any earnings they make in their host societies. Thus, even when they are separated, they have to react to their migrant situation as members of a family group rather than as individuals, feeling a strong impact from their families — in both positive and negative ways.

Lin, Tazuma, and Masuda (1979) studied the adaptation of Vietnamese refugees in the Los Angeles area of the United States. Among other variables, they found that the family types (or structures) of the refugees after migration had a direct influence on their levels of adjustment. Four types of family were identified: young single men, living alone; individuals who lived in a nuclear family unit; individuals who had extended family networks in the host society; and women, divorced or separated, who were also heads of households. At the time of a 2-year follow-up, the investigators found that the widowed or separated female heads of households had less desirable adjustments, as reflected by higher scores on the Cornell Medical Index (CMI), whereas households composed of single young men had the best adjustments, with the lowest CMI scores. Among the four different family types, the divorced–widowed female heads of household appeared to be the least resourceful and most distressed. In contrast, households with single young men benefited from having less responsibility and more free energy to adapt to the highly individualistic society.

6. Premigratory Expectations

What the migrant expects from migration often is a significant factor in shaping the outcome of migration. For instance, McKelvey, Mao & Webb (1993) examined Vietnamese Amerasian youth and reported that those with higher premigratory expectations tended to report fewer symptoms of anxiety and depression after their settlement in the hosting society. Ebata, Tseng, and Miguchi (1996, pp. 56–57) carried out a 3-year follow-up study of a group of Japanese war orphans who moved to Japan from China. They were left in China as orphans at the end of World War II and were adopted and raised by Chinese foster parents. Almost 40 years later, when Chinese–Japan relations were normalized, the orphans, married to Chinese spouses and with adolescent children, were given the opportunity to "return" to Japan with their Chinese families. Ebata and colleagues found that among their adolescent children, those who were highly motivated to migrate transculturally with their parents, in contrast to those who were reluctant to migrate, had fewer mental health problems at an early stage of postmigratory adjustment — 3 months after the migration took place.

B. Different Natures of Migration Groups that Relate to the Process of Adjustment

It is a salient fact that the background of the migrant, coupled with his or her reason for moving to live in a foreign society, will determine the different processes and outcomes of migration. Several identifiable groups of immigrants deserve discussion.

1. Upward Economical Migration

This is the most common form of migration observed in the past and present. The immigrant chose to move from one society to another with the primary intention of seeking a better job and better economic conditions, aiming for an improved quality of life. This kind of migration usually takes place from a rural to an urban area within the same society, or from an economically developing to a developed society. Migration from many parts of Asia, southeast Asia, or south Asia to North America and from eastern Europe, the Mideast, or Africa to western Europe during the past several decades is the kind that is motivated primarily by economic reasons.

2. Political Exile

This occurs when a person, with or without his or her family, is forced to leave his or her home setting and live in another part of the same country (usually a remote area with less favorable conditions), or a foreign society, mainly for political reasons. The person is usually a member of an intellectual group that has been intensely involved in a political movement. He or she is considered to be against his or her own government, and exile is deemed necessary. Thus, migration is involuntary, the connection with the home society is completely disrupted, and the outcome of the migration, in terms of the duration of living in a foreign place, and the final solution regarding the move are uncertain. In other words, there is no definite plan and perspective for the person migrating, and he or she usually suffers from the bereavement associated with separation (Munoz, 1980). Political exile was not only physical expulsion but also psychological rejection. Through his experience caring for many Chilean exiles, Perez (1984) pointed out that they were subject to aggression toward their opponent, who was no longer before them. Therefore, their fight was unfinished and the only means of dealing with it was by turning to the past.

3. War Refugees

As a result of war, either civil or international, people may have to take refuge in other societies. They may have already experienced psychological traumas associated with the war, including being wounded, raped, tortured, or having their families or friends killed or wounded. While a person may become a refugee by himself or with his immediate family, there is usually separation from or loss of a family member or members so that the integrity of the family is seriously damaged. Because migration occurs during wartime, the number of material assets that can be moved is limited, and there is usually severe financial loss, resulting in limited resources after the migration.

Most of the emigrants from southeast Asia as a result of the Vietnam War belong to this category. They had to cope with the psychological traumas of the war, in addition to the challenges of adjusting to a foreign society. Based on their investigation of southeast Asian refugees in the United States, Chung and Kagawa-Singer (1993) reported that premigration traumatic events and refugee camp experiences were significant predictors of psychological distress even 5 years or more after migration.

4. Transient Travelers

Associated with increased international communication and interaction, this form of migration is becoming more frequent than before. It includes students going abroad for study or people living in foreign countries to conduct international business. The duration of living in the foreign societies in these situations is relatively short. Also, the immigrants usually have the clear perspective that they are returning to their home societies eventually. Therefore, there is no need for them to make radical cultural adjustments to suit their host societies.

Several studies have pointed out that the housewives of international businessmen or students tend to encounter more psychological stress than their husbands. The reason is that the businessmen or students have outside contact while they are working at their companies or studying at school, whereas the housewives usually confine themselves to home and are socially isolated. This is particularly true if they have relatively young children and have to be involved in caring for them at home (Armes & Ward, 1989).

After a person or a family has lived in a foreign society for a while — at least 1 or 2 years — when he returns to his home society, readjustment is necessary from a cultural point of view. This is called reentry adjustment or reverse culture shock, indicating that considerable effort is needed to readjust to the home country.

C. Natures of Stress, Supporting Resources, and Coping Styles

From the standpoint of psychology and mental health, migration can be viewed as a process of adjustment to the stresses and difficulties encountered in the new cultural setting. Contemporary concepts of stress and coping take the view that stress does not act alone on an individual in a simple manner, but as a part of an interactional system. Conceptually, it can be grasped from several perspectives, i.e., the nature of the stress encountered by the subject, the stress perceived by the subject, the support systems available, the environmental conditions within which the stress needs to be coped, and the coping mechanisms utilized by the subject. Thus, all of these factors need to be considered in discussing the process of adjustment.

1. Common Stresses Encountered

The usual stresses faced by an immigrant are various in nature. They may be practical, such as difficulty finding a place to live, obtaining a job, arranging for education, establishing a social network, and being accepted by the host society. If the language is different from the home country, there is the additional challenge of learning a new language. Establishing basic security and functioning as an individual or as a family are the main tasks for the new immigrant in the early stages of settlement.

Simultaneously with practical stresses, the immigrant also has to face psychological stresses. These involve the feeling of separation from the home setting, a sense of nostalgia, and a sense of strangeness or unfamiliarity in the new setting. Even though some immigrants may be delighted with and enjoy the new things in the host society, and become busy incorporating the new conditions into their lives, learning new behavior patterns, and accepting the new value systems, there is still a process of change. Such change is always accompanied by hemostatic pressure and requires a process of adjustment at the intrapsychic level.

The matter of ethnic or culture identification may become an issue and a challenge after settlement in the foreign society. This may occur after some time, or soon after the move. A person needs to go through a delicate, ambivalent process, including debating and negotiating with his or her own mind. The process may take forever, without any final settlement.

2. Support Systems

These are the means that are available to provide support and assistance when a person faces a problem. Family members, friends, colleagues, neighbors, or various social organizations can be the resources of support. The support can be given at the psychological level, such as empathy, emotional encouragement, or advice, or at a mechanical and practical level, such as providing a loan, introducing the migrant to a social network, offering assistance in the search for a job, and so on. Support systems can be discussed from two different perspectives: the availability of resources and the utilization of resources. Different resources for support are offered in different societies, depending on their structures and systems. In some societies, resources are more personal and private, whereas in others, they may be more public and official. However, it is quite true that cultural background will significantly influence the pattern of utilization of the

supporting systems, in turn, making a difference on the resulting adjustment. For instance, some people only feel comfortable relying on family members or personal friends to solve their problems, whereas for others, it is easy to make use of public and social institutions, such as banks, occupational guidance, welfare institutions, attorneys, and so on for solving the problems encountered. Whether the immigrant knows about the existence and availability of supporting social systems is one thing; that is often a matter of information and knowledge. However, whether they will approach and make use of them appropriately and efficiently is another thing; that is usually an issue of social experience and cultural attitudes that influence their help-seeking behavior.

McKelvey and Webb (1996), in their survey of Vietnamese-Americans, found that the availability of like ethnic community support was critically important in preventing depressive symptoms in this group of immigrants.

3. Patterns of Coping Adjustment

Very much determined by individual personality, group relations, and social environment, immigrants may follow different patterns and courses of adjustment. For instance, a group of immigrants may congregate among themselves in terms of residential patterns, using their maternal language, and socializing and doing business mainly with people of their ethnic kind. This is exemplified by the formation of a "Little Italy," "Little Tokyo," or "China town" in some cities in the United States. Through such local congregations, the immigrants try to recreate and maintain their original sociocultural settings. Although such communities may provide a place where the immigrants can retreat or regress into their cultures of origin as needed, adherence to such a nest of their original cultures will certainly delay the process of assimilation into the larger host society. Even after several generations, the immigrants may still not be able to speak the language of the host society effectively or properly.

In contrast to this, some individuals may choose a course of isolation from (or even rejection by) their original cultures. They try to move far away from people of their own ethnic groups, trying to mix in the middle of the majority of the host society. They make an effort not to speak their own maternal languages in order to become fluent as soon as possible in the new language. They may try not to observe any cultural behavior from their homeland. Instead, they try to learn and imitate as quickly as possible their new way of life. If they are successful, they will experience a relatively rapid acculturation; if not, they may encounter cultural imbalance and emotional frustration.

Another pattern is to take a guarded position in the new environment. The immigrants may become suspicious, defensive, and have difficulty relating with the majority people in the host society. This pattern of adjustment is occasionally observed among immigrants who are faced with less favorable situations in the host societies, such as illegal immigrants, reacting in this way to avoid being deported. Paranoid phenomena are common in some immigrant groups (Ndetei, 1988).

D. Preexisting Conditions that Affect Migration Outcomes

1. Migrant's Status in the Host Society

The preexisting relations between the immigrant's background and the host society will predetermine the course and outcome of the migration to some extent. A good example is the rather unusual situation in Jamaica. As pointed out by Hickling (1996), when white immigrants moved to Jamaica, a predominantly black country, they do not develop more mental problems than the local black people (as usually happens to immigrants in other situations). Actually, white immigrants in Jamaica usually move into social class positions at a significantly higher level than those of their (white) parents, with whom they grew up in their home country. Hickling explained that the political and economic situation that exists in black postcolonial countries such as Jamaica provides a protective social environment for white immigrants.

2. Migrants' Attitudes toward their Own Culture and the Host Society

The attitudes of immigrants regarding their own and the host culture often have a significant impact on the results of migration. For example, if people have a high degree of pride in their own culture, and are biased toward the cultures of others, they may feel that migration to another culture is not a desirable act and be reluctant to learn the culture of the host society. This creates a resistance to the acculturation process. However, some people do not respect their own cultures and only admire the cultures of others. With this attitude, they tend to assimilate themselves into the host society readily when they migrate.

3. Relations between the Host Society and the Society of Origin

The process of cultural adjustment will vary depending on the circumstances and relations existing between the homeland and the new society. For example, if there are open and friendly relations between the original and the host society, and consequently the immigrant is permitted to come and go freely between the two societies, it will certainly make it much easier for the immigrant to adjust to the host society. The immigrant is allowed to make a gradual shift between the two cultures without the feeling of being blocked, or without a choice.

However, if, after migration takes place, the immigrant has no way to return to his or her homeland, this one-way process of migration will put a great strain on him. This is not only a matter of whether there is an actual opportunity for the subject to return to his or her home culture, it is also a matter of psychological opportunity, which a person is allowed to feel and experience inside of his own mind. For any person, it is desirable to have the chance for "cultural retreat" or "cultural regression" whenever he or she feels the situation is too difficult in the foreign culture. The availability of the mechanism of "cultural time-out" is very important from a psychological perspective.

4. Hospitality of the Host Society toward Immigrants

Host societies may have different attitudes toward immigrants. If a society maintains an aloof attitude about its own culture and looks down upon other people's cultures, it will certainly have difficulty accommodating immigrants. If a society considers it very important to maintain the purity of its ethnic roots and cultural background, insisting that immigrants be assimilated unconditionally into it or creating obstacles that do not allow them to become equal members, the society will never become integrated.

About 1.8 million people came to Britain in 1950–1970 from the West Indies and the Indian subcontinent. Rack (1988) described Britain as not having a liberal, cosmopolitan culture in which newcomers are welcomed, and the situation has deteriorated in response to high unemployment, constant public expenditure, and widening gulfs between income groups. Minority groups are made scapegoats, and racial prejudice is more apparent than ever. A similar situation is observed in Germany, where many minorities have migrated from east Europe or southeast Asia. The people in the host society, particularly the radical groups, tend to show negative and even hostile attitudes toward these new immigrants. In Japan, during World War II, many young men and women from Korea were drafted to Japan as laborers. At present, there are about 1 million Koreans living in Japan. More than half a century has passed, and three generations have emerged of these "Korean-Japanese," yet they are still treated as "non-Japanese" psychologically and politically by the Japanese nationals. Because of this psychological discrimination, the "Korean-Japanese" are reluctant to be naturalized as "Japanese nationals."

In reality, a society that is composed of multiple ethnic or cultural groups seldom becomes a "melting pot" within a short period of time. A society needs to accept that it will never become pure and homogeneous. It is beneficial to have a heterogeneous component and to learn to live together in harmony and integration. This point of view needs to be considered in the search for mental health.

IV. MIGRATION AS A PROCESS OF ADJUSTMENT

A. LONGITUDINAL PROCESS OF ADJUSTMENT

It is common sense that adjustment to migration is not a static phenomenon but a dynamic process. Studying the patterns of adjustment at any given time only reflects a cross-sectional facet of the truth. A meaningful insight can be obtained only through a longitudinal investigation of the process. Thus, a longitudinal follow-up study of a targeted group of subjects becomes almost necessary in examining the process of cultural adjustment associated with migration.

B. DIFFERENT STAGES OF ADJUSTMENT

Based on clinical observations and experiences, as well as the results of investigations, most scholars consider migration to involve different stages of adjustment. Although different investigators have proposed different time periods for each stage of adjustment (Scott & Scott, 1989; Sluzki, 1986), in general, the process of adjustment can be subdivided into the following stages for discussion from the perspective of time.

1. Premigration Stage

This is the stage prior to migration. Based on limited information and actual experience of the society to which he or she is going to migrate, the subject might develop a fantasy speculation about it. The fantasy might be full of idealized dreams or expectations or, conversely, unrealistic fears and concerns. No matter how the subject tries to anticipate the new place, the knowledge is always limited and fragmented, and needs correction after migration. For refugees, such as those from southeastern Asia, it is often an extended time in a second country after they leave their own country and prior to settling in a third. It is a stage full of confusion, uncertainty, and anxiety.

2. Initial Stage

This stage is usually observed several months to half-a-year after entry into the foreign society. At this acute stage, the immigrant may experience a euphoric condition, if he or she is relieved from a stressful refugee status (Sluzki, 1986). It is also the stage in which the immigrant has to start coping with many practical problems in reality. These include learning a new language, searching for a place to live, finding a job, and developing a social network. Depending on the nature of the new society, the experience in this initial stage may be exciting for the subject, as if it were a honeymoon stage, or it may be confusing and frustrating. Pernice and Brook (1996) studied southeast Asian refugees who migrated to New Zealand and reported that, in the initial stage, they were not free from symptoms and their mental health conditions deteriorated for the following 6 months to 6 years of residence. As for the Japanese war orphans and their Chinese families who "returned" to Japan after nearly four decades, the longitudinal follow-up study (Ebata et al., 1995) revealed that their mental health symptom scores were highest in the initial 3-month stage.

3. Middle Stage

This might last for 3 to 5 years before settlement is gradually achieved. During this stage, the initial problems of finding a residence, securing an occupation, and developing a social network might be more or less resolved; however, it is a time during which the subject needs to work on cultural adjustment continuously and vigorously. This might include discovering basic differences in value systems, life customs, and interpersonal relationship patterns between the original and the new host culture. The process involves a constant struggle to maintain some part of the immigrant's original culture and, at the same time, to learn and acquire new life patterns. In this process, the immigrant might change names, alter ethnic–cultural identification, and even develop a sense of loyalty toward the new society. A delicate psychological balance is usually required in this stage of integration.

In some host societies, new immigrants might be expected to acquire only a minimal level of proficiency in the host language and to fulfill only the basic responsibilities of a citizen, such as paying taxes and obeying ordinary laws. However, some societies may expect the newcomers to learn all the behaviors of the society, thinking and acting in the same way as the natives. The latter situation requires a considerable psychological effort on the part of the new settlers (Ebata et al., 1995).

4. Final Stage

This is the balanced stage of adjustment, which might occur 10 or even 20 years after migration. If the process of adjustment has gone smoothly, it is the time when the immigrants will normally experience the feeling of being a member of the host society and begin to feel at home. There will be a gradual occurrence of psychological weaning from the homeland from which they came. However, for many, it is still a time for them to continue to work on the process of adjustment, with different problems to be encountered. These might include developing a feeling of belonging and identification at the deep level of personal emotion.

It needs to be pointed out that the adjustment of immigrants or refugees into a host society is a dynamic process that varies from individual to individual, group to group, situation to situation. For this reason, a point A and point B type of study may be incomplete. However, a general pattern of adjustment might be grasped from the perspective of stages.

C. Studies Relating to the Longitudinal Process of Adjustment

Bauer and Priebe (1994) examined the psychopathology and social adjustment of immigrants from East Germany to West Germany through follow-up assessments over a period of 2.5 years. The immigrants migrated to West Germany just prior to or shortly after the breaching of the Berlin Wall in autumn 1989. The refugees who sought crisis intervention after arrival were used as subjects for the follow-up studies. Although many of them had been exposed to prolonged situations of stress in East Germany and suffered from initial crises with psychiatric symptoms within the first 6 months after settlement, the psychiatric symptoms had decreased significantly in the follow-up period. This raised the view that initial crises are not necessarily associated with poor long-term adjustment after migration. It should be pointed out that the subjects investigated in this study migrated within their home country of Germany. Even though there were radical changes in terms of political and economic conditions, coupled with different past life experiences, there was no language barrier involved.

Focusing on the different natures of immigrants and host societies, namely Vietnamese refugees in the United States, K.M. Lin and colleagues (1979) did 2 years of follow-up investigations. They used the CMI to evaluate the mental health status of the refugees. They reported that the responses on the CMI at the end of the first and second years indicated a high and continuing level of physical and mental dysfunction. In terms of differences between the first year and the second year, in the second year of assessment, there was an increase in anger and hostility, with reductions in feelings of inadequacy. Their findings support the notion that it takes several years after migration to recover mental health, at least among war refugees settling down in quite different sociocultural settings.

Sack, Him, and Dickson (1999) completed a 12-year follow-up study of Khmer youths who migrated to Oregon in the United States. Forty Khmer adolescent youths who had survived the horrors of the Pol Pot regime (1975–1979) as children were initially interviewed in high school in 1983–1984 (Kinzie, Sack, Angel, & Clarke, 1989). The 3-, 6-, and 12-year follow-ups were carried out in 1987, 1990, and 1996, respectively. Twenty-seven were followed-up through these four stages of interviews. The results, according to Sack and colleagues, despite the persistence of posttraumatic stress disorder (PTSD), showed that most of these Khmer youths appeared to make the

transition into American culture quite successfully — pursuing either occupational or educational goals. The persistence of PTSD over time is well noted in this follow-up period in reaction to a "single blow" trauma in children and adolescents, which is different from other kinds of trauma (such as traffic accidents and hurricanes) studied and reported by other investigators. Further, the rate of depression had dropped significantly since the 6-year follow-up (from 41% in the third year to 6% in the sixth year). It was explained that, for this group of youths, depression was related to recent rather than past stressors. Thus, depression followed different pathways over time than PTSD.

Westermeyer, Neider, and Calliew (1989) and Westermeyer, Neider, and Vang (1984) carried out a longitudinal study of Hmong refugees on three occasions after their settlement in Minnesota in the United States. A total of 100 refugees were initially examined in 1977 (at an average of 1.5 years postmigration) restudied in 1979 (at an average of 3.5 years postmigration), and followed-up again in 1983 to 1985. Results indicated considerable evidence of acculturation and greatly reduced symptom levels for several complexes. From the symptom checklist (SCL-90) and the Zung scale for depression administered, it was revealed that depression, somatization, phobia, and self-esteem symptoms improved the most with time and acculturation. However, anxiety, hostility, and paranoid symptoms changed little. Even almost a decade after the migration a large portion of the refugees remained illiterate, unable to speak English, and generally involved with other Hmong but not with the majority society.

In Japan, Ebata and colleagues (1995, 1996) carried out prospective investigations regarding the adjustment of Japanese war orphans and their Chinese families after they moved from China to Japan. They reported that life stress increased abruptly when the availability of support resources declined sharply immediately after migration (at the 3-month postmigration stage) and showed signs of improvement gradually after the 3-year postmigration stage. Individual mental symptom scores reflected in the brief symptoms questionnaire showed that the scores rose sharply in the initial third month, continued to increase in the second year, and started to show signs of decrease in the third year. Family mental health, as reflected by family function and satisfaction, deteriorated considerably in the third month, improved slightly after the first and second years, but did not return to the original baseline even in the third year. On the whole, this study illustrated that in this transcultural migration, after the initial crisis in the third month, the situation started to improve after 1 or 2 years, but had not returned to the original level of mental health, for either the individual or the family, at the end of third year. This indicated that a long process of mental health adjustment was required if the migration took place transculturally, even when the immigrants and the host populations were of the same racial backgrounds.

D. Reentry Adjustment

Recently, many people have begun to recognize the phenomenon of "reentry adjustment." This refers to when a person is away from his or her home society for a while, experiences some difficulty when returning, and has to make some effort to adjust. This occurs particularly when a person has been abroad in a different cultural setting for some period of time. It is also called "reverse culture shock" (toward one's own culture) upon reentry into one's society of origin.

Uehara (1986) investigated reentry adjustment experiences of American students after extended sojourns abroad. Domestic travelers were used for comparison. Results confirm that the returnees from abroad experienced much greater reentry adjustment problems. Changes in the individuals' value structures were considered important factors associated with the reverse cultural adjustment.

Raschio (1987) studied college students who went abroad to western Europe (Italy, France, Spain, Germany) or South America (Peru) for 3 months to 1 year and then returned to the United States. Even though the period abroad was relatively short, the returning students described some changes in their friendships and peer interactions. They attributed the changes to personal growth stemming from their time away, which increased their objectivity and independence and gave them a more global perspective.

Hertz (1984) listed various factors that contributed to the severity of reentry problems, including duration of absence, extent of alienation (from the home society), previous individual and family pathology, and previously existing home or family ties. Reentry problems may involve various areas, including cognitive dysfunction, (disorientation toward the setting), disturbed affect (feeling of detachment from one's home people), or value systems (incongruence and disillusionment).

V. THE EFFECTS OF MIGRATION ON THE FAMILY

A. Influence on the Family as a Whole

Transcultural adjustment does not merely affect the individual, but also the family. A family is a unique group of members who are bound together by marriage, birth, and intimate relations. It is not only the basic unit of society, but also the nest in which a person grows and lives. A family is not merely composed of a group of family members who happen to live together, but is a special kind of social group, within which all members interact, develop private and intense emotional ties, form certain group structures and perform particular roles, and share responsibilities in their emotional, as well as practical, lives. Needless to say, families are the basic social units through which cultural systems are transmitted from generation to generation. When problems or stress are encountered either from inside or outside the family, all family members are affected as a system and react together toward the stress, seeking a solution.

In the process of migration, the family as a group reacts to the process of transcultural adjustment. This may involve changes in hierarchical structure and adjustment of roles and responsibilities between husband and wife, parents and children, or among siblings. The patterns and efficiency of communication within the family might be affected, and the nature of the affect altered, depending on the stress the family encounters. To what extent support is available and provided within the family is a crucial factor in determining the outcome of adjustment.

As pointed out by J.D. Kinzie (personal communication, October, 1999), when there is a family member or members who suffer from a mental disorder(s), a common situation among refugees, then the effects on the family are significant. For instance, a family member who suffers from PTSD will have increased irritability and aggression, which greatly increases the stress between husband and wife and parents and children. Depression, or serious mental disorders, such as schizophrenia, or alcohol and drug abuse, will greatly exacerbate the problems of adjustment for the family as a whole.

A unique phenomenon observed among refugees is that sometimes refugees will create "families" in refugee camps. A group will call itself a family in order to be sent more easily to another country. These pseudo-families live together without a history, traditions, or knowledge of each other. Some Jewish families did this after the Holocaust; Cambodian-refugees have also done this (J.D. Kinzie, personal communication, October, 1999).

Another phenomenon that deserves mention is the sequence and process of migration taken by family members. For one reason or another, a family may not migrate together as a whole, but, instead, one member migrates first and is joined by the remaining family members later. This causes family separation and also creates stresses and burdens on members. For instances, a husband may go abroad to study. After obtaining a degree and securing a job, he will be joined by his wife and children, from whom he has been separated for many years. Some families will send an older son to the host society with the expectation that he will find work and sponsor the entire family. This puts a tremendous burden on the individual.

B. INTERPERSONAL RELATIONS WITHIN A FAMILY

1. Husband–Wife Relations

a. Role Division

Culture plays a significant role in shaping the patterns of role divisions between husband and wife. Thus, when cultural change occurs in association with migration, the role divisions between spouses usually need adjustment. For example, a Japanese man who has enjoyed a certain status as a husband, expecting his wife to serve him at home, may need to give up this superior position if they move to the United States, where husband and wife treat each other more as equal partners, in both domestic and social settings. In order to comply with the new culture and be similar to American husbands, the Japanese husband would have to learn how to help his wife do some domestic chores and expect his wife to have certain input and status in social settings. He would even have to learn how to open a car door for his wife, an etiquette he never practiced in his homeland of Japan. In contrast, if an American couple chose to live in Japan, the wife would need to learn that she may not be invited with her husband (as his partner) to social occasions. She would also need to remember not to speak too outwardly "as a wife" in a social setting with her husband. Otherwise, her behavior may be interpreted as "unsophisticated" or "uncultivated."

b. Work Conditions

In many societies, as a new settler, it is easier for a woman to find a job than a man. This is particularly true in some industrialized societies or in urban settings. There are more nonlabor, unskilled (and perhaps low paying) job opportunities for women than there are suitable opportunities for men. Consequently, a wife may work outside the home, and the husband may become a jobless "house-husband." The responsibility for moneymaking would be reversed between husband and wife, requiring a psychological adjustment, even if the situation were only temporary.

2. Parent–Child Relations

a. Handicaps in Communication

Many things could happen in terms of parent–child relations in a migrated family. If there is a need to learn a new language, it is usually the children who learn faster than their parents. Also, children tend to lose the original language in which they communicated with their parents. Because the parents usually acquire the new language more slowly, limitations in communication occur. This is usually coupled with matters of knowledge. The youngsters acquire new information from the outside, while their parents lag behind. This usually creates handicaps in communication and information exchange between parents and children.

b. Wider Generation Gap

Based on differences in personal experience associated with different backgrounds in time, it is usual to have a certain gap between children and their parents. This generation gap usually becomes much wider when a family migrates to a new cultural setting. The young people acculturate faster than their parents, and they begin to hold different sets of knowledge, views, and values, as if they belonged to different cultures. As mentioned earlier, the generation gap is often worsened by communication handicaps and limitations in cultural sharing.

c. Role Reversal

When, as described earlier, the younger people acquire new knowledge faster than their parents, become more skilled in the language, and more familiar with the rules and situations of the host society, they become more "capable" than their parents in many ways. As a result, a role reversal is created in which parents have to rely on their children's assistance in adjusting to the new culture, and lose their power and ability to discipline them.

C. EFFECTS ON DIFFERENT GENERATIONS OF FAMILY MEMBERS

1. Adjustment of Adolescents

The effects of postmigration mental health adjustment of adolescents in a family can be of two kinds. As young people, they are generally more privileged than their parents or grandparents in learning the new language and adjusting to the host society. This, in turn, helps them absorb the new knowledge needed for adjustment. Their minds and behavior are flexible enough to change and adjust. However, as adolescents, they may suffer from cultural confusion and ethnic identity problems. This is particularly true when their parents lose their ethnic or cultural confidence and find their authority and ability to raise and deal with their children reduced as a result of cultural change after migration.

Brindis, wolfe, McCarter, Ball, and Starbuck-Morales (1995) carried out a comparative study of Latino and non-Hispanic white high school students in northern California. The Latino adolescents were further divided into two groups: Latinos who had immigrated to the United States (Latino immigrants) and Latinos who were born in the United States (native-born Latinos). Eight different risk-taking behaviors were compared among the three groups, which included alcohol, cigarettes, marijuana, illicit drug use, self-violence, drunk driving, unintended pregnancy, and violence. As a result, Brindis and colleagues reported that the mean number of risk behaviors was highest for Latino immigrants (1.78), followed by native-born Latinos (1.71) and native non-Hispanic whites (0.99). A t test revealed that non-Hispanic whites were statistically different from both Latino populations in all levels of risk-taking behavior ($p < 0.050$). The investigators concluded that immigrant Latino students appeared to be vulnerable to risk-taking behaviors and were not protected by their culture.

Focusing on different subjects and situations, Sam and Berry (1995) studied the acculturation stress encountered by young immigrants in Norway. They reported that among adolescent immigrants from the Third World to Norway, mental health conditions as measured by depressive tendencies, poor self image, and psychological and somatic symptoms were found to be related to close and supportive parents, marginality, integration, and number of friends.

2. Adjustment of Young Adults

While, in general, it is considered easier for young adults to adjust to a foreign society, if they are parents with children, and have elderly people in the home, their psychological responsibilities and burdens are higher. As mentioned previously, parents, in contrast to their teenage children, tend to be slower in the process of acculturation and encounter the phenomenon of role reversal with their children. If the adult parents are not psychologically mature, they may have a hard time adjusting to life in the new setting.

3. Adjustment of the Elderly

The elderly members of a family usually face a less privileged situation than other family members in adjusting to the host society, particularly if the language is different and the culture is radically dissimilar to their original culture. They often have difficulty learning the new language. As a result, they are deprived of sources of information and knowledge and are also hindered in socialization. Consequently, they tend to face social and cultural isolation. They are not only isolated from the external world, but also from other family members in the household, primarily due to a language gap and, later, by a cultural gap as well. For instance, many grandparents find it difficult to talk to their grandchildren because there is no common language between them. Any advice that they wish to offer to their grandchildren may become irrelevant, or at least unsuitable, to the grandchildren, who are more or less assimilated into the new cultural setting. This makes the elderly feel lost and unwanted in the new culture.

D. IMPACT ON DIFFERENT GENERATIONS OF IMMIGRANTS

From a long-term perspective, the process of transcultural adjustment needs to be reviewed from the point of view of different generations: the first generation that migrated to the new environment, the second generation, descended from the first generation, and the third generation, which follows the second. All go through different courses and outcomes of adjustment. It is generally believed that different generations of immigrants have different obstacles to overcome. The first generation tends to face the practical problems of adjusting to the new environment, such as learning the new language, securing their lives, and raising their children in the new setting. There is usually a psychological struggle in trying to retain the original culture and acquiring the new one. The second generation faces the problems of balancing the bicultural setting created for them, i.e., the original culture that exists at home and is reinforced by the parents, and the new culture that is experienced in the community outside of the home.

VI. UNIQUE EXPERIENCE OF REFUGEES

By definition, refugee refers to an individual or a group of people who, in order to escape from the dangers in their home countries, seek temporary safety elsewhere, including foreign countries far away, in times of war or persecution. In a way, they experience a special kind of migration. What has been said about migration in the previous sections can be applied generally to the refugee; however, because of his unique nature, the refugee differs from ordinary migrant in many ways.

First of all, a refugee usually migrates to escape from risk or dangers, often related to political, religious, ethnic, or racial persecution, civil or international war, or natural disasters. Second, the seeking refuge usually occurs suddenly, without proper planning and preparation. Third, in many cases, the refugees have encountered killing, robbing, rape, death, and other serious situations that may lead to psychological trauma. Family members are often separated or lose contact. It is thus often grave hardship, suffering and starvation, endless fear, or risk of life that leads to taking refuge. Finally, after arriving in the place of refuge, the problems do not end; rather, new difficulties begin — associated with adjusting to a foreign place. Generally, refugees face more difficulties than ordinary migrants, who planned to migrate. The challenges include adjusting to their new lives from practical social perspectives: finding a place to live and resources for living, and worrying about the family members from whom they are separated or with whom they have lost contact. Thus, there is a series of psychological traumas and burdens that they have to face at different stages of pre-, during, and postrefuge (Beiser, Turner, & Ganesan, 1989). If they take refuge in a foreign culture, dealing with transcultural adjustment presents another level of problems they have to face and with which they have to cope.

One group of refugees is the asylum-seekers. These are people who come into a country without legal protection and are seeking asylum. While their request is being processed, they are in a clearly unprotected no man's land. This group of people tends to suffer from severe psychological stress and tends to manifest serious psychiatric symptoms, as illustrated in the study carried out by Silove, Sinnerbrink, Field, Manicavasagar, and Steel (1997) in Australia.

VII. SOME EXPERIENCES OF WAR REFUGEES

In the history of humankind, there have been countless refugees in almost every corner of the globe, either due to political or religious persecution, territorial conflict, interracial or interethnic conflict, civil or international war. There are still refugees at present, and there will unfortunately continue to be in the future. Based on the circumstances, the situation of refugees differs to some extent. Here, a few examples

will be briefly elaborated to help us understand the nature of such human experiences. Most of these refugee situations took place not too long ago.

A. REFUGEES FROM THE VIETNAM WAR

Perhaps this situation of Vietnamese refugees is the most familiar to Americans as the war had such a strong impact on America. As Boehnlein and Kinzie (1995, p. 229) described, many south Asian refugees who left their native lands after 1975 carried with them memories of brutal war, escape, or concentration camp experiences. Cambodians brought memories of the Khmer Rouge era between 1975 and 1979, during which over 1 million Cambodians died of disease, starvation, or execution. Vietnamese refugees described seeing their family members killed, their possessions confiscated, and their villages destroyed. Ethnic Laotians, Mien and Hmong, also witnessed irreparable damage to their societies and cultures. Clinical investigations have shown that southeast Asian refugees are at great risk of developing psychiatric illness associated with their war experiences.

B. REFUGEES FROM THE CIVIL WAR IN CHINA

A unique situation occurred in China in the 1940s when the Communists took over the mainland. Nearly a million soldiers and civilians were forced to evacuate to Taiwan. Many of them left their immediate family members, parents, spouses, and children behind. Due to the hostile relations between the Communist and the Nationalist governments, there was complete disruption of communication for almost four decades. When the door was opened for communication and visits in 1990, the young soldiers who had fled to Taiwan were 60 or 70 years of age. Many of them returned to the mainland to visit their families, and almost one-third of them developed depression after the reunions (Tseng, Chen, Cheng, Hwang, & Hsu, 1993). Many veterans, after visiting their hometowns and learning of the suffering that their parents, spouses, or children had gone through during and after the civil war and the cultural revolution that took place later, felt guilty that they could not do anything for them. Many of them become depressed after their return to Taiwan. This illustrated that family reunions after long-term separations do not necessarily bring psychological healing, but often cause a reexperiencing of emotional pain.

C. Refugees from the Interethnic Conflict in former Yugoslavia

The situation in Yugoslavia occurred very recently, and most people are familiar with it from daily news reports. According to Weine and colleagues (1995), the recent war in Bosnia–Herzegovina was marked by what the Serbians euphemistically called "ethnic cleansing," a genocidal campaign by the Serbian nationalists against the Bosnian Muslims and other non-Serbs. The war has produced the greatest refugee crisis ever experienced in Europe, with more than 3 million former Yugoslavians being displaced. By assessing some Bosnian refugees who have resettled in the United States, Weine and colleagues reported that ethnic cleansing has caused high rates of PTSD and depression, as well as other forms of psychological morbidity among the newly resettled Bosnian refugees.

VIII. WORKING WITH TRAUMA-EXPERIENCED REFUGEES

Clinicians and scholars are newly interested and concerned with understanding the specific nature of the problems encountered by refugees, including those who have been tortured and experienced other traumas, and providing them with suitable care. However, knowledge and experience regarding culturally relevant treatment for these specific populations are still lacking and await further study and improvement (Draguns, 1996; Friedman & Jaranson, 1994; Varvin & Hauff, 1998; Vesti & Kastrup, 1992).

A. Basic Considerations: Various Traumas Experienced

The first thing that needs to be recognized by clinicians is that most refugees have gone through terrible psychological traumas, either prior to, during, or even after they seek refuge. This is true whatever the main reason for taking refuge. The trauma is often caused by war, associated with interethnic conflict, political torture, and fleeing from dangerous places, or is the result of transcultural migration (Jaranson & Popkin, 1998). Mostly the traumas are multiple, severe, and chronic, beyond what ordinary human beings could take (Kinzie, 2001). Witnessing family members, friends, or neighbors being severely threatened, persecuted, raped, injured, or murdered causes most of these refugees to suffer from posttraumatic stress disorders (Kinzie et al., 1990). Many studies report that nearly 80 to 90% of the refugees manifest such clinical conditions. Treating posttraumatic stress disorders becomes almost synonymous with dealing with refugees.

B. Treatment Issues

1. Basic Cultural Appreciation for Therapy

a. Concept of Severe "Trauma" and Beliefs about "Healing"

Psychiatrists tend to take the general view that a person has the potential to recover from psychological trauma if proper care and treatment are provided. However, such an optimistic view is not held for many war refugees. These people, who have encountered multiple, repeated, severe psychological trauma, have difficulty improving even with long-term, intensive treatment. It needs to be understood that when the trauma is so severe, a person could suffer from it for the rest of his or her life. This means that clinically the therapist should not build false hope for himself or expectations for the patient. He needs to be realistic.

It needs to be understood that severe psychological trauma will take a very long time to heal — if healing ever occurs. The clinical condition will be up and down, depending on the condition of the individual and the situations he encounters in life. Any trivial matter may provoke a stressful reaction and they may become vulnerable. Therapy could be offered mainly in the form of support and guidance, rather than trying to push the patient for a "cure."

b. Adequate Support and Understanding of Trauma

Although it is basic for the therapist to provide support for the patient under treatment, this is particularly true when the treatment is for patients who have suffered from severe trauma. Based on his clinical experience with southeast Asian refugees, Boehnlein (1987, p. 527) commented on the key issues involved in therapeutic work with such patients. The therapist can communicate a sense of warmth, genuineness, and competence by being direct, yet compassionate; by being assertive in the recommendation of a treatment approach, yet responsive to possibly conflicting cultural concepts of illness and healing; and by allowing the patient to report difficult historical information or express intense emotion without a sense of shame.

After working with torture victims, Somnier and Genefke (1986) suggested that by penetrating his most painful experiences, the victim has an opportunity to work with them in a new context. When the victim eventually comes to understand what was done to him and that he was broken down in a predictable way by torture, distorting normal psychological mechanisms, the memories no longer cause the victim the same fear as before.

c. "Self" and Utilization of "Others" for Healing

Because of the severity of the traumas that they have encountered, these refugees need all the support they can get. This includes the support of family, friends, public services, the welfare system, and so on, in addition to that of the therapist, who plays a small role in the process of healing. In other words, psy-chosocial intervention in a broad sense is more useful than individual, traditional psychotherapy in a narrow sense.

d. Inclusion of Team Members of the Same Ethnic Background

It has been learned from clinical experiences that the key element in a successful treatment program for the refugees, as pointed out by Kinzie and Manson (1983), is to have mental health counselors who possess the necessary linguistic, cultural, and psychotherapeutic skills to bridge the gap between therapists and refugee patients. This is particularly true when southeast Asian refugees are to be treated by American therapists. Mental health workers of southeast Asian backgrounds could provide needed social support and cultural interpretation for the refugee patients, who are already burdened by their psychiatric disorders and overwhelmed by the problems of adapting to life in a new culture. Certainly, they would minimize the initial suspicions, mistrust, and mixed feelings that the refugees harbor toward the American therapists associated with the war experiences in southeast Asia. Therapists of the same ethnic background would help involve the refugees in a mental health program that is unfamiliar to most of them.

2. Applicability of Particular Psychotherapeutic Approaches

a. Model of Therapy

It has been emphasized by Kinzie and colleagues, whose clinical services have focused on Indochinese refugees for many years, that instead of a conventional psychiatric approach, the medical approach of a physician, familiar to Indochinese patients, works better for them (Kinzie, Tran, Breckenridge, & Bloom, 1980).

Even though many models of psychotherapy are available for caring for the general population, including intrapsychic, behavioral, cognitive, interpersonal, family, group, or social rehabilitation approaches, experiences working with southeastern refugees have pointed out that family and group-oriented approaches, which focus more on occupation, recreation, or other activities, work better for them. There are many reasons for this. These patients are not familiar with individual psychotherapy, not to mention the language obstacle that limits such an approach. They feel more comfortable in a group, as it is in line with their culture to do things together as a group. It not merely provides mutual group support, and sharing the same life experiences and traumas, they also feel more safe exploring and examining their traumas in group therapy. Groups of the same gender and similar ages work better. Any recreational or social activity, including cooking, sewing, or learning how to prepare things for a cultural festival, for instance, helps them to work together and feel and identify themselves as a group — more important elements for therapy for them than exploring their traumas simply by "talking." Working with these refugees certainly requires bold ideas and revised approaches from a cultural point of view.

b. Major Therapeutic Work

Another clinical debate among clinicians is whether a past trauma needs to be psychologically "explored" or whether the patient should simply be encouraged to "repress" the traumatic experience. This is certainly a clinical judgement that needs be applied case by case. However, from a cultural point of view, particularly for those patients who are not used to expressing their private feelings in public, or to strangers, including a therapist, and who suffered from traumas of a very severe nature without the possibility of resolution for the past, it is considered inappropriate to try to explore the trauma if no resolution can be offered for it. For many kinds of trauma, the goal of therapy is to help the patient suppress or repress the trauma rather than bring it up to a conscious level. This is true for patients suffering from certain kinds of psychopathology, such as psychoses or borderline disorders. The same thing could be said for people of certain cultural backgrounds. In many cultures, repression and suppression are regarded as

more suitable, if not more "mature," coping mechanisms.

c. Cardinal Healing Mechanism Utilized

Very different from the "ordinary" psychotherapy advocated in general (by contemporary Western psychotherapists), in which the major thrust is on psychological awareness in the form of insight, acceleration of maturity of the self, and active resolution of problems, is the treatment of patients of other culture backgrounds in which many other issues could be stressed and utilized. For instance, in the care of southeastern refugees, it was realized that the philosophical acceptance of life and traumatic experience, religious help, or social reintegration were some of the issues that would be culturally appropriate, clinically effective, and relevant, and deserved full utilization.

What is the meaning of life, what is the sense of self, what is the implication of having repeated traumas, what is left for the future, how to live a damaged life, and so on are philosophical questions that could be touched upon and for which certain answers and guidance could be offered to refugee patients. They are questions that contemporary therapists tend to avoid, but they are very relevant and useful to address for people who have encountered many disasters or traumas in their lives.

d. The Need for Much Support, Help, and Care

Many refugees suffer from multiple problems: severe, and often repeated, traumas prior to taking refuge; stress and danger encountered during the process of fleeing from risk or persecution; loss of or separation from family members; arriving in host societies with minimal resources and support; and facing the challenges of transcultural immigration. There is a need for amelioration of the severe and socially crippling psychiatric symptoms of depression and posttraumatic disorder, but in most situations, there is also a need for active support and help to resolve major social difficulties; including poor housing, inadequate medical care, unemployment, financial difficulties, and so on (Mollica & Lavelle, 1988). The refugees not only need psychiatric care in the form of medication and psychotherapy, they are also badly in need of social services.

The situation does not necessarily improve for these refugees after the initial stage of settlement. Their psychological traumas may be stirred up frequently even by minor and unexpected things. Among the list of seemingly endless problems the refugees face, and for which they need continuing professional care and assistance, are how to contact their separated family members, how to react to the news of loss or tragedies of family members left in their home country, and how to face the problems of raising the younger generation in the host society (Kinzie, 2001).

3. Therapist–Patient Relational Issues

a. Boundaries for Confidentiality

The matter of confidentiality is an issue in treating war refugees, including those from southeast Asia. This is not merely because the number of refugees in the community is relatively small, but because are often related, or at least known to each other, and they tend to be concerned with news of what they say spreading to their friends or relatives. The explanation and observation of confidentiality become very important. If the refugees were involved in a civil war, or any intra- or interethnic conflict, the situation could be much more complicated. For instance, who was an enemy sympathizer, who was an antigovernment revolutionist, who worked as a spy, and so on, even though the situation is past, is still of serious concern to members of refugee groups. These are very delicate and sensitive areas to explore (Bernstein, 1998). Unless the information is crucial to therapy, revealing political secrets relating to conflict or war should not be attempted. Sometimes, it can become a matter of death and life, if not revenge, when the secrets are revealed. Closely related to this is the concern with immigration officers. Because some of the refugees may have entered the country illegally, they will always be concerned with revealing their past histories

and personal status. It is always necessary for a clinician to give proper consideration to such issues.

b. Matching of Therapist–Patient

A common question that has been raised, as in other clinical situations, is whether it would be more beneficial to match the therapist with patients who are traumatized refugees. Certainly, some consideration might be helpful. For instance, it might be easier for female patients who are traumatized by sexual abuse to have a female therapist, or for mature males, who have encountered many war traumas, to be cared for by a male rather than a female therapist, who may be considered (by the patient) to know nothing about the cruelty of war. In reality, it is not easy to match the therapist and the patient. This may be simply because there are not enough therapists available with the same ethnic and racial, as well as refugee, background. Further, the traumas of most war refugees are multiple, and there is no way to predetermine and select the therapist by gender. However, it would definitely be very useful to have staff of the same ethnic or racial background on the therapeutic team who may be able to assist in bridging the gap between the therapist and the patient.

c. Philosophical Reaction as Countertransference

Finally, it needs to be mentioned that many therapists who have worked with refugees with massive traumas year after year, hearing all the miserable and traumatic events that they have encountered, become "infected" by the hopelessness of their patients and feel overwhelmed by the horror of their personal stories (Mollica & Lavelle, 1988). Many therapists develop a certain countertransference, not toward the patients as persons, but toward their lives as human beings. They begin to wonder how life could so full of pain, trauma, injury, damage, and why so many people have to suffer repeatedly from severe traumas, which are almost impossible to bear (Kinzie, 2001). It is not a matter of the therapists becoming "numb" to human experiences, but "nihilistic" to some extent in their worldview. Taken to a severe degree, the therapist might become discouraged and his clinical work with traumatized patients compromised. This is a challenge for clinicians to face. As usual, therapists are advised to share such experiences with their colleagues and to offer mutual support among team workers.

IX. CLOSURE: MIGRATION AND REFUGEES

As elaborated early in this chapter, migration is a complex phenomenon that needs to be comprehended from multiple levels, including the individual, family, group, and social. When migration takes place transculturally, extra and special cultural considerations are required.

Variable factors contribute to adjustment to migration, such as personal psychological factors (including personality, motivation for migration, and expectations of migration), personal demographic background (such as occupation, family size and type, and financial condition), and the social environment of the new setting. Therefore, there is a need to recognize the different situations that could exist in migration. Simple overgeneralization should be avoided.

It is better not to examine the impact of migration on mental health at the occurrence of a mental disorder — the direct relation between them is rather thin. Instead, it is more meaningful to investigate psychological adjustment on personal and family levels.

Regarding refugees, as discussed in the latter part of this chapter, taking refuge is understood as a unique kind of migration that occurs when people are fleeing from a threat or danger, particularly from ethnic persecution. It is unfortunate that interethnic conflicts continue to be observed around the globe. Many people will suffer, and even lose their lives, while many others will escape from persecution. It is certainly a tragedy for human beings to encounter dangers in their lives from which they must take refuge. There is great suffering, pain, and trauma involved in such experiences. Clinically, it is a challenge for us to learn how to understand and offer care for refugees who have encountered grave suffering and drastic changes in their lives.

Migration and refugees are appropriate subjects for investigation from a cultural point of view, not only because they provide opportunities to examine the effects of culture on human experience in special social and cultural circumstances, but also because they open the door for clinicians on how to care for and prevent the mental health problems associated with migration and refugees.

REFERENCES

Akiyama, T. (1996). Onset study of English-speaking temporary residents in Japan. *Social Psychiatry and Psychiatric Epidemiology, 31*(3–4), 194–198.

Al-Issa, I., & Tousignant, M. (Eds.). (1997). *Ethnicity, immigration, and psychopathology.* New York: Plenum Press.

Armes, K., & Ward, C. (1989). Cross-cultural transitions and sojourner adjustment in Singapore. *Journal of Social Psychology, 129*(2), 273–275.

Astrup, C., & Ödegaard, Ö. (1960). Internal migration and mental disease in Norway. *Psychiatric Quarterly, Supplement, 34*, 116–130.

Bauer, M., & Priebe, S. (1994). Psychopathology and long-term adjustment after crises in refugees from East Germany. *International Journal of Social Psychiatry, 40*(3), 165–176.

Beiser, M., Turner, R.J., & Ganesan, S. (1989). Catastrophic stress and factors affecting its consequences among Southeast Asian refugees. *Social Science and Medicine, 28*(3), 183–195.

Bernstein, D. (1998). *Psychotherapy with Southeastern Asian refugees.* Presented at the Culture and Psychotherapy Symposium, organized by University of Hawaii School of Medicine, Department of Psychiatry.

Boehnlein, J.K. (1987). Culture and society in post-traumatic stress disorder: Complications for psychotherapy. *American Journal of Psychotherapy, 16*, 519–530.

Boehnlein, J.K., & Kinzie, J.D. (1995). Refugee trauma. *Transcultural Psychiatric Research Review, 32*, 223–252.

Brindis, C., Wolfe, A.L., McCarter, V., Ball, S., & Starbuck-Morales, S. (1995). The associations between immigrant status and risk-behavior patterns in Latino adolescents. *Journal of Adolescent Health, 17*(2), 99–105.

Chung, R.C.Y., & Kagawa-Singer, M. (1993). Predictors of psychological stress among Southeast Asian refugees. *Social Science of Medicine, 36*(5), 631–639.

Draguns, J.G. (1996). Ethnocultural considerations in the treatment of PTSD: Therapy and service delivery. In A.J. Marsella, M.J.

Friedman, E.T. Gerrity, & R.M. Scurfield (Eds.), *Ethnocultural aspects of posttraumatic stress disorder: Issues, research, and cllinical application* (pp. 459–482). Washington, DC: American Psychological Association.

Ebata, K., Miguchi, M. Tseng, W.S., Hara, H., Kosaka, M., & Cui, Y.H. (1995). Migration and transethnic family adjustment: Experiences of Japanese war orphans and their Chinese spouses in Japan. In T.Y. Lin, W.S. Tseng, & E.K. Yeh (Eds.), *Chinese societies and mental health* (pp. 123–137). Hong Kong: Oxford University Press.

Ebata, K., Tseng, W.S., & Miguchi, M. (Eds.). (1996). *Migration and adjustment: The study of the adjustment process of Japanese war orphans returning to Japan from China* (in Japanese). Tokyo: Nihon Hyoronsha.

Ebata, K., Yoshimatsu, K., Miguchi, M., & Ozaki, A. (1983). Impact of migration on onset of mental disorders in relation to duration of residence. *American Journal of Social Psychiatry, 3*(4), 25–32.

Friedman, M., & Jaranson, J. (1994). The applicability of the post-traumatic stress disorder concept to refugees. In A.J. Marsella, T. Bornemann, S. Ekblad, & J Orley (Eds.), *Amidst peril and pain: The mental health and well-being of the world's refugees.* Washington, DC: American Psychological Association.

Hertz, D.G. (1984). Psychological and psychiatric aspects of remigration. *Israel Journal of Psychiatry & Related Sciences, 21*(1), 57–68.

Hickling, F.W. (1996). Psychopathology of white mentally ill immigrants to Jamaica. *Molecular Chemistry and Neuropathology, 28*(1–3), 261–268.

Jaranson, J., & Popkin, M. (Eds.). (1998). *Caring for victims of torture.* Washington, DC: American Psychiatric Press.

Kinzie, J.D. (1999). Personal communication. October.

Kinzie, J.D. (2001). Southeast Asian refugees: Legency of trauma. In W.S. Tseng, & J. Streltzer (Eds.), *Culture and psychotherapy: A guide for clinical practice* (pp. 173–191). Washington, DC: American Psychiatric Press.

Kinzie, J.D., Boehnlein, J.K., Leung, P., Moore, L., Riley, C., & Smith, D. (1990). The prevalence rate of posttraumatic stress disorder and its clinical significance among Southeast Asian refugees. *American Journal of Psychiatry, 147*(7), 913–917.

Kinzie, J.D., & Manson, S. (1983). Five-years' experience with Indochinese refugee psychiatric patients. *Journal of Operational Psychiatry, 14*(2), 105–111.

Kinzie, J.D., Sack, W.H., Angel, R.H., & Clarke, G. (1989). A three-year follow up of Cambodian young couples traumatized as children. *Journal of the American Academy of Child and Adolescent Psychiatry, 28,* 501–504.

Kinzie, J.D., Tran, K.A., Breckenridge, A., & Bloom, J.D. (1980). An Indochinese refugee psychiatric clinic: Culturally accepted treatment approaches. *American Journal of Psychiatry, 137*(11), 1429–1432.

Lin, K.M., Tazuma, L., & Masuda, M. (1979). Adaptational problems of Vietnamese refugees: I. Health and mental health status. *Archives of General Psychiatry, 36,* 955–961.

Malzberg, B. (1935). Mental disease in New York State according to nativity and parentage. *Mental Hygiene, 19,* 635–660.

Mavreas, V., & Bebbington, P. (1989). Does the act of migration provoke psychiatric breakdown? A study of Greek Cypriot immigrants. *Acta Psychiatrica Scandinavica, 80*(5), 469–473.

McKelvey, R.S., Mao, A.R., & Webb, J.A. (1993). Premigratory expectations and mental health symptomatology in a group of Vietnamese Amerasian youth. *Journal of the American Academy of Child & Adolescent Psychiatry, 32*(2), 414–418.

McKelvey, R.S., & Webb, J.A. (1996). Premigratory expectations and postmigratory mental health symptoms in Vietnamese Amerasians. *Journal of the American Academy of Child & Adolescent Psychiatry, 35*(2), 240–245.

Mezey, A.G. (1960). Psychiatric aspects of human migrations. *International Journal of Social Psychiatry, 5,* 245–260.

Mollica, R.F., & Lavelle, J. (1988). Southeast Asian refugees. In L. Comas-Díaz & E.E.H. Griffith (Eds.), *Clinical guidelines in cross-cultural mental health* (pp. 262–304). New York: Wiley.

Munoz, L. (1980). Exiles as bereavement: socio-psychological manifestations of Chilean exiles in Great Britain. *British Journal of Medical Psychology, 53*(3), 227–232.

Murphy, H.B.M. (1965). Migration and the major mental disorders: A reappraisal. In M.B. Kanter (Ed.), *Mobility and mobility health.* Springfield, IL: Charles C. Thomas.

Murphy, H.B.M. (1973). The low rate of hospitalization shown by immigrants to Canada. In C.A. Zwingmann & M. Pfister-Ammende (Eds.), *Uprooting and after.* New York: Springer-Verlag.

Murphy, H.B.M. (1977). Migration, culture and mental health. *Psychological Medicine, 7,* 677–684.

Ndetei, D.M. (1988). Psychiatric phenomenology across countries: Constitutional, cultural, or environmental? *Acta Psychiatrica Scandinavica Supplementum, 344,* 33–44.

Ödegaard, Ö (1932). Emigration and insanity: A study of mental disease among the Norwegian-born population of Minnesota. *Acta Psychiatrica Neurologica, Supplementum 4.*

Perez, M.M. (1984). Exile: The Chilean experience [Special issue]. *International Journal of Social Psychiatry, 30*(1&2), 157–161.

Pernice, R., & Brook, J. (1996). The mental health pattern of migrants: is there a euphoric period followed by a mental health crisis? *International Journal of Social Psychiatry, 42*(1), 18–27.

Rack, P.H. (1988). Psychiatric and social problems among immigrants. *Acta Psychiatrica Scandinavica Supplementum, 344,* 167–173.

Raschio, R.A. (1987). College students' perception of reverse culture shock and reentry adjustments. *Journal of College Student Personnel, 28*(2), 156–162.

Sack, W.H., Him, C., & Dickson, D. (1999). Twelve-year follow-up study of Khmer youths who suffered massive war trauma as children. *Journal of the American Academy of Child and Adolescent Psychiatry, 38*(9), 1173–1179.

Sam, D.L., & Berry, J.W. (1995). Acculturative stress among young immigrants in Norway. *Scandinavian Journal of Psychology, 36*(1), 10–24.

Schwab, J.J., & Schwab, M.E. (1978). *Sociocultural roots of mental illness: An epidemiologic survey.* New York: Plenum Medical Book Company.

Scott, W.A., & Scott, R. (1989). *Adaptation of immigrants: Individual differences and determinants.* Oxford: Pergamon Press.

Silove, D., Sinnerbrink, I., Field, A., Manicavasagar, V., & Steel, Z. (1997). Anxiety, depression and PTSD in asylum seekers: Associated with pre-migration trauma and post-migration stressors. *British Journal of Psychiatry, 170,* 351–357.

Sluzki, C.E. (1986). Migration and family conflict. In R.H. Moos (Ed.), *Coping with life.* New York: Plenum Press.

Somnier, F.E., & Genefke, I.K. (1986). Psychotherapy for victims of torture. *British Journal of Psychiatry, 149,* 323–329.

Tseng, W.S., Chen, T.A., Cheng, Y.S., Hwang, P.L., & Hsu, J. (1993). Psychiatric complication of family reunion: After four decades of separation. *American Journal of Psychiatry, 150,* 614–619.

Uehara, A. (1986). The nature of American student reentry adjustment and perceptions of the sojourn experience. *International Journal of Intercultural Relations, 10*(4), 415–438.

Varvin, S., & Hauff, E. (1998). Psychotherapy with patients who have been tortured. In J. Jaranson & M. Popkin (Eds.), *Caring for victims of torture.* Washington, DC: American Psychiatric Press.

Vesti, P., & Kastrup, K. (1992). Psychotherapy for torture survivors. In M. Basoglu (Ed.), *Torture and its consequences: Current treatment approaches.* Cambridge, UK: Cambridge University Press.

Weine, S.M., Becker, D.F., McGlashan, T.H., Laub, D., Lazrove, S., Vojvoda, D., & Hyman, L. (1995). Psychiatric consequences of "ethnic cleansing": Clinical assessments and trauma testimonies of newly resettled Bosnian refugees. *American Journal of Psychiatry, 152,* 536–542.

Westermeyer, J. (1989). *Psychiatric care of migrants: A clinical guide.* Washington, DC: American Psychiatric Press.

Westermeyer, J., Neider, J., & Calliew, A. (1989). Psychosocial adjustment of Hmong refugees during their first decade in the United States: A longitudinal study. *Journal of Nervous and Mental Disease, 177*(3), 132–139.

Westermeyer, J., Neider, J., & Vang, T.F. (1984). Acculturation and mental health: A study of Hmong refugees at 1.5 and 3.5 years postmigration. *Social Science Medicine, 18*(1), 87–93.

Wittkower, E.D., & Prince, R. (1974). A review of transcultural psychiatry. In S. Arieti (Ed.-in-chief), *American handbook of psychiatry,* (2nd ed., Vol. 2), & G. Caplan (Ed.), *Child and adolescent psychiatry, sociocultural and community psychiatry* (pp. 535–550). New York: Basic Books.

Zilber, N., & Lerner, Y. (1996). Psychological distress among recent immigrants from the former Soviet Union to Israel. I. Correlates of level of distress. *Psychological Medicine, 26*(3), 493–501.

45

Minority by Ethnicity, Gender, and Other Factors

I. INTRODUCTION

A. WHAT DO WE MEAN BY "MINORITY?"

"Minority" refers to a group of people that is customarily treated as less important, with less privilege, in the social system. It is considered of lower status and may even be discriminated against by other groups for various reasons, such as its political, religious, socioeconomic, ethnic/racial, or cultural background, unusual physical conditions (including handicaps), or merely because it has fewer numbers or is "different." Minority is a term used in oppositional relation to "majority," which implies a group of people of remarkably larger size, an inherited more dominant or higher social position, customarily with the tendency to exercise privilege and power over the minority group. Thus, it is a social and political term that has significant mental health implications.

People usually associate the term minority with ethnic or racial groups because they are most obvious and problematic from a social perspective. Minority status in relation to gender or sexual orientation has attracted conscious attention since the 1970s, even though there has been unfair treatment of such groups

around the world for a long time. Historically, social caste systems have existed in many societies that have involved publicly accepted discrimination; such systems are still observed in some societies today. People with physical defects or handicaps suffer because they are different from the "ordinary" majority. They live differently and are much less privileged in many ways; however, the majority of people seldom give them special consideration or attention. In a broader sense, youngsters are more powerless and vulnerable to physical or sexual abuse or neglect by adults. Children who were not properly protected and nurtured by their parents belong to a minority group determined by age factor. Similarly, aged persons with physical or mental handicaps tend to become victims of neglect or abuse by their adult children or care providers. Thus, there are various reasons for being regarded and treated as members of a minority — some of them are temporary (those associated with age), but most are long-lasting (those associated with ethnicity, race, caste system, or physical handicap, for example). In other words, there are many people who are not "equal" to the majority and belong to a less privileged minority group for one reason or another.

When people of a minority group are treated unfairly by the majority and severely discriminated against for a long time, they tend to suffer from psychological feelings of inferiority, inadequacy, or powerlessness. They often have unspoken feelings of fear and resentment toward the majority, which looks down on them and treats them as inferior. Members of the minority tend to be deprived of opportunities for progress and achievement in the social environment. This may affect their self-image and confidence, resulting in negative group identification (Lott & Maluso, 1995).

Caution is necessary not to regard the minority as having more psychiatric disorders than the majority. It depends on the kinds of psychiatric disorders that are concerned. For instance, females (as the less privileged gender), in general, have a higher rate of suicidal attempts, but lower rates of suicide than males. African-Americans (as a minority group in the United States) have lower suicide rates in contrast to the majority Caucasian-Americans. The status of a minority may not necessarily have a more negative effect on psychology. In contrast, persecution of the minority group (by the majority) may lead to a tight bond among minority group members, such as the Irish response to the British or bombing by Basque separatists. The challenges in the lives of the minority may stimulate more creativity in them (Griffith, 1998; Harris, Blue, & Griffith, 1995).

However, a minority may be associated with certain kinds of mental health problems, may be vulnerable to particular behavior problems, and may tend to show certain kinds of psychopathology that warrant special attention (Moffic & Adams, 1983). At the same time, its members often underutilize the mental health care system that is set up for the majority and may not be treated properly and adequately by mental health services. Thus, it is relevant to pay attention to people of such backgrounds from social and cultural perspectives.

II. VARIOUS REASONS FOR MINORITY STATUS

Many different kinds of people are perceived and treated as "minorities" by others. For the sake of con-

venience, they can be subgrouped according to the main reasons that led them to become minorities.

A. MINORITY BY ETHNICITY OR RACE

This is one kind of minority commonly recognized socially and politically. Ethnicity or race is a powerful factor that leads people to identify certain groups as unique, with their members treating themselves or being treated by others as such. This is particularly true if the group emphasizes a distinct way of life, including the way in which they address themselves or their unique appearance (such as Armenian people, a group that originally migrated from Germany, living in some parts of the United States, which emphasizes a very conservative way of life; or orthodox Jewish people in many parts of the world), or obvious physical characteristics such as different facial or physical features, including color of skin. Racism is based on racial difference. Ethnicity or race is one of the main factors for distinguishing one group from another and is often associated with negative treatment. It has been pointed out that racism is more than prejudice. Racism is associated with the overt and covert forceful establishment and maintenance of power by one social group over another (Moore, 2000).

It is not only external appearance that identifies a race as a "different" group, but, most importantly, it is the history associated with the group and their past relations with the so-called "majority." For instance, that African-American people's were brought by Caucasian-Americans to the United States as slaves was the historical root for segregation and discrimination: they were not allowed to use the same restrooms or enter the same restaurants and were required to sit in the back of the bus, for example — phenomena that were still observed not too long ago in a country that was originally built on the spirit of freedom and the fundamental principles of human rights and equality.

Native Americans are associated with the historical fact that they, as the original inhabitants of the American continent, which was "discovered" by a European (Columbus) several centuries ago, followed by the "invasion" of European people, lost their land and their way of life, as well as their dignity. Even though they were the native people, the newcomers, with greater (military) power, not only forced them to move and live on remote reservations, but treated them as people of lower status, not socially but culturally. For instance, as children, many of them were taken away from their homes and placed in boarding schools for the sake of their "education" and health, were not allowed to speak their own native language, or to live their indigenous ("savage") style of life (Jilek-Aall & Jilek, 2001). They were programmed to lose (or be uprooted from) their culture.

In China, despite their long, civilized history, the Chinese were treated unfairly by Westerners at the end of the Qing Dynasty, around the end of the 18th or the beginning of the 19th century, when the Chinese political system collapsed and the land was invaded by several Western countries (including Britain, Germany, and America). In the Western-occupied section of Shanghai, a major city in China, a sign was put up in a public park that said: "Chinese and dogs are not allowed in this park!" Even many generations afterward, Chinese people still remember how they were treated by the Western "imperialists" and "colonialists."

When there has been a negative relationship or severe discrimination between different ethnic or racial groups, the anger, hate, and fear last for a long time, transmitted from generation to generation. Unless special efforts are made to resolve the damage or scars that have resulted, the negative relationship will persist. There are often long-term effects associated with racism on educational and employment opportunities, which, in turn, induce a feeling of chronic despair and unhealthy ways of living — as exemplified by the West Indians in Britain (Burke, 1984). Ethnism or racism will even seriously affect mental health service, particularly in terms of the utilization of service and the therapist–patient relationship (Willie, Rieker, Kramer, & Brown, 1995).

B. Minority by Social Caste

In many societies, people are divided into distinct subgroups with different statuses, hierarchies, and social privilege. The groups are not determined by economic factors, but by heritage. In such a caste system, not only are clear boundaries recognized, but there is no possibility of moving between castes. A person is born in a particular caste and is restricted to it for life. In ancient times, Egypt was well known for such a social caste system, which distinguished among priests, administrators, ordinary people, and slaves, in hierachical order. A similar caste system was observed in most of the Pacific island societies, including Hawaii. It was only a century ago, after the arrival of Westerners, that the caste system was abandoned in Hawaii.

However, the artificial subdivision of castes is still practiced in many societies. For instance, in India, there was news from a rural area that a young man of a lower caste had eloped with a young woman of a higher caste — and intercaste marriages there were still forbidden (particularly for a woman to marry down to a lower caste). When the father of the young woman found out, he expressed his anger by raping and murdering the mother of the young man, while the villagers watched. Nobody tried to stop him until the police arrived because his actions were considered permissible against a person of a lower caste. Although this is a rare instance occurring in a remote, rural area, it reflects in an extreme way how a caste system may become the source of discrimination and mistreatment.

Instead of recognized social castes, there are invisible subdivisions among people according to different economic and social status or other factors in many societies. There are many stories in the East and West describing marriages that were obstructed because of a wide gap in financial status or personal past history. In Japan, the very popular movie, *Aizenkatsura*, written at the end of the Meiji era, described the love story between a doctor and a nurse. The affair met with strong disapproval from the doctor's family because he was the eldest son of the superintendent of a private hospital and was expected to inherit the post. The woman, while she was very pretty and nice, was a widow with a son. Her ex-husband had died in a traffic accident. A wife who had previously had another man and a stepson by another man were considered unacceptable for an important man in traditional Japanese culture. Thus, culturally, the woman was considered unfit to be the wife of a physician and superintendent-to-be. Strong psychological factors associated with cultural beliefs made her an "unqualified" person. This is quite different from the modern Western movie, *Pretty Woman* a love story with a happy ending between a wealthy young man and a pretty, charming prostitute.

C. Minority Associated with Migration

A group of people may be treated as a minority when they migrate to a host society. Simply because they are newcomers, not yet assimilated into the host society, they suffer from less privilege in education and occupation and are even denied opportunities due to potential competition with the original inhabitants. "Minority" versus "majority" status can result simply from migration, without other factors, such as ethnicity or race. This is best exemplified by the Hakka and Bendi distinctions in Guangdong, China. Many centuries ago, there was a war in central China. As refugees of the war, a group of people, mostly well-educated and intelligent, migrated southward to the Guangdong area. As a result of competition and the threat of economic factors, there was tension between the local people and the immigrants, even though they were all Han Chinese. Because the local people mostly inhabited the plains, the migrants had no choice but to reside in the mountain areas. The local people addressed the migrant people as Hakka ("guest family" in Guangdongnese) and themselves as Bendi ("local" people). They spoke distinctly different dialectics (Hakkanese and Guangdongnese). Furthermore, there were slight differences in their lifestyles: for example, the local women normally did not work

in the fields, while the guest women did, and the Hakka valued intellectual education more than the Bendi, who were primarily farmers and merchants. Intermarriage was not encouraged between the two groups. It is interesting that, after more than a century, when both groups migrated as Chinese to Hawaii, they still kept their identification and distinction as Hakka and Bendi, even though they both were "guest people" in their new host country. Intermarriage between them was not practiced until very recently.

Usually this situation is aggravated if the migrants are of different ethnic or racial backgrounds than the majority people in the host society. Difficulties in language, differences in faith, and different ways of observing social rules and etiquette make it more difficult for them to adjust to the majority. The combined effects are the formation of an invisible or apparent wall between the migrants and the host society. The migrants are often treated as "aliens" and are even severely discriminated against or persecuted by the majority in the host society.

With the improvement of transportation, the ease of moving far distances, the need for sociopolitical refuge, and a search for better economic or educational opportunities, there is an increase in migration in many parts of the world. The recent increase of migrants from eastern Europe, the Mideast, and Africa to western Europe is causing new social tensions between the migrating minorities and the host majorities. This has certainly raised mental health concerns (Littlewood & Lipsedge, 1989). The problems are not centered around only the adult migrants, but often extend into and are magnified in the next generation calling for special attention to younger migrants (Powell, 1983; Vargas & Koss-Chioino, 1992) (cross-reference to Chapter 38: Working with Children and Adolescents).

D. Minority for Obscure Reasons

The existence of the *Burakumin* in Japan is a unique example of a group of people that is collectively treated as an "untouchable minority," and regarded by the majority as outcasts, not for ethnic or racial reasons, but simply based on social factors (DeVos & Wagatsuma, 1969). This group was originally called *Eta,* a slang term meaning "excessively dirty," or *Hi-ning,* which literally means "not a person." Some scholars have speculated that they might have originally belonged to a certain lord who lost a war and had to escape from persecution by his enemy. Others think that the prejudice came from the occupations of the group's members; the earliest *Eta* were butchers, tanners, saddle makers, caretakers of the dead, or grave diggers. They touched dead bodies or flesh. In Shinto belief, death was the worst form of pollution; therefore, the *Eta* were regarded as polluted. Later, the group of prejudicial occupations was expanded and the "no person" status became hereditary. The classification was abolished by law in 1870, and the term *Buraku-min* (literally, people of the village) was used more often, but the social discrimination continued. Some Japanese "believe" they can identify a *Burakumin* merely by looking at him or her. In fact, these people look exactly like the rest of the Japanese, except that they tend to have certain family names. Even today, many Japanese parents check the ancestry of a child's prospective spouse for *Buraku-min* taint. The young people, and occasionally even their parents, do not know how the *Burakumin* became outcasts, yet many believe that *they* are mentally inferior, immoral, and aggressive. In this case, the sad outcome of centuries of external scorn, isolation, and discrimination was that the victims believed what others thought of them. They had incorporated the judgment of others and saw themselves as meriting scorn, discrimination, and social punishment. They limited their own educational and occupational opportunities and had a high incidence of delinquent and criminal behavior (DeVos & Wagatsuma, 1969). Recently, there has been a movement among them to improve their own self-image.

E. Minority by Religion

There is no shortage of stories about how people regard others as different, inferior, or improper because of differences in religion. Instead of treating people of other faiths as merely different, sometimes actions of opposition and conflict, discrimination, and even elimination may take place. Many interethnic or interracial conflicts have occurred in the past and still occur today, in every corner of the globe, that originated with differences of religion. The Crusades, which started in the begining of the 11th century in eastern Europe and continued in several waves over a couple of centuries, are obvious examples. The elimination and crucifixion of Christians in Japan before the Meiji era and the persecution of Jewish people in Italy in Roman times and in Nazi Germany are well-known parts of history. It cannot be denied that the present, ongoing conflict in the Mideast is rooted in religious matters in addition to historical interethnic relationships and politics. One of the major reasons people in Tibet were persecuted by Chinese soldiers was that they would not give up their religious beliefs and practices in compliance with the communists' atheistic ideology.

F. Minority by Gender

Differences in treatment between men and women have perhaps existed from the beginning of the history of humankind. They are basically related to the physical and physiological differences between them. The revision of role and function is primarily for the sake of adjustment for survival. However, there are associated psychological factors that make one regarded as superior to the other. Men are mostly regarded as more powerful, warranting a dominant position (not only physically but psychologically), whereas women are considered more vulnerable and therefore assume a subordinate status. Although it is considered almost universal that men have more powerful positions than women, this is not true in some cultures. For instance, in matrilineal societies, such as Micronesia, women enjoy certain unspoken privileges that men do not because the lineal system is identified through the female and property is transmitted accordingly.

However, historically, in many societies, women were, and still are, treated as less favorable than men. There are many examples, which do not necessarily occur as open discrimination, but as unequal treatment. For instance, in Asia, young girls can be sold to others (to serve as maids or prostitutes) for money to help the family resolve financial debts or crises. In China, before the modern revolution, feet binding was practiced for several centuries. For some reason, women with bound feet were considered beautiful (by men), if not sexually appealing (for men). Besides, it enforced women as bound inside the house so that they could belong only to their husbands or male masters. Based on this, young girls of the upper social class were forced to start binding their feet when they were very young, suffering from almost intolerable pain for the sake of men.

In India, women who become widows are not permitted to have a social life outside of the household for the rest of their lives. They are bound only to take care of their children and to serve their parents-in-law. They are forbidden to have any contact with men, except their fathers-in-law and brothers-in-law. No matter how young they are, they are not permitted to remarry.

In many societies, women are considered significant only for bearing children, particularly sons. If they fail, their husbands have a legitimate reason to dismiss them as their spouses or to have other women. There are no guarantees of "wifely status" in a modern sense.

It is well known that even in a society that emphasizes basic equality, wages for women have always been less than those of men, even though their professional performance and experiences are the same. There is no need to mention that it is women who are usually subject to physical and sexual abuse by men, rarely the other way around. Politically the inequality between men and women is decreasing in most modern societies; however, psychologically, the treatment of women as less important persons by men is still prevalent in many places. There is a need to understand the gender differences in psychiatric problems and to treat women patients differently — with con-

sideration of the biopsychological–cultural aspects of life, including the role and function of women in contrast to men (Nadelson & Zimmerman, 1993). This is particularly true of minority group women who suffer from double minority status (Commas-Díaz & Greene, 1994).

In an extreme way, women are often abused by men. Violence against women takes many forms, such as battery, sexual harassment, prostitution, pornography, or rape. Female infanticide is another form of discrimination and abuse of females at the beginning of life. Violence by police and security forces in ordinary times and during armed conflict or war are common occurrences. Violence against women refugees and asylum seekers is another example. However, violence against women in intimate relations is a rather common phenomenon observed cross-culturally. After reviewing research findings from various societies, Krane (1996) reported that 20% to nearly 70% of women have experienced violence in intimate heterosexual relationships.

G. MINORITY BY SEXUAL ORIENTATION

One social phenomenon that has been observed since the 1970s is advocacy for people with different sexual orientations. In the past, gay and lesbian people were regarded as sick. Even psychiatrists categorized them as mentally disordered. It was only in the 1970s that such categories were removed from the official classification system (DSM-III) and in 1980 from the internal classification system (ICD-9). However, there is still a stigma attached to homosexuality, and some negative attitudes are manifested by laymen as well as professionals (Cabaj & Stein, 1996; Greene, 1997; Krajeski, 1993). This was partly the reason the newly arisen AIDS crisis in Europe and North America was associated with gay people and their sexual practices.

Campbell, Hinkle, Sandlin, and Moffic (1983) pointed out that as long as there are social pressures against homosexuality, certain adaptational demands will continue to be made on the members of this minority. The quality of mental health care traditionally provided to this group has often been inferior, resulting in the determination of many homosexuals to provide better care for themselves through growing numbers of gay-staffed and gay-oriented mental health centers. Campbell and colleagues suggested that much remains to be learned about homosexuality. However, the most important recent development is a growing trend toward the reexamination of counter-transference distortions influencing the basic attitudes of the psychiatric profession toward homosexuality. Kitzinger (1997) stressed the importance of promoting the study of lesbian and gay psychology and seeking to counter discrimination and prejudice against lesbians and/or gay men.

In most societies, transvestite are regarded as odd. However, in most Asian societies, people generally tolerate women who dress as men. Actually, there were several well-known operas in China in which a woman dresses as a man to perform a social role that was not open to a woman. The famous story of Hua-mulan, who dressed as a man to serve in the army as a substitute for her father and later became a successful "general," is known not only to the Chinese but also to Westerners, now that Hollywood has made it into an animated movie. Another Chinese opera is the popular love story of Liang Sanbo and Zhu Yingtai. It describes how, in ancient times, when formal education was open only to men, Zhu Yingtai, a girl, disguised herself as a man so that she could enter school. She secretly fell in love with her roommate, Liang Sanbo, who did not detect that Zhu Yingtai was actually a girl until the end of the story. These stories are amazing, but reflect that men and women were assigned distinctly different roles by society. It takes a special person to cross the forbidden gender boundary.

In contrast, men who dress as women are often not tolerated well by people in many societies. The only exception is found on stage. In Japan, as well as in China, some famous "actresses" were actually men — with the profession transmitted from generation to generation in the family. This situation originated because, in the past, it was not convenient for women to tour with a theatre group. Therefore, men were trained to perform as women, even married men. The audience enjoyed "his" skillful performance as a woman and was even attracted by the pretty "actress," although it knew she was actually a he. In the name of art, professional transvestism was (and is even now) accepted by laymen. Despite such exceptions, in real life in most societies, men who dress as women are often teased and even abused. However, there are some exceptions. In some societies, male transvestites are accepted without too much prejudice. Samoa in the Pacific is one such example.

H. Minority by Physical Condition

Some minorities are based on biological causes, such as people who are deaf or blind, or have other conditions they are either born with or have acquired. People with physical handicaps or deformities often suffer from limitations of sensation, communication, or the ability to move around freely. They have to endure different kinds of socialization and life experiences. Unfortunately, some of them are mistreated by ordinary people. The majority people are beginning to pay more attention and give more consideration to them in ordinary life, for instance, building roads in such as way that a handicapped person can get around by wheelchair or having braille in public facilities, such as elvators or automatic bank tellers, for blind people. However, not too many ordinary people know how to use sign language to communicate with deaf persons. The reality is that very few, if any, psychiatrists are trained to provide special services for deaf patients.

I. Minority by Sickness

Due to limitations in medical knowledge and lack of proper and effective treatment, patients with certain communicable diseases, such as leprosy and tuberculosis, were historically treated badly by ordinary people out of fear. Severe psychiatric disorders were no exception. Isolation and segregation were often effected by institutions built in remote areas for custodial care. Even family members were reluctant to visit the patients, not to mention friends. In Asian countries, when arranged marriage was practiced, it was the responsibility of the matchmakers to check and assure the families that there was no history of severe illness or problems such as drinking, gambling, or criminal behavior.

J. MINORITY BY AGE

Finally, without noticing it, young children or aged persons are often treated by adults as minorities due to their age. Young children are powerless to protect themselves if they are abused or neglected by their parents. They can be sold as if they are the property of the adults. They may be forced to serve as laborers without proper consideration of their health. Similarly, aged persons, when they become unable to take care of themselves, can potentially be neglected or abused either by their own family members or by care providers in public facilities. They are a minority and less protected in that sense.

Thus, there are many reasons that persons can be treated unfairly, with discrimination, and even persecution. As a minority group, in a broad sense, they share one thing in common: they are considered less important and less favorable by others and, often, as a result, they perceive themselves in the same way. This leads to an unfavorable mental condition.

III. THERAPEUTIC IMPLICATIONS

A. UTILIZATION OF PSYCHIATRIC SERVICE

Existing mental health services are generally established primarily for the care of people of the majority. This situation may not be intentional, but it often results in unsuitable conditions for minority people. For instance, the language used is not familiar to migrants from other countries, and often there are no staff available for translation. Because there are almost no staff who understand sign language, there is no way to communicate with deaf people. The existence and function of the services are often not familiar to people from foreign countries or indigenous people. It is almost impossible for financially underprivileged people to follow the appointment system involved in care delivery because they do not have telephones and no access to transportation.

The unfamiliarity, unsuitability, and inaccessibility of the services make the existing mental health facilities underutilized by people of minority backgrounds. While some improvements have been made recently in many facilities, with instruction in multilanguages, the utilization of interpreters for certain languages, outreach programs that offer services in the community rather than at a clinic, and so on, there is still a lot of room for improvement.

B. THERAPIST–PATIENT RELATIONSHIP

The therapist–patient relationship is characterized by a wide gap and certain transference/countertransference issues in relation to the treatment of minorities. Most therapists belong to the "majority." This is not merely because they belong to the ethnic or racial background of the majority, but because they are successful in educational, occupational, financial, and social achievements. Often they grew up in families with "ordinary" — if not "affluent" — backgrounds, never suffering from starvation or the problems of homelessness. They speak and use the language of the majority fluently, but may never speak languages other than their native one. They may never live in other cultures and appreciate the differences among cultures. In other words, when they treat a "minority" patient, in the eyes of the patient, the therapist is distinctly perceived as a person of the "majority." Thus, a majority–minority relationship often occurs (develops or repeats itself) in the therapist–patient relationship.

Depending on the nature of the existing majority–minority relationship, the therapist–patient relationship may be characterized by problems of trust, feelings of inequality, resentment, or hatefulness. Certainly it involves the displacement of the social majority–minority situation into the therapeutic relationship. It is a special kind of transference and countertransference that could have a negative impact on therapy and needs to be clarified, managed, and resolved from the very beginning. If the negative ethnic or racial transference and countertransference is very intense and negative, a change of therapists may need to be considered.

Occasionally the therapist–patient relationship is reversed in terms of majority and minority status. That is, the therapist may come from a minority background and the patient from a majority background. This situation often results in similar problems of trust in addition to problems of identification. The patient's identification with the therapist — an important force for successful therapy — may be disrupted.

The gap or differences between therapist and patient is certainly an important issue that cannot be ignored. Often an extra effort is required to minimize potential obstacles. If the obstacles are attributed to issues related to majority–minority status, beyond personal, educational, or socioeconomic differences, they need be brought up openly and managed carefully from the very beginning of such interethnic, -racial, or -cultural therapy (cross-reference to Chapter 26: Therapist and Patient: Relations and Communication; and Chapter 36: Intercultural Psychotherapy).

C. PROCESS OF THERAPY

When a therapist of a majority background treats a patient of a minority background (whether the minority is based on ethnicity, race, gender, sexual orientation, physical handicap, age, or sickness), it is critical to work out the gap and differences between the therapist and the patient. An effort needs to be made by the therapist to develop *empathy* for the patient and, by the patient, to develop *trust* in and *identification* with the therapist.

In clinical practice, therapists often treat patients who are different from themselves: with different kinds of early childhoods, traumas, degrees of problems, or pathologies. Developing empathy for the patient is a basic skill that the therapist must learn. For instance, a therapist who has never been raped or physically abused must learn to understand the suffering of a patient who has. In the same way, when a therapist is treating a patient of a minority background, he needs to understand the life experiences and perceptions of the world held by the patient. How would he feel if he had migrated to a new host society, without knowing much about the social system or how to obtain social support or make a living, when he hardly spoke the language of the society; how would he perceive the world, relate to others and communicate with them, if he were not able to make a sound or to talk, or if he were not able to see or to hear; or how would he manage his daily life, how would he survive and find meaning in his life, if he were bedridden every day, unable to move and needing others' assistance even to go to the bathroom.

In summary, these are issues that the therapist has to deal with, to learn, understand, and feel, so that proper empathy can be developed for the sake of treatment and relevant care can be provided for patients of different backgrounds. This is a challenge for the therapist — one that needs to be undertaken whenever there is a gap between the therapist and the patient in terms of personal conditions, privileges of various kinds, life experiences, social status, culture, or race (Carter, 1995). This basic issue was elaborated previously in a broader sense in the chapter on intercultural psychotherapy (Chapter 36), which, in principle, can also be applied to the treatment of minority patients. It is a basic assumption that there are certain psychological issues associated with being a "minority" — beyond social, economic, ethnicity, race, or cultural differences — that deserve special attention and management in psychiatric therapy (Ho, 1987; Powell, 1983).

REFERENCES

Burke, A.W. (1984). Racism and psychological disturbance among West Indians in Britain. *International Journal of Social Psychiatry, 30*(1&2), 50–68.

Cabaj, R.P., & Stein, T.S. (Eds.). (1996). *Textbook of homosexuality and mental health.* Washington, DC: American Psychiatric Press.

Campbell, H.D., Hinkle, D.O., Sandlin, P., & Moffic, H.S. (1983). A sexual minority: Homosexuality and mental health care. *American Journal of Social Psychiatry, 3*(2), 26–35.

Carter, R.T. (1995). *The influence of race and racial identity in psychotherapy: Toward a racially inclusive model.* New York: Wiley-Interscience.

Commas-Díaz, L., & Greene, B. (Eds.). (1994). *Women of color: Integrating ethnic and gender identities in psychotherapy.* New York: Guilford Press.

DeVos, G.A., & Wagatsuma, H. (1969). Minority status and deviance in Japan. In W. Caudill & T.-S. Lin (Eds.), *Mental health research in Asia and the Pacific* (pp. 342–357). Honolulu: East-West Center Press.

Greene, B. (Ed.). (1997). *Ethnic and cultural diversity among lesbians and gay men.* Thousand Oaks, CA: Sage.

Griffith, E.E.H. (1998). *Race and excellence: My dialogue with Chester Pierce.* Iowa City: University of Iowa Press.

Harris, H.W., Blue, H.C., & Griffith, E.E.H. (Eds.). (1995). *Racial and ethnic identity: Psychological development and creative expression.* New York: Routledge.

Ho, M.K. (1987). *Family therapy with ethnic minorities.* Newbury Park, CA: Sage.

Jilek-Aall, L., & Jilek, W. (2001). A woman who sings spirit songs. In W.S. Tseng & J. Streltzer (Eds.), *Culture and psychotherapy: A guide for clinical practice* (pp. 43–56). Washington, DC: American Psychiatric Press.

Kitzinger, C. (1997). Lesbian and gay psychology: A critical analysis. In D. Fox & I. Prilleltensky Eds.), *Critical psychology: An introduction.* London: Sage.

Krajeski, J.P. (1993). Cultural considerations in the psychiatric care of gay men and lesbians. In A.C. Gaw (Ed.), *Culture, ethnicity, and mental illness* (pp. 553–572). Washington, DC: American Psychiatric Press.

Krane, J.E. (1996). Violence against women in intimate relations: Insight from cross-cultural analysis. *Transcultural Psychiatric Research Review, 33*(4), 435–465.

Littlewood, R., & Lipsedge, M. (1989). *Aliens and alienists: Ethnic minorities and psychiatry* (2nd ed.). London: Unwin Human.

Lott, B., & Maluso, D. (1995). *The social psychology of interpersonal discrimination.* New York: Guilford Press.

Moffic, H.S., & Adams, G.L. (Guest Ed.). (1983, Spring). The psychiatric care of "minority" groups [Special issue]. *American Journal of Social Psychiatry, 3*(2).

Moore, L.J. (2000). Psychiatric contributions to understanding racism. *Transcultural Psychiatry, 37*(2), 147–182.

Nadelson, C.C., & Zimmerman, V. (1993). Culture and psychiatric care of women. In A.C. Gaw (Ed.), *Culture, ethnicity, and mental illness* (pp. 501–515). Washington, DC: American Psychiatric Press.

Powell, G.J. (Ed.). (1983). *The psychosocial development of minority group children.* New York: Brunner/Mazel.

Vargas, L.A., & Koss-Chioino, J.D. (1992). *Working with culture: Psychotherapeutic interventions with ethnic minority children and adolescents.* San Francisco: Jossey-Bass.

Willie, C.V., Rieker, P.P., Kramer, B.M., & Brown, B.S. (Eds.). (1995). *Mental health, racism, and sexism.* Pittsburgh: University of Pittsburgh Press.

46

Intercultural Marriage: Problems and Therapy

I. INTRODUCTION

"Intercultural marriage" refers to a marriage formed by partners with relatively diverse cultural backgrounds so that different cultural factors, including different views, beliefs, value systems, and attitudes toward couples, become the main issues in their marital adjustment. The term "intercultural" (rather than "cross-cultural") is used to signify that the **interaction** of the cultures of both partners tends to occur. From a psychological point of view, men and women are different enough that there is always a need for a husband and wife to adjust to each other from the standpoint of gender alone. This is true even in an ordinary "homocultural marriage" — when the husband and wife have the same cultural background. The need for adjustment to differences is much greater in a "heterocultural," or "intercultural marriage," as addressed in this chapter, when the cultural differences between the husband and wife are considerable or remarkable.

In general, the differences between a husband and wife can be differences in age, gender, educational background, occupational training, personality endowment, family upbringing patterns, or social class. These differences can be magnified if the husband and wife also have different faiths or religious backgrounds, different life experiences or personal histories. A marriage can be seen as an "intermarriage" if one of the couple has a different physical condition, such as deafness or blindness by birth. A blind person has a different perception of an orientation to the outside world from that of a nonblind ("ordinary") person. His or her experiences relating to others are uniquely different also. Even belonging to the same society and ethnicity, a deaf person uses a different language (sign language) and relies on a different means of perceiving the outside world. Thus, when a hearing and sighted person marries a deaf or blind person, there is a great need to understand the differences in each other's internal worlds and the ways each relates back to the outside world.

As an extension of this, if marriage partners belonging to different ethnic or racial backgrounds were raised by radically different language systems and oriented to different ways of thinking and belief systems — namely diverse cultural systems — they need to adjust to their cultural differences (Blount & Curry, 1993; Tseng, McDermott, & Maretzki, 1977). Even though they may have many similarities, including hobbies, interests, and occupations, and have a strong affection for each other, they will potentially encounter difficulties, adjustment to which will require a special effort and search for resolutions of the differences between them.

A scientist, C. Clulow (1993), has correctly pointed out that, in a way, intercultural marriage, particularly mixed racial marriage, is a marriage across frontiers. The social, political, and religious implications of individuals exercising their choice to marry across frontiers are marked when communities feel their resources are at risk, their belief systems are under attack, and their security is at stake. Based on its history and cultural background, a society will react to intercultural marriage in a diversity of ways. For instance, the Japanese, based on their traditional concept of maintaining "pure" Japanese and encouraging ingroup marriage toward that goal, tend to see outside marriage as unacceptable, particularly to someone of another race, with distinctly different physical characteristics. Japanese society is very reluctant to recognize the offspring of Japanese-black parents as "Japanese." In contrast, in Hawaii, very much rooted in the traditional Hawaiian spirit of "aloha" toward members of outside groups, people tend to view everybody as a member of their *hanai* family (family members connected to the same roots), as long as they are willing to be considered as such. Thus, any offspring from an interracial marriage can be considered a member of a Hawaiian family. Therefore, the attitude toward intermarriage is very lenient.

The prevalence of intermarriage is influenced strongly by historical, social, and environmental factors in various societies. For instance, comparing the prevalence of outmarriage among the Asian ethnic groups of Chinese, Japanese, and Korean, Kitano, Yeung, Chai, and Hatanaka (1984) reported that, in Los Angeles in 1979, the Japanese rate of outmarriages was the highest (60.6%), followed by the Chinese (41.2%) and the Korean (27.6%). The figures were different for Hawaii in 1980, with the Korean the highest (83%), followed by the Chinese (76%) and then the Japanese (59%). In general, females of all three groups outmarried at a higher rate than males.

Among many variables examined, generation was found to be the most important related to outmarriage rate, with the third generation outmarrying at a higher rate than the first. This was supported by data from other sources, indicating that the outmarriage rate for Japanese-Americans in Hawaii was originally only 5–10% in the 1940s, increasing remarkably to 50–60% in the 1990s, almost five times greater after two generations.

It is important to point out that when we are discussing the problems and adjustments among interethnic, interracial, or intercultural spouses, one thing that must be taken into consideration is the effect of different combinations of ethnic/racial/cultural backgrounds coupled with gender. For instance, in a white–black interracial marriage, the husband being white and the wife black could result in a different situation than the husband being black and the wife white; or a Euro-American husband married to an Asian wife is different from an Asian husband married to a Euro-American wife. In general, there is a certain hierarchy of relations in different ethnic groups, intermixed with the dominant–submissive relations between husband and wife. Therefore, the ethnic, racial, and cultural backgrounds of the husband and wife will bring about different combinational effects. These will be influenced further by the environment in which the couple lives, depending on how people in the society perceive their marriage and react to them. Thus, it cannot be generalized that all intermarried couples are in the same situation; there is a need to consider specific factors, including their sociocultural backgrounds, community reactions, and their gender combination, in addition to individual factors.

Even though intermarriage as a social phenomenon is complicated, and not given to simple generalizations, from culture and mental health points of view, intercultural marriage is regarded as an interesting subject for investigation and discussion. It provides a laboratory situation for microscopic analysis, allowing us to examine, at intrapsychic and interpersonal levels, how two "cultures" interact with each other through two "individuals" and how two different cultures can adjust at a personal level.

II. ANALYSIS OF MOTIVATION FOR INTERCULTURAL MARRIAGE

Whether there is a particular motivation for a person to choose a marriage partner of a different ethnic, racial, or cultural background is an often raised and investigated question. Clearly there are many couples that marry interculturally for the same reasons that couples marry homoculturally — simply because they become intimate, find themselves compatible, share a mutual affection, enjoy being together, and so on. However, there are some couples who marry interculturally for special reasons or unique motivations. In speaking of motives, one must appreciate that the conscious reasons given for a culturally mixed marriage might not be the actual ones, and that it is often the result of a combination of several factors, both conscious and unconscious.

Chance and availability are very important factors in the process of mate selection. This is true in all marriages, but probably more so in intercultural marriage. For example, a white American soldier stationed in Korea may marry a Korean girl simply because of the factors of availability and propinquity in a setting where it seems appropriate. A Japanese scholar would not have married a French girl if he were not abroad in France to study or an Indian doctor would not have married his American nurse wife if they had not met and worked together in the same hospital.

Beyond such nonspecific factors, there are often special psychological factors that lead people to marry partners of diversely different ethnic, racial, or cultural backgrounds. For instance, Davidson (1992) raised some ulterior motives for marrying interracially (specifically blacks and whites), such as rebelling against their families, being sexually curious about people of a different race, seeking economic or class gains, or satisfying the need for exhibitionism. Cohen (1982) mentioned the problems relating to their parents and feeling a great sense of empathy with the foreign partner.

Let us examine some of the special psychological factors that may lead people to choose to marry interculturally.

A. THE NEED TO BE DIFFERENT

Being "different" may be a characteristic of the flexible, adventurous, often highly intelligent person, or it may identify the exhibitionist. Some people seek an enlarged horizon; they are interested in new ideas, new people, and new places. They are more apt to marry into another culture than their tradition-minded counterparts. An extreme of this need to be different is exhibitionism. A narcissistic, exhibitionistic person may marry outside of his race in order to be different and to attract attention. His motivation is more, "Hey, everybody, look what I've done now!"

B. PROJECTED BELIEFS ABOUT OTHER CULTURES

People have projected beliefs about other cultures that may or may not be founded on reality. Based on such beliefs, an intercultural marriage may result. For example, a white male might marry an Asian woman because he believes that she can better satisfy his desire for a wife who is willing to wait on him. In the reverse of this, an Asian woman might marry a white male because she believes that he is more apt to respect women and be kind to her than someone from her own group. If such beliefs are merely based on projected stereotypes of people of other cultures and have nothing to do with the particular mates that are chosen, they lead to frustration and disappointment when it is discovered that the fantasies are not true.

Sexual fantasies may also contribute to the decision to marry interculturally. Based on ethnic-related stereotypical sexual fantasies, a person may marry a partner of a particular ethnic background to resolve personal psychosexual problems. For instance, a white male who feels sexually inadequate with white females, who he sees as being very demanding, might deliberately seek an Asian women as a sexual object, believing that she is more submissive. A Jewish male who neurotically sees his mother as a pure Madonna and can function sexually only with a devalued woman may seek a nonwhite, sexy female for a mate.

C. FEELINGS OF SUPERIORITY AND INFERIORITY

Although we may consciously deny it, there is a strong tendency for people to rank ethnicities, races, and cultures as being superior or inferior to one another. If a person has a sense of inferiority, for either physical or psychological reasons, it may lead him to feel that he can find acceptance and feel adequate only with people of a less valued ethnic, racial, or cultural background. For instance, a woman with a child born out of wedlock, even if she would prefer to marry someone in her own group, may marry someone outside her ethnic group, usually a member of a less valued group, because he is the only one that is willing to marry her and support her child.

In contrast, another person may feel superior to another ethnic group and prefer to marry someone of an "inferior" ethnic, racial, or cultural background in order to fulfill a rescue fantasy. For instance, an American GI felt pity for a Korean girl who suffered from tuberculosis and was in need of emotional and financial support. He married her with the intention of "rescuing" the helpless girl.

D. SOLVING THE PARENT–CHILD TRIANGULAR COMPLEX

Based on psychoanalytic concepts, one of the psychological reasons for outmarriage is to solve the unresolved triangular complex with parents, particularly with parents of the opposite sex (Char, 1977). According to the psychoanalytic theory of personal development, every person needs to resolve the Oedipus complex encountered during the phallic stage of development. The Oedipus complex refers to the situation when a child of about 3 to 5 years develops intense positive feelings toward the parent of the opposite sex. Associated with this is the development of strong negative feelings toward the parent of the same sex who the child sees as a competitor for the affection of the parent of the opposite sex, thus creating a so-called triangular conflict. Normally, the child overcomes this conflict by identifying with the parent of the same sex and becoming interested in heterosexual objects other than his own opposite-sex parent. However, for various reasons, a child may not be able to resolve his Oedipal conflict successfully, which will influence his choice of a mate later in life. One of the ways to cope with this unresolved Oedipal conflict is to choose a special type of mate for marriage. If a child was strongly attached to his parent of the opposite sex, he might later choose a close relative who resembles that parent for his wife, resulting in an extreme situation of "inmarriage." If he is phobic of incest, he is then driven to choose a mate who is very different from his opposite-sex parent, resulting in the extreme situation of "outmarriage."

Outmarriage with a compound psychological complex can be illustrated by the following unique case vignette. A Japanese girl in Tokyo deliberately dated a black American GI to upset her father. Her father used to say that black men were no good, and she wanted to prove to him that this was not true. Her relationship with her black boyfriend was eventually discovered by her father, who forced their relationship to end. In reaction to this, the girl moved to Hawaii. With the excuse that she was studying abroad, she got her affluent father to send money regularly to "support" her. However, she secretly married a black man she met in Hawaii and had a baby. For several years, she continued to let her father believe that she was still pursuing her college education and relied on his financial support. She needed financial assistance from her father to support her husband, who had drinking problems and difficulty in keeping a job. Her personal history revealed that she was very close to her father when she was little. After puberty, she was sexually involved with her father for several years without the situation being discovered by her mother. Her repeated choice of a nonapproved black mate was a way for her to rebel against her father and, at the same time, try to work out her guilt feelings over having incestuous relations with him. Having a relationship with a man who was physically different from her father was the only way she could allow herself to become sexually aroused. This is a unique case that illustrates complex psychological mechanisms that can lead someone to marry a person of a different race, that is, feelings of superiority–inferiority toward another race, the psychological need for revenge against one's own parent, and the unconscious attempt to resolve a deep-seated Oedipal complex.

III. PROBLEM AREAS OF INTERCULTURAL MARRIAGE

Marital problems can occur between interculturally marriage partners for various reasons. Many are the same reasons observed in homoculturally married couples, but some are closely related to cultural factors. These culture-related causes of marital problems have been discussed briefly in a previous chapter (cross-reference to Chapter 39: Working with Couples and Spouses). Here, those culture-related causes of marital problems observed more frequently in interracial marriages will be elaborated in detail from four standpoints: how culture impacts the marriage system, the relationship of the couple itself, society's reaction toward intermarriage, and child rearing.

A. Impact of Culture on the Marriage System

1. Different Concepts, Expectations of, and Commitments to Marriage

"Marriage" means different things to people from different societies. It can mean the permanent union of a man and woman, no matter what difficulties they encounter, whether they are sick or healthy; once they wed, they are bound for life. For others, it may merely indicate that a man and a woman love each other and want to have an intimate relationship that is formally recognized. If their affection fades, there is the possibility of separation, divorce, and marriage with a new partner(s) (McGoldrick & Preto, 1984). Associated with this is the matter of faithfulness. In some societies, affairs outside of the marriage are absolutely not permitted, whereas in others, they are. If a man and woman marry with these different concepts of marriage, commitment to the husband–wife relationship, or expectations of their union, then there are potential problems.

The tragic opera *Madame Butterfly* shows how an intimate relationship and commitment were viewed entirely differently by a Japanese woman and an American man. From an aesthetic point of view, it may be a beautiful story, but culturally, it reflects misunderstandings regarding expectations of and commitment to "marriage" and "man–woman" relations.

2. Various Defined Relations with Families of Origin

How a person relates to his own parents or siblings after marriage is defined by cultures in various ways. A common problem encountered in intercultural marriage is confusion about what is expected from the relationship and the obligations of the married couple toward their families of origin. From their experiences counseling Korean–American couples at a military base in Korea, Ratliff, Moon, and Bonacci (1978) pointed out that, among many problems, one of the most frequent was that Korean wives expected their American husbands to offer financial and other support to their families — something taken for granted in Korean culture that was considered "absurd" and "unacceptable" by the American husbands.

B. Impact of Culture on a Couple's Own Relations and Interaction

1. Problems in Communication

The difficulty in communication between people of different cultures stems from the practical fact that they may speak different native languages and the common language between them is limited or even nonexistent. Language is a tool not only to communicate meaning but also to transmit feelings and to express emotions, including intimate affection. In a native language, deep-rooted emotions and delicate meanings can be expressed properly. However, this function of language is reduced or limited in a second or foreign language.

In addition to limitations in communication, another barrier of different languages involves the subtleties of message sending and receiving. To what extent self-opinion should be expressed openly or subtlety, in what ways delicate feelings should be described and communicated, and through what patterns intimate affection should be expressed or concealed are some of the basic issues. The following examples illustrate various difficulties in communication that are often encountered by interculturally married couples.

In a American–Japanese intermarriage, an American wife complained that her Japanese husband failed to thank her for a gift. The husband, she learned, followed the traditional Japanese pattern, according to which verbal thanks were given in fairly formal, outside-the-home situations, but were not expected among members of the family.

In several Chinese–American marriages, the nonspecific, nonconfronting style of Chinese communication has caused problems. "We never quarrel," said one American wife, "but we also never have a frank discussion — about finances or sex, or what he likes or does not like about my cooking, or how I dress, or whether he really wants to take a vacation trip or not. Through the years, I've just learned to 'sense' what other couples learn by discussing."

Another American wife complained that when her Japanese husband went back to Japan for a family visit, he never wrote that he loved her and missed her. The man said that he had sent this message in every letter. When the letters were examined carefully, numerous, almost poetic references to moonlight, scenic beauty, whispering pines, and a certain vague mood of wistfulness were found. To this educated, traditional Japanese, the unspoken message "but you are not here with me, beloved" was clear. He also explained that to put his feelings into definite words would "spoil things."

2. Problems in Couple Interrelations

How a husband and wife relate to each other is a private and personal matter. However, there is a subtle but strong cultural element at work behind the scenes. Although, in general, a man is expected to be dominant in his relationship to a woman in many societies, the nature of the dominance is different in different cultures. In matrilineal societies, where inheritance is from mother to daughter, rather than from father to son, a woman has certain privileges. In such societies, a man is not dominant over a woman. The kind of dominant–submissive relationship in a marriage is very much based on ethnic–racial background. If a husband and wife are from the same culture, they have a common, unspoken idea of how to relate to each other according to the ideal dominant–submissive relationship of their culture. However, it is confusing if the husband and wife are from different cultures, and there is no clear-cut, well-defined relationship pattern to follow. The couple needs to explore, experiment, and decide the kind of relationship they want to build.

3. Problems in Role Division

Closely related to the basic pattern of a relationship is how roles are divided and performed between husband and wife. Although it sounds like common sense that the husband is expected to work outside, hunting, farming, or fishing, while the wife is expected to work inside, cooking, cleaning, and raising the children, such role divisions are not necessarily universal from an anthropological point of view. Even among some ethnic groups in south Asia, it is a cultural norm for women to work in the rice fields while the men stay at home.

It is well known that in the traditional Korean household, the kitchen is the wife's territory, and the husband is not permitted to "intrude" into it. In contrast, the Chinese husband, particularly among the Cantonese in the south, is fond of cooking. Particular occasions, such as festival days, are a man's opportunities to cook elaborate meals. What would happen if a Chinese man married a Korean woman, or vice versa? Confusion could result, requiring the couple to redefine and establish new role divisions regarding who was permitted to enter the kitchen and do the cooking.

For a woman from Micronesia, a matrilineal society in which the family lineage and power is recognized through the mother, daughter, and granddaughter, a wife may delegate her power to her husband to execute the family authority. At the time, for major events in life, such as deciding which daughter is allowed to marry which man or whether they should live in another place, the woman will consult with her own brother rather than her husband for a final decision. If the husband is from a patrilineal culture, he will have difficulty accepting the role of a "husband" who has no authority over all the matters in the household.

4. Problems in Boundary Establishment

In order to function as husband and wife, a man and a woman need to develop certain bonds between them and, at the same time, establish certain boundaries toward the outside, including their families of origin. The boundaries that need to be established after marriage are more or less defined in many traditional cultures and vary cross-culturally. This can lead to confusion in intermarriage situations, causing certain problems.

In Hawaii, a Hawaiian husband visited his own parents almost every weekend. From a Hawaiian cultural point of view, there was nothing wrong with that. However, to his American wife, it was an unwelcome situaton: the husband was too close to his family of origin and neglecting the bond between husband and wife — the primary axis of the family according to her cultural view. An American–Filipino couple quarreled over how a sister-in-law should be seated in the car. The Filipino husband suggested that his sister be seated next to him so that she, as a visitor, would have a better view of the scenery. The American wife insisted that she, as the wife, should sit next to him while he was driving. She complained that he was too close to his sister, allowing her to take the "spouse's seat." A Korean wife secretly sent money to her parents without telling her American husband until one day he discovered what she was

doing and became furious. These cases all illustrate how important it is to respect the bond between husband and wife (as the primary axis within a family) and the boundaries that should be established with people outside of the marriage, including families of origin. For interculturally married couples, establishing boundaries is a matter that needs to be clarified, or it can lead to explosive conflicts.

5. Differences in Values, Moral Convictions, or Customs

Problems in intercultural marriages may arise from differing value systems, religious and moral convictions, or merely from variations in manners and styles of living. An American woman, Fay Calkins, who married a Samoan, tells of conflicting concepts of property in her book, *My Samoan Chief* (1962). The couple's car was, in Calkins' (American) view, their personal property. To the many Samoan relatives, the car — as indeed all property — belonged to the whole extended family.

The Filipino culture (like the Spanish) demands virtue of wives, but is tolerant of husbands' infidelities. Here is fertile ground for conflict in a Filipino–non-Filipino union. An English woman married to an ultraconservative Mexican was both wryly amused and irritated at the social role thrust upon her. Even in modern Mexico City, her husband expected her to "stay with the women" and "make woman talk" at parties. In some Middle Eastern cultures, women are expected to be silent or absent themselves when male guests arrive — a situation that might infuriate a Western wife or embarrass a Western husband.

Money, as in any marriage, can cause conflicts for intercultural couples. One culture may advocate the accumulation of wealth; another may place financial solvency second to enjoying life. One may consider that all earnings are to be pooled in a joint bank account; another may feel that only the male household head should handle finances. In middle-class France, women are expected to spend substantial amounts at the hairdresser, on beauty treatments, and on clothing; such expenditures might horrify a Dutch husband.

Various customs are observed by different cultural groups, particularly related to certain religious occasions, ceremonial events (such as weddings or funerals), or observed holidays. Such culture-related customs are usually bound with cultural meaning and emotion. Whether to have a tree for Christmas, whether to worship ancestors on their memorial day, whether to have a baby baptized according to Christian customs, whether to observe 1-month postpartum confinement as expected for Chinese mothers, what kind of funerals to have for parents, who should be invited for what occasions, and so on are potentially explosive subjects that husbands and wives of different cultural backgrounds may argue about, insist upon, and come into conflict over.

6. Adjustment in Sexual Life

There are few studies that examine the sexual life between husbands and wives who are interracially rather than homoracially married to see if any differences may exist between them. Song, Bergen, and Schumm (1995) investigated 100 couples with non-Asian American husbands and Korean wives from the Midwestern United States with respect to sexual satisfaction. They found, in general, that the responses of the spouses correlated highly, and that the husbands were more satisfied with the quality of the sexual relationships than the wives. If there were conflicts over sexual practices related to cultural differences, they would relate to sexual satisfaction for both husbands and wives. For husbands only, marital conflict over cultural differences and rejection by relatives and friends were related negatively to sexual satisfaction.

C. Impact of Society's Reaction toward Intermarriage

1. Prejudices and Stereotypes

Every society has its own attitude toward its people and people from outside it. Some are very friendly and accommodating toward outsiders, whereas others are not. When one spouse in an intermarried couple has a different color skin or the physical features of an "outsider," he or she may be treated differently by the society at large. A Japanese woman married to a black husband with a dark-skinned, curly-haired son declared that there was no way for them to be accepted by her fellow Japanese in Japan. She speculated that if she were walking with her son on the streets of Tokyo, the Japanese people would look at her son with a discriminating eye. Japanese people are so concerned about the "pure" Japanese race that they have a hard time accepting her "black" son as "Japanese." She refused the idea of living in Japan and chose to stay in Hawaii, where most of the people are of "mixed" ethnic backgrounds.

How your family is perceived and welcomed by the people in the society is a serious matter. It will certainly affect your personal life, your relationship, and your happiness. It may take a long time to ignore, adjust to, or overcome the community's reaction toward your intermarriage.

2. Dislocation between Culture of Origin and Host Culture

If a person not only marries a heterocultural partner, but also, as a result, migrates to that partner's home society, additional factors will be involved. For instance, as reported by Hall (1987), many Japanese war brides married to American GIs following World War II encountered discrimination and alienation in both Japanese and American society. In Japan, they were shunned for marrying "gaijin," or foreigners; in America, they faced abuse and nonacceptance as Asian women in a white society. Thus, they felt they did not belong in either their home or their host society.

D. Problems in Childbearing and Child Rearing

Many intercultural couples have few real adjustment difficulties until their first child is expected. Then, for both parents, dormant culturally based conflicts often surface. The pregnant woman's resurgent emotional ties to her own mother can bring about a renewal of old childhood feelings, including racial and ethnic prejudices. If the marriage partners are of different races, anxiety and tensions center around the coming baby's appearance. Will he or she be black or white? Will his or her eyes be round and blue, or black and somewhat slanted? How will the woman's family and friends feel if the baby is not her color? And, a more painful thought, how will she feel about the baby if he or she is black and the mother is white (or vice versa)? These troubling concerns may arise even when a couple has previously discussed having a racially mixed child. How will the baby be named, Mary (Anglo-Saxon) or Marie (French) — even though they both mean the same; Akiko (Japanese) or Qiuhua (Chinese) — even though they are both girls names having something to do with autumn? The battle over naming a baby according to a husband's and wife's ethnic heritage may start even before the baby is born. The reality of approaching parenthood brings fears, doubts, and hidden prejudices into sharp and painful focus.

With the baby's birth, cultural differences in child rearing often arise. For many Asian parents (including Japanese, Korean, and Chinese), small children are allowed to sleep in their parents' bedroom even when they have reached preschool age. Nobody is concerned with early separation and individualization from the parents. In contrast, many Occidental parents (particularly Americans) arrange for the baby to sleep in his or her own bedroom from several days after birth. Small children are encouraged to search for their own autonomy and are expected to sleep in their own bedrooms. Thus, how soon a child should be separated from his or her parents in sleeping arrangements may be viewed differently by intermarried spouses of Asian and Occidental backgrounds.

The essential issues in child rearing may be different even between homoculturally married parents, and could be more divergent in intercultural marriages. The Chinese father who follows tradition believes children should be obedient, respectful, and study hard, whereas the mother whose culture embraces the American idea of individuality and assertiveness may

want the children to attend a relatively "liberal" school and "be creative." She may consider mischief and speaking out to teachers as "self-expression," whereas the father may be shamed and embarrassed.

The Okinawan mother believes in liberal praise and little physical punishment. She discourages aggression and encourages socialization and integration with the group; the Anglo-Saxon husband may believe, especially if the baby is a boy, that the mother is encouraging the child to be "soft," a "sissy," or unable to "stand on his own two feet."

The mother from Micronesia may casually bare her breast to feed her infant in public, embarrassing her Anglo-Saxon husband. How soon to start toilet training, how strictly the child should be encouraged to clean his own room, or how early teens are allowed to date and to stay out late at night are among the issues that can spark husband–wife conflicts. Relatives often add to the stress, as grandparents (of different cultural backgrounds) on each side insist the child should be brought up "their" way, in "their" religion, or as in-laws accept the child as "one of us" or reject him because he is "different."

IV. ADJUSTMENT IN INTERCULTURAL MARRIAGE

A. CORE ISSUES IN CULTURAL ADJUSTMENT

In order to cope with the problems or adjust to the differences that result from the differences in the cultural backgrounds of two people, there are some basic issues that need to be worked out. First, there is a need for both sides to recognize the cultural gaps that exist between them, which are beyond personal differences or individual psychological issues. Cultural understanding and empathy are needed next. This means that each partner should try to learn and understand why the other partner thinks, believes, and behaves in certain ways. What is the past experience or life background that makes your spouse behave and react in a way that is different from yours? This requires not only cognitive understanding but also empathy at an emotional level. Cultural empathy refers to psychologically taking the position of the person of the other culture to try and understand how he or she perceives and feels about the issues. Needless to say, it is a fundamental requirement that one should respect one's partner's ways of viewing things and the emotions attached to them — no matter how they may seem from your point of view, "silly," "strange," or "nonsensical." There is no correct or wrong or good or bad from a cultural point of view. There are merely different patterns of thinking, behaving, and reacting. If both partners could take this kind of understanding attitude and culturally egalitarian position, a door would always be open for negotiation and resolution of differences. This would particularly be so if there were a strong affection between the husband and the wife that bound them together and motivated them to work out their problems.

B. PATTERNS OF ADJUSTING TO DIFFERENCES

The basic challenge in intercultural marriages is to work out any problematic differences that disturb the couple's lives or interfere with their relations. There are several recognized patterns of solving the problems arising from cultural differences. We could label these "ignoring," "one-way," "alternating," "midpoint," and "creative" adjustments.

1. Ignoring Adjustment

This is simply denying the existence of troublesome differences between the partners. As described by Cohen (1982), some couples may attempt to solve their problems by distancing themselves from each other.

2. One-Way Adjustment

Basically this is asymmetric adjustment. One partner gives up his or her own cultural behavior and takes

on that of the other. Frequently, the proximity to relatives of the dominant culture, relocation to the country of the dominant culture, or previous liking or fascination with the partner's culture helps determine this adjustment. In some cases, one partner already dislikes and feels separated from his or her own background. Sometimes the dominant culture demands the one-way solution: One partner must adopt the other's language and religion.

3. Alternating Adjustment

This is the situation when a wife and husband adopt each other's cultural ways on a trade-about basis. The Jewish partner takes an active part in Christmas festivities, and the Christian partner joins in observance of the High Holy Days. The white partner eats soul food; the black enjoys lean broiled meat; the Japanese attunes his ear to Beethoven; the American symphony goer discovers the nuances of the gamelan orchestra. The Oriental–Occidental intermarried couple chooses to prepare Oriental food one weekend and Occidental dinners on alternate weekends so that no one has to stick only to the other partner's kind of food. The alternating adjustment is more apt to succeed in intellectual and social matters and in style of living than in deeply felt religious convictions. Even with today's ecumenical spirit, there are Catholics who cannot in good conscience attend Mass one Sunday and their partner's services the next, and Jews who feel they disfavor their religious heritage when they attend Christian churches.

4. Midpoint Adjustment

This kind of compromise is applicable to specific issues. If an Asian husband feels he must give $400 a month to his parents, and the thrifty French wife argues that this strains the household budget, the compromise may be to give $200 a month to the parents. If the Caucasian bride wants a wedding reception with dainty sandwiches and champagne, and the Polynesian husband says this is embarrassingly "stingy" and that a feast with roast pig should be held, a substantial buffet may provide a compromise. What is significant is the attitude behind the compromise — whether both partners are willing to respect each other's needs and feelings and compromise so both find satisfaction, or whether one partner merely assents for expediency, but clings to grudges and resentments.

5. Parallel Adjustment

Sometimes the nature of the differences is such that there is no room for compromise and differences can only be accepted as they are, allowing parallel existence. For example, a Chinese husband married a Muslim Chinese wife. Although they were both Chinese in the sense that they both spoke Chinese, there was a remarkable difference in their faiths. The "ordinary" Chinese husband ate pork as his main meal, whereas from a religious standpoint, it was taboo for the Muslim Chinese wife to eat pork — she was not even allowed to eat food prepared in a pot in which pork was cooked. The only one solution for this couple was to have two separate sets of cooking utensils. The wife prepared "ordinary" Chinese food in the husband's cooking pot and served it in the husband's bowl, whereas she prepared her Muslim food with her own set of utensils, serving it in her own bowl so that there would be no "contamination" of her food. This sounds rather complicated, but it was their only solution. In a similar way, if a husband and wife have different faiths and it is difficult to compromise, the husband goes to his church and the wife to her temple, allowing both to keep their own faith without disturbing each other.

6. Creative Adjustment

This type of adjustment takes place when both partners give up certain individual, cultural behaviors and evolve a new behavioral pattern. Or it may be a merging of cultural influences — his, hers, and those absorbed from travel, friends, and intellectual and emotional experiences — so that a totally new way of living gradually ensues. Finding a creative adjustment to a specific behavior problem is a conscious procedure. It may be chosen because there is too much conflict or competition between the two cultures and the partners cannot negotiate. Trying a new way bypasses the conflict. Although it may include conscious decisions to solve specific problems, the evolution of a totally new lifestyle is the ultimate adventure for a flexible, emotionally and intellectually receptive couple. Perhaps this should not be called an "adjustment," but rather a "creation."

B. Process of Adjustment

1. Adjustment as a Sequential Process

From a psychological point of view, it is essential to recognize that the process of intercultural adjustment goes through sequential stages. Similarly to adjusting to a foreign society after migration, the intermarried couple will go through an initial stage characterized by a mixture of excitement and confusion. Excitement is brought about by the curiosity of a new experience. Confusion is the result of the unknown and a lack of preparation. This initial stage will be followed by the next stage, in which the couple tries to separate reality from fantasy, making adjustments according to practical needs. This is the stage in which the spouses discover the differences that exist between them and try to adjust them. Many efforts are needed for this adjustment. Finally, the marriage will reach the stage where a certain balance will be obtained. Certain differences will be tolerated and accepted, while many will be compromised and adjusted.

It is important to point out that the process of adjustment does not necessarily progress steadily and smoothly all the time. It usually has ups and downs and may be exacerbated at certain critical times, when there are more direct encounters with the families of origin, more exposure to demands to observe cultural values, etiquette, and customs. Examples are when families get together for birthday celebrations, weddings, memorials, funerals, or other occasions. These are times that people expect you to behave according to certain customs and etiquette, to follow certain rules, and avoid certain taboos. There is no shortage of examples of how families have ended up in unhappiness even though the original intention was to get together for a happy occasion.

2. Adjustment as a Dynamic Process

As psychiatrists, we know that the process of adjustment is always dynamic. It involves both cognitive and emotional levels; it is not only conscious thoughts that count, but also unconscious motives. It takes psychological work to change oneself and to adjust cognitively and emotionally.

From a cultural point of view, it is useful to know that instead of continuous and steady adjustment, it is desirable to have the choice of periodical retreats to one's culture of origin. By allowing a person to return to his or her culture of origin occasionally — a so-called cultural regression, retreat, or vacation — he or she will be removed temporarily from the tension of adjustment and, through regratification or reenjoyment of his or her original lifestyle, will regain the strength for further adjustment and reintegration.

3. Adjustment as a Lifelong Procedure

It is useful to realize that the process of adjustment is a long one. It may involve many, many years — a never-ending lifetime process. However, if there is a good start, it will continue to get better. From a theoretical point of view, it is necessary to have a follow-up study of adjustment so that we know what happens many years later.

Salgado de Snyder and Padilla (1982) did a study of Mexican-American subjects who married non-Mexican spouses two decades after they married in 1963. They found that the participation in Mexican cultural activities decreased between the first and third generations. However, the majority of both male and female subjects of all generations self-identified as being of Mexican origin and believed that their offspring also self-identified as Mexican. Children of female subjects (namely Mexico-American mothers who married non-Mexican husbands) spoke more Spanish and more often had a best friend who was Mexican than did offspring of male subjects (namely Mexico-American husbands who married non-Mexican wives). This study illustrates how the issues of ethnic identity are manifested two decades after intermarriage between Mexican-Americans and non-Mexicans.

V. FACTORS CONTRIBUTING TO SUCCESSFUL INTERMARRIAGE

Even though intercultural marriage is defined as a marriage between two persons of divergently different cultural backgrounds who theoretically need to make more of an effort to adjust to each other, many people are very successful in their adjustment (Crohn, 1995). Advantages and contributions of intermarriage have been noticed, such as a greater degree of commitment, self-other differentiation, the ability to accept, tolerate, and respect each other's differences, and broader opportunities for learning and growth (Ho, 1990). Several factors are essential for success in intermarriage adjustment.

A. SOUND MOTIVATION AND POSITIVE RELATIONS AS FOUNDATIONS FOR MARRIAGE

The concept of marriage may be different in different societies and may vary at different times. Nevertheless, the elemental nature of marriage is that a man and woman who are emotionally fond of each other decide to live together with the mutual goal of forming a family to stabilize and improve the quality of their lives. When a couple gets married for this reason, we consider it a sound motivation. However, people sometimes get married for other reasons, resulting in a so-called "neurotic marriage." For example, a person may get married simply for material benefit, or just to escape from his or her original home or country. This is not only true for ordinary marriages, but also for some intercultural marriages. For an Asian girl to marry an American GI or businessman as a way of getting a ticket out of her country or for a black man to marry a white woman and mistreat her to gratify his individual psychology of resentment toward white people are examples of "neurotic" motivations. A marriage in which certain conditions of marriage are demanded is another example of a neurotic marriage. Marriages based on such motivations are not likely to end up happily.

Just as in homocultural marriages, there should be a positive affection between husband and wife in intercultural marriages. They should know each other for some time before deciding to marry, appreciate each other's qualities and strengths, and know how to relate to each other in private life. Jeter (1982) stresses that whether it is a "straight" marriage or an "intercultural" marriage, the crucial point is whether the union provides the necessary warmth, love, affection, excitement, caring, intimacy, and solidarity that all humans require. Such basic elements of marriage are even more necessary in intercultural marriages, which need sound motivation and strong forces behind them, based on which a lifelong relationship can be built.

B. Mature Personalities with Dynamic Qualities for Adjustment

Because so many changes and adjustments have to be made in marriages, particularly in intercultural marriages, it is very important that the couple be open-minded enough to see that there are many different ways of living in the world and be willing to try new things and make changes if necessary instead of being rigid and resistant to change. A high tolerance for confusion, an acceptance of areas of dissatisfaction, and a knowledge of how to appropriately change one's attitudes according to the situation are equally important. All these qualities are essential for any kind of marriage, but, again, they are especially important in an intercultural marriage.

Because the marriage depends on two people rather than one, it is very important that these two people be a good match in terms of sensitivity to each other's needs. They need to realize that differ-

ences will always occur in the periphery of life but that a basic similar centrality of thought about life is held between them, and that they have a mutual consideration of what is important to each other, respect each other's points of view, and have an attitude of "fairness" for both. The most important thing is that they share a common goal, toward which they are strongly motivated.

C. Welcoming Family and Friends Who Support the Marriage

Even though the nuclear family is the popular family unit in many contemporary societies, the families on both sides still have a lot of input in the marriage, not only in fact, but also at the psychological level, either directly or indirectly. How the marriage is accepted and welcomed by the families of origin still has a significant impact on the marriage. There will be less of a shadow of doubt and insecurity if the marital union is blessed by both families and friends. The husband and wife will not only feel happy about their being together but could receive needed support from their close families and friends in times of daily life crisis.

If the intercultural marriage is not blessed by parents, families, and close friends, there remains a gray shadow in the marital relationship no matter where the couple lives. A very negative impact could occur if the families of origin put pressure on a couple regarding how they should live their cultural lives, and there is always unexpected intrusion and harmful influences from parents, siblings, and other relatives. It is better not to have such nonsupportive family influences even in ordinary marriages, and more so in intercultural marriages.

D. Accommodating Environment That Accepts the Marriage

The environment, which affects our lives in many visible and invisible ways, becomes crucial in an intercultural marriage. If the community tends to accept the intercultural marriage with little discrimination, then it will be a lot easier for the couple to live in that setting, to make friends, and to have a satisfying social life. It is particularly important, when they are raising children, to see that they are accepted by the neighborhood, school, and peer group.

It is clear that some societies have a good tolerance for people of different ethnic and cultural backgrounds, whereas some hold negative or unfriendly attitudes toward them. In general, a multiethnic society is used to living with neighbors and friends of different ethnic or racial background. Living in such a social environment there is less of a tendency to emphasize the majority or minority — everybody is regarded as "majority." In such a social environment, intercultural marriage is viewed and accepted as "ordinary" rather than "strange" or "unusual." Interculturally married couples tend to survive and flourish better in such welcoming environments.

In contrast to many decades ago, black–white interracial marriage is becoming accepted by U.S. society. As a result, there are less discriminating attitudes shown by people toward them. Associated with the increase of this liberal atmosphere in society, the nature of black–white marriage is becoming more "ordinary" than "unusual." According to Kouri and Lasswell (1993), who examined 29 black–white couples living in the greater Los Angeles metropolitan area, the couples married mainly because they were attracted to each other because of overall compatibility — the "normal" reason to get married. The majority of the couples studied also stated that their families had accepted their marriages, although black families were somewhat more likely to accept the relationships from the beginning. This study illustrates that there is a close relation between the attitude in the community and the nature of the interracial marriage. The more accepting the attitude of the community toward the interracial marriage, the more "normal" the motives for such marriages.

VI. SOME THERAPEUTIC CONSIDERATIONS

When a therapist is going to work with an interculturally married couple who has culturally related problems, some considerations are necessary (Hsu, 2001).

A. CAREFUL HANDLING OF RELATIONS WITH SPOUSES OF DIFFERENT ETHNICCULTURES

When a therapist is working with an interethnically or interracially married couple, it is very important to pay attention from the very beginning to how the ethnic or racial backgrounds of the three partners — the therapist, the husband, and the wife — are going to be involved in and affect the therapeutic interaction. The ethnic or racial factor will have a significant impact on the relations that will occur between the therapist and the two married people seeking therapy (Baptiste, 1984).

For instance, when a black therapist is treating a white husband and a black wife, there is a strong possibility that the white husband will suspect the therapist of favoring his black wife in therapy; in the meantime, the black wife may feel unhappy that the black therapist does not take her side when she needs extra help. Sometimes, the black therapist may overidentify with the black wife's problem or, in an opposite way, downplay her problems. No matter which direction the relationship may go, it is potentially problematic what is going to distort the therapeutic relationship in a counterproductive way (Brown, 1987).

An ethnically intermarried couple with a Caucasian husband and a Chinese wife intentionally sought professional help from a Chinese marital therapist. The Chinese wife did not speak fluent English and it was considered a good choice to have a therapist who spoke Chinese. After the session started, even the therapist tried to carry out the session in English — the "common" language for them — so that there would be no communication problems. However, very soon, it was found that the Chinese wife preferred to use Chinese to describe her view of the problem, particularly when she wanted to complain about her (Caucasian) husband. The therapist was sucked into carrying on a "private" conver-

sation with the Chinese wife, and exclude the Caucasian husband on and off during the session. In
order to minimize this awkward and undesirable situation, the therapist made an effort to also function
as an interpreter, translating what the Chinese wife
said in Chinese into English so that the Caucasian
husband could understand. Needless to say, playing
this extra role took more time and effort on the part
of the therapist, but it facilitated the communication
between husband and wife on their psychological
problem and, most importantly, it avoided an unnecessarily unbalanced relationship with either of them
— a basic element needed for successful marital
therapy.

As a rule of thumb, the matter of different ethnic or
racial background should be pointed out from the very
beginning of the treatment, any possible effects should
be laid out on the table openly, and ways to minimize
potential complications should be suggested and carried out (Faulkner & Kich, 1983). Otherwise, the couple in treatment may react strongly to the unbalanced
relationship with the therapist and discontinue the
therapy.

B. Proper Management of Ethnic/Cultural Transference and Countertransference

"Ethnic transference" refers to a patient developing
a displaced relationship with a particular feeling
toward the therapist based on the therapist's ethnic,
cultural, or racial background. The displaced relationship is the result of the projection of what the patient
knows about the ethnic, culture, or race (of the therapist). This projection may or may not reflect reality,
depending on the kind of knowledge or experience the
patient has had in the past, as well as the stereotypical
image that people in the society may have about the
ethnicity, culture, or race concerned, but when it is
associated with a strong (distorted) feeling or (incorrect) bias, it certainly affects the therapeutic relationship between the patient and the therapist. Thus, there
is a need for careful management.

The occurrence of cultural transference is observed
in individual as well as martial therapy. However, in
the latter, the phenomena become more complicated if
the couple are interethnic or interracially married.
Because the ethnic, cultural, or racial background of
the partners is different, they may develop different
kinds of cultural transferences that create a compound
situation for the therapist to manage. For instance, a
black husband and a Filipino wife were seeing a white
therapist for marital problems. The black husband
developed a (negative) cultural transference against
the white therapist, feeling that he was looking down
on him, did not understand him, and would not take
his side. In contrast, the Filipino wife developed a
(positive) cultural transference toward the white therapist, believing that he was a superior person who, as
an able authority, would rescue her from her problems. The different nature of cultural transference
occurring here would certainly affect the relationship
between the therapist and the couple, aggravating the
possibility of an unbalanced relationship with the husband and wife. If the therapist was concerned with the
possible occurrence of cultural transference, or
detected its occurrence, it would have been desirable
to bring the issue out in the open and examine, clarify,
and correct it to avoid any undesirable effects on the
therapy.

The reverse of cultural transference may develop as
"cultural countertransference." In this case, the therapist develops a certain displaced view or feeling
toward the patient based on the patient's ethnic, culture, or racial background. If the views were distorted
or biased with intense feelings, it would certainly
interfere with the therapy process, requiring special
attention and management. Such cultural countertransference may occur in couple therapy, particularly
if the couple is interculturally married. For instance, in
the case of the black husband married to a Filipino
wife, the white therapist may develop a different kind
of cultural countertransference toward the black husband and Filipino wife depending on the therapist's
knowledge, attitude, or prejudice toward a black or
Filipino person. Such ethnic or racially based countertransference would certainly affect the therapist's rela-

tionship with the husband and wife, and require proper care and management.

C. Clear Awareness of the Therapist's Own Cultural Position

When a therapist is working with an interculturally married couple, an important consideration is the therapist's own ethnic–cultural background, examining and managing the therapist's own ethnic views and cultural beliefs (Baptiste, 1984). This is particularly true when the therapist is going to offer suggestions for solutions. The therapeutic suggestions made by the therapist are very likely to be influenced by his or her culture, either consciously or unconsciously. The therapist needs to make an effort to examine his or her cultural position all the time. It is necessary for the therapist to maintain his neutrality without personal (cultural) bias as much as possible, and in the meantime avoid being trapped into the cultural conflict between the interculturally married husband and wife and taking sides emotionally and conceptually with either of them.

D. Proper Performance of the Therapist as a Cultural Broker

1. Promote Awareness and Understanding of Differences between Partners

It is the general goal for couple therapists to promote communication between troubled married partners who tend to under- or misunderstand each other. This is more necessary when the therapist is working with an interculturally married couple. There may be a problem with language or communication. The partners may not share the same primary language so that there is a need for assistance in clarifying and understanding the meaning of what has been said between them. The therapist needs to serve as an interpreter or facilitator. Sometimes, the problems originated by not fully communicating with each other even though they

were emotionally intimate. In some cultures, it is a cultural assumption that, in the intimate relationship of husband and wife, there is no need to express everything in spoken language. It is considered awkward to express appreciation or request in words. It is culturally expected that the partner should be able to perceive the meaning not said.

One of the major problems encountered by intermarried couples is the lack of understanding and appreciation of each other's culture. Specifically, people are unaware that their contrasting viewpoints and behaviors are often based on their different cultural upbringings rather than some problem in the relationship or with them as individuals. It is important for a couple to be able to communicate their complex personal thoughts and deep feelings. Misunderstandings are likely when there is a failure to appreciate the different cultural aspects present in each of the individuals.

2. Reinforce Mutual Respect and Cultural Empathy

The therapist needs to help the couple to be curious about each other's culture and to discover, discuss, and understand the differences in their beliefs, values, concepts, expectations, and attitudes about many things. The couple must appreciate how such differences affect their interaction and cause conflict. Openly discussing these matters can help the couple be conscious of and attuned to the cultural differences between them. Often this alone can result in a greatly improved relationship. Once the couple is attuned to each other's cultural aspects, they should be further encouraged to accept and appreciate the positive attributes of each other's culture and be proud to participate in it as well. The partners need to be encouraged to be empathic about each other's perceptions, feelings, and attitudes toward his or her own cultural beliefs or customs. Through it, appropriate communication, trust, intimacy, and problem solving can be facilitated (Ibrahim & Schroeder, 1990). It is useful for the therapist to stress that there is no right or wrong between various cultures, only differences. The therapist can help the couple to understand not only that their differences are acceptable, but also that they can have a positive impact on the relationship.

3. Encourage Negotiation and Compromise for Resolution of Differences

The therapist needs to function as a cultural broker to both encourage the appreciation of and adaptation to the partners' cultures, and to liberate them from rigid cultural restraints. The couple needs to be encouraged to negotiate and compromise to resolve their differences. They can find a modified middle path that suits both their cultures, or at least find a path that does not conflict with either. A new, more liberated family tradition can also be formed (Eaton, 1994). The therapist can help the couple develop concrete steps to adjust to each other's culture, such as taking language lessons and participating in cultural programs or activities.

The therapy will benefit when the advantages of multiculturism in a family are emphasized: differences do not always create conflict; they can also generate broader perspectives, greater knowledge, and multiple ways to enjoy life, to deal with problems, and to meet challenges. Instead of assigning negative traits to each partner's culture, the couple can attribute positive qualities to their different cultural values and patterns, and learn to appreciate and enjoy the differences.

C. SUITABLE INCORPORATION OF SPECIAL CULTURAL CONSIDERATION

1. Allowance of Time for Gradual Change of Culture-Related Emotion

The couple needs to be educated that there is no quick way to change culture-rooted behavior and emotion. They are built in deeply and intrapsychically and will take a long time to change. The couple needs to be advised that there should be allowance of time for gradual change. Trying to make change hastily

will only result in negative effects. This is particularly true if it involves deeply rooted emotions and attitudes. Time is always the best solution.

2. Permit Cultural Holidays for Each Side as Needed

One way to deal with diverse differences between couples would be for the couple to alternately practice the customs of both cultures at different times and on separate occasions. In other words, they are encouraged to have "cultural holidays." Each spouse is allowed to have a cultural holiday, or cultural regression, during which that spouse is encouraged to practice the rites, rituals, activities, behaviors, and traditions of his or her culture of origin. Such occasional and transient cultural regression will help them resume their newly formed joint lives.

VII. SUCCESSFUL INTERCULTURAL MARRIAGE

Finally, a word needs to be said about the positive aspects of intercultural marriage. In the past, an intercultural marriage tended to be conceptualized as one with potential problems and difficulties in adjustment. A positive aspect has been neglected if we do not consider that our lives are a continuous process of change and improvement, not only originating from the inside, but also from contact with and stimulation from the outside; thus, intercultural marriage should be seen as a means of bringing in new stimuli from the outside and a challenging way of introducing adjustments. Actually, couples who intermarry may be considered pioneers who are brave enough to allow adventure into their lives by breaking from traditional patterns. Couples who intermarry even against resistance and succeed in overcoming problems have strong common goals, act as a positive balance to each other, and demonstrate the ability to adjust. Thus, the successful intercultural marriage should be considered a good example of masterful intercultural adjustment.

Associated with the increase in transportation, migration, working internationally, and living in multiethnic societies, there is an increased tendency for people to meet people of different racial, ethnic, and cultural backgrounds. There is a natural, increased tendency for people to marry interracially and interculturally. This pattern is encouraged by contemporary people becoming more liberal in their attitudes and more tolerant and accepting of differences among people. Within this sociocultural environment, the number of intercultural marriages will continue to increase. There is thus a great need for mental health workers to become familiar with intercultural marriages and learn how to provide assistance if it is needed (cross-reference to Chapter 3: Marriage and the Family, and Chapter 39: Working with Couples and Spouses).

REFERENCES

Baptiste, D.A. (1984). Marital and family therapy with racially culturally intermarried step-families: Issues and guidelines. *Family Relations Journal of Applied Family and Child Studies, 33*(3), 373–380.

Blount, B.W., & Curry, A. (1993). Caring for the bicultural family: The Korean-American example. *Journal of the American Board of Family Practice, 6*(3), 261–268.

Brown, J.A. (1987). Casework contacts with Black-White couples. *Social Casework, 68*(1), 24–29.

Calkins, F. (1962). *My Samoan chief.* Garden City, NY: Doubleday.

Char, W. (1977). Motivations for intercultural marriage. In W.S. Tseng, J.F. McDermott, Jr., & T.W. Maretzki (Eds.), *Adjustment in intercultural marriage.* Honolulu: University of Hawaii School of Medicine, Department of Psychiatry.

Clulow, C. (1993). Marriage across frontiers: National, ethnic and religious differences in partnership. *Sexual & Marital Therapy, 8*(1), 81–87.

Cohen, N. (1982). Same or different? A problem in identity in cross-cultural marriages. *Journal of Family Therapy, 4*(2), 177–199.

Crohn, J. (1995). *Mixed matches: How to create successful interracial, interethnic, and interfaith relationships.* New York: Fawcett Columbine.

Davidson, J.R. (1992). Theories about Black-White interracial marriage: A clinical perspective. *Journal of Multicultural Counseling and Development, 20*(4), 150–157.

Eaton, S.C. (1994). Marriage between Jews and non-Jews: Counseling implications. *Journal of Multicultural Counseling and Development, 22*(4), 210–214.

Faulkner, J., & Kich, G.K. (1983). Assessment and engagement stages in therapy with the interracial family. *Family Therapy Collections, 6,* 78–90.

Hall, C.C.I. (1987). Japanese war brides. *Asian American Psychological Association Journal, 12*(1), 3–10.

Ho, M.K. (1990). *Intermarried couples in therapy.* Springfield, DL: Charles C. Thomas.

Hsu, J. (2001). Marital therapy for intermarried couples. In W.S. Tseng & J. Streltzer (Eds.), *Culture and psychotherapy: A guide to clinical practice* (pp. 225–242). Washington, DC: American Psychiatric Press.

Ibrahim, F.A., & Schroeder, D.G. (1990). Cross-cultural couples counseling: A developmental, psychoeducational intervention. *Journal of Comparative Family Studies, 21*(2), 193–205.

Jeter, K. (1982). Analytic essay: Intercultural and interracial marriage. *Marriage & Family Review, 5*(1), 105–111.

Kitano, H.H., Yeung, W.T., Chai, L., & Hatanaka, H. (1984). Asian-American interracial marriage. *Journal of Marriage & the Family, 46*(1), 179–190.

Kouri, K.M., & Lasswell, M. (1993). Black-white marriages: Social change and intergenerational mobility. *Marriage & Family Review, 19*(3–4), 241–255.

McGoldrick, M., & Preto, N.G. (1984). Ethnic intermarriage: Implications for therapy. *Family Process, 23*(3), 347–364.

Ratliff, B.W., Moon, H.F., & Bonacci, G.A. (1978). Intercultural marriage: The Korean-American experience. *Social Casework, 59*(4), 221–226.

Salgado de Snyder, N., & Padilla, A.M. (1982). Interethnic marriages of Mexican Americans after nearly two decades. *Spanish Speaking Mental Health Research Center Occasional Papers, 15,* 1–18.

Song, J., Bergen, M.B., & Schumm, W.R. (1995). Sexual satisfaction among Korean-American couples in the midwestern United States. *Journal of Sex & Marital Therapy, 21*(3), 147–158.

Tseng, W.S., McDermott, J.F., Jr., & Maretzki, T.W. (Eds.). (1977). *Adjustment in intercultural marriage.* Honolulu: University of Hawaii School of Medicine, Department of Psychiatry.

47

Religion, Psychopathology, and Therapy

I. RELIGION: OVERVIEW

Religion is one of the ways we understand the world and give meaning to our lives. There are numerous religions in different societies and even within the same society that directly or indirectly shape our lives and influence our thought and behavior. They also impact psychopathology, on the one hand, and influence therapy, on the other. Thus, it is essential for clinicians to understand the nature of religion and how to deal with the important cultural aspects of belief and faith. For this reason, there is a renewed interest among psychiatrists and behavior and social scientists in the interrelation of religion, psychiatry, and mental health (Bhugra, 1996; Boehnlein, 2000a; Koenig, 1998; Neeleman & Persaud, 1995; Pattison, 1984). It is very natural for cultural psychiatrists to be concerned with the religious aspects of our lives and behavior, as they are closely tied to culture.

In this chapter, the nature of religion will be reviewed from anthropological, sociological, and psychiatric perspectives.

A. ANTHROPOLOGICAL VIEW

1. Definition and Commonly Used Terms

Anthony F.C. Wallace defined **religion** from an anthropological perspectives as "belief and ritual concerned with supernatural beings, powers, and forces" (1966, p.5). Another anthropologist, Clifford Greetz (1973), defined religion more elaborately as "a system of symbols that acts to establish powerful, persuasive, and long-lasting moods and motivations in men by formulating concepts of a general order of existence and clothing these concepts with such an aura of factuality that the moods and motivations seem uniquely realistic." It is believed that religion exists in almost all human societies; however, different cultures conceptualize supernatural entities very differently. Also, religion, like ethnicity or language, may be associated with social divisions within and across societies and nations (Kottak, 1999, pp. 192–193).

Several terms and concepts that are closely associated with religion deserve clarification. **Magic** refers to supernatural techniques intended to accomplish specific aims; **rituals** are formal sets of social behavior that are stylized, repetitive, and stereotyped, performed in special places and at set times, to convey information about the participants and their traditions (Kottak, 1999, pp. 200–201). **Sacred belief** refers to a conception of the world, historically and culturally determined, that defers the power of human intentions to a superior power that is unmoving in time and transcends human action (Bartocci, Frighi, Rovera, Lalli, & di Fonzo, 1998, p. 322).

Animism is a term derived from the Latin word *anima,* meaning soul or spirit. The English anthropologist Sir Edward Tylor (1871/1958) used this term to describe a belief in spirit beings. It is used interchangeably with the English term **spirituality,** which acknowledges the existence of a transcendent being, power, or reality greater than ourselves. It is the belief that every individual, in addition to a bodily self, has a spiritual self, the soul. Often associated with this is the belief that a person can communicate with the souls of deceased ancestors — the root of ancestor worship. Many people believe that living beings, including animals (specially identified tatoic animals) or plants (particularly large trees), have souls. Cults deifying various aspects of nature also abound in many societies. For instance, gods of land, rivers, stone, or mountains are worshiped. Sun and rain deities are outstanding among agricultural people. Tylor proposed that religion evolved through stages, beginning with animistic beliefs in souls. It then extended into the belief in multiple gods (polytheism), and later the belief in a single, all-powerful deity (monotheism).

A **cult** is simply a system of religious worship or ritual, particularly one that is not established and organized. It should be remembered that most contemporary, mainstream religions started as cults before they were formally recognized and accepted. Sometimes, cults refer to the devoted attachment to, or extravagant admiration for, a principle or person (such as the cult of nudism or the cult whose members believe that their emperor is a descendent of god and are willing to die for him), without being a religion in a general sense. Today, the term cult is often used negatively for groups whose leaders are considered to have unusual, strange, or pathological qualities, resulting in ill effects on the members or society at large (Schwartz & Kaslow, 1982). The boundary between such negatively conceived (pathological) "cults" and (healthy) "regular religion" is often an arbitrary, gray area. A clear distinction is not made easily. This will be elaborated further in the following section on religion and pathology.

2. Different Types of Religions

Religions are parts of cultures, and cultural differences show up systematically in religious beliefs, practices, and institutions. In a cross-cultural comparison, Wallace (1966) identified four types of religion: shamanic, communal, Olympian, and monotheistic. Shamanic religion is the simplest. The shamans are part-time religious figures who, in times of need, perform ceremonies to mediate between people and supernatural beings and forces. Shamanic religions are often found in hunting and gathering societies, particularly those in the northern latitudes, such as Siberia.

Communal religions also utilize part-time religious specialists, with community rituals performed periodically for special occasions, such as harvests or rites of passage. Some hunter–gatherers have communal religions, but they are more typical of farming societies.

Olympian religions are named after Mount Olympus, home of the classical Greek gods. They arose with the organization of nation-states and have full-time religious specialists who are organized hierarchically and bureaucratically. Olympian religions are polytheistic, with many gods. They were found in ancient times in Greece and Rome and exist today in many nonindustrial nation-states in Mexico, Africa, and Asia.

Monotheistic religions are characterized by the belief that all supernatural phenomena are manifestations of a single, omnipotent, supreme being. They have a priesthood. Christianity and the Muslim faith are representatives of monotheistic religions.

3. Purpose of Religion

What is the purpose of religion? According to anthropologist Roger M. Keesing (1976, pp. 386–387), religions offer explanations. They answer existential questions, such as how the world came to be, how humans are related to natural species and forces, why humans die, what happens after their deaths, and why their efforts succeed or fail. Religions provide validation. They posit controlling forces in the universe that sustain the moral and social order of a people. Ancestors, spirits, or gods reinforce rules and give validity and meaning to human acts. Religions provide assistance. They reinforce the human ability to cope with the fragility of life, and events such as death, illness, disaster, or failure.

B. Sociological View

1. Major Religions around the World

At present, there are several major religions around the world that are recognized as mainstream and have a relatively strong impact on the people who believe in them. They are Hinduism, Buddhism, Taoism, Islam, Judaism, and Christianity (Kinzie, 2000; Smith, 1958, 1991).

a. Hinduism

Hinduism has a long history and is tied to the metaphysical concepts of Indian mythology. It took its original form in pre-Vedic times, dominated by animistic beliefs and the belief that an extensive world of demons and evil spirits causes illness to humankind. It is characterized by the symbols, myths, and multiple images of gods. As a new religion during the post-Vedic period (about 600 B.C. to A.D. 1000), Hinduism addressed man's need to take charge of his own destiny and to decrease the importance of the gods that he worshiped. According to orthodox Hinduism, man may desire the acquisition of wealth or sensual pleasures, but they cannot really satisfy him. He needs to tap into the infinite power, which may be accomplished through yoga, a method of training to help unite the power within. Hinduism traces an individual's journey through reincarnation. A person's present life is the product of what he has done in the past. Thus, every action has an inexorable consequence that affects even future life cycles. Indian society subdivides and ranks people hierarchically in a rigid caste system. However, Hinduism believes that through multiple reincarnations all souls migrate through all the castes.

b. Buddhism

Buddhism began with the son (Siddhartha Gautama, born 563 B.C.) of a ruler of a small kingdom in Nepal. Despite his wealth, he became aware of human pain, suffering, and death. At the age of 29, he left home to search for the truth. After his Great Awakening, he taught his path of enlightenment, namely: life is suffering; desire for fulfillment is the cause of the suffering; and suffering can be relieved by release from narrow self-interest. In reaction to the rituals and traditions of Hindu society, Buddha taught a religion devoid of authority, ritual, and the supernatural. The primary goal of enlightenment is wisdom. Although Buddhism originated in Nepal, in northern India, it had little impact on the Indian continent and spread to Asia (China, Japan, and Korea), south Asia (Thailand, Burma, Cambodia), and Sri Lanka.

c. Taoism

Taoism is said to have been originated by Lao Zi (or Lao Tzu, born 604 B.C.), a legendary scholar who is credited with writing the *Dao De Jing* (or *Tao Te Ching,* translated *The Way and Its Power* in English), Taoism's basic text. The key concept of Dao (or Tao, literally, the Way) is the principle of the ultimate reality of the universe and of human life. It emphasizes naturalness, encourages spontaneity, and stresses the search for that which is beyond human affairs. In a strict sense, Lao Zi's teaching is not a religion (it does not refer to a supernatural being), it is a philosophy (its concern is only complying with the laws of the nature). It views the world as complimentarily composed of oppositions, symbolized by ying and yang. Simplicity in thought and action and attunement to nature are valued, while self-assertiveness and competition are rejected. This is called philosophical Taoism. Separate from this is religious Taoism, which is rooted in the indigenous religions of China, and took form in the second century, borrowing the name of Taoism. It is characterized by a multitude of deities and sacred texts. The Taoist priest tries to maximize the power of Tao, often with magical and occult techniques. Such rudimentary practices are observed in present Taiwan.

d. Islam

The prophet Mohammed was born in A.D. 570 in the leading tribe of Mecca in Koreish. He came to believe that Allah, the high God of the Arabic pantheon, was the one and only God. The classic of Islam teaching, the Koran, proclaimed the omnipotence and mercy of God and man's total dependence on Him. Islam brought a vast change to the moral and social order of Arabia and established a specific social order in which faith, politics, and society were joined. At present, the believers of Islam comprise nearly one-quarter of the world's population.

e. Judaism

The Jewish God, Yahweh, evolved from a personal and tribal deity to the ultimate and only God. This God is described as passionate and very involved in human affairs. Judaism conceives God and His creations, the world and its people, as good and righteous. Therefore, our present life is considered important and humanitarian activities are emphasized. The Jewish culture has a strong moral code that emphasizes justice as a basic value. Jewish people emphasize practices and traditions that are rooted in sharing life with God.

f. Christianity

Christianity began with Jesus, a Jewish carpenter who was born in Palestine about 2000 years ago. He stressed Yahweh's compassion and preached to all members of society across social barriers. He opposed the holy codes of the Jewish authorities, which he felt created social division. His teachings were parallel to the Old Testament, but were fresh and appealed to ordinary man's imagination. The Christian religion was institutionalized, and the theology of the church developed over several centuries. It hinges on several key concepts: the original sin of sexuality; God's relief from sin; how God became human; and the Trinity concept of God as the Father, the Son, and the Holy Ghost.

It has been pointed out by Chinese-American cultural anthropologist Francis L.K. Hsu (1967) that Western anthropologists have never made any serious moves in the direction of the study of Christianity, but their view of religion everywhere is the Western folk view of Christianity and religion. For instance, it is assumed that religions in which one God alone prevails are higher (therefore more "civilized," or "rational") than others (which are considered "primitive"). However, examining Christianity from an anthropological perspective, Hsu pointed out several characteristics. Because Christians see their own supernatural being as the only true God and their theology as the only true or pure scripture, they are in essence intolerant of other views and practices. Christianity is prone to missionary activities — with a strong motive to "save" others — while the believers of other creeds have no such need. Christianity is characterized by the extensiveness of its theology, while many other believers are less concerned about elaborating their theologies — they are only interested in receiving blessings, luck, and foreknowledge of personal vicissitudes to come rather than learning the "truth" from the scriptures.

Some Western scholars (such as Smith, 1958) included Confucianism as one kind of religion, while in reality it is not. Confucius was a scholar and teacher of humanity respected (and perhaps worshiped as a great teacher) by people for his ideas regarding human nature and proper behavior. However, his teachings have nothing to do with supernatural power, in fact, he refused to discuss any matter that was related to the supernatural and not associated with concepts of spirituality.

Finally, from a cross-cultural perspective, it should be pointed out that many people have an atheistic worldview and live without religions. This is attributed to their lifestyle and beliefs, on a voluntary basis; rooted in their childhood encultural experiences; or related to official ideology and policy, such as in mainland China, where more than one-fifth of the world's population lives. As an extension of the traditional Confucian atheistic view and present political ideology, the Chinese people are instructed not to believe in any supernatural beings.

2. Syncretism, Variations, Change, and the Rise of Religion

As explained by Hughes and Wintrob (2000), it would be simplistic to consider all "religions" as always self-contained, historically and internally consistent sets of beliefs and practices. In human affairs, diffusion, borrowing, and incorporation of formerly alien traits have been universally observed; the same is true of religion. Hughes and Wintrob went further to give several examples, such as the fusion of animistic, Muslim, and Christian religions in Liberia, West Africa, and the practice of *candomblé* in Brazil — a set of beliefs that incorporates an elaborate pantheon of gods and possessing spirits derived from Africa, the Caribbean, and indigenous Brazilian tribes, along with traditional European-derived religious movements.

A new religion may emerge in revolt against a traditional one. We know that Christianity was established within the historical context of traditional Judaism, adding the New testament to the Old Testament; Protestantism developed in revolt against orthodox Catholic Christianity. Religious practices are frequently modified to accommodate the local sociocultural environment. In Taiwan, people are officially permitted to worship their ancestors, even when they are Catholic; African-Americans attending Christian churches incorporate a lot of physical movement in their singing, borrowed from their African heritage;

and in Micronesia, the people dress up to attend church on Sunday as if they were attending a village meeting in old times.

Religion often faces the dilemma of whether or not to adjust to a changing social environment and culture. For example, it is a challenge for the Catholic church to deal with the contemporary concepts of family planning and the demands of some women to enter the priesthood.

From a social standpoint, it has been noticed that new religions tend to arise in times of social instability — as if starting a religion was a way of dealing with the anxiety associated with social change and confusion or economic distress (Boisen, 1939). A cultural psychiatrist from Korea, Kwang-Iel Kim (1972), reported that nearly 240 new religions have arisen in Korea since the middle of the 19th century. These new religions have appeared in times of social turmoil, such as in the 1860s, during the Tonghok Revolution, which tried to eliminate foreign influences from the country; after the Japanese occupation in 1910; after independence in 1945; after the Korean War in 1950; and after the Student Revolution in 1960. Kim also pointed out that, interestingly enough, these new religions share certain common characteristics: being a syncretism of the past and present (a union of the established religions and elements of shamanism, Confucianism, Taoism, Buddhism, and Christianity) and promising the beginning of a new world after the end of this one.

Cultural sociologist Takie Sugiyama Lebra (1970) reported the religious conversion of Japanese-Americans in Hawaii as a breakthrough in acculturation. It was her interpretation that new religious sects tend to arise in times of social turmoil as ways of coping with the general anxiety experienced by the people in the society.

3. Different Patterns of Religious Practice

It has been suggested that from religious and sociological perspectives, there is a need to distinguish among religious faith, affiliation, and practice, as they imply different aspects of religious behavior. Different patterns of religious practice are illustrated in Japan and China. In Japan, many people choose to have Shinto wedding ceremonies or to be married in Christian churches (even if they are not Christian), while they prefer their funerals to be Buddhist. Thus, disregarding their faiths, they practice different religious rituals based on their preferences (or the fashion). Similarly, a majority of Chinese, for the sake of convenience, may claim that they are Buddhist; however, they may visit different kinds of temples, whether they worship Taoist gods, Buddha, or legendary heroes; and they perform ancester worship at home on various occasions. Therefore, there is no concern with consistency between faith and practice.

From a sociological point of view, participation in common rites may affirm and maintain the social solidarity of a religion's adherents. Religious differences may also be associated with bitter enmity and are often the source of intergroup conflicts and wars. Historically, on a small scale, physical fights have occurred between monks of different denominations, out of rivalry or conflict over property (as observed in some Asian countries, such as China, Japan, and Korea, in the remote or recent past); on a large scale, long, organized wars have been fought between countries (such as the Crusades in Europe from 1096 to 1272). Persecution of people for religious differences has occurrred frequently throughout history in both the East and West.

C. Psychological View

American psychologist David M. Wulff (1996) has reviewed extensively the way in which religion was conceived by influential psychologists in the West during the 20th century. According to Wulff, James Leuba gathered experimental evidence and concluded that mystical experiences may be accounted for adequately in terms of the basic principles of psychology and physiology; challenged traditional theistic religion; and criticized religion as irrationality and pathology. B.F. Skinner, through animal laboratory experience, demonstrated "superstitious" behavior. He explained religion as reinforced behavior, maintaining the view that, like all other behaviors, religious behaviors occur because they have been followed by reinforcing stimuli. George Vetter interpreted religion as a response to unpredictable situations. In contrast to these scholars, who tended to see religion as a liability, Wulff pointed out that there was another group of scholars who saw religion as an asset. For instance, William James provided a model of a more balanced assessment of religion, seeing it as way to human excellence. C.G. Jung suggested that religion was a way to wholeness, and Erik Erikson saw religion as hope and wisdom.

D. Psychiatric View

Some psychiatrists have attempted to explain the nature of religion by utilizing psychiatric theories. For instance, the founder of psychoanalysis, Sigmund Freud, explained that a firm belief in an ominiopotent supernatural being was a projection of the need for an authority figure for security. For Freud, religion was fulfillment of an infantile wish.

The issue of whether very religious people, particularly leaders, are normal or unusual has attracted some interest from a psychiatric point of view. There is a handful of reports concerning the psychiatric examination of religious leaders. For instance, Sasaki (1969) studied the personal history of shamans in Japan. He reported that the first episode of spirit possession for 40 of the 56 shamans studied occurred after self-training to become a shaman; the remaining 16 experienced spirit possession spontaneously prior to deciding to become shamans. Sasaki diagnosed 7 of the shamans as suffering from schizophrenia, 10 from personality disorders, and 2 from other psychiatric disorders. Only 38 out of the 56 were without evident psychiatric symptoms.

In Burma, one of the centers of Theravada Buddhism, almost every village contains at least one monastery with at least one resident monk. According to cultural anthropologist Melford E. Spiro (1965), the monks live an exclusively otherworldly existence. The monastery is outside the village gates, and the monks' interaction with laymen is confined to occasional ritual situations. Although living in a state of absolute dependence on the laymen, the monks have withdrawn both physically and psychologically from the social world, and even from their own selves, through the practice of meditation. This extreme withdrawal from reality might be taken as a manifestation of severe pathology. Spiro notes that James Steel (1963) analyzed Rorschach samples from these monks and reported that there was a very high degree of "defensiveness"; "pathologically regressed" expression of aggressive and oral drives; cautious avoidance of "emotionally laden" situations as a means of obviating the necessity of handling affect; a "hypochondriacal self-preoccupation"; latent homosexuality; and above-average fear of females or mother figures. According to Steel, the Rorschach protocols of these monks are similar to the protocols of Burmese laymen. Thus, Spiro indicated that monks differ from laymen, not because they have different problems, but because they have more of the same problems. In other words, monks are Burmans in extremis. Their religious lives serve as culturally constituted defense mechanisms.

II. RELIGION AND PSYCHOPATHOLOGY

A. Distinction between "Healthy" and "Pathological" Religion

While it is difficult to distinguish between "healthy" and "pathological" religion, there is a practical need for such a distinction. Perhaps it would be easier to examine certain cults that society has considered to be clearly "unusual," "strange," or "pathological."

Still fresh in our memories is the collective suicide of 39 members of the Heaven's Gate cult, who lived in a rented mansion in Rancho Santa Fe, California. Following their leader, Marshall Applewhite, a former mental patient, the cultists ended their lives in a planned, organized way: taking sleeping pills mixed in pudding and lying on their bunkbeds with plastic bags over their heads to await the holy spaceship. This incident occurred when the comet Hale-Bopp appeared in the sky in March 1997. The members believed that they were escaping a revamping of the Earth by hitching a cosmic ride to heaven.

Another tragic religious incident was the massive suicide of the members of the People's Temple in late 1978. Following the Reverend Jim Jones, their religious leader, nearly 900 members moved from California to Guyana, South America, to establish a new life in the jungle. Following their leader's order, as a part of a routine religious ritual, all of them swallowed the fatal substance, cyanide, and died together.

The belief in death as one of the ultimate ways to fulfill their religious mission was found in other cults as well, such as the Sun Cult in Europe. This cult tends to keep its religious affiliations and activities secret, and is not well known to outsiders. Occasionally, a small group of members commits ritual collective suicide as a part of its religious practice.

There is no shortage of examples of cult leaders predicting the end of the world and persuading their believers to prepare for salvation. Many believers sell their properties, quit their jobs, and make all necessary "preparations" for the end of the world. These kinds of religious episodes have occurred in the East as well. In Korea in 1997, a cult leader predicted the end of the world and caused social turmoil. This also happened in Taiwan. In early 1999, several hundred people followed their leader to the United States to await the appearance of God on television on a certain day for his instructions on how to deal with the end of the world.

Another kind of cult involves sexual relations between cult members, or with cult leaders, as part of its religious rituals in the belief that such sexual acts will enhance the blessings of God (Kim, 1972). It was suspected that the leader of the Branch Dividiens had sexual relations with female children of cult members. However, the most terrifying aspect of the Branch Dividiens was their plan to start an antigovernment military movement. They purchased and stored a huge number of weapons in their attempt to achieve their religious goal, and the plan ended in tragedy in Waco, Texas.

In ancient times, it was common for people to sacrifice human beings in religious rituals to please a supernatural power, particularly when the society suffered natural disasters, believing it would relieve the god's anger or induce his favor. Stories are heard in many places of human sacrifices made to appease a supernatural power, such as throwing a young virgin into an erupting volcano or into a river during a flood, or killing someone when there was a drought. Such rituals would be despised by contemporary, humanistic men, but they were practiced by many cults in the not too distant past.

What are the common characteristics of these cults that are easily labeled "pathological?" Usually, there is a charismatic leader who is very powerful and convincing, and demands absolute obedience from the members. The cult is often tightly organized and members' behavior is strictly controlled. The goal of the religion is rationalized in such a way that it is convincing to the members, who have a strong faith in their leader. As a result, the members lose their ego functions and their rational judgment, and are willing to follow the leader's orders blindly.

Aside from extremely pathological cults, there is a borderline normality in many religious groups. For instance, a cult leader matching marital partners (as in the Unification Church, or the so-called Moonies) raises a question from a modern mental health perspective. A religious group fighting with different sects of the same religion, with other religious believers, or with nonbelievers — whether in occasional physical fights or formal wars institutionalized at a national level — poses questions from humanistic and religious points of view. Religious involved in politics, politicized religious movements, or religious organizations that seek economic gain are some examples.

The question is: What are the requirements of a "healthy" religion? What about people who choose not to believe in any religion? Are they right in taking an atheistic view of the world? These are questions that deserve careful consideration before any subjective or biased judgment is made.

B. Religion and Mental Disorders

Concerning the relationship between religion and serious mental illness, Koenig, Larson, and Weaver (1998) reported that religious delusions are not rare in psychotic disorders and may be present in as many as 10 to 15% of patients hospitalized with schizophrenia. Wilson (1998) commented that these delusions, however, are thought to be culturally driven: a manifestation of psychotic illness rather than a cause of it.

Mental phenomena that are significantly colored by religion and require judgments from both religious and psychiatric perspectives may present a real challenge. For instance, if a person believes that he has a mission to deliver a message from God, or claims that he is sent from God, it is difficult to assess whether this is a religious delusion or a religious phenomenon based on the belief alone. The presence of other mental symptoms or signs indicating a mental breakdown often serve as clues for clinical diagnosis.

A traditional healer, such as a shaman, often enters a possessed state, claiming that he or she is possessed by a supernatural being for the purpose of healing. He or she is able to leave the state of possession and return to an ordinary mental state when the healing ritual is over. This is in contrast to a mental patient, whose possession by a supernatural being may be beyond his control, occurring at any time. He may have difficulty coming out of the possessed state, which may last days or months.

C. Experience of Religious Conversion

Religious conversion refers to the phenomenon of a person often rather suddenly obtaining religious enlightenment, with or without mystical mental experiences (such as a twilight state, hallucinatory experiences, or a sense of possession), resulting in the adoption of a new, all-pervasive worldview. This phenomenon is often described by religious leaders who were motivated to establish new religions, as well as members of religions who decided to join in certain religious activities.

According to Galanter (2000), William James (1902/1929) wrote about religious conversion as a process through which an individual, "divided and consciously wrong, inferior and unhappy," becomes "unified and consciously right, superior and happy" as a consequence of achieving a hold on religious reality. Some kind of psychological need is clearly fulfilled for a person who claims that he or she has benefited from religious conversion. It should also be pointed out that, from a clinical point of view, some mental patients report similar religious experiences at the beginning of their mental breakdowns or as a part of their mental disorders.

D. Psychological Impact of Joining a Charismatic Group

Although some religious groups led by charismatic leaders seem "bizarre," "unhealthy," or even "pathological" from an outsider's point of view, they are reported to be beneficial for many of the members who join them.

It was pointed out by Galanter (1982) that most of the people who join charismatic religious sects tend to come from middle- and upper-middle-class backgrounds and troubled families. Psychological distress is a frequent antecedent to joining a sect. The members often have limited social ties before joining the sect.

Galanter (2000) reviewed various studies and summarized that members of charismatic groups often state that joining the group had a positive effect on their psychological states. The members report new strength and spiritual resources, increased feelings of calm and happiness, reduced self-hatred, a capacity for better relationships with others, and so on. It is suspected that individuals who have difficulty with self-identification and self-confidence, and are unable to relate to others (particularly authority figures) in a meaningful way, may benefit from joining a group with a charismatic leader who operates in a firm and organized way.

Followers of an American guru, calling themselves "the Family," were interviewed by Deutsch (1975) in Central Park in New York to determine their psychological states. Results showed that virtually all of the followers had histories of chronic unhappiness and unsatisfactory parental relationships. After becoming involved with the guru and their new "family," they experienced greater well-being and periods of bliss, and their acceptance of mystic Hindu beliefs was solidified. It was postulated that a psychological characteristic of the devotees was a strong underlying wish for union with a powerful object. Deutsch (1980) carried out a follow-up study of the group, which dissolved almost 4 years after its inception. The group moved from New York to a mountaintop in a northeastern state, forming an agricultural commune called "the Hill." However, its leader became increasingly bizarre, and even cruel to his followers. The devotees used denial, rationalization, and other defense mechanisms to maintain the fantasy that their leader was acting for their benefit. The group was finally dissolved after the leader deteriorated mentally.

Interested in the outcome of people who marry a mate assigned by their sect leader, Galanter (1986) carried out a 3-year follow-up study of 305 members of the Unification Church. He found that 95% were still active in the church 3 years later. Eighty-five percent had been married in the interim to mates designated by their religious leader. Several psychological instruments were used to assess mental health and marital adjustment. Results showed that the members' scores on a measure of psychological well-being were below those of the general population. Despite the unusual nature of the marital arrangements, the respondents' scores on the Marital Adjustment Scale were not different from data obtained from a community study. It was speculated that affiliating ties with the sect counteracted the possible distress produced by the unusual marital experience.

E. Deprogramming Cult Members

They are gone now, but in the 1970s many cults arose in European–American societies that not only inducted young members, but also suggested that they cut all ties with their families of origin. Many members were forbidden to contact their parents. As a result, their anxious parents struggled to rescue them from the cults and tried hard to help them return to normal lives. There was often resistance from the brainwashed children, who required "deprogramming" by professionals.

Based on her clinical research, Singer (1979) identified specific cult-related emotional problems with which ex-members had to cope during their reentry into society. Among them were blurring of mental acuity — with indecisiveness and cognitive inefficience; uncritical passivity — accepting almost everything they heard, taking simple remarks of others as commands; slipping into altered states — easily returning to trance-like states in response to stress or depression; and fear of the cult itself — fearing retaliation, some ex-members got unlisted telephone numbers, changed their addresses, even took other names. In therapy for ex-members, Singer suggested that the therapists, friends, and family needed to have at least some knowledge of the content of a particular cult's program in order to grasp what the ex-member was trying to describe. It was also important to understand the whole phenomenon, not merely as a religious conversion, but as the result of high-pressure recruitment tactics and intense procedures that the cults use to attract and keep members. Despite the fear that the ex-members would never recover their full functioning, it was encouraging that most of them eventually come to feel fully competent and independent through proper support.

III. RELIGION AND THERAPY

A. RELIGION AND MENTAL HEALTH

Aside from its negative aspects, religion may have certain positive elements from the standpoint of mental health. Frequent claims are made, particularly by those who are devoted to religions, that religious beliefs are beneficial to mental health, providing faith, hope, and calm to a person's mind.

Larson, Milano, Weaver, and McCullough (2000) pointed out that numerous national surveys established the central role of religion in the lives of many Americans. Nearly 95% of Americans reported a belief in god (of whatever nature). They also indicated that many studies found that higher levels of religious commitment are associated with enhanced feelings of well-being and a lower prevalence of mental illness (particularly evidenced by self-destructive behaviors such as drug and alcohol abuse). Religion has also been identified as a potential buffer against stress. Religious commitment also often plays a role in reducing suicide rates.

According to Griffith and Mahy (1984), the Spiritual Baptist Church is a black Christian movement of long standing in the English-speaking West Indies. Recently, its religious activities have blossomed among African-Americans in urban communities in the United States. Its members engage in a ceremony called "mourning," which involves prayer, fasting, and the experiencing of dreams and visions while in isolation. Members who had undergone these special experiences cited the benefits of the practice: relief of depressed moods; the ability to foresee and avoid danger; improvement in decision-making ability; heightened facility to communicate with God and to meditate; a clearer appreciation of their racial origins; identification with the church hierarchy; and physical cures. Griffith and Mahy commented that mourning appears to be a viable psychotherapeutic practice for these church members.

Despite the general belief that religion is the fountainhead of all the moral tenets of a society, Sanua (1969) pointed out that a number of empirical studies do not support this view. He commented that religious education as it is taught in the United States today does not seem to ensure healthier attitudes, despite its emphasis on ethical behavior.

B. RELIGIOUS COUNSELING

It is common for religious persons to provide mental healing practices for believers. This is observed in different types of religions, from ancient shamanism to contemporary religions. In many Western societies, Jewish and Christian clergy are often called upon to act as front-line mental health providers, especially regarding personal problems. In America, many clients who consulted clergy were satisfied with the service that they received and felt they were helped, even though most clergy are not trained to offer professional counseling (Larson et al., 2000).

American cultural psychiatrist Joseph Westermeyer (1973), after working in Laos, indicated that there were no mental health professionals in Laos when he was there. He pointed out that in the absence of mental health workers, the people of Laos effectively supported one another through crises and role changes. They accomplished this by employing their social institutions and traditions. The main social resources were religious rituals, community elders, and home-centered religious activities involving the extended family, neighbors, and friends, indicating the contribution of religion to the mental health of the people.

Clinical experiences generally indicate that patients prefer to be counseled by therapists who share the same religious background. After an intensive review of the literature on religion and psychotherapeutic processes and outcomes, Worthington, Kurusu, McCullough, and Snadage (1996) pointed out that nonreligious and religious counselors shared most counseling-relevant values, but differed in the value they placed on religion. They commented that these religious differences affected clinical judgment and behavior, especially with religious patients.

Perhaps the comments just described apply differently to various religious groups under different circumstances. When Wikler (1989), through semistructured, in-person interviews, examined the preferences of Orthodox Jewish clients in the New York area regarding the religious identities of their therapists, he found a wide range of meanings attached to a therapist's religious identity; some clients did not care about the religious backgrounds of their counselors. Keating and Fretz (1990) found that religiously committed patients often had more reservations about being counseled by therapists with nonreligious or different religious backgrounds because they feared that the therapists would ignore their spiritual concerns and view their religious or spiritual beliefs as bizarre, if not pathological, rejecting the idea of communicating with a higher power.

C. Religion and Psychotherapy

Lukoff, Lu, and Turner (1995) stressed the importance of cultural considerations in the assessment and treatment of religious and spiritual problems in clinical settings. Beyond that, they also stressed that clinicians need to have religious knowledge and orientation in their clinical work.

Understanding a patient's supernatural belief-related problems and providing relevant psychotherapy was well illustrated in a case report by Jilek-Aall and Jilek (2001). A Native American woman in Canada was mistakenly thought by police to be an insane patient because she could not stop singing a "spiritual song." Applying culturally sensitive attitudes, Jilek-Aall, a female psychiatrist with a European background, was able to understand the patient's depression associated with emotional problems in her life. Singing a spiritual song was merely the patient's way of expressing her sorrow. Based on the trust established in the therapeutic relationship, it was suggested that the patient seek help from traditional healers to relieve her depression.

Counseling psychologists Fukuyama and Sevig (1999), through their clinical experiences, pointed out that there are positive and negative expressions of spirituality among people. Pastoral counselor Clinbell (1995) defined spiritual growth as that which "aims at the enhancement of our realistic hope, our meanings, our values, our inner freedom, our faith systems, our peak experiences, and our relationship with God." Further, Clinbell described pathological or unhealthy religion or spirituality as growth blocking and resulting from rigidity, idolatry, authoritarianism, and practices that constrict life or deny reality. A therapist needs to help his clients distinguish between healthy and unhealthy spirituality — an essential part of therapy that involves religion.

In ordinary psychotherapy, therapists need to consider patients' religious beliefs. This is particularly true for clinicians working in multiethnic, multireligious societies. Turbott (1996), a psychiatrist from New Zealand, pointed out that recent psychiatric literature suggested a need to reconsider the place of religion and spirituality in the practice of psychiatry. He explained that, in New Zealand, the politically mandated bicultural approach to mental health demanded an understanding of the spirituality of the indigenous Maori. He suggested that psychiatry would benefit if the vocabulary and concepts of religion and spirituality were more familiar to trainees and practitioners.

IV. CLOSING: PSYCHIATRY AND RELIGION

As pointed out by Boehnlein (2000b), psychiatry and religion both draw upon rich traditions of human thought and practice. Although it is a branch of medicine, in contrast to the main trend of medicine's reliance on natural science, psychiatry incorporates the humanities and social sciences in its scientific base to understand and treat mental illness. Psychiatry often needs to go beyond the world of natural science into the philosophical realm. However, in the past, in general, psychiatrists have shied away from religion.

As an extension of cultural psychiatry, which emphasizes the importance of understanding and respecting a patient's lifestyle and value system, it is natural to consider the religious aspects of a patient's life and respect the patient's beliefs, whether spiritual or atheistic, rather than imposing the views and judgements arising from the therapist's own religious views and attitudes (Post, 1993). In order to meet the demands of patients of diverse cultures, it is essential to add the dimensions of religion and spirituality to the training of future psychiatrists.

REFERENCES

Bartocci, G., Frighi, L., Rovera, G.G., Lalli, N., & di Fonzo, T. (1998). Cohabiting with magic and religion in Italy: Cultural and clinical results. In S.O. Okpaku (Ed.), *Clinical methods in transcultural psychiatry* (pp. 321–335). Washington, DC: American Psychiatric Press.

Bhugra, E. (Ed.). (1996). *Religion and psychiatry: Context, consensus and controversies.* London: Routledge.

Boehnlein, J.K. (Ed.). (2000a). *Psychiatry and religion.* Washington, DC: American Psychiatric Press.

Boehnlein, J.K. (2000b). Introduction. In J.K. Boehnlein (Ed.), *Psychiatry and religion* (pp. xi–xvii). Washington, DC: American Psychiatric Press.

Boisen, A.T. (1939). Economic distress and religious experience: A study of the Holy Rollers. *Psychiatry, 2,* 185–194.

Clinbell, H. (1995). *Counseling for spiritually empowered wholeness: A hope-centered approach.* New York: Haworth Pastoral Press.

Deutsch, A. (1975). Observations on a sidewalk Ashram. *Archives of General Psychiatry, 32,* 166–175.

Deutsch, A. (1980). Tenacity of attachment to a cult leader: A psychiatric perspective. *American Journal of Psychiatry, 137*(12), 1569–1573.

Fukuyama, M.A., & Sevig, T.D. (1999). *Integrating spirituality into multicultural counseling.* Thousand Oaks, CA: Sage.

Galanter, M. (1982). Charismatic religious sects and psychiatry: An overview. *American Journal of Psychiatry, 139*(12), 1539–1548.

Galanter, M. (1986). "Moonies" get married: A psychiatric follow-up study of a charismatic religious sect. *American Journal of Psychiatry, 143*(10), 1245–1249.

Galanter, M. (2000). A psychological perspective on cults. In J.K. Boehnlein (Ed.), *Psychiatry and religion* (pp. 89–104). Washington, DC: American Psychiatric Press.

Greetz, C. (1973). *The interpretation of culture.* New York: Basic Books.

Griffith, E.E.H., & Mahy, G.E. (1984). Psychological benefits of spritual baptist "mourning." *American Journal of Psychiatry, 141,* 769–773.

Hsu, F.L.K. (1967). Christianity and the anthropologist. *International Journal of Comparative Sociology, 8*(1), 1–19.

Hughes, C.C., & Wintrob, R.M. (2000). Psychiatry and religion in a cross-cultural context. In J.K. Boehnlein (Ed.), *Psychiatry and religion* (pp. 35–65). Washington, DC: American Psychiatric Press.

Jilek-Aall, L., & Jilek, W. (2001). A woman could not stop a spiritual song. In W.S. Tseng & J. Streltzer (Eds.), *Culture and psychotherapy: A guide to clinical practice* (pp. 43–56). Washington, DC: American Psychiatric Press.

Keating, A.M., & Fretz, B.R. (1990). Christians' anticipations about counselors in response to counselor descriptions. *Journal of Counseling Psychology, 37,* 293–296.

Keesing, R.M. (1976). *Cultural anthropology: A contemporary perspective.* New York: Holt, Rinehart & Winston.

Kim, K.I. (1972). New religions in Korea: The sociocultural consideration. *Korean Neuropsychiatric Association, 11*(1), 31–36 (in Korean). (Reviewed in *Transcultural Psychiatric Research Review, 10,* 30–31 [1973]).

Kinzie, J.D. (2000). Historical relationship between the major religions and psychiatry. In J.K. Boehnlein (Ed.), *Psychiatry and religion.* Washington, DC: American Psychiatric Press.

Koenig, H.G. (Ed.). (1998). *Handbook of religion and mental health.* San Diego, CA: Academic Press.

Koenig, H.G., Larson, D.B., & Weaver, A.J. (1998). Research on religion and serious mental illness. *New Directions for Mental Health Services, 80,* 81–95.

Kottak, C.P. (1999). *Mirror for humanity: A concise introduction to cultural anthropology.* Boston: McGraw-Hill College.

Larson, D.B., Milano, M.G., Weaver, A.J., & McCullough, M.E. (2000). The role of clergy in mental health care. In J.K. Boehnlein (Ed.), *Psychiatry and religion* (pp. 155–178). Washington, DC: American Psychiatric Press.

Lebra, T.S. (1970). Religious conversion as a breakthrough in transculturation: A Japanese sect in Hawaii. *Journal for Scientific Study of Religion, 9,* 181–196.

Lukoff, D., Lu, F.G., & Turner, R. (1995). Cultural considerations in the assessment and treatment of religious and spiritual problems. *Psychiatric Clinics of North America, 18*(3), 467–485.

Neeleman, J., & Persaud, R. (1995). Why do psychiatrists neglect religion? *British Journal of Medical Psychology, 68*(2), 169–178.

Pattison, E.M. (1984). Towards a psychosocial cultural analysis of religion and mental health. In R.C. Nann, D.S. Butt, & L. Ladrido-Ignacio (Eds.), *Mental health, cultural values, and social development: A look into the '80s.* Dordrecht, The Netherlands: Reidel.

Post, S.G. (1993). Psychiatry and ethics: The problematics of respect for religious meanings. *Culture, Medicine and Psychiatry, 17*(3), 363–384.

Sanua, V.D. (1969). Religion, mental health, and personality: A review of empirical studies. *American Journal of Psychiatry, 125*(9), 1203–1213.

Sasaki, Y. (1969). Psychiatric study of the shaman in Japan. In W. Caudill & T.-Y. Lin (Eds.), *Mental health research in Asia and the Pacific* (pp. 223–241). Honolulu: East-West Center Press.

Schwartz, L.L., & Kaslow, F.W. (1982). The cult phenomenon: Historical, sociological, and familial factors contributing to their development and appeal. In F. Kaslow & M.B. Sussman (Eds.), *Cults and the family* (pp. 3–30). New York: Haworth Press.

Singer, M.T. (1979, January). Coming out of the cults. *Psychology Today,* pp. 72–82.

Smith, H. (1958). *The religions of man.* New York: Harper & Row.

Smith, H. (1991). *The world's religions: Our great wisdom traditions.* San Francisco: Harper.

Spiro, M.E. (1965). Religious systems as culturally constituted defense mechanisms. In M.E. Spiro (Ed.), *Context and meaning in cultural anthropology.* New York: Free Press.

Turbott, J. (1996). Religion, spirituality and psychiatry: Conceptual, cultural and personal challenges. *Australian and New Zealand Journal of Psychiatry, 30*(6), 720–727.

Tylor, E.B. (1958). *Primitive culture.* New York: Harper Torchbooks. (Original work Published 1871).

Wallace, A.F.C. (1966). *Religion: An anthropological veiw.* New York: McGraw-Hill.

Westermeyer, J. (1973). Lao Buddhism, mental health, and contemporary implications. *Journal of Religion and Health, 12*(2), 181–188.

Wikler, M. (1989). The religion of the therapist: Its meaning to Orthodox Jewish clients. *Hillside Journal of Clinical Psychiatry, 11*(2), 131–146.

Wilson, W.P. (1998). Religion and psychosis. In H.H. Koenig (Ed.), *Handbook of religion and mental health.* San Diego: Academic Press.

Worthington, E.L., Jr., Kurusu, T.A., McCullough, M.E., & Snadage, S.J. (1996). Empirical research on religion and psychotherapeutic processes and outcomes: A 10-year review and research prospectus. *Psychological Bulletin, 119*(3), 448–487.

Wulff, D.M. (1996). The psychology of religion: An overview. In E.P. Shafranske (Ed.), *Religion and the clinical practice of psychology.* Washington, DC: American Psychological Association.

Section I
Research, Theory, and Training

Cultural psychiatry has established its own scope and objects and has been recognized as a unique subfield of general psychiatry. It has reached the point where sophisticated issues need to be addressed at academic levels, beyond clinical concerns. In this section, three subjects are addressed: academic research, the need for theoretical elaboration, and formal training in this special field.

Chapter 48 discusses cross-cultural research in the field of cultural psychiatry, specifically in terms of methods, scope, and goals. Chapter 49 focuses on theory: how social and cultural factors, in addition to professional and other variables, shape theory in psychiatry, and how various existing theories derived primarily from the West need to be modified or revised for cross-cultural application. Finally, Chapter 50 discusses formal training for clinicians in training, as well as advanced training in the area of cultural psychiatry.

48

Cross-Cultural Research

I. BASIC ISSUES AND CONSIDERATIONS

It is a basic requirement that the two dimensions (or variables) of "culture" and "mental health" be examined side by side so that the essence of "culture and mental health" can be grasped as a whole. Canadian cross-cultural psychologist J.W. Berry (1980, pp. 2–5) has correctly pointed out the core of the scientific method: "Without comparison, differences, similarities, covariation, and cause cannot be observed or inferred" for cross-cultural study. Due to the nature of the phenomena, comparative studies are typically nonmanipulative. However, as Berry said, "the selection of natural phenomena for comparison may constitute a quasimanipulation of some variables." As a culture-concerned study, cross-cultural research is not concerned with individual differences, but with natural group differences. Its goal is to comprehend the systematic covariation between culture and behavioral variables, including psychopathology.

American cultural psychologist Michael Cole (1996, pp. 327–331) indicated that various psychologists have sought to implement a scientific approach to the study of culture based on cross-cultural comparisons. However, it has proven very difficult for psychologists to keep culture in the study of the mind. When psychology has treated culture as an independent variable and mind as a dependent variable, it has broken apart the unity of culture and mind and ordered them temporally — culture as stimulus, mind as response. According to Cole, the difficulty was that when psychology became institutionalized as a social behavioral science, the constituent processes of mind were divided among several sciences: anthropology, psychology, sociology, linguistics, history, and so on; each of these disciplines developed methods and theories appropriate to its own domain. In psychology, the major methods depended on the use of standardized tests, experimental tasks, questionnaires, and so on. This was very different from anthropological methods, which primarily use observation and participation in unobtrusive and nonreactive ways to study and understand cultural behavior. Cole suggested the importance of combining psychological and anthropological methods in studying culture in the mind.

In order to comprehend the cultural aspects of mental health or psychiatry from a methodological point of view, the following issues need to be elaborated.

A. Different Basic Approaches to Study Culture and Mental Health

1. Multiple Cross-Cultural Comparisons Using a Specific-Topic Approach

This approach focuses on a selected topic and cross-compares a number of different cultural samples so that, based on resulting similarities and differences, cultural dimensions may emerge. This topic-focused, cross-cultural comparative approach is often used in the field of cross-cultural psychology (Marsella, Tharp, & Ciborowski, 1979) or cross-cultural psychiatry (Murphy & Leighton, 1965), including comparative epidemiology (Murphy, 1982; Yap, 1974). Comparative studies of life events, emotional adjustment, frequency of psychopathology, or particular disorders, such as suicidal behavior, drinking problems or culture-related specific psychiatric disorders (Jilek and Jilek-Aall, 2000), among different societies are some examples.

One advantage of this approach is that information obtained through comparison is relatively objective. It is useful in examining the phenomena — mainly from the standpoint of frequency and mode of difference. A disadvantage, however, is that only a selected area of mental illness/health is compared. For instance, a comparison of the prevalence of suicide in societies can only provide a limited picture of the mental health condition of a society as a whole. As a social science, it is better not to take single traits out of their sociocultural settings, but, rather, to isolate and compare complexes of traits (such as frequency of substance abuse, violent behavior, criminal behavior). Further, unless the source of data is carefully investigated from a methodological point of view, the validity of cross-cultural comparison may be severely limited (Brislin, Lonner, & Thorndike, 1973), for instance, how suicide is recognized and reported in societies, which may differ based on peoples' attitudes toward suicide. Also, unless the impact of culture is studied and analyzed, with careful elaboration and validation, similarities or differences may be prematurely attributed to cultural factors. For instance, differences observed in sexual behavior problems in different societies cannot be attributed to cultural factors unless cultural attitudes toward or related to sexual matters are first investigated carefully and any possible links between such attitudes and the observed sexual behavior problems are clarified.

2. Holocultural Comparisons of the Specific-Topic Approach

An extension of cross-comparison is the hologeistic (whole earth) comparison approach, i.e., a study using data from worldwide samples of entire societies or cultures. Therefore, it is also called a pan-cultural or holocultural study. By utilizing the information gathered and recorded by anthropologists on existing cultural units worldwide, the information concerned is sampled from all available societies. Mathematical statistics are utilized to test associations and significance levels of the variables in question (Naroll, Michik, & Naroll, 1980). The association between the complexity of society and the phenomenon of altered consciousness, for instance, trance being more associated with simple societies and possession trance with more complex ones (Bourguignon, 1976); or the association between degrees of social organization and the nature of institutionalized healing processes either focusing on catharsis or control (Kiev, 1964) are examples of pan-cultural analysis.

The advantage of this approach is that worldwide samples, as far as they are available, are included so that universalities versus cultural uniqueness can be examined more explicitly. However, this approach suffers severely from its reliance on existing recorded information. How the information is collected by the informants or reporters is not controlled and the subject concerned may not have been included in the original investigations. This is particularly true regarding mental illness/health issues, which require psychiatric knowledge and skill beyond that of behavior scientists (anthropologists) as primary observers.

3. Unique Subject-Focused Intensive Study Approach

The third approach is not as concerned with comparison but is more focused on special issues or topics that are highlighted by cultural impact and are worthwhile for study from a mental health point of view. This kind of investigation, frequently adopted by medical anthropologists and clinical cultural psychiatrists, is based on the intensive study of selected unique subjects observed within a culture, with or without comparison with other culture units. The study of culture-related specific psychiatric syndromes, or collective (epidemic) mental disorders, is an example. A microscopic analysis of the "top of ice mountain" is intended to enlighten, or at least produce speculation, about the macroscopic society within which the unique phenomena occurred.

4. Mono-Cultural, Multiple-Subject Examination Approach

Instead of examining a selected unique subject occurring within a society, as described earlier, the fourth approach focuses on a single culture and thoroughly examines various issues of mental illness/health in relation to that culture. Some examples of this approach are the study of the Mohave group (Devereux, 1961/1969), the Japanese group (Lebra & Lebra, 1974, 1986), and the Chinese group (Lin, Tseng, & Yen, 1995; Tseng & Wu, 1985). Various mental health-related subjects (such as the folk view of mental problems, help-seeking behavior, various kinds of psychopathology, and folk treatment) are examined and studied within a selected single culture. The advantage of this approach is that cultural factors are carefully examined from numerous perspectives, and the various ways in which the culture impacts on the multiple dimensions of mental illness/health can be comprehensively studied. The weakness of this monocultural approach is that, since there are no direct cross-cultural comparisons with other cultural groups, there are limitations on assessing findings and reaching conclusions regarding cultural impact from a comparative perspective. The description of culture is meaningful only by relative comparison. Despite this limitation, this monocultural examination approach is justified if the society is a large one or if the culture is very unique and deserving of special attention. If the monocultural investigation is combined with cross-cultural comparison, or compared indirectly through multiple monocultural studies of other societies, such a shortage can be minimized and the usefulness increased.

5. Multiple-Culture, Multiple-Subject Comparison Approach

Clearly, this approach is closely related to the monocultural, multiple-subject examination approach described earlier, except that more than one study is carried out in multiple cultures so that the information can be examined for its implication across cultures. Because of its complexity, very few studies of this kind have been attempted; however, they deserve to be undertaken. The comparison of various mental health indexes (as reflected by the divorce rate, alcohol consumption, substance abuse, criminal behavior, and suicidal rates) among many Asian societies (including China, Japan, Korea, Singapore, and Malaysia) is one such approach used to understand how Asian societies are coping with modernization in terms of mental health (Tseng et al., in press).

B. Basic Methodological Considerations

1. About the Investigator: Insider and Outsider Positions

It is becoming common knowledge in the field of cross-cultural study that whether the investigation is undertaken from an **etic** or **emic** point of view will significantly influence data collected and the interpretation given (Brislin, 1980, 2000). The terms etic and emic are derived from the linguistic terms pho**netic** for universal vocal utterance and phon**emic** for culturally unique sounds. Concerning perspectives in research, **etic** refers to the study of a culture from the outside by an outsider, whereas **emic** means a study from within a culture by an insider. It is clear that each way has its own advantages and shortcomings. An investigation undertaken by an outsider can enhance objectivity, but may suffer from a lack of meaningful cultural interpretation. In contrast, an investigation by a member of the cultural unit may have the advantage of the insider's insight, but will face a subjective bias. Theoretically, it would be desirable to have a combination of investigators so that the study can be checked carefully from both the insider and outsider's points of view. These are issues that need careful consideration in carrying out culture and mental health investigations.

2. Sampling

The success of a cross-cultural study is often related to how the samples (i.e., cultural units) are chosen for investigation. According to Berry (1980, p. 14), there are two distinct goals in a cross-cultural study, and the method of sampling needs to be selected accordingly. For the purpose of studying the cause between cultural and behavioral variables, referred to as "systematic covariation," it is important only to sample cultures and behaviors that display sufficient variation to allow an examination of the systematic relationship between them. The other purpose, referred to as "universal generalization," requires that the sampling takes into account not only the range, but also the representativeness of the culture and behaviors concerned. For the selection of a representative sample for universal interpretation, caution is needed regarding "Galton's problem." This means that there is the potential existence of sample cultures that are related to each other within a similar culture system so that they are in fact not of independent representative cultural units. Thus, the investigators need to have adequate anthropological knowledge of the cultural samples that they are choosing for investigation, for the specific purposes they have in mind.

3. Information Gathering

There are numerous ways to collect information for the purpose of investigation. A massive survey by questionnaire is one of the most frequently applied methods. Interviews of individuals from the targeted group are another approach. Pareek and Rao (1980) have elaborated on interviewing as a research method from a cross-cultural perspective. They have pointed out that variables in the interviewer's background, the respondent's background, the setting in which the interview takes place, and the way the interview is conducted, including the interaction between the interviewer and the respondent, are all factors that are subject to cultural impact and will significantly influence the results of the information gathering.

For instance, imagine the following two circumstances. In one, a male investigator interviews a female respondent, surrounded by other people, on the subject of sexual matters in a society that is very concerned with the relations between men and women, with an emphasis on concealing private matters from outsiders. In the other, a female interviewer carries out an interview with a female respondent in a private setting, without the presence of others, in a society with liberal attitudes toward revealing personal matters, even to outsiders. Data gathered from these two circumstances are not equivalently comparable for obvious reasons. For meaningful comparison, the factors affecting the process of information gathering need mindful attention and appropriate manipulation.

4. Concerning Measurement: The Issue of Equivalence and Validity

Brislin (2000, pp. 94–107) raised a basic consideration that is needed in cross-cultural investigation regarding the equivalence of concept. It concerns the question, "Do the concepts being investigated, and especially the way the concepts are being measured, have the same meaning in different cultures?" The example given was related to the concept of "aggression." When a child is bullied by an older, heavier boy on the playground, what are possible responses the child might make and when is a behavior considered "aggressive" in coping with such a situation? Based on the cultural attitude toward "aggression," there were different concepts to define aggressive behavior. Brislin pointed out that a number of approaches to dealing with the equivalence issue have been developed, such as translation equivalence, conceptual equivalence, and metric equivalence [cross-reference to Chapter 29: Psychological Testing and Measurement (Section II, D)].

Berry (1980, pp. 17–20) warned that the basic problem that often exists in cross-cultural studies is the matter of validity: how do we know we are actually measuring what we think we are measuring? According to him, problems of validity can occur from at least three sources. The first bias is derived from the investigators (particularly outsiders), who are often inherently ambiguous due to their own cultural backgrounds, and it is not known whether the obtained information reflects real phenomena or is a function of the observer's bias. The second bias originates from problems in communication, when it is not certain that the task that is communicated is the task that is responded to. Finally, there is the bias related to the problems of validation techniques. Thus, numerous methodological issues need to be considered carefully and managed properly in order to conduct meaningful cross-cultural studies.

II. METHODOLOGICAL APPROACH

A. Different Methodologies for Studying Culture and Behavior

1. Analysis of Cultural Products

Psychiatrists and anthropologists share common interests and methods for exploring culture and behavior by examining and analyzing cultural products, such as plays, fairy tales, legends, and so on (Barnouw, 1963; Mead & Wolfenstein, 1955). These are convenient ways to study targeted cultures, even from a distance. The weakness is that there are problems regarding how the cultural products are selected for study. The question always encountered is how the selected cultural product fairly represents or reflects the situation actually observed in the culture.

2. Direct Observation of Behavior under Natural Conditions

This is one of the traditional methods utilized by anthropologists in their field studies. Namely, the investigator visits and lives in a selected society and,

as a participant–observer, disturbing the natural setting as little as possible, gathers information on daily-life targeted behavior. This method relies heavily on the personal skill and experience of the investigator–observer, and also the chance for the occurrence of the targeted behavior. Naturally, it takes time, and obtained data are often subjectively inferred. The socialization behavior among children of six cultures carried out by a research team (Whiting & Whiting, 1975) is one representative study.

A modification of this approach is an observation carried out in a stratified selected time span in which the observed behavior is recorded through a pre-designed coding system so that statistical measurement can be performed, minimizing subject influence. The direct observation of mother–infant interaction in residential settings by investigator–observers, carried out in Japan and America (Caudill & Weinstein, 1969) for cross-cultural comparison, is a typical example of such an approach.

3. Survey of Subjects by Interview

This is another method commonly used by anthropologists. Either by direct interview or through interpreters, information gathering is carried out in face-to-face situations with individuals in a targeted group. This process allows for an informal and flexible exploration of targeted areas of information. It is suitable for respondents who are not familiar with pen-and-paper surveys. However, there are many issues that need careful consideration and management in the use of this method. These include cultural factors in interview and response style, and comparability, as elaborated previously.

4. Massive Survey by Testing or Questionnaire Measurement

This is the most commonly used method in cross-cultural studies by psychologists. Samples of individuals are drawn from disparate populations for testing. Culture and personality are often investigated by applying personality questionnaires for respondents of different ethnic/cultural groups for the purpose of comparison. The core problems requiring attention are usually the construct validity in the cross-cultural use of measurements [cross-reference to Chapter 29: Psychological Testing and Measurement (Section II, D)].

5. Manipulative Experiments

Asking respondents in different groups for certain responses according to an experimental design is an approach used by some behavior scientists, although it has been employed infrequently cross-culturally. Family psychiatrists have tried to videotape the interaction patterns of families for cross-ethnic or -cultural comparisons. Following the experimental design, family members are asked to respond to certain tasks. The manifested interactional behavior is observed by a group of raters (Hsu, Tseng, Ashton, McDermott, & Char, 1985; Lewis & Looney, 1983). The advantage is that the observed behavior can be assessed objectively according to a rating scale specially designed for various dimensions of family functioning. It is necessary to train the raters to ensure reliability. The main shortcoming of this approach is that the observed family interaction is provoked to occur in a laboratory setting rather than in a natural situation. There is no way to know the differences that may exist between the behavior in the experiment setting and the behavior in the natural setting at home.

6. Utilization of Existing Ethnographic Archives

This is a unique approach utilized by behavior scientists. As mentioned previously, this method utilizes information that was already gathered through field work and recorded by anthropologists on existing cultural units worldwide. The subjects are sampled from all available societies. Then, mathematical statistics are applied to examine associations and significance levels of the variables in question (Naroll et al., 1980). The disadvantage of this approach is that it relies on already recorded information. How the information was originally collected by the informants is beyond the investigators' control. Further, the subjects concerned may not have been included in the original field investigations.

Behavior and social scientists have utilized the various approaches just mentioned in studying culture and behavior. There is no best approach among them. The appropriate approach depends on both the questions being asked and the cultural groups that are being studied (Berry, 1980, p. 22).

B. Various Ways to Study Culture and Psychopathology

Based on clinical need, psychiatrists have carried out investigations on culture and psychopathology using slightly different approaches than behavior scientists. Most of the studies have been conducted in the following ways.

1. Studying Frequency: Epidemiological Study

In order to find out whether cultural factors affect the occurrence of mental disorders, cross-cultural epidemiological studies have been carried out in the past, mainly by epidemiologists. Methodologically, there is often a problem as to whether a similar methodology is utilized for cross-societal comparison. This includes how data are obtained and the kind of criteria that is used. In many investigations in which the same method was not used, the value of the comparison was limited. However, even when a similar method is used, from a cultural perspective, other problems still remained. Namely, using a standardized method skewed the results because of the problem of "netting effects." That is, only one segment of information is gathered through a standardized method of comparison, leaving out other parts of information that could be very valuable from a cultural standpoint. For instance, when studying the prevalence of certain disorders through uniform criteria, focusing on a so-called "typical" case may leave out an "atypical case" that represents culture-shaped disorders.

Another issue that limits the value of epidemiological studies is that often the samples included are not culturally diversified enough to reflect the impact of cultural factors. For instance, a comparison of prevalence between Caucasian-Americans and Japanese-Americans is not "different" enough to compare with Japanese Nationals. Similarly, comparisons among different ethnic groups in Europe are not culturally divergent enough to cross-compare with ethnic groups from Africa or Asia. This is related to the problem of sampling (from a cultural perspective).

Finally, most of the epidemiological studies include social demographic variables, but seldom involve cultural variables. Thus, the obtained findings cannot be examined and interpreted from cultural perspectives, and only provide information on the basis of which possible cultural influences can be speculated.

No matter how sophisticated the methodology that is planned for an epidemiological study, there are still many issues that need to be considered from a cultural perspective in order for the study to be culturally sensitive and relevant. This is true when conducting a survey with subjects of different ethnic–cultural backgrounds in a multiethnic or -racial society, or in a foreign setting where people use different languages, live quite different lifestyles, and are not used to community surveys. As pointed out by Rogler (1994), several areas need special consideration and careful management in culturally sensitive epidemiological studies. These are the areas of language, the setting of the examination (with or without the presence of family members), the style of interviewing the subject, possible cultural patterns in the subject's reaction toward the interview and the questionnaire survey, confidentiality, the choice and revision of the questionnaire to be used, and the analysis and interpretation of data obtained.

2. Examining Manifestation

Another direction taken by clinicians is the cross-cultural study of the manifestation of disorders. Comparing the symptomatology of the same disorders between or among different cultures allows us to examine possible cultural psychopathoplastic effects on psychopathology. The cross-cultural investigations of the symptomatology of schizophrenia, depression, and other disorders are some examples. Again, basic methodological problems similar to those encountered in epidemiological studies need to be considered.

3. Analyzing Help-Seeking Behavior

How the patient reacts to his illness and the help-seeking pattern that is manifested are serious questions of interest to cultural psychiatrists and culture-concerned mental health workers. Several studies conducted on these subjects have begun to shed light on the help-seeking behavior of people in different cultures (Canino, Lewis-Fernandez, & Bravo, 1997).

4. Comparing Treatment Results

It is reasonable for clinicians to ask whether there are any differences in clinical results when the patient seeks help from various modes of therapy — both contemporary and folk healing practices, for instance — that are available in the same society or in different cultures. Only a handful of studies have been carried out on this subject. Methodologically there are many obstacles in this kind of study, such as how to track the patients, how to investigate the patient-respondents, what kind of criteria should be used for the assessment of the clinical results, and so on. Most of the problems encountered in treatment studies are further complicated in cross-cultural comparisons.

III. SOME SUBJECTS INVESTIGATED: TRACING THE TREND

It is the nature of research that one study always leads to another study and that there is improvement in the methodology used to search for answers to questions. Thus, research often occurs as a series of progressive investigations. Here two selected subjects are presented in terms of how they have been explored by scholars or clinicians in the past. The study of culture-related specific psychiatric syndromes (cross-reference to Chapter 13) is more related to clinical issues; while the investigation of migration and mental health (cross-reference to Chapter 44) is related to social and cultural phenomena.

A. INVESTIGATIONS OF CULTURE-RELATED SPECIFIC PSYCHIATRIC SYNDROMES

1. Case Report

Historically, literature on culture-related specific psychiatric syndromes was only found in the form of case reports. Many travelers, ministers, and anthropologists, who encountered "exotic" or "peculiar" mental disorder in foreign or "primitive" societies, reported their observations. Although the syndromes were not investigated and described carefully from a clinical point of view, they certainly caught the attention of clinicians as evidence of the existence of "culture-bound syndromes."

2. Nosological Elaboration

In addition to reporting the existence of culture-related specific syndromes, attempts have been made by clinicians and mental health-related scientists to evaluate how to categorize the specific syndromes from the standpoint of nosology. The efforts of Simons and Hughes (1985) are one such example.

3. Clinical Study in the Field

Next, some cultural psychiatrists went to certain cultural fields to study certain culture-related specific syndromes. One psychiatrist's clinical study and report of the *imu* phenomenon among the Ainu ethnic group in northern Japan (Uchimura, 1956) was a pioneering affort. Ron Simons' field study (1980) of the *latah* phenomenon in Malaysia is another classic example. From intensive field observation, a comprehensive report was made, including a videotaped record of cases for illustration. It is very helpful to

scholars and clinicians in learning about special syndromes to have not only clinical reports made by psychiatrists, but also videotaped records that go beyond the descriptions of literature. The use of videotapes was certainly a big improvement in the study of such special phenomena.

4. Questionnaire Investigations of Cases

A questionnaire investigation was conducted that not only involved intensive study, as had been done in the past, but utilized a formal questionnaire survey that was designed and carried out specifically for the study of the *koro* epidemic in southern China by a group of investigators (Tseng et al., 1992). Further, a group of *koro* cases was compared with a group of neurotic patients and a normal group in the same geographic area where the epidemic occurred in order to gain a more meaningful understanding of the occurrence of the epidemic.

Thus, many approaches have been undertaken historically to explore the unique phenomena of culture-related specific psychiatric syndromes.

B. INVESTIGATIONZS OF MIGRATION AND MENTAL DISORDERS

How migration is related to psychiatric problems is another subject that has attracted the interest of investigators. It provides another example of the trends in the investigation of such topics. Migration itself, as a sociocultural phenomenon, has been examined in detail previously (cross-reference to Chapter 44: Migration, Refuge, and Adjustment). Here, it will be focused on primarily to show how research approaches and methods have evolved over time.

1. Migration and Psychiatric Disorders

a. Reviewing the Prevalence of Disorders Related to Migration

Psychiatrists started to pay attention to the possible association between migration and mental disorders more than a century ago. Originally, attention was focused on the prevalence of mental disorders among immigrants. According to Murphy (1977), as early as the end of the 19th century (1855), Javis, the superintendent of an insane asylum in Massachusetts, based on his clinical impressions, commented that there were more immigrants admitted to the mental hospital than local people. Perhaps stimulated by this, Norwegian psychiatrist Ö.Ödegaard (1932) conducted an investigation to compare the rates of admission of Norwegian-born immigrants and native-born Americans to the state hospital in Minnesota in the four decades between 1889 and 1929. He reported that the ratio of admission was higher for the former than the latter. He also compared Norwegians born in Minnesota and the population of Norway. He reported that there was more insanity among the Norwegian immigrants in Minnesota than in their home country. The difference was too large to be explained by discrepancies in hospital facilities or modes of commitment. Based on these two sets of findings, he interpreted that the differences were not due to race or stock, but to immigrant status.

Subsequently, an American psychiatrist in New York carried out similar investigations in mental institutions in the New York area and obtained similar findings, i.e., that rates of admission were higher among immigrants than among the native-born. Based on these findings, it has been speculated that migration across cultures might bring about mental stress and cause mental disorders (Ranney, 1850). An alternative hypothesis has been made that those who are mentally vulnerable might have difficulty staying in their own society or have less attachments to their native community and tend to wander and migrate to foreign places (Ödegaard, 1932).

It needs to be pointed out that these studies concerned severe mental disorders and relied on hospitalization rates, which might be influenced artificially by many social and clinical factors, including diagnostic and service utilization patterns.

Later, careful epidemiological studies revealed that the relation between migration and mental disorders was not necessarily a single correlation. For instance, Astrup and Ödegaard (1960) reported that, in Norway,

although internal migrants moving to the capital city had higher rates than nonmigrants born in that city, migrants moving to other parts of the country tended to have lower rates than nonmigrants there. Canadian physician Murphy (1965) reviewed the situation among Jewish immigrants to Israel. He revealed that Jewish immigrants from Asia and Africa had higher mental hospitalization rates than the local-born Jewish population, whereas Jewish immigrants from Europe did not.

The many conflicting results obtained from various investigations prompted scholars to realize that migration is not a single phenomenon. For instance, the person who migrates, the motives for and circumstances of migration, the relation between the host society and the original society, and the ways they were received by the new society are all factors that significantly affect the results of a migrant's adjustment (Murphy, 1977). Further, it is understood that while the process of migration, as a psychological stress, might be a precipitating factor in the development of certain mental disorders, it may not be the main reason a person becomes mentally ill.

b. Examining Different Categories of Psychiatric Disorders

Originally, due to the convenience of data, most of the investigations focused on the hospital admission rates of psychoses. However, it was realized that the etiology of certain mental disorders, such as psychoses, were related more predominantly to biological factors and were not suitable for studies of the psychological and sociocultural effects of migration. Other mental disorders, which were known to be more susceptible to social factors, such as drinking problems, substance abuse, and behavior disorders, were more suitable. This view was supported by an investigation by Burnam, Hough, Karno, Escobar, and Telles (1987). They studied Mexican-Americans residing in the Los Angeles area: one of the selected populations for the Epidemiological Catchment Area project. They assessed the level of acculturation and its relation with the lifetime prevalence of psychiatric disorders. Results revealed that among eight most common

DIS/DSM-III difined psychiatric disorders, only phobia, alcohol abuse/dependence, and drug
abuse/dependence were significantly correlated with
the level of acculturation. That is, the more acculturated a person was to mainstream American culture, the
more the rate of these disorders increased. There were
no significant correlations with other mental disorders, such as major depression, dysthymia, obsessive-
compulsive disorder, or panic disorders.

In another investigation, Mavreas and Bebbington
(1988) compared rates of psychiatric disorders in
three general populations: an English sample in Camberwell, London, and two Greek samples — those living in their home country, Athens, and those living in
Camberwell as immigrants. Results suggested that the
prevalence of minor psychiatric disorders overall was
greater among the Greek populations (it did not matter whether they were in Athens or immigrants in London) than among the British-born general population.
The excess of minor psychiatric disorders appears to
be due to differences in the prevalence of anxiety
states. If the native Greek sample in Athens and the
migrated Greek sample in London were compared, the
syndrome of simple depression was significantly more
frequent only in the immigrant sample. This was interpreted to be possibly due to the sense of loss and separation created by living in a foreign land, as well as
to problems of adjusting to a foreign culture.

These two investigations differed distinctly from
previous investigations in that they focused on the
general population rather than on hospitalized patients
and that they examined various categories of psychiatric disorders rather than only severe mental disorders. Results of such investigations have indicated that
the impact of migration on mental disorders is found
mainly in certain categories of disorders whose occurrence is more or less closely related to social and cultural factors.

c. Exploring the Time Span in the Onset of Disorders

Another way to explore the possible effects of
migration on mental disorders is to trace the time span

in the onset of the disorders. Few such studies have
been carried. Ebata, Yoshimatsu, Miguchi, and Ozaki
(1983) in Japan have reviewed the medical records of
outpatients with diagnoses of schizophrenia, affective
disorders, and neurotic disorders in order to examine
the relationship between the onset of mental disorders
and the duration of residence after internal migration.
The subjects had moved from other parts of Japan to
live in densely populated downtown Tokyo. It was
revealed that the onset of mental disorders was found
to occur in three stages. There was a high risk for
mental disorders within a 1-year period; the risk
declined after that, but rose again after several years,
depending on the gender of the migrant and the disorder. Among rural-to-urban internal migrants, only 10
to 18% of mental disorders were found to occur within
1 year of migration. The rest tended to occur many
years later, indicating that the link with migration was
rather weak where internal migration was concerned.

Mavreas and Beggington (1989) examined the time
span in the onset of disorders among Greek Cypriot
immigrants in London, and concluded that there was
no evidence that the risk of mental breakdown was
increased in the immediate aftermath of migration.

The different approaches to investigating the possible relation between migration and mental disorders
described earlier have revealed much information on
the possible effects of migration on mental disorders.

2. Migration and Psychological Adjustment

The direction of the investigation of migration and
mental health has shifted considerably in the present
time. The major trend is to examine the impact of
migration through the study of psychological reactions or mental adjustment rather than mental disorders. Instead of examining the impact of sociocultural
factors on the development of mental illnesses of any
particular kind, efforts are focused on the study of
psychological difficulties encountered, the emotional
process experienced, and mental problems or symptoms manifested, rather than investing the occurrence
of mental disorders. Studies are more concerned with
the kinds of mental stress that might be encountered,

the psychological coping that is adopted, the resources and support that are utilized, and the outcomes of mental health from the standpoint of the process of adjustment. This might include the matters of ethnic–cultural identification, psychological equilibrium, and mental integration associated with the process of cultural assimilation and acculturation.

Associated with this shift in the focus of investigations, several issues become important. First, it becomes clear that it was important to examine the personal factors that may affect the process of cultural adjustment. These may include individual background, age, and gender. How much these personal factors, interacting with the sociocultural environment, might affect the outcome of the transcultural adjustment was and still is a challenging subject for investigation.

3. Longitudinal Process of Adjustment

The next issue that calls for attention is the process of migration, rather than a cross-section of phenomena at any given point. It is becoming common sense that the adjustment to migration is not a static phenomenon, but is a dynamic process. Studying the pattern of adjustment at any given point in time only reflects a cross-sectional facet of the truth. Meaningful insight can be obtained only through a longitudinal investigation of the process. Thus, a longitudinal follow-up study of a targeted group of subjects becomes almost a necessity in examining the process of cultural adjustment associated with migration (Ebata et al., 1995).

Clinical experience tends to point out that short-term adjustment is very different from long-term adjustment. Actually, the process of adjustment migration might be subdivided into several stages from the perspective of time. These include the premigration stage, the initial stage, the middle stage, and the final stage.

4. Studying Adjustment from the Perspective of the Family as a Whole

Another issue that is important to examine is the process of transcultural adjustment not merely from the point of an individual, but from the perspective of the whole family. A family is a unique group of members who are bound together by marriage, birth, and intimate relations. If problems or stress is encountered either from inside or outside the family, all family members are affected, according to a systems point of view, and react together toward resolution of the stress.

In the process of migration, the family as a group reacts to the process of transcultural adjustment. This may involve a change in the hierarchical structure of the family, and adjustments in the roles and responsibilities between husband and wife, parents and children, or among siblings. The pattern and efficiency of communication within the family might be affected and the nature of the effect altered, depending on the stress encountered. To what extent support is available and provided within the family is a crucial factor that determines the outcome of adjustment.

In general, it is difficult to study the behavior of a family. Although a family as a group may be observed and analyzed by an outsiderobserver, this is time-consuming and not practical. Studying individual family members, either by interview or questionnaire survey, is one frequently applied method of investigation. An attempt can be made to derive a general picture of the whole family by studying the responses given by its individual members (Ebata et al., 1995). However, caution is necessary not to interpret that such findings actually reflect the behavior of the family as a group.

An extension of this issue is the examination of the process of transcultural adjustment through different generations. Namely, the first generation, which migrated to the new environment; the second generation, which is the descendent of the first generation; and the third generation, which follows the second. It is generally believed that different generations of immigrants are faced with different difficulties to overcome.

5. Exploring Help-Seeking Patterns and Service Models Provided

As described earlier, from the standpoint of psychology and mental health, migration is generally considered to be a process of coping and adjustment to the stress and difficulty encountered in the new cultural setting.

Contemporary concepts of stress and coping take the view that stress does not act alone on an individual in a simple manner, but is part of a complicated chain reaction. From a conceptual point of view, at least, stress can be grasped from several perspectives, i.e., the actual stress that is imposed on the subject, the stress perceived by the subject, the potential of the subject to cope with the stress, the support systems available around the subject, the environmental conditions in which the stress needs to be dealt with, and the coping mechanisms utilized by the subject to deal with the stress. All of these factors need to be considered in discussing the process of adjustment to immigration.

The support system refers to the means that are available to provide support and assistance when a person faces a problem. Family members, friends, colleagues, neighbors, and various kinds of social organizations can be resources for providing support. The support can be given at the psychological level, such as empathy, emotional encouragement, or advice, or at a mechanical and practical level, such as providing a loan, introducing a person to a social network, or offering assistance in the search for a job, and so on. Support systems may be discussed from two different perspectives: the availability of resources and the utilization of those resources. Based on the structure and system of the society, different kinds of resources may be available for support. In some societies, support is found mostly in personal, private resources, whereas in other societies, it may be found more in public and official organizations. It is quite true that cultural background significantly influences the pattern of utilization of the available support system, in turn making a difference on the resulting adjustment. Whether the immigrant knows about the existence and availability of social support systems is one thing. This is often just a matter of information and knowledge. However, whether he will approach them and make use of them appropriately and efficiently is another. It

is usually social experience and cultural attitudes that influence help-seeking behavior.

In summary, the study of immigrants and the effects of migration on mental health has gone through the stages of exploring the possible relations between the migration and the occurrence of psychiatric disorders, and concern with the outcomes of psychological adjustment. The focus has shifted to an examination of migration as a process, and longitudinal follow-up investigations have been applied. Based on the realization that migration impacts not only the individual but also the family as a group, investigations have been expanded into the area of family adjustment. The process of adjustment to migration is seen as a dynamic one, occurring as the integrated result of coping with encountered stress, and the utilization of support systems, with models for service explored, as well.

IV. SOME SUGGESTIONS FOR FUTURE INVESTIGATION

There are countless subjects that are worthy of investigation from a cross-cultural point of view. It is impossible to list all of them, but some are mentioned briefly here, merely as suggestions for consideration.

A. STUDY REGARDING THE PSYCHOLOGY OF HUMANS

Historically, most theories about human psychology used in modern psychiatry were based on Western people. To what extent such theoretical concepts can be applied to people of other cultures is a question still awaiting cross-cultural validation and modification. Such an investigation may include fundamental structural theories about the "self," theories about personality development, and theories about defense mechanisms, which have direct relevance to mental health work [cross-reference to Chapter 49: Culture and Psychiatric Theories (Section V, A–C)] It is time to begin such an investigation at a theoretical level.

B. Research Concerning Certain Psychopathologies

Many cultural psychiatrists still follow the old pattern of examining psychopathology cross-culturally, focusing on the content of symptoms, particularly concerning major psychoses. This is merely chasing psychopathoplastic effects without a significant contribution to transcultural clinical practice. It is the time to move on to study more minor psychiatric disorders, psychologically related problems, focusing more on the psychopathogenetic or psychopathoreactive effects that directly impact clinical practice and service from cultural perspectives.

Concerning culture-related specific syndromes, instead of discovering and labeling more, it is necessary now to conduct indepth investigations of cases, including clinical examinations and psychological measurement and assessment. If it is suitable, the studies will involve groups of the normal population and groups with other ordinary psychiatric disorders from the same geographic area so that meaningful comparisons can be made and a better understanding gained of the nature of the disorders.

C. Investigation of Drug Treatments for Patients of Different Ethnic Groups

It is becoming common knowledge that people of different racial or ethnic groups will respond to medication differently from psychopharmacological perspectives. However, as of now, studies have involved only normal people. There is an immediate need to examine the clinical population so that direct application can be made in actual clinical situations [cross-reference to Chapter 31: Culture, Ethnicty, and Drug Therapy (Section II, A–C)].

D. Study Relating to Psychotherapy

1. Effects of Ethnic Matching of Therapist and Patient

While the notion exists that it is desirable to have patients treated by therapists of the same ethnic, racial, or cultural background, not too many sophisticated empirical studies have been carried out to validate such a notion. While studies of the effects of treatment are not easy, especially if the situation is compounded by ethnic, racial, or cultural issues, the challenge of examining the possible effects of the ethnic or cultural matching of therapists and patients needs to be met so that more proper policies and care can be developed.

2. Culturally More Effect Therapeutic Approaches

There is an academic and clinical need to find out whether there are specific therapeutic modes or approaches that are more culturally suitable and effective than others. A systematic comparison of different approaches used for patients of different ethnic groups could help us obtain empirical evidence that we can follow in the future. This is a complicated study, but one that deserves undertaking.

V. FINAL COMMENTS

It is impossible, in this one chapter, to cover all the issues relating to research in the field of culture and mental health. Only basic matters are elaborated, and some examples are given to provide a bird's eye view of this complicated field of research. For more detailed discussions of methodological and technical issues, readers are advised to refer to publications by experts on those topics (Berry, 1980; Brislin et al., 1973).

Although many psychiatrists devoted to clinical work may not conduct research activities, the basic issues that are raised regarding cross-cultural studies can be considered and utilized in transcultural clinical work. This is true regarding how to communicate with patients (as clinical informants) and how to relate to them properly from a cultural perspective so that more meaningful and valid information can be solicited. Last, but not least, is the matter of how to interpret the obtained clinical information to determine its validity, including the consideration of the therapist's own cultural bias. In other words, many of the principles obtained and lessons learned from cross-cultural investigations can be applied directly to transcultural situations in clinical practice.

REFERENCES

Astrup, C., & Ödegaard, Ö. (1960). Internal migration and mental disease in Norway. *Psychiatric Quarterly, Supplement, 34,* 116–130.

Barnouw, V. (1963). *Culture and personality.* Homewood, IL: Dorsey Press.

Berry, J.W. (1980). Introduction to *Methodology.* In H.C. Triandis & J.W. Berry (Eds.), *Handbook of cross-cultural psychology: Vol. 2. Methodology* (pp. 1–28). Boston: Allyn & Bacon.

Bourguignon, E. (1976). Possession and trance in cross-cultural studies of mental health. In W.P. Lebra (Ed.), *Culture-bound syndromes, ethnopsychiatry, and alternate therapies.* Honolulu: University Press of Hawaii.

Brislin, R.W. (1980). Translation and content analysis of oral and written material. In H.C. Triandis & J.W. Berry (Eds.), *Handbook of cross-cultural psychology: Vol. 2. Methodology* (pp. 389–444). Boston: Allyn & Bacon.

Brislin, R.W. (2000). Some methodological concerns in intercultural and cross-cultural research. In R.W. Brislin (Ed.), *Understanding culture's influence on behavior* (2nd ed., Chap. 3) Fort Worth, TX: Harcourt.

Brislin, R.W., Lonner, W.J., & Thorndike, R.M. (1973). *Cross-cultural research methods.* New York: Willey.

Burnam, M.A., Hough, R.L., Karno, M., Escobar, J.I., & Telles, C.A. (1987). Acculturation and lifetime prevalence of psychiatric disorders among Mexican Americans in Los Angeles. *Journal of Health and Social Behavior, 28,* 89–102.

Canino, G., Lewis-Fernandez, R., & Bravo, M. (1997). Methodological challenge in cross-cultural mental health research. *Transcultural Psychiatry, 34*(2), 163–184.

Caudill, W., & Weinstein, H. (1969). Maternal care and infant behavior in Japan and America. *Psychiatry, 32,* 12–43.

Cole, M. (1996). *Cultural psychology: A once and future discipline.* Cambridge, MA: Harvard University Press.

Devereux, G. (1969). *Mohave ethnopsychiatry: The psychic disturbances of an Indian tribe.* Washington, DC: Smithsonian Institute Press. (Original work published 1961)

Ebata, K., Miguchi, M., Tseng, W.S., Hara, H., Kosaka, M., & Cui, Y.H. (1995). Migration and transethnic family adjustment: Experiences of Japanese war orphans and their Chinese spouses in Japan. In T.-Y. Lin, W.S. Tseng, & E.K. Yeh (Eds.), *Chinese societies and mental health* (pp. 123–137). Hong Kong: Oxford University Press.

Ebata, K., Yoshimatsu, K., Miguchi, M., & Ozaki, A. (1983). Impact of migration on onset of mental disorders in relation to duration of residence. *American Journal of Social Psychiatry, 3*(4), 25–32.

Hsu, J., Tseng, W.S., Ashton, G., McDermott, J.F., Jr., & Char, W. (1985). Family interaction patterns among Japanese-American and Caucasian families in Hawaii. *American Journal of Psychiatry, 142,* 577–581.

Jilek, W.G., & Jilek-Aall, L. (2000). Kapitel 14: Kulturspezifische psychische störungen (Chapter 14: Culture-specific mental disorder). In H. Helmchen, F. Hern, H. Lauter, & N. Sartorius (Eds.), Psychiatrie spezieller lebenssituationen (Psychiatry of specific life situations). Berlin: Springer.

Kiev, A. (1964). *Magic, faith, and healing: Studies in primitive psychiatry today.* New York: Free Press.

Lebra, T.S., & Lebra, W.P. (Eds.). (1974). *Japanese culture and behavior: Selected readings.* Honolulu: University Press of Hawaii.

Lebra, T.S., & Lebra, W.P. (Eds.). (1986). *Japanese culture and behavior: Selected readings.* (Rev. ed.). Honolulu: University Press of Hawaii.

Lewis J.M, & Looney, J.G. (1983). *The long struggle: Well-functioning working-class Black families.* New York: Brunner/Mazel.

Lin, T.Y., Tseng, W.S., & Yeh, E.K. (Eds.). (1995). *Chinese societies and mental health.* Hong Kong: Oxford University Press.

Marsella, A.J., Tharp, R.G., & Ciborowski, T.J. (Eds.). (1979). *Perspectives on cross-cultural psychology.* New York: Academic Press.

Mavreas, V.G., & Bebbington, P.E. (1988). Greeks, British Greek Cypriots and Londoners: A comparison of morbidity. *Psychological Medicine, 18,* 433–442.

Mavreas, V.G., & Bebbington, P.E. (1989). Does the act of migration provoke psychiatric breakdown? A study of Greek Cypriot immigrants. *Acta Psychiatrica Scandinavica, 80*(5), 469–473.

Mead, M., & Wolfenstein, M. (Eds.). (1955). *Childhood in contemporary cultures.* Chicago: University of Chicago Press.

Murphy, H.B.M. (1965). Migration and the major mental disorders: A reappraisal. In M.B. Kanter (Ed.), *Mobility and mobility health.* Springfield, IL: Charles C. Thomas.

Murphy, H.B.M. (1977). Migration, culture and mental health. *Psychological Medicine, 7,* 677–684.

Murphy, H.B.M. (1982). *Comparative psychiatry: The international and intercultural distribution of mental illness.* Berlin: Springer-Verlag.

Murphy, J.M., & Leighton, A.H. (Eds.). (1965). *Approaches to cross-cultural psychiatry.* Ithaca, NY: Cornell University Press.

Naroll, R., Michik, G.L., & Naroll, F. (1980). Holocultural research methods. In H.C. Triandis & J.W. Berry (Eds.), *Handbook of cross-cultural psychology: Vol. 2. Methodology* (pp. 479–521). Boston: Allyn & Bacon.

Ödegaard, Ö. (1932). Emigration and insanity: A study of mental disease among the Norwegian-born population of Minnesota. *Acta Psychiatrica Neurologica, Supplementum 4.*

Pareek, U., & Rao, T.V. (1980). Cross-cultural surveys and interviewing. In H.C. Triandis & J.W. Berry (Eds.), *Handbook of cross-cultural psychology: Vol. 2. Methodology.* Boston: Allyn & Bacon.

Ranney, M.H. (1850). On insane foreigners. *American Journal of Insanity, 7,* 53–63.

Rogler, L.H. (1994). Culturally sensitive research in mental health. In J.E. Mezzich, M.R. Jorge, & I.M. Salloum (Eds.), *Psychiatric epidemiology: Assessment concepts and method.* Baltimore: Johns Hopkins University Press.

Simons, R.C. (1980). The resolution of the *latah* paradox. *Journal of Nervous and Mental Disease, 168*(4), 195–206.

Simons, R.C., & Hughes, C.C. (Eds.). (1985). *The culture-bound syndromes: Folk illness of psychiatric and anthropological interest.* Dordrecht, The Netherlands: Reidel.

Tseng, W.S., Ebata, K., Kim, K.I., Krahl, W., Kua, E.K., Lu, Q.Y., Shen, Y.C., Tan, E.S., & Yang, M.J. (in press). Asian mental health: Improvement and challenges. *International Journal of Social Psychiatry.*

Tseng, W.S., Mo, K.M., Hsu, J., Li, L.S., Chen, G.Q., Ou, L.W., & Zheng H.B. (1992). Koro epidemics in Guandong, China: A questionnaire survey. *Journal of Nervous and Mental Disease, 180*(2), 117–123.

Tseng, W.S., & Wu, D.Y.H. (Eds.). (1985). *Chinese culture and mental health.* Orlando, FL: Academic Press.

Uchimura, V.Y. (1956). Imu, eine psychoracktive Erscheinung der ainu-Frauen [*Imu,* a psychoactive phenomena of Ainu-women]. *Nervenarzt, 12,* 535–540.

Whiting, B.B., & Whiting, J.W.M. (1975). *Children of six cultures: A psycho-cultural analysis.* Cambridge, MA: Harvard University Press.

Yap, P.M. (1974). In M.P. Lau & A.B. Stokes (Eds.), *Comparative psychiatry: A theoretical framework.* Toronto: University of Toronto Press.

49

Culture and Psychiatric Theories

I. SOCIOCULTURAL IMPACTS ON THEORETICAL VIEWS

Psychiatrists have developed numerous theoretical views for understanding the nature of human behavior, comprehending the core of psychopathology, and directing the practice of treatment. At the same time, patients and their families also utilize certain theoretical orientations, either conventional or folk ones, to perceive the mental problems from which they are suffering and to guide their illness behavior for coping with such problems. These theoretical conceptions and orientations are mostly based on professional knowledge and clinical experiences; however, they are subject to many other variables, including sociocultural impact. This impact, directly or indirectly, shapes the overall theoretical ground and can be elaborated in several dimensions as follows.

A. INFLUENCE FROM THE PAST: TRADITIONAL MEDICINE

Theories usually do not arise in a vacuum; they are frequently influenced by the theoretical views that have already existed in the past. If a society has a relatively well-established system of traditional medicine, it could continue to influence contemporary medical concepts to some extent.

China is one society that has had its own traditional medicine since ancient times. The core of Chinese traditional medicine is based on the theories of yin and yang, the five elements, the ideas of correspondence between microcosm and macrocosm, the structural and functional orientation of the visceral organs (at a time when the empirical knowledge of anatomy and physiology was still absent), and the concept of vital energy *(Jing)*, which functions as the force of life. All these medical theories probably existed for many thousands of years before they were summarized in the first medical document, the *Classic of Internal Medicine,* presumably written by the legendary Yellow Emperor. The theories were regarded as the backbone of all other medical documents that appeared later and thus continue to affect medical and psychiatric concepts even in the present. For instance, the psychosomatic view is strongly held as a concept without dichotomizing psychic from somatic. Also, the idea of preservation of life force for maintaining health is still strong in the professional and laymen's minds with regard to psychiatric treatment [cross-reference to Chapter 9: Mental Illness: Folk Categories and Explanation (Section III, A)].

India is another example of a society that is very much influenced by its traditional medicine. It is the belief of Ayurvedic medicine that health is conditioned by the balance of three primary fluids in the body: wind, gall, and mucus. There are five separate winds (or "breaths") that control the main bodily functions. "Balancing" these fluids, or winds, is a major concern. The culture-related specific psychiatric syndrome of *dhat* (anxiety over the excessive loss of semen, which results in a deficiency of soul, or *dhat*) is very much rooted in traditional Ayurvedic medical concepts.

Contemporary Western medicine is historically rooted in Greek-Romanic medicine. As elaborated in the Hippocratic writings in 4th century B.C., the medical concept of mental disorders was based on the interactions of the four bodily humors blood, black bile, yellow bile, and phlegm — which resulted from the combination of the four basic qualities in nature — heat, cold, moisture, and dryness. According to temperaments, or the prevailing emotional orientation, persons were classified into four types: sanguine, choleric, melancholic, and phegmatic. When there was appropriate interaction of internal and external forces, an optimal level of functioning, called "crasis," could be reached; conflict between these forces resulted in "dyscrasia," indicating the presence of excessive bodily humor, which had to be removed by purging (Mora, 1975, p. 15). The practice of Mesmerism, initiated by French physician Franz Anton Mesmer at the end of the 18th century, was based on the hypothesis that man was endowed with a special magnetic fluid that, when liberated, could produce amazing healing effects.

B. IMPACT OF THE TIMES: PHILOSOPHICAL AND PROFESSIONAL BACKGROUNDS

Chinese traditional medicine was not merely influenced by ancient medical knowledge and folk clinical experiences, but was also shaped intensively by the philosophical thoughts that existed at the time. The concept of yin and yang is clearly related to Daoism, and the theory of the five elements was the prevalent worldview. Everything in the universe was interpreted as being reducable into the five elements of metal, wood, water, fire, and earth, which have a circular impact on each other and, at the same time, demonstrate paired antagonisms among them. The concept is used to explain the complicated phenomena that exist in nature as well as in human beings (a part of the macrocosm). Thus, the five major visceral organs (heart, lung, liver, spleen, and kidney) correspond to the five elements. Furthermore, it is conceived that the five basic emotions (joy, anger, worry, sorrow, and fear) occur in relation to these five organs. Clearly, these philosophical theories are symbolic. They probably have their roots in the *Yi-Jing (Oracle of Change)* and are not to be interpreted mechanically. They reflect the prevalent philosophical views that existed and were faithfully believed in by the people of the time.

It is obvious that the basis of psychoanalytic theory was impacted by Newton's absolute physics, which was prevalent at the end of the 19th century. Therefore, there arose a dynamic hypothesis relating to "drive" (equivalent to "energy") that needed to be discharged properly (or it might result in an explosion from accumulated pressure — "libido"). It was also evident that analytic theory was influenced by Darwin's evolutionary theory in biology, which significantly affected the professional field then. The concept of psychological development through stages, associated with the concepts of development, fixation, regression, or progression, was apparently impacted by evolutionary theory.

When many cultural anthropologists, in collaboration with psychoanalysts, enthusiastically carried out numerous field investigations in the early 20th century, testing cultural aspects of child development in relation to personality, gathering dream contents to explore the unconscious, or studying mythology and folklore, exemplified by the psychoanalysis and the social sciences study led by Géza Róheim (Muensterberger & Axelrad, 1960–1967), they were obviously influenced by the psychoanalytic theories that flourished at the time.

For some time, psychoanalytical theory in its early stages has been criticized by many professionals as too strongly reflective of the cultural views of Victorian Vienna, and very much biased by "man"-oriented views. For instance, in terms of personal development, the Oedipus complex was developed primarily for males, and penis envy for "inferior" females. The psychology of women was often ignored or left unexplored.

It has been pointed out by scholars that the split between mind and body in symptomotology in contemporary Western psychiatry is a reflection of the dualism that is prevalent in Western philosophy.

C. Bias of Political Ideology

Surprisingly, professional theories (including psychiatry) sometimes cannot escape the influence of political ideology. It is rather rare, but it can and does happen. Among the best examples observed were the situation in the USSR and in communist China in the 1950s and 1960s. As mentioned previously [in Chapter 28: Classification of Disorders (Section I, E, 1)], in the USSR, in order to comply with the demands of the political administration and ideology, the psychiatric diagnoses of antisocial and narcissistic personality disorders were removed from the official classification system. It was considered that such disorders "should" not exist in a communist society, where every individual should devote his life to the collective good. Instead, the concept of "vague schizophrenia" was invented with loose and broad diagnostic criteria for labeling and institutionalizing those accused of political offenses.

In communist China, from the establishment of the regime to the end of the Cultural Revolution, psychoanalytic theories and practices were politically forbidden. The excuse was that psychoanalysis (then prevalent in America) was the product of capitalism: a service provided only for affluent individuals rather than the majority of the people, who are the primary focus of socialism. Instead, theoretical views associated with conditional theory (which originated in Russia) were encouraged, and politically oriented group therapy was practiced rather than individual therapy.

It is also well known that during the Nazi regime, psychotherapy was discouraged in Germany. It was politically believed that the members of the nation needed to rely on the Nazi party to guide their lives, and nothing else.

D. Influence of the Western *Emic* View

It cannot be denied that modern psychiatry has its roots in Euro-American experiences and that many professional concepts and theories are influenced by Western views. The best example to illustrate this point is the professional concept of culture-related specific syndromes (or culture-bound syndromes) that is derived from a Euro-American clinician's perspective. It refers to any "exotic," "unusual," or "unclassifiable" psychopathology that is not observed in Western societies. It takes the professional position that only "other" or "foreign" societies have a cultural impact on certain kinds of psychopathologies — to the extent that they manifest special psychopathologies that cannot be classified according to existing diagnostic categories (which are derived from Western experiences) [cross-reference to: Chapter 13: Culture-Related Specific Syndromes (Section I, A)]. This *emic* view is in need of correction in the sense that culture in every society has an impact on clinical conditions, including "dominant" or "Euro-American" cultures (Littlewood & Lipsedge, 1986). How to take this broad view and recognize culture-related (or -bound) syndromes in every culture is a new challenge for *etic*-oriented scholars.

From the elaboration just given it is obvious that, in the field of psychiatry, professional theories are not determined merely by academic knowledge, but are often influenced by many other factors, including philosophical, political, and sociocultural ones.

II. CROSS-CULTURAL KNOWLEDGE REVISES PROFESSIONAL KNOWLEDGE

A. REVISION AND EXPANSION OF EXISTING CLINICAL VIEWS ABOUT PSYCHOPATHOLOGY

It cannot be denied that most contemporary psychiatric knowledge and hypotheses have been derived historically from clinical data and experiences gained by working with Caucasian populations in Europe and North America, where modern psychiatry developed. By comparing and including clinical information and findings from cross-cultural investigations of populations of other ethnic groups in other cultural settings around the world, the existing knowledge and hypotheses can be revised, corrected, or expanded for scientific accuracy and proper application to humankind as a whole. Following are some examples to illustrate this point.

1. Revised Views Regarding Suicidal Behavior

a. Male/Female Ratio

Regarding committed suicide, based on data available from numerous parts of the world, psychiatrists in the past believed that males tended to commit suicide more often than females (while the numbers for attempted suicide were reversed, with more female than male attempts). It was interpreted that males tended to take more serious action using more lethal methods to end their lives. However, this view was forced to change after epidemiological data became available from China — a country that has nearly one-fifth of the world population — where the situation was the opposite, i.e., females not only attempted more, but also tended to commit suicides more than males (Pritchard, 1996) [cross-reference to Chapter 22: Suicide Behavior (Section II, A, 3). Based on this cross-cultural information, views about gender and suicide needed revision. It was recognized that it was not the gender itself, but the distress encountered in association with the role of

gender that contributed to the taking of suicidal action.

Regarding attempted suicide, it has been the general view that females have a much higher number of attempted suicides than males. This has been attributed to females being more emotional and impulsive than males. However, reports from India, a country with a huge population, indicate that males tend to attempt suicide more often than females (Latha, Bhat, & D'Souza, 1996) [cross-reference to Chapter 22: Suicide Behavior (Section IV, B, 3)]. Although the number of subjects studied for this report was relatively small, we do not know to what extent it represents the total situation in India. If it is representative of the total population, this cross-cultural information certainly stimulates us to reconsider male/female ratios regarding suicide attempts — a behavior not so much determined by gender, but by the stress associated with the role of that gender in the society.

2. Lessons from the Epidemiological Study of Schizophrenia

Because schizophrenia is one of the major and gravest psychiatric disorders, it has been widely investigated by clinicians and scholars, including cultural psychiatrists, with regard to possible sociocultural contributions to its occurrence. However, data gathered from epidemiological studies around the world in various cultural settings have illustrated that the range of prevalence for schizophrenia is very narrow, only varying within two to five times [cross-reference to Chapter 19: Schizophrenia (Section III, D)]; whereas for other disorders, particularly minor psychiatric disorders, as well as substance abuse, alcoholism, or suicide, the range of prevalence is often very large and may vary between 10 and 20 times or even more among different cultures. The cross-society and -cultural epidemiological study of schizophrenia indirectly confirms the view that such a disorder is attributed more biologically and that the impact of sociocultural factors is minimal, i.e., it shows psychopathoplastic and psychopathoreactive effects, but not psychopathogenic effects.

3. Universality and Culture Specificity of Somatic Complaint Syndrome

During the early stages of the development of cultural psychiatry, many scholars, primarily based on clinical experiences in their own cultural settings (mostly in Asia, India, or Africa), made bilateral comparisons with experiences in Western societies, and proposed that somatic complaining among psychiatric patients was more prevalent in their cultural settings, and even that it was rather "unique" and "culture-rooted" clinical behavior. However, with an increase in such reports and the accumulation of knowledge from multiple societies, including various cultural samples, it is becoming clear to scholars that the tendency of psychiatric patients to make somatic complaints is not "culturally unique," but is commonly observed in many societies and cultures (Kirmayer & Young, 1998). Culture may influence the kind of somatic complaints the patient makes, the attention the complaints receive, and the patient's family's and therapist's reactions to them, but making somatic complaints (in addition to psychological complaints) is universally observed illness behavior.

B. Challenge to Expand and Revise the Classification System

1. Depression

Associated with the revitalization of the phenomena-oriented psychiatric classification system, mainly introduced by the American DSM system, psychiatric disorders are defined by so-called "objective" diagnostic criteria. However, it needs to be pointed out that the criteria and primarily based on clinical experiences with American patients (predominantly majority Americans). Thus, it tends to be arbitrary (particularly regarding the duration of the disorder as the criteria for diagnosis) and may not be applicable to patients of different ethnic–cultural backgrounds. This is exemplified by depression. Clinical experiences with Native Americans have disclosed that the duration of depression for them is relatively shorter than the duration that has been

defined arbitrarily by the DSM (Manson, Shore, & Bloom, 1985). Thus, revision of such diagnostic criteria is needed for cross-cultural application. Furthermore, it has been pointed out that depression among Native Americans is often not manifested as a "mood" disorder, but is commonly shown as behavior disorders, drinking problems, or substance abuse, calling for an expansion of diagnostical considerations for people of different ethnic and cultural backgrounds.

2. Neurasthenia

As elaborated previously [cross-reference to Chapter 16: Somatoform Disorders, Including Neurasthenia (Section III, B)], the diagnostic term "neurasthenia" was abandoned by American psychiatry, but is still prevalent in China and other countries. The justification for keeping such a nosological term has been argued by Chinese and other Asian psychiatrists, not because such a diagnosis is still applied frequently, but because of the academic view that there exists such a unique clinical entity that cannot be rediagnosed into depression or anxiety disorders, as claimed by some Western psychiatrists.

C. Modifying Speculation about the Cause of Psychopathology

1. Depression

Very much influenced by analytic theories, clinicians used to consider depression as being derived from the intrapsychic problems of guilt, in addition to being a reaction to loss trauma. Stimulated by these theories, the study of guilt versus shame as the cause of depression was explored by scholars in the early stages of cultural psychiatry. Actually, the father of modern psychiatry, Krepelin, after a visit to Indonesia to try his psychiatric classification system there, reported that guilt is seldom noticed among depressive patients in Indonesia. He even speculated that this situation was possibly related to the people being of the Muslim faith, rather than Christians.

However, a cultural psychiatrist originally from Egypt, M. Fakar El-Islam (1969), based on his clinical comparative study between depressed Christian and non-Christian patients there, reported that there was no difference in the occurrence of guilt between these two groups. In his interpretion, guilt was not necessarily closely related to Christian ideology.

It has also been speculated that the cause of depression is low self-esteem. However, after studying depressed persons of various cultural backgrounds in Hawaii, Yanagida and Marsella (1978) reported that low self-esteem was not necessarily closely related to depression in all cultures. There is still a lot of room for speculation about the psychological causes of depression from cross-cultural perspectives.

2. Drinking Problems

Another good example of how a cross-cultural study may expand and revise a hypothesis of psychopathology is found in the problem of alcoholism. Originally a psychoanalytic concept, it has been speculated that people's indulgence in drinking is related to an "oral" fixation. However, a cross-cultural study of alcoholism has clearly demonstrated that the problems of excessive drinking are related to many other variables besides the individual problem of oral fixation. Cultural background, particularly religious attitudes toward drinking, will certainly have a significant impact on people's drinking. For instance, Muslim people, based on their religious rules, practice strict abstinence from drinking, and alcoholism is almost nonexistent among them. In Japan, cultural attitudes toward male/female discrimination decreased after World War II, and alcohol consumption for women in contemporary Japan has increased almost seven times within a couple of decades.

The biological deficiency of an enzyme among some Asian people has been speculated to be one reason for discouraging Asian people from indulging in alcohol. However, alcohol consumption is surprisingly high in Korea, particularly among male adults. The prevalence of alcoholism has been claimed to be low among the Chinese in the past. However, associated with economic improvement and changes in culture

and lifestyle, a remarkable increase in alcohol drinking problems has been observed in Taiwan (but not yet in mainland China). Thus, many social and cultural factors contribute to drinking problems; individual psychological complexes may only be a part of them.

D. BROADENING THE BASIC ORIENTATION OF THERAPY

The psychoanalytic influences that have dominated American approaches to psychotherapy are characterized by the theme "to help clients to change themselves, to improve their coping skills, to remove the obstacles in their lives, and to help them adjust actively to reality." This theme is supported and enhanced by the American spirit and cultural emphasis. In a subtle but strong way it influences the therapists' as well as patients' orientations and expectations of therapy. It is assumed without question.

However, a study of psychotherapy (particularly folk therapy) developed and carried out in other cultures (primarily non-Western societies, such as Asian) showed that the primary goals of therapy could be entirely different. For instance, "acceptance of the self and problems as they are" is the basic emphasis of Morita therapy, which originated in Japan and is based on Zen concepts. The emphasis on the resolution of problems or removal of obstacles is not there. Change of self is encouraged to allow the patient to learn how to accept and live with his problems and symptoms.

Thus, examining the theories and concepts utilized in various forms of psychotherapy around the world will certainly shed light for clinicians and scholars on the meaning and purpose of therapy.

III. CONTRIBUTIONS OF SPECIFIC THEORETICAL CONCEPTS

Based on their clinical work and cross-cultural field studies, many specific theoretical concepts or views have been developed by cultural psychiatrists or mental health workers. These new concepts definitely impact psychiatric theories and practice in general.

A. Regarding Psychopathology

1. Conceptual Distinction between "Disease" and "Illness"

American social psychiatrist Leon Eisenberg (1977) has emphasized the conceptual distinction between "illness" and "disorder," which has become an important landmark for cultural anthropologists and cultural psychiatry. It helps clinicians understand the potential existence of a gap between physicians and the patients under their care. It addresses the need for attention and understanding from the patient's perspective of his illness rather than a preoccupation with the physician's medical view of the disorder [cross-reference to Chapter 9: Mental Illness: Folk Categories and Explanation (Section V, A)]. It promotes the physician's comprehension of the patient's complaining patterns, including the language used for describing the symptoms (Good, 1977), and improves the quality of care from cultural perspectives (Kleinman, Eisenberg, & Good, 1978).

2. Different Ways Culture Affects Psychopathology

The progress in cultural psychiatry has advanced our understanding of culture and psychopathology. Instead of simply considering that culture has an impact on psychopathology, we have now come to know that the impact of culture on psychopathology is multiple and includes pathogenic, pathoselective, pathoplastic, pathoelaborative, pathofacilitative, and pathoreactive effects [cross-reference to Chapter 11: Culture and Psychopathology (Sections II, A–F)]. This helps us discuss and comprehend the various ways that culture contributes to psychiatric pathology.

3. Different Kinds of Cultural Impact within the Spectrum of Psychopathology

Closely related to the concepts just given is the understanding that culture has a different degree of impact on different kinds of psychopathology. In general, its impact on organic psychiatric disorders (such as psychoses), which are predominantly attributed to biological factors, is minimal, while it is rather great on minor psychiatric disorders, such as adjustment disorders or substance abuse. It is useful to know that culture has a different kind of influence on different kinds of psychopathologies within its spectrum [cross-reference to Chapter 11: Culture and Psychopathology (Sections III, A–E)].

4. Clusters of Psychopathologies Relating to the Same Cultural Theme

Instead of splitting psychopathology into distinctively subdivided nosological entities, cultural psychiatry began to understand that a cluster of psychopathologies may occur from the same psychological cause or etiological theme that could be tied together by a common cultural theme, yet manifested as various kinds of psychopathologies.

For instance, as pointed out by Chinese cultural psychiatrists J.K. Wen (1995), closely associated with the traditional medical concepts of yin and yang, as well as the need to balance and conserve energy, in mainland China and Taiwan, there is a group of disorders labeled in folk terms: *nao-shenjing shuairuo* (brain-nerve weakness syndrome), *shenkui* (kidney deficiency syndrome, or neurasthenia), *pa leng* (frigophobia), and *suoyang* (or *koro,* genital-shrinking anxiety disorder). Closely related to the underlying traditional medical concepts and beliefs, clusters of psychopathologies emerged, connected to the kidneys, sexual organs, and the brain. Even though they have different degrees of severity and different clinical manifestations, they belong to a cluster of pathologies centered around the themes of losing vitality and the imbalance of yin–yang forces.

American medical anthropologist Good (1977) has described another example from Iran. He reported a folk illness observed there called *narahatye qalb* (heart distress). According to classic humoral theory, the backbone of traditional Galenic-Islamic medicine, the illness arises from an excess or deficiency of the humors, or the basic qualities of life. The heart is perceived as an organ of emotional functioning or the seat of the vital soul, providing "innate heat" and "vital breath" to the body. The attention of individuals on the heartbeat establishes causal links between irregularities in heartbeat and specified personal and social conditions. Heart distresses clinically range along a continuum from mild excitation to chronic sensations of irregularities to fainting and heart attack. Thus, a cluster of emotional disorders is linked by the distress of the "heart" organ.

The existence of a culture-related cluster of psychopathologies, as illustrated earlier, is not necessarily observed in every society. It may be discovered only in a society where there are prominent medically related cultural beliefs that profoundly affect the thoughts of the people, even in the area of psychopathology. Without such traditional beliefs, the phenomenon of clustered psychopathologies may not be found [cross-reference to Chapter 11: Culture and Psychopathology (Section III, D)].

However, from a clinical point of view, Western psychiatrists began to understand that many psychiatric disorders, even those with distinctly different diagnostic terms, such as depression, substance abuse, and alcoholism, as well as violent, homicidal and suicidal behavior, are often interrelated. This is explicitly evident among Native Americans in the manifestation of chronic massive frustration by a related cluster of such disorders (Manson et al., 1985).

5. Horizontal Cross-Cultural Perspective

Parallel with the view just described is the concept that certain culture elements (or traits) could relate to the occurrence of various kinds of stress within the same society or among different societies, which in turn produce different kinds of psychopathologies not closely related to them at all.

For instance, the emphasis on educational achievement, as a cultural element, which could promote competition among students and produce academic stress and anxiety in one society, may induce depression and suicide due to academic failure in another society, and, in still another, may become a useful stimulation for healthy competition without the occurrence of any psychopathology. Another example is the cultural emphasis on male dominance over females. In some societies, the female accepts the subordinate

role, and it is acepted part of the pattern of man–woman relationships without significant interpersonal problems. In another society, it could become the source for emotional frustration for the female, who then suffers from chronic depression, psychosomatic conditions, or drinking problems.

In other words, life is complicated. Due to numerous interacting factors, problems may be perceived, reacted to, and managed in various ways, resulting in different mental health outcomes (Fairbank & Hough, 1981). These cultural variations in the interaction between stress and psychopathology may be observed often in horizontal, cross-cultural examinations, i.e., conducting studies and analyses over multiple cultural examples.

6. Longitudinal Evolutionary Perspectives

Associated with this is the concept of the longitudinal evolution of psychopathology. It is derived from the longitudinal study of psychopathology observed in history, or in different societies at different stages of change. It illustrates that some identified psychiatric disorders have certain patterns of viscidity, emerging or fading in longitudinal aspects. The fate of hysterical conversion, catatonic disorder, or certain kinds of substance abuse are some obvious examples [cross-reference to Chapter 11: Culture and Psychopathology (Section III, E)]. While some scholars may regard such phenomena simply as the result of sociocultural change that determines the rise and fall of certain disorders, some scholars may interpret them as associated with the process of human evolution: change and development of the mind (Clements, 1932). This is an issue that deserves further study and understanding.

B. REGARDING THERAPY

By studying various kinds of therapy practiced in different cultures, Jerome Frank (1963) discovered that there are universal elements across various schools of psychotherapy and cultures. This view certainly invites us to understand the basic nature of psychotherapy. In contrast to this, many scholars and clinicians are concerned with and emphasize the importance of providing culture-relevant and -effective therapy for patients of divergent ethnic and cultural backgrounds, stimulating us to comprehend the nature and function of psychotherapy from another angle [cross-reference to Section F: Culture and Psychological Therapy (Chapters 32–37)].

C. Regarding Social and Cultural Dimensions of Human Behavior

Finally, among the contributions of culturally interested scholars are the socioculturally based, fundamental concepts that a person cannot be understood merely in terms of individual psychological aspects and that a society cannot be comprehended simply as an extension or multiplication of personal behavior. A person, in addition to his or her individual psychology, is constantly under the influence of society and culture, while a society or a culture functions as a unique entity of its own character and nature beyond the collective input of its members. These are the basic thoughts that need to be grasped in studying culture and human behavior.

IV. THEORIES AWAITING CROSS-CULTURAL REVISION

There are endless lists of theories or conceptual issues that are awaiting cross-cultural investigation in order to validate cross-cultural application and/or the need of cultural modification and revision. Following are some examples that deserve future attention from theoretical perspectives, particularly regarding theories about the psychology of humans.

A. Structural Theory of the "Self"

The structural theory of the self (dividing the psychology of the self into the id, ego, and superego), derived from analytical concepts, is useful for under-

standing human psychology. However, it is challenged in terms of cross-cultural expansion by cultural anthropologist Francis L.K. Hsu (1973). Hsu, from a cultural perspective, indicated that the boundary of the "self" does not end with the superego, but extends and merges into the surrounding environment of *society* in a concrete sense (including interrelation and interaction with people such as immediate family, friends, neighbors, or members of society at large) and of *culture* in abstract terms (including ways of thinking, attitudes, and value systems). Thus, as illustrated by Fig. 49-1, the structure of "self" could be expanded into sociocultural layers, and the boundary of the self as an individual could become blurred for persons from various cultures. This view was echoed by Korean-American cultural psychiatrist Suk Choo Chang (1988), who stated that the idea of the self was experienced, defined, and used among the cultures of the world between two conceptual poles. At one extreme, the self as individual was emphasized; the self was seen as independent and separate from the social group. At the other extreme, the self was viewed as integrated with the whole. The dominant premise in Western tradition exemplifies the former idea of the self; the latter is characteristic of the East (Roland, 1988). Validation of this view is awaiting more cross-cultural empirical study.

B. Psychosexual Developmental Theory

The developmental theory originally proposed by Sigmund Freud focused on the psychosexual aspects of individual development. Because it concerns biological instinct, it is regarded as applicable universally. However, due to the individual's unique developmental course, it is reasonable to speculate that the drive that emerges in each developmental stage may be subject to variations. In particular, it has been pointed out by scholars that the intensity of the triangular parent–child relationship conflict that occurs at the phallic stage, called the Oedipus complex, will depend on the sexual attitudes that exist in the environment. It also will be subject to variations based on the family system and structure within the society.

(a)   Self In Individual-Oriented Society   **(b)**   Self In Situation-Oriented Society

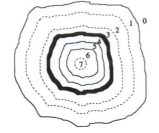

7 unconscious
6 preconscious
5 unexpressible conscious
4 expressible conscious

3 intimate society and culture
2 operative society and culture
1 wider society and culture
0 outer world

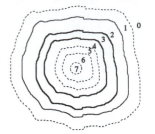

7 unconscious
6 preconscious
5 unexpressible conscious
4 expressible conscious

3 intimate society and culture
2 operative society and culture
1 wider society and culture
0 outer world

FIGURE 49-1   Psychosociogram of man in different societies. (a) Ego boundaries are distinctly defined in individual-oriented societies. (b) Ego boundaries are relatively blurred and extend to include the surroundings in situation-oriented societies. Revised from F.H.L. Hsu, Ph.D., presented at APA annual meeting, Honolulu, 1973.

Anthropologist B. Malinowski (1927), based on his field study of the Trobriand Islands in Melanesia near Australia, reported that in a matrilineal society, where the family lineage is traced from mother to daughter (rather than from father to son as in a patrilineal system), the relationship between the son and the mother's brother (maternal uncle) is more intense than between the son and his own biological father. Also in the matrilineal family system, the bond between brother and sister is an important one. Malinowski reported that in such a society, a boy-child tends to have dream wishes of the death of his brother — his potential rival subject. Thus, based on the family system, the persons involved in the triangular relationship will vary. Based on cross-cultural knowledge, Chinese-American anthropologist Hsu (1972) proposed different primary bonds or dyads within different families, such as the husband–wife dyad in European-American families, the father–son dyad in Asian families, the mother–son dyad in Hindu families, and the brother–sister dyad in matrilineal societies (such as those in Micronesia). Based on the emphasis of different dyads existing within different families, Hsu suggested that different personality patterns may be observed. As an extension of this, it may be speculated that the nature of the triangular conflict may be subject to variation. Echoing this, cultural psychiatrists Abel and Metraux (1974) pointed out that the social structure will also influence the nature of the Oedipus complex.

Furthermore, the cultural impact on the Oedipus complex has been discussed in terms of the solution pattern that may be proposed for it. For instance, the Chinese solution to the conflict, as reflected in opera and fairy tales, sometimes has the son being killed by the father (rather than the father being killed by the son, as in the Western Oedipus story) — an appropriate solution for the parent–child triangular conflict in a society that emphasizes parental respect and authority (Tseng & Hsu, 1972).

B. Psychosocial Development Theory

The psychosocial development theory developed by Erik H. Erikson (1963) deserves cultural adjustment as well. Erikson, as an analyst and child psychiatrist, proposed a theory based on his field work with two Native American tribes, in addition to his clinical experiences with Caucasian child patients. Thus, from a cross-cultural perspective, there are no sufficient and divergent cultural samples, and the theory is subject to expansion and improvement — a need that is even recognized by Erikson himself [cross-reference to Chapter 4: Child Development and Enculturation (Section III, B)]. Based on clinical experiences by cultural psychiatrists from divergent cultural backgrounds, it has been realized that the major theme emphasized in each stage of development warrants cross-cultural expansion or revision, and the pace of development from stage to stage needs cross-cultural adjustment and modification.

1. Concerning the Major Theme in Each Stage

There are many suggestions for expansion and revision in this area. Regarding the oral stage, instead of establishing *basic trust,* as described by Erickson, the need for obtaining a sense of *security* is more important for children who are living in societies where people suffer from a lack of adequate basic living conditions and struggle for daily survival. This is the current situation in many societies in Africa, India, some parts of Asia, and for aboriginal people in Australia.

Regarding the muscular-anal stage, it has been pointed out that for many Asian children, a sense of *dependence* and *indulgence* is permitted, while the emphasis on *autonomy* is rather delayed in association with the prolongation of the oral stage. For the majority of Chinese living in rural-agricultural settings, anal discipline through toilet training is less strict, whereas there is greater stress on behavior control through *shame* (Tseng & Hsu, 1969–1970).

During the locomotor-genital stage, *initiative* is not necessarily stressed in many cultures. Instead, *collaterality,* i.e., how to live with others harmoniously and interdependently, and not "stick out" from others in the group, is the ethos that receives more emphasis. This is exemplified by people living in small island societies with limited resources, such as Micronesia, where mutual dependency and collaterality are vital.

At the stage of latency, *industry* is valued in many societies. However, in addition, in many societies, particularly agricultural or so-called underdeveloped societies, *responsibility* is stressed. For instance, the emphasis is not so much on studying at school, working in a factory (as a junior laborer), or joining the adults working diligently in the field. Rather, the emphasis is on taking full responsibility, almost as an adult substitute, for performing many important tasks,

such as taking care of younger siblings, tending the cows or sheep (important sources of food for the family), or even learning to cook for the family. In other words, the youngsters are expected to learn to take responsibility in association with their rapid entry into adult life and taking part in production.

In the stage of puberty and adolescence, the degree of emphasis on gender identity varies cross-culturally. For instance, David D. Glimore (1990) conducted a survey of ideas about manhood in various cultures. He found that in many societies there is an *exaggeration* of masculinity for men, and a good many take this emphasis to extreme. It was speculated that the emphasis on gender identity (namely, emphasis on masculinity), in addition to occurring as a defense against close mother–son ties, may arise as the result of socioeconomic conditions. Thus, the harsher the environment and the scarcer the resources, the more manhood is stressed as an inspiration and a goal.

In contrast, in many societies that are conservative in sexual matters, there is a delay and *discouragement* of gender identity among youngsters. Any appearance, behavior, or activities that provoke man–woman relations are greatly inhibited until later. For instance, students are required to wear uniforms at school (with no sexually exhibiting dressing allowed) and any individual man–woman interaction (such as social dating between individual boys and girls) is strongly prohibited.

As an extension of this, during the stage of young adulthood, *intimacy* between man and woman and enjoyment in social life are not greatly stressed in many societies. Particularly in societies that still practice arranged marriages, intimacy between couples is not expected until later in their married lives, sometimes after middle age. Instead, *accountability* in work (economic achievement, domestic work, raising children, and so on) are considered the primary issues for young adults. Also, social isolation is not feared if the society is characterized by strong social bonds.

Generally speaking, *generativity* is important throughout adulthood, and striving for progress in life is critical in many societies, particularly achievement-oriented cultures, so that no stagnation results. However, in many cultures, an *obligation* to work, to support one's family, and to raise children are the basic tasks stressed for adults. Later, in many cultures, instead of aged people being concerned with *ego integrity* and avoiding despair, old age is considered the stage in which a person experiences a sense of *belonging* to family and being cared by his or her children. *Comfort* in life is the essential issue in this final stage of life.

2. The Pace of Development from Stage to Stage

It is not merely the major theme in each stage of development, but also the pace from stage to stage that is considered from a cross-cultural point of view. For instance, how long a child is permitted to stay in the oral stage may be determined by child-rearing patterns, including the way in which the infant is viewed and cared for.

In contrast to the contemporary American way of raising children, with a great emphasis on growing up fast, in general, many other societies take a more laid-back attitude toward their babies. Small children are allowed to stay babies, indulged by their parents, grandparents, and siblings, and there is no pressure for them to move into the next stage of development.

However, the pace after that can change rather abruptly. Among the Chinese, it has been pointed out that diligence is stressed for youngsters in the latency period, with the inculcation of the desire to achieve. This is a drastic shift in developmental requirements from earlier stages of indulgence. However, drastic psychological turmoil is not often noticed. This might be because the stage of puberty and adolescence is relatively prolonged and the entry into young adulthood is delayed (Bond, 1991). Related to this, intense relations and bonds with same-sex peers are permitted and maintained during latency, while heterosexual relations are suppressed as long as possible (Tseng, 1995).

Concerning the adolescent stage, Margaret Mead's study of adolescent turmoil outside of Euro-American societies was a landmark investigation. Based on her anthropological field work in Samoa in the South Pacific, she claimed that the psychosocial lives of adolescents there (at the time) were not as tumultuous as those observed in many Western societies, exemplified by contemporary American society. According to Mead, youngsters in Samoa usually went through a relatively calm transition from childhood to adulthood, without drastic changes in the adolescent period.

Thus, there is a need to consider the cross-cultural adjustment and revision of psychosexual development that were originally proposed by Erikson. The basic concept of development by stages is universally applicable; however, the main themes emphasized in each stage and the pace of the transition from stage to stage are certainly subject to cross-cultural revision, as illustrated by Fig. 49-2.

In addition to the psychosexual and psychosocial developmental theories elaborated earlier, there is an increasing awareness among cross-cultural psychologists that the cognitive development theory proposed by Piaget needs sociocultural adjustment as well, at least concerning the rhythms of the stages of development (Segall, Dasen, Berry, & Poortinga, 1990, pp. 143–159). Concerning ego development, Charles Pinderhughes (1974) offered hypotheses that culture will shape ego attitude, emotional attachments, and cognitive styles in the process of development. He stressed that although a person, as a human being, will follow certain universal rules of individual development, the pattern of ego development, in terms of the themes emphasized and the process followed, will vary according to the sociocultural environment.

C. THEORY OF DEFENSE MECHANISMS

Similarly to developmental theories, a theory of defense mechanisms has been developed by psychoanalysts and has made a significant contribution to clinicians and behavior scientists in terms of the in-depth understanding of human psychology. Various defense mechanisms have been identified by scholars historically (Vaillant, 1986) and have been categorized

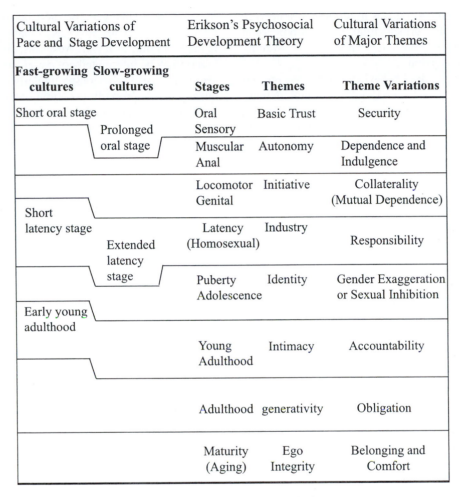

Cultural Variations of Pace and Stage Development		Erikson's Psychosocial Development Theory		Cultural Variations of Major Themes
Fast-growing cultures	**Slow-growing cultures**	**Stages**	**Themes**	**Theme Variations**
Short oral stage		Oral Sensory	Basic Trust	Security
	Prolonged oral stage	Muscular Anal	Autonomy	Dependence and Indulgence
Short latency stage		Locomotor Genital	Initiative	Collaterality (Mutual Dependence)
	Extended latency stage	Latency (Homosexual)	Industry	Responsibility
		Puberty Adolescence	Identity	Gender Exaggeration or Sexual Inhibition
Early young adulthood		Young Adulthood	Intimacy	Accountability
		Adulthood	generativity	Obligation
		Maturity (Aging)	Ego Integrity	Belonging and Comfort

FIGURE 49-2 Cultural modifications of personality development theory. Variations on stages and themes of development.

according to a hierarchy of defense mechanisms (Vaillant, 1971). In principle, the concept of defense mechanism is considered universally applicable, and empirical studies of ego mechanisms of defense have been undertaken (Vaillant, 1986). However, there is a rising voice calling for cross-cultural study and possible revisions from cultural perspectives (Tseng, 1994). The concern is with whether any particular set of defense mechanisms might be utilized more or less frequently by people of particular cultural groups and whether there are any unique defense mechanisms applied in certain cultures that are not described in the present list of defense mechanisms.

As early as the 1940s, Chinese-American anthropologist F.L.K. Hsu (1949) had already brought up the differences between repression and suppression that are commonly utilized in different cultures. Based on his behavioral observation of two groups of people from four cultures, the Chinese and Japanese in the East and Americans and Germans in the West, he claimed that suppression was used more as a defense mechanism by the former group, whereas repression was used more by the latter. This view is awaiting empirical investigation.

"Passive-aggressive" behavior as a defense mechanism is generally considered an "immature" defense by contemporary Western psychiatrists (Gabbard, 1995), whereas such behavior is considered an "adaptive" coping mechanism in many non-Western societies. This is particularly true in relations with authority figures. Direct confrontation (especially with administrative authority figures) is viewed as "unwise" behavior. In China, several decades ago, a well-known writer, Lu Xun, portrayed an imaginary individual (with the psudoname A-Q, or mister Q) in a short story. He used A-Q's behavior ("passive-aggressive rationalization," addressed as A-Q's spirit in the story) as a reflection of the Chinese way of dealing with problems. Politically, it was used to criticize the Chinese way of dealing with Westerners' invasive and insulting behavior in China at the time. However, A-Q's spirit has been consciously recognized among the Chinese as a means of understanding Chinese behavior. In fact, in developing a personality inventory for the Chinese, the behavior cluster of A-Q's coping patterns was incorporated into other clusters in the questionnaire (Cheung et al., 1996). It was found that it was actually one of the characteristic personality traits revealed in the survey. In short, "passive-aggressive rationalization" is a common defense mechanism utilized by the majority of ordinary Chinese and therefore needs to be listed as one of their "mature" (if not "frequently used") defenses.

Humor is among the mature defenses listed by Western psychiatrists at present. It is defined as a mechanism that deals with emotional conflict and internal or external stressors by emphasizing the amusing or ironic aspects of conflict or stressors (Vaillant, 1986, p. 135). It is considered a sophisticated and skillful way of expressing feelings, as it does not produce unpleasant effects on others. Even high-ranking officers feel free to use humor in dealing with public situations. In contrast, it can be interpreted as awkward to do so in societies where the dignity of authority may be challenged by such behavior. In short, humor may not be perceived as a "mature" mechanism in other cultures as it is in Western societies. Actually, humor may be interpreted not merely as improper, but also as sarcastic behavior, particularly if it is used frequently and improperly in certain social settings.

While nervous laughing is a kind of defensive mechanism not described in the existing list of defense mechanisms for Westerners, it is one kind of coping mechanism commonly used by some Asian people. When a person is nervous, particularly in an embarrassing situation, instead of manifesting feelings and gestures of nervousness or embarrassment, he may laugh nervously. By bursting into laughter, a person could save himself embarrassment by concealing his feelings of nervousness. This culturally shaped behavior may look awkward or strange to outsiders, who are not familiar with it, and might interpret it as odd, while actually it is a culturally shaped defense mechanism.

In summary, there are many psychiatric theories that developed originally in the belief that they concerned the "basic" nature of human psychology and were "universally" applicable. However, the progress of transcultural clinical experiences and cross-cultural investigations has begun to challenge such professional "beliefs" held in the past. Certainly, there is a need to examine each psychiatric theory critically and to make cross-cultural revisions for transcultural application.

V. CLOSING REMARKS

In the beginning of the 20th century, cultural psychiatry emerged as a discipline of *research,* interested simply in exploring how culture affects personality development (particularly among so-called "primitive" people) and psychopathology (especially "exotic" syndromes). It was only less than three decades ago, around the 1960s, associated with an increase in knowledge and the demands of reality, that cultural psychiatry began to pay attention to and emphasize cultural aspects of *clinical practice* (mainly among ethnic minorities). However, the concern with providing culturally relevant service, not merely for minorities, but for every patient, is rising, taking cultural psychiatry beyond the scope of minority psychiatry. Thus far, the examination of the cultural aspects of *theory* has been almost ignored. It is time to begin to pay attention to theoretical issues: how culture may affect psychiatric theories, what theories need modification, and what new views and concepts can be developed from cultural psychiatry and contribute to general psychiatry.

Human behavior and mental disorders are broadly attributed to biological, psychological, and sociocultural factors. Although the primary mission of cultural psychiatry is to focus on cultural dimensions, as Paris (1994) warned, cultural psychiatry at times runs the risk of becoming unidimensional. A narrow focus on the cultural variability of mental illness may lose sight of the universals rooted in biology and influenced by individual psychology. The social and cultural dimensions of human behavior and mental problems become more comprehensive when understood in terms of their interactions with biological and psychological factors. Furthermore, the time has passed for arguing about universality versus cultural specificity. We need to move on to examine how the psychiatric theories developed in the past might be culturally biased or skewed, what theories can be universally applied, and what theories need to be developed for transcultural utilization. Focusing attention on these issues is a primary mission for cultural psychiatry.

REFERENCES

Abel, T.M., & Metraux, R. (1974). *Culture and psychotherapy* (p. 127). New Haven, CT: College & University Press.

Bond, M.H. (1991). *Beyond the Chinese face: Insights from psychology.* Hong Kong: Oxford University Press.

Chang, S.C. (1988). The nature of the self: A transcultural view. Part I: Theoretical aspects. *Transcultrual Psychiatric Research Review, 25*(3), 169–203.

Cheung, F., Leung, K., Fan, R.M., Song, W.S., Zhang, J.X., & Zhang, J.P. (1996). Development of the Chinese Personality Assessment Inventory (CPAI). *Journal of Cross-Cultural Psychology, 27*(2), 181–199.

Clements, F.E. (1932). Primitive concepts of disease. *University of California Publications in American Archaeology and Ethnology, 32,* 185–252.

Eisenberg, L. (1977). Disease and illness: Distinctions between professional and popular ideas of sickness. *Culture, Medicine and Psychiatry, 1*(1), 9–23.

El-Islam, M.F. (1969). Depression and guilt: A study at an Arab psychiatric clinic. *Social Psychiatry, 4,* 56–58.

Erickson, E.H. (1963). *Childhood and society,* (2nd ed.). New York: Norton.

Fairbank, D.T., & Hough, R.L. (1981). Cross-cultural differences in perception of life events. In B.S. Dohrenwend & B.P. Dohrenwend (Eds.), *Stressful life events and their contexts.* New York: Prodist.

Frank, J.D. (1963). *Persuasion and healing.* New York: Schocken Books.

Gabbard, G.O. (1995). Theories of personality and psychopathology: Psychoanalysis. In H.I. Kaplan & B.J. Sadock (Eds.), *Comprehensive textbook of psychiatry/VI,* 6th ed., Vol. 1, pp. 451–452. Baltimore: Williams & Wilkins.

Glimore, D.D. (1990). *Manhood in the making: Cultural concepts of masculinity.* New Haven, CT: Yale University Press.

Good, B.J. (1977). The heart of what's matter: The semantics of illness in Iran. *Culture, Medicine and Psychiatry, 1*(1), 25–58.

Hsu, F.L.K. (1949). Suppression versus repression: A limited psychological interpretation of four cultures. *Psychiatry, 12,* 223–242.

Hsu, F.L.K. (1972). Kinship and ways of life: An exploration. In F.L.K. Hsu (Ed.), *Psychological anthropology.* New Edition. (pp. 509–567). Cambridge, MA: Schenkman.

Hsu, F.L.K. (1973, May 7). *Psychosocial homeostasis (PSH): A sociocentric model of man.* Presented as William P. Menninger Memorial Lecture at the annual meeting of the American Psychiatric Association, Honolulu.

Kirmayer, L.J., & Young, A. (1998). Culture and somatization: Clinical, epidemiological and ethnographic perspectives. *Psychosomatic Medicine, 60,* 420–430.

Kleinman, A., Eisenberg, L., & Good, B. (1978). Culture, illness, and care: Clinical lessons from anthropologic and cross-cultural research. *Annals of Internal Medicine, 88,* 251–258.

Latha, K.S., Bhat, S.M., & D'Souza, P. (1996). Suicide attempters in a general hospital unit in India: Their socio-demographic and clinical profile — emphasis on cross-cultural aspects. *Acta Psychiatrica Scandinavica, 94,* 26–30.

Littlewood, R., & Lipsedge, M. (1986). The 'culture-bound syndromes' of the dominant culture: Culture, psychopathology and biomedicine. In J.L. Cox (Ed.), *Transcultural psychiatry* (pp. 253–273). London: Croom Helm.

Malinowski, B. (1927). *Sex and repression in savage society.* New York: Harcourt.

Manson, S.M., Shore, J.H., & Bloom, J.D. (1985). The depressive experience in American Indian communities: A challenge for psychiatric theory and diagnosis. In A. Kleinman, & B. Good

(Eds.), *Culture and depression: Studies in the anthropology and cross-cultural psychiatry of affect and disorder* (pp. 331–368). Berkeley: University of California Press.

Mora, G. (1975). Historical and theoretical trends in psychiatry. In A.M. Freedman, H.I. Kaplan, & B.J. Sadock (Eds.), *Comprehensive textbook of psychiatry* (2nd ed., Vol. 1). Baltimore: Williams & Wilkins.

Muensterberger, W., & Axelrad, S. (Eds.). (1960–1967). *The psychoanalytic study of society* (Vol. 1–4). New York: International Universities Press.

Paris, J. (1994). Evolutionary social science and transcultural psychiatry. *Transcultural Psychiatric Research Review, 31*(4), 339–367.

Pinderhughes, C.A. (1974). Ego development and cultural differences. *American Journal of Psychiatry, 131,* 171–175.

Pritchard, C. (1996). Suicide in the People's Republic of China categorized by age and gender: Evidence of the influence of culture on suicide. *Acta Psychiatrica Scandinavica, 93,* 362–367.

Roland, A. (1988). *In search of self in India and Japan: Toward a cross-cultural psychology.* Princeton, NJ: Princeton University Press.

Segall, M.H., Dasen, P.R., Berry, J.W., & Poortinga, Y.H. (1990). *Human behavior in global perspective: An introduction to cross-cultural psychology.* New York: Pergamon Press.

Tseng, W.S. (1995). Psychotherapy for the Chinese: Cultural adjustment. In L.Y.C. Cheng, H. Baxter, & F.M.C. Cheung (Eds.) *Psychotherapy for the Chinese* (2nd vol.) (pp. 1–22). Hong Kong: Chinese University of Hong Kong.

Tseng, W.S., & Hsu, J. (1969–1970). Chinese culture, personality formation and mental illness. *International Journal of Social Psychiatry, 16*(1), 5–14.

Tseng, W.S., & Hsu, J. (1972). The Chinese attitude toward parental authority as expressed in Chinese children's stories. *Archives of General Psychiatry, 26,* 28–34.

Vaillant, G.E. (1971). Theoretical hierarchy of adaptive ego mechanisms. *Archives of General Psychiatry, 24,* 107–118.

Vaillant, G.E. (1986). Introduction: A brief history of empirical assessment of defense mechanisms. In G.E. Vaillant (Ed.), *Empirical studies of ego mechanisms of defense* (pp. viii–xx). Washington, DC: American Psychiatric Press.

Wen, J.K. (1995). Sexual beliefs and problems in contemporary Taiwan. In T.-Y. Lin, W.S. Tseng, & E.K. Yeh (Eds.), *Chinese societies and mental health* (pp. 219–230). Hong Kong: Oxford University Press.

Yanagida, E., & Marsella, A.J. (1978). The relationship between self-concept discrepancy and depression among Japanese-American women. *Journal of Clinical Psychology, 34,* 654–659.

50

Cultural Psychiatry Training

I. HISTORICAL TRENDS

When scholars of various professional backgrounds, including anthropologists, psychologists, and psychiatrists, began to show an interest in culture and its relation to behavior, mental health, and psychiatric disorders in the early 20th century, cultural psychiatry was not yet recognized as a special subfield, and there was no formal training program available for it. In fact, cultural psychiatry developed simply because some Western psychiatrists had the opportunity to work with indigenous people of different cultural backgrounds in foreign settings — mostly in non-Western societies — and, through their encounters, began to experience and appreciate the impact of culture on psychiatric disorders and clinical practice.

Conversely, many non-Western psychiatrists who traveled abroad for psychiatric training in Europe or America encountered problems of transcultural practice with their Western patients. Later, when they returned to their home countries, they faced the challenge of applying the psychiatric knowledge and clinical experience they had received in the West to the indigenous people in their own cultural settings. Thus, encountering a culture or cultures other than one's own is key to becoming sensitive to and appreciative of different cultures. Experiencing the transcultural practice of psychiatry and incorporating knowledge and theories obtained from cultural anthropology and cross-cultural psychology, as well as contribution from the psychoanalysis, regarding cultural aspects of human behavior and mind, promoted the development of cultural psychiatry as a scientific subfield [cross-reference to Chapter 1: Cultural Psychiatry (Sections II, A–F)]. In the early stages of its development, there was no formal training, and the careers of many pioneer cultural psychiatrists developed mainly through their own transcultural clinical experiences.

Later, there were some psychiatrists who formally studied anthropology, and some anthropologists who received formal training in medicine and psychiatry. With academic degrees in both areas, they became experts in cultural psychiatry. However, there are only a handful of such scholars and clinicians.

Associated with the rising awareness of and concern for human rights and minority movements, there is an increasing emphasis on the need for providing ethnic- or minority-relevant mental health care. Related to this new consciousness, is the demand for culture-oriented training and what is now called cultural competence for psychiatrists and all other mental health practitioners (Lefley & Pedersen, 1986). Beyond the movement of minority psychiatry, there has been increased academic recognition that, for proper cultural psychiatry, the professional field must move beyond a focus on minorities and address culture in an overall sense. Examining the different cultures around the world, and studying how culture impacts on psychiatric practice in similar or different ways in diverse cultural settings, will stimulate the development of theoretical concepts and clinical experiences of cultural psychiatry in a broad sense with a solid foundation. There is a cultural dimension to treating every patient — not only minority patients, but those with other ethnic backgrounds, including members of the majority group. This was elaborated in the beginning of this book [cross-reference to Chapter 1: Cultural Psychiatry (Section II, E)]. Thus, it is desirable for all clinicians to have cultural psychiatric training included in their general clinical training to enable them to provide treatment for patients of diverse ethnic or cultural backgrounds. Knowing this, there is an increased demand to include such formal training. It should be a basic requirement for all psychiatrists-in-training, not just for those who plan to specialize in cultural psychiatry.

Despite the need for such training, in the late 1970s when Jeffress (1968) carried out a survey on training in cultural psychiatry in the United States, he found that less than half of the residency programs reported any training at all. Similarly, Rogers, Ponterott, Conoley, and Wiese (1992) conducted a national survey of school psychology programs, and reported that 40% of those surveyed did not offer specific multicultural courses. As pointed out by Moffic, Kendrick, Lomax, and Reid, (1987), actual training and education in cultural psychiatry in the United states in the 1980s seemed to be decreasing, even though the knowledge in the area was significantly increasing. Among various speculations, Moffic explained that while biological psychiatry had grown in influence, concern for cultural issues may have decreased. It was rather recently that there was an official request to incorporate cultural psychiatry training into the curriculum of general

psychiatric training, as well as culture competency training (ACGME. 2001), which is expected nowadays, even for medical students and medical residents (AMA, 1999).

In addition to general resident training programs, some institutions have provided special programs in cultural psychiatry at advanced levels. However, there is no concurrence among experts in the field on how to offer cultural psychiatric training to all psychiatric residents. Work is currently being done to formalize and implement such a program. For instance, there is a task force group in the Society for the Study of Psychiatry and Culture working on a proposal on how to provide such training. Recently, cultural psychiatrists Foulks, Westermeyer, and Ta (1998) gave detailed suggestions for a model curriculum for medical students, psychiatric residents, and fellows in cultural psychiatry. In the fourth edition of *Diagnostic and Statistical Manual of Mental Disorders* (DSM-IV) of the American Psychiatric Association (1994), Appendix I includes a formal guideline for cultural formulation [cross-reference to Chapter 27: Clinical Assessment and Diagnosis (Section V)]. As stressed by Lu, Lim, and Mezzich, (1995), it offers suggestions on how to assess cultural dimensions in clinical practice — another indication of the official recognition of the importance of cultural psychiatry.

II. BASIC QUALITIES FOR CULTURAL COMPETENCE

It is becoming common opinion that beyond being "clinically competent," every clinician needs to be "culturally competent." "Cultural competence" is being aware of and sensitive to the patient's as well as the therapist's (own) cultural background, having the needed cultural knowledge, empathy, and skill to carry out appropriate clinical work, including communication, relationship, assessment, care, and treatment, and having the desirable culture attributes of being comfortable, relevant, meaningful, and efficient in working with patients of diversified ethnic-cultural backgrounds. In other words, a psychiatrist needs to be competent in biological psychiatry, psychological psychiatry, and cultural psychiatry to ensure that the whole spectrum of psychiatry is covered in effective clinical work. Cultural competency has been suggested as a basic requirement. It is particularly important when clinicians are working in multiple ethnic–cultural societies, providing care for patients of diverse backgrounds (Gopaul-McNicol & Brice-Baker, 1998). Even in mono–ethnic–cultural societies (such as Japan and Korea in the east, or Finland and Poland in the West), when closely examined, there is no difficulty finding many subgroups based on social class differences and geographic differences, or minority groups created by social or psychological factors (rather by ethnicity or race), or the presence of foreigners associated with education, business, diplomatic work, or transient travelers who may need mental health care at some times or another. The diversified populations in these socieites require training in cultural psychiatry for clinicians.

Based on the degree to which ethnic background and cultural factors are regarded in clinical service, Jordan (1995) presented a continuum of levels of cultural competence, a process that starts with *cultural destructiveness* followed by *cultural incapacity* (clients segregated by ethnicity), *cultural blindness* (patients selected for treatment with no regard to their ethnic or cultural background), *cultural precompetence* (patients distributed by ethnicity is understood to be an issue, but nothing is done to change policies), *cultural competence* (patient distribution matches the demographic base), and *cultural proficiency* (full awareness of needs and solutions regarding comprehensive coverage of all ethnic groups).

Alarcón, Westermeyer, Foulks and Ruiz (1999) have described five independent, but interrelated, clinical dimensions that identify and define culture as: an interpretive/explanatory tool, a pathogenic/pathoplastic agent, a diagnostic/nosological factor, a therapeutic/protective element, and a service/management instrument. This stresses the clinical relevance of contemporary cultural psychiatry in a broad sense, rather than being merely concerned with single aspects of it.

From a clinical point of view, several basic qualities are required to become a culturally competent cli-

nician, at which training must aim (Foulks, 1980; Lu et al., 1995; Moffic, Kendrick, & Reid, 1988; Tseng & Streltzer, 2001; Westermeyer, 1989, 1990). They are:

A. SHARPENING OF CULTURAL SENSITIVITY

The clinician needs to have the clinical quality of cultural sensitivity. This is fundamental to being able to appreciate the existence of various lifestyles among human beings, diverse views and attitudes toward patterns of living, different natures of stress encountered, and dissimilar or unique coping patterns utilized for adaptation. Actual experience encountering cultures other than one's own can facilitate and stimulate the development of cultural awareness and sensitivity.

Beyond awareness, the clinician needs to be able to perceive and sense cultural differences among people and know how to appreciate them without ignorance, bias, prejudice, or stereotyping. For instance, if a patient complains that his "heart is vacant," another that she is "feeling cold on her back," another that he has "butterflies in the stomach," and another that he has "lost his soul," the clinician needs to develop a cultural curiosity about what the patients are trying to communicate through such sayings. If a mother scratches her baby's body with a coin, causing infections and scars, or if a patient wears cloth rings on her wrist, a culturally sensitive clinician would try to find out whether these actions reflect the patients' own idiosyncratic style; are culturally patterned, unique ways of expressing emotional problems; or are culturally common and accepted ways of coping with crises. The clinician would further try to find out whether there is any symbolic meaning behind the patients' symptoms and behavior.

The clinician or therapist needs to be willing to communicate and to learn as much as necessary from his patients and their families about their beliefs, attitudes, values systems, and ways of dealing with problems. It is not merely a matter of sensitive perception, but is also an attitude of wanting to learn others' lifestyles rather than being trapped in one own's subjective perception and interpretation of others' behavior. Sometimes, we are ignorant in the sense of not knowing that we do not know something. In cultural matters, this is referred to as "cultural blindness" — not knowing the existence of certain cultural areas and not even being aware of our ignorance. This is common when we encounter very divergent, unfamiliar, foreign cultural systems. If we are culturally sensitive, such cultural ignorance or so-called "cultural scotoma" is minimized. Being sensitive in our perceptions, maintaining curiosity about differences, being willing to learn and understand the nature of uniqueness, and having an understanding attitude that appreciates cultural differences are all qualities needed for cultural sensitivity.

B. Acquiring Cultural Knowledge

Beyond sensitivity, a clinician needs to have a certain base of cultural knowledge about humankind as a whole and of the particular patient and family concerned. It is difficult even for well-trained professional anthropologists to know about every cultural system. They tend to choose certain cultural areas for their field studies and become knowledgeable about certain cultural systems. Clinicians are not anthropologists and, therefore, it is impossible to expect them to know about all the cultural systems that exist. It is, however, desirable for them to have some basic anthropological knowledge about how human beings vary in their habits, customs, beliefs, value systems, and illness behavior, in particular. They should know more about the cultural systems of their patients so that culture-relevant assessment and care can be delivered. For instance, it is important to know that Asian people scratch the skin of babies to create scar tissue is an attempt to stir up the yong (fire) element to resist (or counteract) sickness; that a concern with feeling cold is based on the cold–hot theory of sickness, according to which feeling cold on the trunk of the body is a serious sign of losing the yang element; that butterflies in the stomach is an Anglo-Saxon symbol for irritated anxiety; that the loss of soul is a Latin American expression describing absentmindedness, loss of will, or emotional instability; and that cloth rings worn around the wrist are Micronesian charms against sicknessevil. Such knowledge will help the clinician distinguish between the normality and pathology of behavior from a cultural perspective — extremely useful cultural knowledge in relation to illness behavior.

Reading books and other literature is one way to obtain such cultural information. Consulting with medical anthropologists on general issues or with experts on a particular cultural system is another approach. If material or consultations is not easily available, the patient and his family or friends of the same ethnic–cultural background may be used as resources, even though careful judgment is needed in determining their accuracy or relevance.

C. Enhancement of Cultural Empathy

Cognitive information about a patient's culture alone is not sufficient to reach the patient transculturally. There is another quality needed, namely, being able to feel and to understand at an emotional level from the patient's own cultural perspective. Otherwise, a gap in understanding will remain, and the therapist will be unable to participate in the emotional experience of the patient — an ability that is important to the quality of therapy (Pinderhughes, 1984). This ability is known as "cultural empathy," the ability to have empathy in therapeutic situations, with an emphasis on the cultural level.

For example, knowing cognitively that a patient's concern with "feeling cold on her back" or "fearing his penis is shrinking into his abdomen" is related to a hot–cold folk theory is not sufficient. The clinician needs to be able to sense, to feel, and to share the patient's anxiety about his bodily symptoms as matters of life or death — based on the patient's folk beliefs. The symptoms are not merely somatic symptoms derived from folk medical concepts, but are critical signs of impending death (from the patient's cultural perspective), as much as if a person were having a heart attack (from the physician's medical perspective). The clinician must show concern, comfort, and offer assurance to the patient, as if he were treating a serious condition (and it may be serious indeed!).

If a parent becomes extremely upset about someone hitting his young child on the head, it is necessary to understand cognitively that the parent is so upset because, according to his folk belief, the head is where the soul is located. A physical examination to rule out the possibility of any head injury is not enough. The clinician also needs to comprehend, feel, and share the parent's fear that the child may lose his soul — a very serious possibility (according to the parent's belief system), much more serious than a severe concussion, in the physician's medical view. Assurance that the soul is intact is the central issue in the care of the parent. Being able to demonstrate empathy for the patient from a cultural perspective is an important quality for the clinician.

D. Adjustment of Culturally Relevant Relations and Interactions

In a clinical setting, particularly in a psychotherapeutic situation, the therapist is greatly concerned with maintaining a proper professional relationship with the patient. The aim is to achieve therapeutic effects and minimize any complications or ill effects. The age, gender, and personality of the patient; the nature and severity of the psychopathology; and the purpose of therapy are some of the elements to consider in adjusting patient–therapist relations. An extension of this is a need to incorporate cultural attributes. That is, the relation and interaction between the therapist and the patient need to take into consideration the cultural background of the patient, the therapist, and the setting in which the therapy takes place.

More specifically, it is always necessary to consider the proper relation between an authoritative and a subservient figure and persons of different genders, and whether it is a professional or a social occasion. Such cultural knowledge, in addition to clinical judgment, will lead to a proper therapist–patient relationship and interaction, aimed at both cultural relevancy and therapeutic effect.

Involved here are not only the nature of the relationship between therapist and patient, in terms of role, status, and level of intimacy, but also issues of interaction, including communication, understanding, and giving and receiving between therapist and patient.

A practical example is determining the proper and therapeutic way for a male therapist to relate to a female patient from a culture in which a submissive role and passive behavior is the norm for females. Shall the therapist expect and encourage the female patient to have "good" eye contact with the male therapist, or would that violate the cultural norms of the patient? Is it possible for the therapist to give a "wrong" message to the patient by asking her to maintain direct eye contact with the therapist, or would it serve as a "therapeutic" maneuver, encouraging the female patient to be more assertive and relate to males on an equal basis?

What does it mean when a patient keeps saying, "Yes, yes, doctor" to the therapist? Is it the culturally patterned behavior toward an authority figure (the therapist) of a patient from a culture that emphasizes hierarchy? Does saying "yes" merely acknowledge "I am listening" rather than express agreement? For therapeutic purposes, should the therapist encourage the patient to feel comfortable negotiating or even disagreeing with the therapist? These are issues that need careful consideration before action is taken.

How to detect, comprehend, and manage ethnic or race-related transference and countertransference is another level of concern in dealing with patients of distinctly different ethnic or racial backgrounds. This is particularly true when negative and even hostile relations preexist between the ethnicity or racial backgrounds of the patient and the therapist. The same applies to the association of a minority group member and a majority group member when discrimination and an imbalanced power preexist between them.

These are issues that significantly influence the process of therapy. The willingness of the therapist to give careful consideration to these issues, in order to properly manage and make appropriate adjustments to therapy, is an important quality for cultural competence (cross-reference to Chapter 36: Intercultural Psychotherapy and Chapter 37: Culture-Relevant Psychotherapy).

It is certainly a challenge to learn how to establish a relevant therapist–patient relationship and interaction with consideration for clinical as well as cultural perspectives. Further, it is necessary to pay attention to the ethical aspects of clinical practice — a cultural perspective beyond general clinical consideration. Although the basic principles of medical ethics apply universally and cross-culturally, certain cultural modifications or variations are necessary to adapt to the culture of the patient and the environment in which the clinical care takes place.

E. ESTABLISHMENT OF ABILITY FOR CULTURAL GUIDANCE

It is important for the therapist to be able to select clinically suitable and culturally relevant ways of treatment that will work best for the patient. It is becoming clear among cultural psychiatrists that there are no specific treatment models for particular ethnic groups. There are so many kinds of problems even within one ethnic group that there is a need to apply different therapeutic approaches accordingly. However, a certain therapeutic approach may be better suited to a certain ethnic group depending on that group's understanding of psychiatric service, style of relating to the therapist, and pattern of working on psychological problems. For instance, directive, educational, cognitive therapy is suited better for ethnic people who welcome such an approach, in contrast to an emotion-oriented, analytic approach. Besides, even within the same ethnic group, there are various subgroups that deserve careful evaluation when selecting a therapeutic approach [cross-reference to Section G: Culture and Therapy with Special Subpopulation (Chapter 38–42)]. However, there is accumulated clinical knowledge on the basic rules and principles that need consideration in the proper selection of a treatment approach to match cultural style as well as therapeutic effect. This is a part of the cultural competence necessary for successful clinical care by every clinician.

Moreover, a clinician needs to be able to make proper judgements on the extent to which and in what way the patient's problems are related to cultural factors, and to comprehend dynamically how to provide culturally relevant advice for patients in dealing with their problems. This may involve choice of coping style, ways of dealing with problems, and the ultimate goal of resolving the conflict. Culturally determined norms, values, and goals may need to be challenged and adjusted in order to treat problems or resolve conflicts. Culturally sanctioned coping mechanisms may need reinforcement or, if ineffective, may need to be confronted. Alternatives to culturally defined solutions may need to be proposed. It takes not only clinical judgment but cultural insight to find relevant and optimal solutions (Tseng & Streltzer, 2001).

For instance, if a young patient is facing the dilemma of establishing his or her independence to meet contemporary cultural emphasis on the one hand and complying with filial obedience to his parents and following traditional cultural expectations on the other, finding a suitable way to deal with this complicated situation is a challenge in cultural guidance. Another example is finding a way for a woman to strive for self-reliance, either personally or professionally, and still maintain a subordinate status toward her husband to fulfill cultural demands of the husband–wife roles, a delicate matter needing sensitive and proper guidance. It is the task of the clinician to comprehend the whole situation within the biological, medical psychological, social, and cultural spectrum.

Finally, it is vital to know that psychiatric treatment, particularly psychotherapy, involves the interaction of two value systems: the patient's and the therapist's. Therapeutic interaction provides opportunities for exposure, exchange, and incorporation of differing cultural elements between therapist and patient (Tseng & Hsu, 1979). Cultural insight allows regulation of this core interaction and the overall therapeutic process in a culturally competent manner.

The just-described basic professional qualities — cultural sensitivity, cultural knowledge, cultural empathy, culturally relevant relations and interaction, and cultural guidance — are essential for performing culturally competent clinical work. It is the goal of training in cultural psychiatry for clinicians.

III. GENERAL CULTURAL PSYCHIATRIC TRAINING

It is becoming the common view that every psychiatrist needs cultural psychiatric training as part of his formal curriculum so that culture-relevant care can be provided for patients of diverse cultural backgrounds. The same view is held regarding training in ethnic and cultural diversity for professional psychologists to increase treatment efficacy (Toia, Herron, Primavera, & Javier, 1997; Yutrzenka, 1995). This is a contemporary clinical demand in many societies, particularly multiethnic societies.

In the United States, effective January 2001, the revised accreditation standards set up by the Accreditation Council for Graduate Medical Education Program Requirements for Residency Training in Psychiatry include several key innovations in cultural psychiatry training (ACGME, 2000). They include the following:

Regarding the scope of education, it is now stated: "The didactic and clinical program must be of sufficient breadth and depth to provide residents with a thorough and well-balanced presentation of psychological, sociocultural, and neurobiological observations and theories and knowledge of major diagnostic and therapeutic procedures in the field of psychiatry.

Objectives of training for residents second through fourth year now include "sensitivity to cultural diversity."

Concerning curriculum, the didactic components "should include such issues as gender, race, ethnicity, socioeconomic status, religion/spirituality, and sexual orientation.... Understanding cultural diversity is an essential characteristic of good clinical care."

"Didactic exercises must include resident presentation and discussion of clinical case material at confer-ences attended by faculty and fellow residents. This training should involve experiences in integrative case formulation that includes neurobiological, phenomenological, psychological, and sociocultural issues involved in diagnosis and management of cases presented."

As for the evaluation of resident competencies, there is a new section that requires programs to assess a resident's performance in six core competencies: patient care, medical knowledge, practice-based learning and improvement, interpersonal and communication skills, professionalism and systems-based practice. Cultural issues can be seen in the patient care, interpersonal and communicaiton skills and professionalism competencies.

In general, many cultural psychiatrists consider that the practical aspects of providing culture-competent training for psychiatry residents can be elaborated from several perspectives, as follows.

A. FORMAT OF TEACHING

1. Formal Didactic Seminar

In the same way as basic clinical psychiatry, cultural psychiatry could be taught through a formal didactic seminar. The advantage of this approach is that comprehensive topics relating to cultural psychiatry could be reviewed in a given period of time. Ideally cultural psychiatry should be taught from the very beginning of the training and throughout the entire course of training program. Competing with the need for teaching other subjects, it would be practical to have the didactic seminar within an intermediately short period of time (about 3 to 4 months for 12 to 16 weekly sessions, for example). It would be preferable to have the didactic seminar in the second or third year of training, while there is a more urgent need for a basic seminar on general psychiatry in the early part of the program, in the first or second year.

2. Bedside Clinical Teaching

This form of teaching should be provided from the very beginning of the training program to the end. The need for incorporating cultural dimensions into clinical assessment and care should be a focus from the beginning clinical training, rather than waiting until a didactic seminar in the later stages. The emphasis needs to be on how to distinguish among biological, psychological, social, and cultural impacts on clinical issues. The broad impact of culture on stress, the formation of pathology, as well as clinical care could be addressed in many cases. It is important to develop the attitude that cultural orientation and attention are needed for every patient, not because he or she happens to be part of an ethnic minority or a foreigner. It is more essential to learn to distinguish to what extent sociocultural dimensions need proper consideration due to the nature of the problems rather than underemphasize, or overstress, cultural factors in every case. In addition to biological and psychological dimensions, learning how to incorporate the sociocultural dimension in case formulation is an important task to master.

3. Cultural Psychiatry Conference or Round

Based on the availability of clinical material and the overall structure of the training program, it is desirable to periodically hold cultural psychiatry case conferences or rounds. These will provide the opportunities to elaborate on and discuss cultural issues in detail and depth. Suitable cases should be selected for discussion. Medical anthropologists, cross-cultural psychologists, and other culture-related disciplines, as well as a culture resource person, may be invited to participate in the discussion.

4. Cultural Psychiatry Supervision or Consultation

As in regular clinical teaching, clinical supervision or consultation is essential. The availability of supervision or consultation from culturally competent supervisors or experts will make the learning process much more efficient and effective.

It may often be the case that qualified and experienced cultural psychiatrists are not available in a train-

ing setting. It may also be difficult to get faculty (even part-time or affiliated faculty) with backgrounds in medical anthropology or cross-cultural psychology who could expose trainees to cultural psychiatry from a broader perspective. It may be necessary for trainees to rely on temporary visiting consultants. Even if a clinical supervisor does not have expertise as a cultural psychiatrist, as long as he or she is sensitive to and oriented toward the cultural dimensions of human behavior and mental disorders, he or she can still be of value to a student.

5. Other Teaching Strategies

There are many other ways to help the trainees learn to better appreciate the impact of culture on our lives and mental health and on clinical practice. For instance, if the seminar were composed of participants from different ethnic/racial groups, their life experiences and cultural views could be shared so that the impact of culture on them could be more vividly expressed. Knowing you own culture as well as others' is important in becoming culturally sensitive.

Besides suggested reading material for topics to be covered, audio-visual materials could be utilized to maximize the actual impact. Showing films from other cultures, followed by discussions of the cultural aspects in them, would be useful for those who have never had life experiences outside of their home countries or exposure to other cultures. Family conferences that expose trainees to the folk beliefs of the family members and their cultural interpretation of the illness involved would also be valuable. These are merely examples of many possible teaching strategies.

B. Subjects to be Covered in Training

Based on the professional opinions and backgrounds of the faculty, the subjects that are included in cultural psychiatric training could vary greatly. There is currently no consensus of what areas should be covered, even among cultural psychiatric experts. The rule of thumb is to include subjects that are relevant to the clinical setting, the interests of the trainees, and the experience of the faculty.

1. Topics to be Covered

The core subjects to be included in training are those that cover the scope of cultural psychiatry broadly rather than in too much detail only in certain areas. It is more important for the trainees to gain a sense of the way in which cultural factors have an overall impact on clinical psychiatry. For this reason, it is suggested that the following subjects (as reflected on the contents of this book) be considered for inclusion.

a. The impact of culture on human behavior in general. This may include how culture contributes to personality formation, behavior, the family system, and life cycle.
b. Cultural influences on mental health. This refers to how culture contributes to stress and coping, the recognition and perception of problems, and illness behavior, including help-seeking behavior in folk as well as conventional medical systems.
c. The effects of culture on psychopathology. This concerns the way culture influences the formation and manifestation of psychopathology. Besides general concepts, the impact of culture on various mental disorders could be examined.
d. Culture contributions to the clinical practice of psychiatry. This refers to the way in which culture impacts clinical practice in terms of making assessments and diagnoses of various psychiatric disorders according to descriptive classification, and delivery of care. It also includes how minorities, racism, folk beliefs, traditional medical knowledge, attitudes toward the mentally ill, and other factors influence the treatment of mental patients.
e. Cultural modeling of psychological treatment. This covers the kinds of folk or indigenous healing practices that are available and utilized

by people; how the theory and practice of psychotherapy, even contemporary, mainstream therapy, are shaped by the culture in which it is practiced; and how to provide culture-relevant psychotherapy in transcultural situations.
f. Culture-related special social phenomena. This concerns certain special social phenomena, such as cultural change, migration, refugees, minority issues, religion and spirituality, and so on, that are closely associated to clinical practice and about which clinicians need to have some knowledge and understanding.
g. Cultural knowledge regarding particular ethnic or cultrual groups. Since it is impossible to study and learn about the cultural systems of all ethnic groups that exist in the world, there is a need to obtain at least basic cultural knowledge of any ethnic groups that are to be served in their clinical setting. This may include their ethnic histories, commonly held folk beliefs, attitudes toward mental illness, help-seeking behavior, coping patterns, and so on.

2. Material for Reading

The volume of published articles and books in the area of cultural psychiatry is expanding rapidly, providing abundant reading material for teaching. It is difficult to provide a comprehensive list of reading material, as teaching depends on the interests and level of sophistication of the trainees, as well as the trainer's professional judgement. Based on these considerations, the individual trainer could select reading material. (Chapter references and books relating to culture, psychiatry, and mental health, listed in the Appendix, could serve as resources for selection.)

C. Stages of Training

Successful clinical training needs to take into consideration the various stages and progression of effective training. It is commonly understood that clinical training in any field should start early to orient and familiarize the trainees with the issues concerned; however, it is also practically impossible to focus on everything from the start. This is the dilemma faced in any training program, including cultural psychiatric training. Thus, a general map of the stages of training is needed.

1. Initial Stage

Generally speaking, at the very beginning of the training, the focus should be primarily on increasing the awareness that culture shapes human behavior, even illness. Then the focus can move on to cultural aspects of clinical assessment and establishing professionally correct and culturally relevant working relations with the patient and his or her family. In this stage, training could be conducted mainly in brief introductory (or orientation) seminars, through bedside clinical teaching and supervision.

2. Middle Stage

This stage could proceed to an understanding of how culture contributes to the nature of stress and the various manifestations of psychopathology. It would include culturally suitable diagnosis and case formulation — a comprehensive and dynamic understanding of the nature of the problems. Formal didactic seminars and cultural case conferences or rounds could be utilized in this stage. Additionally, emphasis could be placed on how to provide clinically and culturally appropriate and effective treatment for the patient. This would include ethnic–racial–cultural aspects of biological, psychopharmacological, psychological, and environmental approaches of treatment.

3. Later Stage

This final stage of training should focus on learning more about cultural psychiatry-related knowledge in other cultural settings and international circumstances. The subjects of cross-cultural comparisons of psychopathology, including culture-related specific syndromes and various forms of indigenous healing practices, could be introduced. The emphasis should

be on understanding the nature of human behavior and the mental health situation worldwide, beyond one's own society.

D. Model Curricula for Specific Focus

Based on actual experiences in clinical teaching, different model curricula have been proposed by several clinicians and scholars during the past several years for particular topics or for specific ethnic groups. For instance, Garza-Trevino, Ruiz, and Varegos-Samuel (1997) have proposed a teaching program for the care of Hispanic patients, Thomson (1996) one for American Indians and Alaskan natives. Larson, Lu, and Swyers (1997) have suggested model curriculum focused on religion and spirituality in clinical practice; Spielvogel, Dickson, and Robinson (1995) on gender and women's issues; and Stein (1994) on homosexuality, gay men, and lesbians. Thus, the scope and focus of teaching of cultural psychiatry through formal curricula has been continuously expanding.

IV. ADVANCED TRAINING FOR CAREER DEVELOPMENT

Beyond basic cultural psychiatric training for all psychiatrists-in-training, there is a need to form an advanced training program for those who are interested in cultural psychiatry as a professional specialty or for their career development. Those trainees might consider the following several suggestions.

A. Working Professionally in Foreign Cultures

It is a very valuable personally and professionally to live and practice in foreign countries or societies with very different cultural systems than one's own. The cultural dimensions of psychiatry will certainly be highlighted when a trainee directly and practically experiences the impact of culture on psychiatric practice. It was through such experiences that many pioneer cultural psychiatrists became interested and knowledgeable in this field. It is difficult to expect all psychiatrists-in-training to have this kind of unique cultural experience; perhaps it could be substituted by audio-visual materials on other cultures. However, personal experience is very desirable for those who are pursuing cultural psychiatry as a professional career. While it is better to spend a longer period of time gaining a deep understanding of one of two cultural settings, it is also useful to have encounters with multiple, diverse cultural systems. It certainly will help trainees to learn the differences between universally observed human behavior and culture-molded, specific behavior. It will not merely be a valuable life experience, but would stimulate trainees to study cultural systems as a whole, in addition to learning about clinically related issues through reading and field encounters.

For practical reasons, living in remote areas with unique cultural settings is not easy, and sometimes impossible. However, it should be mentioned that even within one's own country or neighborhood, there are many culturally diverse people, often not too far away. They may be immigrants or refugees from other cultures, indigenous people, or socioculturally deprived people who live in different socioeconomic–cultural settings. Working with such diversified subcultural groups could have a learning effect similar to actually living in another society. This kind of experience may be supplemented by short-term travel or visits to other countries to experience the cultures in their home settings.

B. Mentoring with Senior Cultural Psychiatrists

Merely being exposed to other cultures is not enough. It would also be desirable to have experienced, senior cultural psychiatrists who are willing to offer trainees guidance and suggestions for learning. Through such mentorships, the training would be strengthened and learned much faster and in a more correct direction. If possible, it is recommended that

trainees have several mentors with different expertise to gain broader views. For example, one mentor could be an expert on a particular cultural or ethnic group, and another on the psychological consequences of severe trauma and forced migration among refugees.

C. Taking Culture-Related Academic Courses

In order to obtain in-depth knowledge and insight, cultural psychiatry could be approached through other related scientific fields, such as cultural anthropology, medical sociology, cross-cultural psychology, or community healing. Although it would be more comprehensive to take courses formally and obtain an academic degree for them, this could be time-consuming. Taking some courses and reading, as well as consulting with scholars in these related fields, are alternative choices.

D. Participating in Cross-Cultural Research Efforts and Programs

Participating in research programs would provide actual opportunities to learn how culture contributes to human behavior and mental health, as well as to mental problems. Research projects in other societies or foreign cultures would be desirable; but even within one's own societies, there are ample opportunities to carry out research that directly relates to cultural matters. Such field work would certainly enrich our clinical and scientific experience.

E. Involvement in Advanced Cultural Psychiatry Workshops

Because there are few formal programs for advanced training, an alternative way of pursuing a career in this field is to become involved in any advanced cultural psychiatry workshops or study courses available. Joining a cultural psychiatry study group or association would certainly be beneficial. It would not only provide the chance to gain a wide range of advanced knowledge, but also the opportunity to meet and relate to experts in the field — a valuable experience in this special area at this stage of development.

F. Participating in an International Cultural Psychiatry Conference

Finally, it would be desirable to participate in a cultural psychiatry conference that was organized and held at an international level, either as an independent event or as a workshop or seminar at a larger convention. This would offer professionals the opportunity to meet colleagues from various countries and obtain a general sense of and a broader perspective on various issues studied in different countries of distinctly divergent cultural settings.

V. CLOSING: THE FUTURE OF CULTURAL PSYCHIATRY

Cultural psychiatry as a special subfield of psychiatry emerged only a few decades ago. It started with a primary interest in research into how culture impacts psychopathology. Gradually, it focused on clinical aspects; how to provide culture-relevant clinical service for patients of diverse cultural backgrounds. It is gradually moving away from a narrow attention on minority issues to address culture broadly in terms of world perspectives. It is predicted that, in the future, cultural psychiatry as a special subfield of general psychiatry will move forward in the following directions.

A. Clinical Application beyond Academic Research

Cultural psychiatry has been moving in this direction for a couple of decades, and will continue to do so. It is not merely a field of research, but is clinically oriented. Any study will end with the benefit of contributing to our knowledge of how to provide culturally relevant, effective therapy for patients of diversified ethnic or cultural backgrounds. More clinical research will, or should, be undertaken to explore whether there is any particular mode of therapy or emphasis in treatment that will better suit a patient of a particular cultural background. This issue will be considered not only at the level of ethnic minorities within societies, but also at cross-societal and cross-national levels for majority groups.

B. Move from an Ethnic-Minority Focus to Worldwide Cultural Concern

Although the emphasis on how to develop and improve culturally relevant care for underserved and unsuitably cared for ethnic minorities needs to be addressed from a practical perspective, from an academic point of view, the focus of cultural psychiatry needs to move and expand to include more worldwide aspects. This will give the field a broader base of information and knowledge and enable it to establish a sounder academic foundation. Comparing situations in distinctly divergent cultural settings and examining lifestyles and mental health problems that have more obvious and wider differences will stimulate us to comprehend the impact of culture on mental health and psychiatry at higher levels. It will certainly help us understand universal aspects as well as culture-specific or -modified situations.

C. Theoretical Elaboration beyond Clinical Concerns

It is time for cultural psychiatrists to move into the areas of theoretical examination and elaboration beyond clinical issues. This is not simply due to the increase in information from worldwide sources, which has contributed to a better understanding of the issues of universality versus culture specificity. It is also because cultural psychiatrists, joined by many non-Western, nonmainstream professionals, are becoming free from ethnic- or culture-centered views, explanations, and theories of human behavior and mental illness. It offers opportunities to reexamine established theories and revise or even develop new theories of interpreting and understanding the nature of human behavior and personality formation, the occurrence of stress and problems, coping styles, the development of psychopathology, mechanisms of therapy, and so on.

D. BALANCING OVEREMPHASIZED BIOLOGICAL PSYCHIATRY

With the remarkable progress in biological psychiatry over the past several decades, there has been significant improvement in understanding the psychopathology and treatment of mental disorders. At the same time, the whole field of psychiatry has been so colored by the overemphasis on biological psychiatry that psychological psychiatry, including the psychological understanding of human behavior and mental health, as well as psychological therapy, has been seriously neglected. This has resulted in an imbalance in psychiatry from practical as well as academic perspectives.

Sociocultural psychiatry will help the field regain a balance in concerns, orientations, knowledge, and theories. At the opposite end of the spectrum from a biological orientation, a cultural orientation will help psychiatrists maintain a holistic view of and approach to the human mind and the care of the mentally ill. In this regard, cultural psychiatry could make a significant contribution through its specific focus and concern.

E. CONTRIBUTIONS TO GENERAL PSYCHIATRY AS A WHOLE

In addition to correcting the present imbalance in emphasis in contemporary psychiatry, cultural psychiatry will continue to make a useful contribution to general psychiatry. It will stimulate psychiatrists to examine the extent to which the knowledge, experience, and theories of psychiatry are locally or culturally bound, versus what is universal for humankind. Such a broad world perspective will enrich and strengthen the nature and quality of psychiatry. This is one of the significant contributions that cultural psychiatry offers to psychiatry in general and is one of its most important, ultimate, and timeless goals.

REFERENCES

Accreditation Council for Graduate Medical Education (ACGME). (2000). *Program requirements for residency training in psychiatry.* Chicago: Accreditation Council for Graduate Medical Education.

Alarcón, R.D., Westermeyer, J., Foulks, E.F., & Ruiz, P. (1999). Clinical relevance of contemporary cultural psychiatry. *Journal of Nervous and Mental Disease, 187,* 465–471.

American Medical Association (AMA). (1999). *Cultural competence compendium.* Chicago: American Medical Association.

American Psychiatric Association. (1994). *Diagnostic and statistical manual of mental disorders* (4th ed.). Washington, DC: APA.

Foulks, E. (1980). The concept of culture in psychiatric residency education. *American Journal of Psychiatry, 137,* 811–816.

Foulks, E., Westermeyer, J., & Ta, K. (1998). Developing curricula for transcultural mental health for trainees and trainers. In S.O. Okpaku (Ed.), *Clinical methods in transcultural psychiatry* (pp. 339–362). Washington, DC: American Psychiatric Press.

Garza-Trevino, E.S., Ruiz, P., & Varegos-Samuel, K. (1997). A psychiatry curriculum directed to the care of the Hispanic patient. *Academic Psychiatry, 21* (1), 1–10.

Gopaul-McNicol, S.A., & Brice-Baker, J. (1998). *Cross-cultural practice: Assessment, treatment, and training.* New York: Wiley.

Jeffress, J.E. (1968). Training transcultural psychiatry in the United States: A 1968 survey. *International Journal of Social Psychiatry, 19*(1), 69–72.

Jordan, D. (1995). Cultural competence and desistance of planning care model: Consolidation of two planning strategies. Presented at the *Cultural Competence Summit:* San Francisco, November 2.

Larson, D., Lu, F., & Swyers, J. (1997). *Model curriculum for psychiatry residency training programs: Religion and spirituality in clinical practice,* revised edition. Rockville, MD: The National Institute for Healthcare Research.

Lefley, H.P., & Pedersen, P.B. (1986). *Cross-cultural training for mental health professionals.* Springfield, IL: Charles C. Thomas.

Lu, F., Lim, R., & Mezzich, J. (1995). Issues in the assessment and diagnosis of culturally diverse individuals. In P. Ruitz (Ed.),

Annual review of psychiatry (pp. 477–510). Washington, DC: American Psychiatric Press.

Moffic M.S., Kendrick, E.A., Lomax, J.W., & Reid, K. (1987). Education in cultural psychiatry in the United States. *Transcultural Psychiatric Research Review, 24*(3), 167–187.

Moffic M.S., Kendrick, E.A., & Reid, K. (1988). Cultural psychiatry education during psychiatric residency. *Journal of Psychiatric Education, 12,* 90–101.

Pinderhughes, E. (1984). Teaching empathy: Ethnicity, race, and power at the cross-cultural treatment interface. *American Journal of Social Psychiatry, 4,* 5–12.

Rogers, M.R., Ponterott, J.G., Conoley, J.C., & Wiese, M.J. (1992). Multicultural training in school psychology: A national survey. *School Psychology Review, 21,* 603–616.

Spielvogel, A., Dickson, L., & Robinson, G. (1995). A psychiatric residency curriculum about gender and women's issues. *Academic Psychiatry, 19* (4), 187–201.

Stein, T.S. (1994). A curriculum for learning in psychiatry residencies about homosexuality, gay men and lesbians. *Academic Psychiatry, 18* (2), 59–70.

Thompson, J. (1996). A curriculum for learning about American Indians and Alaska Natives in psychiatry residency training. *Academic Psychiatry, 20* (1), 5–14.

Toia, A., Herron, W.G., Primavera, L.H., & Javier, R.A. (1997). Ethnic diversification in clinical psychology graduate training. *Cultural Diversity and Mental Health, 3*(3), 193–206.

Tseng, W.S., & Hsu, J. (1979). Culture and psychotherapy. In A.J. Marsella, R.G. Tharp, & T.J. Ciborowski (Eds.), *Perspectives on cross-cultural psychology.* New York: Academic Press.

Tseng, W.S., & Streltzer, J. (2001). Integration and conclusion. In W.S. Tseng & J. Streltzer (Eds.), *Culture and psychotherapy: A guide for clinical practice* (pp. 265–278). Washington, DC: American Psychiatric Press.

Westermeyer, J. (1989). *The psychiatric care of migrants: A clinical guide.* Washington, DC: American Psychiatric Press.

Westermeyer, J. (1990). Working with an interpreter in psychiatric assessment and treatment. *Journal of Nervous and Mental Disease, 178,* 745–749.

Yutrzenka, B.A. (1995). Making a case for training in ethnic and cultural diversity in increasing treatment efficacy. *Journal of Consulting and Clinical Psychology, 63*(2), 197–206.

Appendix: List of Books Relating to the Subject of Culture, Psychiatry, and Mental Health

A. CULTURAL PSYCHIATRY IN TEXTBOOK STYLE

Kiev, A. (1972). *Transcultural psychiatry*. New York: Free Press.

Pfeiffer, W.M. (1970). *Transkulturelle psychiatrie: Ergebnisse und probleme* [Transcultural psychiatry: Results and problems]. Stuttgart: Thieme. (Reviewed in *Transcultural Psychiatry Research Review, 7,* 113–118 [1970])

Pfeiffer, W.M. (1994). *Transkulturelle psychiatrie: Ergebnisse und probleme* (Transcultural psychiatry: Results and problems) (2 ed.). Stuttgart: Thieme. Reviewed in *Transcultural Psychiatry Research Review, 32,* 59–64 [1995]

Tseng, W.S., & McDermott, J.F., Jr. (1981). *Culture, mind and therapy: An introduction to cultural psychiatry*. New York: Brunner/Mazel.

B. CULTURAL PSYCHIATRY OR ETHNOPSYCHIATRY WITH MIXED TOPICS

de Reuck, A.V.S., & Porter, R. (Eds.). (1965) *Transcultural psychiatry* (Ciba Foundation Symposium). Boston: Little, Brown.

Devereux, G. (1980). *Basic problems of ethnopsychiatry*. Chicago: University of Chcago Press.

Fernando, S. (1988). *Race and culture in psychiatry*. London: Croom Helm.

Fernando, S. (1991). *Mental health, race and culture*. New York: St. Martin's Press.

Foulks, E.F., Wintrob, R.M., Westermeyer, J., & Favazza, A.R. (1977). *Current perspectives in cultural psychiatry*. New York: Spectrum.

Gaines, A.D. (Ed.). (1992). *Ethnopsychiatry: The cultural construction of professional and folk psychiatries*. Albany: State University of New York Press.

Gaw, A. (Ed.). (1993). *Culture, ethnicity, and mental illness*. Washington, DC: American Psychiatric Press.

Gopaul-McNicol, S.A., & Brice-Baker, J. (1998). *Cross-cultural practice: Assessment, treatment, and training*. New York: Wiley.

Hoffmann, K., & Machceidt, W. (Eds.). *Psychiatrie im kulturvergleich* [Psychiatry in cross-cultural comparison]. Berlin: Voriae für Wissenschaft und Bildung.

Littlewood, R. (1998/2000). *The butterfly and the serpent: Essays in psychiatry, race and religion*. London: Free Association Books.

Marsella, A.J., & White, G.M. (Eds.). (1982). *Cultural conceptions of mental health and therapy*. Dordrecht, The Netherlands: Reidel.

Mezzich, J.E., & Berganza, C.E. (Eds.) (1984). *Culture and psychopathology*. New York: Columbia University Press.

Murphy, J.M., & Leighton, A.H. (Eds.). (1965). *Approaches to cross-cultural psychiatry*. Ithaca, NY: Cornell University Press.

Okpaku, S.O. (Ed.). (1998). *Clinical methods in transcultural psychiatry*. Washington, DC: American Psychiatric Press.

Opler, M.K. (1967). *Culture and social psychiatry*. New York: Atherton Press.

Rack, P. (1982). *Race, culture, and mental disorder*. London: Tavistock.

Westermeyer, J. (1976). *Anthropology and mental health: Setting a new course*. Paris: Mouton.

C. Cultural Psychiatry Issues from Worldwide Multiple Regions

Al-Issa, I. (Ed.). (1995). *Handbook of culture and mental illness: An international perspective.* Madison, CT: International Universities Press.

Brown, B.S., & Torrey, E.F. (1973). *International collaboration in mental health.* Rockville, MD: U.S. Department of Health, Education, and Welfare, National Institute of Mental Health.

Cox, J.L. (Ed.). (1986). *Transcultural psychiatry.* London: Croom Helm.

Leff, J. (1987). *Psychiatry around the globe: A transcultural view.* London: Gaskell.

Price, R.K., Shea, B.M., & Mookherjee, H.N. (Eds.). (1995). *Social psychiatry across cultures: Studies from North America, Asia, Europe, and Africa.* New York: Plenum Press.

D. Cultural Psychiatry with Particular Issues

Favazza, A.R. (1987). *Bodies under siege: Self-mutilation and body modification in culture and psychiatry.* Baltimore: Johns Hapkins University Press.

Favazza, A.R. (1996). *Bodies under siege: Self-mutilation and body modification in culture and psychiatry* (2nd ed.). Baltimore: Johns Hopkins University Press.

Kleinman, A. (1980). *Patients and healers in the context of culture: An exploration of the borderland between anthropology, medicine, and psychiatry.* Berkeley: University of California Press.

Kleinman, A. (1988). *Rethinking psychiatry: From cultural category to personal experience.* New York: Free Press.

Szasz, T.S. (1961). *The myth of mental illness: Foundations of a theory of personal conduct.* New York: Hoeber-Harper.

Townsend, J.M. (1978). *Cultural conceptions of mental illness.* Chicago: University of Chcago Press.

E. Culture and Mental Health Issues

Comas-Díaz, L., & Griffith, E.E.H. (Eds.). *Clinical guidelines in cross-cultural mental health.* New York: Wiley.

Desjarlais, R., Eisenberg, L., Good, B., & Kleinman, A. (1995). *World mental health: Problems in low-income countries.* New York: Oxford University Press.

Gamwell, L., & Tomes, N. (1995). *Madness in America: Culture and medical perceptions of mental illness before 1914.* Ithaca, NY: Cornell University Press.

Nann, R.C., Butt, D.S., & Ladrido-Ignacio, L. (Eds.). (1984). *Mental health, cultural values, and social development: A look into the 80's.* Dordrecht, The Netherlands: Reidel.

F. Cultural Anthropology and Medical Anthropology

Bourguignon, E. (Ed.). (1973). *Religion, altered states of consciousness, and social change.* Columbus: Ohio State University Press.

Devereux, G. (1978). *Ethnopsychoanalysis: Psychoanalysis and anthropology as complementary frames of reference.* Berkeley: University of California Press.

Helman, C.G. (1994). *Culture, health and illness: An introduction for health professioals* (3rd ed.). Oxford: Butterworth-Heinemann.

Hernandi, P. (1995). *Cultural transactions: Nature, self, society.* Ithaca, NY: Cornell University Press.

Hoebel, E.A. (1972). *Anthropology: The study of man.* New York: McGraw-Hill.

Hsu, F.L.K. (Ed.). (1972). *Psychological anthropology.* Cambridge, MA: Schenkman.

Ingham, J.M. (1996). *Psychological anthropology reconsidered.* Cambridge, UK: Cambridge University Press.

Jaoda, G. (1992). *Crossroads between culture and mind: Continuities and change in theories of human nature.* New York: Harvester Wheatsheaf.

Johnson, T.M., & Sargent, C.F. (Eds.). (1990). *Medical anthropology: Contemporary theory and method.* Westport, CT: Praeger.

Keesing, R.M. (1976). *Cultural anthropology: A contemporary perspective.* New York: Holt, Rinehart & Winston.

Kottak, C.P. (1994). *Cultural anthropology,* (6th ed.). New York: Mcgraw-Hill.

Kottak, C.P. (1999). *Mirror for humanity: A concise introduction to cultural anthropology.* Boston: McGraw-Hill College.

Landy, D. (Ed.). (1977). *Culture, disease, and healing: Studies in medical anthropology.* New York: Macmillan.

Mascie-Taylor, C.G.N. (Ed.). (1993). *The anthropology of disease.* New York: Oxford University Press.

Nanda, S. (1980). *Cultural anthropology.* New York: Van Nostrand.

Romanucci-Ross, L., Moerman, D.E., & Tancredi, L.R. (Eds.). (1991). *Anthropology of medicine: From culture to method,* (2nd ed.). Westport, CT: Bergin & Garvey.

Spiro, M.E. (Ed.). (1965). *Context and meaning in cultural anthropology.* New York: Free Press.

G. Culture and Personality

Barnouw, V. (1963). *Culture and personality.* Homewood, IL: Dorsey Press.

Inkeles, A. (1997). *National character: A psycho-social perspective.* New Brunswick, NJ: Transaction.

Kaplan, B. (Ed.). (1961). *Studying personality cross-culturally.* New York: Harper & Row.

Kluckhohn, C., & Murray, H.A. (Eds.). (1953). *Personality in nature, society, and culture* (2nd ed.). New York: Alfred A. Knopf.

Wallace, A.F.C. (1970). *Culture and personality* (2nd ed.). New York: Random House.

H. Culture and Social Psychiatry

Bergen, B.J., & Thomas, C.S. (Eds.). (1966). *Issues and problems in social psychiatry: A book of readings.* Springfield, IL: Charles C. Thomas.

Cockerham, W.C. (2000). *Sociology of mental disorder* (5th ed.). Upper Saddle River, NJ: Prentice Hall.

Ginsburg, S.W. (1963). *A psychiatrists's view on social issues.* New York: Columbia University Press.

Kato Price, R.K., Shea, B.M., & Mookherjee, H.N. (Eds.). (1995). *Social psychiatry across cultures.* New York: Plenum Press.

Sorel, E., Favazza, A., et al. (Eds.). (1993). *Social psychiatry in the late twentieth century: Selected proceedings – 12th World Congress of Social Psychiatry.* Brooklyn, NY: Legas.

Vanneman, R., & Cannon, L.W. (1987). *The American perception of class.* Philadelphia: Temple University Press.

Willie, C.V., Rieker, P.P., Kramer, B.M., & Brown, B.S. (Eds.). (1995). *Mental health, racism, and sexism.* Pittsburgh: University of Pittsburgh Press.

Zubin, J., & Freyhan, F.A. (Eds.). (1968). *Social psychiatry.* New York: Grune & Stratton.

I. Cross-Cultural Psychology

Adler, L.L., & Gielen, U.P. (Eds.). (1994). *Cross-cultural topics in psychology.* Westport, CT: Praeger.

Berry, J.W., Dasen, P.R., & Saraswathi, T.S. (Eds.). (1997). *Handbook of cross-cultural psychology:* 2nd ed., Vol. 2. *Basic process and human development.* Boston: Allyn & Bacon.

Berry, J.W., Poortinga, Y.H., & Pandey, J. (Eds.). (1996). *Handbook of cross-cultural psychology:* 2nd ed., Vol. 1. *Theory and method.* Boston: Allyn & Bacon.

Berry, J.W., Poortinga, Y.H., Segall, M.H., & Dasen, P.R. (1992). *Cross-cultural psychology: Research and applications.* Cambridge, UK: Cambridge University Press.

Berry, J.W., Segal, M.H., & Kagitçibasi, C. (Eds.). (1997). *Handbook of cross-cultural psychology: 2nd ed., Vol. 3. Social behavior and applications.* Boston: Allyn & Bacon.

Brislin, R.W. (Ed.). (1990). *Applied cross-cultural psychology.* Newbury Park, CA: Sage.

Brislin, R.W. (2000). *Understanding culture's influence on behavior* (2nd ed.). Fort Worth, TX: Harcourt.

Cole, M. (1996). *Cultural psychology: A once and future discipline.* Cambridge, MA: Harvard University Press.

Fox, D., & Prilleltensky, I. (1997). *Critical psychology: An introduction.* London: Sage.

Javier, R.A., & Herron, W.G. (Eds.). (1998). *Personality development and psychotherapy in our diverse society: A source book.* Northvale, NJ: Jason Aronson.

Kazarian, S.S., & Evans, D.E. (Eds.). (1998). *Cultural clinical psychology: Theory, research, and practice.* New York: Oxford University Press.

Marsella, A.J., Tharp, R.G., & Ciborowski, T.J. (1979). *Perspectives on cross-cultural psychology.* New York: Academic Press.

Rokeach, M. (1980). *Beliefs, attitudes, and values: A theory of organization and change.* San Francisco: Jossey-Bass. [Original work published 1968]

Roland, A. (1988). *In search of self in India and Japan: Toward a cross-cultural psychology.* Princeton, NJ: Princeton University Press.

Segall, M.H. (1979). *Cross-cultural psychology: Human behavior in global perspective.* Monterey, CA: Brooks/Cole.

Segall, M.H., Dasen, P.R., Berry, J.W., & Poortinga, Y.H. (1990). *Human behavior in global perspective: An intro-*

duction to cross-cultural psychology. New York: Pergamon Press.

Triandis, H.C. (1994). *Culture and social behavior.* New York: McGraw-Hill.

Triandis, H.C., & Berry, J.W. (Eds.). (1980). *Handbook of cross-cultural psychology: Vol. 2. Methodology.* Boston: Allyn & Bacon.

Triandis, H.C., & Brislin, R.W. (Eds.). (1980). *Handbook of cross-cultural psychology: Vol. 5. Social Psychology.* Boston: Allyn & Bacon.

Triandis, H.C., & Draguns, J.G. (Eds.). (1980). *Handbook of cross-cultural psychology: Vol. 6. Psychopathology.* Boston: Allyn & Bacon.

Triandis, H.C., & Heron, A. (Eds.). (1980). *Handbook of cross-cultural psychology: Vol. 4. Developmental psychology.* Boston: Allyn & Bacon.

Triandis, H.C., & Lambert, W.W. (Eds.). (1980). *Handbook of cross-cultural psychology: Vol. 1. Perspectives.* Boston: Allyn & Bacon.

Triandis, H.C., & Lonner, W. (Eds.). (1980). *Handbook of cross-cultural psychology: Vol. 3. Basic process.* Boston: Allyn & Bacon.

Warren, N. (Ed.). (1977). *Studies in cross-cultural psychology.* London: Academic Press.

J. Psychological Measurement and Research

Brislin, R.W., Lonner, W.J., & Thorndike, R.M. (1973). *Cross-cultural research methods.* New York: Wiley.

Cronbach, L.J., & Drenth, P.J.D. (Eds.). (1972). *Mental tests and cultural adaptation.* The Hague, The Netherlands: Mouton.

Dana, R.H. (1993). *Multicultural assessment perspectives for professional psychology.* Boston: Allyn & Bacon.

Irvin, S.H., & Berry, J.W. (Eds.). (1983). *Human assessment and cultural factors.* New York: Plenum Press.

Lonner, W.J., & Berry, J.W. (Eds.). (1986). *Fields methods in cross-cultural research.* Newbury Park, CA: Sage.

Ratner, C. (1997). *Cultural psychology and qualitative methodology: Theoretical and empirical considerations.* New York: Plenum Press.

Samuda, R.J. (1998). *Psychological testing of American minorities: Issues and consequences* (2nd ed.). Thousand Oaks, CA: Sage.

Sodowsky, G.R., & Impara, J.C. (Eds.). (1996). *Multicultural assessment in counseling and clinical psychology.* Lincoln, NE: Buros Institute of Mental Measurement.

Spielberger, C.D., & Dias-Guerrero, R. (Eds.). (1976). *Cross-cultural anxiety.* Washington, DC: Hemisphere.

Suzuki, L.A., Meller, P.J., & Ponterotto, J.G. (Eds.). (1996). *Handbook of multicultural assessment: Clinical, psychological, and educational applications.* San Francisco: Jossey-Bass.

K. Clinical Assessment, Diagnosis and Classification

Cooper, J.E., Kendell, R.E., Gurland, B.J., Sharpe, L., Copeland, J.R.M., & Simon, R. (1972). *Psychiatric diagnosis in New York and London.* London: Oxford University Press.

Mezzich, J.E., Honda, Y., & Kastrup, M. (Eds.). (1994). *Psychiatric diagnosis: A world perspective.* New York: Springer-Verlag.

Mezzich, J.E., Kleinman, A., Fabrega, H.J., & Parron, D.L. (Eds.). (1996). *Culture and psychiatric diagnosis: A DSM-IV perspective.* Washington, DC: American Psychiatric Press.

Tseng, W.S., & Streltzer, J. (Eds.). (1997). *Culture and psychopathology: A clinical guidance for assessment.* New York: Brunner/Mazel.

L. Comparative Psychiatry

Calloway, P. (1993). *Russian/Sovient and Western psychiatry: A contemporary comparative study.* New York: Wiley.

Lenz, H. (1964). *Vergleickende psychiatrie* [Comparative psychiatry]. Wien, Germany: W. Maudrkh Verlag.

Murphy, H.B.M. (1982). *Comparative psychiatry: The international and intercultural distribution of mental illness.* Berlin: Springer-Verlag.

Yap, P.M. (Edited by Lau, M.P., & Stokes, A.B.) (1974). *Comparative psychiatry: A theoretical framework.* Toronto: University of Toronto Press.

M. Psychiatric Epidemiology

Mezzich, J.E., Jorge, M.R., & Salloum, I.M. (Eds.). (1994). *Psychiatric epidemiology: Assessment concepts and methods.* Baltimore: Johns Hopkins University Press.

Robins, L.E., & Regier, D.A. (Eds.). (1991). *Psychiatric disorders in America: The Epidemiologic Catchment Area Study.* New York: Free Press.

Schwab, J.J., & Schwab, M.E. (1978). *Sociocultural roots of mental illness: An Epidemiologic Survey.* New York: Plenum Medical Book Company.

Srole, L., Langer, R.S., Michel, S.T., Opler, M.K., & Rennie, T.A.C. (1962). *Mental health in the metropolis.* New York: McGraw-Hill.

Templer, D.I., Spencer, D.A., & Hartlage, L.C. (1993). *Biosocial psychopathology: Epidemiological perspectives.* New York: Springer.

Tsuang, M.T., Tohen, M., & Zahner, G.E.P. (Eds.). (1995). *Textbook in psychiatric epidemiology.* New York: J Wiley.

Üstün, T.B., & Sartorius, N. (Eds.). (1995). *Mental illness in general health care: An international study.* Chichester: Wiley (on behaef of WHO).

N. PSYCHOPATHOLOGY IN GENERAL

Al-Issa, I. (Ed.). (1982). *Culture and psychopathology.* Baltimore: University Park Press.

Al-Issa, I. (Ed.). (1995). *Handbook of culture and mental illness: An international perspective.* Madison, CT: International University Press.

Bartocci, G. (Ed.). (1990). *Psicopatologia cultura e pensiero magico* [Psychopathology, culture and magic thought]. Napoli: Liguori Ed.

Ghadirian, A.M.A., & Lehmann, H.E. (Eds.). (1993). *Environment and psychopathology.* New York: Springer.

Leff, J. (1981). *Psychiatry around the globe.* New York: Dekker.

Linton, R. (1956). *Culture and mental disorders.* Springfield, IL: Charles C. Thomas.

Mezzich, J.E., & Berganza C.E. (1984). *Culture and psychopathology.* New York: Columbia University Press.

Pfeiffer, W., & Schoene, W. (Eds.). (1980). *Psychopathologie im kulturvergleich* [Psychopathology in cross-cultural comparison]. Stuttgart: Enke Verlag.

Seeman, M.V. (1995). *Gender and psychopathology.* Washington, DC: American Psychiatric Press.

O. PSYCHOPATHOLOGY OF SPECIAL KIND

1. Culture-Related Specific Syndromes

Friedmann, C.T.H., & Faguet, R.A. (Eds.). (1982). *Extraordinary disorders of human behavior.* New York: Plenum Press.

Rubel, A.J., O'Nell, C.W., & Collado-Ardon, R. (1984). *Susto: A folk illness.* Berkeley: University of California Press.

Simons, R.C. (1996). *Boo! — Culture, experience, and the startle relfex.* New York: Oxford University Press.

Simons, R.C., & Hughes, C.C. (Eds.). (1985). *The culture-bound syndromes: Folk illness of psychiatric and anthropological interest.* Dordrecht, The Netherlands: Reidel.

Winzeler, R.L. (1995). *Latah in Southeast Asia: The history and ethnography of a culture-bound syndrome.* Cambridge, UK: Cambridge University Press.

2. Anxiety Disorders, Including Posttaumatic Stress Disorder

Friedman, S. (Ed.). (1997). *Cultural issues in the treatment of anxiety.* New York: Guilford Press.

Marsella, A.J., Friedman, M.J., Gerrity, E.T., & Scurfield, R.M. (Eds.). (1996). *Ethnocultural aspects of posttraumatic stress disorder: Issues, research, and clinical applications.* Washington, DC: American Psychological Association.

Wilson, J.P., & Raphael, B. (Eds.). (1993). *International handbook of traumatic stress syndromes.* New York: Plenum Press.

Yamashita, I. (1993). Taijin-Kyofu *or delusional social phobia.* Sapporo, Japan: Hokkaido University Press.

3. Somatoform Disorders

Ono, Y., Janca, A., Asai, M., & Sartorius, N. (Eds.). (1999). *Somatoform disorders: A worldwide perspective.* Tokyo: Springer.

4. Dissociation and Possession

Daiguji, M. (1993). *Psychopathology of possession: Modern clinical study* (in Japanese). Tokyo: Seiwa.

Spiegel, D. (Ed.). (1994). *Dissociation: Culture, mind, and body.* Washington, DC: American Psychiatric Press.

Suryani, L., & Jensen, G. (1993). *Trance and possession in Bali.* Oxford: Oxford University Press.

Ward, D. (Ed.). (1989). *Culture and altered state of consciousness.* Beverly Hills, CA: Sage.

5. Depression

Kleinman, A., & Good, B. (Eds.). (1982). *Culture and depression: Studies in the anthropology and cross-cultural psy-

chiatry of affect and disorder. Berkeley: University of California Press.

Sartorius, N., Davidain, H., Ernberg, G., Fenton, F.R., Fujii, I., Gastpar, M., Gulbinat, W., Jablensky, A., Kielholz, P., Lehmann, H.E., Naraghi, M., Shimizu, M., Shinfuku, N., & Takahashi, R. (1983). *Depressive disorders in different culutres: Report on the WHO collaborative study on standardized assessment of depressive disorders.* Geneva: World Health Organization.

6. Schizophrenia

Jablensky, A., Sartorius, N., Ernberg, G., Anker, M., Korten, A., Cooper, J.E., Day, R., & Bertelsen, A. (1992). *Schizophrenia: Manifestations. incidence, and course in different cultures — A World Health Organization ten countries study* (Psychological Medicine Monograph Suppl. 20). Cambridge, UK: Cambridge University Press

World Health Organization. (1973). *The international study of schizophrenia.* Geneva: WHO

World Health Organization. (1979). *Schizophrenia: An international follow-up study.* New York: Wiley.

7. Alcoholism:

Babor, T.F. (Ed.). *Alcohol and culture: Comparative perspectives from Europe and America.* New York: New York Academy of Sciences.

Group for the Advancement of Psychiatry. (1996). *Alcoholism in the United States: Racial and ethnic considerations.* (Formulated by the Committee on Cultural Psychiatry, Report No. 141). Washington, DC: American Psychiatric Press.

Helzer, J.E., & Canino, G.J. (Eds.). (1992). *Alcoholism in North America, Europe, and Asia.* New York: Oxford University Press.

Helzer, J., Canino, G., & Chen, C.N. (1998). *Cross-national studies of alcoholism.* New York: Oxford University Press.

MacAndrew, C., & Edgerton, R.B. (1969). *Drunken comportment: A social explanation.* Chicago: Aldine.

Pittman, D.J., & Snyder, C.R. (Eds.). (1962). *Society, culture, and drinking patterns.* New York: Wiley.

Ritson, E.B. (1985). *Community response to alcohol-related problems: Review of an international study.* Geneva: World Health Organization.

8. Abuse of Substance Other Than Alcohol

Botvin, G.J., Schinke, S., & Orlandi, M.A. (1995). *Drug abuse prevention with multiethnic youth.* Thousand Oaks, CA: Sage.

Edwards, G., & Arif, A.E. (Eds.). (1980). *Drug problems in the sociocultural context: A basis for policies and programme planning.* Geneva: World Health Organization.

Edwards, G., Arif, A.E., & Jaffe, J. (Eds.). (1983). *Drug use and misuse: Cultural perspectives.* London: Croom Helm.

Gordon, J.U. (Ed.). (1994). *Managing multiculturalism in substance abuse services.* Thousand Oaks, CA: Sage.

McDonald, M. (Ed.). (1994). *Gender, drink and drugs.* Herndon, VA: Berg Publishers.

Trimble, J.E., Bolek, C.S., & Niemcryk, S.J. (Eds.). (1992). *Ethnic and multicultural drug abuse: Perspective on current research.* New York: Harrington Park Press.

9. Suicide

Farberow, N.L. (1975). *Suicide in different cultures.* Baltimore: University Park Press.

Group for the Advancement of Psychiatry (GAP). (1990). *Suicide and ethnicity in the United States* (GAP Report No. 128). New York: Brunner/Mazel.

Kok, L.P., & Tseng, W.S. (Eds.). (1992). *Suicidal behavior in the Asia-Pacific region.* Singapore: Singapore University Press.

10. Eating Disorders

Gordon, R.A. (1990). *Anorexia and bulimia: Anatomy of a social epidemic.* Cambridge, UK: Basil Blackwell.

11. Personality Disorders

Alarcón, R.D., Foulks, E.F., & Vakkur, M. (1998). *Personality disorders and culture: Clinical and conceptual interactions.* New York: Wiley.

12. Child Abuse/Sexual Abuse

Fontes, L.A. (Ed.). (1995). *Sexual abuse in nine North American cultures: Treatment and prevention.* Newbury Park, CA: Sage.

Korbin, J.E. (Ed.). (1981). *Child abuse and neglect: Cross-cultural perspectives.* Berkeley: University of California Press.

P. Folk Healing and Unique Psychotherapy

Adler, L.L., & Mukherji, B.R. (Eds.). (1995). *Spirit versus scalpel: Traditional healing and modern psychotherapy.* Westport, CT: Bergin & Garvey.

Frank, J.D. (1961). *Persuasion and healing: A comparative study of psychotherapy.* New York: Schocken Books.

Frank, J.D., & Frank, J.B. (1991). *Persuasion and healing: A comparative study of psychotherapy.* Baltimore: Johns Hopkins University Press.

Harvey, Y.S. (1979). *Six Korean women: The socialization of shamans.* New York: West Publishing.

Heinze, R.I. (1988). *Trance and healing in Southeast Asia today.* Bankok: White Lotus Co.

Heise, T. (1999). *Qigong in der VR China: Entwicklung, theorie und praxis* [Qigong in China: Development, theory and practice]. Berlin: Verlag fur Wissenschaft und Bildung.

Jilek, W.G. (1982). *Indian healing: Shamanic ceremonialism in the Pacific Northwes today.* Surrey, BC, Canada: Hancock House.

Kakar, S. (1982). *Shamans, mystics, and doctors.* New York: Knopf.

Kendall, L. (1985). *Shamans, housewives and other restless spirits: Women in Korean ritual life.* Honolulu: University of Hawaii Press.

Kendall, L. (1988). *The life and hard times of Korean shaman.* Honolulu: University of Hawaii Press.

Kiev, A. (1964). *Magic, faith, and healing: Studies in primitive psychiatry today.* New York: Free Press.

Nathan, T., & Hounkpatin, L. (1996). *La guérison Yoruba* [Yoruba healing]. Paris: Odile Jacob.

Reynolds, D.K. (1980). *The quiet therapies: Japanese pathways to personal growth.* Honolulu: University Press of Hawaii.

Reynolds, D.K. (1983). *Naikan psychotherapy: Meditation for self-development.* Chicago: University of Chicago Press.

Rosenbaum, R. (1999). *Zen and the heart of psychotherapy.* Philadelphia, PA: Brunner/Mazel.

Torrey, E.F. (1986). *Witchdoctors and psychiatrists: The common roots of psychotherapy and its future.* New York: Harper & Row.

Q. Culture, Psychotherapy, and Cross-Cultural Counseling

Abel, T.M., & Metraux, R. (1974). *Culture and psychotherapy.* New Haven, CT: College & University Press.

Acosta, F.X., Yamamoto, J., & Evans, L.A. (1982). *Effective psychotherapy for low income and minority patients.* New York: Plenum Press.

Aponte, J.E., & Wohl, J. (Eds.). (2000). *Psychological interventions and cultural diversity* (2nd ed.). Boston: Allyn & Bacon.

Chin, J.L., De La Cancela, V., & Jenkins, Y.M. (1993). *Diversity in psychotherapy: The politics of race, ethnicity, and gender.* Westport, CT: Praeger.

Devereux, G. (1951). *Reality and dream: Psychotherapy of a Plains Indian.* New York: International Universities Press.

Fine, R. (Ed.). (1987). *Psychoanalysis around the world.* New York: Haworth Press.

Fish, J. (1996). *Culture and therapy: An integrative approach.* Northvale, NJ: Jason Aronson.

Foster, R.P., Moskowitz, M., & Javier, R.A. (Eds.). (1996). *Reaching across boundaries of culture and class: Widening the scope of psychotherapy.* Northvale, NJ: Jason Aronson.

Helms, J.E., & Cook, D.A. (1999). *Using race and culture in counseling and psychotherapy: Theory and process.* Boston: Allyn & Bacon.

Higginbotham, H.N., West, S., & Forsyth, D. (1988). *Psychotherapy and behavior change: Social cultural and methodological perspectives.* New York: Pergamon Press.

Kareem, J., & Littewood, R. (Eds.). (1992). *Intercultural therapy: Themes, interpretations and practice.* Oxford: Blackwell Scientific Publications.

Lauterbach, W. (1984). *Soviet psychotherapy.* Oxford, UK: Pergamon Press.

Leman, J., & Gially, A. (Eds.). (1991). *Therapies interculturelles* [Intercultural therapies]. Brussels, Belgium: Editions Universitaires De Boeck.

Locke, D.C. (1992). *Increasing multicultural understanding: A comprehensive model.* Newbury Park, CA: Sage.

Marcella, A.J., & Pederson, P.B. (Eds.). (1981). *Cross-cultural counselling and psychotherapy.* New York: Pergamon Press.

Nathan, T. (1994). *L'influence qui guérit* [The healing influence]. Paris: Odile Jacob.

Paniggua, F.A. (1998). *Assessing and treating culturally diverse clients: A practical guide* (2nd ed.). Thousand Oaks, CA: Sage.

Pedersen, P.B., Draguns, J.G., Lonner, W.J., & Trimble, J.E. (Eds.). (1989). *Counseling across cultures* (3rd ed.). Honolulu: University of Hawaii Press.

Pedersen, P.B., Draguns, J.G., Lonner, W.J., & Trimble, J.E. (Eds.). (1996). *Counseling across cultures* (4th ed.). Thousand Oaks, CA: Sage.

Pedersen, P.B., Lonner, W.J., & Draguns, J.G. (1976). *Counseling across cultures.* Honolulu: University Press of Hawaii.

Perez, R.M., Moskowitz, M., & Javier, R.A. (Eds.). (1996). *Reaching across boundaries of culture and class: Widening the scope of psychotherapy.* Northvale, NJ: Jason Aronson.

Pfeigger, W.M., & Schoene, W. (1980). *Psychotherpie im kulturvergleich* [Psychotherapy in cultural comparison]. Stuttgart: Ferdinand Enke.

Pope-Davis, D.B., & Coleman, H.L.K. (Eds.). (1997). *Multicultural counseling competencies: Assessment, education and training, and supervision.* Thousand Oaks, CA: Sage.

Ramirez, M. (1991). *Psychotherapy and counseling with minorities: A cognitive approach to individual and cultural differences.* New York: Pergamon Press.

Rivera-Ramos, A.N. (1984). *Hacia una psycoterapia para el peurtorriqueno: Enfoque psico-social* [Toward a psychotherapy for the Puertorican: A psychosocial approach]. San Juan, PR: Centro para el Estudio y Desarollo de la Personalidad Puertorriquena.

Samuda, R.J., & Wolfgang, A. (Eds.). (1985). *Intercultural counselling and assessment.* Toronto: C.J. Hogrefe.

Sue, D.W., Carter, R.T., Casas, J.M., Fouad, N.A., Ivey, A.E., Jensen, M., LaFromboise, T., Manese, J.E., Ponterott, J.G., & Vazquez-Nutall, E. (1998). *Multicultural counseling competencies: Individual and organizational development.* Thousand Oaks, CA: Sage. *Publications*

Sue, D.W., & Sue, D. (1999). *Counseling the culturally different: Theory and practice.* New York: Wiley. [Original work published 1990].

Tseng, W.S., & Streltzer, J. (Eds.). (2000). *Culture and psychotherapy: A guide to clinical practice.* Washinton, DC: American Psychiatric Press.

R. Psychiatric Assessment and Treatment

Aponte, J.F., Rivers, R.Y., & Wohl, J. (Eds.). (1995). *Psychological interventions and cultural diversity.* Boston: Allyn & Bacon.

Chin, J.L., De La Cancela, V., & Jenkins, Y.M. (1993). *The politics of race, ethnicity, and gender.* Westport, CT: Praeger.

Comas-Díaz, L., & Griffith, E.E.H. (Eds.). (1988). *Clinical guidelines in cross-cultural mental health.* New York: Wiley.

Cuellar I., & Paniagua, F.A. (Eds.). (1999). *Handbook of multi-cultural mental health: Assesment and treatment of diverse populations.* San Diego: Academic Press.

Lin, K.M., Poland, R.E., & Nakasaki, G. (Eds.). (1993). *Psychopharmacology and psychobiology of ethnicity.* Washington, DC: American Psychiatric Press.

Paniagua, F.A. (1994). *Assessing and treating culturally diverse clients.* Thousand Oaks, CA: Sage.

Ruiz, P. (Ed.). (2000). *Review of Psychiatry, vol. 19: Ethnicity and Psychopharmacology.* Washington DC: American Psychiatric Press.

Sartorius, N., de Girolamo, G., Andrew, G., German, G.A., & Eisenberg, L. (Eds.). (1993). *Treatment of mental disorders: A review of effectiveness.* Washington, DC: American Psychiatric Press (on behalf of WHO).

Vargas, L.A., & Koss-Chiono, J. (Eds.). (1992). *Working with culture: Psychotherapeutic interventions with ethnic minority childlren and adolescents.* San Francisco: lossey-Bass.

S. Mental Health Service Delivery

Higginbotham, H.N. (1984). *Third world challenge to psychiatry.* Honolulu: University Press of Hawaii.

Pedersen, P., Sartorius, N., & Marsella, A. (Eds.). (1984). *Mental health services: The cross-cultural context.* Beverly Hills, CA: Sage.

T. Culture and Psychiatry Subcategory (or Population Subgroup)

1. Children and Adolescents

Canino, I.A., & Spurlock, J. (1994). *Culturally diverse children and adolescents: Assessment, diagnosis, and treatment.* New York: Guilford Press.

Hernandez, M., & Isaacs, M.R. (1998). *Promoting cultural competence in children's mental health services.* Baltimore: Paul H. Brooks.

Ho, M.K. (1992). *Minority children and adolescents in therapy.* Newbury Park, CA: Sage.

Johnson-Powell, G., Yamamoto, J., Wyatt, G.E., & Arroyo, W. (1997). *Transcultural child development: Psychological assessment and treatment*. New York: Wiley.

Powell, G.J., Yamamoto, J., Romero, A., & Morales, A. (Eds.). (1983). *The psychosocial development of minority group children*. New York: Brunner/Mazel.

Stiffman, R., & Davis, L.E. (Eds.). (1990). *Ethnic issues in adolescent mental health*. Thousand Oaks, CA: Sage.

Tobin, J.J., Wu, D.Y.H., & Davidson, D.H. (Eds.). (1989). *Preschool in three cultures: Japan, China, and the United States*. New Haven, CT: Yale University Press.

Vargas, L.A., & Koss-Chiono, J.D. (1992). *Working with culture: Psychotherapeutic interventions with ethnic minority children and adolescents*. San Francisco: Jossey-Bass.

Whiting, B.B. (Ed.). (1963). *Six cultrues: Studies of child rearing*. New York: Wiley.

Whiting, B.B., & Whiting, J.W. (1975). *Children of six cultures: A psycho-cultural analysis*. Cambridge, MA: Harvard University press.

2. The Aged

American Psychiatric Association. (1994). *Ethnic minority elderly: A task force report of the American Psychiatric Association*. Washington, DC: APA.

Aponte, J.F., Rivers, R.Y., & Wohl, J. (Eds.). (1995). *Psychological interventions and cultural diversity*. Boston: Allyn & Bacon.

Bergener, M., Hasegawa, K., Finkel, S.I., & Nishimura, T. (Eds.). (1992). *Aging and mental health disorders: International perspectives*. New York: Springer.

Berger, A., Badham, P., Kutscher, A.H., Berger, J., Perry, M., & Beloff, J. (Eds.). (1989). *Perspectives on death and dying: Cross-cultural and multi-disciplinary views*. Philadelphia: Charles Press.

Duffy, M. (Ed.). (1999). *Handbook of counseling and psychotherapy with older adults*. New York: Wiley.

Padgett, D. (1995). *Handbook on ethnicty, aging, and mental health*. Westport, CT: Greenwood Press.

3. The Family

Ariel, S. (1999). *Culturally competent family therapy: A general model*. Westport, CT: Greenwood.

Boyd-Franklin, N. (1989). *Black families in therapy: A multisystem approach*. New York: Guilford Press.

Falicov, C.J. (Vol. Ed.). (1983). *Cultural perspectives in family therapy*. Rockvill, MD: Aspen.

Hansen, J.C. (Ed.). & Falicov, C.J. (Vol. Ed.). (1983). *Cultural perspectives in family therapy*. Rockvill, MD: Aspen.

Ho, M.K. (1987). *Family therapy with ethnic minorities*. Newbury Park, CA: Sage. (Reviewed in *Transcultural Psychiatry Research Review 30*(4), 373–374.]

Ho, M.K. (1990). *Intermarried couples in therapy*. Springfield, IL: Charles C Thomas.

Levinson, D. (1989). *Family violence in cross-cultural perspectrive*. Newbury Park, CA: Sage.

Lewis, J.M., & Looney, J.G. (1983). *The long struggle: Well-functioning working-class Black families*. New York: Brunner/Mazel.

McAdoo, H.P. (Ed.). (1993). *Family ethnicity: Strength in diversity*. Newbury Park, CA: Sage.

McGoldrick, M., Giordano, J., & Pearce, J.K. (Eds.). (1996). *Ethnicity and family therapy* (2nd ed.), New York: Guilford Press.

McGoldrick, M., Pearce, J.K., & Giordano, J. (Eds.). (1982). *Ethnicity and family therapy*. New York: Guilford Press.

Mindel, C.H., & Habenstein, R.W. (Eds.). (1981). *Ethnic families in America: Patterns and variations*(2nd ed.). New York: Elsevier.

Nuckolls, C.W. (1993). *Siblings in South Asia: Brothers and sisters in cultural context*. New York: Guilford Press.

Rosenblatt, P.C., Karis, T.A., & Powell, R.D. (1995). *Multiracial couples: Black and White voices*. Thousand Oaks, CA: Sage.

Tseng, W.S., & Hsu, J. (1991). *Culture and family: Problems and therapy*. New York: Haworth Press.

4. Minority Groups

Jones, E.E., & Korchin, S.J. (Eds.). (1982). *Minority mental health*. New York: Praeger.

Lott, B., & Maluso, D. (1995). *The social psychology of interpersonal discrimination*. New York: Guilford Press.

Wilkinson, C.B. (Ed.). (1986). *Ethnic psychiatry*. New York: Plenum Press.

U. SPECIAL CULTURE GROUPS/AREAS

1. North America, Including Native American and Other Ethnic Minorities

Devereux, G. (1969). *Mohave ethnopsychiatry: The psychic disturbances of an Indian tribe*. Washington, DC:

Smithsonian Institute Press. (Original work published 1961)

Grob, G.N. (1983). *Mental illness and American society: 1875–1940.* Princeton, NJ: Princeton Unversity press.

Jilek, W. (1974). *Salish Indian mental health and cultural change.* Toronto: Holt, Rinehart & Winston.

Lee, E. (Ed.). (1997). *Working with Asian Americans: A guide for clinicians.* New York: Guilford Press.

Manson, S.M. (Ed.). (1982). *New directions in prevention among American Indian and Alaska native communities.* Portland: Oregon Health Sciences University.

Neighbors, H.W., & Jackson, J.S. (Eds.). (1996). *Mental health in Black America.* Newbury Park, CA: Sage.

2. South (Latin) America, Including Hispanic Americans

Becerra, R.M., Karno, M., & Escobar, J. (Eds.). (1982). *Mental health and Hispanic Americans.* New York: Grune & Stratton.

Figge, H. (1973). *Geisterkult, poessessenheit und magie in dos Umanda-religion Brasilieus* [Spirit cult, possession and magic in the Umbanda religion of Brazil] Freiburg: Verliae Kar; Alber.

Garcia, J.C., & Zea, M.C. (Eds.). (1997). *Psychological interventions and research with Latino populations.* Needham Heights, MA: Allyn & Bacon.

Gaviria, M., & Arana, J.D. (1987). *Health and behavior: Research agenda for Hispanics.* Chicago: University of Illinois at Chicago, Hispanic American Psychiatric Research and Training Program.

Hollweg, M.G. (1991). *Locura, cultura y magia: Aspectos transculturales de la psycologia y la psicopathologia Boliviana* [Madness, culture and magic: Transcultural aspects of Bolivian psychology and psychopathology]. Santa Cruz de la Sierra, Bolivia: Centro de Salud Mental, Casilla. (Reviewed in *Transcultural Psychiatry Research Review 29*(2) [1992]

Malgady, R.G., & Rodriques, O. (Eds.). (1994). *Theoretical and conceptual issues in Hispanic mental health.* Malabar, FL: Krieger.

Padilla, A.M. (Ed.). (1994). *Hispanic psychology: Critical issues in theory and research.* Newbury Park, CA: Sage.

Perales, A., Montoya, A., & Sogi, C. (1995). *Social and cultural landmarks for community mental health.* Lima: Peruvian University "Cayetano Heredia" and National Institute of Mental Health "Honorio Delgado–Hideyo Noguchi."

de Rios, M.D. (2000). *Brief psychotherapy with the Latino immigrant client.* Binghamton, NY: The Hawarth Press.

Rogler, L.H., & Hollingshed, A.B. (1985). *Puerto Rican families and schizophrenia.* Maplewood, NJ: Waterfront Press.

Rogler, L.H., Malgady, R.G., & Rodrigues, O. (1989). *Hispanics and mental health: A framework for research.* Malabar, FL: Krieger.

Segun, C.A. (Ed.). (1979). *Psiquiatria folkorica* [Folk psychiatry]. Lima: Instituto Peruano de Psiquiatria Social.

Segun, C.A. (1988). *Medicinas tradicionales y medicinal folklorica* [Traditional medicine and folk medicine]. Lima: Banco Central de Reserva da Peru Fondo Editorial.

Telles, C.A., & Karno, M. (Eds.). (1994). *Mental disorders in Hispanic populations.* Los Angeles: University of California Los Angeles (UCLA).

Villaseñor Bayardo, S.J. (Ed.). (1996). *Encuentros Franco-Mexicanos de etnopsiquitria y de psiquiatria: 1994–1996 actas* [French-Mexican encounter of ethnopsychiatry and psychiatry: 1994–1996]. Mexico: Centro Científico y Técnico de la Embajada de Francia en Mexico, Instituto Francés para América Latina, & Revista del Residente de Psyquitría.

3. Asia, Including Asian Americans

Bond, M.H. (1991). *Beyond the Chinese face: Insights from psychology.* Hong Kong: Oxford University Press.

Bond, M.H. (Ed.). (1996). *Handbook of Chinese psychology.* Hong Kong: Oxford University Press.

Caudill W., & Lin, T.Y. (Eds.). (1969). *Mental health research in Asia and the Pacific.* Honolulu: East-West Center Press.

Cooper, J.E., & Sartorius, N. (Eds.). (1996). *Mental disorders in China.* London: Gaskell.

Doi, T. (1973). *The antomy of dependence.* Tokyo: Kodansha International.

Johnson, F.A. (1992). *Dependency, independency, and amae: Psychoanalytic anthropological observations.* New York: New York University Press.

Kimura, B. (1995). *Zwischen mensch und mensch: Strukture Japanischer subjektnität* [Between man and man: Structure of Japanese subjectivity] Darmstadt: Wssenschaftliche Tsuchqisaschft.

Lebra, T.S. (1976). *Japanese patterns of behavior.* Honolulu: University Press of Hawaii.

Lebra, T.S., & Lebra, W.P. (Eds.). (1974). *Japanese culture and behavior: Selected readings.* Honolulu: University Press of Hawaii.

Lebra, T.S., & Lebra, W.P. (Eds.). (1986). *Japanese culture and behavior: Selected readings.* (Rev. ed.). Honolulu: University Press of Hawaii.

Lebra, W. (Ed.). (1972). *Mental health research in Asia and the Pacific: Vol. 2. Transcultural research in mental health.* Honolulu: University Press of Hawaii.

Lebra, W. (Ed.). (1974). *Mental health research in Asia and the Pacific: Vol. 3. Youth, socialization, and mental health.* Honolulu: University Press of Hawaii.

Lebra, W. (Ed.). (1976). *Mental health research in Asia and the Pacific. Vol. 4. Culture-bound syndromes, ethnopsychiatry, and alternate therapies.* Honolulu: University Press of Hawaii.

Lin, T.Y., & Eisenberg, L. (Eds.). (1986). *Mental health planning for one billion people: A Chinese perspective.* Vancouver: University of British Columbia Press.

Lin, T.Y., Tseng, W.S., & Yeh, E.K. (Eds.). (1995). *Chinese societies and mental health.* Hong Kong: Oxford University Press.

Sue, S., & Morishima, J.K. (1982). *The mental health of Asian Americans.* San Francisco: Jossey-Bass.

Tseng, W.S. (Ed.). (1997). *Chinese mind and therapy* (in Chinese). Beijing: Beijing University Press.

Tseng, W.S., & Wu, D.Y.H. (Eds.). (1985). *Chinese culture and mental health.* Orlando, FL: Academic Press.

Watson, C.W., & Ellen, R. (Eds.). (1993). *Understanding witchcraft and sorcery in Southeast Asia.* Honolulu: University of Hawaii Press.

4. South Asia

Charkarborty, A. (1990). *Social stress and mental health: A social-psychiatric field study of Calcutta.* New Delhi: Sage.

Mohebali, A. (1987). *Socio-psychological study of mental health in India and Iran: A cross-cultural study.* Agra: Agra Psychological Research Cell.

Suryani, L.K., & Jensen, G.D. (1993). *Trance and possesion in Bali: A window on Western multiple personality, possesion disorder, and suicide.* Kuala Lumpur: Oxford University Press.

Wagner, N.N., & Tan, E.S. (1971). *Psychological problems and treatment in Malaysia.* Kuala Lumpur: University of Malaya Press.

5. Mideast

Racy, J. (1970). *Psychiatry in the Arab East.* Munksgaard, Copenhagen: Munksgaard. (As *Acta Psychiatrica Scandinavica, Supplemetum, 211*)

6. West Europe

Boroffka, A., & Pheiffer, W.M. (Eds.). (1977). *Fragen der transkulturell-vergleichenden psychiatrie in Europe* [Problems of transcultural comparative psychiatry in Europe]. Münster: Westfälische Wilhelms-Universität.

7. East and North Europe

Calloway, P. (1992/1993). *Russian/Soviet and Western psychiatry: A contemporary comparative study.* New York: J Wiley.

8. Africa/African-American

Carothers, J.C. (1970). *The African mind in health and disease: A study in ethnopsychiatry.* New York: Negro University Press. (Original work published 1953)

Erinosho, O.A., & Bell, N.W. (Eds.). (1982). *Mental health in Africa.* Ibadan, Nigeria: Ibandan University.

Fierman, S., & Janzen, J.M. (1992). *The social basis of health and healing in Africa.* Berkeley: University of California Press.

Field, M.J. (1962). *Search for security: An ethnopsychiatic study of rural Ghana.* Chicago: Northwestern University Press.

Friedman, S. (Ed.). (1994). *Anxiety disorders in African Americans.* New York: Springer.

Leighton, A.H., Lambo, T.A., Hughes, C.C., Leighton, D.C., Murphy, J.M., & Macklin, D.B. (1963). *Psychiatric disorder among the Yoruba.* Ithaca, NY: Cornell University Press.

Mulling, L. (1984). *Therapy, ideology, and social change: Mental healing in urban Ghana.* Berkeley: University of California Press.

Okpaku, S. (Ed.). (1991). *Mental health in Africa and the Americas today.* Nashville, TN: Chrisolith Books.

Onwuzurike, C.A., & Enekwechi, E. (Eds.). (1984). *Clinical psychology in the Nigerian society.* Jos: Nigerian Association of Clinical Psychologists.

Orley, J. (1970). *Culture and mental illness: A study from Uganda.* Nairobi: East African Publication House.

Ortigues, M.C., & Ortigues, E. (1966). *Oedipe Africain* [African Oedipus]. Paris: Plon.

Peltzer, K. (1987). *Some contributions of traditional healing practices towards psychosocial health care in Malawi.* Eschborn bei Frankfurt am Main: Fachbuchhandlung für Psychologie Verlagsabteilung.

Peltzer, K. (1995). *Psychology and health in African cultures: Examples of ethnopsychotherapeutic practice.* Frankfurt: IKO-Verlag für Interkulturelle Kommunication.

Pelzer, K., & Ebigbo, P.O. (1989). *Clinical psychology in Africa.* Enugu, Nigeria: Work Group for African Psychology.

Ruiz, D. (Ed.). (1990). *Handbook of mental health and mental disorder among Black American.* New York: Greenwood Press.

Sow, I. (1980). *Anthropological structures of madness in Black Africa.* New York: International University Press.

Staewen, C., & Schonberg, F. (1970). *Kulturwandel und angstentwicklung bei den Yoruba Westafikas* [Cultural change and the development of anxiety among the Yoruba of West Africa]. Miich, Germany: Weltforum Verlag.

Swift, C.R., & Asuni, T. (1975). *Mental health and disease in Africa.* London: Churchill-Livingstone.

Westley, D. (1993). *Mental health and psychiatry in Africa: An annotated bibiography.* London: Hans Zell.

9. Australia, New Zealand, and Papua New Guinea

Burton-Bradley, B.G. (1973). Long long: *Transcultural psychiatry in Papua and New Guinea.* Port Moresby, P.NG.: Public Health Department.

Burton-Bradley, B.G. (1975). *Stone age crisis: A psychiatric appraisal.* Nashville, TN: Vanderbilt University Press.

Cawte, J. (1974). *Medicine is the law: Studies in psychiatric anthropology of Australian tribal societies.* Honolulu: University Press of Hawaii.

Jilek, W.G. (Ed.). (1985). *Traditional medicine and primary health care in Papua New Guinea.* Geneva: World Health Organization & University of Papua New Guinea.

10. The Pacific Island Groups

Robillard, A.B., & Marsella, A.J. (Eds.). (1987). *Contemporary issues in mental health research in the Pacific islands.* Honolulu: University of Hawaii, Social Science Research Institute.

Tseng, W.S. (Ed.). (1986). *Culture and mental health in Mcronesia.* Honolulu: University of Hawaii School of Medicine, Department of Psychiatry.

11. Multiple Ethnic/Cultural Groups

Gaw, A. (Ed.). (1982). *Cross-cultural psychiatry.* Boston: Wright-PSG.

McDermott, J., Jr., Tseng, W.S., & Maretzki, T. (Eds.). (1981). *People and cultures in Hawaii: A psychocultural profiles.* Honolulu: University Press of Hawaii.

V. Special Subject Groups

1. Minorities

Littlewood, R., & Lipsedge, M. (1989). *Aliens and alienists: Ethnic minorities and psychiatry* (2nd ed.). London: Unwin Human.

Moffic, H.S., & Adams, G.L. (Guest Eds.). (1983, Spring). The psychiatric care of "minority" groups [Special issue]. *American Journal of Social Psychiatry, 3*(2).

2. Immigrants and Refugees

Al-Issa, I., & Tousignant, M. (Eds.). (1997). *Ethnicity, immigrantion, and psychopathology.* New York: Plenum Press.

Arpin, J., Comba, L., & Fleury, F. (Eds.). (1988). *Migrazione e salute mentale* [Migration and mental health]. *Anthropologia Medica,* [Special issue], *4* (in French, Italian, & English).

Holtzman, W., & Bornemann, T. (Eds.). (1990). *Mental health of immigrants and refugees.* Austin, TX: Hogg Foundation.

Koch, E., Özek, M., & Pheiffer, W.M. (Eds.). (1995). *Psychologie und pathologie der migration: Deutsch-Turkische perspetiven* [Psychology and pathology of migration: German-Türkish perspectives]. Freiburg im Breisgau, Germany: Lambertus-Verlag.

Marsella, A.J., Bornemann, T., Ekblad, S., & Orley, J. (Eds.). (1994). *Amidst peril and pain: The mental health and well-being of the world's refugees.* Washington, DC: American Psychological Association.

Peltzer, K. (1996). *Counselling and psychotherapy of victims of organised violence in sociocultural context.* Frankfurt, Germany: IKO-Verlag fü Interkulturelle Kommunication.

Scott, W.A., & Scott, R. (1989). *Adaptation of immigrants: Individual differences and determinants.* Oxford, UK: Pergamon Press.

Van der Veer, G. (1992). *Counselling and therapy with refugees: Psychological problems of victims of war, torture and repression.* Chichester: Wiley.

Westermeyer, J. (1989). *Mental health for refugees and other immigrants: Social and preventive approaches.* Springfield, IL: Charles C. Thomas.

Wesermeyer, J. (1989). *Psychiatric care of migrants: A clinical guide.* Washington, DC: American Psychiatric Press.

Williams, C.L., & Westermeyer, J. (Eds.). (1986). *Refugee mental health in resettlement countries.* Washington, DC: Hemisphere.

3. Homosexuality

Cabaj, R.P., & Stein, T.S. (Eds.). (1996). *Textbook of homosexuality and mental health.* Washington, DC: American Psychiatric Press.

Greene, B. (Ed.). (1997). *Ethnic and cultural diversity among lesbians and gay men.* Thousand Oaks, CA: Sage.

Whitam, F.L. (1986). *Male homosexuality in four societies: Brazil, Guatemala, the Philippines, and the United States.* New York: Praeger.

4. Women

Comas-Díaz, L., & Greene, B. (Eds.). (1994). *Women of color: Integrating ethnic and gender identities in psychotherapy.* New York: Guilford Press.

5. Medical Patients

Qureshi, B. (1994). *Transcultural medicine: Dealing with patients from different cultures* (2nd ed.,). Dordrecht, The Netherlands: Kluwer Academic Publishers.

W. Special Issues, Social Phenomena, and Mental Health

1. Cultural Change and Adjustment

Chance, N.A. (Ed.). (1968). *Conflict in culture: Problems of developmental change among the Cree.* Ottawa: Canadian Research Centre for Anthropology.

Niehoff, A.H. (1966). *A casebook of social change.* Chicago: Aldine.

Pedersen, P. (1995). *The five stages of cultural shock: Critical incidents around the world.* Westport, CT: Greenwood Press.

2. Religion, Culture, and Psychiatry

Bartocci, G. (Ed.). (1994). *Psicopathologia cultura e la dimensione del sacro* [Psychopathology, culture, and the dimension of the sacred]. Roma: Edizioni Universitarie Romane.

Bhugra, E. (Ed.). (1996). *Religion and psychiatry: Context, consensus and controversies.* London: Routledge.

Boehnlein, J.K. (Ed.). (2000). *Psychiatry and religion.* Washington, DC: American Psychiatric Press.

Bourguignon, E. (Ed.). (1973). *Religion, altered states of consciousness and social change.* Columbus: Ohio State University Press.

Fukuyama, M.A., & Sevig, T.D. (1999). *Integrating spirituality into multicultural counseling.* Thousand Oaks, CA: Sage.

Koenig, H.G. (Ed.). (1998). *Handbook of religion and mental health.* San Diego, CA: Academic Press.

Kaslow, F., & Sussman, M.B. (1982). *Cults and the family.* New York: Haworth Press.

Pargament, K.I. (1997). *The psychology of religion and coping: Theory, research, practice.* New York: Guilford Press.

Schumaker, J.F. (Ed.). (1992). *Religion and mental health.* Don Mills, Ontario: Oxford University Press Canada.

Shafranske, E.P. (Ed.). (1996). *Religion and the clinical practice of psychology.* Washington, DC: American Psychological Association.

Wulff, D.M. (1991). *Psychology and religion: Classic and contemporary views.* Rexdale, Ontario: Wiley.

3. Ethnic Identity and Mental Health

De Vos, G., & Romanucci-Ross, L. (Eds.). (1975). *Ethnic identity: Cultural continuities and change.* Palo Alto, CA: Mayfield.

Harris, H.H., Blue, H.C., & Griffith, E.E.H. (Eds.). (1995). *Racial and ethnic identity: Psychological development and creative expression.* New York: Routledge Press.

Thompson, C.E., & Carter, R.T. (Eds.). (1997). *Racial identity theory: Application to individual, group, and organizational interventions.* Mahwah, NJ: Erlbaum.

4. Race, Racism, Mental Health, and Therapy

Bowser, B.P. (Ed.). (1995). *Racism and antiracism in world perspective.* Newbury Park, CA: Sage.

Carter, R.T. (1998). *The influence of race and racial identity in psychotheapy: Toward a racially inclusive model.* New York: Wiley.

Griffith, E.E.H. (1998). *Race and excellence: My dialogue with Chester Pierce.* Iowa City: University of Iowa Press.

Harris, H.W., Blue, H.C., & Griffith, E.E.H. (Eds.). (1995). *Racial and ethinc identity: Psychological development and creative expression.* New York: Routledge.

Hirschfeld, L.A. (1996). *Race in the making: Cognition, culture, and the child's construction of human kinds.* Cambridge, MA: MIT Press.

Holmes, R.M. (1995). *How young children perceive race.* Newbury Park, CA: Sage.

Pinderhughes, E. (1989). *Understanding race, ethnicity, and power: The key to efficacy in clinical practice.* New York: Free Press.

Thomas, A., & Sillen, S. (1972). *Racism and psychiatry.* New York: Brunner/Mazel.

Willie, C.V., Rieker, P.P., Kramer, B.M., & Brown, B.S. (Eds.). (1995). *Mental health, racism, and sexism.* Pittsburgh: University of Pittsburgh Press.

5. Sexual Behavior across Cultures

Abramson, P.R., & Pinkerton, S.D. (Eds.). (1995). *Sexual nature/Sexual culture.* Chicago: University of Chicago Press.

Irvine, J.M. (1995). *Sexual education across cultures: Working with differences.* Scarborough, Ontario: Prentice Hall Canada, Jossey-Bass.

Laumann, E.O., Gagnon, J.H., Michael, R.T., & Michaels, S. (1994). *The social organization of sexuality: Sexual practices in the United States.* Chicago: University of Chicago Press.

Liu, D., Wu (Ng), M.L., & Chou, L. (1992). *Sexual behavior in modern China: A report of the nation-wide "sex culture" survey on 20,000 subjects in China.* In Chinese Shanghai: Joint Publishing. (Reviewed by M.P. Lau in *Transcultural Psychiatry Research Review, 32*(5) [1995])

Ruan, F.U. (1991). *Sex in China: Studies in sexology in Chinese culture.* New York: Plenum Press.

X. CULTURE, MEDICNE, AND HEALTH CARE DELIVERY

1. Traditional Medicine Systems

Leslie C. (1976). *Asian medical systems: A comparative study.* Berkeley: University of California Press.

Bannerman, R.H., Burton, J., & Ch'en, W.C. (1983). *Traditional medicine and health care coverage.* Geneva: World Health Organization.

Kutumbiah, P. (1962). *Ancient Indian medicine.* Calcutta: Orient Longmans.

2. Culture and Health Care

Kavanagh, K.H., & Kennedy, P.H. (1992). *Promoting cultural diversity: Strategies for health care professionals.* Newbury, CA: Sage.

Leininger, M.M. (Ed.). (1991). *Culture care diversity and universality: A theory of nursing.* New York: National League for Nursing Press.

Leininger, M.M. (1995). *Transcultural nursing: Concepts, theories, research and practices* (2nd ed.). New York: McGraw-Hill.

Lipson, J.G., & Steiger, N.J. (1996). *Self-care nursing in a multicultural context.* Thousand Oaks, CA: Sage.

Stein, H.F. (1993). *American medicine as culture.* Boulder, CO: Westview Press.

3. Culture and Mental Health Service

Dean, C., & Freeman, H. (Eds.). (1993). *Community mental health care: International perspectives on making it happen.* London: Centre for Mental Health Services Development.

Pedersen, P.B., Sartorius, N., & Marsella, A.J. (Eds.). (1984). *Mental health services: The cross-cultural context.* Beverly Hills, CA: Sage.

4. Culture, Ethics, and Psychiatry

Okasha, A., Arboleda-Florz, J., & Sartorius, N. (Eds.). (2000). *Ethics, culture, and psychiatry: International perspectives.* Washington, DC: American Psychiatric Press.

Y. Cross-Cultural Training and Training in Cultural Psycihatry

Lefley, H.P., & Pedersen, P.B. (1986). *Cross-cultural training for mental health professionals.* Springfield, IL: Charles C. Thomas.

Z. Culture–Psychology–Medicine–Psychiatry-Focused Serial Publications

1. Periodical Books

Jahrbuch fur transkulturelle Medizin und Psychotherapie [Yearbook of cross-cultural medicine and psychotherapy]. Berlin: Verlag fur Wissenschaft und Bildung. (1990~)

The psychoanalytic study of society. New York: International University Press. (1960~).

2. Journals (by Alphabet Order)

Cultural Diversity and Ethnic Minority Psychiatry. (1999~). [Previously: *Cultural Diversity and Mental Health.* (1995~1998).]

Culture, Medicine and Psychiatry. (1977~).

International Journal of Social Psychiatry. (1955~).

Transcultural Psychiatry. (1999~). [Previously: *Transcultural Psychiatry Research Review* (1963~1999).]

Zeitschrift für Ethnomedizin und Transkulturelle Psychiatrie [Journal for Ethnomedicine and Transcultural Psychiatry] (Curare). (1978~).

3. Journals Related to Culture, Behavior Sciences, and Health (by Alphabet Order)

Cross-Cultural Research. (1993~)

Culture and Psychology. (1995~)

Journal of Cross-Cultural Psychology. (1970~).

Journal for the Psychoanalysis of Culture and Society. (1996~)

Journal of Psychological Anthropology. (1978~1980).

Journal of Transcultural Nursing. (1982~)

Author Index

Subject Index

ISBN 0-12-701632-5

90038

9 780127 016320

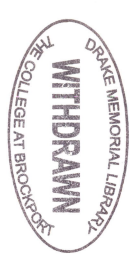

DATE DUE

GAYLORD   PRINTED IN U.S.A